D1242140

The Reverse Effect

"He who knows only his side of the case, knows little of that."
—John Stuart Mill

"Anyone who has begun to think places some portion of the world in jeopardy."
—John Dewey

A *Reverse Effect* .... HIV (the AIDS virus) May Cause Immunodeficiency or Immunostimulation

As this book neared completion, John J. Wright et al. published a study in the *New England Journal of Medicine* (Dec. 10, 1987) 317, no. 24: 1516-1520 that suggests HIV may be able to act as a cure for the primary problem it often causes, i.e., immune deficiency. They reported on a single case of a 36-year-old bisexual man who had received a diagnosis of common variable hypogammaglobulinemia in 1974. During the subsequent five years the patient suffered many types of infections and the diagnosis of hypogammaglobulinemia was reconfirmed, in 1979, at the National Institutes of Health. He was found to be seropositive for HIV in 1982 but not in 1981. At least one of his sexual contacts during the early 1980's died of AIDS. For the past two years he has been healthy without evidence of complications associated with either hypogammaglobulinemia or HIV infection. Thus HIV may be able to show a *reverse effect* by working to cause either immunodeficiency or immunostimulation.

The Reverse Effect

How Vitamins and Minerals Promote Health and CAUSE Disease

by

Walter A. Heiby

Technical Consultants:

Robert D. Piersanti
Josephine R. Szczesny

It is well known that x-rays can both cure and cause cancer. Vitamins and minerals also exhibit *reverse effects* and can cure a n d cause disease. Laymen should not, however, construe the ideas in this book to be medical advice. Consult your physician regarding specific health problems.

MediScience Publishers, P.O. Box 256A, Deerfield, IL   60015

"Yes, it is crazy, but it is not crazy
enough!"
—Niels Bohr. Said to Werner
Heisenberg, creator of quantum
mechanics and of the *uncertainty
principle* and, like Bohr, a Nobel
Laureate. Quoted by Gerard Piel in
Science (Jan. 17, 1986) 231: 201.

UND
QP771
H45
1988

Furthermore, Niels, our intelligence
keeps us from making it crazy enough!
—Walter A. Heiby

First Edition.

Printed in the United States of America.

Library of Congress Cataloging-in-Publication Data

Heiby, Walter A.
     The reverse effect.

     Bibliography: p.
     Includes indexes.
     1. Vitamins in human nutrition. 2. Minerals in human
nutrition I. Title. [DNLM: 1. Diseases—etiology. 2. Health
Promotion. 3. Minerals. 4. Vitamins. QU 160 H465r]
QP771.H45   1988   615'.58   87-7829
ISBN 0-938869-01-9

Dedicated to the person who, while refusing to uncritically accept every hypothesis as being tenable, remains open to the great possibilities that are beyond the scope of current orthodoxies whether of the medical, nutritional, faddist, or eclectic varieties. No one has all the wisdom, but each of us has a portion of the truth and each of us has some ability to catch wisdom's fire from others, brighten it, and pass it on. Dedicated also to those scientists and clinicians that are beginning to recognize that a great challenge of nutrition and of medicine in the 21st century will be to optimize nutritional and drug intakes in terms of dose-response relationships with full cognizance of the *reverse effect.*

VI

"I did not arrive at my understanding of
the fundamental laws of the universe
through my rational mind."
—Albert Einstein

Our life purpose should be to change for the better
ourselves and the world.
—Walter A. Heiby

The Rising Price of Science Books

Each year, *Science* reports the average per page price of books in the natural sciences reviewed during the previous year. During 1987 (as reported on page 81 of the Jan. 1, 1988 issue) the average per page price was 12.5¢. At this rate, an 800-page book would cost about $100.00 and one of 1200 pages about $150. The current cost of scientific journals is also astonishing. The price of an annual subscription to *Brain Research* is now $3826.00 and that of *Chemical Abstracts* $8400.00. (Constance Holden, *Science* [May 22, 1987] 236: 908-909). Regrettably, few individuals and few libraries can afford this price of education.

VIII

"There often is darkness at the foot of a lighthouse."
—Old Spanish proverb

"Truth lives in the cellar; error on the doorstep."
—Austin O'Malley

"Wise men argue causes; fools decide them."
—Anacharsis (c. 600 B.C.)

A scientific concept is valuable not to the extent it is true but to the extent it is fruitful in leading to new ideas.
—Walter A. Heiby

"Progress is the result of some person's discontent put into action. Things as they are are never the best."
— Walter A. Heiby, *Live Your Life* (New York: Harper and Row, 1964) p. 51.

The Author and the *Reverse Effect*

Walter A. Heiby is the instructor of literature research seminars in medicine, dentistry, and nutrition convened at the University of Illinois under the auspices of the *Nutrition for Optimal Health Association*. This has proved to be the ideal setting for development of his *theory of the reverse effect*.

The *theory of the reverse effect* states that there is a good probability that the activity of any substance that is health-promoting or health-destructive in a given concentration may reverse its role and become respectively health-destructive or health-promoting at a different concentration. The author presents numerous examples of vitamins and minerals that reverse their customary action at different concentrations. He speculates that the *reverse effect* may be used to our advantage in finding new therapies for cancer and other diseases. Both *The Reverse Effect: How Vitamins and Minerals Promote Health and CAUSE Disease* and the

x

introductory sampler *Better Health and the Reverse Effect* are replete with creative speculations—new ways of looking at nutritional and medical phenomena. Now, in the big 1216-page volume, the wealth of research support for the theory is being made available to scientists, physicians, nurses, dietitians, nutritionists and intelligent laymen. Its list of 4821 references is believed to be a record number for a single-author book.[*]

---

[*] The single-author book with the greatest reference density (references per page) is believed to be *Hormesis with Ionizing Radiation* by T.D. Luckey (Boca Raton, Florida: CRC Press, 1980). It is a 222-page book with 1299 references or 5.85 references/page. (Luckey's book contains 168 pages of text or 7.73 references/text page.)

Markers and Underlying Causes

Distinguishing between markers and underlying causes is not sufficiently recognized as a problem of various sciences. Cholesterol (an essential chemical required for metabolic processes), for example, may be merely a marker, rather than a cause, of cardiovascular disease. If true, reducing cholesterol would have little bearing on cardiovascular health. Cholesterol could be the body's patching material to correct for free-radical damage. If so, our objective should be to reduce free-radical damage instead of just working to reduce the mere marker of that damage. Let's concern ourselves with causes, rather than just with markers, of physiological problems.

If This Book Is Yours—Mark It Up!

A book becomes truly yours when you mark it up and list key page numbers at either the front or the rear for later review. Mark up this book unless, of course, you have borrowed it from a friend or from the library in which case turn to page 1197 and order your personal copy.

XII

"The creation of a thousand forests is in one acorn."
—Ralph Waldo Emerson

"Have patience. All things are difficult before they become easy."
—Saadi (1190-1291)

"What I admire in Columbus is not his having discovered a world, but his having gone to search for it on the faith of an opinion."
—A. Robert Jacques Turgot

"Columbus was the last to discover the New World, but his was the first *effective discovery.*"
—J.W. Stephenson, *Insight* (Nov. 16, 1987) 3, No. 46:4

"It is quite possible to misinterpret what appear to be obvious, easily-explained facts. Listen carefully and you can hear the words of an archaeologist of 100,000 A.D., who is excavating the Vatican. Across the millennia, our time machine brings us the words: 'This was obviously an art school.'"
— Walter A. Heiby, *The New Dynamic Synthesis* (Chicago: The Institute of Dynamic Synthesis, 1967)

Table of Contents

The importance of controlling stress in animal studies • Factors scientists sometimes improperly ignore

Doctrine of sufficient challenge • Amative individuality • *Reverse effects* common but unrecognized • Small dosages sometimes more dangerous than large ones • The *reverse effect* as a new therapeutic paradigm • Pleasure and a substance's physiological effect • Recommended Dietary Allowances

XVI

Search out the wildernesses
    in which strange voices are crying.
Would that each Socrates
        had at least a lone Plato!
—Walter A. Heiby

Acknowledgments

In my small way I am trying to play "Plato" for thousands of scientists whose data and discoveries form the basis of the *theory of the reverse effect*. My efforts, in turn, have come to fruition in this book only through interaction with the many "Platos" who have aided me. A special word of gratitude is due America's outstanding health activist, Josephine R. Szczesny, who has been called "the Paul Revere of the Health Movement." She is a perspicacious health consultant, the editor of *Health Happenings* and moderator of the radio program of the same name. Jo has helped acquaint me with many of the informational byways that lead to better health and has made very valuable contributions to this book.

My indebtedness to my good friend Robert D. Piersanti is especially great. Bob not only applied his tremendous knowledge to the editing of the manuscript, but he criticized the text with unusually high sensitivity and creativity. Bob was also the stimulus for much of the literature research behind this work. This is a much better book because of him. Bob and Moreen Piersanti, along with Jo Szczesny, were also of tremendous assistance in creating the book's index. (Only those who have indexed a book can know the magnitude of such an undertaking.) The huge project of indexing was made feasible only through their loyal dedication.

My deepest appreciation is felt for Fred Glotzer who located most of the many thousands of studies that were perused while this book was in preparation. (Even though a record total of 4821 citations appear in the reference list, a far greater number of studies were considered but not used.) My thanks also go to Roland Glotzer who skillfully assisted Fred in this massive endeavor. The work of locating obscure references often involved considerable insight and dedication.

I am indebted to Henrietta Leary who edited an early edition of the manuscript. My gratitude also goes to Lynn McEwan for her highly-perceptive work in copyediting and proofreading, and to Robin O'Connor who introduced me to Lynn. My thanks also go to Eunice Strehlow Heiby, Pamela A. Heiby Roesner, Thomas F. Roesner, C. Elizabeth Reisner Heiby and Ronald W. Heiby for their help. I thank my late father, Albert H. Heiby, for instilling in me a love of science and my late mother, Laura Heiby, for giving me the energy to effect its pursuit. My gratitude also goes to my sister Myrtle G. Shaw, as well as to Robert W. Shaw, Howard L. Taylor, Frank S: Hauser, Earle D. Strehlow and Betty J. Stribling whose encouragement over a period of years has been very inspiring.

Many scientists, physicians, dentists and nutritionists have assisted me with this project. Some of those that were especially helpful are Barbara Sachsel, Cynthia Hrisco, Ralph Hovnanian, Richard A. Strehlow, Ph.D., John J. Miller, Ph.D., Irwin Fridovich, Ph.D., Oscar Rasmussen, Ph.D., Irwin Stone, Ph.D., Denham Harman, M.D., Ph.D., Tim Roads, M.D., Jeremiah J. Morrissey, Ph.D., Alexius J. Crowley, D.D.S., Seymour Gottlieb, D.D.S. and Joseph Phillips, D.D.S. Thousands of other scientists, nutritionists, doctors and dentists, although not assisting me on an individual basis, were invaluable in that their research findings have been incorporated in my text.

No book of this scope can come into existence without the help of dedicated reference librarians. Jack Hicks and his associates—Angela Platt, Peggy McCabe, Cynthia Wargo, Elaine Kinney, Joan Bairstow and Rick Bean of the Deerfield, Illinois Public Library; Bill Hagedorn of Central Serials; Rita Obuchowski of the North Suburban Interlibrary Loan Service; Ed Vladas of John Crerar Library; and James Parrish and his associates of the University of Illinois Library of the Health Sciences, Chicago, Illinois have been especially helpful.

I am grateful to Margie Schroeder for an art concept used on the book's cover. Special thanks are due my loyal typists, Lenore Garcia and Margie Schroeder, who laboriously prepared the manuscript for publication. My gratitude also goes to Jo Szczesny, Marie Szczesny, Helen Monaghan, Lisa Dianovsky, Helen Sherbondy, Chris Lattig and Penny Leary who assisted them. The dedicated artisans who converted the manuscript into a book are acknowledged in the colophon on the book's final page.

Are You an Index Reader?

Relatively few persons are avid index readers. To most, the suggestion that one read an index straight through from A to Z will seem equivalent to the idea of reading the telephone directory from cover to cover. Index reading, nevertheless, can point out subtleties of a book that may not be found readily with an attentive reading or even several re-readings. A thorough reading of a good index may result in a better learning experience than that provided by a cursory perusal of the book itself.

Right after finishing the Preface of this book, you might like to turn to the Subject Index (which starts on page 1077) for what could be an interesting experience. You may desire to look especially at the large number of subentries under *Reverse effects*. Physicians and medically-oriented scientists may be interested in noting that drug-related *reverse effects* are indexed under *Drugs*. (I view this listing, along with the concepts, theories and speculations on pages 73-74, 164, 260, 326, 786 and 868, as the start of a book someone will write, perhaps entitled *The Reverse Effect in Medicine*. Physicians know much about side effects—little, generally, about *reverse effects*.) A careful reading of the index may suggest the possible existence of *reverse effects* that have not yet been demonstrated. For example, the index shows that on page 752 there is a suggestion selenium may exacerbate arthritis while on page 755 is an indication that selenium may *alleviate* arthritis. Large dosages are often more dangerous than small ones. You may, however, find it intriguing to look in the index under "Dosage" to find examples of large dosages that may be safer than small ones.

Possibly you'll want to check the entries under *Circadian rhythms* for the daily variations in body concentrations of various nutrients. Reading the index will yield such possibly-intriguing entries as the dangers not only of vitamins and minerals but also the dangers of fiber, exercise, peanut butter and water. Readers of the index also will be presented with such possibly-curious entries as the benefits of smoking, caffeine, sugar, obesity and hypertension. Will this be the day you become a confirmed and avid index reader?

> "I always had the feeling that the surgeons should have read one more book."
> — President John F. Kennedy (in regard to the recurrent problems with his back). Quoted by Kenneth S. Warren, *Coping with the Biomedical Literature* (New York: Praeger Publishers, 1981), p. 18

> "Scientific revolutions are very interesting. The way they happen is that most people deny them and resist them. And then there's more and more of an explosion; and there's a paradigm shift."
> — Candace Pert, *Science 85* (November, 1985) 6, no. 9: 96

A Preface to be Read

Over the past 15 years I have uncovered a massive amount of information vital to health and longevity. Many of the facts I have discovered are virtually unknown to the public whether they are laymen, medical doctors, dieticians or nutritionists. Much of the information has remained hidden even from scientists themselves except, of course, for the material that relates to their respective specialties. The facts presented in this book were turned up through intensive study of tens of thousands of articles from scientific journals published throughout the world. The monumental project of finding the key material was made possible by doing both manual and computer searches involving *Index Medicus, Biological Abstracts, Chemical Abstracts, Excerpta Medica,* the *Toxicology Data Bank of the Oak*

Ridge National Laboratory, and *Citation Abstracts.** The task I set for
myself was the deciphering of this huge number of technical studies
into language understandable by nonspecialists whether they are
scientists, dieticians, nutritionists, medical doctors or intelligent
laymen.

I hope this book will help you—whether you are a doctor, a
scientist, a dietician, a nutritionist or a layman—to learn how to sort out
mere popular notions about health from those ideas that are supported
by clinical or laboratory evidence. After reading this book—and
especially the final chapter—I think you will have a better concept of
how information is sometimes managed for profit. Furthermore, it is
likely you will by then have increased your ability to not only detect
such managed information, but to discover when the popular media are
merely acting as progenitors of nutritional nonsense.

Some of the things you are about to learn will shock you. Can the
time of day one takes mineral supplements be a factor in health and
sexuality (Chapter 7)? Is it possible that vitamin C *causes* cancer
(Chapter 6)? What recent research suggests that vitamin D might help
cure cancer (Chapter 4)? Could it be that vitamin E, widely
recommended to make men more potent, may actually cause
degeneration of the sex organs (Chapter 2)? Is it possible that the
vitamin B complex could *reduce* one's energy level (Chapter 5)? When
is vitamin A effective in preventing breast cancer induced in animals by
carcinogens and when does it show a *reverse effect* by increasing
mammary carcinomas (Chapter 4)? Under what circumstances will zinc
work to suppress immunity and when will it strengthen the immune
system (Chapter 7)? Instead of being a cancer cure, is it possible that
laetrile might be carcinogenic (Chapter 5)? Can it be that lead, a poison
in large amounts, is essential for growth in small amounts (Chapter 8)?
Could strenuous exercise be a cause of cancer and reduced longevity

---

* *Citation Abstracts* (available in libraries of the health sciences) makes it possible to follow up
on any given study (including the 4,821 references cited in this book) as future researchers cite
these earlier studies. One of the great treasures of a study is likely to be its list of references. The
references cited in those references may, in turn, be consulted and so *ad infinitum*. Thus, an
endless chain reaction of ever-increasing knowledge can proceed backward in time just as
Citation Abstracts permits an endless chain reaction perusal of future research relevant to your
chosen topic.

(Chapter 10)? Can chemicals called antioxidants—including the much-maligned BHT—give us better health and increased longevity (Chapter 9)?

In addition to presenting new research findings throughout the book, I have developed some of my own health-related hypotheses. My proposed *theory of the reverse effect* may make it possible, via "armchair chemistry" to predict which substances may be therapeutically useful for treating cancer and other diseases. The *reverse effect* may, however, be masked by the very way in which science is so often performed with experimental parameters that have been set too narrowly, along with an improper use of extrapolation. It is sometimes argued that extrapolation is a valid procedure when there exists a theory regarding the functional relationship between variables. I argue, on the contrary, that the theory may be false and that data should be gathered covering wide parameters. In this way it becomes possible not only to prove or to disprove any existing theory, but to allow for the possibility of a new discovery.

Suppose a set of experimental data involving the varying concentrations of a test substance (shown on the X-axis) and the values of a dependent physiological variable (shown on the Y-axis) is properly graphed in this way:

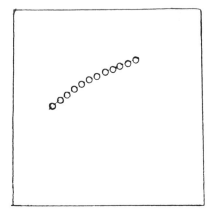

Often a scientist will improperly extrapolate and will presume that the function would graph as follows:

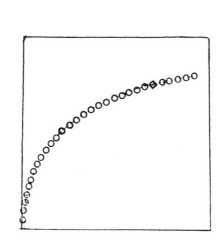

Reality might involve, unknown to the scientist, a *reverse effect* at lower concentrations of the test substance:

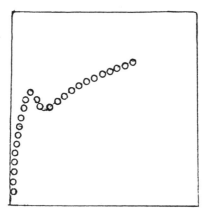

Or, a *reverse effect* might exist at the upper end of the data:

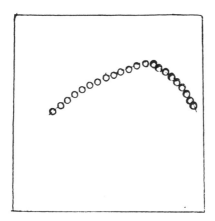

Or, a *reverse effect* might be present at each end:

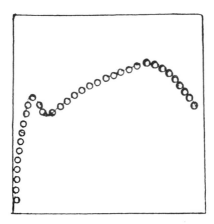

Since, in this example, three reversals exist (two peaks and one trough), we have what I call a *triphasic reverse effect* . (Without the last turn downward the effect would be *biphasic*.) It is possible that at higher concentrations of the substance being tested there could be a fourth reversal to exemplify a *polyphasic reverse effect*. A scientist should extend the parameters of his experiment in order to discover, rather than to hide, new phenomena exemplified by *reverse effects.* Throughout this book we will be examining *reverse effects* of vitamins and minerals as well as, in a few cases, those involving drugs, exercise, x-ray phenomena, etc.

I have referenced virtually every statement unless it is clearly indicated to be my own idea or is a fact or opinion that is widely held. My information is in many cases so unbelievable that I want you to not only question my facts, but I want you to be able to easily check their validity. The citations make it possible for you to ask your local librarian to order for you photostatic copies of the relevant research material. Then you can read the original studies for yourself and come to your own conclusions.

All of us tend to be tree-minded, ignoring the vast forest that lies beyond our immediate perceptions of reality. Some will find in this book merely a few new trees of knowledge about health and longevity. The rare person will use this book as a guide to comprehending the forest of health and longevity perceptions that extends to infinity in all directions. For some, this book may help foster a healthy skepticism in the midst of the noise of nutritional evangelists bent on fostering their own polarized views. But remember, skepticism is healthy only if it allows for the possibility of truth emerging from each of many opposing positions. Truth is always *quasi,* never *absolute.*

Many of the nutritional suggestions that follow will be based on animal experiments and in drawing conclusions for human applications we will sometimes feel less than completely confident. However, we can't wait for everything in nutrition to be proved conclusively. (Of course, nothing ever is.) Those of us with just one life to live are willing to proceed on the basis of probability.

Mankind faces no more intriguing problem than that of how to improve health and increase longevity. I hope you will be as enthralled as I am with the answers now coming from the research centers of contemporary science.

"If we would have new knowledge,
we must get us a whole world of
new questions."
— Susanne K. Langer, *Philosophy
in a New Key* (Cambridge:
Harvard University Press, 1948)

Introduction

How to Read Biomedical Literature

I want to encourage you, as you read this book, to ask your librarian to obtain for you photostatic copies of interesting references. Remember, a study that questions the validity of one of your own firmly held opinions may be especially rewarding.

Take cognizance of the fact that prospective studies (ones involving future developments, e.g., after administering a given nutrient) are more apt to lead to reliable conclusions than are retrospective ones (where conclusions are drawn based on past, thus uncontrolled, events). Epidemiological studies may offer reliable suggestions but conclusions drawn from them may not be applicable to individuals who have health parameters greatly deviating from mean values.

When reading a journal article, note whether the purposes of the study are clearly defined. Is it apparent what hypothesis is to be tested or what question is to be answered? In reading the study, be wary of confused writing that should have been corrected by the scientist's editor. If the investigator writes that he fed each mouse 10 mg./kg., does he mean he fed the animal 10 mg. of the test substance per kg. of chow or per kg. of body weight? I think one is proper in downgrading the importance of studies containing unresolved confusion. Is the experimental protocol given in detail? In analyzing the scientific literature, one must especially be on guard against the possibility that the protocol of a study itself may lead to doubtful conclusions no matter how well the study was otherwise done. In analyzing a given study, examine its protocol to determine if the experiments were performed in a double-blind, controlled manner. In a controlled experiment neither the scientist who is to interpret the results nor the subjects know whether the test substance or a placebo has been administered. That information is known only to a third party, with the results to be decoded only upon termination of the experiment. In many cases, experimenters believe it is unethical (or at least contrary to the dictates of their own conscience) to withhold a thought-to-be-efficacious therapy to, say, one-half of a test group.* Thus, they may administer a test substance to all and then compare the results against their opinion of how patients treated with a standard therapy would have responded. In analyzing such studies we must be aware of the power of patients to help cure themselves when given loving care regardless of the efficacy of whatever is being tested. Furthermore, in such cases the scientist/physician may overoptimistically interpret the power of his new therapy. The results of controlled double-blind experiments are more believable, but even those are subject to possible defects in the manner in which they are conducted.

In many cases the results of a triply-blind experiment, as discussed by Adolph Grünbaum,[1a] may be even more reliable than results of one that is double-blind. In a triply-blind experiment the patients are unaware of the group to which they have been assigned, the dispensers do not know what they are administering and those assessing the outcome do not know which were the patients and which were the controls. In some cases, e.g., surgery or psychotherapy, the dispenser cannot be blind and so, at best, we have a double-blind study. (By the way, the cited reference 1a

---

* Peter McCullagh[1] quotes the Helsinki Code, which states that "Concern for the interests of the subject must always prevail over the interests of science and society." (Paragraph I.5) Furthermore, this Code also states, "In any medical study every patient—including those of a control group, if any—should be assured of the best proven diagnostic and therapeutic method." (Paragraph II.3)

contains a very valuable discussion of the placebo concept. You may want to request this article from your local library.)

When analyzing an experiment involving human subjects, see if the protocol clearly discloses how they were selected and try to form an opinion whether such selection was valid in terms of the experiment's objectives. Note also how the dropouts were handled. Be wary of the scientist's conclusions if he simply excluded them from his analysis or (far worse) added them to his control group. Keep in mind that many variables (e.g., blood pressure or cholesterol level) will fluctuate over time and the extreme values will tend to regress to the mean values.[1b] Especially low values will tend to rise, and particularly high values will tend to fall, quite irrespective of any given therapy being tested, because of the undue influence of random variation. Such values, if remeasured, are likely to be closer to the mean, a phenomenon called "regression toward the mean."

There are many other considerations in analyzing the appropriateness of an experiment's design. Philip W. Lavori et al.,[2] in discussing prognostic factors other than the treatment itself, says, "If patients who are assigned to separate treatment groups differ before treatment in factors that affect prognosis, such as age, extent of disease or concurrent medical problems, the observed results may be affected by this difference as well as by treatment." Such factors are called "confounding variables," "prognostic factors" or "covariates" and they must be considered or the assessment of the value of the treatment will be biased. Lavori points out that randomization reduces the effects of confounding variables. He says: "Randomization confers several benefits on a study. It protects the rules for treatment assignment from conscious or unconscious manipulation by investigators or patients. Randomization may include the various forms of 'blindness,' but it always ensures that the assignment to treatment groups is left to an objective and indifferent procedure that cannot be predicted. Randomization is not the only way to achieve such protection, but it is the simplest and best understood way to certify that one has done so."

Randomization, however, never provides complete protection, as Thomas A. Louis[3] observes, "against the possibility of producing a trial with unacceptable balance." Louis[3] says, regarding randomization: "Statistical theory tells us that we can expect balance on the average, but provides no iron-clad guarantees for any particular trial. It also tells us that if we check for imbalance on enough covariates (risk factors), we will find some that are significantly out of balance, even if 'perfect' randomization were used." In considering the design and interpretation of studies, John C. Bailer, et al,[4] make the point that "in the absence of a well-defined sampling plan or other support for inference, a finding of 'statistical significance' may be misleading or impossible to interpret, whereas a finding 'not statistically significant' may be meaningless." Valuable suggestions regarding experimental design, appropriateness of subjects and statistical concepts—along with an excellent list of references—will be found in an article by Louis[3] entitled "Critical Issues in the Conduct and Interpretation of Clinical Trials" and in a recent review by Lincoln E. Moses.[5]

Sometimes a purely methodological procedure can be of far greater importance than the experimenter might imagine. Plaut tells about an experiment of S. A. Barnett and J. Burn,[6] who clipped the ears of pups in a rat litter in order to identify the animals. They found that the mothers treated the clipped and unclipped pups differently, thus affecting the results of their study. If they had not been especially alert, a false conclusion based on a defective protocol could have resulted.

The reader of scientific literature must be aware of the possibility that a scientist may not always be studying what he thinks he is studying. If research involves, for example, human intake of high- vs. low-fiber foods, is it possible that the results may have been influenced by the additional milk or cream taken with the bran cereal or by the increased butter used with the bread? Suppose a study is being made of the effects of drinking coffee. Coffee drinkers tend to do more smoking than noncoffee drinkers. Unless the effect of this confounding variable is appreciated and smokers excluded from the study, caffeine could get the blame which might more properly be ascribed to nicotine.

In animal experiments, especially, there may often be little if any appreciation for how the central nervous system can modulate body processes. In particular, Robert Ader[7] points out that it is not a universally accepted premise, even among behavioral scientists, that the central nervous system and immune functions are interrelated.* Without such an appreciation, is a scientist apt to adequately insure that the psychological problems of his animals are not affecting their immune responses in addition to any possible effect of the substance he is testing? Marvin Stein et al.[8] showed that hypothalamic lesions have a significant effect on the immune processes of animals. Nicholas Pavlidis and Michael Chirigos[9] reported that stress inhibited the ability of macrophages to kill tumor cells. Jay R. Kaplan et al.,[10] experimenting with monkeys, reported that "psychosocial factors may influence atherogenesis in the absence of elevated serum lipids." R. H. Gisler et al.[11] say,"Animals used for immunological studies should certainly not be exposed to stressful situations before or during experimentation." It is up to us, the readers of scientific literature, to form a judgment as to the appropriateness of the scientist's protocol which will be disclosed in his published study.

To illustrate the point that the ways in which a scientist works with his animals may (perhaps unbeknownst to him) affect his results, let's cite some studies showing the importance of stress:

1.   Stanford B. Friedman et al.[12] reported that when adult mice were inoculated with Coxsackie virus and/or given an electric shock, animals died when both inoculum and the shock were administered, but not when either inoculum or shock was given

---

* In the five years since Ader made that comment there have been many relevant articles, an international symposium (under the auspices of the Princess Liliane Cardiology Foundation in Brussels, Belgium, October 27 and 28, 1983) whose proceedings were published as a book,[7a] as well as other books[7b-f] relating to psychoneural effects on immunity. Other recent studies showing how the immune and neuroendocrine systems are interrelated have been published by J. Edwin Blalock[7g] and by Jean L. Marx.[7h]

alone.* Experimental conditions do not generally offer, unknown to the scientist, factors that may be as upsetting as an electrical shock, but still they could be serious enough to affect the results.

2. Contrary to the Friedman study above, Benjamin H. Newberry et al.[13] found that severe electrical shock stress applied to rats in which mammary tumors had been chemically induced (by DMBA) caused a significant reduction in tumor count. On the other hand, Lawrence S. Sklar and Hymie Anisman[13a] reported that a single session of inescapable shock resulted in earlier tumor appearance, exaggeration of tumor size and decreased survival time in mice with syngeneic P815 mastocytoma. Escapable shock, however, had no such effects. In fact, Madelon A. Visintainer, et al,[13b] found that while only 27% of rats receiving inescapable shock rejected a transplanted tumor, 63% of rats receiving escapable shock and 54% of rats receiving no shock rejected the tumor. Lack of control over stress, a psychological variable, seems to sometimes reduce tumor rejection and decrease survival. Stress, while often detrimental, can sometimes be beneficial; the point is that stress should be minimized in a nutritional study.

3. Benjamin H. Newberry et al.[14] demonstrated that chronically administered restraint inhibited the development of DMBA-induced rat mammary tumors. It seems that our perception of what is "good" and "bad" stress may need modification.

4. Andrew A. Monjan and Michael I. Collector[15] reported that daily auditory stress applied to mice for varying lengths of time can,

---

* Is it possible that human inoculation is less likely to produce negative side effects if it is performed in the absence of a second perturbing influence? Could the scream of another child be such a second perturbational factor? (The tremendous stress that noise can cause in animals will be discussed soon.) A scream may or may not be stressful. Steven Greer [12a] says, however, in regard to stressful events: "It is the individual's appraisal of and response to an event rather than the event per se which is the nub of the matter."

depending on conditions, either suppress or enhance immune response. Malcolm P. Rogers et al.[16] found that noise stress significantly increased the prevalence of arthritis in rats. Marcus M. Jensen and A. F. Rasmussen[17] reported a progressive hypertrophy of the adrenal glands under the influence of daily three-hour exposures to high intensity sound. They also reported that leukopenia (a decreased white blood cell count) existed during the period of sound stress while leukocytosis (an increase in the number of white blood cells) followed the termination of the stress period. In another study, I. S. Chohan et al.[17a] reported that blood coagulation in rats can be affected by continuous exposure to loud noise. Various blood parameters were changed, including the development of significantly prolonged bleeding time. Ernest A. Peterson[18] says that "noise commonly found in the human environment can cause sustained changes in laboratory animals."* He goes on further to state, "...it is reasonably likely that self-generated noise in dog and monkey quarters is sufficiently high to merit abatement measures." If an experiment is conducted in a noisy laboratory, will results be affected? Possibly, but probably the experimenter would innocently avoid commenting on the condition of his lab. (In the interest of space, a scientist is forced to limit description of his protocol, eliminating possibly important factors.)

There is a kind of "noise" that is often ignored by scientists—that of animal communication. When animals are handled, injected or treated in other ways, they may send supersonic signals[19] to their cagemates or to animals in other cages (where perhaps a different experiment is in progress). The increased corticosterone levels that might result could affect the experimental results.

5. The time at which stress is introduced can have an important bearing on experimental results. We have just noted some effects

---

* The health of humans is also affected by noise. Baird cites a study by P. Rachootin and J. Olsen[18a] showing occupational exposure of women to noise resulted in hormonal disturbances and reduced fertility.

of sound stress. In another study, Marcus M. Jensen and A. F. Rasmussen[19a] reported that susceptibility of mice to intranasally inoculated vesicular stomatitis virus was significantly altered by daily exposure to three-hour periods of high intensity sound. However, animals inoculated before stress were more susceptible, whereas those inoculated after stress were more resistant to the virus than were the controls. Another study showed the importance of the relative time at which surgical stress occurred. A. R. Turnbull et al.,[19b] in studying the effects of cholecystectomy on guinea pigs after a lethal injection of leukemic cells, found that surgery before the injection of the tumor cells *prolonged* mean survival time by 77%. Surgery one day after the tumor dose did not significantly affect survival, but surgery nine days after the injection of the leukemic cells shortened survival time by 35%. In another study, George F. Solomon et al.[19c] found that when mice, after being given an intravenous injection of Newcastle disease virus, were stressed by repeated random electric shocks preceded by a warning buzzer their interferon response was not altered compared to controls. However, when such stress was given five hours prior to virus inoculation, interferon production was significantly enhanced.

6. The laboratory lighting may influence the experimental results, possibly through involvement of the pineal gland.[20] J. F. Spalding et al.[20] report that black and white mice differ markedly in their reactivity to light of different hue. The importance of laboratory lighting as an experimental variable has been reviewed by John Ott.[21] In a given study you may be examining, did the scientist use the same lighting for his experimental group and for his controls, or was one of the groups housed in a different corner of the room where the lighting (and perhaps the temperature and noise level) differed?

7. Earlier, we noted some benefits of stress. Another benefit of stress is shown by the work of James T. Marsh et al.[22] Eleven

monkeys were subjected to avoidance stress for 24 hours. (They learned to press a telegraph key at a steady rate to avoid a shock that would be delivered every 10 seconds if the lever were not pressed.) After the 24-hour period they were inoculated with type I poliovirus. Twelve control monkeys were similarly inoculated. Seven of the eleven stressed animals survived the infection, whereas only one of the control animals survived. Marsh et al. point out that this study contrasts with findings of *reduced* resistance in mice to virus infection if they are subjected to a different kind of stress called "shuttle box stress." The Marsh study also contrasts with observations of increased susceptibility to poliovirus in hamsters and mice given cortisone before inoculation.

8. The stress of a cold temperature may be beneficial or detrimental. Susan R. Burchfield et al.[23] reported that singly housed male and female rats stressed by cold only before receiving an injection of tumor cells developed significantly smaller tumors than an unstressed group. Rats stressed with cold only after injection of tumor cells developed slightly smaller tumors than the unstressed group. Benjamin H. Newberry and Lee Sengbusch[24] cite other studies showing noxious environmental conditions can either facilitate or inhibit tumor development. When studying the protocol of a given study, try to determine if the scientist minimized stress on his animals unless it was his purpose to stress them.

9. Malcolm P. Rogers[25] reported that if rats that had been immunized with type II collagen were exposed to a cat for a ten-minute period four times a day at six-hour intervals, the stress of that exposure abrogated development of arthritis. They cautioned, however, that the stress may have merely delayed onset of arthritis. The study helps remind us, however, that many types of stress may be beneficial and emphasizes the importance of the scientist minimizing stress in his animals to help assure reliable experimental results.

10. Housing conditions under which animals live may present stresses which could affect an experiment. Either isolation or crowding may generate stresses that can affect experimental validity. Male rats housed together, for example, are prone to fighting (which according to H. M. Weiss et al.[26] may not be bad for them since it prevents stress-related pathology, such as ulceration)* but, on the other hand, group housing confounds the experiment because the less dominant animals may be unable to participate. George F. Solomon et al.[29] observed that mixed-sex group housing at high male-female ratios increases the severity of adjuvant-induced arthritis in the male rat. Vernon Riley[30] reported that 92% of female mice carrying an oncogenic virus developed mammary tumors under conditions of extreme stress, including crowded housing and other detrimental environmental circumstances, as contrasted with only 7% in a protected environment. Tumors appeared earliest when females were housed with males, when housed in the vicinity of disturbed mice having elevated corticosterone values (presumably due to contagious anxiety) and when exposed to dust, odor, noise and pheromones.** Animals housed more than one to a cage may compete for food. The less aggressive ones may get less food and consequently live longer (or less long if starvation results)—thus negating the "experimental results." Mice housed alone are significantly less susceptible to certain parasites but, on the other hand, show depressed immunity to the parasite *Hymenolepis nana*.[8] In some cases, even humans living

---

* Fighting between male rats has other consequences. Henry reported that F. H. Bronson and B. E. Eleftheriou[27] have found such fighting for a few minutes each day leads to an increased adrenal content of cortical hormone. B. L. Welch and A. S. Welch[28] showed that five to ten daily five-minute bouts increase brain noradrenaline and adrenaline.

** Riley did not report on the longevity of male mice housed with females relative to male mice housed with other males. However, P. Ebbesen and R. Rask-Nielsen,[31] in studying various types of mice, found that "survival time was much shorter in sex-segregated males of all strains than in nonsegregated males, whereas the survival time was long in all groups of females. (Perhaps sexual intercourse is a longevity factor for male, but not for female, mice.) One variety of sex-segregated male mice (DBA-2) developed a progressive normocytic anemia and reticulocytosis.

alone may show benefits. For example, in a study of prison inmates, David A. D'Atri et al.[32] found that those housed in multiple-occupancy dormitories had significantly higher blood pressures than those housed alone. Crowded conditions may be stressful to men or to animals. Friedman and Glasgow[33] cite animal studies showing that fighting (among males under crowded conditions) may have great influences upon resistance through changes involving the pituitary-adrenocortical axis, reproductive organs and other endocrine functions. However, in favor of crowded housing, they point out that, in another study, such conditions increased the resistance of mice to tuberculosis.* Furthermore, yet another study cited by Stanford B. Friedman and Lowell A. Glasgow[33] showed that female mice housed in groups lived significantly longer after inoculation with encephalomyocarditis virus than when housed alone. Earlier, Howard B. Andervont[35] had reported that virgin mice that were isolated into separate cages at 4 and 20 weeks of age developed mammary tumors at an average age of 9.6 months, while those housed 8 to a cage developed such tumors only after an average age of 11.9 months.** About seven years later, O. Muhlbock[36] did a study related to that of Andervont and achieved similar results. LaBarba, writing about this study, cited Muhlbock as reporting that "animals housed in larger groups consume less food and that caloric intake may be of some importance in tumorigensis." Another study, this one by J. L. Barnett et al.,[37] found that individual penning of pigs resulted in a chronic stress response. Similarly, Vernon Riley[38] reported that female mice had greater

---

* The study referred to, one by Ethel Tobach and Hubert Bloch,[34] in which a Tween albumin culture of M_1 tuberculosis strain was injected intravenously into mice, indicates that "males which were crowded before or after injection of bacilli showed less resistance to tuberculosis than the control mice, whereas females which were crowded before or after injection survived longer than the controls." (Tween solvent may introduce problems as discussed in Chapter 2. Disclosing, in the protocol, the fact that Tween solvent was used allows us to speculate that Tween may have exacerbated any effect caused by the T.B. bacilli.)

** Andervont, writing almost a half-century ago, expressed his concern with the protocol of experiments in these words: "The primary purpose for placing this work on record is to show that in studies on the occurrence of mammary tumors in mice the cages of control and of experimental animals must contain equal numbers of mice."

ability to reject a tumor challenge when housed in groups compared
to their single-animal-per-cage counterparts. Joseph T. King et
al.[38a] showed that male mice housed 2 per cage or 20 per cage also
lived significantly longer than those housed alone. Doreen Berman
and Barbara E. Rodin[39] reported on an experiment following dorsal
rhizotomy in 44 male rats. (They surgically made a unilateral
intradural section of dorsal roots.) Each of 10 isolated animals self-
mutilated to an extreme degree with 7 cannibalizing the denervated
limb. In contrast, only one of 34 that were housed with female rats
showed any sign of self-biting. In any experiments such as this one
involving chronic pain, housing conditions may have important
bearing on the results. G. S. Wiberg and H. C. Grice[40] reported
that rats isolated for long periods became nervous and aggressive
and developed caudal dermatitis (scaly tail). They also reported that
isolated rats had heavier thyroid glands in addition to heavier
adrenals, but lighter spleen and thymus glands compared to group-
housed animals. Obviously, colony living is not always stressful
for the animals. Such living can be stressful, however, if the
colony is disturbed. James P. Henry et al.[41] found that if newborns
are removed from a socially organized mouse colony, the social
order breaks down. There is fighting among the males and the
young are lost due to neglect and injury by the females. James P.
Henry et al. reported that there was a high incidence of mammary
tumors in such socially disorganized colonies.

Mixing sexes of animals within the same vicinity, although
housed in separate cages, can, according to Riley,[38] distort
immunological parameters and affect growth of tumors. James
Rollin Slonaker[42] had reported, even earlier, that "the activity of
male rats in cages near a female tended to follow the rhythm of the
female activity." E. P. Durrant[43] also found that the activity of
males housed near a female "took on a rhythmic variation agreeing
in 95 per cent of instances with that of the associated female." It
may be necessary, however, for the males to see the females if
such increase in activity is to occur. David R. Lamb et al.[44] reported
that when adjacent animals were positioned so they could not see
each other, the heterosexual odors and sounds did not result in a

significant increase in male activity. H. M. Bruce,[45] however, reports that many animal responses are stimulated by pheromones. He states there is "convincing evidence that the notorious aggression between male mice is released by olfactory signals alone." He also cites a study showing that the domestic cat will display estrus behavior if placed in a cage which recently held a male cat unless the cage has been washed.

Housing conditions often provide a confusing element in the attempt to judge an experiment's protocol. However, in making judgments regarding a given study, I think it proper to be suspicious of an experiment performed under extremely crowded conditions. The resulting stresses could negate the conclusions being drawn by the scientist in charge. Nevertheless, it may not be the crowding per se that is negative but simply the resulting physical contact. S. Michael Plaut et al.[46] reported that in studying mice infected with *Plasmodium berghei,* which produces malaria in rodents, cage size did not affect the mortality rate. They concluded that "the housing effect is dependent upon population size, rather than density." The investigators went on to say, "grouped mice separated by screening died as slowly as individuals, suggesting a role of physical contact in the high mortality rate of grouped mice." Chevedoff et al. cite a study by V. Riley and D. Spackman[47] who, "using cage densities from 1 to 20 animals/cage, failed to repeat earlier results in mice in which tumor incidence was found related to cage density. They concluded that crowding per se is not stressful provided that the overall housing environment is not stressful." Earlier, June Marchant[48] concluded one of her own studies by saying: "It is impossible to make any definite statements about the effect of particular social conditions on susceptibility to breast tumor induction by this or that carcinogen. Each genetic type responds in its own way to a particular carcinogen and may respond in a somewhat different way to another carcinogen. Different social conditions with their accompanying hormonal disturbances do not always have the same kind of effects on breast tumor induction in different genetic types of mice." A study by Patricia F. Hadaway et al.[49] bears out the importance of housing considerations if animals self-administer substances. When morphine-sucrose solutions were self-administered by rats, isolated females drank 5 times as much as colony rats and isolated males 16 times as much. The scientists commented: "If this housing effect proved to be a general phenomenon, it would suggest that the influence of laboratory conditions per se must be emphasized more in the interpretation of self-administration studies." Either excessive crowding or isolation can sometimes influence the results of an experiment. Experimental animals and controls must be housed under "identical" conditions. If this has not been done we should rightfully downgrade the reliability of a scientist's "results."

11. Were animals "handled" as infants and/or were they handled during the course of the experiment? George F. Solomon[50] observes that there are conflicting results regarding handling of infant rats and their later experience with respect to tumor growth. He notes that G. Newton et al.[51] found that rats held and stroked for 10 minutes daily after weaning and implanted with Walker carcinoma 256 two days after cessation of handling survived significantly longer and had smaller adrenals than nonhandled controls. In contrast, Solomon et al. cite the work of S. Levine and C. Cohen[52] where mice handled for the first 24 days of life showed shorter survival times after transplantation of leukemia as adults. Riley[30] found that merely handling mice for tumor inspection provides stress that increased tumor production. Stanford B. Friedman et al.[53] similarly found that simply placing rats in experimental cages increased their plasma corticosterone levels. These studies contrast with those of Robert M. Nerem and Murina J. Levesque,[54] reported in more detail in Chapter 1, that showed rabbits held, petted, talked to and played with had better health. Of course, there is a big difference

between "handling" and "petting" and the results of handling may vary with species and with the disease being studied. Solomon et al.,[50] even though they cited studies showing detrimental effects of handling, say: "It seemed possible that one of the chief consequences of infantile stimulation is to endow the organism with the capacity to make fine discriminations concerning the relevant aspects of the environment. This view seems to be supported by evidence that manipulated animals showed less adrenal response to a new situation and quicker habituation." Robert Ader and Stanford B. Friedman[54a] reported that rats handled during the preweaning period showed a reduced rate of tumor development relative to unmanipulated controls. Ader[55] also found that, "among individually housed animals, handling experience during the first 3 weeks of life decreased susceptibility to gastric erosions." He concluded that "early life experiences can modify a genetically determined susceptibility to disease."

12. We have already noted some housing-related effects on hormone levels. Stephen H. Vessey[56] cites many other studies showing the effect of various stressors on the production of adrenocortical hormones. Grouped mice not only had heavier adrenal glands, but lower numbers of circulating eosinophils relative to isolated mice. Rats housed in colonies had higher levels of plasma corticosterone than those housed in groups of four. Another study cited by Vessey showed groups of 20 had higher corticosterone levels than did those housed alone. Interestingly, David E. Davis and John C. Christian[57] found that group-housed male mice ranking low in their social "pecking" order have heavier adrenal glands than high-ranking mice (Figure 1). Davis and Christian concluded that these findings suggest low-ranking mice are subjected to more physical and psychological stressing stimuli. Furthermore, male mice housed in groups have heavier adrenal glands than those kept in isolation. This contrasts, however, with the finding reported by Paul Brain[58] that isolated female rats have relatively smaller adrenal glands than those housed in groups. (Brain also cites many studies

that show isolation increases gonadal activity in males and that isolated males have heavier sex accessories than group-housed rats. Brain notes that this also may be true of female rats.) Brain[58] cites several studies showing that the turnover rate of neurotransmitters in the brain of isolated mice is lower than in those that are group-housed. Friedman and Glasgow[33] speculate that "the adrenocorticosteroids, and probably other hormones, might act either alone or in conjunction with other physiological processes to modify host susceptibility as a result of psychologic stress." They point out that the modified resistance might be due to the known influence of adrenocortical hormones upon antibody levels[59] and interferon production.[60] They quote I. E. Bush[61] as saying: "Our whole concept of the adrenal cortex as a gland the secretions of which regulate an as yet undiscovered metabolic process that affects the metabolism of carbohydrate, protein and other substances is thrown into confusion by the suggestion that the most important natural stimulus to the activity of the gland is psychological stress." Histamine may also be influenced by stress. W. Cassell et al.[61a] reported that mice exposed to a group environment had a high tissue concentration of histamine. This is in line with a finding by B. Jencks [61b] showing that mice reared in groups had larger numbers of subcutaneous mast cells than isolated animals. (Is it possible that a copious histamine response to stress might be an unsuspected influence in studies using vitamin C—a vitamin that destroys histamine?) When analyzing an experiment, ask yourself if the scientist took cognizance of the problem of insuring the psychological health of his subjects (animal or human) by minimizing stressful conditions.

In studying the protocol of an experiment, be cognizant of the possibility that the scientist may have improperly ignored still other factors:

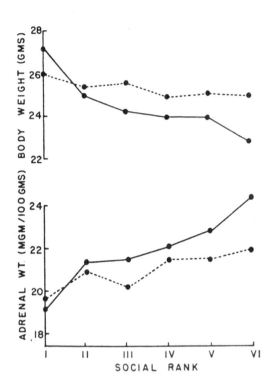

Figure 1. Relation of body weight and rank (upper lines) and adrenal size and rank (lower lines) to social rank in mice. Dotted line refers to weight at start and solid line refers to weight at end of ten days. Reproduced from David E. Davis and John J. Christian, *Proc. of the Society for Experimental Biology and Medicine* (1957) 94: 728-731, with permission. Is it not conceivable that stress might have such an overwhelming influence on adrenal action as to unduly influence a nutritional study? Stress must be controlled if one is to draw valid nutritional conclusions.

1. Did the experimenter take precautions to avoid a conditioned response in his animals that might have affected his results?

Mason tells about a study by F. H. Bronson and B. E. Eleftheriou[62] which showed that merely exposing a subordinate mouse to fighters—especially if the subject mouse has a previous history of defeat in combat—can produce adrenal cortical responses as great as if he had been attacked and defeated. J. W. Mason[63] states that a study he did with J. V. Brady and M. Sidman "showed that a conditioned emotional response, elicited simply by presentation of a mild clicking noise that had been previously paired with electrical shock, was associated with marked plasma 17-hydroxycorticosteroid elevations in the monkey." There are other examples of conditioned responses. Robert Ader and Nicholas Cohen[64] administered to rats the drug cyclophosphamide (the unconditioned stimulus), a substance known to cause immunosuppression. Simultaneously, they gave a distinctly flavored drinking solution of saccharin (the conditioned stimulus), a substance that has no such effect. After training in this manner, the rats were allowed to recover. Then later, when saccharin was given alone, an immunosuppressive effect was produced, illustrating a conditioned response.*

Michael Russell et al.[65] recently showed that histamine, so important in allergic reactions, may be released as a learned response. When an immunologic challenge was paired with the presentation of an odor, guinea pigs showed a plasma histamine response. Later, those guinea pigs showed a plasma histamine response when presented with the odor alone. The experimenters concluded that the study "suggests that the immune response can be enhanced through activity of the central nervous system." Is it possible that, in a study you may be investigating, the animals

---

* More recently, Ader et al.[64a] reported that such conditioning can reduce by 50% the amount of cyclophosphamide needed to control the murine version of the human autoimmune disease lupus erythematosus. Such a finding may eventually lead to human conditioning therapies that might permit similar reductions in drug dosages. Recalling Pavlov and his dogs, need we be limited to using chemicals to potentize drugs? Could we condition the immune system of a lupus patient to be depressed when given just half of the normal amount of an immune-suppressing drug if that drug were given coincidentally with the ringing of a bell? Could we, on the other hand, condition the immune system of a cancer patient to greater stimulation with an immuno-stimulating drug administered to the sound of a bell?

might have been conditioned to the injection procedure, or to the body odor of the caretaker, or to a certain food, or to the mere opening of their cage doors to react with an increase in plasma corticosteroid regardless of any nutrient or drug the scientist was testing? S. Michael Plaut[66] states, "In many cases, the effects of an early life experience are not apparent until the animal is faced with an appropriate stimulus situation later in life." This suggests that scientists must know their animal supplier and know the precautions he takes for avoiding conditioned responses in his animals. As readers of scientific literature we have to assume the scientists are cognizant of the possibility of such conditioned responses and that they have discussed this problem with their animal supplier. Could it be, however, that laxity in this matter may sometimes be a reason results of different, but similar, experiments are not always the same?

2. We saw earlier that the time at which stress is introduced can greatly affect the results of an experiment. Is it possible that, in a study you may be analyzing, the sequence in which drugs or nutrients were administered or the sequence in which procedures were performed might have influenced the results? Peraino et al.[66a] reported, for example, that phenobarbital administered to rats having liver cancer that was induced by 2-acetylaminofluorene either inhibited or enhanced growth of the cancer, depending on when the phenobarbital was given. If the phenobarbital was given simultaneously with the carcinogen, there was no protective effect; if given after the rats had been exposed to the carcinogen, there was an enhancing effect on tumor incidence.

3. Could one or more circadian rhythms be at work that might influence the experimental results? Ader,[67] studying group-housed rats who were sacrificed sequentially at 90-second intervals, found that "the elevation in plasma corticosterone levels shown by the rats sampled at the crest in the daily cycles is relatively slight as compared to the nearly 5-fold increase in the

corticosterone levels shown by the last animal to be sampled at the trough in the adrenocortical cycle." In another study, Ader [68] reported that rats immobilized at the peak as compared with the trough in the 24-hour activity cycle were more susceptible to gastric erosions. In yet another study, Robert Ader and S. B. Friedman [69] observed that "the time course of the plasma corticosterone response to environmental stimulation depends on the duration of the stimulation and the point in the 24-hour adrenocortical rhythm upon which the stimulation is superimposed." In other research, Alexander H. Friedman and Charles A. Walker [70] reported that histamine levels in the caudate nucleus and midbrain of rats undergo a circadian rhythm and are maximal when body temperature and motor activity are maximal. M. P. Rogers et al. [71] have reported a diurnal variation in natural killer cell activity. If a test substance were to be administered at the time of day when natural killer cell activity was low, would a possible increase in animal death rate be due to that substance or due to the time of day during which it was given? Does the study's protocol consider the possibility that the diurnal variation of plasma coricosterone, of histamine and of natural killer cell activity could be relevant to the experiment being performed?

Friedman et al. [72] point out that sometimes a nutritional deficiency can weaken a microorganism, but sometimes such a deficiency can strengthen other microorganisms (while probably weakening the host).* A scientist, while perhaps taking cognizance of such facts, may improperly ignore the possible chronicity of an infection due to such microorganisms. [73] Studying an experiment's protocol tells us if the scientist in charge is aware of the possible influence of circadian rhythms on his work. Ader [74] cautions that:

---

* Friedman et al. [72] say: "It cannot be predicted whether a specified experimental stimulation will increase, decrease, or not influence host resistance on any a priori grounds. Rather, it has been our view that whether or not a given form of stimulation is detrimental to the host depends upon the particular infectious agent (or disease process) to which the animal is subsequently subjected. Therefore, it seems best to avoid, whenever possible, the very use of the word 'stress,' since it connotes, to many, a deleterious effect on the organism."

The results and interpretation of any study on the effects of the adrenocortical system on conditioned emotional responses (and, perhaps, other conditioned responses) would be determined by the time of day at which different experimenters decided it was convenient to observe their animals. Moreover, unless the light-dark schedule and the time in this schedule were specified, discrepancies between studies would be impossible to evaluate fully. On the basis of these data it does not seem facetious to ask how many discrepancies in the literature are attributable not to who is right and who is wrong but to when the behavior was sampled.

Then, too, the time of day a nutrient or drug is administered may have a great effect on animals, including humans. The science of chronobiology has had its own journal (called *Chronobiologia*) since 1974. Examples of chronobiological effects of potassium, iron, zinc and of other nutrients can be found throughout this book.

4. Was an appropriate animal species used in the study? E. A. Emken[74a] points out that rats have enzyme systems capable of synthesizing many fatty acid isomers which humans may not be able to produce. If so, rat studies in this area might be misleading if extrapolated to man. If it is desired to learn something conceivably applicable to human male sexuality, the rat may be a better experimental animal than the mouse. Morton Rothstein[75] relates that basal levels of testosterone do not decrease with age in mice but do decline in the rat (as in the human male). However, S. Mitchell Harman et al.[75a] reported that the Leydig cells in the testes of aged rats respond to gonadotrophin stimulation far better than do those of aged men. Thus the rat may, as Harman et al. say, "be a poor species in which to attempt to elucidate the nature of age-acquired defects of Leydig cell function."

If an experiment involves use of penicillin with guinea pigs, has the fact, as stated by G. Miescher and C. Böhm,[76] that penicillin is 1000 times more toxic to these animals than to mice been taken into consideration? The cardiac drug digitoxin is toxic at very low levels in the cat, but only at very high levels in the guinea pig. The dosage of oral LD50—at which 50% of the animals will live and 50% will die—is just .18 mg./kg. in the cat, but a much larger 60 mg./kg. in the guinea pig.[76a] Mankind's use of foxglove *(Digitalis purpurea)* that contains this drug goes back hundreds of years so that history was able to guide physicians in establishing therapeutic dosages. If we had relied on the cat or the guinea pig reaction to this drug, we could have been badly misguided.

All scientists know, if they are conducting a vitamin C experiment, the difference between using an animal species that makes vitamin C (such as the rat) and one that does not (such as the guinea pig). But when doing a study involving the effect of honey, does the experimental protocol involve an animal that does not naturally eat honey (such as the rat or mouse) or one that does (such as the bear, sloth bear, ratel or kinkajou)? The ancestors of these latter animals have, like those of contemporary human beings, been eating honey for thousands, perhaps for millions of years, and should therefore be more appropriate experimental subjects.

John B. Jemmott, III et al.[77] have shown that academic stress may affect the immune system of students, as measured by the secretion of salivary immunoglobulin. If the protocol of an experiment discloses the fact that students were used as subjects, were academic pressures considered by the scientist in charge? Students may not be appropriate "animals" for some studies. Other persons under the stress of a large number of life-change events show, as Jemmott, III et al. note, an increased incidence of infectious disease, allergic responses, as well as cardiovascular and psychiatric symptoms. Ziad Kronfol et al.[78] have shown that mood states and immunity may be related. They found defective lymphocyte function in patients with primary depressive illness. (In such studies it is very difficult to separate cause and effect. Did the depression lead to lowered lymphocyte levels, as Kronfol implies, or did the depressed lymphocyte levels lead to depression?) Stanley M. Bierman[79] has developed the concept that recurrent genital herpes may have a psychoneuroimmunologic basis. Similarly, emotional stress factors in the development of multiple sclerosis are discussed by Sharon Warren et al.[80] while psycho-social risk factors in the development of infectious mononucleosis are covered by Stanislav V. Kasl et al.[81] Studies by Richard B. Skekelle et al. [82] and by Cary L. Cooper[83] and by others[84] suggest that psychological depression and other social psychological factors are related to the impairment of mechanisms preventing the establishment and spread of cancer cells. Lawrence E. Hinkle, Jr. et al.[85] make the point, however, that their findings suggest, in regard to the determinants of genetic and environmental illness, the actual life situations encountered are less important than the way in which these situations are perceived. Nevertheless, persons undergoing many life-change events or who are psychologically depressed might be inappropriate subjects for some nutritional studies. Different affective states can be a factor in causing various physiological responses. How carefully does the experiment's protocol minimize such perturbations?

5. Assuming an appropriate animal species has been used, did the experimenter take the necessary precautions to achieve his objective? Many animals are coprophagic—they eat their own feces or the feces of their cagemates. Coprophagic animals normally eat 30 to 50% of their feces.[86] When they are not allowed to engage in this practice, detrimental effects are observed.[86-91] B. K. Armstrong and A. Softly[92] reported that growth was inhibited (as shown in Figure 2) in rats prevented from coprophagy. (Since the animals eat directly from the anus, jackets,[92] collars[92a] or anal caps[92b] must be attached to the animals when it is desired to stop coprophagy.) In consuming feces, the

animals get large amounts of the vitamin B complex, a fact that must be considered in the protocol of an experiment that involves any of these vitamins. If this nutritional source is not controlled, the experimental results may be subject to misinterpretation. Coprophagy can, however, cause animals to develop intestinal infections,[93] and so the experimenter must also be on guard against this eventuality. When you analyze the protocol of any animal experiment involving members of the vitamin B complex, decide whether or not coprophagy might negate the conclusions. On the other hand, if the experimenter restricted coprophagy, did he consider the possibility that in doing so, he may have worsened the condition of his animals?

Another factor in influencing the results of an experiment is the health of the experimental subjects. Vernon Riley et al. [93a] warn that it is essential to the control of inadvertent stress to eliminate the generally unrecognized LDH-virus contamination for experimental mice, tumors and oncogenic virus preparations. Riley and his associates further caution that changes occur in plasma corticosterone levels, the thymus, macrophages, T cells and B cells, as well as in other immunological factors of mice infected with this ubiquitous virus. When the results of a seemingly identical experiment fail to replicate those of an earlier experiment, it may be that sick mice were inadvertently used in one of the studies.[*]

6. If experiments are being done with chromium, zinc or copper, were wood, galvanized metal, stainless steel or plastic cages used? It seems possible that chromium obtained from gnawing on stainless steel cages might affect nutritional studies involving chromium. Studies regarding zinc may be invalid if the animals received the metal by gnawing on the galvanized metal cage in

---

[*] It would be inappropriate to consider here the ethics of how animals are treated in the laboratory. Those interested are referred to a recent article, "The Use of Animals in Research," by John K. Inglehart[93b] and another titled "Regulation of Animal Experimentation" by Thomas D. Overcast and Bruce D. Sales. [93c] Entirely apart from ethical considerations, however, when animals are mistreated to the point they become ill, the results of experiments become unreliable.

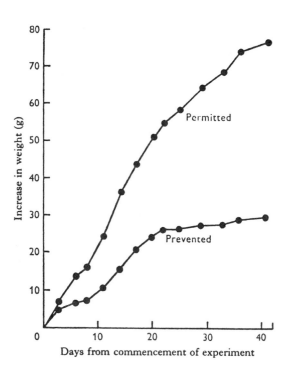

Figure 2. Increase in mean weights over six weeks of rats in whom coprophagy was permitted or prevented on the same diet. Graph reproduced from B. K. Armstrong and A. Softly, *British Jrl. of Nutrition* (1966) 20: 595-598. Reprinted with permission of the publisher, Cambridge University Press. Experiments not considering coprophagy as a nutritional source of the vitamin B complex may be subject to misinterpretation.

addition to the measured amounts received in their diet. For that matter, the zinc received through gnawing on the cage might depress absorption of the dietary copper or selenium that may be factors in the study. Research by Douglas K. Obeck[94] did, in fact, show that four rhesus monkeys and their infants kept in galvanized enclosures had significantly depressed plasma copper values and significantly elevated plasma zinc and liver zinc levels. They developed achromotrichia (absence of hair pigment), alopecia (baldness) and weakness that varied from moderate to severe, while three infants kept in stainless steel cages were clinically normal. As we will see in Chapters 3 and 7, zinc is a factor in prostaglandin metabolism. Some prostaglandin studies conducted using animals housed in galvanized cages might, therefore, lead to questionable results.

7. Scientists may sometimes improperly experiment with nutrients, such as vitamins and minerals, as if they were unessential. Maxine Briggs[94a] points out, in reference to ascorbic acid (AA) studies, that:

> Unlike other drugs used against infectious diseases, AA is also a nutrient, though being used at nonphysiological doses. Nevertheless, in double-blind studies, especially where there is no cross-over, it is essential to be certain that nutrient intake is adequate in both groups, so that high-dose AA is not being used merely to correct a deficiency of vitamin C that could have been corrected with a much lower dose. Very few of the published studies have determined either the dietary vitamin C intake of their volunteers, or any laboratory index of vitamin C status (such as leukocyte concentrations or 24-hour urinary output).

In your study of scientific literature, look at the experiment's protocol and ask yourself this question: Were adequate steps taken to assure that the experimental subjects being given a certain nutrient were not deficient in that nutrient before the experiment began? If they were deficient before the study began, simply giving them enough of the nutrient to satisfy the RDA (Recommended Dietary Allowances of the National Academy of Sciences) might have produced the same good results that the experimenter may have attributed to the megadoses he administered.

8. What other factors may have been ignored that might modify the experimental results? (You may never know. Scientists are often lax in disclosing details of an experiment's protocol.) M. W. Fox[95] says:

> Color of clothing most likely has little effect on rats, but the odors of different caretakers may be important. I think cage position is a serious question in rat colonies. If you don't regularly change the cage positions, rats at the top of the rack would have very different experiences from those on the bottom rack. You might note that those on the bottom are under a different light intensity, temperature, and so on; such variables can be controlled by rotation of the cages.*

9. Could the nature of a laboratory animal's diet lead the experimenter to false conclusions regarding the probable human effects of the nutrients or toxins being studied? A. Wise and D. J. Gilburt[95b] noted B. H. Ershoff[95c,d] and D. Kritchevsky [95e] have shown that fiber in the diet of laboratory animals affected the toxicity of many test chemicals. Such effects could conceivably sometimes lead to erroneous conclusions regarding the safety of certain chemicals in the human environment.

Fiber in the human or animal diet is widely considered to be protective against colon cancer. However, as recently as 1986, David M. Klurfeld et al.[95f] cautioned that isolated cellulose, which is the standard fiber source in semipurified diets for biomedical research, may not give results comparable to feeding intact dietary fiber. They found that rats fed a fiber-free diet had a

---

* Friedman and Ader[95a] reported, however, that "merely placing rats in a new environment resulted in a significant rise in corticosterone levels," the magnitude of which "depends upon when during the 24-hour adrenocortical rhythm such stimulation is imposed."

71% incidence of colon cancer after six weekly gavages of the chemical 1,2-dimethylhydrazine (DMH). On the other hand, those fed 5%, 10% or 20% powdered or microcrystalline cellulose for six months following similar gavages of DMH had colon tumor incidences of, respectively, 75%, 92% and 100%.

Then too, Victor Herbert,[95g] also writing in 1986, cited a study by L. R. Jacobs[95h] showing that, "A 20 percent wheat bran dietary supplement increased by more than three times the numbers of colonic adenomas and adenocarcinomas in rats given 1,2-dimethylhydrazine." Furthermore, Hugh J. Freeman et al. [95i] reported that when mice were administered 1,2-dimethylhydrazine, a diet containing 4.5% or 9.0% purified cellulose was protective against colon cancer (rather opposite to the results of the Klurfeld group). On the 9% pectin diet, the number of small bowel tumors was increased. Other studies cited by Hugh J. Freeman[95j] and done by K. Wakabayashi et al.[95k] and by K. Watanabe et al.[95l] showed that carrageenan (a polysaccharide fiber derived from red marine algae that is used in food as a stabilizing, jelling or viscosity agent) enhanced chemically-induced colon carcinogenesis and even caused rodent colon cancer.

Obviously, it is simplistic to categorize various fibers simply as "fiber." Different fibers consumed under varying circumstances have diverse effects. To conclude that modest amounts of fiber in the human diet may be dangerous based on experiments with animals that had been fed either large amounts of cellulose or of wheat bran and administered DMH would be improper, but the questioning attitude that asks "why the difference" could lead to good discoveries. Many studies continue to suggest, of course, that fiber used in modest amounts is protective against colon cancer. For now, our primary concern is that, when studying the protocol of an experiment involving animals, we ask ourselves if the diet fed them might have contained enough fiber to influence the outcome and to affect the conclusions that were drawn. Furthermore, various fibers contain different proportions of celluloses, hemicelluloses, pectin and lignin. Therefore, a conclusion regarding a given fiber at a certain concentration in one animal system must not be presumed valid for another fiber at a different concentration in another human or nonhuman animal system.

10. Much animal research is performed in order to draw conclusions that might benefit the health of humans. However, one must always be cautious about extrapolating animal results to man. In reading scientific papers, observe whether the author made such extrapolations cautiously. Plaut quotes R. A. Hinde[96] as writing, "Apparently close similarities between species may prove to be merely paralleled evolutionary adaptations to a similar environment, and rest on quite different causal bases." Plaut goes on to cite S. A. Barnett[97] who wrote, "Choose the right animal species and you can 'prove' anything you like." Animal diseases are not always similar to the corresponding disease in man. Animal muscular dystrophy is not. Absorption of a given nutrient in an animal may be greater or less than it would be in man. The amount of zinc taken up by the rat and reaching internal organs in five hours was found to be four to six times greater when vitamin C was present.[96a] In humans, however, vitamin C seems to neither enhance nor inhibit the biological availability of orally ingested zinc.[96a] One must be cautious about assuming that a useful nutrient/body weight dosage in an animal is anything more than suggestive of what might be a useful dosage in man.* Furthermore, one must not assume that

---

* In Chapter 1 we will discuss the recommended dietary allowances (RDA) for various nutrients as determined by the National Academy of Sciences. However, requirements for laboratory animals, even if they are primates, may be far different. For example, the National Academy of Sciences[98] recommends that nonhuman primates obtain 10,000-15,000 I.U./kg. of vitamin A from their diet. (Man eats about one kg. of food daily, yet his RDA is only 5,000 units.) The Academy recommends that nonhuman primates receive 2 mg./kg. diet of iodine, 180 mg./kg. diet of iron and 40 mg./kg. diet of manganese. This contrasts with a human RDA of a mere 150 mcg. (1/14 as much) for iodine; 10 mg. for men and 18 mg. for women (1/18 and 1/10 as much respectively) for iron; and 2.5 to 5 mg. (1/16 to 1/8 as much) for manganese. Not only absorption differences but the generally higher metabolic rates in nonhuman primates are factors in the recommendation that laboratory animals receive a higher vitamin and mineral intake than is suggested for humans.

absorption and utilization of a given substance will be the same
for different persons. (A difference in stomach acid concentration
might have a big influence.) Then too, the method of
administering a nutrient or drug has a great bearing on its
effectiveness. In analyzing an experiment, observe whether the
studied substance was administered orally, by injection,
sublingually (under the tongue), buccally (through the buccal
glands in the cheeks), rectally or nasally. Usually, injection of a
given substance will, for example, be far more potent than if the
same amount were administered orally. Generally, oral
administration puts the least amount of nutrient or drug into the
body since the substance has to not only contend with the often
destructive action of the gastric and pancreatic juices, but then
has to find its way past the brush border into the body proper.
(An exception to this rule is given by Lowell A. Glasgow et al.[99]
They found that murine— i.e., mouse—cytomegalovirus, which
is a relative of human cytomegalovirus, is far more effectively
combated when the drug acyclovir is administered orally than
when it is injected intraperitoneally. To cite a second example,
laetrile is active, for better or for worse, when taken orally, but is
without effect when administered by injection.[99a] (Laetrile's
action is discussed in Chapter 5.) Thus, even if the same animal
(or human) model and the same dosage of the same nutrient or
drug were to be used in two experiments, but the method of
administration differed, the results might not be comparable. Be
wary of articles in popular magazines that may analyze a study
involving injection of a vitamin and then report that the vitamin
was "administered"—leaving the reader to erroneously assume
that the substance was taken by mouth.

The results of one study will sometimes be found to contradict
those of another. In such a case, it is likely that the experimental
protocols of those experiments differ in seemingly extraneous, but
actually important, factors that the respective scientists may, or may
not, have disclosed. John C. Bailar III[99b] discusses some of the

implications of well-done studies whose results are in conflict with each other.

It is not to be expected that a scientist will always be cognizant of the defects in the protocol of his study. What is important is that experimental details be fully disclosed so others may criticize the implications of that protocol. For example, a scientist doing studies of BHT-induced physiological damage in rats might not know that the cedarwood shavings used as bedding on the floor of the animal's cage could, through the sublimation of terpenes, and via an effect on the liver enzyme system, prevent BHT-caused lung damage.[100]* Thus, he might falsely conclude that BHT was innocuous from the standpoint of lung damage. Scientists making use of the possibly dangerous vehicles polysorbate 20, polysorbate 80, Tween 20 or Tween 80 for carrying vitamin E or other vitamins may improperly ascribe fetal malformations,[101] depressed immune response[102] and other outward effects[103] to the vitamin rather than to the vehicle. (More about the dangers of the polysorbates will be found in Chapter 2. Our concern at this point is only to point out that the toxic effects of the polysorbates could sometimes cause scientists to draw erroneous conclusions.) As long as a scientist fully discloses his protocol, others will have the opportunity to point out, in criticizing his research, that sesqui terpenoid compounds emanating from the cedar shavings might have protected the animals' lungs or that polysorbates may have caused toxic effects, contrary to the conclusions of the scientists conducting the respective studies.

As you read scientific literature, not only be on guard against possibly defective experimental protocols but beware of the experimenter's prejudices. A researcher may be so intent on proving

---

* Many physiological effects such as this occur through influences on the liver enzymes. Vesell et al.[100a] reported that not only aromatic hydrocarbons from cedarwood bedding, but also eucalyptol from aerosol sprays and chlorinated hydrocarbon insecticides can induce activity in the hepatic (liver) microsomal enzymes (HME). On the contrary, ammonia generated from feces and urine accumulated in unchanged pans under wire cages can inhibit HME activity. Rats in wire cages where the pans were changed infrequently had only one-third the aniline hydroxylase activity, a little more than one-half the ethylmorphine N-demethylase activity and two-thirds the cytochrome P-450 content of rats in wire cages where the pans were cleaned frequently. Vesell and his colleagues state that variations caused by the various above-noted factors in control animals can be so large as to obscure the effects being investigated in an experimental group.

his hypothesis that he could overlook alternate explanations of the phenomenon he is observing. Plaut quotes T. C. Chamberlin,[104] writing almost a century ago, who said, "The moment one has offered an original explanation for a phenomenon which seems satisfactory that moment affection springs into existence, and as the explanation grows into a definite theory his parental affections cluster about his offspring and it grows more and more dear to him." Be aware also that the scientist may have set his experimental parameters so as to make it impossible to discover a *reverse effect* (something we will be continuing to discuss throughout this book).

I hope this study of experimental protocol will help guide you. In order to sharpen your own talent for the criticism of experimental protocol, visit a medical library and consult *Citation Abstracts*. These volumes permit you to discover articles by various scientists that have referenced the study in which you are especially interested. The authors of these more recent articles may have comments on the validity of the study that concerns you.

This excursion into ways to more meaningfully read biomedical literature has two more subtle purposes. The first is to caution scientists about exposing their subjects (animals or humans) to stressful conditions that are not essential to the purpose of their studies. Secondly, and more important, I want to emphasize the fact that a person's health or illness is influenced (as are the health or illness of an animal in a laboratory cage) by many factors that may ordinarily escape our attention and the attention of our physicians.

> "Nutritional questions have about them an air of reasonableness that often belies their intrinsic complexity. Nutrition is direct and personal for everyone, and nearly everyone, it seems, has an opinion on the subject. It is not surprising that controversy abounds, to say nothing of faddism, exploitation, and outright charlatanism."
> — R. P. Heaney[1]

CHAPTER 1

How to Use the *Reverse Effect* and the *Pleasure Concept*

What is *health*? According to the constitution of the World Health Organization (WHO), health is a state of complete physical, mental and social well-being, not merely the absence of disease or infirmity.* Health is also a high-energy state accompanied by a feeling of being at peace with oneself and with others. To achieve and maintain good health we must have good nutrition. However, good health depends on far more than good nutrition.

For one thing, mental attitude can be extremely important. A study of four decades by George E Vaillant[4] showed the effect of mental health on physical health and longevity. A total of 204 men were selected as adolescents for continued study. Of the 59 men with the best mental health assessed from the age of 21 to 46 years, only two became chronically ill or died by the age of 53. Of the 48 men with the worst

---

* F. C. Redlich[2] disagrees with the WHO definition of health. He maintains that health is "nothing more than the absence of disease." Obviously, I am pro-WHO and anti-Redlich on this issue. Those who are philosophically inclined will want to read not only Redlich, but other articles in the same issue that carried Redlich's article and also one by Michael H. Kottow.[3] Kottow, in turn, cites references for additional study.

mental health assessed from the age of 21 to 48, 18 became chronically ill or died by the age of 53. Vaillant concludes that "good mental health retards midlife deterioration in physical health." The positive mental attitude toward one's illness and toward one's doctor is also of great therapeutic importance. S. Greer et al.[5] reported that, in a study of 69 breast cancer cases, the patient's psychological response was a significant factor in the course of the disease. They reported that, "Recurrence-free survival was significantly common among patients who had initially reacted to cancer by denial or who had a fighting spirit than among patients who had responded with stoic acceptance or feelings of helplessness and hopelessness." In a followup of the same patients about five years later, Keith W. Pettingale, Steven Greer et al.[5a] found that recurrence-free survival continued to be significantly more common among those who reacted with denial or "fighting spirit." Greer has quoted J. Paget[6] as saying (over 100 years ago), "The cases are so frequent in which deep anxiety, deferred hope and disappointment are quickly followed by the growth and increase of cancer, that we can hardly doubt that mental depression is a weighty addition to the other influences favoring the development of the cancerous constitution." Lawrence LeShan[7,8] has reviewed many studies showing the influence of mental state on the development of malignant disease. Additional studies involving the mind-cancer connection have subsequently been reviewed by Constance Holden.[9] Interestingly, Phillip Shaver et al.[10] reported that certainty of religious beliefs (either strong religiousness or confident nonreligiousness) was associated with better mental and physical health. It is apparent that good health and bad health are functions of the mental state.

The living of a healthy, vigorous life and the attainment of longevity will not simply occur. We must maintain a happy, friendly, confident attitude. We must like ourselves; we must give and receive love. We must eat good foods and when necessary, use additional nutrients in the form of supplemental vitamins and minerals and perhaps take them at certain times of the day or night. We must exercise regularly throughout our lives—and the exercise should, ideally, include regular, loving sexual activity. Furthermore, to live long, healthy lives our days must be filled with joy...not only with the joy of sex,* but also with the pleasure of eating and drinking, including perhaps an occasional cup of coffee, an alcoholic drink or a banana split. If one experiences great pleasure in eating or drinking a proscribed treat, I believe the benefit to the psyche will in many cases offset the negative nutritional aspects. In addition to the psychic value, there is the physiological effect of increased enzyme flow when eating or drinking is accompanied by feelings of pleasure. I call this idea the *pleasure concept.* Do not, however, eat or drink questionable foods at every meal and in between your meals.**

Hedonic capacity—the ability to experience pleasure—is a measure of health and can be important in influencing more usual ways of analyzing health status. Anhedonia—a severely limited capacity to experience pleasure—has been described as a characteristic of schizophrenia by many psychopathologists.[15-25a] A number of true-false type tests, including those of Loren J. Chapman et al.,[15] have been devised to measure anhedonia. More recently, Robert H. D. Dworkin and Kathleen Saczynski[21] have constructed scales of hedonic capacity from the Minnesota Multiphasic Personality Inventory and the California Psychological Inventory. Dworkin and Saczynski found significant positive correlations between hedonic capacity and responses to daily events such as feelings of elation/pleasure, playfulness, leisureliness and friendliness. They found significant negative correlations between hedonic capacity and feelings of anger, fear, sadness and annoyance. The *pleasure concept,* as I have

---

* Erik Agduhr[11] found that sexual activity increases resistance of both male and female rats, mice and rabbits to toxic substances. (Perhaps the rationale for this finding relates to stimulation of gonadotropin. Agduhr found that injecting gonadotropic hormone into unmated mice poisoned with arsenic also resulted in an antitoxic effect.) D. Drori and Y. Folman[12] reported significantly increased longevity in rats who had the opportunity to mate at least once a week. The results of a subsequent study by Drori and Folman[13] are shown in Figure 1.

** Nevertheless, let's not lose sight of the doctrine of "sufficient challenge."[14] Muscles, brains and sex organs are made stronger through challenges and perhaps other organs may also be benefitted. Might not small amounts of coffee or alcohol strengthen the liver? H. F. Smyth, Jr.[14] reported that rats inhaling small amounts of the poison carbon tetrachloride grew better and were more fertile than controls.

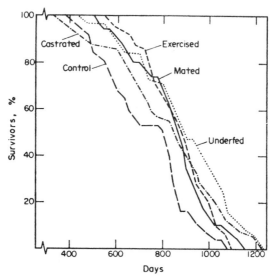

Figure 1. Survival of mated, exercised, underfed, castrated and untreated (intact) control male rats. Castration and underfeeding produced more *late* survivors, but exercise and mating prolonged life better while the males were young. Graph reproduced from D. Drori and Y. Folman, *Experimental Gerontology* (1976) 11: 25-32, with permission of the authors and of the publisher, Pergamon Press, Ltd.

presented it, suggests (to me) that the Dworkin and Saczynski scales of hedonic capacity will eventually be related to a great multitude of health-related problems other than depression and schizophrenia, and including longevity itself. Paul E. Meehl[22] has said: "I am convinced that 'high joy' people do exist; and I should be surprised if my readers, in contemplating their range of acquaintances, disagree with me. There are persons who seem able to take considerable pleasure from almost any circumstance not distinctly loaded with aversive components and for whom the most ordinary experiences appear to be a source of considerable gratification. I conjecture that these people are the lucky ones at the high end of the hedonic capacity continuum." In characterizing individual differences in hedonic capacity, Paul E.

Meehl[22] cites the Wild West maxim, "Some are born three drinks behind." Meehl goes on to say: "I think people with low hedonic capacity should pay greater attention to the 'hedonic bookkeeping' of their activities than would be necessary for people located midway or high on the hedonic capacity continuum. That is, it matters more to someone cursed with an inborn hedonic defect whether he is efficient and sagacious in selecting friends, jobs, cities, tasks, hobbies, and activities in general."

To many persons the search for good nutrition has become an unhealthful neurosis. To maximize health, I believe that the search for good nutrition must become not a neurosis, but a way of life. It must be a way of life in which one generally eats healthful food in pleasant surroundings with a congenial person or persons. But it will also be a way of life in which no guilt is attached to the occasional eating of a not-so-healthful fun-food just for the sheer pleasure of it.

Learn to intensify the pleasures of eating by savoring your food. Enjoy its color; note its texture. As you bring the food slowly to your mouth, excite your nostrils with its aroma. Good eating, like good sex, should have a loving period of foreplay. Chew every bite far more times than is usually considered to be necessary. Revel in the taste sensations. Make each act of eating an adventure in sensuality. Long-staying eating and long-staying sex have more benefits in common than is generally realized. There is an added advantage to super-enjoyment of food beyond this increase in psychic joy. Through getting all this additional pleasure from the food you eat, satisfaction is achieved sooner and overeating becomes merely a problem of yesterday.

It is widely believed, and I also hold this view, that fried foods are less healthful than the same foods prepared differently. However, a contrary view regarding the unhealthfulness of fried foods is suggested by some data from the *Hammond Report on Smoking in Relation to Mortality and Morbidity* that was presented by E. Cuyler Hammond, Sc.D. of the Medical Affairs Department of the American Cancer Society, New York, N.Y. to the American Medical Association in 1963.[26] This material was brought to my attention through reading an interesting book, *Wine of Life,* by Harold J.

Morowitz. The *Hammond Report* provides longevity data of a group of 442,094 men aged 40-89, over a period of 34.3 months. It indicates that both smoking and nonsmoking men who regularly eat fried foods seem to live longer than those who do not! Observe this interesting data at age-standardized death rates per 100,000 man-years during the 34.3 month period that was studied:

Age-Standardized Death Rates

Weekly Frequency of Eating Fried Food	Subject Never Smoked Regularly	Subject Smoked 20 Cigarettes or More Daily
No Fried Food	1,208	2,573
1-2 times	1,004	1,694
3-4 times	642	1,714
5-9 times	781	1,520
10-14 times	722	1,524
15 or more times	702	1,399

Reproduced from E. Cuyler Hammond, *Jrl. of the National Cancer Institute* (May, 1964) 32: 1161-1188.

I think it quite premature, however, to conclude that fried foods are more healthful.* This data from the *Hammond Report* provides, I believe, an example of the *pleasure concept* in operation. It is probable that persons who avoid fried foods may do so because they already have bad digestive systems and might tend to die earlier whether or not they ate such foods. Nevertheless, I believe the data also suggest, but of course do not prove, that those more casual about their eating habits—even if life-shortening foods are consumed—will generally live longer than those eating only healthful

---

* Stephen L. Taylor[27] of the University of Wisconsin, Madison, has found that foods deep-fried are far less mutagenic than foods cooked on a grill. The deep-fried foods, with their surfeit of fat, may add to heart problems, but it is the grilled foods that may pose a greater threat of cancer.

foods if the orientation of the latter group is such that pleasure is reduced.*

I suggest that those overly concerned about their eating habits have less fun in life. Those eating fried foods 15 or more times per week may, as a group, experience more joy in eating. Perhaps in other ways also they may find more pleasure in living *which is an approach to life that, I believe, promotes longevity.* Those who, on the other hand, can minimize their intake of fried foods without becoming overly concerned about such restrictions to the point that pleasure is reduced might, I think, live still longer. I believe it important that healthful foods be eaten more often and the consumption of unhealthful ones (including perhaps fried foods) be reduced *without one's pleasure being reduced.* In line with this reasoning, I suspect that an overconcern for eating presumably healthful foods such as yogurt, wheat germ and brewer's yeast on a rigidly regular basis could actually be life-shortening if it takes too much pleasure out of life. Eat healthful foods and avoid unhealthful ones, but only to the extent that such eating does not reduce the fun of living!

The beneficial effect of love in experiments with rabbits implies that love is also very important for human health and longevity. Robert M. Nerem et al.[28] reported that rabbits, on a 2% cholesterol diet, when petted, held, talked to and played with on a regular basis had improved health. Compared to control groups given the same diet, the experimental groups showed more than 60% reduction in percentage of aortic surface having sudanophilic lesions even though serum cholesterol, heart rate and blood pressure were comparable.**

---

* The beneficial effects of eating fried foods (like the benefits of modest drinking of alcohol) may also involve stimulation of the liver's microsomal enzymes, collectively called cytochrome P-450. (This will be discussed in Chapter 3.)

** B. S. Gow et al.[28a] and M. J. Legg et al.,[28b] using different strains of rabbits, were unable to replicate these results. (Nerem and his associates used the Sudan strain of New Zealand White rabbits while the Gow and Legg groups used Canadian and Australian strains of New Zealand White rabbits.) The "love-factor" in the development of atheroma in cholesterol-fed rabbits seems to depend on the strain of rabbits used. Perhaps the "love-factor" in human health may vary from person to person just as do the effects of vitamins and drugs. The concept of what I propose to call *amative individuality* may be just as valid as that of *biochemical individuality* which was popularized by Roger J. Williams and which we will be considering frequently in the pages ahead.

(When two scientists get conflicting results, could it sometimes be that only one is taking cognizance of the *pleasure concept?*)

When Michael Plaut et al.[28c] deprived rat litters of their mother at the age of 13 days, 90% of the adult-deprived pups died between 18 and 21 days of age. But, the scientists say, "most mortality was prevented by the presence of a nonlactating adult." They go on to comment, "Survival could be attributed largely to the opportunity for tactual contact between pups and the adult, even though a significant amount of mortality could be prevented even by housing maternally deprived pups with a female from whom they were separated by a double wire screen." Not the lack of mother's milk, but the absence of loving contact, or the absence, at least, of a nearby female, is what seems to have been the major cause of death. Elsewhere, Plaut [28d] has this to say in regard to undernutrition in young rodents:

> These studies provide support for the hypothesis that offspring physiology and behavior can be affected by adult-litter interactions which are not related to nutritional factors. This hypothesis is contrary to the tacit assumption, made in many studies of undernutrition, that the effects of maternal deprivation can be related only to nutritional factors. The hypothesis is substantiated by some studies of early weaning in which an additional group of pups is left with a mother whose nipples have been cauterized to prevent suckling. Where this was done, the effects of maternal deprivation were not seen in the offspring of the cauterized mothers.

Love and physical contact are "nutrients" essential to the well-being of rodents (and humans). The need for love can be readily seen in lower animals such as birds. It is interesting to speculate, since I believe the relevant studies have not yet been made, whether the need for love exists in worms, amoebae, bacteria and plants.

In a related study, W. B. Gross and P. B. Siegel[29] habituated chickens to human beings by talking to them, offering them food and gently handling them, a process called *socialization*. After seven weeks of socialization the birds were challenged by an exposure to *Escherichia coli*. Compared with ignored chickens, the socialized birds showed a 60% reduction in pericarditis and death. In another study, Gross and Siegel [30] found that when socialized chickens were stressed by fasting and then exposed to *Staphylococcus aureus* their resistance was good. However, when unsocialized chickens were given a similar treatment, their resistance was less.

Jay R. Kaplan et al. [31] performed a related experiment with monkeys. Thirty animals were assigned to six groups, each of which contained five members, and all were fed a moderately atherogenic diet. Group members were changed continually among three groups of five monkeys to create an unstable social condition, while the other three groups of five were allowed to remain in a stable social condition. Each of the 30 monkeys was classified as dominant or subordinate based on patterns of aggression or submission. Both dominant and subordinate animals in unstable social groups had significantly greater coronary artery atherosclerosis than those housed in stable social groups.

Social isolation among human groups can be similarly related to disease. John N. Edwards and David L. Klemmack[32] "found that the best predictors of life satisfaction are socioeconomic status, perceived health status and informal participation with nonkinsmen." Judith G. Rabkin and Elmer L. Struening[33] state that sheer size of a given group, called *ethnic density,* has been found to be inversely related to psychiatric hospitalization rates.

Michael G. Marmot and S. Leonard Syme[34] found that among men of Japanese ancestry, the gradient in occurrence of coronary heart disease (CHD) was lowest in Japan, intermediate in Hawaii and highest in California. They maintain that "this gradient appears not to be completely explained by differences in dietary intake, serum cholesterol, blood pressure and smoking." Marmot and Syme hypothesized that social and cultural values may account for the CHD differences between Japan and the United States. They classified 3,809 Japanese Americans according to the degree to which they maintained a traditional Japanese culture. The investigators found that in the most traditional group the prevalence of CHD was as low as that in Japan. The group most acculturated to Western living had a three- to five-fold excess in the prevalence of CHD. Marmot and Syme concluded that "this difference in CHD rate between most and least acculturated groups could not be accounted for by differences in the major coronary risk factors."

Analogous studies in the town of Roseto, Pennsylvania, which is ethnically homogenous, have also related inversely the prevalence of CHD with social support and close family ties. John G. Bruhn et al.,[35] who have analyzed nine of these studies, give us the lesson Roseto teaches:

> The major lesson from Roseto is that we all have a
> need for a safety net. We all have a need for ties that
> bind us to the social fabric. We need someone to talk
> to, to listen; we need social institutions, clubs,
> organizations, and informal groups to provide us with
> a sense of purpose for living; we need close personal
> ties with a loved one, with family members, and with
> others who care beyond listening; we need a
> philosophy or point of view of life to help us set
> personal goals and assess our personal ability to share,
> to give, and to take; and finally we need to select a
> physical and social environment in which to live that
> will provide a meaningful mixture of opportunities and
> security.

Pleasure can be affected by changes in life events, for better or for worse. Loss of a loved one, divorce or loss of a job can sometimes have negative effects on our health. Other life change events may (but will not necessarily) represent beneficial stresses, and some of these might be marriage, a new job or a vacation trip. Many studies[36-38] have found that clusters of events are associated with illness. Rafaella M. A. Osti et al.[39] reported that stressful life change events were associated with the occurrence of hypertension. Carol W. Buck and Allan P. Donner[39a] have also associated life change events with hypertension. Life change events have also been related to ischemic heart disease, myocardial infarction and stroke.[39b-e] Those making high scores on the Holmes-Rahe Social Readjustment Rating Scale[40] and on the UCLA Loneliness Scale have been reported by Janice K. Kiecolt-Glaser et al.[41] to have decreased immuno-competence as indicated by significant declines in natural killer cell activity and in total plasma IgA. In a subsequent study, Steven E. Locke et al.[42] found that life change stress and natural killer cell activity were not significantly correlated, but they reported that "good copers" had significantly higher natural killer cell activity than those who were not "good copers." R. W. Bartrop et al.,[42a] studying the effects of severe stress on the immune system of 26 bereaved spouses, found that the response to phytohemagglutinin and to concanavalin A was significantly depressed, but only after a delay of six weeks. S. J. Schleifer et al.[42b] reported, on the other hand, that lymphocyte function was immediately depressed after bereavement and persisted for two months or more.* Harold Levitan[42ba] recently reported that intense grief seemed to be a key psychological factor contributing to the onset of asthma. Life change events have also been associated with the development of *alopecia areata* (a kind of baldness),[43a] yeast infections,[43b] late onset manic-depressive disorder,[43c] rheumatoid arthritis,[43d] colds,[43e] gastric (but not colorectal) cancer,[43f] and appendicitis.[43g]

Kenneth P. Matheny and Penny Cupp[44] found that not only could negative life changes lead to illness but, in the case of females (but not of males), desirable events (if unanticipated) were also positively related to illness. Matheny and Cupp note that one of the factors that may contribute to the degree of life change stress is whether or not a given change was anticipated. Those who doubt their ability to cope may increase the negative effect of the anticipated change. On the

---

* Studies of widows and widowers show an increase as high as 40% in mortality rates compared to married men and women of the same age.[42c] Knud J. Helsing et al.[42d] reported that mortality rates among widowed males who remarried were much lower than among those who did not remarry. However, they found no significant difference among widowed females who did or did not remarry. Interestingly, Marian Osterweis et al. cite W. P. Cleveland and D. T. Gianturco[43] as reporting that age-specific mortality rates among widowed males who remarried were lower than the rates among married males.

other hand, self-confident persons may make plans to meet the anticipated change and thus reduce its stressing effect. Paul J. Rosch[45] points out that "pleasurable experiences may be powerful stressors, and winning a race or an election may evoke the same or greater secretion of epinephrine or hydrocortisone as losing; getting married is likely to be as stressful as becoming divorced." Therefore, "desirable" or "undesirable" events may have a stressing effect. We must not assume, however, that stress is always detrimental. Hans Selye[46] coined the word "eustress" to designate pleasurable stress as distinguished from "distress," meaning painful stress. It is not the type of stress, but the demands it places on us and our perceived capability of meeting those demands that are the determining factors. It is not so much the nature of stress nor whether the stress was or was not anticipated that detrimentally or beneficially affects our lives, but our perception of each of those stressors and our reactions to them. The support of family and friends and of our communities, and especially support of what Rickey S. Miller and Herbert M. Lefcourt[46a] call a "current intimacy" is vital to our well-being. Their offering consolation during times of bad stress and congratulations in times of beneficial stress add to life's pleasure and are health-fostering. When bad events occur, one with a "healthy personality" tends to express feelings such as anger,* hate, fear and sorrow if he has such feelings. The less healthy personality has similar feelings

---

* W. D. Gentry et al. [46b] found that those who showed a tendency to express the anger they felt had lower rates of hypertension than those who suppressed their anger. Steven Greer and Maggie Watson[46c] reported that independent groups of scientists[46d,e] have found expression of anger to be significantly less among breast cancer patients than among controls. Greer and Watson[46c] noted that similar findings have been reported by Watson et al.[46f] in patients with malignant melanoma. Anger, in my opinion, ideally should be directed against what was done rather than against the one who did it. One might say: "What you did has made me angry. Why did you do this?" Airing the grievance is, I believe, more healthful and gives the other person an opportunity to explain and perhaps to apologize. Aristotle is credited with saying, "Anyone can become angry—that is easy; but to be angry with the right person, and to the right degree, and at the right time, and for the right purpose, and in the right way—that is not within everybody's power and is not easy." Anger can modify many physiological parameters, including even the composition of the intestinal flora. L. V. Holdeman et al.[46g] have reported a variation of the composition of fecal bacteria in those under emotional stress. Specifically, during periods of anger or of fear stress there is a rapid increase in the level of *Bacteroides fragilis,* subspecies *thetaiotaomicron* in the ascending colon (perhaps arising, I presume, from action in the cecum). Subsequently, these bacteria are found throughout the colon.

but does not know in which direction to take those feelings. To have a good sense of personal worth, to feel in control of life rather than being controlled by life, to love more, to laugh more and to cry more when appropriate and to do "crazy" things sometimes—these are important for better health.[*]

We have seen many examples of the *pleasure concept* in action. Whether it is the rabbits being petted, chickens being socialized, monkeys living in stable groups or human beings living in socially close, loving communities, pleasure is a health-fostering factor. The nutritive power of love and pleasure is just as needed as are other forms of nutrition if we are to live healthfully and long. However, we have also seen that the golden mean of moderation, even in matters of pleasure, may be important in order to avoid psychological *reverse effects* just as it will be shown to be important in avoiding physical *reverse effects.*

In further relation to pleasure, the studies of Reubin Andres[48] and of A. R. Dyer et al. (the Chicago Peoples Gas Co. study)[49] indicate that a modest degree of overweight may be life-lengthening.[**] The favorable longevity effect of moderate drinking of alcohol has also been reported in several studies (as cited in Chapter 7). *The Boy Scout Handbook* gave (and perhaps it still gives) the advice, "Eat to live; don't live to eat." There is, of course, much to be said in favor of that statement. Although one should not live only to eat, I believe

---

[*] Many studies confirm the influence of mental attitude on health and disease while a few deny or minimize its importance. In keeping with the attitude expressed throughout this book, I want to encourage readers to investigate positions contrary to my own. If you are interested in studying denials of mental effects on physical health, ask your librarian to obtain an article by Marcia Angell[46b] and also some of the studies cited therein, especially those by Robert B. Case et al.[46a] and by Barrie R. Cassileth et al.[47] Recent reviews by Austen Clark[47a] and by Edward R. Friedlander[47b] are also interesting.

[**] R. J. Garrison et al.[50] have, however, criticized various weight-longevity studies because of failure to control for smoking. Leanness and smoking tend to be correlated. Thus, the factor of not smoking rather than the factor of overweight, itself, may have resulted in increased longevity. (Refer to a 1987 review by Manson et al.)[50a] Ulf Smith[50b] maintains that overweight persons with big abdomens are health-threatened more than those of similar weight and height whose fat is distributed around the hips and limbs. The abdominal fat pattern, according to Smith, carries a three- to five-fold increased risk of myocardial infarction or stroke. He says that a waist-to-hip ratio of over 1.0 in men or over .8 in women has a significant impact on prognosis.

that, unless one receives joy from eating, the lack of pleasure could be life-shortening. Pleasure, in moderation, is life-extending.*

Perhaps you have never felt the full intensity of the pleasure that you are capable of feeling. As an experiment, eat your food while concentrating on the sensations and compare the feelings you have with those experienced in ordinary eating. Try giving total concentration to smelling a flower, to looking at a painting—or to making love with such intensity that you are cognizant of nothing other than you and your lover's** oneness. I speculate that greater pleasure, whether attained in these or in other ways, will lead to less tension and increased health.

I speculate that some of us will be more healthy if our lives are filled with the joys of play, of travel and of being tuned in to the world of art, music, poetry, sports, politics and science. Others, however, will find that fixing their car, going to a bar or picking up women (or men) to be more pleasurable, and I speculate that for such persons these actions are health-fostering. I hold that laughter, conversation with friends, the wonder and delight shown by children, the smell of a rose or of dinner, sexual and nonsexual touching and hugging, red raspberries picked and immediately eaten, the face of a sleeping child, doing a good turn for someone with my role in the action being discovered only by accident, and a sense of unity with all of creation are joys that add to my pleasure. I believe that such experiences are, for me, health-fostering. Not just the experiences, but the memory of those experiences, add to the delight I take in living. I recall, as a 12-year-old, buying all the 5¢ Jamestown, U.S. postage stamps of 1907 I could find in dealer stocks at 25¢ each and the economic power I felt in selling them next year for $1.00 apiece. (I thus discovered for myself the profit-

---

* Bernard Fisher et al.,[51] in a randomized study involving 1,843 women, reported that segmental mastectomy (lumpectomy), *with or without radiation*, led to a higher disease-free survival rate than total mastectomy. (Segmental mastectomy with radiation was, however, greatly superior to the same operation without radiation.) Does this argue lumpectomy patients may feel happier than those who have had a breast removed? Is this yet another example of the longevity-increasing effect of pleasure?

** When I use the word *lover*, I do not exclude lovers married to each other. The term *lover*, as I use it, simply refers to one who loves.

making power behind what I call the *Law of Current Supply and Future Demand*.) I remember the intellectual "coming of age" that occurred through winning, against nationwide rivals, the University of Chicago's six-hour scholarship competition. I recall, as a young adult beginning to develop *dynamic synthesis,* how I used my entire "fortune" of $180 to trade stocks until my account was worth $5,000 (at which point I started a business). I remember the excitement, a few years later, in seeing a featured photo in the Decatur, Illinois, newspaper of one of my oil wells gushing uncontrolled over a field of soybeans. I recall the delight at the birth of my son Ron and of my daughter Pam. I remember my late wife and I designing our home and the subsequent pictures of our library that appeared in the *New York Times* and in other national media. I recall the flowers and wines of Madiera, the Great Pyramid of Cheops cutting a wedge of blackness in the star-filled Saharan sky, sunset behind the Parthenon and the visual treasury of a sunrise with Venus still shining through the already-blue sky. All of us have experienced our own versions of pleasure-yielding events, but do you and I extract all the pleasure possible from these life experiences?

To live most healthfully we must seek to live life more fully. Living life for some persons may mean a denial of most of what has been said above. For some, pouring a concrete sidewalk on a beautiful Sunday afternoon is just as pleasurable as a trip to an art institute may be for another. A photographer might derive more pleasure from working in his darkroom than he would from going on a picnic. The editing of this chapter is being done on a beautiful Sunday and is giving my editor and me a pleasurable sense of accomplishment. I speculate that for better health it is important to engage in pleasure-yielding activity enthusiastically—with maximization of its pleasurable possibilities.

Pleasure is a culturally-defined concept. It is based on society's concept of normative values. What is pleasurable today in socially unacceptable ways may, in the future, become socially acceptable. In the 1940s, oral sex was illegal in many states but now many enjoy it even though it is still on the books as being illegal. Nude sunbathing is similarly growing in acceptability. Our concept of pleasure today should not be unduly limited.

An important key to living healthfully and youthfully all one's life is to maximize the number of experiences that are apt to be worth experiencing. Perhaps to be most healthy we must continually experience the greatest joys of all. And what are the greatest joys of all? Each of us will have different ideas of such joys, but perhaps you'll agree with mine: the giving and receiving of love to and from a very special person and helping that person and all others with whom I come in contact to live happier, more meaningful lives. (If the health benefits of love could be provided by a pill, that pill would outsell all the vitamins and drugs on the shelves of drugstores and of health food suppliers.) In our giving and receiving happiness we should strive to achieve in ourselves, and foster in others, peace of mind.*

The *pleasure concept* of health deserves our attention not only in terms of *thought* but in terms of *action*. A most important prescription for health and longevity is to *determine what you like to do—what makes you very happy—and then find lots of opportunities to do it!*

Pleasure must, however, be subject to the dictates of the Greek principle of the *golden mean*. The *golden mean* recognizes that there is a position between "too little" and "too much" that is often superior to either extreme. Not only in the case of pleasure but in the case of various other phenomena, including the action of toxins and of nutrients, there is a *golden mean* that may be more healthful than either extreme. Science has a lot to learn about the quantities of nutrients or of toxins which are likely to lead to either health benefits or health threats. Like the love-hate duality to which human love affairs are subject, so there is a love-hate body reaction that may be exhibited by foods, vitamins, minerals, alcohol, coffee and other substances.

---

* An important step toward achieving and maintaining peace of mind is to keep a list of jobs to be done. Work on each item in the sequence of its time-order importance. Keep at the top of the list the never-finished project entitled: "Make love, not war."

The *Reverse Effect*

The *theory of the reverse effect* states that there is a good probability that any activity or any substance that is health-promoting or health-destructive in a given concentration may, on occasion, reverse its role and become respectively health-destructive or health-promoting at a different concentration. Furthermore, the same activity or the identical dosage of a substance may sometimes show an opposite effect in different persons or animals. What I term a *reverse effect* is not always a matter of going from enhancement to inhibition, but may simply be a trend reversal from increased enhancement to lesser enhancement or from increased inhibition to lesser inhibition. The action will be modulated* not only by the amounts of the chemical or other entity being considered but by the species involved, its health-disease state and its environment. In some cases (e.g., vitamins C and E) the *reverse effect* may involve a change in role from that of antioxidant to pro-oxidant. Perhaps the *theory of the reverse effect* will remind some of my readers of the statement of J. B. S. Haldane: "Nature is not only queerer than we suppose, but queerer than we *can* suppose."

The toxicologist, M. Alice Ottoboni[52] is referring to the phenomenon I call the *reverse effect* when she writes:

> Every toxicologist who has been engaged for any period of time in research into chronic toxic effects of chemicals has observed, more often than not, that animals in the group with the lowest exposure to the test chemical grew more rapidly, had better general appearance and coat quality, had fewer tumors, and lived longer than the control animals. I know from personal experience that novice

---

* Note my use of the word *modulated*. If the *reverse effect* concept proliferates, I suspect that, in the absence of dose-response data on a given substance relative to a given disease, scientists and physicians will increasingly employ the words *modulate* or *modulated* when an effect is apparent but it is not known if a given dosage works as a cause or as a cure or acts to exacerbate or to molify.

toxicologists usually consider such observations as aberrations in their data or the result of some flaw in their experimental design or conduct. They are usually loath to call attention to such findings, perhaps because to do so might bring their competence into question, or because they are unable to explain the reason for such findings. It is only with the confidence that comes with experience that the research toxicologist can comfortably acknowledge the occurrence of such results in his own experiments and broach the subject with his colleagues. The reaction from his fellow toxicologists is usually one of, "You, too?"

The phenomenon of beneficial effects from trace exposures to foreign chemicals, although often a subject of conversation among toxicologists, particularly with regard to why such effects occur, is rarely mentioned in the scientific literature. If the phenomenon does occur in a chronic toxicity experiment, the text of the paper reporting the results will seldom mention the fact. It is only by careful perusal of the data tables and figures presented in the body of the text that the phenomenon is revealed. Such subtleties are lost on people who read only the abstracts of scientific papers. Unfortunately, there are some scientists who may be counted among the abstract-only readers.

The doctrine of "sufficient challenge" of H. F. Smith, Jr.[14] was introduced in a subnote earlier in this chapter. This doctrine is based on the concept that an unused function atrophies. Ottoboni[53] quotes Smith as saying: "I think that most of the small non-specific responses which we measure in chronic toxicity studies at low dosages are readjustments or adaptations to sufficient challenge. I interpret them as manifestations of the well-being of our animals, healthy enough to maintain homeostasis. They are beneficial in that they exercise a function of the animal. Only when challenge becomes overwhelming does injury result." The doctrine of "sufficient challenge" obviously casts doubt on the attitude expressed by the Delaney Clause. The Delaney Clause is based on the idea that if a substance is carcinogenic in large dosages it may also be dangerous in small dosages and it should therefore not be permitted as a food additive. *The Federal Register*[54] perpetuates the line of reasoning behind the Delaney Clause by saying, "The exposure of experimental animals to toxic agents in high dosages is a necessary and valid method of discovering possible carcinogenic hazards in man." Those fostering the Delaney Clause are not concerned with the possibility that such "carcinogens" might, at certain dosages, constitute a "sufficient challenge" and offer protection against cancer. We will consider the Delaney Clause again later in this chapter.

In this book I will report on much research suggesting that large amounts of vitamins and minerals may at times be harmful. Conversely, I speculate that small quantities of toxins may beneficially stimulate the liver to be more efficient just as muscles become stronger when they are occasionally exercised.[*] The advice to eat a well-balanced diet may be good information not only in order to achieve a broad spectrum of needed nutrients but because it introduces the body to a well-balanced but minor intake of toxins, at least some of which in small amounts might actually be beneficial. Nutrition and pharmacology must become sciences, not merely of nutrients, drugs and toxins, but sciences of dose-response relationships.

Thus, I am suggesting that we do not always know which constituents are good and which are bad for the body. *That which is good may be bad; that which is bad may be good.* It depends on the circumstances and one of the circumstances is the quantity of the presumed nutrient or presumed poison that is involved. W. W. Duke,[55] three-quarters of a century ago, tested the effects on blood platelets of many different agents such as toxins, bacteria, a chemical

---

[*] The rationale for this proposed action may involve stimulation of the liver's microenzyme cytochrome P-450. This will be discussed in Chapter 3 (references 129b-d of Chapter 3).

poison and x-rays. He observed that agents causing rapid and large rises in the platelet count (diphtheria toxin and benzol) were the ones producing the most rapid and extreme falls in the count. It was an early recognition of the presence of a *reverse effect.*

Several decades later, Lawrence P. Garrod[56] gave examples of bacterial growth being stimulated when small dosages of chemotherapeutic agents were used. Among those examples he cited was a study of G. E. Foley and W. D. Winter[57] which showed that penicillin increased the mortality of chick embryos inoculated with *Candida albicans.* Garrod noted that "superinfections" sometimes occur clinically during penicillin treatment. On the other hand, T. D. Luckey[58] has reported that antibiotics such as sulfa drugs, succinylsulfathiazole, streptomycin and 3-nitro-4-hydroxyphenyl-arsonic acid can be used in very small quantities to support life and to promote growth in animals.*

About a quarter-century ago, N. V Medunitsyn[58e] found that various painful stimuli given rabbits had an influence on immunological reactivity. A weak stimulus increased phagocytic activity of the leucocytes and increased the antibody titer in the blood while strong painful stimuli showed a *reverse effect* and suppressed these processes. Alcohol in moderation can add to the joy of life and may possibly bring improved health and greater longevity. In excess, alcohol can produce liver cirrhosis and death. A high dose of not only alcohol, but also of sodium pentobarbital, acts as a behavioral depressant, while a low dose of either drug produces behavioral activation.[59] Small amounts of vitamin D are good—they help put

---

* However, antibiotics stimulate growth not only of the animals, but of the biota they are meant to oppose. In 1978, 48% of the antibiotics produced were designated for use in animal feeds.[58a] They are used not only for growth promotion but for better feed conversion, prophylaxis and the treatment of certain diseases.[58b] However, there is a danger in the practice. It appears that antimicrobial-resistant bacteria from animals can cause infection in humans and there have been a number of investigations of epidemics that may have been caused by these bacteria.[58c] Scott D. Holmberg et al.[58d] have identified 18 persons in four midwestern states that have been infected by *Salmonella newport,* a strain resistant to antibiotics. The onset of the illness was often triggered by the taking of amoxicillin or penicillin. They concluded that "antimicrobial-resistant bacteria of animal origin can cause serious human disease, especially in persons taking antimicrobials, and that the emergence and selection of such organisms are complications of subtherapeutic antimicrobial use in animals. We advocate more prudent use of antimicrobials in both people and animals."

calcium in the bones. Large amounts are bad—they pull calcium out of the bones and dump it in the soft tissues, including those of the kidney and of the joints.

Sometimes antivitamins can fulfill some of the functions of the vitamins they ordinarily oppose. Pantoyl taurine can, according to Robert E. Hodges et al.,[60] both cause a pantothenic acid deficiency or reverse that effect and mimic some of the properties of the vitamin. Hodges also reports that the antagonist *omega methyl pantothenic acid* may possibly act as a substitute for pantothenic acid in aiding production of antibodies, thus reversing its generally antagonistic nature. The two-faced nutritional and antinutritional properties of vitamins and their antagonists make the science of nutrition far more subtle than it was once thought to be.

Reverse effects are very common, albeit often unrecognized. Prolactin stimulates milk secretion in lactating women. Prolactin appears also to facilitate processes associated with sperm capacitation (the process, occurring in the vagina, by which sperm become capable of fertilizing an ovum).[61,62] A deficiency of prolactin may be associated with benign prostatic hypertrophy and nominal amounts seem to be required for prostatic health.[63] Rubin et al.[64] reported that prolactin seems to be capable of increasing plasma testosterone in adult men. Furthermore, according to S. P. Ghosh et al.,[65] rat experiments suggest that prolactin acts with testosterone to regulate acid phosphatase activity in the male accessory sex organs.* On the other hand, excessive prolactin, hyperprolactinemia, shows a *reverse effect* compared with normal amounts of prolactin and (like a deficiency of prolactin) is often associated with impotence, hypogonadism, decreased semen volume and reduced spermatic

---

* Interestingly, unless prolactin secretion increases in young (but not in older) men during sleep, their testosterone production is unlikely to follow its normal tendency to peak the following morning.[66] The herb yohimbine from bark of the evergreen tree yohimbe, often used as an aphrodisiac, may stimulate prolactin secretion.[67] (Scientists for many years have declared aphrodisiacs to be nonsense. Experiments at Stanford University by John T. Clark et al.[68] have shown that yohimbine has both immediate and more lasting effects in increasing the sexual appetite of male rats. Experiments are now underway at Stanford to test yohimbine's effect in men. Perhaps the results will confirm what African natives have maintained for centuries about the effects of using the bark of the yohimbe tree.)

density in men and lessened orgasmic capacity in women. [69-72] (Bromocriptine is often used to reduce prolactin levels and for bringing on a restoration of potency and of orgasmic capacity.) Thus, too little or too much prolactin may lead to dire sexual effects.

John Bancroft[72a] reported that L. Lidberg [72b,c] and, later, Lidberg and Sternthal[72d] found that oxytocin may enhance sexual responsiveness in men. Bancroft noted that two of the three studies showed the effect was greater at lower dosages and he refers to the results as "these surprising findings." It is another example of the *reverse effect*.

Pharmacists preparing anticancer drugs may become victims themselves according to a study at the M. D. Anderson Hospital, Houston, Texas.[73,74] The urine of nine pharmacists preparing such drugs became highly mutagenic showing that somehow they absorbed substances that mutate cells, leading possibly to cancer and thus exemplifying the *reverse effect*. A number of other studies[75-78] have reported that urine of nurses and other hospital personnel handling cytotoxic drugs showed positive mutagenicity. Smoking may potentiate the hazard.[77] Recently, Marja Sorsa et al. [77a] published additional evidence of the hazards of occupational exposure to anticancer drugs. Many others have commented on the problem. [79-82*] Then too, a *reverse effect* of the cytotoxic drugs may be shown in the cancer patients themselves after they have been "cured." Robert Hoover and Joseph F. Fraumeni, Jr.[82c] observe that various alkylating agents (including not only cyclophosphamide but also melphalan and chlorambucil) used in treating malignant neoplasms can all *cause* cancer (perhaps, in part, because they break chromosomes). Lancet[81] comments, "In patients who have been cured of malignant disease, clinicians gloomily accept that further neoplasia may arise as a late effect of treatment." Would this occur as

---

* The antineoplastic drugs (cyclophosphamide, diethylstilbestrol, fluorouracil, methotrexate and vincristine) show teratogenic and mutagenic *in vivo* effects in animals. Selevan et al., [82a] in a case-control study involving 17 hospitals in Finland, found that pregnant nurses exposed to antineoplastic drugs had a statistically significant increase in fetal loss. Nurses who lost their fetuses were twice as likely to have been exposed to antineoplastic drugs during the first trimester as those who gave birth. In a related article, Bingham[82b] has observed that, "Institutions such as hospitals and university laboratories have not been in the forefront of occupational-disease prevention."

often if the therapies took full cognizance of dose-related *reverse effects?*

Small amounts of an allergen may stimulate Immunoglobulin E (IgE) antibody production, whereas larger amounts of that allergen may suppress such production.[83] E. R. Stiehm et al.[84] reported that the alpha, beta and gamma families of interferons, which are produced when mammalian cells are stimulated in the inflammatory process, can augment the immune function or can show a *reverse effect* by suppressing immunity. Interferon has the ability to inhibit growth of some malignant cells. On the other hand, a study by Gene P. Siegal et al.[84a] showed that at least three types of interferon can *increase* the ability of Ewing sarcoma cells to invade healthy tissue, which also exemplifies the *theory of the reverse effect.* And so it is in the case of many other drugs, vitamins and minerals.

Foods can also display *reverse effects.* Frederick Hoelzel and Esther DaCosta,[85] in reporting that a protein-deficient diet caused ulcers to form in the stomach and duodenum of mice, observed that an excess of protein also tended to produce gastric lesions. Then too, water sustains life and also displays the *reverse effect* of causing death by drowning.*

Reverse effects are also very common where radiation is concerned. T. D. Luckey[86] relates that small amounts of radiation seem to increase the reproduction rates of protozoa. Fecundity of higher animals may also increase with increased radiation, hens may lay more eggs and sterility rates may be reduced. Luckey cites studies showing that irradiated mammals have increased cerebral blood flow, brain development, audio and visual acuity and learning ability. Large amounts of radiation show a *reverse effect* and cause a decrease in various life functions; still larger amounts result, of course, in death. Many studies, also cited by Luckey, indicate that background radiation can reduce deaths attributed to cancer, while

---

* Even excessive amounts of drinking water may be dangerous to epileptic patients. White[85a] observes that hydration has long been known to induce seizures. He calls attention to a diet plan which advocates drinking of eight to twelve 8-ounce glasses of water per day and cautions that epileptic patients should be aware of the possible dangers.

larger amounts show a *reverse effect* and, as is well known, can cause cancer.*

The *Encyclopaedia Britannica*[87] states that, "A sample of nearly 100,000 survivors of Hiroshima and Nagasaki yielded the anomalous result that groups exposed to doses between 11 and 120 rads actually had a lower death rate in the ensuing 15 years than those receiving a lesser dose." (It is anomalous only in the sense that there is little appreciation for how common the *reverse effect* really is.) A more recent analysis by G. W. Beebe et al.[88] found similar but somewhat different results. Beebe et al. showed a death rate during the 25-year span of 1950-1974 of 23.3% for persons who received no radiation, then rising death rates up to 25.5% at a dose level of 99 rads. At a level of 100-199 rads a *reverse effect* set in and death rates declined to 23.8%, declined further to 22.6% at 200-299 rads, and further yet to 21.6% at 300-399 rads. Then a second *reverse effect* occurred and at dosages of about 400 rads the death rate was highest at 28.4% (as expected). It is interesting to note that the death rates for those exposed between 200 and 399 rads were lower than controls that received no radiation.

Exposure of plants and animals to x-rays and other ionizing radiation shows many beneficial effects. L. P. Breslavets et al. [89] reported that irradiating dry seeds of the radish and the carrot at 2,000 to 4,000 rads before sowing increased radish production by 11% and that of carrots by 26%. The carotene content of the carrots increased by 57%. L. D. Carlson et al.[90] found that rats exposed to low total-body irradiation of .1 rad/hour for 8 hours daily from 4 months to 16 months of age had increased life spans. They speculated that mild injury may be beneficial by stimulating renovation processes. Radiation may even be useful in human therapies. Carolyn Ferree[90a] has reported that the occurrence of gynecomastia (abnormal growth of breasts) secondary to estrogen

---

* Radiation from the sun and from the rest of the cosmos has been bombarding life on earth for the two billion years life has existed. Recently, the intensity of some types of radiation that reach earth has diminished due to the presence of particulates from industrial pollution. Other types of radiation have probably increased due to reduced protection provided by the ozone layer. Could it be that optimal radiation for living things are those levels existing before man fouled the atmosphere?

therapy for prostatic cancer can be largely prevented by irradiating each breast with 900 to 1,000 rads before estrogen therapy.

Roy E. Albert et al.[91] reported many interesting dose-response relationships of beta-ray-induced skin tumors in rats. Figure 2 shows

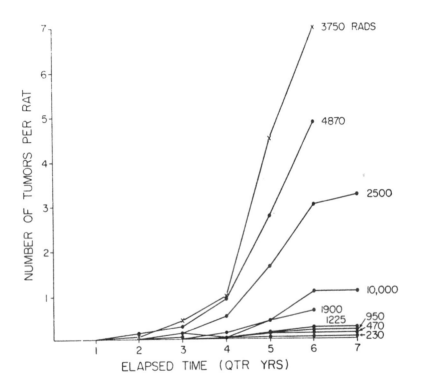

Figure 2. Cumulative incidence of adnexal tumors in rats versus elapsed time after irradiation. Note that the number of tumors increased up to an irradiation level of 3,750 rads and then showed a *reverse effect* by declining at 4,870 rads and declining further at 10,000 rads. Graph reproduced from Roy E. Albert et al., *Radiation Research* (1961) 15: 410-430, with permission of the publisher, Academic Press. (This graph exemplifies the fact that sometimes data can be presented in such a way as to mask the *reverse effect*. See Figure 3.)

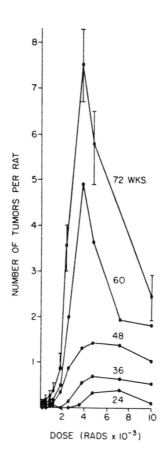

Figure 3. Skin tumors of all types (adnexal, epidermoid carcinoma, etc.) per rat versus skin irradiation dose at the indicated post-irradiation times. Bar lines indicate standard error. Data presented in this form more clearly show the *reverse effect* than do the data presented in Figure 2. Graph reproduced from Roy E. Albert et al., *Radiation Research* (1961) 15: 410-430, with permission of the publisher, Academic Press.

the cumulative incidence of adnexal tumors per rat at three-month intervals for various dosages of radiation. Note that the smaller dosages from 230 to 1,900 rads produced very few tumors. The most tumors developed at a level of 3,750 rads. Then a *reverse effect* set in with fewer tumors being produced at 4,870 rads and fewer still at 10,000 rads. Figure 3 shows the total number of skin tumors of all types as a function of radiation dosage. It is a method of presentation that more clearly shows the *reverse effect*.

Wheeler P. Davey[92] similarly observed that beetles exposed at two different moderate dosages of x-radiation lived longer than controls not exposed at all, those exposed at low dosages and those exposed at high dosages. Many such experiments are cited by T. D. Luckey.[93]

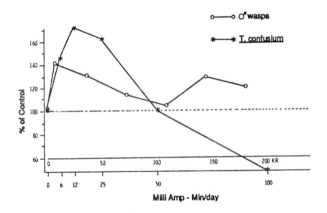

Figure 4. Increased longevity in invertebrates exposed to x-rays followed by a *reverse effect* and lowered longevity. The data of Davey exhibit the response of *T. confusium* to mA/min/day of radiation. The abscissa for the data of Sullivan and Grosch with male wasps is given in kR as one acute exposure. Graph reproduced from T. D. Luckey, *Hormesis with Ionizing Radiation* (Boca Raton, Florida: CRC Press, 1980), with permission of the publisher.

T. D. Luckey's book[93] contains some very interesting graphs, three of which are shown here. Figure 4, using data from Davey[92] and from R. L. Sullivan and D. S. Grosch,[94] shows that the life span of the insect *Tribolium confusum* increased to a maximum at an x-ray exposure of about 12 milli amp/min/day and then a *reverse effect* set in, reached par with controls at 50 milli amp/min/day, and then continued to show longevity decreases. The same figure illustrates the response of male wasps to radiation expressed as kR and given

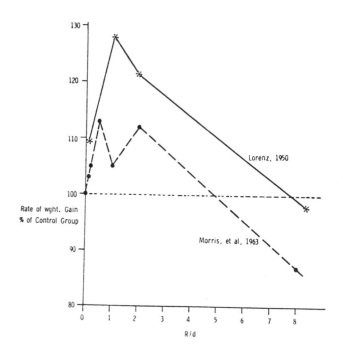

Figure 5. Increased growth rates in irradiated mice were comparable in experiments of different laboratories. In both cases, after an initial surge, a *reverse effect* set in, followed by decreased growth rates. Graph reproduced from T. D. Luckey, *Hormesis with Ionizing Radiation* (Boca Raton, Florida: CRC Press, 1980), with permission of the publisher.

as one acute exposure. Here, the life span increased at an exposure of about 10 kR, then showed a *reverse effect* by declining almost to a par with controls at about 55 kR. At this level a *biphasic reverse effect* set in with longevity increasing again as the radiation dosage was raised.

Figure 5, again from Luckey,[93] illustrates different experiments by E. Lorenz et al.[95] and by J. J. Morris et al.[96] on growth rates in mice irradiated with x-rays. These experiments indicate maximum growth as the radiation increased from .1 to .5 or 1 R/day. At about .5 or 1 R/day (depending on the study) *reverse effects* occurred and rate of weight gain declined, reaching par of the control group at 5 to 7.5 R/day and then continued to worsen.

Figure 6, the final illustration from Luckey,[93] shows yields of grain and of strawberries in terms of x-ray dosages based on data from studies by L. P. Breslavets and A. S. Afanasyeva,[97] by R. K. Schulz[98] and by I. Fendrik.[99] Growth increased as x-ray dosage rose and reached maxima (in some cases doubling the yield of the controls) between 10^2 and 10^3 R/day. Then *reverse effects* took place and, between a radiation level of 10^3 and 10^4, the yield declined to par of the controls and then continued to decline as dosage increased.

Concern has been expressed about the dangers of electromagnetic waves emanating from high tension wires and questionable tales have been told about the Russians using such waves to "zap" our embassy in Moscow. One of the effects of electromagnetic waves on cells is to affect the glucose content. Crediting the work of Budho, A. S. Pressman[100] of the Department of Biophysics, Moscow University, Moscow, U.S.S.R., has illustrated the phenomenon with two graphs (Figures 7 and 8). Note (in Figure 7) as the frequency of the waves increases glucose content of cells declines, but at 30 k Hz a *reverse effect* sets in and thereafter the glucose content rises. A similar effect is shown as the field strength varies. Glucose content declines as field strength increases up to about 15V/cm, then shows a *reverse effect* and rises as the field strength continues to increase (Figure 8). From these examples it should be apparent that *reverse effects* are common when life forms interact with radiation.

The Reverse Effect

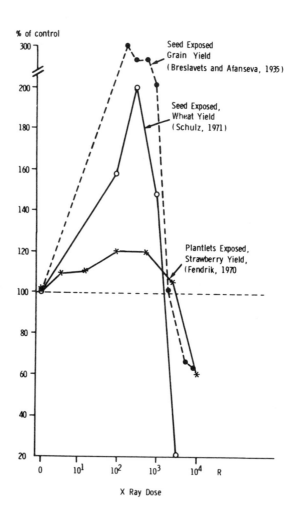

Figure 6. Changes in yield as seeds and plants are irradiated. In each case, a *reverse effect* is apparent. Graph reproduced from T. D. Luckey, *Hormesis with Ionizing Radiation* (Boca Raton, Florida: CRC Press, 1980), with permission of the publisher.

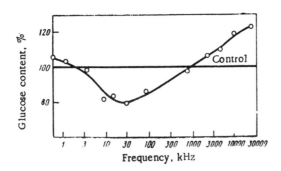

Figure 7. Change in glucose content of isolated rat liver due to low- and high-frequency EmFs. Note the *reverse effect* at about 30 kHz. Graph reproduced from A. S. Pressman, *Electromagnetic Fields and Life* (New York: Plenum Press, 1970) pp. 156-157, with permission of the publisher.

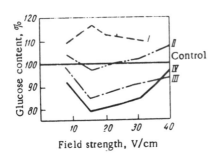

Figure 8. Change in glucose content of isolated rat liver in relation to EmF strength. I) 9.5 MHz; II) 730 kHz; III) 85 kHz; IV) 29 kHz. Note the *reverse effect* at about 15 V/cm. Graph reproduced from A. S. Pressman, *Electromagnetic Fields and Life* (New York: Plenum Press, 1970) pp. 156-157, with permission of the publisher.

Paracelsus, back in the 1500s, is credited with the statement, "Dosis sola facit venenum—Only the dose makes the poison." Then in the 19th century, a principle in pharmacology was developed that came to be known as the *Arndt Law* or the *Arndt-Schultz Law*. This law states: *weak stimuli excite physiologic activity, moderately strong ones favor it, strong ones retard it, very strong ones arrest it.* T. D. Luckey has been a key factor in the development of the related sciences of *hormology* and *hormoligosis*. Luckey has defined *hormology* as the study of excitation and includes in it not only the effect of *hormones* but the effect of other chemicals, radiation, heat, cold and other agents on cells. Hormoligosis is the part of hormology which includes the entire phenomenon of the stimulatory effect of a small amount of an agent on living organisms. *Hormesis* is the subdivision of hormoligosis which deals with the stimulatory amount of toxins, and the compounds involved are called *hormetics.** In connection with hormology, Luckey has modified the Ardnt-Schultz Law to read: *subharmful doses of any harmful agent may stimulate organisms in suboptimum condition.* Luckey[102] predicts, by the way, that "over half of all toxic compounds would be hormetics if appropriately low doses were administered."

The *theory of the reverse effect* differs from the Arndt-Schultz Law and from hormology in that it relates to organisms that are not necessarily in a suboptimum condition and it recognizes that the effect of a "high dosage" is often not simply a matter of retardation or arrest, but one of producing an opposite effect. Weak or moderate sexual activity may increase the functional ability of a man's prostate gland. Too much sex, on the other hand, might not merely arrest the prostate's ability to perform (as the Arndt-Schultz Law might suggest), but could induce a pathological condition that might be attended by symptoms of pain and bleeding. Vitamins C and E can not only act as antioxidants (as is well known) but, as we noted earlier, can show a *reverse effect* by acting as pro-oxidants. (See Chapters 2 and 6.) Many examples of the *reverse effect* can be found throughout this book.

---

* The word *hormesis* was neologized by C. M. Southam and J. Ehrlich who reported [101] that an extract of tree bark stimulated bacteria at low levels but was bacteriostatic at high levels. Luckey has expanded their definition.

As I said, a chemical or other entity (e.g., exercise or pleasure-yielding activity), which at a given dosage causes a certain physiological reaction, will often cause a *reverse effect* at either a much greater or a much smaller dosage. Mild exercise (a "nutrient") may lead to a stronger heart, stronger arms, etc. Too much exercise, however, may at times bring on a heart attack and "tennis elbow" and, as we will see in Chapter 10, may even be life-shortening. Modest amounts of sunshine can foster health; large amounts can promote sunburn, leathery skin and melanoma. Other "nutrients" and "toxins" that exemplify *reverse effects,* in addition to exercise, drugs, herbs, vitamins, minerals, foods and pleasure-yielding activity, will probably occur to the reader.

With this line of reasoning, I am, of course, casting doubt on the multitude of experiments in which huge doses of a given substance are fed animals in order to produce, say, cancer and then those experiments are used to predict the possibility that the substance may cause cancer in man. I am not, right now, concerned with the dubious assumption that a chemical in the diet of man will act as that chemical does in the diet of a mouse. I am concerned, instead, with something I believe to be far more important. The procedure of estimating low-dose human response based on experiments involving high-dose animal response could be an improper extrapolation of dose-response relationships. The famous Delaney Clause,* as we noted earlier, is based on the presumed validity of this extrapolation that I am questioning. Extrapolation of any data outside the observable range can be an error-fraught exercise. M.

---

* Since the Delaney Clause was enacted in 1958, it has been interpreted to mean that no substance known to cause cancer in animals may be added to food. (It might be naturally present, but may not be added.)[103] Saccharin was subsequently given a legal exemption. In June, 1985, Dr. Frank Young, FDA commissioner, stated that his reading of the law permits use of the legal concept known as *de minimus,* meaning "the law does not concern itself with trifles."[103a] Young maintains that a *de minimus* risk does not mean the substance must be banned. Two articles by Marjorie Sun,[103b,c] one by Kessler[103d] and one by Flamm[103e] discuss some of the problems occasioned by the Delaney Clause.

Alice Ottoboni[104] tells about a "megamouse" study of the National Center for Toxicological Research (NCTR)[105] involving more than 24,000 mice and the carcinogen 2-acetylaminofluorene (AAF). A committee of the Society of Toxicology [106] reviewed the NCTR report.[105] Ottoboni, in citing from this review, said:

> The Society's review points out that the statistical model used for extrapolating effects from very low doses "provides statistically significant evidence that low doses of a carcinogen are beneficial...."
>
> "If the time-dependent low-dose extrapolation models are correct," the Society states, "then we must conclude that low doses of AAF protected the animals from bladder tumors." However, the Society also asserts, "...not only is the simple model used by NCTR statisticians inappropriate to the data, but most of the models that have been proposed in the statistical literature are also inappropriate." They urge a "profound rethinking of the entire problem of chemical carcinogenesis and low-dose extrapolation."

The *theory of the reverse effect* suggests just the opposite of the standard line of reasoning. Small doses of a huge-dose cancer-causer might protect against cancer! Tomorrow's statements of physiological interactions with drugs and nutrients are likely to be elucidated in dose-response tables rather than in simple sentences.

Then too, the fact that many drugs have side effects corresponding with the same condition for which they are curative provides many examples of the *reverse effect*. This fact also serves as a warning that drugs must be carefully studied for dose-responses and possible *reverse effects* that can be exacerbative rather than curative. If you study several drugs in the *Physicians' Desk Reference* [107] you will probably discover that, for at least a few of them, the list of side effects contains a symptom for which the drug

is sometimes curative. The diazepam, Valium® is one such drug.*
Among the indications for its use is included "management of anxiety
disorders or for the short-term relief of the symptoms of anxiety."
Among its adverse reactions are included "hyperexcited states" and
"anxiety."[107b] The barbiturate, Nembutal® Sodium is used as a
"sedative hypnotic." Among its side effects are "agitation,"
"nightmares," "nervousness" and "anxiety."[107c] Quinidine sulphate
(Quinora®) is used for "paroxysmal atrial tachycardia" and
"paroxysmal atrial fibrillation" and "paroxysmal ventricular
tachycardia when not associated with complete heartblock." Among
its adverse effects are "ventricular tachycardia and fibrillation" and
"paradoxical tachycardia."[107d] The rauwolfia product, Harmonyl® is
employed for its "antihypertensive effects" and it also displays
"sedative and tranquilizing properties." Among its adverse effects are
"nervousness," "paradoxical anxiety" and "nightmares."[107e] To cite a
final example, Asellacrin®, a growth hormone (somatropin or
somatotrophin) which is used in treating short children in the attempt
to increase their height, may sometimes be subject to a *reverse effect*.
The *Physicians' Desk Reference* relates that "bone age must be
monitored annually during Asellacrin® administration, especially in
patients who are pubertal and/or receiving concomitant thyroid
replacement therapy. Under these circumstances, epiphyseal
maturation may progress rapidly to closure."[107f] In other words,
sometimes there is a *reverse effect* and, instead of the child growing
taller, his epipheses close and he completely stops growing.

In each of these drugs the normal action shows a *reverse
effect* at some concentrations in some persons. A *reverse effect* of
the drug diphenylhydantoin (Dilantin®), alias phenytoin, involving
vitamin D is shown in Chapter 4 and, in connection with
hypertension (in the potassium section of Chapter 7), we will note
the *reverse effect* shown by hydrochlorothiazide. At a given dosage a

---

* The patent on Valium® has recently run out, so there are likely to be many more
diazepam drugs to offer it competition. Horrobin [107a] speculates that diazepams and
possibly the benzodiazepines, including chlordiazepoxide hydrochloride (Librium®), may
promote tumor growth. (Tumor promoters do not usually cause cancer when used alone but
can enhance the effect of a cancer initiator.) Is it possible that diazepams and/or
benzodiazepines at some dosage might show a *reverse effect* and act to cure cancer?

drug may *cause* in one person the same condition which the same dosage *cures* in another. A different dosage will often show a *reverse effect* and be curative to the first but detrimental to the second. The side effects of many of the drugs listed in the *Physicians' Desk Reference* give testimony to the reality of the *reverse effect*. Medicine, like nutrition, must study dose-response relationships and, by administering individually determined dosages in therapeutic applications, strive to eliminate iatrogenic *reverse effects.** (The research-minded reader will discover other *reverse effects* in the *Physicians' Desk Reference* and may also desire to search for additional examples in *AMA Drug Evaluations* [107fa] or in *Drug Facts and Comparisons.* [107fb] Some libraries also have on-line data base information regarding recently discovered drug-associated problems. If your local library does not have *Drug Facts and Comparisons* and its monthly supplements, your pharmacist may let you look at his.)

Let me caution against quickly concluding that small doses of a given substance may often be beneficial with large doses of that substance being dangerous. As we will see in Chapter 6, small amounts of vitamin C detrimentally encourage lipid peroxidation, larger amounts beneficially act as an antioxidant and still larger amounts may once again act detrimentally as a pro-oxidant. Studies show that estrogen can promote carcinogenesis. On the other hand, Joseph Meites et al.[107g] have shown that a large dose of estrogen (20 mg. of estradiol benzoate) effectively inhibited growth of DMBA-induced mammary tumors in rats. Meites also cites the work of C. Huggins[107h] and of R. I. Dorfman[107i] that also showed large doses of estrogen resulted in tumor regression in rats. In addition, Meites cites a study of J. Hayward[107j] in which large doses of estrogen (or of androgen) induced remission of human breast cancer in more than 20% of treated patients. In further regard to estrogen, Hoover and Fraumeni[82c] cite three studies that suggest oral contraceptives may

---

* Studying the *Physicians' Desk Reference (PDR)* at intervals of a decade or more, I get the impression that drugs reported by the *PDR* as having a "paradoxical effect" are associated with a tendency to be retired. However, a phenomenon is paradoxical only until the paradox is resolved. Would it be beneficial to keep using some of these retired drugs but more clearly define dose-response relationships?

offer some protection against ovarian cancer. Perhaps in the case of the ovary, estrogen may show a *reverse effect* at the dosage of the Pill and provide protection. Obviously, more (in the case of estrogen) may sometimes induce a beneficial *reverse effect.*

Large amounts of dihomo-gamma-linolenic acid (DGLA), a substance which is present in human milk and which is metabolized in the body (especially if evening primrose oil is consumed), can inhibit the growth of malignant cells *in vitro.* However, Robinson and Botha (as discussed in Chapter 3) found that a small amount (50 µg. per ml) of DGLA, on the other hand, can produce a *reverse effect* (my language) and promote cancer. Here again, a large amount of a substance may work for our benefit while a small dosage may be dangerous. (Since evening primrose oil is widely sold, it is important that any possible *reverse effect* be precisely delineated. In Chapter 3 we will consider evening primrose oil—its benefits and possible dangers—in greater detail. The *reverse effect,* as we will see throughout this book, can be very subtle indeed.)

Physicians must learn that the answer to ineffectiveness of a therapy is not necessarily to increase the dose. A decreased dose, instead, might produce the desired result. Similarly, scientists must learn to construct experimental protocols that make it possible to discover *reverse effects.* Often experiments are done with dosage increments that make it impossible to discover what, if any, phenomena might exist at intermediate levels.

Could the *theory of the reverse effect* have implications as a research tool, e.g., in the search for anticancer agents? Podophyllotoxin from the herb *American mandrake (mayapple)* is reported to cause cancer. It is reported to also actively inhibit carcinoma and sarcoma in animals. Perhaps it might prove rewarding to look for cancer-treating substances among factors known to be mitogenic, mutagenic or carcinogenic. Such a search might be a valuable application of the *theory of the reverse effect.* Mary E. Caldwell and Willis R. Brewer[108] recently published a list of 50 plant extracts from 42 species that have been shown to significantly enhance tumor growth. A total of 300 extracts were found to exhibit prominent enhancement of tumor growth. The work was well done in terms of its objectives and tests were performed at various toxic and nontoxic levels. However, I think the entire group of 300 extracts should be studied for *reverse effects* and possible antitumor action at some yet-to-be-discovered dosages.*

The *Reverse Effect* as a New Therapeutic Paradigm

Thomas S. Kuhn has thrown interesting new light on the ways in which various sciences evolve. Paramount to Kuhn's viewpoint is the role in scientific research played by "paradigms" which he defines as "universally recognized scientific achievements that for a time provide model problems and solutions to a community of practitioners."[108c]

Kuhn develops the thesis that "normal science," as he calls it, presupposes one or more paradigms which are accepted by practicing scientists as being beyond questioning. Thus, research tends to be looked upon as an act of puzzle-solving that occurs within the bounds set by a paradigm rather than as a free-wheeling exploration of the unknown. Kuhn, in his thought-provoking book *The Structure of Scientific Revolutions,* says:

> ...normal science repeatedly goes astray. And when it
> does—when, that is, the profession can no longer
> evade anomalies that subvert the existing tradition of
> scientific practice—then begin the extraordinary
> investigations that lead the profession at last to a new
> set of commitments, a new basis for the practice of
> science. The extraordinary episodes in which that

---

* D. R. Stoltz et al.[108a] found that 22 fruits and vegetables had mutagenic activity. Grapes, onions, peaches, raisins, raspberries and strawberries showed the most potent mutagenicity. Could components (perhaps flavonoids) from these six be concentrated to act as anticancer agents, as the *reverse effect* suggests? Many flavonols found in foods are mutagenic and references for this finding are found in Chapter 6. I have not seen studies indicating that 3,4'-dimethoxy-3'5,7-trihydroxyflavone and centaureidin are mutagenic and/or carcinogenic. However, S. Morris Kupchan and E. Bauerschmidt[108b] found that these flavonols from the plant *Baccharis sarothroides* showed significant inhibitory activity against cells derived from human carcinoma of the nasopharynx carried in cell culture.

shift of professional commitments occurs are the ones known in this essay as scientific revolutions. They are the tradition-shattering complements to the tradition-bound activity of normal science.[108d]

Kuhn, in further development of his view of "normal science," goes on to say:

Few people who are not actually practitioners of a mature science realize how much mop-up work of this sort a paradigm leaves to be done or quite how fascinating such work can prove in the execution. And these points need to be understood. Mopping-up operations are what engage most scientists throughout their careers. They constitute what I am here calling normal science. Closely examined, whether historically or in the contemporary laboratory, that enterprise seems an attempt to force nature into the preformed and relatively inflexible box that the paradigm supplies. No part of the aim of normal science is to call forth new sorts of phenomena; indeed those that will not fit the box are often not seen at all. Nor do scientists normally aim to invent new theories, and they are often intolerant of those invented by others. Instead, normal-scientific research is directed to the articulation of those phenomena and theories that the paradigm already supplies.[108e]

Thus, dramatic new breakthroughs can occur only through the process of overthrowing well-established doctrines. The doctrine that extrapolation can predict effects in nutrition and in medicine must be viewed as being obsolete. A *reverse effect* might be present and produce a reaction quite the opposite from what data extrapolation would suggest—perhaps even a cure from a known disease-causer. I propose that the *theory of the reverse effect* as a tool for developing new therapies is a revolutionary paradigm.

Orthodox nutrition and orthodox medicine have played too many tricks on those relying on the efficacy of extrapolation for predicting effects out of the range of available data. Nature is always a formidable opponent. John Pfeiffer, in his excellent book regarding radio astronomy, has this to say about the battle between nature and science:

> Science is an intricate guessing game with nature as the adversary. The rules and regulations of the game are known somewhat loosely as the scientific method; the moves and strategies are our experiments and theories. Nature is continually fooling us, outguessing us, surprising us by doing the things we least expect of her. But every time we are fooled, we learn another one of her tricks. She is infinitely resourceful, of course, and we might as well face it.
>
> But we are fairly resourceful, too. When nature outguesses us, when we find our theories inadequate to account for the facts, we must be ready to shift and vary our attack as cleverly as a prizefighter exploring the strengths and weaknesses of his opponent.[108f]

So, it is time to conclude that the possibility of *reverse effects* should be employed in devising nutritional and medicinal approaches for the creation of new therapies.

Much "mop-up" work, as Kuhn would call it, will be needed to determine *reverse effect* levels of different therapeutic agents for various diseases. If, for example, mutagenic agents may work not only to *cause* cancer but, at different dosages work to *cure* cancer, what are the critical dosages for each such agent? Specifically, what might be the cancer-fighting dose of each of the bioflavonoids that, at a different dosage, show mutagenicity? Are "miracle" cures a possibility? St. Augustine (354-430A.D.) said, "Miracles are not contrary to nature but only contrary to what we know about nature." It is time to employ the *reverse effect* as a new therapeutic paradigm. The existence of a vast body of anomalies following from the established paradigm of extrapolation demands a revolutionary approach and this new paradigm providing for possible *reverse effects*.

The *theory of the reverse effect* gives added support to the idea of eating a well-balanced diet: not too much of this, not too little of that. Then too, I think of the *pleasure concept* as being a sub-principle of the *theory of the reverse effect*. Occasional ingestion of coffee and sweet rolls or occasional sex may be psychologically nutritional. Too much coffee, sweet rolls or sex may be toxic. It is an application of the ancient Greek principle of the golden mean: *moderation in all things*. Now that we have speculated about the *reverse effect*, it may be useful to rephrase the *pleasure concept* as follows: *A generally beneficial substance consumed without pleasure or when one is in an angry state or is in unpleasant surroundings may be detrimental to the body. A generally detrimental substance consumed with joy may be beneficial to the body.*

Whenever dosages of nutrients can be shown to display *reverse effects* on body functions, the science of nutrition needs to be rewritten in terms of dose-response relationships. To the extent that relevant *reverse effects* exist, never again will the science of nutrition—whether a "nutrient" be defined as a food or a toxin, a mineral, a vitamin, sunshine or other radiation, sex or other exercise or pleasure, etc.—be the same.

Is there a rationale that might explain the *reverse effect?* A. J. Clark[109] postulated the existence of two types of receptor sites, one producing a positive effect and the second acting in opposition to the first. E. J. Ariens et al.[110] and J. M. von Rossum et al.,[111] as well as W. D. M. Paton[112] developed this idea further. It is theorized that at low concentrations a given substance combines mainly with the activating receptor. At higher concentrations the action of the activating receptor reaches a plateau or continues to increase to only a minor degree. On the other hand, the blocking receptor becomes increasingly more active and eventually the effect is to overwhelm the action of the activating receptor. The peak of the bell-shaped dose-response curve is reached, then passed and we have a *reverse effect*. Some substances may occupy only activating receptors or only blocking receptors. They would, of course, have linear dose-response curves and would not exhibit the *reverse effect*. Such substances that occupy only activating receptors may be far more rare than is now believed to be the case. It might, for example, be argued that aflatoxin, which is toxic in just a few parts per billion, depending on the species, and continues to be toxic at higher concentrations, might be such a substance. However, can we rule out the possibility that, in minute concentrations of say a few parts per trillion or per quadrillion,* aflatoxin might show one or more *reverse effects* and might even be therapeutic? I think much is to be gained from hypothesizing that most substances taken into the body or produced by the body will, at some dosage or dosages, show one or more *reverse effects*.

Scientists often find that for which they look, and I think they should be looking for *reverse effects*.** Even in cases where chemicals are not obviously involved (e.g., exercise and pleasure-activation) they may in actuality be involved. For example, exercise involves adenosine triphosphate (ATP), adenosine diphosphate (ADP), creatine, creatine phosphate, glucose, insulin, lactic acid, glycogen, etc.

---

* Scientists may soon be able to detect a single atom or a single molecule by laser-based analytic methods.[112a]

** In general, scientists find only that for which they are searching, serendipitous discoveries being rather rare. In attempting to set an appropriate dosage for a clinical trial of retinyl acetate for use in treating histopathologic lesions of the cervix, Seymour L. Romney et al.[113] wrote: "The 3 mg. dose was eliminated as part of the empiric effort to establish the maximally tolerated dosage." It seems obvious they gave no thought to the possibility that the 3 mg. dose could be more effective than the 9 mg. dosage they finally decided to use. (That is, no thought was given to the possibility that a *reversal* could exist somewhere between a dose of zero and one of 9 mg.) The scientific literature contains innumerable other examples indicating that the possibility of a *reverse effect* was simply not considered.

Pleasure (or pain which, depending on its intensity, may sometimes be pleasurable) may involve endorphins and enkaphilins. Thus, the binding-site theory may have general application in explaining the *reverse effect*. In the case of cancer applications, mutagens that will modify the DNA of normal cells and sometimes produce cancer, may act reversely to combat cancer by modifying the cancer cell's DNA. Through this mechanism the function of a cancer cell may be inhibited leading, in turn, to its demise. The fact that normal cells may be destroyed concomitantly is regrettable but not crucial since the body can replace them through its normal reparative processes. Other explanations of specific *reverse effects* are suggested throughout the book.

Current nutritional and medical practice frequently ignores not only the possible occurrence of *reverse effects* but also generally ignores the importance of the time of day, time of month or time of year that a nutrient, a drug or other treatment is administered. The developing science of chronobiology is concerned with the fact that the toxicity and/or effectiveness of drugs (and also perhaps of nutrients and other treatment modalities) can vary greatly depending on the time they are administered. The possibly increased effectiveness of vitamins or of drugs administered on a nonuniform time basis is illustrated by studies of Erhard Haus et al.,[114] F. Halberg et al.,[115] L. E. Scheving et al.[116] and Karel M. H. Philippens.[117] Some of these scientists [114] observed that mice inoculated with L1210 leukemia survived for a statistically significant longer span when four courses of arabinosyl cytosine were administered at 4-day intervals—not in courses consisting of 8 equal doses at 3-hour intervals, but in sinusoidally varying 24-hour courses, the largest amount being given at the previously mapped circadian and circannual times of peak resistance to the drug. Other studies have also demonstrated the increased therapeutic effectiveness of sinusoidal dosage schedules. Such research suggests that drugs presumably having an unacceptable toxicity-therapeutic ratio may be useable and of considerable value when administered in accordance with chronotherapeutic principles.

Healthful Thoughts and Other Supplements

This book deals not only with the prevention of *disease*, but also with far more. Beyond just prevention of disease, this book relates to the building of *health*. Health is a state of well-being which is far superior to the mere absence of disease and relates to joy, happiness and the enhancement of life; and remember this: joy, happiness and the enhancement of life cannot only be the *result* of superior health but a *cause* of superior health. Most persons now believe in the reality of psychosomatic disease. Why not also believe in the reality of psychogenic health? You can think yourself into better health. Do it!

Often the comment is heard that if one eats good food, then supplementation is unnecessary. There are several reasons why this doctrine is apt to be false. Try as we can, it is unlikely that all our foods will be grown on rich soil, and thus at least some of these foods are less likely to contain the healthful array of minerals our ancestors enjoyed. Even if our foods were all grown on rich soil, many would still be irrigated with polluted waters and exposed to air pollution. Furthermore, we are breathing that polluted air and we are subjected not only to toxic chemicals in our foods but to those in cosmetics, cleaning compounds, and so on. Then too, our society subjects us to many mental stresses which may, if we let them influence us negatively, deplete vitamin and mineral stores as the body attempts to compensate for those stresses.

G. Brubacher et al.[118] make the point that borderline vitamin deficiency exists in many population groups and in single persons even in industrialized countries. Their studies demonstrated that the avoidance of pork and whole wheat bread can lead to a borderline vitamin B_1 deficiency. Similarly, their studies have shown that avoidance of other items can lead to other vitamin deficiencies. Most persons who have fully operational food-assimilational and enzyme systems can probably get their vitamin and mineral needs from their diet if their objective is an *average* state of health. Those less efficient in food assimilation and in enzyme production or those with unusual diets (such as those who avoid pork and whole wheat bread) or those desiring superlative health may require supplements.* Moreover, R. L. Gross and P. M. Newberne,[119] in citing C. M. Leevy et al.[119a] who studied a selected municipal hospital population, say:

> These studies of isolated vitamin deficiencies lead to the inescapable conclusion that a single nutrient deficiency can result in profound impairment of specific immunologic processes—a concept that has not yet received widespread attention or general acceptance. This inattention may be having important clinical results, since the immunologic defects resulting from even marginal deficiencies may significantly alter disease course and/or therapeutic response. The incidence of hypovitaminosis discovered in a randomly selected U. S. hospital population in the 1960's dramatically illustrates that this is not an exclusive problem of underdeveloped countries. In this study, only 12% of the 120 patients had normal serum levels of all vitamins tested; 88% had at least one deficiency, and 59% had two or more biochemical deficiencies. There appeared to be no consistent trend with regard to sex, age, or racial group. Only 39% of the deficient patients had any history of dietary deficiency, the other 61% consuming what was considered a normal U. S. diet. Clinical signs of deficiency were present in only 38%; the remainder had deficiencies falling into the subclinical or marginal categories.

The elderly may be especially prone to vitamin deficiencies. D. J. Smithard and M. J. S. Langman[120] found subclinical vitamin C

---

* On the other hand, it may be possible that food itself could sometimes supply a dangerous *excess* of vitamins. Certainly, Eskimos consuming bear liver have been known to get dangerous excesses of vitamin A. Kummerow maintains, as we will see in Chapter 4, that foods may contain unhealthful excesses of vitamin D.

deficiency in nearly half of geriatric patients they studied. Vitamin C, through its effect on the P-450 enzyme system (which will be discussed in later chapters), is a factor in drug metabolism. Thus, low levels of vitamin C in many of the elderly may account for their generally slowed rates of drug metabolism. One must, however, use caution in concluding that low levels of vitamins and/or minerals in the elderly are necessarily unhealthful. Remember, in any study of the elderly, the subjects have been selected on the basis of longevity. Some of their characteristics obviously account for that longevity. Which ones?

Vitamins can sometimes correct or partially correct for inborn errors of metabolism. These errors of metabolism involve genetically determined absences of, or reductions of, enzyme activity and almost any biological transformation could be affected. K. Bartlett,[120a] in a very thorough treatment (with over 300 references), takes each vitamin in turn and discusses vitamin-responsive inborn errors of metabolism. S. Harvey Mudd[121] has also discussed various phases of vitamin-responsive genetic disease. In this regard, Charles Scriver[122] tells of some of the ways in which a vitamin dependency caused by gene-dependent nutritional disorders could be operating. First, an abnormal gene product might affect the body's ability to convert a vitamin into its biologically active coenzyme. Secondly, the cells could be impaired in their ability to take up a vitamin to convert it to its coenzyme. Thirdly, the apoenzyme might be altered so as to impair its ability to bind to the coenzyme. The mutant allele (one of a pair, or of a series, of variants of a gene having the same locus on homologous chromosomes) might not completely eliminate activity at a particular step in the biosynthetic pathway. It might still allow some coenzyme to be formed if the precursor vitamin were present in sufficient concentration. Do you or I perhaps have an undiscovered mutant allele affecting a physiological phenomenon that might be helped by extra amounts of one or more of the vitamins?*

An excellent overview relating to gene-dependent disorders was written by S. Harvey Mudd[123] and is entitled "Vitamin-Responsive

---

* In Chapter 5 we will examine the possibility that megadoses of the B vitamins might in some cases play a detrimental role in the formation of enzymes.

Genetic Abnormalities." Mudd says: "...rather than there being a single 'ideal' human with a 'normal' requirement for a vitamin, about which actual persons cluster as imperfect approximations, there may well exist an array of individuals in any population with genetically determined differences in their vitamin requirements spread over a wide range. If this is so, determination of nutritional standards for vitamins takes on an increased complexity to which nutritionists may wish to give a good deal of thought in the years to come."

Every individual, whether or not he has genetic "abnormalities," is unique in his or her nutritional requirements. Drs. E. Cheraskin and W. M. Ringsdorf, Jr.[124] relate that between two healthy young men of the same racial stock, one may require 4.5 times as much calcium as the other and 6.5 times as much of a particular amino acid as the other. For some nutrients the range of minimums is probably much greater. Vitamins A and C are two such examples. One individual might require ten times as much of one or both of these vitamins as another person. However, Drs. Cheraskin and Ringsdorf (and, for that matter, Dr. Roger J. Williams in his many writings over a period of many years) should have observed that "biological individuality" applies inversely as well. The level at which a given vitamin or other nutrient may become toxic could be ten times *lower* in you than it may be in me.

This book should not be construed as giving medical advice. No vitamin, mineral, herb, food, drug or doctor ever "cures" any condition. The body cures itself when it receives the necessary raw materials and/or the necessary treatment. Furthermore, it should be emphasized that one's state of health and potential for great longevity depend on a multitude of factors, among which are: someone to love and be loved by; a good self-concept, an active sense of responsibility for one's own health; a positive attitude; a recognition of the fact that there are always options; a happy, tranquil mind with good ability to cope with stress, including efficient use of anger to get jobs done rather than to cause ulcers and heart trouble; a firm resolve to worry only about things one can conceivably control; a willingness to see problems as being opportunities; crying more, smiling and laughing more and in other ways expressing rather than holding back the emotions; giving attention to the needs of others; adequate exercise; sufficient rest; clean air;* pure water; wholesome food and all the necessary vitamins and minerals. The facts conveyed in this book must speak for themselves and are to be used or ignored in accordance with the independent judgment of each individual reader.

Often we hear criticism of the RDA (Recommended Dietary Allowances) which are set, at five-year intervals, by the Food and Nutrition Board of the National Academy of Sciences. In criticizing the RDA we should keep in mind that the ninth edition of the academy's book states:

> RDA are recommendations for the average daily amounts of nutrients that *population groups* should consume over a period of time. RDA should not be confused with requirements for a specific individual. Differences in the nutrient requirements of individuals are ordinarily unknown. Therefore, RDA (except for energy) are estimated to exceed the requirements of most individuals and thereby to ensure that the needs of nearly all in the population are met. Intakes below the recommended allowance for a nutrient are not necessarily inadequate, but the risk of having an inadequate intake increases to the extent that intake is less than the level recommended as safe.
>
> RDA are recommendations established for *healthy* populations. Special needs for nutrients arising from such problems as premature birth, inherited metabolic disorders, infections, chronic diseases, and the use of medications require special dietary and therapeutic measures. These conditions are not covered by the RDA.[125]

---

* Clean air obviously includes avoidance of smoking and smoke-filled rooms. However, smoking can improve some conditions. Through an anti-estrogenic effect, it reduces the incidence of endometrial cancer in postmenopausal women.[124a-c] Smoking may also help protect against ulcerative colitis[124d] and Parkinson's disease.[124e]

Henry Kamin was the chairman of the Committee on Dietary Allowances of the Food and Nutrition Board in charge of preparing the tenth edition of the book, *Recommended Dietary Allowances,* publishing of which was recently aborted.* Kamin has stressed that the RDA of vitamins and minerals are in accordance with their requirements as nutrients and without consideration of possibly desirable pharmacological effects. He says:

> ...it is not inconceivable that some nutrients, even *within* the limits of a normal varied diet may, by some chemical accident, have some beneficial effect unrelated to its normal biological function. There has been considerable activity recently which suggests that some compounds chemically related to vitamin A—but not necessarily having biological vitamin A activity—may act as anticarcinogens. Future RDA committees and perhaps—even at our limited stage of knowledge—our own, must consider and debate whether there may be benefits, unrelated to normal biological activity, which could accrue by changing the recommended level of a nutrient in a diet while still remaining within the normal dietary. But if it falls outside of those limits, then I think that it's a problem for pharmacologists rather than for RDA Committees. And, as we consider these possible

---

* On October 7, 1985, the National Academy of Sciences killed this report that was five years in the making because of an impasse between the authors and its reviewers in the academy. The report proposed to lower the RDA for vitamins A and C. Eliot Marshall,[126] writing in *Science,* says that Kamin thinks Frank Press, president of the Academy, "caved in to pressure from activists worried about the RDA's." Marshall reports that critics denounced the draft as a threat to welfare programs. A new committee will be formed to again consider possible revisions in the RDA. The failure by the National Academy of Sciences to publish the 1985 RDA Committee's report continues to be discussed. See, e.g., letters by Kamin,[127] by Robert E. Olson[128] and by Frank Press[129] as well as articles by Schneider et al.,[130] by Herbert,[131] and a group of articles by many authors in *Nutrition Today.*[132] A recent statement of the Food and Nutrition Board [133] regarding the scientific issues related to establishing the RDA is especially valuable. (This article also lists names and addresses of the 1986 members of the board.)

secondary benefits, we should also be careful to give
close attention to possible long-term risks.[134]

In the chapters ahead we will be examining the RDA for various
vitamins and minerals and pointing out cases where the RDA might
be set too low (e.g., calcium).* It will become clear that I personally
have no problem with one's decision to use amounts of nutrients that
may, in some cases, exceed the RDA. I also have no problem with a
decision to sometimes take in *less* than recommended amounts of
certain nutrients—examples being fatty acids and protein.** I think
"optimal nutrition" can refer to amounts that may be more or may be
less than the RDA. Pharmacological dosages of vitamins and
minerals in excess of RDA levels may have benefits and may pose
dangers. We will be exploring those benefits and those dangers in
the chapters to come. Now, together, we will examine overwhelming
proof in the case of vitamin after vitamin, mineral after mineral, that
each, depending upon dosage, can either help or harm the body.

---

* The possible need in many persons (especially women) for supplemental calcium is
being actively debated. The dangers as well as the benefits of greater calcium
consumption are discussed in Chapter 7.

** RDA values may vary from country to country. The U.S. RDA for ascorbic acid is just
60 mg., compared with 50 mg. in Holland and only 30 mg. in the United Kingdom.[135]

"It is better to light one small
candle than to curse the darkness."
— Chinese Proverb

"It is better to curse the darkness
than to light the wrong candle."
— Unknown

Light countless candles! The
interplay of light and darkness
writes the poetry of the shadows.
— Walter A. Heiby

CHAPTER 2

Vitamin E—Reputed Miracle Worker—Dangerous in Excess

Vitamin E was discovered in 1922 by H. M. Evans and K. S. Bishop at the University of California. It has been called the "fertility vitamin," the "rejuvenation vitamin" and reputedly in Sweden and Russia is simply known as the "sex vitamin." Such appellations give the false impression that one vitamin, and one alone, can be particularly effective. Many vitamins and minerals work synergistically—that is, they help one another. (For example, vitamin E requires vitamin A and manganese to perform some of its functions.) The body requires a complete array of nutrients to do its work.

Vitamin E is present in the human body in quantities greater than that of any other vitamin. In a study done in 1948, the total tissue mass of an adult woman reportedly contained 8,130 mg. of vitamin E as compared to 3,440 mg. in an adult man. [1] The figures now would likely be higher since vitamin E consumption has risen with the increased intake of polyunsaturated fatty acids.

Tocopherol is carried in the serum by lipoproteins and the tocopherol level here is reported to be a function not only of the amount in the diet but, more importantly, of the level of lipoprotein in the serum.* Unlike vitamin A which is stored primarily in the liver, vitamin E is stored almost completely in the adipose tissue. Vitamin E's popular status as a worker of miracles has continued to grow as vitamin enthusiasts have touted its use in treating an increasing number of health problems.

Members of the vitamin E complex are chromanols consisting of any of, or a combination of, four naturally occurring tocopherols (or tocols) and four naturally occurring tocotrienols plus some other natural, synthetic and semisynthetic forms, as well as the corresponding natural and synthetic esters (e.g., succinate, acetate, palmitate and allophanate). The four tocopherols are named alpha, beta, gamma and delta. Older texts refer to three more—epsilon, eta and zeta. It has been found useful, however, to consider these latter three (plus one more recently discovered member) as belonging to a new chemical group called *tocotrienols*. They are named *alpha* (sometimes *zeta*), *beta* (sometimes *epsilon*), *gamma* (sometimes *eta*) and *delta* (sometimes *8-methyl*) *tocotrienol* and are found in nature associated with vitamin E.[2]

The various tocopherols are found in the "dextro" or "d" form (which designation indicates that the product sometimes turns polarized light to the right, i.e., in the "dextro" direction) and in the "levo" or "l" form (meaning it is different from the "d" form, but not that it turns polarized light to the left, i.e., in the "levo" direction). The d-alpha variety of vitamin E turns polarized light in the "dextro" direction if it is in a solution of ethanol. However, if the d alpha

---

* More alpha tocopherol is found in low density lipoproteins (LDL) than in high density lipoproteins (HDL) in males, but the opposite is true in females. The variance in distribution is apparently due to the different proportions of HDL-LDL, females generally having higher amounts of HDL than males.[1a] Subsequently, Behrens and Madere [1b] reported that gamma tocopherol appeared to be transported nonspecifically by lipoproteins. Haddad et al.[1c] found that, in feeding 14 hyperlipidemic men a low cholesterol diet for 20 days, plasma α tocopherol decreased as the plasma cholesterol levels declined, but the ratio of α tocopherol to cholesterol remained constant. Interestingly, as plasma α tocopherol levels declined there was a significant *increase* in the α tocopherol content of the red blood cells.

tocopherol is in a benzene solution its rotation is opposite, i.e., in the "levo" direction. Oddly, the epimer (the other stereoisomer) of d-alpha tocopherol, prepared synthetically and designated l-alpha tocopherol, does not turn polarized light in the "levo" direction if it is in an ethanol solution, as might have been guessed, but, like the d form, turns polarized light in the "dextro" direction.[3] Obviously, the d and l designations are far from satisfactory. The common variety of synthetic vitamin E is labeled "dl" which indicates that both dextro and levo isomers (also called *enantiomorphs, epimers* or *epimerides*) are present and chemists would call it a *racemic mixture*. As we shall soon see, a given weight of d-alpha tocopherol has much more vitamin E activity than the dl-alpha tocopherol form of the vitamin. All types of vitamin E are, however, adjusted in terms of international units,* so a given number of units of the "dl" variety will have the same so-called vitamin E activity as that number of units of the "d" type.

In addition to the tocopherols (they are alcohols, as shown by the ending in "ol"), vitamin E is also available as tocopheryls—the ester forms (shown by the "yl" ending) which result when the alcohols react with acids. These ester forms are less subject to oxidation and resultant spoilage, but, according to some, may not be as efficiently assimilated if the body is deficient in pancreatic enzymes. Actually, all forms of vitamin E require both bilary and pancreatic secretions for efficient absorption.

In a report that seems to be lost in the archives of science, Erling F. Week et al.,[4] based on experiments with 10 men and 10 women in normal health, concluded that dl-alpha tocopherol gave 35% more biological response than dl-alpha tocopheryl acetate. As we will soon see, rat experiments (which are given considerable publicity) show just the opposite, i.e., that the ester form is more potent. However,

---

* The 1980 edition of the *Recommended Dietary Allowances* suggested a change in international units (I.U.) to tocopherol equivalents (T.E.), one T.E. being equal to 1.5 I.U. The RDA is (sometimes) now expressed as 10 T.E. instead of 15 I.U. which, of course, represents no change in the actual amount. Confusion has resulted and Herman Baker[3a] pointed out that even H. Kamin, chairman of the committee to consider revisions of the RDA (defunct since September, 1985), erroneously referred to a "1/3 drop in the RDA for vitamin E."

Week et al. report that the acetate is much more efficiently hydrolyzed to the tocopherol form by the rat than by humans even if they have no shortage of pancreatic enzymes. (It's apparently one of many examples of problems in applying animal research to human physiology. By the way, E. E. Edwin et al.[5] state that the rat is able to take up large amounts of alpha tocopherol, a characteristic not found in all species. In at least two ways then, the rat may not be the ideal animal for experiments with vitamin E, yet this is the animal that is almost always used.)

Ever since 1972 and 1973, when the IUPAC-IUB Commission on Biochemical Nomenclature of the World Health Organization recommended changes in the names of various stereoisomeric vitamin E compounds, there has been a slow conversion to modern nomenclature.[6-8] The approved name of d-alpha tocopherol is now *RRR-alpha tocopherol,* l-alpha tocopherol is now called *SSS-alpha tocopherol* and dl alpha tocopherol is now *all-rac-alpha tocopherol.* (As suggested by the term "all-rac," it is a mixture of the four racemates—alpha, beta, delta and gamma forms—in unspecified proportions.) There are newly discovered forms that bear only the new names. One isomer is called *2-epi-alpha tocopherol,* a semisynthetic is called *2-ambo-alpha tocopherol** and another semisynthetic is known as *4'-ambo-8'-ambo-alpha tocopherol.* ("Ambo," akin to "ambi," is Latin for "both" and refers to the presence of both "d" and "dl" stereoisomers.) Modern names for the various tocotrienols (and for compounds sometimes called *mono, di* or *trimethyltocols* or *tochochromanol-3)* are covered in the references cited.[6-8] Corresponding forms exist, at least in some cases, for the acetate and succinate tocopheryl and tocotrienyl esters. The vitamin E family is quite large and I will ignore the complexities. Furthermore, I will use either the old or the new nomenclature in accordance with the usage of each study we will be considering.

The American Pharmaceutical Association has now dropped the concept of international units (I.U.) in favor of weight/potency factors called USP Units. The I.U. are still widely used (and I will

---

* Formerly, this mixture was known as *dl-alpha tocopherol,* but now the use of the name dl-alpha tocopherol is restricted to all-rac alpha tocopherol.

continue to use them) because of their numerical equivalence with the USP Unit as given in the *U.S. Pharmacopeia:* [9]

> 1 mg. dl-alpha tocopheryl acetate = 1 USP Unit
> 1 mg. dl-alpha tocopheryl acid succinate = 0.89 USP Unit
> 1 mg. dl-alpha tocopherol = 1.1 USP Units
> 1 mg. d-alpha tocopheryl acetate = 1.36 USP Units
> 1 mg. d-alpha tocopherol = 1.49 USP Units
> 1 mg. d-alpha tocopheryl acid succinate = 1.21 USP Units

These values are based on multitudes of experiments using many different assaying methods involving a wide variety of biological responses, some of which we will consider at this time. Inclusion in the *U.S. Pharmacopeia* does not, however, mean that these values are universally accepted. Stanley R. Ames[9a] and Max K. Horwitt et al.,[41a] for example, have presented evidence supporting different values for d-alpha tocopherol acetate instead of the generally accepted 1.36. However, H. Baker et al.,[9b] using a double-blind trial of two groups of 12 male subjects, confirmed the accepted biopotencies of 1.0 I.U./mg. and 1.36 I.U./mg. respectively for dl- and d-alpha tocopheryl acetate.

The biological activity of the various tocopherols and tocotrienols has been examined by many investigators. Various techniques will yield somewhat different values for biopotency. Even when the same assaying method is employed, the details of the methodology will vary in the different laboratories or even between experiments in the same laboratory. Furthermore, when using bioassays, i.e., in experimenting with animals rather than with just "test tubes," dietary levels of other vitamins, of minerals, of amino acids and proteins, of lipids and of other factors such as thyroid status will all make uniformity quite impossible. Then too, as Rao V. Panganamala et al.[10] pointed out in another connection, the effects of administering vitamin E could reflect its various roles as antioxidant, lipidoxidase inhibitor or membrane stabilizer. Perhaps even the vitamin E status of the experimental animals' antecedents may affect the bioassay of vitamin E. A related and possibly very important experiment was conducted by C. W. Birky and J. A. Power.[11] Birky and Power showed that the effect of administering vitamin E to female rotifers can be transferred to their granddaughters who received no vitamin E. Based on this experiment, M. K. Horwitt[12] has speculated that if there is merit to the claim that vitamin E is involved in some genetic or biochemical regulations, that may have to be considered in evaluating the differences between the various isomers.

The Many Ways of Measuring Vitamin E Activity

Philip L. Harris was among the early pioneers in evaluating the potency of vitamin E. Philip L. Harris et al.[13] first reported some 40 years ago that d-alpha tocopherol possessed 50% more activity than dl-alpha tocopherol.* The determination was based on vitamin E's ability to prevent the resorption of fetuses in the pregnant rat.

A few years later, Harris and Ludwig[15] reported values for various vitamin E compounds. Note the inclusion of an acetate and a succinate:

Table 1

Form of Vitamin E	Relative Potency I.U. per mg.
alpha tocopheryl acetate	1.00
alpha tocopherol	0.68
alpha tocopheryl acetate	1.36
alpha tocopheryl succinate	1.21
alpha tocopherol	0.92

Subsequently, there have been numerous evaluations of the activities of the various members of the vitamin E family.

---

* Comparing 59% with 80% in Table 2 indicates that the correct value for the superiority of the d (natural) form over the dl (synthetic form) of the alpha tocopherol is about 36%. A more recent study by T. Leth and H. Sondergaard confirmed the 36% superiority of natural alpha tocopherol.[14]

Using the fetal resorption test, Torben Leth and Helge Sondergaard[16] reported activity values as follows based on a 100% value for dl-alpha tocopheryl acetate:

Table 2

Form of Vitamin E	Relative Potency
dl-alpha tocopheryl acetate	100%
d-alpha tocopherol	80%
dl-alpha tocopherol	59%
d-alpha tocopheryl acetate	136%
d-alpha tocotrienol	13%
d-delta tocotrienol	under 4%

Note that the acetate forms have more activity (using the rat fetal-resorption bioassay) than do the tocopherols themselves (although we have already cited the work of Week et al. suggesting this may not be true in humans). Observe also that the dl (synthetic) forms have less activity than the d (natural) forms and that the tocotrienols have minor activity. Note also that the ratio between the synthetic (dl) acetate and the natural (d) acetate is 1.36 which many experiments have demonstrated. (A study by H. Weiser and M. Vecchi[17] recently verified this 1.36 figure.) However, J. Bunyan et al.[18] reported a much higher activity value of 29% for d-alpha tocotrienol. Generally, nevertheless, the above values are corroborated by other researchers.

An interesting sidelight in regard to the resorption-gestation assay is that several other antioxidants (among which are selenium, BHT, ethoxyquin, propyl gallate and methylene blue) will substitute for vitamin E in producing viable offspring. Bernard Century and M. K. Horwitt[19] cite many of these studies and relate that methylene blue and another antioxidant, N, N-diphenyl-p-phenylene diamide (DPPD), have maintained reproduction for two and three generations of rats without vitamin E.

A second way of measuring biological activity uses vitamin E's ability to resist the hemolyzing action of allox and its derivatives, especially dialuric acid, using *in vitro* experiments. Leo Friedman et al.[20] reported activity values based on this ability to resist breakup of red blood cells:

Table 3

Form of Vitamin E	Relative Potency
dl-alpha tocopheryl acetate	100
dl-alpha tocopherol	101.6
d-alpha tocopherol	132.8
d-alpha tocopheryl acetate	147.4
d-alpha tocopheryl succinate	113.5
d-gamma tocopherol	21.7
d-gamma tocopheryl acetate	18.9

More recently, M. K. Horwitt[21] reported that the peroxide-hemolysis test was used with vitamin E-depleted, adult male prisoners. Horwitt found that the synthetic all-rac-alpha tocopheryl acetate may have no more than half the biological potency of the natural d-alpha tocopheryl acetate.

In comparing Table 2 with Table 3, we can make some interesting observations. The natural acetate and succinate esters are generally more potent than the corresponding tocopherols (as they were in a Leth and Sondergaard study)[14] but not so with the synthetic dl-alpha tocopheryl acetate, it being slightly less potent than dl-alpha tocopherol. Whereas in the rat fetal-resorption bioassay d-alpha tocopherol was less effective than either acetate form, in the hemolysis assay it was superior to dl-alpha tocopheryl acetate and not greatly inferior to d-alpha tocopheryl acetate. Somewhat later, H. Weiser et al.[22] reported that the rat hemolysis test yielded an activity ratio of 1.36 (rather than 1.47) for the relative activity of d-alpha tocopherol and dl-alpha tocopherol, thus providing good agreement between the fetal-resorption and the hemolysis tests.

Most experiments, using various measuring techniques, have indicated that the gamma form of tocopherol is rather impotent.[22a]

However, hemolytic experiments by Abbas E. Kitabchi and Jay Wimalasena[23] have shown that the concentrations of the tocopherols may vary in their relative power to prevent hemolysis. The d-gamma tocopherol at low concentrations (.5 mcg./ml.) had 50% of the antihemolytic effect of d-alpha tocopherol, but at higher concentrations (5 mcg./ml.) the effects were equal. They also reported that d-alpha tocopherol quinone was inactive in this application and dl-alpha tocopherol nicotinate actually *increased* hemolysis. Note, however, that these were *in vitro* studies. A given amount of the gamma form, although an excellent antioxidant *in vitro,* is more rapidly cleared from the serum so, until recently, had been considered to be far less potent *in vivo.* However, C. J. Dillard et al.,[23a] in studying the ability of alpha and gamma tocopherol to inhibit erythrocyte hemolysis in rats, found that the gamma variety of vitamin E was far more effective *in vivo* than had been reported earlier. They observed that gamma tocopherol had 37% as much antioxidant power as alpha tocopherol. Although a given amount of gamma tocopherol is less potent than the alpha form, large amounts of gamma tocopherol are present in the body. Studies have shown that the ratio of gamma to alpha tocopherol of patients who died in 1973 ranged from 28% to 80% in the liver, from 29% to 98% in the lipids and about 50% in the heart.[24] Obviously, the antioxidant significance of the gamma tocopherol content of the body should not be ignored.

At this time we are not going to consider what might be a reasonable intake of vitamin E for optimal health. However, since we are considering erythrocyte damage as an index to vitamin E activity, let's digress to observe these words by Max K. Horwitt:[24]

> The most important question to be asked is should frank deficiency, a state of pathology obtained only in young animals with essentially zero levels of tocopherols in their blood, be considered the criterion of tocopherol inadequacy, or should one strive for levels in the blood which protect at least 99% of the population from the type of erythrocyte

fragility that can be measured by currently accepted techniques? Admittedly, the healthy hematopoietic system has no apparent difficulty in repairing the damage caused when a few more erythrocytes are destroyed. However, until we know that other cells in the body are not similarly affected, there is little choice but to make a decision on the side of safety.

Protection of erythrocytes from oxidative damage relates to vitamin E's antioxidant power. Dr. Horwitt goes on to say:

> As for the antioxidant function of the tocopherols, one must admit that larger amounts of an antioxidant should protect tissues susceptible to oxidative stress more efficiently than would smaller amounts. In this respect vitamin E differs from vitamins involved in enzymatic reactions, for example thiamin and riboflavin, where increases in the consumption of thiamin- and riboflavin-containing coenzymes beyond the amounts needed for normal rates of reaction do not cause the in vivo rate of the reaction to change.

A third index to vitamin E activity involves the prevention of encephalomalacia in chicks. Using this bioassay technique, H. Dam and E. Sondergaard[25] reported that d-alpha tocopheryl acetate has a biopotency of 1.68 I.U./mg. Similar work was done by W. L. Marusich et al.[26] and, under a recalculation by Stanley R. Ames,[27] the biopotency of d-alpha tocopheryl acetate was given as 1.77.

A fourth way of rating biological activity of the various forms of vitamin E makes use of their ability to cure creatinuria associated with muscular dystrophy in animals. E. L. Hove and Philip L. Harris,[28] using rabbits, found that the various forms of tocopherol show about the same activity relationships as Harris et al. had reported earlier applied to the prevention of fetal resorption. Specifically, among other relationships they observed, the natural d-gamma tocopherol was almost three times as active as the synthetic dl-gamma tocopherol. The synthetic gamma form had about 8.5% the activity of the synthetic alpha variety while the natural gamma had about 20% the activity of the natural alpha.

M. L. Scott and I. D. Desai,[29] and, independently, the team of L. D. Matterson and W. J. Pudelkiewicz[30] reported on the relative antimuscular dystrophy activity (in chicks) of several members of the vitamin E family. Again, the natural forms d-alpha tocopherol and d-alpha tocopheryl acetate were the "winners" over the synthetic forms.

A fifth method for rating "E" activity was introduced by L. J. Machlin et al.[31] This group measured the ability of the natural d-alpha tocopheryl acetate (RRR-alpha tocopheryl acetate) and the synthetic dl-alpha tocopheryl acetate (all-rac alpha tocopheryl acetate) to cure necrotizing myopathy in the rat. The natural form was 141% as active as the synthetic variety.

The ability of various animals to store the various forms of vitamin E in their plasma or in their livers is yet another, and sixth, technique for rating biopotency. Using this methodology, W. J. Pudelkiewicz et al.[32] reported that d-alpha tocopheryl acetate was 1.34 times as potent as dl-alpha tocopheryl acetate when measured by liver storage in chicks. However, somewhat surprisingly, dl-alpha tocopherol was utilized equally as well as its acetate ester (and in this, remembering the work of Week et al., a chicken may be more like a man than like a rat).* Later, L. D. Matterson and W. J. Pudelkiewicz[30] found that the d-alpha tocopherol form is not 1.34, but 1.21 times as effective as the synthetic dl-alpha tocopherol (all-rac alpha tocopherol) in the chick liver storage assay.

Yet another, and seventh, way of measuring biological activity of the "E" family is to use antioxidant ability by measuring the rapidity of *in vitro* oxidation of the various tocopherols by peroxy radicals. G. W. Burton and K. U. Ingold[34] state that alpha tocopherol is the most reactive, chain-breaking, phenolic antioxidant known. They give these values for relative antioxidant ability:

---

* This phenomenon may, perhaps, relate to the fact that birds absorb vitamin E almost entirely via the portal vein (rather than via the two-way portal vein and lymphatic routes of mammals).[33]

Table 4

Form of Vitamin E	Relative Potency
alpha tocopherol	235
beta tocopherol	166
gamma tocopherol	159
delta tocopherol	65

Finally, an eighth way of determining vitamin E activity is by reversal of plasma pyruvate kinase activity in curative myopathy (muscle disease) of rats. (Pyruvate-kinase is an enzyme that catalyzes the conversion of phosphoenolpyruvate to pyruvate. A deficiency of the enzyme is associated with hemolytic anemia.) Using this technique, L. H. Chen and R. R. Thacker[34a] found that the relative potency of RRR-alpha tocopheryl acetate was 1.31, that of 2-ambo-alpha tocopheryl acetate was 1.09, that of RRR-alpha tocopherol was 1.45 and that of d-gamma tocopherol was .21 to .24.

Many workers had reported gamma tocopherol *in vitro* to be superior to alpha tocopherol in antioxidant power and these studies are discussed by Burton and Ingold. C. K. Chow and H. H. Draper[35] cite studies showing that, in linolate-rich substrates, the *in vitro* power of gamma exceeds that of alpha which, in turn, exceeds that of delta. However, regarding antioxidant activity in lard, gamma exceeds delta, which exceeds alpha. At very high concentrations the tocopherols can show a *reverse effect,* that of a pro-oxidant. [35a] The difference between *in vitro* power and *in vivo* potency is obviously tremendous. Forms other than the alpha leave the tissues much more rapidly so their *in vivo* power is less. The consensus is that the relative *in vivo* antioxidant activity of the various tocopherols both *in vitro* and *in vivo* usually follows the same sequence as does their biological activity using other bioassay methods, i.e., alpha>beta>gamma>delta.* Alpha tocopherol reacts more rapidly in trapping free radicals than the beta, gamma and delta forms.[35b] Alpha

---

* We have just seen, however, that antioxidant activity in lard is an exception to this rule.

tocopherol is, therefore, available for a shorter period of time than the more slowly reacting tocopherols. (This suggests an advantage in these latter forms that is generally ignored.) The retention rate of not only the various tocopherols, but of the other forms of vitamin E, is probably the most important factor in their activity.[36-36d]*

We have noted that, in many applications, d-alpha tocopheryl acetate has greater biological activity than other forms of vitamin E. However, when it comes to preventing lipid peroxidation and using *in vitro* (but not *in vivo*) experiments, the d-alpha tocopherol acetate not only fails to be superior but seems to have negligible power. Using *in vitro* experiments with rat brain tissue, V. N. R. Kartha and S. Krishnamurthy[37] reported that d-alpha tocopheryl acetate has very poor power to prevent lipid peroxidation to liposome membranes and concomitant production of malonaldehyde. The poor or nonexistent antioxidant ability of d-alpha tocopheryl acetate *in vitro* (although it has excellent antioxidant power *in vivo*) was confirmed by Kenji Fukuzawa et al.[38] However, tocopheryl acetate is hydrolyzed *in vivo* to the tocopherol form before being absorbed in the intestines and so the ester form after conversion is quite active *in vivo* as an antioxidant.

In this discussion I have ignored still other ways of measuring vitamin E activity such as dystrophy-anemia in the monkey[39] and various other techniques involving secretion in cow's milk, liver storage in the rat and plasma levels in chick, rat, calf and human.[40] It should be quite feasible to develop still other ways of rating biological activity of the vitamin E family such as, for example, their influence on different aspects of the immune function. Various measurement techniques will always lead to differing values of "activity." E. L. Hove and Zelda Hove[41] stressed the point, some 40 years ago, that a distinction should be made between the activity and the potency of an antioxidant. They say: "...the activity of an

---

* John G. Bieri and R. Poukka Evarts[36] found that gamma tocopherol was absorbed from the intestines of rats about as efficiently as alpha tocopherol but it disappears much more rapidly from body tissue. They also reported that gamma tocopherol is now the most common dietary form of vitamin E for humans. This reflects the change in consumption of fat from largely animal fat to increased amounts of vegetable fat (especially soybean oil and its products).[36a]

antioxidant represents a general quantitative expression, the value of which depends upon the characteristics of the ingredients in the system as well as the criterion used as the end-point while the potency of an antioxidant is a more absolute value which probably is represented by its oxidation-reduction potential." What Hove and Hove may have been trying to say (or at least I would say) is that the effects involve more than just antioxidant power. Why, therefore, should we expect uniformity? The preponderance of studies using various measuring techniques seems to show, at any rate, that whether we are dealing with tocopherols, tocopheryls or tocotrienols, and whether they are natural, synthetic or semisynthetic, the alpha form is usually more potent than the gamma, while the delta variety generally has the least activity.

Recent work by Max K. Horwitt et al.[41a] suggests that many of the assay techniques for determining the relative potency of the various forms of vitamin E may not be applicable to humans. They concluded that animal assay data do not correlate with data from studies of absorption and retention in humans. Horwitt found that 24 hours after oral ingestion of 800 I.U. of various forms of vitamin E, 71.2% of the RRR-α tocopherol was in the serum contrasted with 63.3% of the RRR-α tocopheryl acetate (given with apple pectin), 60.9% of the RRR-α tocopheryl acetate (given without apple pectin), 31.6% of the all-rac-α tocopheryl acetate and 41.2% of the RRR-α tocopheryl succinate. The study by Horwitt et al. also indicated that the acetate forms are far more potent relative to d-alpha tocopherol than had previously been thought. They also reported that the natural d-tocopheryl acetate is 2.62 times as potent as the synthetic dl-tocopheryl acetate.

The Horwitt study thus reinforces the superiority of natural vitamin E as shown by earlier research.* However, if supplements

---

* However, vitamin E from natural sources such as wheat germ, if consumed in excessive amounts, could be more dangerous since it contains estrogens derived from the wheat. Synthetic "E" contains no estrogens. Perhaps this is the reason vitamin E capsules are reputed to sometimes function like estrogen (e.g., in the reduction of breast cysts or of "hot flashes" during menopause). Nevertheless, whether natural or synthetic, vitamin E stimulates cytochrome P-450, which is a cofactor in the formation of estrogens and androgens,[68b,165] but this does not necessarily mean such production will be increased.

are used, it might be advisable not to limit consumption to just the d-alpha tocopherol or d-alpha tocopheryl acetate. Even though the beta, gamma and delta forms have less activity than d-alpha tocopherol, if one is going to take vitamin E supplements it might be better to use capsules containing mixed tocopherols or tocopheryls. Franklin Bicknell and Frederick Prescott[42] report on a study that showed a sex difference in muscular storage of vitamin E. In men, gamma and delta tocopherols were present only in the subcutaneous fat, while in women they formed 20% to 40% of the tocopherols in most tissues. However, subsequent changes in dietary habits to include more soybean and corn oil have resulted in gamma tocopherol being a far more prominent feature of tissues than it was when Bicknell and Prescott wrote. The Bicknell and Prescott data suggests, however, that, at least for women, there may be a reason to prefer mixed tocopherols over alpha tocopherol alone. (Incidentally, this same study found that the fat of the testes and of the uterus contain far more vitamin E than does fat elsewhere in the body.)

If we are going to supplement our diet with vitamin E, perhaps we should seek a brand that also contains the tocotrienols. (Natural varieties of "E" probably do contain the tocotrienols since they are generally found in close association with the tocopherols. When the news gets around, companies will probably just change their labels without changing the product.) In lard, the various tocotrienols were found to be more active antioxidants than the corresponding tocopherols.[43,43a]* Is it possible that d-alpha tocotrienol—which most tests show to be a weak form of vitamin E—could be a similarly active antioxidant in the human body? Will commercial supplements some day include a greater concentration of d-alpha tocotrienol? The sales pitch might be a powerful one!

---

* Ascorbyl palmitate increases d-alpha tocotrienol's effectiveness further just as it increases the antioxidant power of other members of the vitamin E family.[43]

Therapeutic Uses for Vitamin E

Since 1933 and until their recent deaths, Drs. Wilfred and Evan Shute studied vitamin E, primarily as an aid to heart treatment (but in other applications also). The Drs. Shute and their staff used vitamin E to treat some thirty thousand patients with what they reported to be highly successful results.

Drs. Shute reported that daily doses of 300 to 600 units of vitamin E reduce the need of the heart muscle (as well as of other body tissues) for oxygen. (It is lack of oxygen that causes angina pectoris.) This means the heart, with its supply of vitamin E, can presumably tolerate increased levels of physical activity. On the other hand, in a double-blind trial of vitamin E, T. W. Anderson[44] found that there was no significant difference among angina patients who used vitamin E and those who did not. Angina is, of course, a very real physical problem. It does, however, have psychogenic characteristics so that some patients may very well be helped to increase their blood flow to the heart regardless of the type of therapy being used. (Similarly, schizophrenia and sexual potency will often be beneficially affected by caring treatment, a fact that makes analysis of results of any given therapy—such as vitamin therapy—somewhat more difficult.)

In addition to using vitamin E to treat angina, the Shutes have also discovered or promulgated many other facts, or what they reported as facts, relating to vitamin E. Let us mention some of the advertised properties of this vitamin. Vitamin E was said by the Shutes to prevent blood clots and to dissolve a clot (called a *thrombus*) in as little as five days. Therefore, they called vitamin E an antithrombin. They recommended that it be taken prior to a surgical operation in order to minimize the danger of clots forming. They also reported that taking vitamin E regularly could minimize the probability of an occurrence of a coronary thrombosis or of a stroke.

There are numerous *in vitro* experiments that show vitamin E has the ability to inhibit aggregation of blood platelets. This could indicate antithrombic power since it is thought that platelet aggregation is one of the first steps in thrombus formation. Manfred Steiner and John Anastasi[45] observed that blood platelet aggregation in human subjects was beneficially inhibited by oral doses of vitamin E. At 1,800 I.U. daily, both plasma and platelets became saturated and failed to show any increase as doses in excess of 1,800 I.U. were administered. The study does not prove, however, vitamin E intake at this level is optimal since it may not be maximally healthful to saturate platelets and plasma. P. C. Huijgens et al.[45a] attempted to determine if these increased plasma and platelet levels of vitamin E had any effect on platelet function. They found that, in healthy persons, a daily dose of 2,000 I.U. did not prolong bleeding time and had no influence on platelet aggregation. A subsequent trial by M. Steiner[45b] of healthy men and women also indicated that vitamin E (in dosages of 400 I.U.-1,200 I.U. daily) is not a very potent antiaggregating agent. They reported, however, that platelet adhesiveness to collagen (which was not affected by aspirin ingestion) was greatly reduced in individuals treated with vitamin E or with vitamin E plus aspirin. They concluded their results suggest that vitamin E administration could be beneficial in treating arterial thromboembolic diseases. A more recent study by Jun Watanabe et al.[45c] of diabetic patients found that in those with proliferative retinopathy the vitamin E content of their platelets was significantly reduced compared to that of age-matched controls. Watanabe et al. suggested that this contributes to the mechanisms of the enhanced platelet thromboxane A, production of which leads to vascular complications.

The inhibition of platelet aggregation by vitamin E was at one time thought to be related to its antioxidant power. M. Steiner[46] subsequently showed, however, that vitamin E's oxidized metabolite vitamin E quinone (which they reported as being without antioxidant power)* has antiaggregating properties fully as powerful as alpha tocopherol. In fact, A. Chadwick Cox et al.[47] reported that vitamin E quinone was five to ten times as potent as alpha tocopherol in inhibiting platelet aggregation. They suggested that it could, therefore, be a better

---

* More recent work by Ozawa and Hanaki [152a] suggests, however, that vitamin E quinone may act as an antioxidant by scavenging superoxide.

antithrombic agent and could possibly be responsible for the *in vivo* antiaggregating effects previously attributed to alpha tocopherol.

There is, by the way, a strong resemblance between the molecule of phylloquinone (vitamin K_1) and vitamin E quinone. If the latter is a competitive inhibitor of vitamin K (the coagulation vitamin)—and D. W. Wooley[48] showed that it is—that could help explain vitamin E's action as an anticoagulant and perhaps also its action as an antithrombin.

J. D. Kanofsky and Paul B. Kanofsky[49] reported on studies by six different groups of scientists in regard to thromboembolism disease in patients treated with tocopherol and in controls. They concluded that pooled estimates of approximate relative risks associated with no vitamin E treatment as compared with vitamin E treatment were 2.12 for peripheral venous thromboses, 5.96 for all pulmonary embolisms and 9.11 for fatal pulmonary embolisms.*

Some (but a small minority) of physicians who work with vitamin E are convinced that it is far more effective than anticoagulant drugs in preventing clots. Furthermore, it is theorized that if an attack should occur in those taking vitamin E, the need for oxygen would be so reduced that survival might be more likely than if large amounts of vitamin E were not present. However, other investigations[51,52] have failed to corroborate the Shute theories. Nevertheless, I think the study by the Kanofsky team is a great vindication for what the Drs. Shute maintained for so many years!

The supposed antithrombin nature of vitamin E should be especially interesting to women taking the Pill. Medical literature is replete with reports of increased danger of thrombophlebitis in women using contraceptive pills. Thrombophlebitis is the inflammation of a vein with the formation of a thrombus (clot) and especially one that is attached to the vein's wall. Regularly taking vitamin E has been reported to virtually eliminate the possibility that thrombophlebitis will occur.   However,   studies   mentioned   earlier   that

---

* E. Agradi et al.[50] studied the *in vitro* effects on platelet aggregation not only of vitamin E but of other antioxidants. They concluded that the ability of various antioxidants to combat platelet aggregation does not correlate directly with their antioxidant power. The Agradi group speculates that the antioxidants may be acting not only as antioxidants but as compounds with detergent or other properties.

were done by R. E. Olson[51] and by Joseph Gomes et al.[52] failed to confirm the antithrombic nature of vitamin E and Hyman J. Roberts[53] found that thrombophlebitis recurred in patients taking the vitamin. In spite of a possible *reverse effect,* vitamin E's apparently real reduction of platelet aggregation that we noted earlier argues, I think, in favor of it possessing an antithrombic property.

The antithrombic nature of vitamin E acts through its influence in reducing the body's production of thromboxane (TX). Like vitamin E, linoleic acid (most sources for which also contain vitamin E) depresses TX production. P. Bostwick and M. M. Mathias[53a] reported that linoleic acid and vitamin E, independently of each other, depress TX formation. They found that when vitamin E is deficient in male rats TX increases. When the vitamin E requirement was met, either a higher level of vitamin E (200 parts per million) or a higher amount of linoleic acid (representing 23% of energy needs) depressed TX production. Interestingly, however, at high levels of both a *reverse effect* set in and the TX depression was abolished.

For a time it was believed that vitamin E might also be beneficial to the health of the heart and of the arteries in its effect on the high density lipoprotein (HDL). William J. Hermann, Jr. et al.[54] reported that, in persons with decreased HDL, beneficial cholesterol redistribution occurs when they are given vitamin E. The HDL reportedly increases and the LDL (low density lipoprotein) and total triglycerides decrease. Subsequently, Hermann[55] observed that vitamin E redistributes cholesterol primarily in those under 35 years of age and having other additional characteristics. However, other studies have failed to substantiate the claim that vitamin E raises HDL. Peter L. Schwartz and Ian M. Rutherford[56] reported that not only did they find no evidence of a rise in HDL, but they found that triglycerides rose. L. J. Hatam and H. J. Kayden,[57] Donald R. Howard et al.[58] and Meir J. Stampfer et al.[59] also found that vitamin E did not modify HDL-cholesterol.

A recent study by W. J. Serfontein et al.[69a] also showed that, in healthy young men, alpha tocopherol (in amounts of 400 mg. daily) did not significantly alter serum total HDL. (Vitamin E did, however, increase the HDL3-v subfraction.) In the same article it was reported that vitamin E significantly increased the LDL-cholesterol concentration and unfavorably affected the LDL-cholesterol/HDL-cholesterol and the HDL_2-cholesterol/HDL_3-cholesterol ratios. (It is the HDL_2 subfraction of HDL that is believed to be of greatest benefit to heart health. The HDL 3 fraction may convey no such benefit, but the matter is far from settled.)[69b]* However, LDL perhaps could offer heart protection to the extent that vitamin E may be a factor in heart health. Maret G. Traber and Herbert J. Kayden[69c] have recently shown that the receptor for LDL functions as a mechanism for delivery of vitamin E to cells. Nevertheless, the fact that W. Marx et al.[60] reported rats fed 150 mg. of vitamin E weekly for six months showed significantly higher liver cholesterol and high incidence of cholesterol deposits and intimal sclerosis of the aorta is more than a little disturbing. Even further disturbing news is provided by O. A. Levander et al.[61] who discovered that rats fed vitamin E in the amount of 500 ppm of food appeared to have increased liver triglycerides (similar to the findings of Schwartz and Rutherford).[56] They also found that liver necrosis induced by alcohol was hastened. (On the contrary, N. R. DiLuzio and F. Costales[61a] observed that ethanol-induced fatty liver was inhibited by prior administration of alpha-tocopheryl acetate. Perhaps this seeming contradiction is due to dose-response *reverse effects* of either alcohol, vitamin E or the combination.)

There is additional evidence that vitamin E may help protect against damages caused by excessive consumption of alcohol. It is believed that the toxic effects of ethanol may be mediated by free radical reactions and, if this is a fact, then vitamin E and other antioxidants should offer some protection. Joyce E. Redetzki et al.[61b] found that when mice were given a single intraperitoneal injection of 2 grams/kg. of ethanol it led to increased lactic dehydrogenase plasma isoenzymes that indicated myocardial damage. When the animals were pretreated with 86 I.U. of alpha tocopherol the changes in isoenzyme patterns were partially prevented, thus reducing the evidence of myocardial damage.

---

* More about the HDL and LDL carriers for cholesterol will be found in Chapter 3.

When administered to a patient who has recently suffered a heart attack, vitamin E is said to open collateral circulation in an area deprived of blood. Vitamin E reportedly dilates capillaries to bring blood to areas requiring it. Vitamin E is also said to help the capillaries to maintain their normal permeability so their function in providing nourishment to cells is not impaired.

Vitamin E may sometimes be able to remove scar tissue. It also is said to prevent formation of scar tissue. (This is why, in treating a burn, it is sometimes recommended that one not only take vitamin E by mouth but that one also pierce a vitamin E capsule with a needle and promptly smear it on the wound and repeat several times a day. The pain is dulled and the probability of scar tissue forming is reportedly reduced.) If it is true that the formation of scar tissue can be reduced, then many diseases or problems exacerbated by scarring, such as arthritis, bursitis and myositis could perhaps be prevented or the conditions aleviated with vitamin E. A study with rats by H. Paul Ehrlich et al.[62] showed vitamin E of use in the beneficial slowing of wound healing through a measurement of the tensile strength and accumulation of collagen. The research suggested that vitamin E may in fact, as Dr. Shute said, be of clinical value in modifying scar formation. In this respect, Dr. Ehrlich observed that vitamin E could be of greater value than corticoids because of its lesser side effects. However, James O. Woolliscroft[63] questions whether the result is cosmetically pleasing.

The scarring of secondary fibrositis, such as present in urethral strictures may also be amenable to vitamin E therapy. Peter L. Scardino and Perry B. Hudson[64] reported that of 22 urethral stricture patients given 200 to 1,200 mg. of mixed tocopherols daily (i.e., 100-600 mg. of alpha tocopherol), 15 had a good response and 4 had a fair response. Vitamin E has also been used for treating Peyronie's disease, a form of primary fibrositis where there is a fibrous replacement of the intercavernous septum of the penis—resulting in a curvature of the organ which may make sexual intercourse painful or impossible. Peter L. Scardino and William Wallace Scott[65] found that, out of 23 patients, the treatment resulted in a complete disappearance of curvature in 4 patients and some favorable change in all but 5. The scientists stated that the patients were treated for 10 months with 300 mg. of mixed tocopherols or 200 mg. of synthetic alpha tocopherols. The treatment was oral, but it seems reasonable (to me) that applying vitamin E topically to the penis might have been even more effective. In a subsequent study, R. J. Morgan and J. P. Pryor[65a] compared a therapy involving the drug procarbazine with a therapy using vitamin E. Of 31 men treated for 12 weeks with procarbazine, only 2 improved. Of 31 men treated with vitamin E for 12 weeks, 2 were considered cured and 10 improved. In spite of these good results, however, Morgan and Pryor note that often Peyronie's disease will improve even when no treatment is given. Thus the use of vitamin E in treating this disease is still problematical. (The dermal graft procedure of Devine and Horton or Nesbit's operation, although more heroic, have a better record of success in treating Peyronie's disease than therapy using vitamin E.)[65b]

Dr. H. J. Roberts[66] reported that his clinical experience has shown a possible association between vitamin E and cystic mastitis. He found that eight patients, all women, complained of sore breasts and two developed cystic mastitis while on vitamin E. However, in a possible example of a *reverse effect,* several investigators have found cystic mastitis to be benefitted by vitamin E. A number of studies by Archie A. Abrams[67] and David Solomon et al.[68] and by G. S. Sundaram et al.[69,70] reported oral vitamin E to have a beneficial effect in treating cystic mastitis and other types of mammary dysplasia. (Furthermore, K. Larry Smith et al.[70a] concluded that vitamin E, and also selenium, was beneficial in treating dairy cows with mastitis.) Solomon[68] ascribed vitamin E's presumably beneficial effects in cases of cystic mastitis to its ability to enhance androgen production in the adrenal glands and androgens are, of course, antiestrogenic. *
Sundaram et al.[70] ascribed their favorable results to raising of the patients' abnormally low progesterone/estradiol ratio. Subsequently,

---

* P. P. Nair and H. J. Kayden,[70b] however, found significant increases in both estrogens and androgens in the urine of persons taking supplementary vitamin E. Might not this prove dangerous, as Briggs[165] has pointed out, for patients with an early hormone-dependent cancer such as carcinoma of the breast or prostate?

however, R. London and G. S. Sundaram et al.[74b] arrived at results that contradicted their earlier work. They studied use of 150 I.U., 300 I.U. and 600 I.U. of dl-alpha tocopherol daily for 2 months in a placebo-controlled study of 128 women with confirmed mammary dysplasia and could find no significant objective effects of the treatment. Furthermore, they found that serum concentrations of estradiol, progesterone, dehydroepiandrosterone sulfate and testosterone were unaffected by the tocopherol treatment. A recent study by Virginia L. Ernester et al.[74ba] found that daily supplementation of 600 I.U. of vitamin E over a 2-month period produced no beneficial effect on benign breast "disease."*

Perhaps the reason for the conflicting results of the use of vitamin E in treating this problem is not a *reverse effect,* as I suggested earlier, but simply the frequent occurrence of symptom remission. Robert V. P. Hutter,[74c] in a recent editorial in the *New England Jrl. of Medicine,* maintains that it is time to say goodbye to fibrocystic disease. Hutter

---

* J. P. Minton et al.[70c,d] have reported success in treating fibrocystic breast disease by restriction of caffeine ingestion. Following Minton's lead, Philip G. Brooks et al.[71] reported 88% improvement in breast symptoms among 66 patients with the problem. Siegfried Heyden,[72] in analyzing Minton's data, concluded that there was no valid evidence associating coffee consumption with fibrocystic disease. A bit more favorably, V. L. Ernester et al.[73] found a minor improvement in fibrocystic breast disease with a decreased caffeine consumption. James Marshall et al.[74] reported that, in a comparison of 323 women with benign breast disease and 1,458 controls, no differences were noted in coffee and tea consumption patterns of the cases and the controls. More recently, however, Collen A. Boyle et al.,[74aa] in a hospital-based case-control study of 634 women with fibrocystic breast disease and 1,066 controls, found that women who consumed 31-250 mg. of caffeine/day had a 1.5-fold increase in the odds to get the disease, whereas women who drank over 500 mg./day had a 2.3-fold increase in the odds. In an even more recent study, this one involving 854 histologically diagnosed cases of benign breast disease and 755 matched surgical controls, Flora Lubin et al.[74aa] found no evidence of an association between advent of the disease and the consumption of coffee or other methylxanthines. Subsequently, Minton[74ab] criticized Lubin's study and continued to maintain that "benign breast disease will resolve after total and complete methylxanthine abstention and will reactivate with resumption of methylxanthine consumption." To this, Lubin et al.[74ac] replied that their objective was to investigate a possible etiological association between methylxanthine intake and benign breast disease. Minton's work refers to *therapy* while Lubin et al. are concerned with *cause.* Michael F. Jacobson and Bonnie F. Liebman,[74ad] in 1986, provided additional valuable input to the problem. (Jason Pozner,[74ae] writing in 1986, makes the point that coffee has antineoplastic effects and so advice regarding coffee abstention in cases of fibrocystic disease may at best be premature.)

quotes S. M. Love et al.[74d] as asking: "Is it reasonable to define as a disease any process that occurs clinically in 50 per cent and histologically in 90 per cent of women?" (Helmuth Vorherr,[74e] on the contrary, believes there are "grave dangers in labeling fibrocystic disease a harmless nondisease." He states further that "in advanced fibrocystic disease, intraductal proliferation often results in epithelial atypia, which in turn may progress to carcinoma.")

Vitamin E and Cancer

Vitamin E may be valuable in preventing cancer since one of its basic functions is reported to be that of protecting the apparatus for the division of cells. Seth L. Haber and Robert W. Wissler[75] found, in experiments with mice, that vitamin E inhibited the carcinogenicity of methylcholanthrene. Interestingly, S. A. Burobina and E. A. Nefakh[76] reported that, in experiments with tumorous mice, vitamin E left the liver, spleen and kidneys and concentrated in the tumors. Burobina and Nefakh did not, however, offer any suggestion as to whether the vitamin E might be combating or feeding the tumors. However, experiments have shown that when malignancies were induced in animals receiving various amounts of vitamin E, those malignancies were fewest, smallest and slowest in developing when the greatest amount of the vitamin was taken. One such example was reported by Gerald Shklar.[77] Shklar found that when the buccal pouches of hamsters were painted with the carcinogen 7, 12-dimethylbenzanthracene (DMBA), vitamin E significantly inhibited tumor formation. Incidentally, he used synthetic dl-alpha tocopherol which, unlike natural vitamin E, is devoid of estrogen, a possible procancer substance.

In a related experiment, Woranut Weerapradist and Gerald Shklar[78] reported that vitamin E caused a significant delay in tumor formation in hamsters, and after 12 to 14 weeks there were fewer tumors and they were of smaller size than in untreated controls. In yet another experiment, Martin G. Cook and Peter McNamera[79] fed one group of mice 10 mg. of vitamin E per kg. diet and another group 600 mg. of vitamin E per kg. diet while injecting members of both groups with the carcinogen 1,2-dimethylhydrazine. The mice fed the excessive "E" had fewer colorectal tumors and fewer carcinomas than those fed just 10 mg./kg. diet. On the other hand, Clement Ip[80] reported that, while a vitamin E deficiency may increase the risk of cancer in rats, a high vitamin E supplementation, by itself, does not seem to have any prophylactic effect on tumorgenesis. However, while Paula M. Horvath and Clement Ip[80a] found that vitamin E alone was not effective in inhibiting mammary tumors induced by DMBA in rats, they reported that vitamin E facilitated the anticarcinogenic action of selenium against such tumors.

Vitamin E also acts as an anticancer agent by inhibiting formation of N-nitroso compounds.[80b] (The acetate and succinate forms were not, however, of use in preventing formation of nitrosamines according to William J. Mergens.[81] On the contrary, C. K. Chow et al.[81a] found that rats fed sodium nitrate with a vitamin E-deficient diet showed a higher mortality rate, a marked increase in liver necrosis, tubular nephrosis and myodegeneration compared to rats fed 200 ppm of vitamin E as dl-α tocopheryl acetate.) Irons and oils (both of which increase the need for vitamin E) have produced far more malignancies in cancer-susceptible mice when vitamin E was absent than when generous amounts of this vitamin were given. Michael P. Kurek and Laurence M. Corwin[82] reported that mice fed 5 grams dl-alpha tocopheryl acetate/kg. diet (equivalent to about 500 I.U. in man) showed decreased incidence of tumors produced by transplanted sarcoma cells. When vitamin E was increased 10-fold the protective effect was no longer observed. The researchers concluded that the direct effect of vitamin E is on the tumor cell rather than on the immune system. Furthermore, they hypothesize that "within several days of tumor cell inoculation, a critical event occurs that determines whether a tumor will develop. This event may involve destruction of the tumor cells or establishment of a dormant state, as suggested by Weinhold et al. Vitamin E is most probably effective at this stage, because once a tumor becomes palpable, its rate of growth is not affected by diet."

Toshima Yasunaga et al.[82a] recently reported that tumor growth of mice, each of whose right footpad had been implanted with Meth-

A tumor cells, was inhibited by vitamin E injected at the rate of 5 to 20 I.U./kg./day (Figure 1). They studied lymphoproliferative responses to mitogens and found that these responses were enhanced in mice injected with 5 to 20 I.U./kg./day of vitamin E. This immunopotentiating effect disappeared in a group treated with 40 I.U./kg./day of vitamin E. Another group treated with 80 I.U./kg./day exhibited a *reverse effect* (reversing the action of the 5 to 20 I.U. doses) with a suppression of mitogen responses. Perhaps a modest amount of vitamin E may be immunopotentiating and cancer inhibiting in man (as in rats) while a large amount of vitamin E may be immunosuppressive.

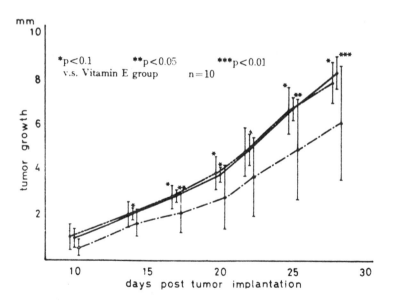

Figure 1. Effect of Vitamin E on Tumor Growth. 2x 10⁵/0.02 ml. of Meth-A tumor cells were implanted in the right footpad and 20 I.U./kg./day of vitamin E (—·—), its solvent equivalent (—··—) or saline solution (—) was injected i.p. daily from the day of tumor implantation until death. Reproduced from Toshima Yasunaga et al., *Nippon Geka Hokan, Archiv für Japanishe Chirurgie* (1984) 53, no. 2: 312-323, by permission of the publisher.

In working with cell cultures, Kedar N. Presad et al.[83] found that not only does vitamin E exhibit anticancer properties, but that it acts synergistically with chemotherapeutic agents in inhibiting the growth of glioma and neuroblastoma cancer cells. Furthermore, anticancer drugs tend to induce lipid peroxidation through the action of free radicals (which we will discuss soon). Vitamin E, through scavenging free radicals, can protect the tissues. Ifor D. Capel et al.[83a] reported that rats receiving vitamin E supplementation along with 5-fluorouracil treatment had significantly lower liver and plasma lipoperoxide levels than those given only the anticancer drug.

A study by Takashi Kohunai et al.[83b] has shown that vitamin E displays significant effects against rat glioma cell cultures. Furthermore, vitamin E produced an additive cytotoxic effect against such cells when used with ACNU, bleomycin and fluorouracil. In addition, vitamin E had a significant synergistic effect on the cytotoxicity of vincristine sulphate to rat glioma cells. Then too, Richard F. Wagner et al.[83c] reported that K. N. Prasad and J. Edwards-Prasad,[83d] in working with *in vitro* B16 mouse melanoma, found that d-alpha tocopheryl succinate induced dramatic, dose-dependent morphological alterations and growth inhibition of melanoma cells.

There seems to be an inverse relationship between the amount of vitamin E (and also of vitamins A and C and of carotene) in the serum and the incidence of lung cancer and of breast cancer. A. Lopez and B. Y. LeGardeur reported that patients with lung carcinoma averaged .84 mg. % vitamin E in their serum compared to 1.06 for other hospitalized patients and 1.19 for matched free-living persons. N. J. Wald et al.,[84a] in a prospective study involving 5,004 women in Guernsey, England, found that low plasma vitamin E levels were associated with significantly higher risk of breast cancer. They reported that the risk of breast cancer developing in women with vitamin E levels in the lowest quintile was about five times higher than the risk for women in the highest quintile.

The use of vitamin E may tie in with irradiation treatment of neoplasms. When vitamin E was injected intramuscularly in doses of 5, 25 or 50 mg./100g. body weight, tumor growth retardation in rats by irradiation was greatly enhanced (Figure 2). Injected (or oral) doses of 100 mg./100g. body weight without irradiation were ineffective.[85]

Cancer-causing agents are very likely to also be mutagens and vice versa. C. Beckman et al.[86] cite many experiments over the years that show genetic damage can sometimes be reduced by treatment with antioxidants. Beckman et al. experimented with fruit flies and studied the effect of vitamin E on sex-linked recessive lethal mutants induced by x-irradiation. In one experiment, males raised on either a culture supplemented with 500 I.U. of alpha tocopheryl acetate per kg. of culture medium or on a nonsupplemented medium were irradiated and mated to virgins raised and subsequently maintained on unsupplemented medium. The percent of lethal mutations was respectively 7.8 and 5.1—not a great difference. However, in a second experiment, males on unsupplemented medium were irradiated and mated to females on either tocopheryl-supplemented or on a nonsupplemented medium and the progeny were examined for lethal chromosomes. Here the difference was tremendous. The progeny of the tocopheryl-supplemented females had just 3.3% lethals while the progeny of the unsupplemented females showed 13.6% lethal chromosomes. Humans are not fruit flies, but perhaps vitamin E taken by women protects against mutations among offspring that might otherwise have occurred because the fathers had been excessively exposed to x-rays. Remember, then, this was not a cancer study but a possibly related study of the beneficial effect of vitamin E in reducing the number of mutations.

The effect of vitamin E on cancer is not always uniformly good. On the contrary, vitamin E may sometimes have a procancer effect. I. R. Telford[87] has reported that the formation of lung tumors in mice induced by dibenzanthracene was retarded by vitamin E deficiency and enhanced by vitamin E excess. Then, too, large amounts of vitamin E are poorly absorbed and are excreted in the feces. M. H. Briggs[88] has pointed out that metabolites of bile salts may be carcinogenic and the antioxidant property of "E" might encourage their formation in the colon. This factor, therefore, may also provide a procancer element in excessive vitamin E intake.

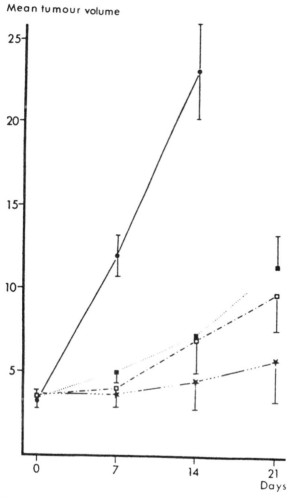

Figure 2. Mean external tumour volumes (cm³) with SEM in nonirradiated controls (circles), irradiated controls (black squares), animals pretreated with placebo (white squares) and animals pretreated intramuscularly with tocopherol in a dose of 5 mg./100 g. body weight 7 days before irradiation (stars). Tumour irradiation on day 0. Retardation of tumour growth rate in all irradiated animals, enhanced tumour growth retardation in animals given tocopherol. Reproduced from A. Kagerud and H. I. Peterson, *Acta Radiologica Oncology* (1981) 20: 97-100, with permission of the publisher.

In 1986, Onatolu Odukoya et al.[88a] reported that vitamin E (as dl-∝ tocopherol) stimulated growth, in culture, of an epidermoid carcinoma cell line. The effect was dose-related up to a maximum stimulatory effect at 10 μM. Then a *reverse effect* set in and at a concentration of 100 μM there was inhibition on both cell turnover and colony formation. The realities of the experiment were, however, far removed from conditions existing *in vivo*.

The Immune System and Vitamin E

Vitamin E may be useful not only in helping to prevent cancer, but in strengthening the immune system in general. Vitamin E protects mice against fatal infection caused by *Diplococcus pneumoniae* according to Rollin H. Heinzerling et al.[89] The mechanism increasing phagocytic activity is thought to be vitamin E's beneficial influence in increasing body synthesis of ubiquinones, especially coenzyme Q_{10}. The ubiquinones are lipid-soluble compounds that function as electron carriers in the cell's mitochondrial electron transport system and K. Folkers[90] has claimed that vitamin E protects ubiquinone. Emile Bliznakov et al.[91] reported and Andria C. Casey and E. Bliznakov[92] also reported that coenzymes Q_4, Q_6 and Q_{10}, administered to rats by injection, beneficially modified parameters in the reticuloendothelial system that controls phagocytosis. Although Casey and Bliznakov found vitamin E ineffective under the conditions studied, Heinzerling[89] subsequently discovered vitamin E to be of value in influencing phagocytosis. Still later, Emile G. Bliznakov[93-93a,b] reported that one of the types of coenzyme Q (Q_{10}) can partially reverse immunological senescence in mice.[*]

---

[*] The many other possible physiological roles of coenzyme Q [94-94c] may give us additional reasons to protect this substance with vitamin E. The ubiquinones are now used in treating periodontitis,[94d-94i] for experimentally protecting animals during ischemic damage to the heart[94j] and the kidney,[94k] and also for lowering human blood pressure (references cited in Chapter 7 under potassium). Several useful 1, 4-benzoquinone analogs of coenzyme Q 10 have also been developed. Of these, two have been shown to inhibit two human tumor cell lines and another showed cures against Walker Carcinosarcoma 256 in rats.[94l] Murine studies suggest Q 10 may also help human muscular dystrophy.[94m-o]

In another study, this one by Toshima Yasunaga et al.,[95] when mice were injected daily with 5 to 20 I.U. per kilogram of body weight of all-rac-alpha tocopherol (formerly called dl-alpha tocopherol) immune response was significantly enhanced. The dosage corresponds with about 350 to 1,400 I.U. in a 70 kg. (150 lb.) person and the fact that injections were used suggests that the oral amount required for an equivalent response would be greater. However, when the dosage was increased to 80 I.U./kg. a *reverse effect* set in, immune responses were inhibited and at 400 I.U./kg. all mice died within three days. (A similar, more recent study by Yasunaga[82a] was discussed earlier in relation to cancer.)

Cheryl F. Nockels[96] has reported that supplementing dietary vitamin E in the form of dl-alpha tocopheryl acetate or dl-alpha tocopherol effectively improves the humoral response of mice, chicks, turkeys and guinea pigs when challenged with nonliving antigens, bacteria and a virus. Resistance to disease was also significantly improved. Many other animal studies showing increased resistance to bacterial infections and stimulation of phagocytosis and mitogen responsiveness through vitamin E supplementation are cited by T. S. Lim et al.[97] More recently, Laurence M. Corwin and Richard K. Gordon,[98] using mice as subjects, also reported that dietary vitamin E in higher than normal doses (50 I.U./kg. of feed) stimulated the response to T cell mitogens as well as the lymphocyte response to murine (mouse) spleen cells. On the other hand, Naoki Inagaki et al.[98a] found that vitamin E (as alpha tocopheryl acetate or alpha tocopheryl nicotinate) suppressed IgE antibody formation in mice immunized with dinitrophenylated ascaris protein and aluminum hydroxide gel. Nevertheless, IgM and IgG formation was significantly enhanced. The results show that vitamin E can work to suppress or to enhance antibody formation.

Various other animal studies[99] indicate that vitamin E may be useful in improving the immune system. These independent studies show that 150 to 300 mg. of vitamin E per kilogram of food (about the amount of food eaten daily by humans) may increase immune response to antigens and improve resistance to microorganisms. T.

S. Lim et al.,[97] in reporting on this effect, noted that supplemental
vitamin E may be of special value during the early period of a low-
protein diet. (Although low-protein diets have been shown by several
studies to increase longevity, immune responses may be suppressed
at the start of such a diet.) As an offset to these good reports, a
negative note regarding vitamin E and bactericidal activity is raised
by J. Siva Prasad.[100] A group of adult males and young boys were
each given a daily divided dosage of 300 mg. (300 I.U.) of dl-alpha
tocopheryl acetate for a period of 3 weeks. Prasad reported a
significant depression in the bactericidal activity of the leukocytes.
Furthermore, Alan C. Tsai et al.[101] found that college student
volunteers orally taking 600 I.U. dl-tocopheryl acetate daily showed
few beneficial or detrimental effects. However, the vitamin E caused
a significant reduction of serum thyroid hormone levels and also an
elevation in triglyceride levels in females. Thyroid function is related
to the immune function so this also indicates that vitamin E can have
both beneficial and negative effects on the immune system. It should
be noted that the beneficial responses seem to generally occur at
lower oral dosage levels than the 600 I.U. used by Tsai. Remember,
the Yasunaga study[95] showed a beneficial immune effect in mice at
modest "E" levels and then a *reverse effect* at higher levels.

Adrianne Bendich et al.[101a] showed, in a 1986 rat study, that
while 7.5 mg. of vitamin E/kg. diet was enough to maintain normal
growth rate, 15 mg./kg. diet was adequate to prevent myopathy, and
50 mg./kg. diet was sufficient to prevent hemolysis of red blood
cells, a level exceeding 50 mg./kg. diet was needed for optimum T-
and B-lymphocyte responses. The T- and B-lymphocyte responses
correlated with plasma vitamin E levels over a range of .04-18 µg/ml.
If the action in humans is at all comparable to that of rats, the human
RDA level may be set too low for optimum immune response. (But
don't forget the *reverse effect* demonstrated by the research of
Yasunaga.)

J. S. Goodwin and P. J. Garry[102] studied the immunological
effects, not only of vitamin E usage, but of general "megadose"
vitamin and mineral supplementation. They compared immunological
functions of healthy elderly persons taking large quantities of

supplements. Those taking vitamin E (or any of several B vitamins) had lower circulating lymphocyte counts than the controls. Those taking megadoses of vitamin C showed increased cell-mediated immune responses as measured *in vivo* by skin test reactivity but not by *in vitro* mitogen responses. Goodwin and Garry reported a relative lack of long-term effect of megadose vitamins on immunological function compared to reports of short-term trials of meganutrients such as we have been discussing. They suggested that the reported immuno-enhancing properties of megadose nutrients may be due to a nonspecific adjuvant effect that disappears with time.

Other Physiological Applications for Vitamin E

There are reported to be many other uses for vitamin E in body chemistry, some of which are based on merely anecdotal evidence. Vitamin E may help facilitate transport of amino acids.[103] Vitamin E reportedly helps regulate fat and protein metabolism and also preserves the health of the capillaries (very much as the bioflavonoids do). Vitamin E may also be useful in preventing atherosclerosis. M. Passeri and D. Provedini[104] enthusiastically state: "The effects of tocopherol on the glyco-lipid metabolism, as well as its hypocholesterolemic and antithrombophylic activities can positively protect the organism from the atherosclerotic damage."

Vitamin E may be useful in preventing arteritis (inflammation of an artery). R. L. Holman[104a] found that if he gave dogs excessive amounts of cod-liver oil and then damaged their kidneys they developed arterial lesions and died of uremia caused by renal insufficiency. However, dogs on the same diet but given by mouth 2.5 to 4.0 mg./kg. wt. per day of vitamin E, beginning either before or after their kidneys were damaged, did not develop arterial lesions.

Rheumatoid arthritis (RA) may also be amenable to treatment with vitamin E. Toshikazu Yoshikawa et al.[105] point out that the fact thiobarbituric acid reactants are found in high concentrations in the synovial fluids of RA patients argues that peroxidation is related to the development of or the aggravation of this disease. Vitamin E, in acting as an antioxidant, inhibits lipid peroxidation (which we will discuss later in this chapter) and thus might be useful in RA therapy. Yoshikawa found that rats in which arthritis had been induced had high synovial levels of thiobarbituric acid reactants, but those levels were lower in rats given supplemental vitamin E. Yoshikawa concludes that vitamin E and other antioxidants may be useful in treating human arthritis.

Vitamin E is also said to aid in the treatment of gangrene, varicose veins, psoriasis, itching skin (pruritis), purpura, cerebral palsy, Parkinson's disease, multiple sclerosis, cystic fibrosis, Down's syndrome, hydrocephalus and epilepsy. It is also reported of value in treating hemorrhoids, chorea, leg ulcers, bursitis, Hansen's disease (leprosy), menopause symptoms (including leg cramps, hot flashes, a shrinking, tender vagina due to aging, leukoplakia of the cervix, etc.), dysmenorrhea (painful menstruation), hay fever, asthma and emphysema. Vitamin E may also be of value in treating diabetes. Diabetics generally have increased platelet aggregation and thromboxane B_2 production. J. Watanabe et al.[105a] found that dl-$\propto$ tocopherol, which is known to inhibit platelet prostaglandin production and aggregation, also worked in diabetics to improve their platelet function. Samuel Ayres, Jr. and Richard Mihan[106] reported that they found vitamin E has even been useful in treating the autoimmune disease, chronic discoid lupus erythematosus. (In this application, and to the extent that vitamin E is beneficial, it seems obvious that it must be suppressing the immune system.)

In those suffering from an overactive thyroid gland, vitamin E is said to act as a tranquilizer. However, this may be a dangerous use for the vitamin. Arthur Vogelsang,[107] who is generally enthusiastic about its use in various therapies, points out that vitamin E taken by a hyperthyroid person can result in cardiac status being impaired. He cautions that atrial fibrillation and attacks of supraventricular tachycardias may be produced. Dr. Vogelsang concludes that no patient with hyperthyroid heart should be given vitamin E.

Vitamin E is said to be useful in treating neurotic or psychotic individuals. There are reports that in chronic malabsorption of fat attended by severe vitamin E deficiency, supplementation with the vitamin may inhibit progressive neurological disorders.[108,109]

Although many vitamin E therapies are in dispute, an increasing number of physicians believe that vitamin E may be efficacious in cases of intermittent claudication, a disease where there is impaired circulation in the legs, causing pain during walking and leading sometimes to gangrene. Knut Haeger[110] reported on a clinical trial of male patients with intermittent claudication and having a mean age of 67 years. One group was given 300 I.U. of d-alpha tocopheryl acetate daily and a control group was treated with either vasodilating agents or an anticoagulant (dicoumarin). After 4-6 months, 54% of the vitamin E group reached the objective' of 1,000-meter uninterrupted walking distance compared with 23% of the control group. After 20-25 months the arterial flow to the lower leg increased approximately 34% in the "E" group, with no change noted in the control group. Phillip M. Farrell [111] cites additional impressive evidence supporting use of vitamin E in treating intermittent claudication. Even here, however, agreement regarding the efficacy of vitamin E therapy is far from unanimous.*

Conor T. Keane and Rosemary Hone[112] and Robert Semple,[113] in independent trials, failed to find vitamin E of use in treating intermittent claudication. Nevertheless, Woolliscroft[114] reports that a linear relationship exists between the amount of vitamin E in the soleus muscle and improvement in walking ability. Thus, vitamin E may be causing changes in the muscle as well as in the musculature. Woolliscroft concludes that, "based on available evidence, megadoses of vitamin E are clinically efficacious in the long-term treatment of claudication resulting from peripheral vascular disease." Nocturnal leg cramps (systremma) are also often amenable to vitamin E therapy. In 125 cases only 2 patients failed to show satisfactory improvement.[115]

Vitamin E may be useful (perhaps because it might stimulate production of sex hormones)[165] in ameliorating the symptoms of premenstrual syndrome. Robert S. London et al. [115a] found, in a

---

* Therapies often involve a judgment of the risk-benefit ratio. The attending physician must decide whether the possible benefit of treating a patient with large dosages of "E" for his intermittent claudication is worth the risk of his contracting a more serious disease because of possible depression of his immune responses.

randomized, double-blind investigation of 75 patients, that treatment with 150, 300 or 600 I.U. of alpha tocopherol daily showed significantly favorable effects for the week preceding the menses. Symptoms of nervous tension, mood swings, irritability, anxiety, headache, craving for sweets, increased appetite, heart pounding, fatigue, dizziness, fainting, depression, forgetfulness, crying, confusion and insomnia were improved. Symptoms of weight gain, swelling of extremities, breast tenderness and abdominal blocking were not improved.

The fact, as reported early in this chapter, that the biological activity of various forms of vitamin E can be measured by their ability to resist the hemolyzing action of allox suggests that this vitamin might be useful in treating erythrocyte-related disorders. Keiji Ono[115b] studied the effects of vitamin E on anemia and the osmotic fragility of red blood cells in dialysis patients. Ono found that after orally administering 600 mg. daily for 30 days the fragility of erythrocytes was significantly reduced. Ono concluded that vitamin E could be of clinical benefit in correcting anemia in regular dialysis patients by reducing fragility of their red blood cells.

Laurence Corash et al.[116] reported that oral administration of high dosages of vitamin E was useful in treating hereditary red-cell disorders caused by a deficiency of glutathione synthetase or of G6PD. But later, this group[117] and Gerhard J. Johnson et al.[118] reported that high-dose vitamin E therapy did not diminish the hemolysis resulting from a severe variant form of G6PD deficiency. Earlier, Johannah G. Newman et al.[119] stated that vitamin E supplementation in individuals with a G6PD deficiency had little or no effect on the response of erythrocytes to oxidative stress. Newman's negativism seems to be unwarranted, but Corash[117] concludes that the role of vitamin E in treating the G6PD disorders "remains largely theoretical." (More about G6PD deficiency can be found in Chapter 6 dealing with ascorbic acid.)

Perhaps related to this discussion is a blood-related condition where vitamin E may work against its cure. The disease is malaria and the mice studies of John W. Eaton et al.[120] suggest that a *deficiency* of vitamin E may be helpful in treating this disease.* Possibly the vitamin E deficiency tends to induce destruction of the malaria-sickened erythrocytes and the cure is effected through the body's manufacture of new, nondiseased blood cells. It is known, at any rate, that sickle-cell anemia protects against malaria and vitamin E combats sickle-cell anemia, and so this may be the relevant mechanism. C. L. Natta et al.[121] reported on treatment of sickle-cell anemia patients with vitamin E. Patients given 250 I.U. of alpha tocopherol daily for 6 to 35 weeks had their percentage of irreversibly sickled red cells decreased from 25% pretreatment to 11% after vitamin E administration. The percentage of irreversibly sickled red cells remained below pretreatment levels as long as the vitamin was administered (up to 35 weeks). Studies published by Danny Chiu et al.[122] also suggest that "vitamin E supplementation to sickle-cell patients could be of clinical benefit."

The incidence of cortical cataracts (those due to the loss of transparency of the outer layers of the lens of the eye), which often occur in older diabetic persons, might conceivably be reduced through use of vitamin E. An experiment by William M. Ross et al.[123] found that the lenses of diabetic rats who continued to be injected with vitamin E showed minimal changes. However, John R. Trevithick and William M. Ross et al.[124] reported that vitamin E, given in the diet at the high level of 125 I.U. daily per rat, was not effective in preventing cataracts in animals receiving large amounts of galactose *ad libitum.* Kailash C. Bhuyan et al.,[124a] hypothesizing that cataracts are triggered by toxic metabolites of oxygen (superoxide, hydrogen peroxide, hydroxyl ion and singlet oxygen), administered vitamin E to rabbits in which cataract had been induced. The cataracts were arrested in about 50% of the animals and reversed in some. Based on experiments with rabbits, P. P. Gupta et al. [125] concluded that ∝ tocopherol can prevent as well as arrest the progress of cataractogenesis. S. D. Varma et al.[125a] found that lipids of rat lenses maintained in organ culture were photodegraded, apparently by light-catalyzed generation of superoxide,

---

* Many animal studies[120a] show that not only a deficiency of vitamin E but also deficiencies of protein, riboflavin, vitamin C or PABA restrict multiplication of malarial parasites.

but the degradation was then thwarted when vitamin E was added to the culture. Varma observes that epidemiological studies point to a higher incidence of cataracts in human populations living in areas of greater sunlight. Thus, vitamin E supplementation (and also vitamin C supplementation, based on other experiments[125b,c]) might be indicated for those doing extensive "beaching" in Florida, California, Hawaii and other sunny locations.

Vitamin E may be of value in treating muscular dystrophy if treatment is begun early. Circumstantial evidence suggests that muscular dystrophy may be caused by free-radical damage.[125d] Regrettably, antioxidants such as vitamin E[25e,f] and superoxide dismutase[125g] have thus far not produced significant benefit in the treatment of this disease. Even when plenty of vitamin E and/or other antioxidants are present, the primary lack is probably that of an enzyme which allows the muscles to use vitamin E. Arthur C. Guyton[126] states it is believed that the muscular dystrophy resulting from vitamin E deficiency is caused by rupture of the cells' lysosomes (the organelles for digesting damaged cells or portions of cells for removal from the body) and subsequent autodigestion (autolysis) of the muscle. It is likely, as Franklin Bicknell and Frederick Prescott say,[127] "that the key to the cure of muscular dystrophy is vitamin E, but we have as yet no knowledge of how to fit the key to the lock."

M. C. Farber et al.[127a] found the compound alpha tocopheramine to be active against muscular dystrophy in vitamin E-deficient rabbits. Later, E. Sondergaard and H. Dam[127b] reported similar efficacy in using various other vitamin E compounds to treat the disease in chicks. Methylene blue, like vitamin E, is effective in preventing cod-liver oil dystrophy in calves.[128] H. H. Draper and A. S. Csallany reported that N, N´-diphenyl-p-phenylenediamine (DPPD) cured muscular dystrophy in vitamin E-deficient rabbits.[129]

There is, however, research that would seem to cast doubt on the Bicknell and Prescott hypothesis. Benjamin N. Berg[130] reported that vitamin E failed to prevent muscular dystrophy in aging rats. Then too, K. L. Blaxter et al.[131] reported that calves with muscular dystrophy that was induced by cod-liver oil have just as much vitamin E in their bodies, including their muscles, as controls. Furthermore, J. W. Safford et al. [132] found no correlation between the disease in lambs and the concentration of vitamin E in their mother's milk. Thus, the possible involvement of "E" in muscular dystrophy is yet to be elucidated. However, the fact that the potency of various vitamin E compounds can be assayed by measuring their effect on the creatinuria levels of dystrophic rabbits, as we saw earlier, argues that a very real relationship exists. Furthermore, M. J. Jackson et al. [132a] have recently presented evidence suggesting that calcium antagonists, phospholipase inhibitors and antioxidants such as vitamin E may be useful in reducing the amount of muscle damage in patients with severe myopathies.

In animal experiments, diets severely deficient in vitamin E and selenium have led to development of liver necrosis. Surprisingly, O. A. Levander et al. [133] have reported that liver necrosis in animals with insufficient vitamin E and selenium is delayed by using a 20% solution of ethyl alcohol in water as their drinking fluid (a *reverse effect* since alcohol causes liver necrosis).

It is postulated that the shortage of vitamin E and/or selenium among bottle-fed babies may be responsible for some of the unexplained crib deaths.* In April, 1974, evidence was presented by Dr. Richard Naeye of the Pennsylvania State University's Medical School at Hershey, Pennsylvania, that indicates a chronic lack of oxygen may be a cause of crib death. The chronic lack of oxygen would seem to suggest that vitamin E may play a vital role in helping to prevent the deaths. However, studies by W. J. Rhead et al.,[134] Gerhard N. Schrauzer et al.[134a] and Sidney L. Saltzstein[134b] have indicated no correlation with vitamin E or selenium inadequacy and sudden infant death.

In the matter of crib death there are, incidentally, many other hypotheses, including strong cases for the theories that shortages of biotin or of magnesium may be among the causes. (This is discussed further when we treat biotin and magnesium in later chapters.) Derrick Lonsdale, M.D., of the Cleveland Clinic views crib death as

---

* Mother's milk contains far more vitamin E than does cow's milk, suggesting that nature intended infants to receive a generous quantity of the vitamin.

being a kind of infant *beri beri* caused by a shortage of thiamin (vitamin B₁). There are probably other causative factors in these tragedies. Ashley Montagu[135] suggests that crib deaths may be due at least in part to inadequate sensory stimulation, particularly tactile stimulation. It is essential that babies be cuddled, kissed and be given other forms of sensory stimulation.* Montagu also suggests the possibility that cradle-raised babies (who receive more sensory stimulation because of the rocking motion) may be less subject to crib death than cot-raised babies. (On April 24, 1975, the Associated Press reported that Dr. Louis Gluck, chief of neonatology at University Hospital, San Diego, California, had installed oscillating water beds for the newly born in the attempt to reduce crib death.) So, although there are many theories as to the cause of crib death, there is a possibility (disputed by the work of Drs. Rhead and Schrauzer) that a shortage of vitamin E is a factor.

I. Gontzea et al.[136a] reported that congenital tocopherol deficiency contributes to neonatal jaundice and recommended that the mother take vitamin E supplementation during the last three months of pregnancy. Malcolm L. Chiswick et al.[136b] found, in a study involving 44 babies born after less than 32 weeks gestation, that the incidence of intraventricular hemorrhage was just 18.8% in supplemented babies versus 56.3% in those not supplemented with vitamin E.

Vitamin E deficiency has been linked to another problem of premature infants. The fetus absorbs vitamin E inefficiently until he reaches gestational maturity.[198] Therefore, if born prematurely, the infant is likely to be deficient in this vitamin. Injected vitamin E has been suggested for the treatment of infants with retrolental fibroplasia. Retrolental fibroplasia (RLF) is very common in premature infants, excessive oxygen therapy in incubators being, at one time, the major cause. Now oxygen levels are carefully monitored and the problem is reduced but not eliminated. Neil N.

---

* Adults need sensory stimulation too. As William J. Goldwag, M.D.,[136] says "...the nutritive value of another's touch may overshadow the benefits from food and medicine." Often we define "nutrition" too narrowly. Loving touches and sounds and words of love and encouragement may be phases of nutrition we ignore to the detriment of our health.

Finer et al.[199] conducted a controlled trial of vitamin E therapy in infants with a birth weight of 750 to 1,500 grams and showed that RLF incidence is not affected by vitamin E, but its use reduces the severity of the problem and reduces subsequent eye damage. This treatment is, however, questioned by Robert E. Kalina,[200] although he probably did not know about the Finer[199] study that was to be published the following month. Solomon Sobel et al.[200a] have also warned about the possibility that parenteral vitamin E may cause necrotizing enterocolitis in premature infants. Neil N. Finer et al.,[200b] in phase II of their study, concluded that vitamin E should be given within 12 hours of birth to infants weighing less than 1,250 grams who require supplemental oxygen. Arnall Patz[200c] and Neil N. Finer et al.[200d] have recently reviewed the current therapy of retrolental fibroplasia. Finer has warned especially about the dangers of necrotizing enterocolitis developing following use of hyperosmolar vitamin E preparations.* David B. Schaffer et al.[200e] reported that, in a randomized study of 545 infants weighing less than 1,501 grams at birth, there was a trend toward less severe retrolental fibroplasia among those that were vitamin E-treated. However, the incidence of retrolental fibroplasia was 6.8% in the placebo-treated infants and 7.2% in those treated with vitamin E.

Vitamin E has been effective in treating itching of the vaginal and anal areas. Dr. Evan Shute suggested that the reason for its success in these applications may be because small blood vessels apparently age more rapidly in the genital and anal regions. Vitamin E, to the extent that it can open up collateral circulation, may be valuable in eliminating itching of these areas. Puncturing a vitamin E capsule and smearing the contents in the anal region can mollify the itching of *pruritis ani*. Vitamin E suppositories are also available for either rectal or vaginal use. This treatment could be yet another example of masking symptoms rather than treating the underlying condition. The basic problem, in some cases, might be irritation caused by toxins coming out of a colon burdened with disease-causing bacteria. If this is the underlying cause, acidophilus and yogurt by mouth and

---

* The dangers might lie in the carrier if polysorbates are used rather than in the vitamin E. Further details are in a subnote later in this chapter.

applied topically, or colonic irrigations, might be indicated. In some cases, *pruritis ani* may be caused by food sensitivity, perhaps especially to alcohol, citrus, sugar, coffee or chocolate, or in yet other cases it may be caused by excessive histamine, in which event vitamin C might be helpful. Another possible cause of *pruritis ani* or vaginitis is fungi *(Candida)* and other appropriate therapy may be required.

Vitamin E, in acting as an antioxidant which inhibits oxygen in combining with lipids to form peroxides, simultaneously conserves oxygen for vital uses. Perhaps this vitamin E effect is at least partially caused by its influence on the production of coenzyme Q 10, an important component of the mitochondrial electron transport processes of respiration.[136c,d] At any rate, E. L. Hove et al.[137] reported on an experiment evaluating survival times of rats exposed to a gradual reduction in available air. They found that anoxia, while being further exacerbated by vitamin A and carotene, was improved by vitamin E. Thus, vitamin E may stretch the oxygen supply available at high altitudes or when engaging in hard work or athletics. Vitamin E may also help protect the body against ozone and nitrogen dioxide.* M. G. Mustapha[139] found that when rats were fed an amount of vitamin E comparable to average American consumption they showed marked lung damage upon being exposed to .1 ppm of ozone for seven days. Another group of rats fed six times as much vitamin E (6.6 mg./100 g. of food) showed virtually no lung damage. On the contrary, as a result of a double-blind, controlled trial, Jack D. Hackney et al.[140] reported that supplemental dl-alpha tocopherol had no meaningful role in the observable responses to ozone exposure in a young, healthy population. The Hackney group did not rule out, however, the possibility that vitamin E supplementation could be of use in other populations or in other types of environmental oxidant insults. In related work, Timtim and McNamara[140a] reported that intramuscular injection of vitamin E provided no protection against oxygen toxicity in

---

* Use of nitrogen dioxide as an anesthetic is probably safe but is questionable. It can damage respiratory epithelial cells, can inhibit vitamin B12 metabolism and can promote formation of nitrosamines. Many references support these statements.[138]

normal rats exposed to a high oxygen environment. As a matter of fact, they found a significant *decrease* in survival time of rats given high dosages of vitamin E, which suggests "a previously unknown toxic effect." Later work by L. N. North et al.[140b] showed, however, that protection against hypoxia in mice was directly related to the level of vitamin E supplementation. As in the case of so much other nutritional research, contradiction is sometimes more prevalent than agreement—which suggests that a *reverse effect,* depending on dosage, could be operating.

Vitamin E has also been used successfully as a deodorant. Bacteria on the skin, interacting with perspiration, cause a rancidity that creates underarm odor. Vitamin E's antioxidant property combats the oxidation. Mennen Company marketed a deodorant containing vitamin E quite successfully until stopped by the Food and Drug Administration because of complaints of a few persons that they experienced allergic reactions.[141] The reactions were probably due to the aerosol propellant rather than to the vitamin E. Some soaps and cleansers also contain vitamin E.

Vitamin E may also be of use in treating some skin conditions. A combination of dl-alpha tocopheryl acetate and vitamin C was reported by R. Hayakawa et al.[142] to be effective in treating chloasma (patchy tan-brown-black hyperpigmentation, especially on brow or cheeks) and pigmented contact dermatitis. A multiclinical, double-blind study showed that vitamins E and C worked synergistically to produce a therapeutic effect superior to either used alone. The proposed mechanism is thought to relate to the ability of both vitamin E and vitamin C to inhibit the formation of melanin from tyrosine.

Vitamin E has been used in the treatment of kidney disease (nephritis), and for the prevention and treating of sterility in men, miscarriages, premature delivery and the possibility of brain damage in full-term infants. An enzyme, hyaluronidase, can thin out the synovial fluid of the joints and vitamin E may protect the body against some of the negative actions of this enzyme. To the extent that vitamin E might prevent thinning of the synovial fluid, it could be helpful in alleviating or preventing arthritis. There is limited evidence that, topically applied, vitamin E may even be of value in treating some types of herpes, specifically *herpes gingivostomatitis*.[143] Sixty units of d-alpha tocopheryl acetate (an enormous amount) administered orally to rats who had received a gingival wound (similar to gingivectomy) caused accelerated wound healing.[144] Robert L. Ruberg,[144a] on the contrary, citing Ehrlich, states that "vitamin E's action is similar to that of steroids: it interferes with collagen synthesis and wound repair." However, according to Ruberg, vitamin E may be theoretically useful in preventing the appearance of hypertrophic scar or keloid. Nevertheless, Ruberg states that "all efforts to date using topical or systemic vitamin E have failed to show a clear-cut practical effect of this theoretical benefit." Vitamin E is reported to be useful for alleviating allergies, for promoting growth of skin over wounds (in addition to gingiva wounds), and for a great number of other applications.

Vitamin E and Aging

Chronological age is irrelevant. It is one's biological or functional age that is an index to his or her health, bouyant spirit, longevity potential and sexual power. How can vitamin E help keep one youthful?

The secret seems to relate to vitamin E's powerful antioxidant nature. It scavenges free radicals, entities with one or more unpaired electrons which sometimes poison the body by flying around and damaging cells. We have learned much about free radicals since the pioneering work done by Nobel laureate Gerhard Herzberg. Some free radicals have a life span of microseconds and act close to their site of production. Others may move over greater distances and live for days before causing biological damage.[144b] These free radicals can damage our foods* before we eat them and can also cause many types of damage within our bodies. After decades of speculation,

---

* If you are dining in a restaurant that appears to have insufficient customers to guarantee fast turnover of the food, avoid foods that may have undergone excessive free-radical reactions and give preference to those coming directly from the freezer.

proof that alpha tocopherol is the major lipid-soluble chain-breaking antioxidant in human blood plasma was finally published by G. W. Burton et al.[145]* Free radicals can be discerned during chemical reactions by pulse radiolysis, by nuclear magnetic resonance techniques and by use of a chemiluminescent probe.[146,146a]

Lipid peroxidation (autoxidation)** occurs when a polyunsaturated fat reacts with an oxidant to form a lipid free radical which, in turn, reacts with oxygen to produce a peroxy free radical.[146c] According to B. Halliwell and J. M. C. Gutteridge,[146d] any free radical species with sufficient reactivity to abstract H· will start off lipid peroxidation. Free radicals that do this include the hydroxyl radical, alkoxy radicals, peroxyradicals and possibly $HO_2·$, but not superoxide. (Some of these types of free radicals will be discussed further in Chapters 3, 6 and 9.)

Among the many "free-radical diseases," Denham Harman[147] includes cancer, atherosclerosis, essential hypertension, Alzheimer's dementia, amyloidosis, immune deficiency of age, osteoarthritis, senile macular degeneration and Parkinson's disease. Oxygen-derived free radicals can also cause tissue damage during ischemia (diminished local blood supply due to obstruction of inflow of arterial blood or its vasoconstriction).[147a,b] Shunichi Fujimoto et al.,[147b] in studies involving dogs, have shown that intravenous pretreatment with 30 mg./kg. of dl-alpha tocopheryl nicotinate can protect the brain from cerebral ischemia. (Oral treatment with vitamin E, compared to controls, did not produce a statistically significant effect.)

---

* Albert A. Barber and Frederick Bernheim[145a] cite studies indicating the amount of vitamin E needed to protect against lipid peroxidation. In one of these studies, E. G. Hill[145b] found that 100 mg. of vitamin E was needed to protect young pigs for every 1% of peroxidized corn oil fed above 4% of the diet. J. G. Bieri and A. A. Anderson[145c] kept chicks healthy for 24 weeks on an E-free diet when it was fat free or when it contained 4% lard (which consists mostly of saturated fat). As we can see from these studies, "E" serves a function in protecting against lipid peroxidation only if polyunsaturates are present. (The term "lipid peroxidation" is inaccurate although commonly used. Lipids include saturated fats, waxes, sterols and other substances that are relatively unaffected by free radicals and, therefore, are not subject to peroxidation. A better term would be *polyunsaturate peroxidation*.)

** Photosensitized oxidation of unsaturated fatty acids proceeds by a different mechanism that does not involve free radicals.[146b]

Richard G. Cutler[149e] speculates that if the maximum life-span potential of a species is related to the ability of the tissues to protect themselves against the toxic effects of oxygen, then the ability of humans (a very long-lived species) to protect themselves from lipid peroxidation should be relatively good. Cutler has graphed the *in vitro* rate of autoxidation of whole brain homogenate in air of various species as a function of their maximum life-span potential (MLSP). Figure 3 shows that the correlation between autoxidation of brain tissue of various mammals and their MLSP is very good, with humans having the lowest rate of autoxidation (lipid peroxidation) and the highest maximum life-span potential.

I do not desire, however, to further the tendency to cast lipid peroxidation in a strictly negative role. Nature is a chemist with physiological concepts of which we may not always be aware. Free-radical lipid peroxidation chain reactions produce hydroperoxy fatty acids at each completed peroxidation. It is not lipid peroxidation as such that may cause the physiological mischief, but its improper control through too little or perhaps through too much of antioxidants such as vitamin E. Properly controlled, however, lipid peroxidation is a beneficial factor used in the metabolic pathways whereby the polyunsaturated fatty acids are converted into prostaglandins, thromboxanes, leukotrienes and prostacyclin.[148] Vitamin E inhibits platelet aggregation,*in vivo*, both by lowering platelet thromboxane, TxA_2, and by raising arterial prostacyclin, PGI_2.[149] Free radicals themselves are essential to many normal body processes. Phagocytosis, for example, is dependent in part on a burst of the free radical superoxide given off by leucocytes (as will be discussed in Chapter 9). Even some of the reactions involving vitamin E occur because "E" itself forms a free radical.[149b] A large number of drugs promote or inhibit the generation of free radicals and some drugs, *in vivo*, do both.[149a] The anticancer drug adriamycin generates free radicals that may aid in curing cancer but can also lead to the undesirable side reactions of cardiomyopathy and cataract![149a]

For many years free radicals and lipid peroxidation have been thought of as causes of cell death. It is now considered likely that

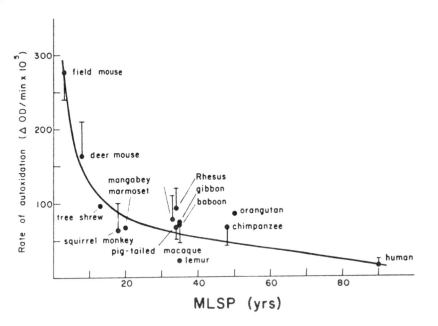

Figure 3. Rate of autoxidation of whole brain homogenate in air from different mammalian species as a function of MLSP. Numbers in parentheses represent number of individuals used in each determination. Reproduced from Richard G. Cutler in *Free Radicals in Molecular Biology, Aging and Disease*, ed. Donald Armstrong et al., (New York: Raven Press, 1984), pp. 235-266, at 260, with permission of the publisher and of the author.

free radical activity may also be a sequel of most types of biological damage.[149c] Rancid fat has been viewed for centuries as a source of deadly tumors. It is now being suggested, however, that some products of rancidification may act to protect the body against the effects of local tissue destruction![149c] Furthermore, Burton et al.[149d] cite studies showing lipid peroxidation is often decreased in tumors compared to normal tissues. Moreover, antioxidants, and in particular alpha tocopherol, are at high levels in the tumor cell. A reduction in the amount of these antioxidants present within the cancer cell might foster lipid peroxidation and thereby reduce the growth of cancer because lipid peroxidation produces substances that inhibit DNA synthesis and cell division. I speculate that it is therefore possible that lipid peroxidation occurring within the cancer cell could be unhealthy for a cancer cell and thus be beneficial to human health. Moreover, the antioxidants, including vitamin E, may be present in the cancer cell to protect it and the processes that foster its life and their presence may be detrimental to the health of the host. However, Rao V. Panganamala and David Cornwell[149da] point out the many paradoxical effects (what I call *reverse effects*) of vitamin E. These effects make it difficult at this time to speculate whether either supplementing with vitamin E or restricting the intake of this vitamin might be therapeutic for the cancer patient. Recall again the statement by Haldane: "Nature is not only queerer than we suppose, but queerer than we *can* suppose." We can't always separate the "good guys" from the "bad guys." In fact, we're not always sure when a "good guy" is being "bad" or a "bad guy" is being "good"—or whether a "guy" is being "good" and "bad" at the same time. We must remain open-minded and await the exciting nutritional discoveries that are about to be made.

To some extent, the body may compensate for our nutritional sins. Richard G. Cutler[149e] has pointed out that when a rat is fed a long-term, vitamin E-deficient diet, the amount of his other antioxidants (glutathione peroxidase, glutathione reductase and superoxide dismutase) will dramatically increase and thus partially compensate for his vitamin E deficiency. On the other hand, excessive supplementation of vitamin E depresses body levels of the other antioxidants, thereby reducing to some extent the protection supplemental vitamin E might be expected to provide. This, Cutler speculates, could explain the relatively equal aging rates of individuals regardless of their dietary intake.* Of course, we all know aging rates are not equal (some 40-year-olds look to be 60 and vice versa). However, real antiaging success will come when scientists discover how to put antioxidants not just within the cells (which was accomplished by nature some two billion years ago), but learn how to place those antioxidants within the mitochondria of the cells.

Lipid peroxidation exemplifies the golden mean—moderation in all things. For example, atherosclerosis is associated with an increased level of lipid peroxides. This leads to a relative decrease in prostacyclin (the powerful antiaggregatory factor) and an increase in thromboxane A_2 (TxA2) which may lead, in turn, to thrombosis.[150] You will note I've had to qualify this statement with the word "may." Actually, we do not know to what extent the platelet aggregation contributes to the formation of thrombi nor the manner in which arachidonic acid and thromboxane control the process. Anyway, too much vitamin E might tend to inhibit the beneficial aspects of lipid peroxidation, while too little might encourage excessive peroxidation and eventual heart trouble. Throughout this book we will see how health is a game of countless teeter-totters of nutrients, exercise, mental effects, etc. A book, a nutritionist or your physician may make suggestions as to how to balance the teeter-totters, but ultimately the decisions will always be yours.

Inhibitors of lipid peroxidation (autoxidation) can be divided into two categories: primary antioxidants which reduce the rate at which free radicals are formed and secondary antioxidants which break free-radical chains by trapping the free radicals. Vitamin E is believed to operate as a secondary antioxidant for lipids by trapping superoxide free radicals (about which more will be said in Chapter

---

* Perhaps the "wisdom" of the body "knows" that antioxidants in excess, unless they can be moved into the cell's mitochondria, might inhibit production of beneficial prostaglandins. Then, too, vitamin E in the blood gives no indication of how the tissues are turning it over and thereby protecting themselves from oxidation. Cutler[149e] says, "Nothing appears to be known of what regulates vitamin E levels in tissues." Contrary to Cutler's findings, however, J. Hallfrisch et al.[149f] reported during 1986 that, in a study of 419 men and women 17-93 years old, SOD levels tended to be higher in multivitamin users and also in men taking vitamin E.

9), lipid peroxyl radicals and methyl linoleate radicals. [150a] It acts as a free radical scavenger by donating a phenolic hydrogen atom to a free radical, thus neutralizing the unpaired electron and oxidizing the vitamin E to its quinone form. [151] Morimitsu Nishikimi et al. [152] discovered that the intermediate reaction product of this free-radical trapping by alpha tocopherol is *8a-hydroxy-alpha tocopherone* and the corresponding compounds for the beta, gamma and delta tocopherols. They further reported that the products change spontaneously to tocopherol quinone. Vitamin E quinone, as well as other quinones such as p-benzoquinone, duroquinone and 1,4-naphthoquinone, can be reduced by the superoxide ion to yield the corresponding semiquinone radicals. [152a] This suggests that vitamin E quinone, like vitamin E, may, in a hydrophobic environment, protect cells from the superoxide free radical. [152a]

When insufficient antioxidants such as vitamin E are present and lipid peroxidation (autoxidation) occurs, this may cause damage to the cell's membrane and impair its function. Then, too, in destroying free radicals, vitamin E and the other antioxidants may slow down cross-linkage in the collagen which could result in a hard, leathery skin and cause the body to take on other characteristics of aging.*

Free radicals can be produced in the body through the effects of nitric and nitrous oxides, excess polyunsaturated fatty acids, alcohol, carbon tetrachloride, ozone, tobacco smoke, auto exhaust fumes and various forms of radiation—x-rays, microwaves, radioactivity, cosmic rays, ultraviolet light and just plain sunlight. Excessive exposure to sunlight may be especially dangerous as is suggested by relative longevity data of blacks versus whites. The life expectancy of whites is greater than that of blacks until the sixties, at which time the life expectancy of blacks relative to whites is reported to improve.

---

* Irwin Fridovich[153] points out, however, that vitamin E acts primarily as a backup defense to scavenge oxygen free radicals that have been missed by enzymes such as superoxide dismutase. He states that it is more efficient for the body to save the vitamin E to minimize damage by free radicals that evade the enzyme scavengers.

Johann Bjorksten[154] speculates that the pigmented skin of the blacks protects them from the radiation that can cause life-shortening cross-linkages. The life-extending benefit of the skin pigmentation of the blacks is operational at all ages, but in the younger age brackets is overshadowed by other effects.

Johann Bjorksten has extended the cross-link theory to apply to large molecules within the cells—perhaps even involving the DNA—so that normal cellular functions are inhibited. If DNA is affected to the extent of producing defective RNA molecules, then the defective RNA would produce defective protein in the ribosomes. This accumulation of defective protein molecules would then bring about inaccurate enzyme synthesis, ineffective cellular action and even death of the cells.

Vitamin E not only works to protect cell membranes and prevent cross-linking of collagen, but may protect the chromosomes themselves. Beverly D. Lyn-Cook and Rosalyn M. Patterson[150a] found that vitamin E inhibited chemically induced chromosomal aberrations in hamster cells *in vitro*. If such chromosomal aberrations are permitted to occur, they could produce defective protein and thus promote aging.

So to work toward the objective of inhibiting the destruction of cells that promote aging, under the presumption that the above scenario has some validity, make sure there is enough vitamin E in your diet. Be sure there is sufficient vitamin E to protect against free radicals and to keep molecules of fat from forming excessive peroxides. The vitamin E will, at the same time, protect valuable substances—among which are carotene, vitamin A and the pituitary, adrenal and sex hormones—from being destroyed by oxygen. Furthermore, as Robert L. Baehner et al.[155] pointed out, vitamin E protects red blood cells against a variety of drugs that generate hydrogen peroxide.

As we noted earlier in this chapter, Kenji Fukuzawa et al.[38] have reported on the protective effect of alpha tocopherol in regard to lipid peroxidation of liposome membranes. You will recall that the Fukuzawa group found that peroxidation (as measured by production of malonyldialdehyde)* was catalyzed by vitamin C and ferrous iron, but was inhibited by alpha tocopherol. They also reported that cholesterol, while not acting as an antioxidant, increased the antioxidative efficiency of alpha tocopherol. (I wonder if "body wisdom" sends cholesterol to an atheroma caused by free radicals so that, together with alpha tocopherol, it combats those free radicals? I speculate that cholesterol, instead of being a promoter of the atherosclerotic process, may be a friendly combatant against that process.)**

A recent study carried out by M. Wartanowicz et al.[156a] in 100 subjects, mainly women aged 60-100 years and living in nursing homes, showed that vitamin E (and to a lesser extent vitamin C) reduced the serum lipid peroxide levels. A daily supplementation of vitamin E (of undisclosed type) in the amount of 200 mg. (100 mg. twice daily) for four months decreased the serum peroxide level by a mean value of 14%. A daily intake of 400 mg. of vitamin C (200 mg. twice daily) for four months decreased the peroxide level by 8%. When subjects were given both vitamins in the above amounts for four months, the serum peroxide level decreased by 20% compared with the control level. After one year the serum peroxide levels decreased by 26% with vitamin E supplementation, by 13% with vitamin C and by 25% when both vitamins were used. (The fact that Wartanowicz et al.[156a] found vitamin C useful in decreasing lipid peroxidation while Fukuzawa[38] found the opposite action,*** suggests a *reverse effect* may be operating and shows the need for dose-response delineation in the respective experiments.) Etsuo Niki et al.,[156b] like Wartanowicz, found that lipid peroxidation of a solution of methyl linoleate was suppressed most efficiently when

---

* Malonyldialdehyde is not only a measure of lipid peroxidation but a sensitive marker of the presence of free radicals.[155a] Hans Nohl and Dietmar Hegner,[155b] however, citing R. O. Recknagel and A. K. Ghoshal,[156] have stated that malonyldialdehyde "cannot be regarded as a reliable index of lipid peroxidation *in vivo*, since it is readily metabolized by mitochondria."

** Vitamin E might play a beneficial role even after an atheroma comes into existence by decreasing platelet aggregation, blood viscosity and thrombosis.

*** The fact that iron was also present in the Fukuzawa study was probably crucial to vitamin C's acting as a pro-oxidant.

vitamin E at a concentration of 290 mM and vitamin C at a concentration of 275 mM were both present. They reported that vitamin E remained almost unchanged with only vitamin C being consumed at the initial stage. Vitamin E was consumed only after vitamin C was exhausted. They concluded that vitamin E trapped the peroxy radical, while the resulting α-chromanoxy radical reacted with vitamin C to regenerate vitamin E.

In spite of the evidence we have been examining, there are some scientists who do not consider the antioxidant theory of aging to be tenable. A. D. Blackett and D. A. Hall,[157] for example, maintained that, although they found vitamin E lowered fatal tumor incidence in mice and lipofuscin levels in heart tissue, the significance of lipid peroxidation in regard to aging was questionable. Those who like to study contrary views may be interested in learning that L. Green[158] covers several viewpoints opposing the prevalent views about the antioxidant effects of vitamin E. More recently, however, William A. Pryor[159] has discussed discoveries that would seem to put free-radical biology on a basis of solid facts. The three key discoveries he emphasizes are the role of superoxide dismutase, the biosynthesis of peroxidic compounds from arachidonic acid and the body of research that points to the conclusion that environmental toxins exert their effects through radical-mediated reactions. Some of the supporting research is discussed in the present chapter, while other relevant research will be discussed in Chapters 3 and 9.

Furthermore, Lloyd A. Witting[160] reports that, when the analogies are correctly stated, there is excellent correlation between lipid autoxidation *in vitro* and lipid peroxidation *in vivo* in various studies including those of Dr. Green. Then too, Robert L. Baehner et al.,[155] five years after Green wrote, state, "It is known that vitamin E is a less efficient antioxidant *in vitro* than it appears to be *in vivo*."

Rather than seeing lipid peroxidation as primarily a cause of tissue damage, B. Halliwell and John M. C. Gutteridge[160a] suggest that, often, a disease or toxin causes cell damage which leads to increased lipid peroxidation. Luis Garcia-Bunuel,[160b] as well as Iswar S. Singh and Jagat J. Ghosh,[160c] have developed and criticized the proposed mechanism of Halliwell and Gutteridge. (Halliwell and

Gutteridge replied in a later issue of *Lancet*.)[160d] It seems apparent that both processes may often be coexistent; the *cause* of lipid peroxidation may be an effect and the effect, in turn, may be causal.

While we are considering the pros and cons of lipid peroxidation let's remember that, whether or not lipid peroxidation negatively affects the course of disease and of aging, it is not fair to imply that peroxidation is all bad. Peroxidation is the first step in the conversion of arachidonic acid to prostaglandins. Laurence M. Corwin and Janet Shloss[161] point out that vitamin E may be involved in the reactions, although A. M. Butler et al.[162] insist that vitamin E has no effect on prostaglandin synthesis. Subsequently, Robert O. Likoff et al.[162a] experimenting with chickens, reported that vitamin E inhibited endogenous prostaglandins PGE_1, PGE_2 and $PGF_{2\propto}$. This was not unhealthful since it protected the chickens from a lethal *E. coli* infection. Nevertheless, the possibility of inhibiting prostaglandins (some of which are, of course, beneficial) gives us a reason not to overdose on vitamin E.

A sign of possible vitamin E deficiency is the ceroid pigment (lipofuscin) that shows up as brown spots on the face, on the back of the hands and elsewhere.* This pigment is the remains of the unsaturated fatty acids that were destroyed by oxygen. It can be found in humans and animals virtually everywhere in the body. Many experiments by A. Tappel and others have shown that feeding animals antioxidants, including vitamin E, reduces lipofuscin accumulation. Vitamin E can be effective in this regard in even young animals. A. Saari Csallany et al.[163a] found that, of several tissues tested, only the liver showed reduced lipofuscin due to dietary vitamin E treatment. However, as a result of more recent work, Patricia Kruk and Hildegard E. Enesco[164] reported that alpha tocopherol injected into mice reduced the lipofuscin in their hearts and brains. Such pigment forms in women during menopause because the need for vitamin E rises so tremendously at this time and especially if estrogen therapy is employed. Although some of the above-cited research suggests that

---

* I and others often use the words "ceroid" and "lipofuscin" interchangeably. Their composition is similar, but ceroid contains more acidic lipid polymers, while lipofuscin has a higher concentration of neutral lipid polymers.[163]

dietary supplementation of vitamin E (and perhaps of other antioxidants) may reduce lipofuscin formation, a 1986 rat study of B. Zaspel Menken et al.[164b] (a group that included Saari Csallany[163a] who was cited above) throws doubt on that possibility. Their conclusions were confined to the lipofuscin concentrations in the heart and brain of the mice (and thus are not necessarily related to the skin of humans). Menken and his associates reported that, although age-related factors played a part in the concentration of lipofuscin pigments, dietary supplementation of vitamin E was without effect.

Vitamin E for Athletes

Supplemental vitamin E may be important for all athletes, including those performing sexual athletics. Vitamin E is reported to dilate the blood vessels, including those supplying the penis, and thus it might help assure a good firm erection. Vitamin E is used by the pituitary gland (where it is more concentrated than anywhere else in the body) in producing gonadotropins. As already reported, when vitamin E is present in red blood cells they do not lose their hemoglobin so fast as do cells deficient in this vitamin and this could also be a factor in erection maintenance. Vitamin E assists in detoxifying the environmental pollutions and can thereby increase the energy level of the body. Vitamin E is reported (by some, but not by others) to raise the sperm count and may increase the volume of semen. Furthermore, vitamin E may reduce the body's oxygen requirement and so minimize heart strain and the "panting effect" (dyspnea) that may occur concomitant with really active sex.[*]

Vitamin E, as Michael Briggs[165] points out, has been shown to stimulate production of cytochrome P-450 in animals. Cytochrome P-450 is a family of isoenzymes possessing catalytic activity toward thousands of substrates.[165a] ("Cytochrome" literally means "cell's

---

[*] This speculation may be questionable in light of an experiment by A. Salminen et al.[164a] that used mice and rats in connection with a daily treadmill training program. Such training did not affect the concentration of vitamin E in the lung sof the mice or rats. Salminen concluded that "increased vantilation and oxygen utilization induced by exercise training do not modify lung antioxidants in contrast to hyperoxia and hypoxia."

color." It is a hemoprotein whose reddish color is derived from the iron it contains.)[165a] Cytochrome P-450 is an essential cofactor in steroid metabolism and so it is likely to enhance production of corticosteroids and sex hormones. Furthermore, D. Lees et al.[166] reported that plasma testosterone and cortisone concentrations in male rats fed a diet deficient in vitamin E for 130 days were significantly lower than in rats fed the same diet supplemented with vitamin E. We should stress, however, that correction of a vitamin deficiency is not a good gauge as to whether a surplus of that vitamin will produce an additional effect. However, the experiment at least suggests the possibility that vitamin E may increase sexuality in both men and women (since sexuality in women is also related to the concentration of blood testosterone).

In addition, J. P. Mather et al.[166a] have recently reported that an *in vitro* experiment with porcine (swine) interstitial cells (leydig cells) of the testes, in a hormone-supplemented medium, showed vitamin E added to the culture resulted in an increased production of testosterone and also lengthened the life span of the cells. *In vitro* is not *in vivo* and porcine leydig cells are not human leydig cells, but, nevertheless, this experiment may offer some support to the thesis that vitamin E increases human sexuality. At the same time, we should note again that supplemental vitamin E might constitute a danger in a person having any early—perhaps undetected— hormone-dependent cancer such as those involving the breast or the prostate gland.

Vitamin E helps protect the seminiferous epithelium in male rats. Prior to maturity vitamin E is not needed to provide such protection. However, with the onset of maturity, sperm is produced and it contains large amounts of the enzyme hyaluronidase. Hyaluronidase is essential if sperm are to retain their fertilizing ability, but when vitamin E levels drop too low the hyaluronidase may attack neighboring tissue.[167] Another somewhat surprising fact is that, while a vitamin E deficiency in male rats causes testicular degeneration and also decreased production of testosterone, a deficiency also causes *increased* production of the reproduction-related folicle-stimulating and leutenizing hormones in female rats.[168]

Vitamin E supplements seem powerless to aid in the generation of sperm. Edmond J. Farris[168a] reported that, in testing four different vitamin E preparations *on human volunteers* in dosages as high as 3,000 mg. and for periods up to 90 days, there was no significant change in the semen. Farris concluded that spermatogenesis was not influenced by supplementary vitamin E.

Excessive amounts of vitamin E may, in fact, have a detrimental effect on the ability of females to reproduce. In an experiment with female rats, N. Y. J. Yang and I. D. Desai[169] found that the fertility of rats was detrimentally affected when fed 10,000 I.U. of dl-alpha tocopheryl acetate per kg. diet. A vitamin E deficiency has long been known to detrimentally affect fertility of female rats.[170] So, we have a biphasic *reverse effect:* infertility reverses to fertility with normal amounts of dietary vitamin E and then fertility reverses to infertility in rats with massive amounts of "E."

In spite of vitamin E's presumed essentiality, a number of studies suggest that it may not be needed for libido or reproductive capacity. Thor W. Gullickson[171] reported that male and female calves fed rations deficient in vitamin E showed full sexual and reproductive capacity. The bulls fed such deficient rations from birth showed, at six months of age, marked libido and their semen samples indicated that all ejaculates were normal in sperm activity, morphology and longevity. Similarly, heifers at the age of seven to nine months showed that their estrus cycles, including ovulation, were normal. Furthermore, breeding records demonstrated that the reproducing ability of the cattle fed vitamin E-poor rations was not adversely affected through three generations. However, many of the animals showed signs of illness and 13 out of 28 animals deficient in vitamin E died suddenly. Thus, health was negatively affected, but not libido or reproductive capacity. F. C. van der Kaay et al.[172] reported that there was no relation between the tocopherol level in the blood of cows and horses and sterility. They cited four references to studies that concluded vitamin E therapy has a favorable effect on sterility of farm animals, but they themselves found no such effects. When it comes to vitamin E and sex, it is obviously quite possible to "prove" whatever position you have set out to prove.

A study in regard to vitamin E and human sexuality was done by Edward Herold et al.[173] This research showed no effects of a daily intake of 1,000 I.U. of alpha tocopherol on sexual arousal in a group of 35 men and women, age 21-50. However, four members of the group taking "E" reported "increased energy" against just one in the placebo group. The authors concluded that a larger and more diverse sample is needed before one can state that vitamin E does not influence sexual functioning. Thus, while vitamin E and sex seem to be only tenuously related, at best, how about nonsexual athletics?

Dr. Evan Shute,[174] in his book, *The Heart and Vitamin E,* gives results of studies made by Lloyd Percival of Canada's Sport College. Percival gave each athlete 300 units of vitamin E daily at breakfast and reported they showed greater endurance, better "wind" and generally improved feeling. In a carefully controlled experiment, on the other hand, I. M. Sharman[175] reported there was no athletic improvement using vitamin E. Sharman used two experimental groups of 13 boarding school boys and fed one group 400 mg. alpha tocopheryl acetate daily and the other group placebos. (Since all were boarding, the diet of each group was very similar.) Sharman reported that training resulted in an improved physiological function but vitamin E did not. A subsequent study by Ivan M. Sharman and Michael G. Down[176] of human swimming performance also found no increased ability after vitamin E supplementation. Sharman pointed out, however, that the earlier work of T. K. Cureton[177] used wheat-germ oil rather than just vitamin E and that Cureton's positive results could have been due to some other component (such as octacosanol) present in the wheat-germ oil. * Many other studies, most of which

---

* Some experiments[178] also suggest sex-promoting properties for wheat-germ oil and octacosanol, although others do not. The work of Cureton[177] has been evaluated by Williams,[178a] who concludes that Cureton established a case supporting wheat-germ oil and octacosanol, but that the evidence is conflicting and the interpretation of results may be open to question. Furthermore, some wheat-germ oil is extracted with ethylene dichloride, a substance which has been found to be carcinogenic.[179,179a] If you purchase oils, lecithin and glandular products involving extractions, ask your supplier for information regarding the extractant used.[179b] Do remnants remain in the oil? One process[182] involves treatment with an alcoholic solution of potassium, hydroxide, activated alumina, acetone and a mixture of hexane and benzene. Exposure to sufficient benzene can cause leukemia (and no one knows what level is "sufficient"). It is

led to results showing no gains in performance using vitamin E, have been analyzed by Roy J. Shephard.[182a] Nevertheless, an unpublished Ph.D. thesis by Y. Kobayaski[182b] is reported to show that 1,200 I.U. of vitamin E taken for six weeks increased aerobic capacity 9% at 5,000 feet and 14% at 15,000 feet with reductions in oxygen debt of 16% and 20% respectively.* In light of such good results, more experiments relating vitamin E to athletic performance should be conducted. Furthermore, A. T. Quintanilha[183] recently found that there was an increased requirement for vitamin E during endurance exercise training.

How Much Vitamin E Should We Take?

If you desire to supplement your diet with vitamin E, it should be taken initially on a very modest basis of perhaps 100 I.U. a day for several days or a week and then gradually the daily intake may be increased to a level of perhaps 400 units. The Shutes recommended slowly increasing vitamin E intake in this manner. Even when this is done it might conceivably result in an increase in blood pressure.** At least, a murine experiment by R. D. Wigley and M. Vlieg[183b] suggests that possibility (Figure 4). They studied blood pressure effects in mice on a low-E diet of 10 mg. daily and those on a high-E diet of 80 mg.

---

frightening and infuriating to contemplate the possibility that even minor remnants of this carcinogen may be in a "health-food" product. A study published by L. G. Rowntree et al.[180] indicated that ether-extracted wheat-germ oil (but not wheat germ) produced intraabdominal cancer (sarcomata) in rats when fed by mouth. However, a follow-up study by L. G. Rowntree and W. M. Ziegler,[180a] as well as other studies by Christopher Carruthers[180b] and by Paul N. Harris, [180c] were unable to replicate the original Rowntree results through feeding crude ether-extracted wheat-germ oil. Nevertheless, Rowntree and Ziegler[180a] produced a substantial number of tumors by injecting rats with wheat-germ oil or other oils. (Werner G. Jaffee[181] found, to the contrary, that wheat-germ oil inhibited the carcinogenic action of methylcholanthrene in rats—a possible *reverse effect.*)

** Wilfrid E. Shute[183a] warned that, while small initial daily dosages of 75 to 100 mg. may lead to a lowering of blood pressure, large dosages of 300 or more mg. daily may cause blood pressure to rise—sometimes for as long as the high dose is continued. (Perhaps surprising to vitamin E enthusiasts, the study shows that the Shutes, in at least one case, prescribed stilbestrol along with vitamin E.)

daily and found that blood pressures rose in those given the greater amounts of "E". At the end of the third month 8 of 16 mice were changed to a low-E diet. At the end of six months the blood pressure of the mice deficient in vitamin E had fallen to that of mice raised continually on the low-E diet (Figure 5). We should note that 80 mg. daily of vitamin E is a huge amount for a little mouse! Then, too, mice absorb vitamin E much more readily than humans do. Thus, a conclusion that use of supplemental "E" by humans must necessarily lead to an increase in blood pressure is not warranted. Furthermore, since "E" acts to prevent platelet aggregation, at some point

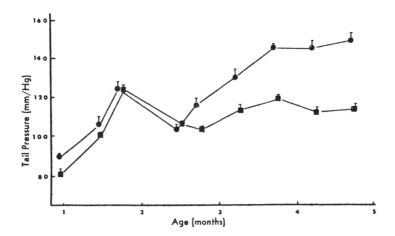

Figure 4. Mice given diets daily supplemented with 80 mg. of vitamin E (high-E, circles) or supplemented with 10 mg. of E (medium E, squares) from weaning. Those given 80 mg. showed a greater rise in blood pressure with age. Equal numbers of male and female mice were used and no sex difference in pressure was shown. The transient rise in blood pressure at 7 weeks coincided with sexual maturation. Reproduced from R. D. Wigley and M. Vlieg, *AJEBAK* (1978) 56, part 5: 631-637, with permission of the publisher.

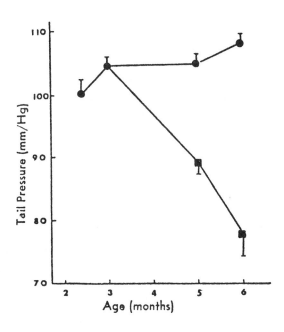

Figure 5. Shows results from 16 mice bred on the high-E diet to three months (circles), when 8 of these were changed to the low-E diet (squares). The pressures of the deficient mice had fallen by six months of age to that of the mice bred on the low-E diet. Reproduced from R. D. Wigley and M. Vlieg, *AJEBAK* (1978) 56, part 5: 631-637, with permission of the publisher.

(with lesser amounts of vitamin E) a *reverse effect* might set in with pressure being favorably affected. At any rate, as far as humans are concerned, an individual report of the blood pressure effects of each of 66 patients by Wilfrid E. Shute et al.[183c] argues convincingly that vitamin E generally works to lower human blood pressures. Whether "E" works at some levels to raise blood pressure and possibly operates at other levels to lower pressure, I think that, if one has a history of rheumatic fever, hypertension or a hyperthyroid condition, vitamin E should be taken only under the care of a physician.*

Some believe that the use of chlorinated water should be minimized (drinking spring water instead) since the chlorine tends to destroy vitamin E. It seems likely, however, that the chloride ion in the stomach's hydrochloric acid is far more destructive of vitamin E. Some acid exists in the stomach at all times but its concentration increases when protein is present. Irrespective of the presence of food, nocturnal and diurnal variations in the acidity of gastric juice have been reported.[185] (Perhaps enteric-coated vitamin E pills will eventually come into common use to overcome the effect of this factor. Meanwhile, consider taking the vitamin on an empty stomach when gastric juice will be at a minimum.) Contrary to the suggestion just given, it is commonly (but perhaps erroneously) held that vitamin E should be taken, not on an empty stomach but with food that contains fat. The theory is that the fat acts as a carrier to put vitamin E into the body. However, M. S. Losowsky et al.[186] found that absorption of tocopherols was not influenced by bodily deficiency, the amount of dietary fat or the vehicle in which they are administered. Furthermore, it is reported that while intestinal absorption of vitamin E is dependent on the presence of bile salts, high concentrations of polyunsaturated fatty acids in the lumen of relevant blood vessels depress the uptake of vitamin E from the intestines.[187,188] Perhaps not surprising in light of these facts, Hugo E. Gallo-Torres[189] cites studies by Schmandke and Schmidt indicating that vitamin E is twice as well absorbed from orally administered aqueous solution as compared to oily solutions. Similarly, L. Jansson et al.,[189a] in studying intestinal absorption of vitamin E in low-birth-weight infants, reported that dl-alpha tocopheryl acetate was absorbed about 1 1/2 times better in a water

---

* Jane Kinderlehrer[184] quotes Dorothy E. Fisher, the head enterostomal therapist at the Pottsville Hospital in Pottsville, Pennyslvania. Ms. Parker, who represents a far less timid view toward vitamin E, says: "When we first started using vitamin E, we were not courageous enough to use high dosages. Now we don't fool around with anything less than 1,200 or 1,600 I.U. daily and it hasn't disturbed anything. There has been no adverse reaction, not even in hypertensive patients." I think such statements may lead many to take what could be dangerous dosages.

dispersible form than when a lipid dispersible form was administered. In like vein, N. E. Bateman and D. A. Uccellini[189b] reported that the absorption of vitamin E (and also A and B2) can be greatly increased if formulated in a liquid vehicle composed of 80% polysorbate 80,* 10% ethanol and 10% propylene glycol. Aquasol® E drops[189h] (vitamin E in an aqueous solution) contains 25% polysorbate 80.[189i] These various studies (and products) would seem to definitively negate the idea that the absorption of vitamin E is promoted by fat. In addition, Fritz Weber[190] cites several other studies showing that polyunsaturated fatty acids adversely affect the intestinal uptake of vitamin E.

Drs. Shute, in their work, have used maintenance dosages of vitamin E as high as 1,600 I.U. per day. Other doctors have reported good results with dosages above 2,000 I.U. daily. However, oil-based vitamins tend to accumulate in the body and so there is danger of overdosage. Franklin Bicknell and Frederick Prescott[191] say: "Nothing is known of where or how excess vitamin E is destroyed, but since it is mostly stored in the muscles it well may be that they not only utilize vitamin E but also destroy any excess. If this is so muscular metabolism might be overburdened by the effort of destroying large amounts. The stimulating effect of large quantities

---

* Use of polysorbates (e.g., polysorbate 80, Tween 20 or Tween 80) may, however, pose some dangers even though polysorbates are widely used in cleaning agents, as food additives and as vehicles for drugs and cosmetics. Tween 20 is reported to be teratogenic in animals, and Ursula Kocher-Becker and Walter Kocher[189c] discovered it "produces malformations with striking similarities to those produced by thalidomide." John B. Barnett[89d] found that Tween 80 depresses humoral immune response in mice. C. M. Brubaker et al.[189e] reported that when rats and monkeys were given Tween 80 orally, degenerative changes in the liver, heart and kidney resulted. In another experiment, the male rat pups of dams who were given Tween 80 in their drinking water showed nervous system disorders. Emanuela Masini et al[89ea] reported that injections in dogs of polysorbate 80 have caused increased plasma histamine accompanied by severe hypotension. Carl J. Bodenstein[89f] asks the question: "Is anyone aware of possible toxicology associated with polysorbate 80 or 20 in neonates, especially small premature infants?" John Butler et al.[89g] discuss the death of five preterm infants treated with intravenous vitamin E supplements containing polysorbate 80. (Intramuscular injections, although often producing tissue trauma at the injection site, are probably safer.) It is hoped that the query of Bodenstein and the infant deaths reported by Butler will not be ignored, but applied not only to the treatment of preterm infants but more widely to question the use of the polysorbates in vitamin E products for adults such as those to promote growth of hair. Astonishingly, several popular nutrition writers are recommending use of these possibly dangerous products.

of vitamin E on phosphorus metabolism in muscle may also be overwhelming."

What about really large dosages of vitamin E? Concerning the possible negative effect of vitamin E on the liver, Evan Shute[192] has said: "I have taken 800 to 1,600 i.u. of vitamin E daily for 40 years and my liver still works well. Others have taken 400 to 8,000 i.u. daily for many years—always with safety." In fact, the *Encyclopedia of Chemical Technology* by R. E. Kirk and D. F. Othmer[193] relates that adult humans have been given 500-600 mg./kg. body weight (i.e., about 35,000 mg. for a 150 lb. person) daily of alpha tocopherol for five months.

Large dosages of vitamin E, as we noted, have been reported to be nontoxic, but Victor Herbert[194] points out that experimental animals injected with large amounts of vitamin E showed a number of ill effects with gonadal degeneration being the most prevalent. Some persons have consumed 40 grams of vitamin E daily for six months without ill effects, but others have shown not only reduced *in vitro* leukocyte bactericidal activity but have also developed headache, nausea, fatigue and blurred vision on the minor intake of just 300 mg./day![194] In another study, 2 to 4 grams/day led to creatinuria, chapping, cheilosis, gastrointestinal disturbances and one case of muscle weakness![194] Consumption of 4 to 12 grams daily for prolonged periods has been suspected of causing interruption in gonadal function (ironic since many men take "E" in hope of increasing sexual potency).[194] If sexual potency is increased by small amounts of "E" and decreased by large amounts, it would, of course, be another example of the *reverse effect.* As reported earlier, natural "E" contains estrogen which might threaten potency and perhaps even be a cancer promoter.

Other studies have shown more numerous examples of muscular weakness following vitamin E ingestion and recovery of strength when the vitamin was discontinued. Harold M. Cohen[195] reported such findings and they were confirmed by Michael Briggs.[196] Dr. Briggs reported that the patients experiencing fatigue showed elevated serum creatine kinase and creatinuria. However, Samuel Ayres, Jr. and Richard   Mihan[197]   reported   that   they   have   given hundreds of patients vitamin E in doses of 400 to 1,600 I.U. daily without observing a single case of muscular weakness or fatigue.

It has been discovered that human lymphocytes seem to be best protected at normal or below normal levels of vitamin E. When human lymphocytes were incubated *in vitro* without vitamin E or with vitamin E at a concentration of 11.6µM (normal concentration in adult blood), there was little effect. Narayanareddy and Krishna Murthy[197a] have discovered, however, that at increasing "E" concentrations the lymphocytes died at an accelerated rate (Figure 6).

There are yet other problems that may be associated with excessive "E" consumption. The processing of vitamin E involves chemical extractants and this can be a very unsettling fact.* Vitamin E is relatively safe but go easy on the megadosages!

I have cited here just a few of the possible problems in consuming excessive amounts of vitamin E. Hyman J. Roberts[201] has written a review concerning both the clinical disorders attributed to excessive vitamin E consumption and the laboratory abnormalities that may be induced by this vitamin. He covers far more problems than I have elected to consider and his article with its 44 citations should be "must reading" for those especially interested in vitamin E. However, the review discusses only detrimental effects and much of the reporting is biased and based on very small numbers of patients. For example, Roberts reports that some patients improved when they stopped taking "E," but he does not mention if those who continued to take "E" failed to improve. On the other hand, Philip M. Farrell and John G. Bieri[202] tell about clinical studies of 28 adults ingesting

---

* Is synthetic vitamin E made under patent number 2,215,398 still processed with benzene? If it is, does it contain any remnants of this leukemia-causing agent? Water-soluble tocopherol derivatives (such as tocopheryl acid succinate) are made under patent number 2,680,749 and may be processed with toluene, ethylene dichloride, benzene or naphtha, at least some of which can be carcinogenic. Ask your health food supplier to find out the extractant used in any vitamin E you are considering for purchase. Information on how vitamins are manufactured (and numerous patent numbers) can be found in *The Vitamins*, vol. 5, 2nd edition, edited by W. H. Sebrell, Jr. and Robert S. Harris. If your curiosity is unbounded, your library can arrange to have *Medline* search for patent numbers relating to any vitamin you specify. After you have the patent numbers, the patents themselves can be obtained for $1.50 each from the Patent and Trademark Office, Washington, D.C. 20231.

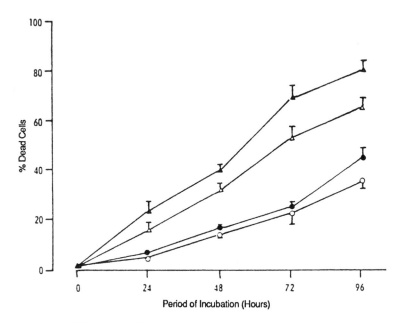

Figure 6. Effect of different concentrations of vitamin E (dl-α-
tocopherol) on the viability of human lymphocytes *in vitro*.
Tocopherol concentrations: (white circles) no tocopherol,
(black circles) 11.6 μM, (white triangles) 116 μM, (black
triangles) 1.16 μM. Approximately 1.5 million human
lymphocytes were incubated in 1 ml. medium in the absence or
presence of vitamin E, and the cell viability determined by
Trypan Blue exclusion. Each point is the mean of five
experiments and the vertical bars indicate standard errors.
Data at 96 hours of incubation are based on four observations
only. Reproduced from K. Narayanareddy and P. Bala Krishna
Murthy, *Nutrition Reports International* (1982) 26, no. 5:
901-906, by permission.

100 to 800 I.U. of vitamin E daily for an average of three years.
Using 20 standard clinical blood tests, they failed to find any
disturbance in liver, kidney, muscle, thyroid gland, erythrocytes,
leukocytes, coagulation parameters or blood glucose. They
concluded that megavitamin E supplements produced no apparent

toxic side effects and the subjective claims for beneficial effects were highly variable.

If, in spite of the possible dangers, one is considering supplementing the diet with vitamin E, how much might it be wise to take? Jeffrey Bland, Philip Madden and Edward J. Herbert[203] reported on some interesting work with vitamin E and the longevity of red blood cells. They found that oxidative damage to the lipids in the membranes of these cells was reduced in human volunteers with an oral intake of 600 units of vitamin E daily. This study might argue in favor of a daily intake of 600 units. However, I think such a conclusion would be premature since, in the Bland study, amounts above and below this level were not studied.

Vitamin, Mineral and Drug Interactions

Vitamin E is widely reported to have a sparing effect on vitamin A and in *small* amounts it does seem to provide an antioxidant effect and thus preserve the latter vitamin. On the other hand, Joseph L. Napoli et al.[203a] have shown, with *in vitro* experiments, that alpha tocopherol affects vitamin A metabolism in several tissues via reduction of retinyl palmitate hydrolase activity. J. C. Somogyi [203b] also reports on experiments that seem to indicate that *large* amounts of vitamin E can have an antagonistic effect on vitamin A. Furthermore, W. J. Pudelkiewicz et al.[204] observed that when chicks were given huge amounts of vitamin A their tissue tocopherol level was greatly depressed. Animal experiments, of course, are not always ideal models for drawing human conclusions. L. Amrich and V. A. Arthur[205] found that vitamin E supplementation in humans increased absorption of a single massive dose of vitamin A but, because of an increased loss in the urine, the net retention of vitamin A in the body was virtually unchanged.

On the other hand, A. L. Tappel suggested, and J. E. Packer et al.[206] directly observed, a favorable free radical interaction between vitamins E and C. The two vitamins operate synergistically, vitamin E radical reacting with vitamin C to regenerate vitamin E.* Thus the Packer group has demonstrated that vitamin C has a "stretching" effect on vitamin E. In other words, less vitamin E is required when sufficient amounts of vitamin C are available. Conversely, when the plasma levels of vitamin C are low, guinea pig experiments have shown it is spared by vitamin E. [206a] E. Ginter et al.[207] also reported that large dosages of vitamins C and E fed simultaneously to guinea pigs on a high-cholesterol diet resulted in greatly enhanced activity of the liver enzyme *aniline hydroxylase*. They concluded that taking vitamins E and C together may greatly enhance the detoxifying ability of the liver. However, when the intake of vitamin C is inordinately increased there could be effects detrimental to the antioxidant action of vitamin E. Linda H. Chen[208] reported that when large amounts of vitamin C were given rats having only marginally adequate amounts of vitamin E *in vitro* erythrocyte hemolysis and liver lipid peroxidation were increased. Thus, the overall antioxidant potential of the animals was lowered. If the analogous phenomenon occurs in man, it might be inadvisable to greatly increase the consumption of vitamin C without also increasing intake of vitamin E. Leung et al.[208a] subsequently reported that when vitamins C and E were present, suppression of peroxidation was approximately equal to the sum of the individual inhibitions. However, at longer time points, there was a synergistic action, i.e., there was an effect greater than the sum of the individual inhibitions. Paul B. McCay[208b] has recently reviewed vitamin E and ascorbate interactions.

Vitamin E should not be taken with iron, copper, estrogen, digitalis, dicumerol or heparin. If you are taking any of the latter three, discuss vitamin E with your physician. Arthur Vogelsang[209] reports a synergism between vitamin E and digitalis that can cause potassium depletion and result in digitalis intoxication. Different studies suggest that other anticoagulant drugs such as warfarin may be potentiated by vitamin E to unduly depress the action of vitamin K.[210,211] If you're a woman on the Pill, or are otherwise taking estrogen, take it 12 hours apart from your vitamin E. Cod-liver oil is

---

* Scarpa et al. (ref. 155b of Chapter 6) has shown that the ascorbate free radical is the active agent in this regeneration of vitamin E.

also an antagonist of vitamin E and it is, in fact, used experimentally to make animals vitamin E deficient.[212,213] Vitamin E-deficiency symptoms were precipitated in rabbits by cod-liver oil even when the oil and the vitamin E were fed on alternate days.[213]

If you use iron or copper supplements, do not take them close to the time you take vitamin E unless you also take vitamin C. * W. M. Cort et al. [214] reported that *in vitro* experiments showed that iron and copper ions degrade both alpha and gamma tocopherol. However, ascorbic acid completely inhibited the action of the metalic ions and protected the tocopherols. Vitamin E in the form of acetate and succinate tocopheryl esters is much more stable, by the way, and is not subject to oxidation by the metals. Nevertheless, in the body these esters convert to the tocopherol form. If metals were taken simultaneously they would oxidize the tocopherol as soon as it formed unless ascorbic acid were also present.

Those, then, are just some of the vitamin E interactions. If your physician has prescribed drugs for you, tell him about any vitamin E or other vitamin or mineral supplements you may be taking. Earlier in this chapter we explored the possibility that vitamin E may be useful in cancer prevention or treatment, but we should also be aware that "E" supplements could interfere with or potentiate the action of anticancer drugs. Adriamycin, for example, is an antitumor drug whose toxicity may be increased by vitamin E according to experiments in treating leukemic mice.[215]

Optimal (as well as potentially dangerous) levels of vitamin E for those also taking vitamin B complex and/or vitamins B2 or B6 may be less than when vitamin E is taken alone. H. A. Nadiger studied plasma vitamin E levels in a group of male volunteers.[216] He found that those taking 100 mg. of vitamin E three times a day had far higher plasma tocopherol levels than those taking the same dosage but also taking the B complex, pyridoxine or riboflavin either singly or in combination. At the end of one month, the plasma vitamin E

---

* Vitamin C may be fine to take with iron, but it can decrease the absorption of copper, as discussed in Chapter 7. The advice here relates only to protecting vitamin E. Best advice probably is to take "E" far away from iron and copper; take "C" with iron but not with copper.

level of those taking only the "E" averaged 1.68 mg./dl. After the same period, the plasma vitamin E level of those taking "E" with vitamin B2 or B6 averaged just 1.13, i.e., about one-third less. A follow-up study reported by H. A. Nadiger et al.[217] found thiamin, nicotinic acid or B12 did not produce similar results. More recently, Nadiger et al.[217a] discovered that 10 mg. of vitamin B6 given twice daily to adult male volunteers along with vitamin E improved $Na^+ K^+$ ATPase activity more than vitamin E alone or B6 alone. The results were interpreted to indicate that simultaneous administration of these vitamins is beneficial to membrane function. Another study, this one by W. V. Applegate et al.,[218] also showed that the actions of "E" and of "B6" are related. They reported that women taking oral contraceptives had lower blood levels of vitamin E. When 1,200 I.U. of dl-alpha tocopheryl acetate were administered for three to four months there was an improvement in hematocrit level as the serum vitamin E level rose. Giving vitamin B6 elevated the mood of 56% of his subjects but almost completely nullified the effect of vitamin E on the hematocrit. This led Applegate to suggest that women on the Pill take both "E" and "B6" but at separate times.

Sources of Vitamin E

Sources for vitamin E, in addition to wheat-germ oil and other polyunsaturated oils, are wheat germ itself, butter, eggs, lettuce, whole grains, milk, spinach, chard, molasses, lima beans, soybeans, beet greens, peanuts, beef, lamb and mutton. The various forms of vitamin E are found primarily in the oil of seeds. Although, as we have seen, alpha tocopherol is the most potent, it is seldom the most common. Sunflower seed oil is an exception; here the alpha form predominates. Wheat-germ oil also contains a large amount of both the alpha and the beta tocopherols. The gamma form is the most common in soybean oil and in corn oil. Delta tocopherol is fairly prominent in both soybean and peanut oils. Oats and barley contain the alpha tocotrienol as the most common form, while the vitamin E in coconut oil is mostly gamma tocotrienol. Margarine contains many of the tocopherols, while butter, on the other hand, has significant amounts of only alpha tocopherol.[219]

Persons taking vitamin E supplements often commonly consume alfalfa tablets. Irvin E. Liener[220] cites the work of E. P. Singsen et al. showing an interference between vitamin E and alfalfa. Later, W. J. Pudelkiewicz and L. D. Matterson found it was an ethanol-soluble fraction in alfalfa that inhibits the absorption of vitamin E. If both alfalfa tablets and vitamin E supplements are taken, it might be wise to separate them by several hours.

The vitamin E molecule is quite large and is absorbed from the intestinal tract with difficulty. When megadoses are being consumed this absorption difficulty, although a waste of money, could be health-serving. Based on animal studies, J. G. Bieri[221] has suggested that tissue levels of vitamin E are proportional to the logarithm of the dosage. If true, this means a 1,000-fold increase in dosage would be required to increase tissue levels just four times. Percentage absorption (as contrasted with tissue storage) is not diminished so dramatically at the larger dosages. In related work, M. S. Losowsky et al.[222] also found that the percentage of vitamin E absorbed falls as the magnitude of the dose increases. More recent absorption studies by Joanna Lehmann[222a] and by Herman Baker et al.[222b] are in substantial agreement with Losowsky. Losowsky's figures suggest that, while percentage of absorption diminishes with increasing dosage, the relationship is certainly not logarithmic. If you are going to supplement your diet with "E", 100 I.U. taken four times a day will put more of the vitamin in your body than will the taking of a single 400 I.U. capsule.

A study by Baker et al.[222b] indicated that higher plasma tocopherol levels were noted after injection of dl-α tocopherol than after the injection of the esterified form, dl-α tocopheryl acetate. They noted that studies by Hugo E. Gallo-Torres[222c] and by M. T. Mac Mahon and G. Neale[222d] showed that bile is needed to emulsify tocopherol preparatory to absorption and so biliary obstruction may lead to a vitamin E deficiency. Baker et al. also cited J. G. Bieri and P. M. Farrell,[222e] who showed that patients with a pancreatic deficiency disease, e.g., cystic fibrosis, may be refractory to treatments with oral tocopheryl acetate since pancreatic juice is required for its hydrolysis preliminary to absorption.

In further regard to vitamin E absorption, Garry J. Handelman et al.[222f] recently reported that oral α tocopherol supplements decrease the plasma gamma tocopherol levels in humans. We noted earlier that gamma tocopherol, which is a common tocopherol in many salad oils, is superior to alpha tocopherol in antioxidant power.

Can Vitamin E Act *In Vivo* as a Pro-Oxidant?

Even though there is no animal or human study showing vitamin E acts *in vivo* as a pro-oxidant, there is evidence that it may act as a pro-oxidant (i.e., show a *reverse effect*) in both nonbiological systems and in cell-culture systems. Perhaps this work will lead to similar studies in animal systems. I think the *reverse effects* that have been shown throughout this chapter suggest that vitamin E may act as a pro-oxidant in the human body.

Telegdy Kovats and E. Berndorfer-Krazner[222g] studied the effects of the antioxidant effects of the alpha, beta, gamma and delta tocopherols in lard. They reported that the antioxidant power of each tocopherol increased as its concentration rose to a level of .01 to .05 mg./100 g. (depending on the temperature) but then showed a *reverse effect* and declined (Figure 7). If the concentration of vitamin E can be too high in lard for maximal antioxidant effect, it seems likely it can also be too high within the human body. Large excesses can obviously cause a loss of power to control lipid peroxidation *in vitro* and perhaps they can also do so *in vivo*.

G. Pongracz[223] reported that *in vitro* experiments with fats have indicated that the optimal effect of tocopherol as an antioxidant occurs at about 200 parts per million. After that, a *reverse effect* (my language) sets in and tocopherol becomes pro-oxidative.[224] The related compound, gamma tocopherylquinone (which is produced in the body from gamma tocopherol) can also act, in nonbiological systems, as an antioxidant at low concentrations. Then, according to Jenifer A. Lindsey et al.,[225] it can show a *reverse effect* (my

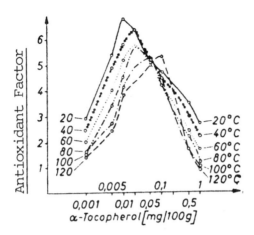

Figure 7. The antioxidant effect of alpha tocopherol in lard at temperatures ranging from 20°C to 120°C. Reproduced from Telegdy Kovats and E. Berndorfer-Krazner, *Nahrung* (1968) 12, no. 4: 407-414, with permission of the publisher. Note that antioxidant power, at various temperatures, rises as the level of tocopherol increases to a range of .01 to .05 mg./100 g. and then shows a *reverse effect* by declining.

language) at higher concentrations and become a pro-oxidant. The Lindsey group found that in a biological system (when cultures of aorta smooth muscle cells were incubated with tocopherols and their quinones) alpha tocopherylquinone enhanced cell growth while the same concentration of gamma tocopherylquinone caused extensive cell death. (This suggests that excessive amounts of gamma tocopherol—so common in salad oils—might be more dangerous than excessive amounts of alpha tocopherol.)

The pro-oxidant effect of alpha tocopherol in grape seed, soybean and cottonseed oils has been discussed by various scientists cited by J. Cillard et al.[226] In studying the autoxidation of linoleic acid, Cillard et al.[227] found the pro-oxidant effect of ∝tocopherol depended on two factors: the concentration of ∝tocopherol($\geq 5 \times 10^{-3}$ mol. ∝tocopherol/ mol. linoleic acid) and the solvent. Subsequently, J. P. Koskas, J. Cillard and P. Cillard[228] reported that ∝ tocopherol in linoleic acid exhibited a pro-oxidant activity at high concentration (3.8% by weight of linoleic acid). Alpha tocopherol at lower concentrations (.38% and .038%) and both gamma and delta tocopherols at high concentrations were antioxidant.* Since vitamin E can act as a pro-oxidant in nonbiological systems, I think it might act, at high dosages, as a pro-oxidant *in vivo* including, perhaps, in the human body.**

Many of the so-called detrimental effects of vitamin E are supported by strictly anecdotal evidence—just as so much pro-vitamin E evidence is anecdotal. We have seen that *in vitro* experiments with fats show that vitamin E's antioxidant action can undergo a *reverse effect* at high concentrations. Furthermore, even at levels where vitamin E is still acting as an antioxidant, an excess could result in inhibition of normal and valuable oxidation processes. Nevertheless, reviewing only what seem to be the better studies, those based on good controls with a reasonably large number of animals or human subjects, it seems that detrimental effects are, in general, associated with daily dosages in excess of 400 I.U. Those who decide to heed the warnings and refrain from using even modest amounts of supplemental "E" will forego its benefits, some of which are well-supported by the evidence. However, the "better studies" are often contradictory, so daily levels should perhaps be kept well below the 400 I.U. level. (Remember, J. Siva Prasad[100] showed that bactericidal activity of leucocytes decreased at a human daily intake level of 300 mg. of vitamin E.)

There is a widespread but false idea circulating among "health nuts," as they like to call themselves, that medical journals ignore nutrition. The many nutritional references from medical journals which I cite throughout this book should help dispel that idea. James

---

* Formation of *trans* fatty acids (*trans, trans* hydroperoxide isomers) was completely inhibited at the highest concentrations of the three tocopherols, independently of their antioxidant or pro-oxidant activity.[228] (*Trans* fatty acids will be discussed in the next chapter.)

** Cillard et al.[227] also reported that BHT, an antioxidant at low concentrations, became a pro-oxidant at high levels. Life-extension studies using BHT are discussed in Chapter 9. I wonder if increased life extension might have occurred if these studies had used lower levels of BHT—levels low enough to make certain the antioxidant effect was operational. Perhaps the use of BHT in life extension is subject to a *reverse effect*.

C. Woolliscroft[114] writes: "Pharmacologic doses of vitamin E may play an important role in future medical therapy. Because of its unique antioxidant properties, scientific investigation is ongoing as to the use of vitamin E in many situations. The future appears to be extremely promising that as our knowledge of vitamin E increases so also will be medical indications for its use as a therapeutic agent."

One could, however, speculate that the future may show that use of vitamin E may not be as promising as Woolliscroft [114] suggested. One should recall that the Sundaram studies (in 1981) [69,70] showed vitamin E to be useful in treating mammary dysplasia. These studies were later contradicted by Sundaram himself (in 1984).[74b] Then too, the former presumed usefulness of vitamin E in immunological responses has been shown to be contradictory.

Recent studies have shown that, in controlled situations, vitamin E is affected by the amount and quality of fat and the amounts of vitamins A, C and B Complex in the diet. Certainly, vegetarians, who normally have a lower fat intake, might conceivably have low vitamin E intakes to which their bodies (including their immune systems) have become accustomed. Vegetarians do not normally use supplements, but if they were to increase their vitamin E consumption via supplementation, might they dangerously reduce their immune responses? Proper dosages of vitamin E and of other nutrients to maintain health or to help cure a disease must be determined with increasing sophistication.

So, then, is the therapeutic use of vitamin E a promising medical tool or is it not? I think the answer lies in determining at what levels vitamin E is likely to exhibit a *reverse effect,* whether that reversal is due to a switch from a role of antioxidant to a role of pro-oxidant or is due to a reversal in some other mode of action. The future for vitamin E may be "extremely promising," as Woolliscroft[114] suggested, but it must be a future based on a dose-response knowledge of the *reverse effect* and not on some idle hope that megadoses are the way to super health.

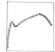

In Vitro Reverse Effects and *In Vivo* Actions

Many of the pages to come will illustrate *reverse effects* using *in vitro* methods. However, it is difficult to relate *in vitro* results to possible *in vivo* actions. The *in vivo* mileau is almost infinitely complex and variable compared with the relative simplicity of *in vitro* conditions. Furthermore, the *in vivo* concentration of each vitamin, mineral, drug, enzyme, hormone or other body chemical may vary from organ to organ. Vitamin C, for example, concentrates in the adrenal gland and zinc in the prostate. Thus, a certain nutrient might show antioxidant action (as vitamins C and E generally do) in most areas of the body. However, in organs concentrating that nutrient a detrimental pro-oxidant action might occur and I speculate that this could be an initiating cause of disease and of side effects. Lipid peroxidation due to vitamin C might conceivably occur even in an organ that does not concentrate this vitamin but instead accumulates iron. An *in vitro* study by David Blake et al.[229] showed that vitamin C in the presence of iron may cause lipid peroxidation in phospholipid liposomes. Could this phenomenon occur *in vivo* in iron-rich organs? Furthermore, vitamin C can concentrate iron in the liver and spleen (of mice) while having no such effect on the heart.[230]

Future physicians will continually face these difficult therapeutic questions: Is it wise to set the dosage of a nutrient or a drug at a level that will promote beneficial actions in most areas of the body while risking a detrimental *reverse effect* in an organ that concentrates that nutrient or drug? How can I set the dosage level to achieve the desired action in my patient while minimizing the risk of side effects caused by a *reverse effect* in a concentrating organ? Much research for generations to come will be required to correlate *in vitro reverse effects* with estimates, organ by organ, of the probable *in vivo* actions of various nutrients and drugs. In the more distant future, *reverse effects* will be controlled by sending nutrients and drugs to specific organs, thereby reducing their entrance into organs in which *reverse effects* might occur. Directed delivery of nutrients and drugs will be achieved by attaching them to carrier molecules with a chemical bond that will be broken only by enzymes in the target organ.

See page 786 for a discussion of side effects.

"When a book doesn't require much thought from its reader, we may be sure it didn't require much from its author, either; when we go through a book 'easily,' it goes through us just as easily.
— Sydney J. Harris, *On the Contrary* (Boston: Houghton Mifflin Co., 1964)

"All history teaches us that these questions that we think the pressing ones will be transmuted before they are answered, that they will be replaced by others, and that the very process of discovery will shatter the concepts that we today use to describe our puzzlement."
— J. Robert Oppenheimer, *The Open Mind* (New York: Simon and Schuster, Inc., 1955)

CHAPTER 3

The Polyunsaturated Fatty Acids (PUFAS)—Formerly Called "Vitamin F"

Fatty acids consist primarily of carbon and hydrogen with small amounts of oxygen. Fats, some common examples of which are butter, margarine, vegetable oils, lard and suet, consist of combinations of three fatty acids and an alcohol named *glycerol* (often called *glycerin*). Fats may be either *saturated, monounsaturated* or *polyunsaturated*.

The fatty acids are long-chain carbon compounds and there are many different kinds. The carbon atoms of the saturated acids are connected by only single bonds, whereas the carbon atoms in the unsaturated ones have a double bond between two or more of the carbon atoms. The carbon atoms with single bonds cannot combine with any more atoms and so they are called *saturated*. Carbon atoms with double bonds, on the other hand, can each combine with one hydrogen atom and so are called *unsaturated*. If there is just one such double bond the fat is called *monounsaturated*. The more double bonds that exist in the molecule, the more polyunsaturated the fatty acid is. If, through the process of hydrogenation, each carbon atom of a vegetable oil is made to take on a hydrogen atom, a saturated product called a *margarine* is created.The percentage of fat in margarine will vary with the degree of polyunsaturation of the initial product and the degree of hydrogenation it has undergone.

The oils contain saturated, monounsaturated and polyunsaturated fatty acids but in different proportions. As indicated in Table 1, safflower oil, for example, is very polyunsaturated with 70.1% linoleic acid, 18.6% oleic (monounsaturated) acid and just 6.8% saturated acid. Sesame oil, on the other hand, has just 40.4% linoleic acid but 45.4% oleic acid and 15.2% saturated acid. Because of its high content of linoleic acid, safflower oil is likely to become rancid more quickly than sesame oil (inside or outside the body). On the other hand, its high content of linoleic acid may stimulate prostaglandin production, as soon will become increasingly clear.

Fatty acids may be consumed with food or may be taken as supplementary capsules or may be absorbed through the skin. Oils rubbed on the skin may be a more rapid way of overcoming a deficiency in essential fatty acids than consuming polyunsaturated oils by mouth. Martin Press et al.[1] reported that in patients having fatty-acid deficiencies because of small-bowel resections, small amounts of linoleic-rich oils rubbed on the skin were very effective. They found that rats fed linoleic acid oxidize about 60% immediately, presumably in the liver. Therefore, a possible explanation of the greater effectiveness of linoleic acid applied to the skin may be that it is incorporated directly into the circulatory lipoproteins.

Fatty acids which are incorporated into soaps and detergents during their manufacture have many antibacterial, antiviral and antifungal properties. Those interested are referred to a book edited by J. Kabara.[2] Included among the topics covered in this volume are two chapters dealing with the anticaries potential of monolaurin Lauricidin®, ester of the saturated fatty acid, lauric acid.

Linoleic, linolenic and arachidonic are the three most important polyunsaturated fatty acids required by the body. The first two are "essential" (meaning the body cannot manufacture them). Arachidonic is not "essential," which does *not* mean that it is of no use to the body. It simply means that the body can manufacture arachidonic acid.

For some body functions linoleic acid and linolenic acid (also called alpha-linolenic acid) will substitute for one another. In other applications, however, linoleic is absolutely essential and linolenic may be essential (although this is still being debated).[3] Linoleic acid is essential, for example, in the sexual development of the male rat. Rats fed either a diet deficient in essential fatty acids or supplemented with only alpha-linolenic acid showed deficient testicular development.[4] Obviously, alpha-linolenic acid cannot replace linoleic acid in the development of rat testes. Brack A. Bivins et al.[5] have recently reviewed the question of the essentiality of alpha-linolenic acid but arrived at no definite conclusion.

These long-chain EPA and docosahexenoic acids are found in plasma and platelets,[7a] as well as in reproductive and nervous tissue, including the retina.[8] Docosahexenoic acid is the most abundant fatty acid in the ethanolamine phospholipids of the retina and of the gray matter in the cerebrum.[8] However, eicosapentenoic and docosahexenoic acid are not as efficiently formed by humans as they are by lower animals.[9] The flesh and oils of fish are rich in these substances and we will consider them and the possible danger of excessive consumption in the next chapter in connection with cod-liver oil.

Alpha-linolenic acid (18:3n-3)[*] is present in flaxseed oil, black and English walnuts, beans, cucumbers, mushrooms, spinach, turnips, bananas and other plant foods.[6] Like linoleic acid, it is used

---

[*] Those untrained in biochemistry (or several years out of school) may appreciate a brief note about nomenclature. All organic acids have a carboxyl (COOH) group in their molecular structure. The designation 18:2n-6 for linoleic acid means that its structure consists of an 18-carbon chain with 2 double bonds, the first of which is located 6 positions away from the methyl end of the molecule, i.e., the end opposite to that containing the carboxyl (COOH) group. Linolenic acid (alpha-linolenic acid) has the formula 18:3n-3, which means it is an 18-carbon chain with 3 double bonds, the first of

as an energy source by the body but, while linoleic acid is stored in fat tissues, alpha-linolenic acid is hardly stored.

Alpha-linolenic acid is a precursor of eicosapentenoic acid (EPA) but probably not to significant amounts in humans. Eicosapentenoic acid (20:5n-3) after further desaturation (i.e., after adding one more double bond) and elongation (i.e., after adding 2 more carbon atoms) becomes docosahexenoic acid (22:6n-3). It had been suggested by J. Dyerberg et al.[7] that humans have very little ability to elongate alpha-linolenic acid to eicosapentenoic acid. Although Dyerburg's conclusion was at one time disputed,[7a] O. Adam et al.[7b] recently reported that α-linolenic acid in the diet did not increase EPA in plasma proteins. (Furthermore, α-linolenic acid inhibited prostaglandin formation and reduced excretion of sodium and creatine when linoleic acid was insufficient.)

The isomer of alpha-linolenic acid, gamma-linolenic acid (18:3n-6), is made in the body from 18:2n-6,*cis* linoleic acid. (Many polyunsaturated acids exist as both *cis* and *trans* forms, terms which will be discussed later in this chapter.) As we will soon see, gamma-linolenic acid (GLA) is very important in the chain of events leading to prostaglandin synthesis. For now, simply note, as I have said, that gamma-linolenic acid (18:3n-6) is formed not from alpha-linolenic acid (18:3n-3), but from *cis*-linoleic acid (18:2n-6). Various omega-3 or omega-6 fatty acids must be synthesized, respectively, from omega-3 or omega-6 precursors or obtained from the diet.

Arachidonic acid is the precursor of many of the prostaglandins, of thromboxanes and of the leukotrienes that we will discuss soon. Some of these products derived from arachidonic acid tend to

---

which is 3 positions away from the methyl end. Gamma-linolenic acid (18:3n-6) and dihomo-gamma-linolenic acid (20:3n-6) are respectively 18- and 20-carbon chain compounds having 3 double bonds; arachidonic acid (20:4n-6) is a 20-carbon chain with 4 double bonds; eicosapentenoic acid (20:5n-3) is a 20-carbon chain with 5 double bonds, the first of which is 3 positions away from the methyl end. Sometimes instead of using "n" in the formula, the Greek letter omega, "ω," is used. Those compounds containing (n-3) or (ω-3) are called "omega-3 fatty acids." "Omega," just as it is the last letter in the Greek alphabet, represents, in this case, the end of the chain of carbon atoms. Thus, "omega-3" means that the first double bond is 3 carbon atoms away from the methyl end of the molecule.

promote platelet aggregation which, more often than not, is a negative factor.* S. Gudbjarnason and J. Hallgrimsson [10] reported that persons dying a sudden cardiac death had a higher content of arachidonic acid in their hearts than did controls. Furthermore, arachidonic acid may engage in a reaction that produces superoxide.[11] As explained in Chapter 9 in connection with superoxide dismutase, superoxide and other free radicals have both good and bad attributes. So, though vital to body chemistry, arachidonic acid should not be consumed to excess.

Free radicals and the lipid peroxides resulting from their actions, while stimulating production of some prostaglandins and leukotrienes, adversely affect synthesis of the valuable prostaglandin PGI2. (PGI2, prostacyclin, beneficially promotes deaggregation of platelets and thus opposes the action of the generally detrimental thromboxane TxA2 that induces platelet aggregation through the release of adenosine diphosphate.)[12,12a] When the concentration of hydroxyl radical scavengers (e.g., DMSO) is high, prostaglandin synthesis (in bovine seminal vesicles, for example) is inhibited. However, at low concentrations of hydroxyl radical scavengers there is a *reverse effect* and biosynthesis of the prostaglandins is stimulated.[13] Hydroxyl radicals stimulate platelet aggregation, and for this reason hydroxyl radical scavengers such as DMSO and glycerol may be of therapeutic benefit in cerebrovascular disease.[13a]

It will soon become increasingly clear that, although arachidonic acid plays many useful roles in body chemistry and is present in body tissues greatly in excess of any other long-chain polyunsaturated fatty acid,[15] I do not think its presence should be encouraged either from dietary sources or via endogenous production.** According to A. L. Willis,[14] arachidonic acid is the most common polyunsaturated fatty acid in most meat products, a

---

* Jacques Maclouf et al.[9a] have presented evidence that arachidonic acid can induce human platelet aggregation not only via the cyclo-oxygenase and lipoxygenase pathways (which will be discussed soon) but also independent of these pathways.

** This statement may be a bit strong. Phosphatidylcholine (available as a supplement in the form of lecithin) is a major source of arachidonic acid and is also a valuable nutrient.[13b]

Table 1
Some Constituents of Some Fats and Oils
In Percentages

Fat or Oil	Palmitic	Oleic	Linoleic	Alpha-Linolenic*	Gamma-Linolenic*	Eicosa-pentenoic	Docosa-hexenoic	Other PUFAS	Saturated
From Land Animals:									
Butterfat	4.6	26.7	3.6	-	-	-	-	8.5	59.0
Lard	2.7	47.5	6.0	-	-	-	-	2.3	41.5
From Marine Animals:									
Cod-Liver Oil	20.1	⟸29.1⟹		-	-	25.4	9.6	-	14.8
From Plants:									
Cocoa Butter	-	38.1	2.1	-	-	-	-	-	59.8
Coconut Oil	.4	7.5	trace	-	-	-	-	-	91.2
Corn Oil	1.5	49.6	34.3	-	-	-	-	-	14.6
Cottonseed Oil	2.0	22.9	47.8	-	-	-	-	-	27.2
Evening Primrose Oil	-	-	72.0	-	10.0	-	-	18.0	-
Linseed Oil	-	19.0	24.1	47.4	-	-	-	.2	9.3
Olive Oil	-	84.4	4.6	-	-	-	-	-	9.3
Palm Oil	-	42.7	10.3	-	-	-	-	-	47
Palm-Kernel Oil	-	18.8	.7	-	-	-	-	-	80.8
Peanut Oil	-	56.0	26.0	-	-	-	-	4.2	13.8**
Safflower Oil	-	18.6	70.1	3.4	-	-	-	-	6.8
Sesame Oil	-	45.4	40.4	-	-	-	-	-	15.2
Soybean Oil	.4	28.9	50.7	6.5***	-	-	-	.1	13.4
Sunflowerseed Oil	-	25.1	66.2	-	-	-	-	-	8.7
Wheat Germ Oil	-	28.1	52.3	3.6	-	-	-	-	16.0

The data above (except for that of evening primrose oil) was taken from the *CRC Handbook of Chemistry and Physics*, ed. Robert C. Wheast (Boca Raton, Florida: CRC Press, 1984) p. D-221. The data was originally compiled for the *Biology Data Book* by H. J. Harwood and R. P. Geyer, 1964, pp. 380-382. Data reproduced here by permission of CRC Press and by the copyright owners of *Biology Data Book*, the Federation of American Societies for Experimental Biology, Bethesda, Maryland. Data for evening primrose oil is from R. B. Wolf et al., *Jrl. of the Amer. Oil Chemists' Society* (Nov., 1983) 60, no. 11: 1858-1860.

---

* Gamma-linolenic acid (GLA) may be more widely distributed than previously thought. Only recently have simple methods come into general use to separate alpha- and gamma-linolenic acids and thus it is possible that some of the alpha-linolenic acid in this table could be GLA.

** Van Duyn et al.[7a] have reported that peanut oil contains a large amount of hexacosanoic acid, a saturated, long-chain fatty acid associated with adrenoleukodystrophy, a disorder of the white matter of the central nervous system and of the adrenal glands.

*** Attempts are being made to improve the stability of soybean oil by reducing the amount of linolenic acid through hybridization among parent plants of low linolenic acid genotypes. Thus, the A-5 cultivar has produced an average yield of 3.8% (compared with the 6.5 in the above table). Ultimate objective is a linolenic acid content of under 1%.[3a] Normal use of soy oil is safe as is moderate supplementary use of vitamin E. However, Paris Constantinides and Martha Harkey[3b] reported that when alpha tocopherol dissolved in soy oil was subcutaneously injected into mice once a week for 10 months it caused development of vigorously growing fibrosarcomata.

WARNING

On page 166, we noted the work of Press et al.[1] showing how readily oils are absorbed via the skin. If you use massage oils over large areas, remember that they will enter your body. These oils, since they are not regulated as foods, could be an unsuspected source of toxins as well as of unwanted calories.

fact that I think lends support to vegetarianism.* Furthermore, N. Chetty and B. A. Bradlow[6b] have demonstrated the platelet deaggregating effects of a vegetarian diet which may be due to the increased concentrations of linoleic and alpha-linoleic acids.

At this time, let's present a brief introduction to prostaglandins and then show how the polyunsaturated fatty acids influence their production. Over 100 natural prostaglandins, isomers and their metabolites are now known to exist.[14] The leukotrienes we will tell about later were discovered just a few years ago and now, as this book was in preparation, the vic-diols (hydration products of several epoxyeicosatrienoic acids) are being studied for their possible effect in calcium metabolism.[14a] In addition, a novel series of compounds, the trihydroxytetrenes, have recently been reported and their biological effects are now being examined.[14b,c] Two groups of Japanese researchers,[14d-f] working with a soft coral plant, have independently isolated the claviridenones, a class of prostaglandins with anti-inflammatory properties. The chemistry and the physiology of prostaglandins and their related compounds are extremely active fields of research. The 1982 Nobel Prize in Physiology or Medicine was awarded to Bengt Samuelsson, Sune Bergstrom and John Vane for their work in this area.

Prostaglandins are hormone-like substances that are manufactured in the membrane of cells. In describing the formation of prostaglandins, Gene Bylinsky[16] says: "Production of prostaglandins can be set off either by muscle stretching or contraction, by injury to the cell, or by the arrival at the membrane of hormones secreted by the various glands. Inside the membrane, prostaglandins act as a crucial signal transmitter, an on-off switch, that passes the hormonal or other message into the cell. There, on the inner surface of the membrane, other messenger substances are manufactured, and those in turn set off

---

* Tropical seafoods also contain significant amounts of arachidonic acid. A report by O'Dea and Sinclair[15a] showed amounts ranging as low as 4.8% of the total fatty acids for oysters to highs of 11.0% for red snapper, 11.1% for catfish and 14.3% for whiting. Cold-water fish, on the other hand, have only trace amounts of arachidonic acid.[15b]

desired cellular activities." Bylinsky wrote this statement well over a decade ago; as we will see, sometimes the prostaglandins and their relatives can set off undesirable activities.

Prostaglandin was discovered way back in 1930 in human semen by two New York gynecologists, Raphael Kurzrok and Charles C. Lieb. They observed that some unidentified substance in the semen was able to stimulate strips of muscle tissue that had been taken from the uterus. It was thought to be produced by the prostate (hence its name), although we now know that it is a product of the seminal vesicles. (Dr. von Euler, who named this substance "prostaglandin," theorized that it had a dual purpose to facilitate the male's ejaculation and to stimulate the muscles of the female's reproductive tract to move in such a way as to aid the sperm in their search for the egg.)[*] We now know that prostaglandins are produced by females as well as males and in almost every part of the body. These substances can lower (or raise) blood pressure, inhibit (or promote) formation of ulcers, open (or constrict) air passages for asthma sufferers, inhibit (or promote) blood clot formation and cause (or alleviate) pain. Enzymes that synthesize prostaglandins have been found in most organs, but some tissues, such as seminal vesicles, kidneys and lungs, have a greater prostaglandin-producing capacity than others.[4] In addition to enzyme-induced production, prostaglandins can be synthesized as a result of simple mechanical stimulation.[16a] Prostaglandins are, in fact, produced in every cell of the body except erythrocytes.[16b] Prostaglandins seem to be paracrine compounds, i.e., they act on cells near their site of origin, rather than endocrine substances that circulate, via the bloodstream, to distant sites of action. They are generally short-lived (with half-lives of 30 seconds to a few minutes) and are converted in most cases to

---

[*] The future sometimes reevaluates the relative importance of a scientist's discoveries. Just as the 1970 Nobel Prize Committee in honoring von Euler failed to mention his work with prostaglandins, so, in 1904, Pavlov was honored with the Nobel Prize for his research on the physiology of digestion while his work on the conditioned reflex was not cited. In granting the 1921 Nobel Prize to Einstein, his discovery of the law of the photoelectric effect was singled out but relativity was not mentioned.

inactive compounds through the action of dehydrogenase and reductase enzymes in the lungs.[16b]*

It has been shown that prostaglandins can bring on missed menstrual periods or induce abortion. (It is thought that the effectiveness of the coil method of birth control lies in the presumed fact that it induces the body to manufacture a prostaglandin which stimulates a spontaneous abortion.) A clinical study by Niels H. Lauerson et al.[16d] has shown that abortion procedures using PGE_2, PGF_2 and 15-methyl analogs, administered through intraamniotic instillation, continuous extraovular infusion, vaginal suppositories or intramuscular injections have a success rate of about 98%. Niels H. Lauerson and Kathleen H. Wilson[17] reported a 98% success rate was also achieved when oral PGE_2 was used to bring on labor.

Prostaglandins affect the release of many of the pituitary hormones, follicle-stimulating hormone, leutenizing hormone and growth hormone. Prostaglandins E_1 and E_2 are also reported to stimulate adenylate cyclase activity, the enzyme that produces cAMP (cyclic adenosine monophosphate) from ATP (adenosine triphosphate).

Kaare M. Gautvik and Mojmir Kriz[17a] studied the effects of prostaglandins E_1, E_2, $F_{1\alpha}$ and $F_{2\alpha}$ and also the effect of thyrotropin-releasing hormone (TRH) on prolactin synthesis in the rat. As dosages of $PGF_{1\alpha}$ or of $PGF_{2\alpha}$ increased up to about 30nM, there was a corresponding increase in prolactin production. Then a *reverse effect* set in and prolactin production decreased (Figure 1). When PGE_1 and PGE_2 were used, an increased production of prolactin resulted up to concentrations of .3 and 30nM respectively, then *reverse effects* set in and prolactin synthesis was inhibited. In the case of TRH, prolactin synthesis declined as TRH was increased

---

* Many of the prostaglandins and the related leukotrienes are available commercially. A report of Nelson et al.[16c] of the Upjohn Co. relates that in the mid-1960s "a million dollars worth of prostaglandin could fit comfortably within a single Petri dish." A 1985 price list of Upjohn Diagnostics shows that today they cost much less but are still far from inexpensive. Ten milligram quantities of the various prostaglandins range in price from $135 to $400. Much smaller 5 mcg. amounts of the leukotrienes range in price from $200 to $300. (A 1,000 mg. tablet of vitamin C, 20,000 times larger than the 5 mcg. leukotriene quantity cited, sells for less than a nickel.)

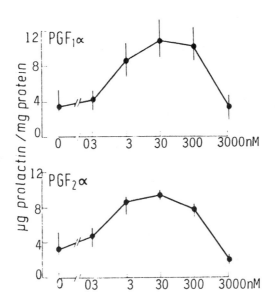

Figure 1. Effects of prostaglandins F₁α and F₂α on extracellular accumulation of prolactin. Reproduced from Kaare M. Gautvik and Mojmir Kriz, *Endocrinology* (1976) 98: 352-358, with permission of the publisher, The Williams & Wilkens Co. Note the *reverse effects* that set in at about 30nM concentrations of PGF₁α and PGF₂α.

from 0 to .2nM and then reversed and rose as TRH concentration increased beyond .2nM (Figure 2). These dose-response effects might have implications not only for lactating women, but in terms of the other effects of prolactin on both women and men.

Not a single prostaglandin can be produced naturally by the body unless one of the polyunsaturated acids is present. Commercially available prostaglandins of many types are or will probably be used for such diverse purposes as inducing therapeutic abortions, bringing on labor at term, providing relief for asthma, normalizing hypertension and kidney function, reducing gastric secretions that in excess can lead to ulcers, relieving glaucoma, increasing fertility,

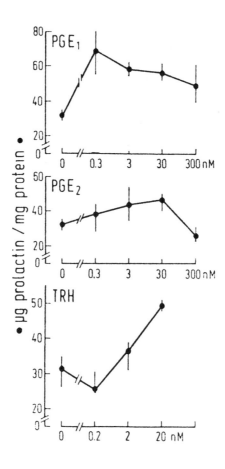

Figure 2. Effects of prostaglandins E₁ and E₂ and of TRH on extracellular accumulation of prolactin. Graph adapted and reproduced from Kaare M. Gautvik and Mojmir Kriz, *Endocrinology* (1976) 98: 352-358, with permission of the publisher, The Williams & Wilkens Co. Note the *reverse effect*, in each case, of prolactin as the concentrations of PGE₁, PGE₂ and TRH changed.

controlling blood clot formation and ameliorating inflammation as in arthritis. They are a group of highly active compounds. Isn't it logical to manufacture sufficient amounts of these prostaglandins in our bodies by consuming adequate (but not excessive) quantities of the polyunsaturated fats? Yes, of course, but optimal quantities for you might be quite different than optimal quantities for me.

The various types of prostaglandins are 20-carbon unsaturated hydroxylated fatty acids with a cyclopentane (5-carbon) ring at the bend in the molecule's hairpin-shaped structure. They are each designated by a letter of the alphabet, A through I, depending on specific combinations of hydroxyl groups and ketone groups on unsaturated carbon atoms of the cyclopentane ring.[17b] The A, E and F series constitute the three major classes. Those with one double bond in their side-chains are called monoenes (the adjective is *monoenoic)* and are known as the PG_1 series; those with two double bonds are called dienes (the adjective is *dienoic* or *bisenoic)* and are known as the PG_2 series; those with three double bonds are called trienes (the adjective is *trienoic)* and are known as the PG_3 series. Note that the subscript, in each case, refers to the number of double bonds in the side-chain of its molecular structure. * An additional subscript α or β is added to F series prostaglandins to indicate the spatial position (stereospecificity) of the hydroxyl group at carbon 9 of the cyclopentane ring.[17b]

Let's observe at this time some of the things that can happen to one of the essential fatty acids, *cis*-linoleic acid, as it engages in body processes leading to the production of prostaglandins. When we consume *cis*-linoleic acid in the form of salad oil or as a supplement, it undergoes desaturation in the microsomes, i.e., each molecule becomes less saturated by the removal of a hydrogen atom through the action of an enzyme called *delta-6-desaturase* with magnesium also participating in the reaction.[17ba]** (Delta-6-desaturase introduces

---

* The primary prostaglandins E_1 and F_1 contain a *trans* double bond between the 13th and 14th carbon atoms, E_2 and F_2 have an additional *cis* double bond between the 17th and 18th carbon atoms. (We will define the terms *cis* and *trans* later in this chapter.)

** The desaturation of linoleic acid undergoes a circadian rhythm (at least in mice). Actis Dato et al.[178] reported two maxima with 32% desaturation and two minima with 15% and 23% desaturation respectively.

a double bond, i.e., removes a hydrogen atom, between the 6th and 7th carbons of the molecular structure.) The result is gamma-linolenic acid (GLA), a substance also obtainable from a diet containing evening primrose oil,[*] mother's milk,[17c] spirulina algae[17d] as well as other blue-green algae,[17aa] or the oil of the salad herb borage.[3a] (Many of the borages[**] are rich sources of GLA, *Nonnea macrospermia* being the most concentrated.[6a] A total of five members of the Boraginaceae are richer sources of GLA than evening primrose[6a] GLA is also present in large amounts in *Scrophularia marilandica* and *Ribes alpinum*.[6a] Other members of the *Ribes* genus are potent sources of GLA. For example, the seeds of gooseberries (*Ribes uva crispa)* and of black currants (*Ribes nigrum)* contain much more GLA than evening primrose seeds.[6c] Yet other sources of gamma-linolenic acid are oil from the seed of the box elder tree,[17e] fungi such as Phycomycetes[17f] and protozoa such as *Tetrahymena pyriformis*.[17f] Gamma-linolenic acid elongates in the body by adding two methyl (CH_3) units, to become dihomo-gamma-linolenic acid.

Observations indicate that the activity of the delta-6-desaturase enzyme system is frequently diminished, thus inhibiting the various transformations leading to the series-1 prostaglandins. There are inhibitors, and also some stimulators, of the transformations that end in series-1 prostaglandin production. D. F. Horrobin et al.[18] cite some of these influences. The conversion of *cis* linoleic acid (via the delta-6-desaturase system) to gamma-linolenic acid (GLA) will be inhibited by fat, by lack of insulin and by aging. The conversion will also be inhibited by oleic acid (as in olive oil), by *trans* linolenic acid (as produced in the hydrogenation process), by saturated fats or by cholesterol. Massive amounts of phenylalanine and tyrosine in the diet are also reported to inhibit Δ 6-desaturase activity.[18a] (Users of

---

[*] The evening primrose (*Oenothera biennis, Oenothera caespitesa* and other Oenothera species), of the family Onagraceae, is also called *tea primrose* and *sun drop*. The bark and leaves have been used for many years as an astringent and sedative. More recently, the seed oil has been found to be a concentrated source of gamma-linolenic acid. It also contains linoleic acid and sterols such as beta sitosterol and citrostadienol.[17bb] Numerous articles regarding the constituents of evening primrose oil appeared during 1983 and 1984 in *Chemical Abstracts*.

[**] Some of the Boraginaceae (e.g., comfrey) contain the poisonous pyrrolizidine alkaloids and consolidine, a central nervous system depressant.

supplements of these amino acids, which are sold by health food suppliers, drugstores and some supermarkets, could be detrimentally affecting this metabolic pathway.) The conversion will, on the other hand, be encouraged by the presence of vitamin B6, or possibly the favorable action of B6 is effective instead at the next step which converts GLA to dihomo-gamma-linolenic acid (DGLA). Body stores of DGLA are also available to be converted to free DGLA and this conversion is promoted by zinc * and prolactin but inhibited by copper and lithium.[18, 18c]** Free DGLA (obtained either from body stores or directly from mother's milk), in turn, can follow either of two pathways. Some of it will immediately form the prostaglandins of the PG1 series. On the other hand, some dihomo-gamma-linolenic acid will be further desaturated to form arachidonic acid through the action of the enzyme *delta-5-desaturase.**** This metabolic pathway, however, is thought to function inefficiently in humans.[20b] Nevertheless, large amounts of arachidonic acid are present in the diet, especially when meat or dairy products are consumed.[14,20b,c]

Arachidonic acid, whether it derives from the Δ 5-desaturase pathway or directly from the diet, follows either the lipoxygenase enzyme pathway (which we will discuss a little later) or, under the influence of the cyclo-oxygenase enzyme system, creates the various prostaglandins of the PGE2 series.[21] The general term "eicosanoid" was coined by E. J. N. Corey to encompass both lipoxygenase and cyclo-oxygenase products of the arachidonic cascade. ("EICOS,"

---

* Simon N. Meydani and Jacqueline DuPont[1b] found that, in rats, zinc was in most cases positively correlated with PGE1 and that either a zinc deficiency or food restriction decreased not only PGE1 but also PGF2α and PGI2 metabolites. (In serum from clotted blood, however, zinc deficiency *increased* the level of the PGF2α metabolite, 13,4-dihydro-15-keto PGF2α. Alan C. Fogerty et al.[1d] however, recently reported that while zinc increased Δ 6-desaturase activity in the liver of rats, it did not do so in the testes.

** Perhaps this is the reason lithium is of value in treating mania, a condition in which the level of PGE1 may be excessive.[19]

*** Arachidonic acid is also produced through the calcium-enhanced action of the phospholipase A2 enzyme acting on phospholipids. Vitamin E is an important modulator of this transformation.[19a,b,20] Triglycerides may be converted, through the action of lipase, directly into arachidonic acid or, instead, into phospholipids for subsequent conversion to arachidonic acid.[19a] While the concentration of arachidonic acid is increased with increasing amounts of linoleic acid, at high levels of linoleic acid there is a *reverse effect* and a slight decline in arachidonic acid is induced.[20a]

Greek for 20, refers to the presence of 20 carbon atoms not only here but in the case of eicosapentenoic acid, etc.) Cyclo-oxygenase products are called "prostanoids" and those made in the lipoxygenase pathway are known as "lipoxynoids."

The Cyclo-Oxygenase Pathway

Cyclo-oxygenase is a heme-requiring enzyme, which is also called *prostaglandin synthetase,* and is associated with membranes. It is inactivated by peroxides and by nonsteroidal anti-inflammatory drugs such as aspirin and this is the basis for aspirin's physiological action.[22] The first of these arachidonic acid products produced via the cyclo-oxygenase pathway (by incorporation of two molecules of oxygen into a molecule of arachidonic acid) is the endoperoxide intermediate, PGG_2. Then, PGG_2, in turn, produces the endoperoxide PGH_2 while generating reactive oxygen species* that may be the cause of inflammation and endothelial damage.[12,12a] A free-radical scavenger, the experimental drug MK-447, acts as an anti-inflammatory without inhibiting the PGG_2-to-PGH_2 reaction and so it seemed logical to assume that free radicals were causing the inflammation. More recently, however, compounds that lack anti-inflammatory ability have been found to scavenge free radicals just as effectively as MK-447. Thus, it now appears that the inflammation may be caused by factors other than free radicals.[17a]

The free radicals, produced during the PGG_2-to-PGH_2 conversion with a life span of only microseconds, probably mediate

---

* F. A. Kuehl et al.,[23] following the lead of R. W. Egan et al., promoted the theory that the oxygen species derived from this reaction is the hydroxyl radical. Daljeet Singh et al.,[24] on the other hand, reported that the cyclo-oxygenase pathway produces relatively small amounts of hydroxyl free radicals compared to those produced in the lipoxygenase reactions. A study by Suthanthiran et al.[24a] also suggests that the hydroxyl radical may be generated by the lipoxygenase reactions, but probably not by those involving cyclo-oxygenase. Then too, the studies of M. Tien et al.[24b] suggest that hydroxyl ions are not active agents in lipid peroxidation. A. Rahimtula and P. J. O'Brien[24c] as well as Richard S. Bodaness and Phillip C. Chan[24d] have, on the other hand, presented evidence implicating singlet oxygen in the action of prostaglandin synthase and the attendant inflammation. On the contrary, Phillip C. Baumann and G. Wurm[24e] recently presented evidence suggesting that neither singlet oxygen nor superoxide anion radicals are related to cyclo-oxygenation. The matter is far from settled.

the further transformation of the endoperoxides. Lipid hydroperoxide seems to be needed to initiate and to maintain this free-radical chain reaction.[24e] Vitamins E and C and also phenol (as found in tea), by serving as free-radical scavengers, act to control prostaglandin synthesis.[23,25]

Prostaglandin PGH_2 then splits into three pathways: it produces the thromboxane TxA_2, with a half-life of only 30 seconds,[27da] which is rapidly transformed to TxB_2; or it produces PGE_2, $PGF_{2\alpha}$ and PGD_2;* or it produces the vasodilator prostacyclin I_2 (PGI_2), formerly called PGX, the major cyclo-oxygenase product in blood vessel walls.** PGI_2, with a half-life of about 3 minutes,[27da] in turn, is converted *in vitro* (and perhaps *in vivo*) to a stable prostaglandin,

---

* PGD_2 spontaneously decomposes under physiological conditions to $PG\ J_2$[27c.] (Although PGJ_2 is about ten times weaker than PGD_2 in its antiaggregatory action, it is more potent than PGD_2 as an inhibitor of L1210 leukemia cultured cells.[27e]

** A vitamin E deficiency is reported to reduce cyclo-oxygenase activity[28a] and therefore reduces PGI_2 synthesis in the aortic walls. This may occur because lack of "E" can cause peroxidation of arachidonic acid, the products of which depress PGI_2 production.[26] These results support the long-existing claim of the Shute brothers that vitamin E is correlated with cardiovascular health. On the other hand, vitamin E (not a deficiency of vitamin E) may inhibit the conversion of arachidonic acid into PGE_2 and $PGF_{2\alpha}$.[26a] In my opinion, this is probably beneficial. *In vitro* experiments by Ali et al.,[26b] using vitamin E with human platelets, showed a 60% inhibition in formation of thromboxane B_2 and prostaglandin D_2 and I think this also may be generally beneficial. Not just vitamin E, but also vitamin C, has been shown, in animal experiments, to increase the production of prostacyclin (PGI_2) in the aorta and elsewhere.[26c,d] (The action of vitamin C depends, however, on the type of cells involved.[27] It activates prostaglandin synthesis in lung fibroblasts. In smooth muscle cells vitamin C activates release, but inhibits synthesis, of prostaglandins. In endothelial cells it has no effect on release, but inhibits prostaglandin synthesis.) A deficiency of selenium has also been reported to suppress formation of PGI_2, probably because insufficient glutathione peroxidase was available to reduce lipid peroxidation.[27a] Respiratory distress in mice that was induced by injections of arachidonate was aggravated in a selenium-deficient group.[27a] More recently, N. W. Schoene et al.[27b] found, in rat experiments, that platelets deficient in glutathione peroxidase produced larger amounts of TxB_2 than did controls.

One must not presume that the action of supplements on fatty acid composition and prostaglandin synthesis in other tissues will be similar to the action in the aortic walls. Elisabeth Schafer and Lotte Amrich[27c] recently reported that dl-alpha tocopheryl acetate supplementation of male weanling rats seemed to have no significant effect on serum prostaglandin synthesis, although the arachidonic acid/linoleic acid ratio was significantly lowered. In the lungs, neither fatty acid composition nor prostaglandin synthesis was affected, probably because of the lung's small lipid content and presumed inability to accumulate excess vitamin E. A study by Mohsen Meydani et al.[27d] found synthesis of PGE_2 in the rats' brain—in the cerebellum, the midbrain and the brain stem, but not in the cerebrum—varied inversely with dietary vitamin E.

6-keto-PGF₁∝. Some of the biological effects attributed to PGI₂ may be due instead to this metabolite.[27f]

Oleic, linoleic, alpha- and gamma-linolenic acids (as found in seeds, nuts and salad oils) inhibit cyclo-oxygenase activity, while saturated fatty acids (lauric, palmitic and stearic acids, as present in meats, eggs and dairy products) do not. The *cis*-polyunsaturated fatty acids (as in salad oils) are more effective inhibitors than their *trans* isomers (as in vegetable shortenings and margarines). The inhibition also depends (in general, directly, but varying with each cyclo-oxygenase product) on the number of double bonds in the acids.[25a] Aspirin, as we noted earlier, is another inhibitor of the cyclo-oxygenase enzyme. The pineapple-derived enzyme bromelain also inhibits the cyclo-oxygenase pathway but is believed to act lower on the arachidonic cascade at the point thromboxane is produced. Thus, it may beneficially inhibit the synthesis of pro-inflammatory prostaglandins while not affecting the anti-inflammatory ones.[25b] Eating onions or garlic can also help to block the synthesis of thromboxane and thus inhibit platelet aggregation.[25c, ca]

Alcohol ingestion may also affect the platelets. D. P. Mikhailidis et al.[25d,29b] found that the coronary protective effect of alcohol may sometimes be due to its inhibiting the release of thromboxane A₂ from platelets. Platelets from alcoholics who were actively drinking were found to be hypoaggregable and to release considerably less thromboxane A₂. Continued abstention was followed by a gradual return to normal platelet aggregation and release of thromboxane A. Prostacyclin release is sometimes affected by ethanol.[25d-dc, 29b] G. G. Fenn and J. M. Littleton[25e] reported that 700 ml. of white wine taken alone by healthy young men had no effect on platelet aggregation. However, when wine was consumed with a meal high in saturated fat (which would otherwise promote platelet aggregation), there was a significant inhibitory effect on platelet aggregation. An epidemiological study by A. S. St. Leger et al.[25f] found that the strong negative correlation between alcohol and ischemic heart disease is accounted for primarily by wine. Consumption of spirits showed only a minor negative correlation, while drinking of beer was positively correlated. On the other hand, consumption of spirits was reported to have the highest negative correlation with hypertensive disease. Studies by Charles H. Hennekens et al.[25g] and by T. W. Meade et al.[25h] support these findings showing that small amounts of alcohol benefit cardiovascular health.

When it comes to *acute* alcohol ingestion, however, it may be another story. Matti Hillbom et al.,[25i] in a study using ten healthy, young male volunteers, concluded that acute ethanol ingestion increases platelet reactivity to produce irreversible aggregation. Hillbom et al. speculate this change in platelet reactivity might sometimes be a factor in causing stroke.

In light of the seeming contradictions, what is a reasonable health-oriented attitude toward alcohol? Whenever there are apparent contradictions, expect a *reverse effect* to be operating. It seems that small, chronically ingested amounts of alcohol (perhaps especially wine) beneficially work to deaggregate platelets. On the other hand, acute ingestion of large amounts (i.e., getting drunk) harmfully hyperaggregates platelets.

The concentration of the many products of the arachidonic cascade will vary with the concentration of arachidonate but not necessarily in a linear relationship. Using an *in vitro* experiment employing a homogenate of beef seminal vesicles, Akio Yoshimoto et al.[25j] found that the rate of formation of PGE$_2$ rose rapidly to a peak at an arachidonate concentration of about $.5 \times 10^{-3}$M and then showed a *reverse effect* by declining as arachidonate continued to increase up to 3×10^{-3}M. (Higher concentrations of arachidonate were not studied.) The amount of oxygen consumed in the reaction followed approximately the same curve (Figure 3).

The nature of the prostaglandin mix that is produced in each tissue will also be determined by the enzyme content of that tissue. For example, thromboxane A$_2$ is concentrated in the platelets and prostacyclin is the principal metabolite of arachidonic acid formed by the vascular endothelial cells in the aorta.[29,29a] The production of prostacyclin may be low in healthy persons but is likely to be increased in those with atherosclerosis as a result of platelet

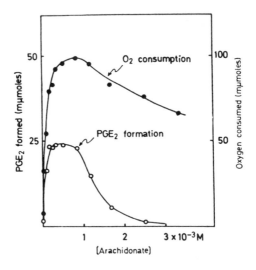

Figure 3. Effects of various concentrations of arachidonate on formation of PGE2 by microsomes of bovine seminal vesicles and the concomitant consumption of oxygen. Reproduced, from Akio Yoshimoto et al., *Jrl. of Biochemistry* (1970) 68:487-499, with permission of the authors and of the publisher, The Japanese Biochemical Society.

interactions with the endothelium. This is in keeping with prostacyclin's role as a local mediator of platelet-vascular interactions.[29a] In human beings, as in rats, PGI2 and PGD2 act antihypertensively and thromboxane A2 and PGF2α develop prohypertensive effects.[29c] When these systems of "checks and balances" get out of alignment, disease may result.

The Lipoxygenase Pathway

Instead of being converted by the cyclo-oxygenase enzyme to yield prostaglandins and thromboxanes, arachidonic acid can come under the influence of the lipoxygenase enzyme. Although "lipoxygenase" is often used in singular form, the lipoxygenases are a group of iron-containing dioxygenases found ubiquitously in plants and animals.[29d,e] Although cyclo-oxygenases from many organs seem to be identical, in contrast there appear to be several different lipoxygenases.[29ea] The lipoxygenases add hydroperoxy groups to fatty acids, but they add them at different locations in the molecule.[29ea] The lipoxygenase will vary from tissue to tissue—the major lipoxygenase in platelets being 12-lipoxygenase and in neutrophils, 5-lipoxygenase.[29e] Each converts arachidonic acid first to a hydroperoxyeicosatetrenoic acid (12-HPETE, 15-HPETE or 5-HPETE) and then into a hydroxyeicosatetrenoic acid (12-PETE, 15-PETE or 5-PETE) and free radicals are formed at this point just as they are when PGG$_2$ is converted from a hydroperoxy to a hydroxy fatty acid.[29e] In turn, 5-HPETE can form the unstable epoxide, leukotriene A$_4$, which is subsequently converted into the other leukotrienes.[29ea]

In the leukocytes, the 5-HPETE, in the presence of reduced glutathione, will tend to take the pathway to 5-HETE rather than the pathway to the leukotrienes.[29f,g] Mark McCarty[29g] speculates that selenium will also foster the conversion to 5-HETE. (Fostering the pathway to 5-HETE rather than to the leukotrienes may have considerable merit in treating those with asthma. In rheumatoid arthritis, on the other hand, there are generally elevated levels of LTB$_4$ in the synovial fluid and of 5-HETE in the synovial tissue.[29h] Favoring one pathway over the other in such cases may be more problematical.) In the platelets, 12-HPETE can similarly follow either of two pathways, the one with reduced glutathione or selenium as probable catalysts going to 12-HETE, and the other giving rise to a group of trihydroxyeicosatrienoic acids (THETE).[29g]

Studies by Ephraim T. Gwebu et al.[29i] found that human platelets preincubated with vitamin E also showed decreased lipoxygenase activity. However, Edward J. Goetzl[30] has shown that the concentration of this vitamin determines lipoxygenase activity. At normal plasma concentrations alpha tocopherol will enhance lipoxygenase activity. However, at higher levels of vitamin E a *reverse effect* occurs and, acting as a hydroperoxide scavenger, it suppresses formation of lipoxygenase products.[30]

Some of the leukotrienes* formed on the lipoxygenase pathway exhibit negative effects such as broncoconstriction[14,33] and this is why I suggested above that, especially for asthma patients, the pathway to 5-HETE might be preferable. Leukotrienes C_4, D_4 and E_4** are components of the "slow-reacting substance of anaphylaxis," which may be an important mediator in asthma and other immediate hypersensitivity reactions.[33a,17a] The leukotrienes also affect leukocyte chemotaxis, lysosomal enzyme release and capillary permeability[33b] (Based on guinea pig experiments, the imidodisulfamides such as SK & F 88046—which is a potent *in vivo* antagonist of LTD_4—are drugs that might be useable in therapy.)[34] Inhibiting the biosynthesis of the leukotrienes may, in fact, be found to be a more effective way of treating asthma than is provided by antihistamines.

Leukotriene B_4 may be a mediator of ulcerative colitis[34c] as well as being a factor in producing acute attacks of gout.[35] Gout is an inborn error of uric acid metabolism, the acute attacks of which are believed to be initiated by crystals of monosodium urate. These crystals are thought to act through their ability to stimulate arachidonic acid metabolism and leukotriene formation in neutrophils.[35] The therapeutic effect of colchicine is believed due to its ability to impair the cell's ability to form LTB_4, which is an active promoter of inflammation.[36] Leukotriene B_4 has also been suggested, by Susan D. Brain et al.,[37] as playing a role in the pathogenesis of psoriasis. Lipoxygenase inhibitors are now used to treat this disease. T. Ruzicka et al.[37a] have reported

---

* The name *leukotriene* is derived from the fact that they were first detected in leukocytes as trienes (compounds whose side-chains have three double bonds). We now know they can be not only trienes but can have four or five double bonds in their side-chains and can be generated not only by leukocytes but by mastocytoma cells, basophils, macrophages, neutrophils, eosinophils, by human lung tissue and probably by other tissues.[30a] The subscript on a leukotriene indicates the number of double bonds in its side-chain. For example, the side-chain of each of the leukotrienes deriving from arachidonic acid, LTA_4, LTB_4, LTC_4, LTD_4 LTE_4[30b] and LTF_4,[30c] contains four double bonds. The leukotrienes of the 3-series, LTA_3, LTB_3, LTC_3 and LTD_3, are lipoxygenase products of dihomo-gamma-linolenic acid metabolism. Leukotrienes of the 5-series, LTA_5, LTB_5 and LTC_5, are lipoxygenase products of eicosapentenoic acid.[31,32]

** Glutathione is used by the body to convert LTA_4 to LTC_4 and the body uses glutamic acid to convert LTC_4 to LTD_4.[33a,c]

LTB[4]-like immunoreactivity in affected skin in atopic dermatitis and suggest that lipoxygenase inhibitors could also be of value in treating this condition.* LTB[4] has also been shown to have many other biological actions.[43] Among these, as shown by Hideki Sumimoto et al.[37d] and by Jeffrey K. Beckman et al.[37e] is the stimulating of superoxide production by human polymorphonuclear leukocytes. (Beckman et al.[37e] have also reported that superoxide can be enhanced by a number of other lipoxygenase products.) W. Martin et al.[37f] in this regard, have shown that superoxide dismutase (which will be discussed in Chapter 9) inhibits LTB[4]-induced leukotaxis. LTD[4] and LTE[4] inhibit appearance of antibody-forming cells in tissue culture,[38] giving added evidence that they could work against the immune system. Sensitive, recently developed radioimmunoassay techniques have permitted detection of leukotrienes in tissues or exudates in several diseases, including not only asthma and psoriasis, but also diverse allergic states, adult respiratory distress syndrome, spondyloarthritis and gout.[43a] The pharmacology of the various leukotrienes has been reviewed by Priscilla J. Piper.[39] Isomers of some of the leukotrienes have now been found and studied.[39a,b] The science is developing rapidly and novel leukotrienes continue to be discovered.[40,41,41a]

If we are tempted to think that the leukotrienes derived from arachidonic acid generally have more physiological "minuses" than "pluses," it may be only a matter of our perception. Leukotrienes and other lipoxygenase products provide many physiological benefits. They are likely to exhibit detrimental effects only if their production becomes excessive. To cite some benefits, R. Reich et al.[41aa] gave evidence supporting the idea that lipoxygenase products may be involved in the process of follicular rupture at the time of ovulation. Then too, M. Chopra et al.[41b] have reported that LTB[4] and LTD[4] act as radical scavengers. Furthermore, C. R. Pace-Asciak and J. M.

---

* Tak H. Lee et al.[37b] recently presented evidence showing that "diets enriched with fish-oil-derived fatty acids may have antiinflammatory effects by inhibiting the 5-lipoxygenase pathway in neutrophils and monocytes and inhibiting the leukotriene B4-mediated functions of neutrophils." Joel M. Kremer et al.[37c] recently reported that, in a double-blind controlled study, patients with rheumatoid arthritis experienced lessening of morning stiffness and of the number of tender joints when they took a dietary supplement of eight grams of eicosapentenoic acid.

Martin[41ba] have reported that pancreatic islets in the presence of 10 nM glucose convert 12 S-HPETE (a hydroxy-epoxide intermediate compound)[41bb] into two hydroxy-epoxides, which they call Hepoxilin A and B, that augment secretion of insulin. Obviously, the leukotrienes and other lipoxygenase products have useful physiological functions. However, their production must be controlled or detrimental effects may occur. Dihomo-gamma-linolenic acid (DGLA) can be converted into a 15-hydroxy derivative that tends to block the conversion of arachidonic acid to the leukotrienes. [14,34a, b] Thus, evening primrose oil, a dietary source of gamma-linolenic acid, the precursor of DGLA, may be an effective way of combating leukotriene-mediated disease.[*]

The fact that leukotrienes C_4 and D_4 can promote the synthesis of the potent vasodilatory agent prostacyclin by human endothelial cells [42] also exemplifies the positive side to their nature. Then too, LTB_4 stimulates the passage of calcium across the cell membrane.[43] Leukotrienes A_4 and B_4, which have been seen to have some negative properties, are reported to stimulate leukocyte formation of cyclic adenosine monophosphate (cyclic AMP)[45] that is needed not only for liberating glucose from glycogen in the liver (glyogenolysis) but for mediating the action of many hormones. [46,47] Furthermore, it seems likely that many additional "pluses" will be found in the actions of the leukotrienes. Nature does not create worthless entities. It would certainly be erroneous to imply that arachidonic acid and its successors are not valuable to body chemistry.

Keep in mind that my quasi-negativity toward leukotrienes refers only to the metabolic family formed from arachidonic acid. Some of the other leukotrienes, on the other hand, may be very beneficial. Those derived from eicosapentenoic acid, for example, may mediate or modulate some of the symptoms of inflammation.[43b] Takashi Terano et al.[43b] reported that an EPA-rich diet not only decreased the inflammation-promoting PGE_2 and the platelet aggregating $Tx B_2$, but

---

[*] If evening primrose oil acts as a drug, and it appears to do so, there may be danger in using it as a "dietary substance." If it is determined to be a drug, it seems likely that the FDA will insist that it be adequately tested for safety and efficacy. Meanwhile, as long as it is commonly available over the counter, caution should be exercised.

increased the leukotriene LTB_5. We will look at EPA further in Chapter 4 in connection with cod-liver oil.

If excessive production of arachidonic acid-derived leukotrienes has, on balance, negative physiological effects, we have yet another reason to make sure our vitamin E intake is adequate. As noted earlier, vitamin E, while not inhibiting the cyclo-oxygenase enzyme that converts arachidonic acid to prostaglandins (and possibly even prolonging its action), at high concentrations inhibits the lipoxygenase enzyme that converts arachidonic acid into the leukotrienes.[20,30]

We have said negative things about some of the metabolic products of arachidonic acid and also cited some good effects. Everything in nature has both a good and a bad side. Certainly, the arachidonic acid product prostacylin is very valuable to body chemistry. It is not only an extremely powerful inhibitor of platelet aggregation, 30 times more active than PGE_1 and 10 times more active than PGD_2, but it also has potent gastrointestinal, anti-ulcer properties.[44] Even an increase in the arachidonic acid product thromboxane A_2, which may contribute to the formation of thrombi and thus will generally be a negative influence, could be life-saving in bleeders who do not form clots readily enough. Various lipoxygenase products of arachidonic acid metabolism also play vital roles in mediating neutrophil, lymphocyte and macrophage functions. Experiments with *in vitro* malignant effusions suggest that patients with cancer may be significantly deficient in 5-HETE and 15-HETE.[44a] The impaired ability of cancer patients to lipoxygenate arachidonic acid may be a factor in their loss of immunity.[44a] As in so many other physiological phenomena, however, it may be difficult to separate cause from effect as well as to separate each from concomitant occurrences.

Tissue Ratios Between Cyclo-Oxygenase and Lipoxygenase Products

Regardless of the "pluses" and "minuses" of arachidonic acid and its metabolites, in a state of disease the proportion of the body's cyclo-oxygenase to lipoxygenase products is likely to be out of balance. Helen G. Morris[48] reported that while the average ratio of cyclo-oxygenase products to lipoxygenase products was 3.24 for platelets from normal subjects, it was only 1.14 for platelets of those with asthma. Males may, in fact, generally produce relatively more cyclo-oxygenase products than do females. At any rate, isolated vessels of male animals have been found to produce more cyclo-oxygenase products compared to the vessels of females.[51b] Furthermore, secretions of the hormone testosterone have been reported to increase as more cyclo-oxygenase products are formed.[51b] Interestingly, in an *in vitro* experiment, this one with rat platelets, a vitamin E deficiency stimulated formation of the cyclo-oxygenase products thromboxane (TxB_2) and $PGF_2\alpha$, but did not affect formation of lipoxygenase products.[52] Another *in vitro* experiment, this one with human platelets, showed that high concentrations of vitamin E depressed formation of the cyclo-oxygenase products TxB_2, $PGF_2\alpha$, PGE_2 and PGD_2.[52a] (However, we saw earlier that vitamin E stimulates the formation of the cyclo-oxygenase product prostacyclin in the endothelial cells of the arterial wall.[26] We must keep in mind, however, that cyclo-oxygenase activity in platelets does not indicate the amount of cyclo-oxygenase activity in the arterial wall.[52b] The effects of vitamin E depend on the tissue involved. A *deficiency* of vitamin E *increases* the platelet-derived prostaglandin level in the serum but *decreases* production of prostaglandins in the muscles, bursas, spleen and testes.)[48a,b] At unphysiologically low concentrations of vitamin E—as in the experiment with rat platelets[52]—there was a *reverse effect* and creation of cyclo-oxygenase products was enhanced.[52a]

We have seen that, along with other physiological entities, arachidonic acid and its products are detrimental or beneficial in terms of their concentration and/or proportional representation in body tissues. Human colonic tissue converts arachidonic acid into both cyclo-oxygenase and lipoxygenase products. When the lipoxygenase products are present in excess, this may lead to inflammatory bowel disease.[52c] Let's not conclude, however, that it is always wise to promote production of cyclo-oxygenase products

(continued on page 193)

Some Speculations on the Treatment of Asthma

Histamine was, at one time, considered to be the main chemical involved in allergic reactions, including inflammation and contraction of the smooth muscle of the respiratory tract. It is now known that leukotrienes can be far more powerful in their allergic effects. Leukotrienes have also been shown to stimulate production of mucus both *in vitro* and *in vivo*.[48c] Furthermore, modulation of the ratio between cyclo-oxygenase and lipoxygenase products of arachidonic acid metabolism could be a factor in the control of these effects.

The work of Helen G. Morris[48] suggests that persons with asthma might benefit from an increase in the proportion of cyclo-oxygenase to lipoxygenase arachidonic acid products. * The sophistication needed, however, to modify such a ratio is indicated by an experiment of Karen G. Rothberg and Margaret Hitchcock.[49] It involved an *in vitro* study using lung tissue of vitamin C-deficient guinea pigs at different levels of arachidonic acid from 10 to 100 µM. They found the biosynthesis of cyclo-oxygenase metabolites (especially $PGF_{2\alpha}$) was high at low levels of arachidonic acid (10 µM), increased further at 20 µM, but then showed a *reverse effect* and was lower at 100 µM. Should the *reverse effect* be taken into account when treating asthma patients? Should we work to achieve an arachidonic acid concentration in the lungs of about 20 µM in the attempt to raise the asthma patients' cyclo-oxygenase products? Perhaps we should, but not *necessarily,* since the experiment was done on vitamin C-deficient guinea pigs—not on vitamin C-replete

---

* Lawrence Levine and Nancy Worth[48d] reported, based on an *in vitro* study, that eicosapentenoic acid (from marine oils) causes a decrease in cyclo-oxygenase products and may slightly increase lipoxygenase products. In asthma control, however, our concern is with the control of arachidonic acid products, not with those of eicosapentenoic acid.

humans. The Rothberg and Hitchcock study and my warning about a possible *reverse effect* could, however, provide guidance for human research. (An earlier experiment by Pugh et al.[49a] found a *biphasic reverse effect* of ascorbic acid in the production of prostaglandin F in guinea pig uterine homogenates. Perhaps varying quantities of vitamin C may affect the prostaglandin F content of other tissues also, not only in the guinea pig but in humans. Asthma patients, remember, often take vitamin C, which could be causing a *reverse effect* in their prostaglandin F production. Such possible *reverse effects* should not be ignored by therapists.

An *in vitro* experiment showed that the antioxidant BHA increased lipoxygenase activity,[50] which is the wrong direction to go in to help asthmatic patients. (At higher concentration, BHA shows a *reverse effect* and depresses both cyclo-oxygenase and lipoxygenase activity.)[50] I think for successful asthmatic treatment we may need to modify the arachidonic acid products in a way opposite to that provided by modest amounts of BHA (i.e., low amounts of this preservative, widely used in foods, could be detrimental to those with asthma, while higher concentrations might possibly be of value). Various selective inhibitors of platelet arachidonic acid metabolism (especially acetylenic analogs) have been studied by Alvin R. Sams et al.[51] and several will inhibit lipoxygenase activity without affecting cyclo-oxygenase activity. Furthermore, Kenneth R. McLeish et al.[51a] and K. Miyazawa et al.[51aa] reported that the antioxidant nordihydroguaiaretic acid (NDGA) inhibits the lipoxygenase activity, while Rao V. Panganamala and David G. Cornwell[20] confirmed an earlier finding by A. L. Tappel that vitamin E also effectively inhibits this enzyme activity. The antioxidant propyl gallate is also known to preferentially inhibit the lipoxygenase pathway compared to the cyclo-oxygenase pathway.[51ba] Yuhei Hamasaki and Hsin-Hsiung Tai[51c] have found that gossypol, the male antifertility drug derived from cotton, is a potent and specific inhibitor of arachidonate 5- and 12-lipoxygenases which initiate biosynthesis of leukotrienes. Tanihiro Yoshimoto et al.[51ca] found that various bioflavonoids (especially cirsiliol) *in vitro* inhibited arachidonate 5-lipoxygenase and, to a lesser degree, 12-lipoxygenase. Then too, J. M. Bailey et al.[34b] have discovered that a 15-lipoxygenase product derived from DGLA is a potent inhibitor of leukotriene biosynthesis. These various substances should therefore be considered by therapists for possible use in alleviating asthma symptoms.

A study by Per Hedqvist et al.,[51d] using the leukotriene synthesis inhibitor piriprost, showed that leukotrienes, but not cyclo-oxygenase products, are mediators of acute airway response to allergen in guinea pigs. This helps support the suggestion that successful manipulation of the products of the cyclo-oxygenase and lipoxygenase pathways may provide effective relief for asthma patients.

(continued from page 190)

over those formed in the lipoxygenase pathway. Cyclo-oxygenase activity appears to be increased in diabetic animals and perhaps is increased in human diabetics also.[29b] Arachidonic acid and its lipoxygenase metabolites, in the presence of glucose, as shown by an *in vitro* study of Stewart Metz et al.,[52d] led to increased insulin release (Figure 4).* Arachidonic acid and the integrity of the lipoxygenase pathway are obviously important for proper use of glucose by the body. It is apparent that it is important to maintain a healthy balance among the metabolites produced in the body's major metabolic pathways. Nevertheless, I think it may often be appropriate to favor production of the 1-series prostaglandins over both cyclo-oxygenase and lipoxygenase products of arachidonic acid as can be accomplished by eating a more vegetarian diet and/or through supplementing with evening primrose oil. But now, after this lengthy excursion relating to arachidonic acid and the delta-5-desaturase

---

* An earlier study of Metz,[52da] however, found that PGE inhibits insulin secretion. Sumer Pek et al.[52db] even earlier, had found that at some concentrations PGE_1, PGE_2 and $PGF_{2\alpha}$ *in vitro* stimulate the release of insulin and glucagon. L. Best and W. J. Malaisse[52dc] comment on the "bell-shaped" dose-response curves of prostaglandin pharmacology and the stimulatory or inhibitory effects on insulin secretion, i.e., *reverse effects.*

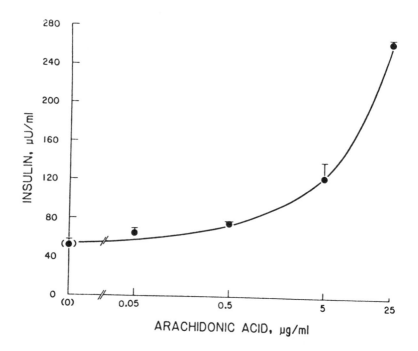

Figure 4. Effect of varying concentrations of arachidonic acid on insulin release in the presence of glucose, 300 mg./dl., over a static, 1-h incubation period. Reproduced from Stewart Metz et al., *Jrl. of Clinical Investigation* (1983) 71: 1191-1205, with permission of the authors and of the copyright holder, The American Society for Clinical Investigation.

enzyme system that led to arachidonic acid, we will return to follow dihomo-gamma-linolenic acid (DGLA) through the body. But this time, instead of traveling the delta-5-desaturase pathway to arachidonic acid, we will follow DGLA as it goes directly to the series-1 prostaglandins.

Prostaglandins and Alcoholic Intoxication

D. F. Horrobin has suggested[19] that the euphoric phase of alcoholic intoxication may be associated with high-PGE_1 production. The depressed phase that follows may be due to low PGE_1 production because of a depletion of DGLA stores. Furthermore, many alcoholics are depressed before they drink because of depleted DGLA and PGE_1. Therefore, they may drink to relieve that depression (which alcohol does by increasing PGE_1). If a deficiency of PGE_1 is a factor in increasing and fostering alcoholism, a supplemental intake of linoleic acid and GLA may be protective.*

On the other hand, a depletion of essential fatty acids can increase formation of fibrous tissue and so this depletion of DGLA by alcohol could be a mechanism for bringing on cirrhosis of the liver. Supplemental PGE_1 is, in fact, reported to prevent alcohol-induced fatty liver in rats.[53] Finally, if the depletion of PGE_1 is an important contribution to alcohol's other physiological effects, then linoleic acid and GLA (as in evening primrose oil) may be useful in alleviating hangovers. J. Lieb[54] has reported preliminary indications that this line of reasoning may be correct. The popular belief that alcohol itself helps cure hangovers can also be explained by its fostering new production of PGE_1. (Perhaps this prostaglandin facilitates production of opioids in the brain, the probable immediate cause of alcohol-induced euphoria.)

---

* GLA, administered as evening primrose oil, greatly reduced the embryopathic activity of ethanol in animals.[52a] Could it protect against the congenital anomalies found in infants of alcoholic mothers?

Transforming DGLA to the 1-Series Prostaglandins

Transformation of the DGLA into PGE₁ and into other series-1 prostaglandins is promoted by reduced glutathione in combination with an antioxidant,[52e] by vitamin C[7], by many other antioxidants and by ethanol (yes, the kind of alcohol some of us drink).* Alcohol's beneficial action in promoting this conversion is, however, offset by its blocking of GLA formation and by its depletion of DGLA stores.[52g] On the other hand, the DGLA-to-PGE₁ transformation is inhibited by wheat, by peptides from milk protein and by opiates. Digestion of several food proteins including gliadin (found especially in wheat and rye) and alpha-casein (found in milk and cheese) produces fragments (peptides) with opiate activity. To the extent they are absorbed, this could be detrimental to the production of PGE₁.[55]

PGE₂, an arachidonic acid product, acts oppositely to PGE₁ in platelets, i.e., PGE₂ promotes platelet aggregation while PGE₁ fosters deaggregation. (In most other tissues PGE₁ and PGE₂ are reported to exhibit similar pharmacological effects.)[56] Since we usually desire to promote platelet deaggregation, this gives us another reason to encourage production of PGE₁. Orally ingested DGLA has considerable power (since it leads to PGE₁ production) to foster platelet deaggregation and thus work to prevent thromboses. Orally ingested DGLA has, in fact, been reported to have considerable potential for preventing and treating human thromboembolic disease.[57]

Both DGLA and arachidonic acid are present in most, if not all, cells of the body. However, the amount of arachidonic acid (AA) greatly exceeds that of DGLA by 10- to 40-fold (except in the human liver where the excess of AA over DGLA is about 4-fold). Thus, when quantities of *cis*-linoleic acid and/or DGLA are inadequate, the free supplies   of   DGLA   will   be   depleted,   while   the

---

* Ethanol also affects arachidonic acid metabolism. *In vitro* studies have shown that when free arachidonic acid is depleted, ethanol caused a *decrease* in arachidonic acid metabolites.[52f] However, both *in vivo* and *in vitro* studies indicate that when exogenous arachidonic acid is added, i.e., when free arachidonic acid is present, ethanol *enhances* production of prostaglandin products, including the leukotrienes.[52f]

amounts of AA will be relatively unaffected. Therefore, our proper concern would seem to be to have sufficient DGLA present and to promote its conversion to PGE$_1$ rather than to worry about the arachidonic acid unless perhaps the concern might be to reduce its presence. PGE$_1$ itself, according to M. B. Feinstein et al.,[57a] may be a regulator of the AA transformations (the arachidonic cascade). At any rate, PGE$_1$ has been shown to block mobilization of free arachidonic acid in blood platelets. Perhaps consumption of strong dietary sources of AA (such as peanut oil) should be reduced.

How can we defend the especially good notice given to PGE$_1$ (and to evening primrose oil that increases its production by the body)? D. F. Horrobin et al.[18] state that PGE$_1$ *in vitro* acts like thymic hormone in causing maturation of T lymphocytes. Horrobin further reports that thymus atrophy in mice can be prevented by treating them with GLA in the form of evening primrose oil. Perhaps this stimulation of the immune function might work synergistically with vitamin C to combat infection but only, of course, if enough DGLA were present to promote production of PGE$_1$.* At high doses of PGE$_1$ there is, however, not only a *reverse effect* in the maturation rate of T lymphocytes but a reduction in lymphocyte-mediated cytotoxicity and a depressing of various types of immune responses.[18,57f,g,58,96] More will be said about PGE$_1$ in relation to the immune system later in this chapter. For now, let's simply note that the overproduction of PGE$_1$ might sometimes be detrimental and this should be kept in mind by members of the public who may be tempted to overdose on evening primrose oil.

Another problem of excess PGE$_1$ is that it may detrimentally affect stomach acid. *In vitro* rat experiments have shown PGE$_1$[57b] or

---

* Perhaps the widely varying reports regarding vitamin C's effect in treating many conditions from colds to cancer may relate to the presence or absence of DGLA available for "C" to help convert it into PGE$_1$. Perhaps it is PGE$_1$ that is causing the presence or absence of effects from vitamin C supplementation. If so, it seems to me that someone should perform experiments in cold-fighting with one group taking mega-C without evening primrose oil and the other group mega-C with evening primrose oil. If the results are interesting, the study should be extended to include experimental treatment of cancer. (I am calling for studies of a substance that has not been adequately tested for safety. I do not desire to encourage the unsupervised use of evening primrose oil by the public.)

PGE$_2$[57c] suppressed gastric acid secretion. Subsequently, R. Befrits and C. Johansson[57d] found that oral PGE$_2$ inhibited gastric acid secretion in five healthy young men. If oral PGE$_1$ acts similarly, this might be another negative for evening primrose oil. Then too, Jan Nilsson and Anders G. Olsson[57e] have found that PGE$_1$ inhibited DNA synthesis in smooth muscle cells of the rat that had been stimulated with human platelet-derived growth factor. These "negatives" suggest that the increased production of PGE$_1$ (and the consumption of evening primrose oil) should generally not be encouraged for those without problems. On the other hand, the "positives" for increased production of PGE$_1$ in those having various problems including high blood pressure suggest that a vegetarian diet or increased use of oils containing linoleic or gamma-linolenic acid (such as evening primrose oil) may be of value.

Some Interesting Prostaglandin Effects

M. S. Manku et al.[58a] found some interesting effects when various concentrations of prostaglandins E$_1$, E$_2$, A$_1$, A$_2$ and F$_{2\alpha}$ ranging from 10 to 10^5 pg./ml. (2.8×10^{-11} to 2.8×10^{-7}M) were perfused through a rat mesenteric vascular bed. As shown in Figure 5, prostaglandins E$_2$, A$_1$ and F$_{2\alpha}$ markedly potentiated responses to noradrenaline at all concentrations studied. (*Reverse effects* could conceivably have taken place at other concentrations.) On the other hand, prostaglandin E$_1$ and A$_2$, up to concentrations of 10 pg./ml. potentiated responses to noradrenaline. Each then showed a *reverse effect* with lessening potentiation and, a bit past 10^3 pg./ml., potentiation turned to inhibition.

In a follow-up study, Manku et al.[58b] again perfused the mesenteric artery of the rat with PGE$_1$ and reported interesting effects on the artery's response to noradrenaline and angiotensin. Since an increase in the action of noradrenaline and angiotensin may be a factor in raising blood pressure, the effect of PGE$_1$ on the artery is of vital concern. At low PGE$_1$ concentrations, responses to

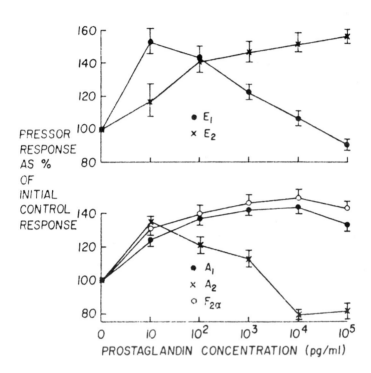

Figure 5. The effects on the pressor response to 10 ng. noradrenaline of adding increasing amounts of PGs E_1, E_2, A_1 and $F_{2\alpha}$ to the perfusate. Each concentration was maintained for 20 minutes and the response amplitude at the end of 20 minutes noted. Responses were expressed as percentages of the responses obtained before addition of any PG to the perfusate. Each PG was tested on six preparations. Each point represents a mean and ± SEM. Also observe the *reverse effects* shown by PGE₁ and PGA₂ are not simply reverses from a greater to a lesser increase in pressor response, but to an actual inhibition of pressor response. (This is shown by the graphs dipping under 100.) Reproduced from M. S. Manku et al., *Prostaglandins* (1977) 13: 701-710, with permission. Note the favorable effects of PGE₁ and PGA₂ (that translate into blood pressure-lowering effects) and the unfavorable effects of PGE₂, PGA₁ and PGF₂α.

noradrenaline and angiotensin were potentiated. Then, at higher concentrations above 10^{-11} M, there was a *reverse effect* and the action of each was decreasingly potentiated (Figure 6) and the potentiation was converted to inhibition above 10^{-7} M. No concentrations of PGE1 had any effect on potassium responses. On the other hand, PGE2 potentiated pressor responses to noradrenaline and potassium (Figure 7) and to angiotensin. (In a subsequent study, Manku et al.[58c] found that prolactin and dihomo-gamma-linolenic acid, like PGE1, each potentiated norepinephrine responses at low concentrations but slowed *reverse effects* at higher concentrations.) Prostacyclin (not shown) inhibited responses to noradrenaline and angiotensin but had no effect on potassium responses.[58b] To reduce hypertension it seems that we should, if possible, increase the arterial concentration of PGE1 to a value well above 10^{-11} M and also increase the concentration of prostacyclin but reduce that of PGE2.

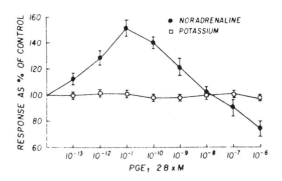

Figure 6. Changes in response amplitude to fixed doses of potassium and noradrenaline in the presence of increasing concentrations of PGE1 Results are expressed as percentages of response amplitudes in the absence of PGE1. Each point represents the mean ± SEM for six experiments. Reproduced from M. S. Manku et al., *Biochemical and Biophysical Research Comm.* (1978) 83, no. 1: 295-299, with permission of the publisher, Academic Press.

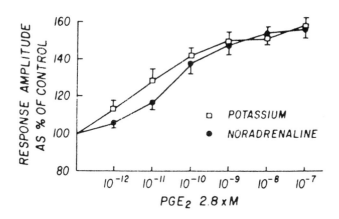

Figure 7. Changes in response amplitude to fixed doses of potassium and noradrenaline in the presence of increasing concentrations of PGE₂. Results are expressed as percentages of response amplitudes in the absence of PGE₂. Each point represents the mean ± SEM for six experiments. Reproduced from M. S. Manku et al., *Biochemical and Biophysical Research Comm.* (1978) 83, no. 1: 295-299, with permission of the publisher, Academic Press.

Linoleic Acid and GLA for Normalizing Blood Pressure

Linoleic acid and gamma-linolenic acid, probably because they foster production of prostaglandin E₁, are important to heart health. F. ten Hoor,[59] summarizing the cardiovascular effects of diet, reported that patients who ate a high-linoleic diet showed a lower cardiovascular death rate. He stated also that salt-induced hypertension in rats could be prevented and cured by a high-linoleic diet. In a study with spontaneously hypertensive rats, P. Hoffman et al.[60] reported that, although the blood pressure of all the rats increased with age, those fed evening primrose oil had the least rise.[*] Linseed oil was next best and then sunflowerseed oil. Rats fed hydrogenated palm kernel oil showed the greatest increase in blood pressure. Furthermore, in man, several experiments including a study by Peter Oster et al.[61] and one by H. U. Comberg et al.[62] showed a decreasing tendency of blood pressure with a diet enriched with linoleic acid.

Scores of studies in animals and in humans have reported similar findings. The results may be due, at least in some degree, to increased urinary sodium concentration and urinary volume.[63] However, a decrease in dietary linoleic acid may result in increased blood pressure (and an increased intake of linoleic acid result in a reduction of excessive blood pressure) regardless of the sodium content of the diet.[64,64a] A. J. Vergroesen et al.[64a] observed significant decreases in diastolic pressures of borderline hypertensives during a period when they were consuming moderately increased amounts of dietary linoleic acid. The investigators also found a significant increase in creatine excretion and clearance. They interpreted this as indicating improvement in kidney function, which might partially explain the blood pressure-lowering effect. In a related study using 24 young adults, Olaf Adam and Gunther Wolfram[64b] compared a linoleic acid intake of zero and one of 20 energy % (i.e., 20% of their energy needs) and found an 8% increase in sodium and 16% in creatine in their 24-hour urine on the fifth day of the high-linoleic-acid diet.

On the other hand, P. Singer et al.[65] reported that genetically determined hypertension in rats could not be benefited by linoleic acid. Furthermore, a study by G. J. Mogenson and B. M. Box[66] seems to contradict the Hoffman study reported above. Mogenson and Box reported that the effect of linoleic acid on spontaneously hypertensive rats was detrimental as compared with a beneficial effect of linoleic acid on rats having salt-induced hypertension. This

---

[*] The potent factor of evening primrose oil is gamma-linolenic acid which is converted in the body to dihomo-gamma-linolenic acid (DGLA). Cedrick H. Hassall and Stephen J. Kirtland[60a] reported that hypertension induced in rats by a diet rich in saturated fat (16% coconut oil, 4% palmitic acid) was reversed by the addition of DGLA at 5% but not at .5% of dietary energy.

warns us that there may be hypertensive humans whose condition bears no relation to salt intake, and such persons might even react detrimentally to an increased intake of linoleic acid. *Reverse effects* are subtle and pervasive!

Other scientists, although finding linoleic acid beneficial in reducing blood pressure, have ascribed a different reason for its favorable action. Rainer Düsing et al.[67] concluded that rats deprived of linoleic acid produced reduced amounts of arachidonic acid and thus deficient amounts of prostacyclin (PGI_2) which, acting oppositely to PGE_2,* works like PGE_1 to lower blood pressure. P. Hoffman et al.[73] found that spontaneously hypertensive rats on a diet deficient in linoleic acid produced relatively high amounts of $PGF_{2\alpha}$ and they concluded that this was a factor in their hypertension. (N. W. Schoene et al.[73a] have stated, in agreement with Hoffman, that a linoleic acid-supplemented diet beneficially shifted the PG synthesis away from $PGF_{2\alpha}$.) Most scientists conclude that an adequate amount of linoleic acid has a beneficial effect on blood pressure, only the relative importance of the various modes of action being debatable.

A study by James M. Iacono et al.[74] of normotensive and mildly hypertensive 40- to 60-year-old men and women showed beneficial blood pressure reductions when the dietary ratio of polyunsaturated fat to saturated fat was maintained at about 1.0 with fat providing 25% of total energy intake. When the diet of the subjects was returned to its former polyunsaturated-to-saturated-fat ratio, their blood pressures returned to their pretreatment levels. In another study,[75] this one done in Finland, a group on a low-fat diet (23% of energy) with a high polyunsaturated-fat/saturated-fat ratio (1:1) showed a

---

* There are many studies showing that PGE_2 elevates blood pressure.[68] However, Christopher L. Melby[69] reports, to the contrary, that PGE_2 acts as a vasodilator and *lowers* blood pressure. Louis Tobian et al.[70] similarly report that PGE_2 lowers blood pressure in rats. Since PGI_2 and PGE_2 are created simultaneously, I wonder if one group of investigators is incorrectly attributing the effects to PGE_2, or perhaps a dose-responsive *reverse effect* might be involved. When arachidonic acid is administered, there is an increased urinary output of prostaglandins, mainly PGE_2.[71] Prostacyclin (PGI_2) is reported to be the predominant metabolic product of arachidonic acid in blood vessels,[72] and as far as blood pressure is concerned this would be of more importance than urinary output. It would be easy, but perhaps incorrect, to attribute blood pressure-lowering effects to PGE_2 that may be due to prostacyclin.

decline in average systolic pressure from 138.4 to 129.5 mm. Hg. and in average diastolic pressure from 88.9 to 81.3 mm. Hg. A second group on a reduced salt intake, and a control group eating their usual diet, experienced little change in mean blood pressure. By the way, suggestions for a multifaceted dietary approach to blood pressure reduction are summarized in the potassium section of Chapter 7.

Treating Other Diseases with Linoleic Acid, GLA and Prostaglandins

Not only blood pressure, but the incidence of coronary heart disease may be favorably influenced by increased dietary linoleic acid. D. A. Wood et al.[76] reported that in 28 men (aged 45-54) recently diagnosed as having coronary heart disease, adipose tissue linoleic acid and dihomo-gamma-linolenic acid were lower than in 336 control subjects. (They did not find, however, significant differences in the linoleic acid content of platelet phospholipids between the two groups.) On the other hand, Ancel Keys[77] observed that a study has shown the Japanese and Greeks had an average intake of only 3% of their dietary calories from linoleic acid compared with an average of 4% to 5% for men in Finland, in the Netherlands and in the U.S., where the coronary death rates are 5 to 10 times greater. Perhaps the high intake of saturated fats offsets any benefit from increased linoleic acid. More studies are obviously needed to determine the possible role of linoleic acid in preventing heart disease. However, many studies have already suggested that linoleic acid can favorably affect the course of experimental atherosclerosis in animals. Furthermore, human prospective studies have shown that diets high in linoleic acid can be beneficial in preventing atherosclerosis.[77a]* Then too, age-adjusted death rates in the U.S. from heart disease reached a peak about 1930 and have been declining for a half-century. At the same time, the consumption of linoleic acid (as in salad oils) has greatly increased.[77b]

---

* Although linoleic acid is effective in lowering cholesterol levels, gamma-linolenic acid (GLA) was calculated to be 163 times more potent in this function.[77aa] GLA has been reported also to be very effective in reducing LDL cholesterol.[77ab]

Perhaps there is a connection between this improvement in heart health and the increase in dietary linoleic acid. Incidentally, there has been a concomitant increase in vitamin E consumption because of this greater use of salad oils (not a decrease because the vitamin is refined out of wheat as the Shutes maintained).

Regarding heart health, it is interesting to note that a number of prostaglandins have been shown to protect against abnormalities of beating that were induced in cultured heart cells.[78] PGE_2 and $PGF_{1\alpha}$ were especially protective against challenges induced by a number of chemical agents.[78] However, in small dosages there is a *reverse effect* and these and other prostaglandins can cause cardiac rhythm disturbances (dysrhythmias).[78a-c,79] The belief is widespread, as I have remarked before, that if a certain dose is beneficial or neutral, then smaller dosages can do no harm. As seen in the example of small dosages of prostaglandins causing heart dysrhythmias while larger dosages benefit heart action, this line of reasoning is sometimes fallacious. *Reverse effects* can act for our benefit or for our harm.

What is the possible role of polyunsaturated fatty acids and of prostaglandins in the prevention and treatment of cancer? David G. Menter et al.[79a] have reported that prostacyclin, PGE_1 and PGD_2 inhibited tumor cell-induced platelet aggregation of several rodent liver tumors *in vitro,* but PGE_2 did not. Prostacyclin has been found especially active in this regard and is reported to partially reverse *in vitro* aggregation of tumor cells. On the other hand, PGE_2 reduced the ability of prostacyclin to inhibit tumor aggregation. The Menter group cited P. H. Rolland et al.[79b] as suggesting that PGE_2 levels in human breast cancer may serve as a marker for metastatic potential. They also cited A. Bennett et al.[79c] who reported that survival time after human breast cancer surgery was inversely related to the level of PGE_2 in the tumor.* P. K. Heinonen and T. Metsä-Ketelä[79cb] have reported that PGE_2 and TxB_2 are also significantly higher in

---

* S. Nigam et al.[79ca] have recently reported that 6-keto-$PGF_{2\alpha}$ and TxB_2 were significantly higher in female patients with malignant or benign breast tumors than in healthy controls. Surgical removal of the primary tumor seemed to have no effect on the plasma concentrations of 6-keto-$PGF_{2\alpha}$ and TxB_2 over a follow-up period of nine days.

metastatic ovarian cancer tissue. Then too, M. Rita Young and Sarah Knies[79d] found when mice that had been implanted with tumors were treated with exogenous PGE$_2$, the result was an increased frequency of tumor establishment. On the other hand, when they were treated with the prostaglandin synthetase inhibitor indomethacin, the result was reduced rates of both tumor establishment and of metastasis. Goodwin[79e] has reviewed the beneficial effects of indomethacin and of other prostaglandin synthetase inhibitors in the experimental treatment of animal cancers.

Prostaglandin E$_2$ obviously gets rather bad notice in regard to cancer in the experiments cited above. R. A. Karmali et al.[79f] found, similarly, that cell proliferation of a Raji lymphoid cell line was stimulated *in vitro* by PGE$_2$ up to a concentration of 1 to 10 picograms/ml. However, as the concentration of PGE$_2$ continued to increase, a *reverse effect* set in and the number of cells decreased relative to a control group (Figure 8). They found that PGA$_1$ showed little effect, but both PGE$_1$ and PGF$_{2\alpha}$ increased cell proliferation up to 10^2 and 10^4 pg./ml. respectively before exhibiting *reverse effects*.

Other experiments using prostaglandins have also been interesting. Kenneth V. Honn[91] has reported that prostacyclin (PGI$_2$) is not only the most potent antithrombogenic agent known, but is a powerful inhibitor of metastasis of B-16 amelanotic melanoma cells. Thomas Simmet and Bernard M. Jaffe[92] announced that PGD$_2$ is a potent inhibitor of B-16 melanoma cell replication *in vitro*. Several other groups have reported inhibition of the growth of melanoma cells in culture through use of PGE$_1$ and PGE$_2$. On the other hand, Popescu[93] found that prostaglandin *inhibitors* (rather than prostaglandins) reduced skin tumor proliferation in animals. These results are not necessarily contradictory. Inhibiting certain prostaglandins (e.g., PGE$_2$) may sometimes encourage production of others (e.g., PGE$_1$). Eric J. Werner et al.[79g] noting that *in vivo* studies have shown that cyclo-oxygenase inhibitors can diminish growth and metastases of certain tumors, reasoned that lipoxygenase products might be agents in this inhibition since lipoxygenase products may be increased as cyclo-oxygenase products are

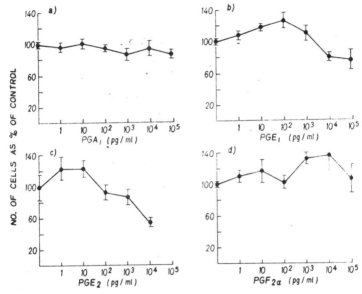

Figure 8. 2 x 10⁵ Raji cells/ml. were exposed to 0, 1, 10, 10^2, 10^3, 10^4, 10^5 pg./ml. of each of the prostaglandins—PGA₁ (a), PGE₁ (b), PGE₂ (c) and PGF₂α (d). Note the *reverse effects* in (b), (c) and (d). Reproduced from R. A. Karmali et al., *Pharmacological Research Communications* (1979) 11, no. 1: 69-75, with permission of the publisher, Academic Press.

inhibited. In experimenting with neuroblastoma cells in culture, they concluded that 12-HETE, a product of platelet lipoxygenase, and 15-HETE, a product of neutrophil and lymphocyte lipoxygenases, can inhibit neuroblastoma cell growth *in vitro*. Werner et al. speculate that they might also do so *in vivo*.

It appears that cancer cells, because of a defective delta-6-desaturase system, cannot convert linoleic acid to GLA, DGLA and PGE₁.[80] Thus, although cancer cells produce 2-series prostaglandins, they do not efficiently make those of the 1-series.* D. F. Horrobin [80]

---

* Presence of PGE₂ and of PGF₂α were found in an extract of Kaposi's sarcoma. When Kaposi tissue homogenates were incubated with arachidonic acid the production of the E and F prostaglandins increased 13.5 and 6.6 times respectively.[81] Similarly, cultures of cells from medullary carcinoma of the thyroid showed considerable PGE₂ and PGF₂α production.[82]

points out that vitamin C might be expected to help counteract this defect since, by using any residual DGLA, cancer cells may increase their production of PGE1, which could possibly help reduce cancer growth. (M. G. Santoro et al.[83] had, in fact, shown earlier, with both *in vitro* and *in vivo* experiments, that PGE1 suppressed tumor growth.) Horrobin[84] reported that transformed cells can be normalized by exposure to PGE1 as well as to certain drugs such as thioproline. Restoring PGE1 synthesis by providing GLA or DGLA may therefore be an effective technique for treating cancer. PGE1 can induce reverse transformation, so Horrobin suggests that not only PGE1 but also other drugs that induce reverse transformation be used with GLA and DGLA as a possible cancer therapy.

Eduardo N. Siguel[85] objects, however, to the above line of reasoning and to using increased DGLA as a cancer treatment. He suggests, on the contrary, that deactivation of the delta-6-desaturase enzyme in cancer may be defensive and that supplemental DGLA might actually increase tumor growth. Nevertheless, laboratory tests seem to suggest that Horrobin's concept of cancer may have validity. Evening primrose oil (a source of GLA, you will recall, which the body converts to DGLA) was reported by Horrobin[86] to cause regression in weight of breast cancers in rats. (Prolactin and penicillin were also effective, but less so than the evening primrose oil.) Nola Dippenaar et al.[87] observed that GLA inhibited *in vitro* mouse melanoma cells. A few weeks later, W. P. Leary et al.[88] reported that GLA caused the death of human esophageal carcinoma cells. Nola Dippenaar et al.[89] announced that GLA produced a significant reduction in growth rate (up to 87%) of a cultured human hepatoma cell line. (These various experiments by Dippenaar et al. and by Leary et al. used GLA itself, not evening primrose oil.) Dippenaar[87] notes that GLA supplementation presumably allows the cells to bypass the need for delta-6-desaturase and synthesize their own PGE1. "Such synthesis of PGE1," Dippenaar[87] speculates, "possibly via improved cAMP production and calcium homeostasis, could be the factor reducing the high proliferation rate of these cancer cells." Then, C. F. van der Merwe[90] published a preliminary clinical study with two male patients, aged 84 and 56, with primary liver cancer. This is a fatal disease with no specific treatment. The patients were given 12 capsules of evening primrose oil daily. Tumors decreased in size in both patients and pain decreased. The results were reported as encouraging, although both patients died, as was expected. More recently, van der Merwe[90a] reported increased duration of survival in other cases of histologically-proven primary liver cancer treated with evening primrose oil. Several foreign patent applications relate to products containing eicosanoids or GLA along with various vitamins and minerals for use in inhibiting tumor growth.[90b]

Nevertheless, Eduardo N. Siguel[85] may be correct in objecting (as we have noted) to the use of DGLA as a cancer treatment and in predicting that it might actually promote growth of tumors. K. M. Robinson and J. H. Botha[90c] have recently reported that while all concentrations of GLA or high concentrations of DGLA inhibited the growth of malignant cells *in vitro,* low concentrations (50 µg. per ml.) of DGLA showed a *reverse effect* (my language) and promoted cancer cell growth. Robinson and Botha point out that the fact DGLA in low concentrations stimulates cancer growth casts doubt on a role for PGE1 as the mediator for those effects observed for GLA and for high concentrations of DGLA. They note further that J. Booyens et al.,[90d] among others, have shown a number of other polyunsaturated fatty acids (linoleic acid, arachidonic acid, alpha-linolenic acid, eicosapentenoic acid and docosahexaenoic acid) inhibit growth and/or cause the death of malignant cells *in vitro* and in these cases PGE1 is probably not involved. To conclude, let's observe that evening primrose oil (which the body metabolizes to DGLA) could sometimes act as a cancer threat and sometimes as a therapeutic agent. This oil should not be in the hands of amateurs until the dose-response *reverse effects* can be precisely delineated.

The polyunsaturated fatty acids and the prostaglandins are involved in the cause, the prevention and the treatment of many other diseases. R. L. Aspinal and P. S. Cammarata[94] reported that injected PGE2 reduced the tibiotarsal swelling in rats with adjuvant arthritis. Then, R. B. Zurier and F. Quagliata[95] found that the PGE1 treatment of rats with adjuvant arthritis resulted in suppression of humoral response (antibody formation to sheep red blood cells) and in enhanced cell-mediated immune response. Severe polyarthritis developed in all controls and in rats treated with prostaglandin A 2 but not in those treated with PGE2. Later, R. B. Zurier and Maurice Ballas [96] reported that PGE1 treatment improved synovitis and halted the progression of arthritis and cartilage destruction. Louis M. Pelus and Helen R. Strausser [97] have speculated that prostaglandins of the E series prevent and suppress adjuvant-induced rat arthritis through increasing adrenal steroid synthesis and by reducing the release of lysosomal enzymes from white blood cells. They noted that considerable evidence suggests prostaglandins act by influencing intracellular cyclic nucleotide levels. Exogenous prostaglandins (especially those of the E series) have been shown to increase or decrease intracellular cAMP (cyclic adenosine monophosphate) levels in various tissues. In spite of these interesting experiments with rats, Troels Mork Hansen et al.[98] reported that 20 patients with rheumatoid arthritis showed no effects when treated for 2 weeks with prostaglandin E1 precursors in the form of eight evening primrose oil capsules per day plus 1 g. ascorbic acid, 200 mg. niacin, 200 mg. pyridoxine and 40 mg. zinc sulphate. This work helps underline the fact that studies on animals only suggest the possibility of corresponding results in human beings.

The effect of PGE1 on immunological response is also shown in other ways. We noted earlier that D. F. Horrobin[18] had reported PGE1 *in vitro* acts like a thymic hormone in promoting maturation of T lymphocytes. Robert B. Zurier and Maurice Ballas[96] found that, although PGE1 treatment seemed to enhance *in vivo* T cell (thymus cell) activity, it suppressed B cell (bursa equivalent cell) activity.* They reported that PGE1 treatment was beneficial in a breed of mice that spontaneously develop a disease similar to lupus erythematosus and have excessive B cell activity but are deficient in T cell activity and cell-mediated immunity. These mice, after treatment with PGE1,

---

* The T cells, which are responsible for cellular immunity, are formed in the thymus gland. The B cells, which govern humoral immunity, are probably formed in the bone marrow. (B cells were first discovered in birds, being formed in the *bursa of Fabricius,* a structure that does not exist in mammals.) T and B cells circulate freely in the blood, filter into the tissues, then enter the lymph and are carried into the lymphoid tissues.[96a]

were protected against development of anemia, clinical nephritis and death.

J. P. Kelly and C. W. Parker[98a] found that arachidonic acid in low concentrations enhanced mitogen-induced lymphocyte transformation, while higher dosages approaching physiological serum levels showed a *reverse effect* and inhibited immunological effects. Of course, suppression of immunological function may sometimes be of value. Certainly this is true not only in autoimmune diseases such as lupus or rheumatoid arthritis but in organ-transplant operations where the immunological function must be suppressed to avoid rejection of the transplanted organ. Then too, B. D. Bower and E. A. Newsholme[98b] reported that two children disabled with idiopathic neuritis began to recover within a week of starting on a diet with increased amounts of polyunsaturated fatty acids (pufas). They suggested that the pufas increased immunosuppressive activity and may have been responsible for the favorable effects. (Suppression of immunological function is, of course, generally unfavorable. Such suppression could be related to the possibility that pufas may be more carcinogenic than saturated fats since a well-functioning immune system is needed if cancer is to be avoided.) Let's stress that polyunsaturated fatty acids and the prostaglandins can promote or inhibit the immunological process, a fact which suggests we continue to observe the Greek principle of the golden mean. A recent review by M. I. Gurr[98c] entitled "The Role of Lipids in the Regulation of the Immune System" is very thorough.

Cis-linoleic acid may be of value in treating diabetes. A. J. Houtsmuller et al.[99] found that a linoleic-acid-rich diet* had an insulin-sparing effect and was beneficial in treating adult-onset diabetes. Then, too, Houtsmuller et al.[100] reported on 102 patients with newly discovered diabetes who were followed for 5 years. Half the patients received a linoleic-enriched diet (20 grams of linoleic acid per 1,000k Cal) and the other half a saturated fat diet (5 grams of linoleic acid per 1,000k Cal). After five years the group fed the

---

* When scientists report on the use of linoleic acid they virtually always mean *cis*-linoleic, not *trans*-linoleic; but, as in these studies, the exact substance used is not always specified.

linoleic-rich diet had significantly less retinopathy and electrocardiographic abnormalities. Furthermore, in female patients—but not in male patients—on the linoleic acid diet, there was an improvement of the glucose tolerance tests and the corresponding blood insulin concentrations.

A number of studies cited by M. Yusoff Dawood[100a] have shown that women having painful periods (dysmenorrhea) excrete large amounts of prostaglandins in their menstrual blood. Increased production of F2∝ and of E 2 seems to be particularly responsible.[100aa] H. P. Zahradnik and M. Breckwoldt[100ab] state that in dysmenorrhea estradiol seems to increase relative to progesterone. This is associated with an increase of PGF2∝ and a simultaneous reduction of PGЕ in uterine tissue that, they suggest, seems to be responsible for dysmenorrheic bleeding. Nulliparous women (those who have never given birth) are more afflicted and the frequency of dysmenorrhea decreases as the number of births increases. Drugs have a good record of suppressing the painful and other unpleasant symptoms. Trials of several of these drugs, which work by inhibiting the cyclo-oxygenase pathway, have been reviewed by James R. Dingfelder [100b] and, separately, by M. Y. Dawood [100c] and by Penny Wise Budoff.[100ca] The fact that not all women find these drugs ameliorate their dysmenorrhea suggests that the leukotrienes, which are unaffected by cyclo-oxygenase depression (or might even be increased by cyclo-oxygenase depression), may account for some of the problems. Studies by R. Carraher et al.,[100d] with an *in situ* preparation of guinea pig uterus, have demonstrated that leukotrienes can contract the uterus. Therefore, they might also be a causal factor in some human dysmenorrhea.

Linoleic acid and evening primrose oil have been used for treating dysmenorrhea and received considerable anecdotal support. Clinical evidence is also good. M. G. Brush[100da] reported on results of treating 68 patients for premenstrual syndrome with evening primrose oil. Most of these women had been treated with various drugs by their family doctors before being referred to Dr. Brush. In almost all cases, Dr. Brush started treatment with two capsules of evening primrose oil twice daily after food. In some severe cases the dosage was increased to three capsules twice daily. Some were concurrently given pyridoxine (vitamin B_6) but in these cases it was known that pyridoxine when given alone did not provide sufficient relief. Of the 68 women treated with evening primrose oil, 61% showed marked improvement, 23% experienced partial relief and only 16% showed no significant change. Patents granted in both the U.S. and Great Britain concern a product containing evening primrose oil (in combination with zinc sulphate) for treating premenstrual syndrome.[100db] Recent studies, one by David F. Horrobin[100dc] and another by Jukka Puolakka et al.[100dd] have also found evening primrose oil to be useful in alleviating premenstrual syndrome generally and depression especially.

Guy E. Abraham and Michael M. Lubran[100e] have reported that a low magnesium level exists in the red blood cells of women experiencing premenstrual tension. Joshua Backon[100f] has pointed out that magnesium is needed for delta-6-desaturase to convert linoleic acid to gamma-linolenic acid (which in turn is converted, as we have seen, to DGLA and PGE_1). It would seem, therefore, the magnesium study gives support to the concept that dysmenorrhea may be treatable, not only with magnesium but with evening primrose oil. The possible role of prostaglandins in releasing gonadotrophin from the pituitary by acting on the hypothalamus and other possible functions of the prostaglandins in reproductive processes have been discussed by Burton V. Caldwell and Harold R. Behrman.[100g]

Evening primrose oil has been found useful not only in treating dysmenorrhea, but N. L. Pashby et al.[100h] reported it to be valuable also in alleviating mastalgia (painful breasts). He conducted a controlled clinical trial of 73 patients with benign breast disease during which evening primrose oil was administered for 3 months. He concluded that evening primrose oil "helps reduce breast pain and tenderness in the non-cyclical group and, although less marked in the cyclical group, some individuals have had striking benefit."

Interestingly, a deficiency of DGLA may be among the possible causes of sudden infant death syndrome (SIDS). Alan C. Fogerty et al.[100i] reported that SIDS infants appeared to have lower levels of

DGLA than non-SIDS infants. Since mother's milk, as we have noted, contains large amounts of GLA, the precursor of DGLA, we are provided with another strong argument in favor of breast feeding.

The polyunsaturated fats and the prostaglandins may be useful in preventing or treating still other problems. Certain neurological abnormalities may be due to a deficiency of alpha-linolenic acid and may be benefited by supplementation.[2,101,102] Prostaglandin E₁ may be of value in treating depression when that depression is accompanied by excessive plasma PGE₂ and thromboxane (TxB₂) since PGE₁ can inhibit the arachidonic acid conversions leading to PGE₂ and TxB₂.[103] On the other hand, in mania, as we noted earlier, PGE₁ is generally produced in excess and in such cases lithium is sometimes prescribed to inhibit production of this prostaglandin.[104] Schizophrenia may also be amenable to prostaglandin therapy. D. F. Horrobin et al.[104-104aa] have proposed that schizophrenia may be due to a deficiency of PGE₁ or, in some cases, to an excess of this prostaglandin. (Under Horrobin's line of reasoning, PGE₁ might show a beneficial effect on schizophrenia at either low or at high concentrations, i.e., it might show what I call a *reverse effect*. Evening primrose oil has been reported by K. S. Vaddadi[107a] as being beneficial in the treatment of schizophrenia. More recently, Parviz Malek-Ahmadi and Margaret A. Weddle[104b] have reviewed the therapeutic implications of prostaglandins in the treatment of this disorder.

Prostaglandins may eventually be shown to be important mediators of osteoporosis. O. Sahap Atik[105] discovered that PGE₂ activity was above normal in patients with osteoporosis. D. F. Horrobin[106] reported that Sjögren's syndrome (one symptom of which is dryness) and Raynaud's phenomenon (intermittent circulation problems in the fingers and/or toes) can be alleviated by raising endogenous PGE₁ production through administering *cis*-linoleic acid, GLA and vitamins B₆ and C. Horrobin[106] was also successful in increasing the deficient tear and saliva production that characterize Sjögren's syndrome. Furthermore, Horrobin[107] met with some success in treating MS patients with evening primrose   oil   in   conjunction   with   colchicine

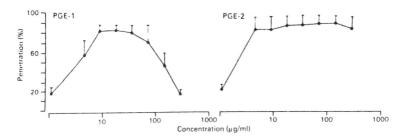

Figure 9. Influence of prostaglandins on the ability of human spermatozoa to penetrate zona-free hamster oocytes: all results corrected to a motile sperm concentration of 5 X 10^6/ml. The dose-response curves were constructed from data obtained from three separate experiments. Points and error bars indicate mean and standard error for the results obtained for each dose. Reproduced from R. J. Aitken and R. W. Kelly, *Jrl. of Reproduction and Fertility* (1985) 73: 139-146, with permission of the authors and of the publisher. Note the *reverse effect* that occurs (at about 10 µg./ml.) in PGE1 but not in PGE2 (at least not in the range of concentrations tested).

but, more recently, Donald N. Paty[107c] found no long-term benefits in treating MS with evening primrose oil. Vaddadi and Horrobin[107b] reported weight loss in some, but not in all, overweight individuals administered evening primrose oil.* Finally, evening primrose oil (with its *cis*-linoleic acid and GLA) was found effective, in a double-blind cross-over study, for treating patients with atopic eczema.[108] M. S. Manku et al.[108a] suggest that atopic eczema is not associated with any deficiency in the intake of essential fatty acids but persons with this problem may have a deficit in their metabolism, probably involving Δ 6-desaturase. (Administering evening primrose oil supplies GLA so that the metabolic step involving Δ 6-desaturase is bypassed.)

---

* S. C. Cunnane et al.[107d] found, however, that of obese mice fed diets iso-energetically supplied with either sucrose, hydrogenated coconut oil, safflower oil or evening primrose oil, weight gain in those fed evening primrose oil exceeded the gain of any other groups.

The many facets of the prostaglandins and of the immune response have recently been reviewed by Johnson and Marshall.[108b] In working to achieve a "golden mean" of endogenous prostaglandin production, keep in mind that the polyunsaturated fats present in salad oils and in other oils and fats are precursors of the prostaglandins. Their consumption can sometimes be excessive. However, it should be noted that the quantity of polyunsaturated fats needed by men is apparently far greater than that needed by women, perhaps at least partially because of the special need of the prostate gland. Then, too, linoleic acid is incorporated into sperm at various stages of their formation.* More importantly, however, men may have a far less efficient pathway for the metabolism of essential fatty acids than women if relevant experiments with rats are applicable to humans.[113]

Let's stress again that prostaglandins can have both good and bad effects, and so the taking of large amounts of evening primrose oil is not recommended except upon a physician's advice. Remember, in beneficially modifying one natural phenomenon (say lowering high blood pressure) we could at the same time be detrimentally affecting other natural processes. Let your physician help guide you in an appropriate course of action.

---

* Essential fatty acids are required throughout the body, including the male and female reproductive organs. The need for small amounts of the essential fatty acids for sexuality has been known for a half-century based on the rat experiments of H. H. Evans et al.[109] Rat studies have shown a great conversion of linoleic to gamma-linolenic acid in the testes, especially at young ages.[110] Testicular lipids also contain large amounts of arachidonic acid and of docosapentenoic acid (which appears only in small amounts or is absent in other tissues). Human semen is also rich in PGE_1, PGE_2, 19-hydroxyprostaglandin E_1 and 19-hydroxyprostaglandin E_2.[111] Penetrating ability of human sperm requires the presence of prostaglandins. Aitkin and Kelly [111a] reported that PGE_2 induced an increase in penetration rates at all tested doses greater than 8.4 µg./ml. Penetration ability increased with PGE_1 up to a plateau at concentrations of 8.4 to 33.3 µg./ml., then showed a *reverse effect* by declining all the way to the control level at a concentration of 270 µg./ml. (Figure 9). There is recent evidence[111b] that rat testes can synthesize fatty acids with chain lengths of 24, 26, 28 and 30 carbon atoms. But the prostaglandins will be produced only if the polyunsaturated fatty acid precursors are present. Furthermore, the ability of testicular microsomes to synthesize polyunsaturated fatty acids declines much more rapidly with age than such synthesis by liver microsomes.[112] Earlier, we noted that a deficiency of vitamin E decreases production of prostaglandins in the testes.[48a,b] Would there be a human fertility and/or libido effect in applying gamma-linolenic acid (as evening primrose oil) and eicosapentenoic acid (as marine oil) to the scrotum?

Problems with Supplementing PUFAS

As we keep noting, polyunsaturated oils and prostaglandins are not unmixed blessings. Diets high in polyunsaturated fats (pufas) but deficient in vitamin E and/or other antioxidants cause animals to show various undesirable symptoms. Such diets have resulted in muscular dystrophy, degeneration of the testes, dental depigmentation and creatinuria. Such diets in chickens have led to encephalomalacia, decreased egg production and reduced egg hatchability.[114]

Health and longevity effects may, however, be related to factors in the oils other than their fatty acid composition. Kaunitz,[114a] in carrying out rat feeding experiments with corn oil, cottonseed oil, soybean oil, olive oil, butter oil, beef fat, lard and coconut oil, reported significant differences in survival times of the various groups. However, he found no relation between fatty acid composition and survival time and suggested that the 2%-4% nontriglyceride materials present in these oils should be more carefully studied for their possible effects. (Kaunitz notes that among these chemical entities are antioxidants such as vitamin E, glycols, phenolic compounds, sterols, hydrocarbons, saponins, hemaglutinins, hormones and hormone-like substances such as goiterogens, enzyme inhibitors, antagonists to vitamins and amino acids, etc.) In a study of the incidence of nonendocrine tumors that H. Kaunitz did with R. E. Johnson[114b], results indicated consumption of chicken fat, lard and soybean oil (i.e., both saturated and unsaturated fats) was associated with much higher incidence of tumors than consumption of butter, cottonseed oil and coconut oil (another group containing both saturated and unsaturated fat). This fact tends to support the statement that factors other than fatty acid content must be operating.

If your decision is to use supplementary polyunsaturated vegetable oils, you may want to give preference to *crude* oils, packaged under nitrogen seal and in dark glass bottles to reduce oxidation caused by light-catalyzed generation of superoxide.

Refining, although it improves the taste and appearance, may remove valuable nutrients while introducing questionable factors. R. G. Ackman and S. N. Hooper[114c] discuss the artifacts that are not present in unrefined or bleached oils but may be introduced in the deodorization process. However, crude oils may not, on balance, be superior to refined oils. Sometimes the presence of chlorophyll is cited as being a beneficial component of unrefined oils. A. Kiritsakis,[114d] nevertheless, found that chlorophyll functioned as a photosensitizer, resulting in rapid oxidation of the oil. He used olive oil, bleached to remove most nontriglyceride components, and added chlorophyll a, pheophytin a and b, α and β carotene, d-α-tocopherol and nickel dibutyldithiocarbamate. (This mixture may or may not have approximately simulated unrefined oil.) Kiritsakis observed that carotenes acted as singlet oxygen quenchers (more on this subject in Chapters 4 and 9), while alpha tocopherol had little apparent effect on the oxidation rate. (This seems surprising in light of vitamin E's antioxidant potential.) Kiritsakis reported that carotenes and tocopherols apparently were destroyed more rapidly when chlorophyll was present. He also found that pheophytin was an oxidation promoter. Furthermore, crude corn or peanut oils may sometimes contain aflatoxin. (Wilbur A. Parker and Daniel Melnick[114e] found, on the other hand, that aflatoxin was completely absent from refined oils.) It seems reasonable that if one is to give preference to crude oil then that preference should not extend to oils which pose a danger of aflatoxin poisoning, i.e., corn oil and peanut oil.

Oils, whether refined or not, may contain detrimental constituents. Wheat-germ oil, rice bran oil, safflower oil and the other oils contain estrogen, with soybean oil being especially high in this questionable factor. Therefore, use a variety of different oils so you don't overdo any particular factor that might be detrimental. Furthermore, I think it preferable to obtain oils by eating the corresponding nut, seed or grain rather than through using the processed oil.

Whatever one's sources of oils may be, such oils and foods containing them should be used only in moderation since fat consumption beyond body requirements is an antilongevity factor. Excessive use of oils may produce flatulence, an increased number of bowel movements and also add to one's obesity problems. If one decides to give preference to the unrefined oils, it may be desirable to select those that are cold pressed.

Actually, the expression "cold pressed" has no legal meaning and can mean whatever the manufacturer wants it to mean. Oils are extracted by one of three techniques:

1. Hydraulic pressed, preferably without heat. In practice the material is ground or rolled and often steam cooked at temperatures as high as 270° F. Only sesame seeds and olives will yield enough oil without first being treated, and the expression "cold pressed" ought to be restricted to such oils but is not. (The words "extra virgin" in regard to olive oil refer to the first pressing by a hydraulic press without added heat. "Virgin" refers to subsequent pressings, again without added heat.)

2. Expeller pressed (using a press with a constantly rotating worm shaft) and temperatures usually ranging between 200° F. and 475° F. The higher the temperature, the better for production and the poorer for leaving nutrients unaffected. In spite of high temperatures such oils are often called "cold pressed."

3. Solvent extracted. Hexane and other petroleum or coal tar-derived chemicals are commonly used. Solvent residues are apt to remain in such oils and so they should be avoided as possibly being carcinogenic.* Extraction using petroleum-derived solvent is, regrettably, a very common method of producing oil and is used by all the big oil processors. It is estimated, for example, that 98%

---

* We must never conclude, by invoking the *reverse effect,* that small amounts of carcinogens may be valuable and cancer-protective. Research must, by studying dose-response relationships, tell us if small amounts of carcinogens may be valuable.

of soy oil produced in the United States is extracted using such solvents.

Confine your purchases to those oils extracted without use of coal tar or petroleum-derived solvents. If the bottle does not say words such as "no solvents used," "mechanically pressed," "cold pressed" or "expeller pressed," assume the worst and avoid it. "Cold pressed" implies (but may not guarantee) that no solvents have been used, whereas "cold processed" implies the use of a solvent which may be ethylene dichloride, a carcinogenic chemical. Ask your supplier what extractant, if any, was used.

Keep oils under refrigeration after opening and use promptly, since even refrigeration will not eliminate the possibility of their turning rancid. That means buying oil in small bottles or, if you purchase a large bottle and will not be consuming the oil promptly, transfer it to several small bottles, completely filled, to minimize oxygen effects. How does an oil become rancid? It becomes rancid by combining with the oxygen in the air to form peroxides. The peroxides, in turn, break up into aldehydes, which give rancid oil its characteristic odor and flavor. Putting the contents of a vitamin E capsule in the oil will help preserve it.

The use of polyunsaturated oils in cooking may be questionable. The polyunsaturated nature of most of the oils means that under the influence of heat they readily combine with oxygen in the air to form peroxides that are implicated as a cause of aging and cancer. Olive oil, as we have indicated, is primarily monounsaturated and therefore will pick up oxygen less readily than polyunsaturated oils, but more readily than saturated varieties.

Let's cite an experiment to suggest the possible dangers in using heated oils. Antti Ahlstrom and Ritva Jarvinen,[115] of the Department of Nutritional Chemistry, University of Helsinki, Helsinki, Finland, fed fresh and aerobically heated (i.e., heated in the presence of air) safflower oil to rats for a three-month period from the time of weaning. Rats fed the heated oil showed some signs of enlargement of the liver and the kidneys. Male rats given heated oil tended to have swollen spleens. On the other hand, Granville A. Nolen et al.[115a]

reported that, although frying in fats causes toxins to form, their toxicity was too low to have dietary significance.

This optimistic view of Nolen et al. is now disputed. Cooking may introduce not only the threat of peroxide formation, but also, in the case of seafood, may result in an increase in amines. Jen-Kun Lin[115aa] reported that frying seafoods decreased dimethylamine content, but diethylamine was increased. Broiling seafoods at 200° C. significantly elevated both dimethylamine and methylamine, so broiling would appear to be more dangerous than frying from the standpoint of nitrosoamine formation. Boiling, as contrasted with broiling, may be a much safer method of cooking (not only of seafood but also of fowl or meat). Boiling seafoods for 20 minutes removed 90% of their dimethylamine.[115aa]*

Using the Ames salmonella test, L. F. Bjeldanes et al.[115b] found that well-done ground beef, beef steak, ham, pork chops and bacon had significant amounts of mutagens. In the case of chicken and beef steak, high temperature broiling produced the most mutagens, while stewing, braising and deep frying produced very little mutagenicity. Eggs produced mutagens only when prepared at high temperatures (the yolk producing more than the white). Spingarn and Weisburger[115ba] reported that mutagens formed rapidly when meat was fried, more slowly when broiled (contrary to Bjeldanes et al.) and only very slowly when boiled. (Hamburgers from commercial franchises were frequently found to be mutagenically active.) Thus, rare meat seems to be safer mutagenically, but it will have a higher fat content and there may be a danger of acquiring toxoplasmosis.

Related studies by S. L. Taylor et al.[115c] have shown that oils used in frying at least some foods—e.g., french-fried potatoes and onion rings—can be used repeatedly (up to at least 44 batches) with no increase in mutagenicity. In the case of fish fillets, however, mutagenicity increased after the seventh batch.[115c] Other studies by Taylor et al.[115d] have found that deep-fried ground beef possessed mutagenic activity but at only one-fourth the level found in surface-

---

* However, if the amines are still in the liquid, fish soup and bouillabaisse might be dangerous.

fried ground beef.* (Deep-fat-frying—done as it is, away from air that could form peroxides—may very well be safer than sautéing, which is contrary to popular opinion.) Other studies cited by Taylor[115c] confirmed that deep-fat-frying chicken, tofu and shrimp produced very little mutagenic activity. On the other hand, it may be possible that volatile decomposition products of fats and oils produced during deep-fat-frying may sometimes be dangerous but, as far as I know, their effect on those inhaling them has not been studied. At least 220 such compounds, however, have been identified![116]

The exhortation to avoid cooking in polyunsaturated oils extends, of course, to foods you purchase. Potato chips and other products fried in polyunsaturated fats should be shunned. Foods of this type may be especially dangerous if unprotected by antioxidants. (Antioxidants, if present, will protect the products, and your body, against the formation of carcinogenic, longevity-decreasing peroxides.)** It is also a good idea to minimize use of margarines. In the hydrogenation process (when hydrogen fills in the open bonds) nutrients may be lost. As another possible negative factor, nickel is used as a catalyst in the hydrogenation process. This impurity probably exists in the finished product. Margarines have also been accused, because of their content of *trans* fatty acids, by F. A. Kummerow[117] and others[117b] of being more damaging to the heart and arteries than cholesterol or natural fats.

---

* Michael W. Pariza et al.[115e] reported that fried ground beef (and also raw beef) contains an unknown substance that modulates bacterial mutagenesis. Pariza et al. noted that it seems to interact *in vitro* with rat liver microsomes that were added to metabolically activate promutagens. The substance has been partially purified and either inhibits, enhances or has no effect on promutagen activation depending on the promutagen under study and the pretreatment of the rat which was the source of the microsomal fraction. (There may be some interesting *reverse effects* here that are yet to be delineated.)

** Commercially canned foods may show varying amounts of mutagenicity. In a study of C. A. Krone and W. T. Iwaoka,[115bb] canned pink salmon exhibited the highest mutagenicity of any canned foods tested, while the researchers could detect no mutagens in sardines or tuna packed in water. In a subsequent interview with *Longevity Letter*,[115bc] Dr. Krone stated that pink salmon had only slightly higher mutagenic activity than red salmon. Furthermore, according to Krone, these levels were well below those found in hamburger and in other cooked meats.

The most common natural structure of a fatty acid is called *cis* (meaning "same side" in Latin) and denotes a geometric isomer having a pair of identical atoms or group attached on the same side of two atoms linked by a double bond. A *cis-cis* fatty acid contains two such formations. The hydrogenation process, however, creates a *trans* form (a geometric isomer having a pair of identical atoms or groups on the opposite sides of two atoms linked by a double bond) or a *trans-trans* form (two such formations) or a *cis-trans* form or a *trans-cis* form.* In every case, the *trans* form of a fatty acid has a much higher melting point than the corresponding *cis* form. *Trans* forms of fatty acids are often said to occur only rarely in nature, so we might suspect that the human body would metabolize such fats only under considerable stress. However, J. B. Ohlrogge et al.[118] have reported that there are 2% to 5.8% *trans* fatty acids in human adipose tissue and similar amounts in ruminant fats that have been in the diets of humans for centuries. For example, butterfat contains 5.0-9.7% *trans* fatty acids.[119]

In attempting to discover whether or not *trans* fatty acids pose dietary dangers, T. Mizuguchi, F. A. Kummerow et al.[117b] found that 7 of 12 swine fed *trans* fatty acids developed raised lesions in the abdominal aorta, whereas only 13 of 92 aortas of swine fed other diets developed raised lesions. However, in criticizing this study, Walter H. Meyer[119a] states that the high-*trans* diet was deficient in essential fatty acids and, in turn, cites many studies showing a lack of adverse effects of *trans* fatty acids. Recently, Steven M. Royce, F.

---

* More recently, in a lecture at the Nutrition for Optimal Health Assn., Winnetka, Illinois, March 9, 1983, Dr. Kummerow related that the manufacturers have now significantly reduced the content of *trans* fatty acids in margarines. Earlier, F. A. Kummerow[117a] had reported European and Canadian fat processors managed to eliminate most of the *trans* isomers from their products. An analysis by J. L. Beare-Rodgers[117c] of eight margarines made in the year 1977 showed two brands had *trans* fatty acids in excess of 60% by weight, while the six others varied in *trans* content from 12.0 to 27.9%. S. P. Kochhar and T. Mutsui[117d] and, independently, H. T. Slover et al.[117e] have recently published in-depth analyses of the various lipids in margarines and in margarine-like foods. M. G. Enig et al.[117f] have tabulated the fatty acid composition (including *trans* fatty acids) in selected food items. (It might be a good project for the FDA to mandate that food labels show the *trans*-fatty-acid content.)

A. Kummerow et al.,[119b] in another swine study, concluded that "when a carefully formulated diet is used, the extent of atherosclerosis in adolescent swine is low, and that neither increasing levels of saturated fatty acids nor increasing levels of isomeric fatty acids influence the development of atherosclerosis." Nevertheless, Royce, Kummerow et al.[119b] found that *trans* octadecenoic acids in hydrogenated fat used in this study (at the 39% level, i.e., much higher than the average amount consumed by Americans) depressed release of prostacylin. Thus, *trans* fatty acids are probably cleared from the standpoint of atherogenicity, but they might still be implicated in heart disease through a possible effect on the induction of thrombi. Thomas et al.[119c] have recently observed that the adipose tissue of heart disease victims contains higher levels of certain *trans* fatty acids. In addition, *all-trans*-linoleic acid inhibits the conversion of *cis*-linoleic acid into gamma-linolenic acid.[18,119d] Relative to this finding, J. E. Kinsella et al.[119d] reported that rat studies have shown high levels of *trans, trans* linoleate can impair the action of Δ 6-desaturase and thus inhibit prostaglandin production. Remi deSchrijver and Orville S. Privett[119e] subsequently confirmed that Δ 6 -desaturase activity was depressed in the liver microsomes by feeding rats a diet containing a mixture of *trans* fatty acids. More recently, Miriam D. Rosenthal and Mark A. Doloresco[119f] found that omega-9 *trans* fatty acids are potent inhibitors of Δ 5-desaturase (although omega-7 *trans* fatty acids are relatively ineffective). Because of this enzyme inhibition, some *trans* fatty acids would seem to have negative physiological implications. A number of studies have also reported a decrease in monamine oxidase (MAO) activity in the livers and hearts of rats.[119g] On the other hand, as we have noted, it has been argued that the metabolism of *trans* fatty acids by the human body may not occasion any special problems. In research with monkeys, David Kritchevsky[120] found that *trans* fatty acids, while being more hypercholesterolemic, were not more atherogenic. A subsequent study by Herbert Ruttenberg et al.[121] indicated that rabbits fed *trans* unsaturated fatty acids also showed elevated cholesterol levels but no increase in aortic atherosclerosis.

So while some animal studies suggest that *trans* fatty acids may be innocuous from the standpoint of being a factor in atherosclerosis, they still seem to bear a relationship to other problems. John J. Kabara,[121a] in an attempt to find an ideal natural germicide, has studied many microbial agents derived from fatty acids. *Cis* isomers were found to be active against microorganisms; *trans* isomers were not. Furthermore, Remi deSchrijver and Orville S. Privett[121b] recently reported that mitochondrial ATP synthesis was reduced in rats fed *trans* fatty acids at both 2% and at 5% levels. The efficiency of metabolizable energy utilization was reduced in rats fed at the 5% level but not in those fed at the 2% level. These studies may give us reasons to avoid *trans* fatty acids.

Could *trans* fatty acids possibly be related to cancer incidence? Mary G. Enig et al.[122] stated that *trans* fatty acids affect the function of cellular membranes and alter enzyme function in the mitochondria of the cells. These factors, Enig speculated, may increase the cell's permeability to carcinogens. However, J. Edward Hunter[123] accused Enig of ignoring studies in which elevated levels of *trans* fatty acids were fed to animals for long periods without adverse effects. In one of these studies, Roslyn B. Alfin-Slater et al.[124] had concluded, "In all the multi-generation and longevity studies, herein reported, no deleterious effects were observed as a result of the ingestion of the small amounts of saturated fatty acids present in the hydrogenated fats." More recently, R. B. Alfin-Slater and L. Aftergood[125] reviewed these and other studies. T. W. Applewhite,[126] in commenting on the various work, said, "In long-term multi-generation studies (over 30 years) with rats fed a margarine fat containing 35% *trans*-fatty acids as the sole dietary fat, no problems were observed in growth, reproduction, survival, plasma and liver cholesterol levels or tissue pathology." Recent work by Kikuko Nishiyama et al.[126a] demonstrated that the geometry of dietary fatty acids (i.e., whether they were *cis* or *trans*) had little effect in modulating the hepatic mixed function oxidase system. One might wonder if the fuss about *trans* fatty acids is much-ado-about-nothing.

Atif Awad,[126b] however, reported that *trans* fatty acids (as elaidic acid) fed to Ehrlich ascites tumor-bearing mice at a level of only 5% in the diet resulted in a reduction of 23% to 45% in host-survival rate. On the other hand, this finding was not replicated in the more recent work of Sandra L. Selenskas et al.[126c] The Selenskas group studied *trans* and *cis* fatty acids compared with corn oil as promoters of mammary tumors induced by dimethylbenz(a)anthracene in rats. They found that rats fed either a 20% *trans* fat or *cis* fat diet had a slightly higher tumor incidence than did those on a 5% corn oil diet. However, rats fed a 20% corn oil diet developed a much greater number of tumors than those fed only 5% corn oil. They concluded that *trans* fat behaves very similarly to saturated fat in modifying mammary carcinogenesis. Furthermore, Kent L. Erickson[126d] recently reported that mice fed *cis* fatty acids in their diets had a higher level of mammary tumor metastasis compared to animals fed the *trans* fatty-acid-containing diets.

Nevertheless, it seems to me that the negatives associated with *trans* fatty acids may outweigh the positives. However, the great bulk of the studies fail to make the distinction between the many varieties of *trans* fatty acids. T. H. Applewhite[127] has pointed out that "this is sloppy science that only serves to confuse and mislead less astute readers." He continues to urge that discussions distinguish between the various lipid classes and their varying physiological properties. It seems clear that the "evidence" against *trans* fatty acids is muddy. The interesterification process, (which changes the distribution of the fatty acids among the triglycerides of fats or mixture of fats) is, however, an alternative to hydrogenation. This process minimizes *trans* fatty acids in the resulting margarine while retaining properties similar to those of hydrogenated products. Interested readers are referred to the work of D. Chobanov and R. Chobanova;[127a] B. Sreenivasan;[127b] D. G. Chobanov and M. R. Topalova;[127c] and Y. C. Lo and A. P. Handel.[127d]

If you prefer to avoid margarine (in order to reduce your consumption of *trans* fatty acids) and also prefer to avoid polyunsaturated fats, what else is left to use in cooking? You might consider using butter, lard, beef fat or olive oil. (Coconut oil, while it is very saturated, seems to pose problems.)* Of these, you might prefer to use olive oil since it is primarily monounsaturated as contrasted with the others mentioned which are mostly saturated. If some of the air near the frying operation is breathed, the peroxides might conceivably be a contributing cause of lung cancer. If you must fry, keep the exhaust fan going and breathe through a gauze mask.

In the interest of presenting a balanced view, I should remind you, however, that some of the data in the Hammond Report (referred to in Chapter 1) suggested that fried foods might be life-lengthening. I indicated there that I questioned such a conclusion, preferring to explain the effect in terms of the *pleasure concept.* At any rate, it may be simplistic to consider fried foods as one class. Specifically, when meat is charcoal grilled, the carcinogen benzo(a)pyrene is produced. Whether this tends to be life-lengthening or life-shortening, however, may not be so obvious. R. F. Heller et al.[129b] reported that when 12 volunteers ate, each day for 9 days, 8-ounce hamburgers and 6-ounce steaks barbecued over charcoal, they had a 25% rise in the mean value of their high density lipoprotein (HDL) cholesterol and a decline in total cholesterol.** (Eating the same quantity of meat under the same

---

* A study by H. Kaunitz and R. E. Johnson[128] was made of the influence of dietary fats on the longevity of male rats. Rats fed coconut oil lived on average just 592 days, while those fed beef fat (suet) lived the longest at an average of 703 days. Those fed chicken fat, butter, lard, cottonseed oil, corn oil and olive oil lived, respectively, averages of 613, 626, 639, 641, 652 and 670 days. Rats are not people but, based on this study (which could subsequently be contradicted by other research), we should reduce consumption of coconut oil and chicken fat, including reduction of their use in cooking. In other research (not with rats, but with primates) that involved feeding with butter and with peanut, coconut and corn oils, the most atherogenic was peanut oil and the next most atherogenic was coconut oil. It is speculated that this negative feature of peanut oil may be due to the presence of the long chain arachidic, behenic and lignoceric saturated fatty acids and bears no relation to aflatoxin content.[129] By the way, Patrick Tso et al.[129a] subsequently reported that randomization (rearrangement of fatty acids to random distribution) of peanut oil significantly reduced its atherogenicity for rabbits and monkeys.

** Heller et al.[129b] cite the work of Durrington[129c] showing that drugs such as phenobarbitone induce hepatic microsomal enzymes (collectively called cytochrome P-450) that produce a rise in HDL-cholesterol. Heller et al. cite a study by A. H. Conney et al.[129d] showing that men fed charcoal-broiled beef for four days had an increase in microsomal-enzyme induction. This increase in cytochrome P-450 presumably was due to the consumption of benzo(a)pyrene and/or other polycyclic aromatic hydrocarbons associated with such meat.

conditions but cooked in an electric oven did not produce the effect.) Although increased HDL and lowered total cholesterol is associated with heart health, more must be learned about the possible cancer-causing effects of benzo(a)pyrene before charcoal broiling can be recommended as a health measure.

It is interesting to note that microwave-cooked meat was found to contain no extractable mutagenic activity, nor did it contribute to urinary mutagenicity.* This beneficial lack of mutagenic activity may be due to the paucity of browning reactions. Such browning reactions constitute a possible threat when meat is cooked in more usual ways.[130]

The saturated fats went into disrepute many years ago when fears about cholesterol began to circulate. We should return to using them whenever heat is involved. The body requires both saturated and unsaturated fats (although not in the quantities consumed by most of us). A high incidence of cancer, liver disease, muscular dystrophy, intestinal irritation, hypertension, elevated uric acid levels in the blood and damaged ovaries and testes have been found in animals permitted to consume only unsaturated fats. A principal cause of such morbidity may be lipid peroxidation-caused erythrocyte hemolysis due to a deficiency of vitamin E. S. Krishnamurthy et al.[130a] found that a vitamin E-deficient diet containing saturated fat yielded the same pattern of lipid peroxidation and erythrocyte hemolysis one sees when unsaturated fat is fed.

(Continued on page 245)

---

* Meat, although an excellent source of iron, zinc and complete protein, can hardly be recommended as a "health food." David A. Snowdon et al.,[129e] studying the meat consumption habits of 25,153 California Seventh-Day Adventists, discovered a dose-response relationship between meat consumption and heart-disease risk. They reported that the association was apparently not due to confounding by eggs, dairy products, obesity, marital status or cigarette smoking. The association between meat consumption and fatal ischemic heart disease was stronger in men than in women. There was approximately a 3-fold greater risk for 45- to 64-year-old men who ate meat daily and those who did not eat meat at all.

Cholesterol and its Carriers—HDL and LDL

Cholesterol is required for cells to function normally. It is a precursor of steroid hormones and bile acids. On the negative side, it is an important constituent of gallstones and atherosclerotic plaques. J. Szepsenwol[130b-d] has even reported that cholesterol, extracted from eggs, may be a cause of murine (mouse) cancer.

Cholesterol is an unsaturated monohydric alcohol in the class of sterols. Though often associated in the mind with saturated fats, cholesterol is unsaturated. It may, therefore, be subject to oxidation (as will be discussed later) and it is possible that oxidized cholesterol, rather than cholesterol itself, may be the cause of the bad effects that have been reported.

The Nobel Laureate Konrad Bloch, in collaboration with D. Rittenberg, showed that cholesterol is synthesized in the body from acetic acid. This synthesis, which occurs in the liver as well as in extra-hepatic tissues, is probably controlled through a feedback mechanism. Cholesterol synthesis is likely to increase or decrease inversely with the cholesterol derived from the diet.[131] However, this mechanism is generally not operative on a one-for-one basis. That is, a given decline or increase in dietary cholesterol is not apt to invoke an inverse response in endogenous cholesterol production to the same degree.[131] If it is desirable to decrease serum cholesterol, a reduction in the dietary intake of cholesterol is probably indicated.

Intracellular metabolism of cholesterol esters in the arterial wall proceeds by means of several enzymes, acyl-CoA: cholesterol acyltransferase (ACAT), lecithin-cholesterol-acyltransferase (LCAT), cholesterol ester hydrolase, acid cholesterol hydrolase and cholesterol esterase.[131a] Suckling and

Stang have cited the work of P. Helgerud et al.[131b] showing that ACAT activity is subject to a diurnal cycle, being at a maximum (at least in rats) at the start of their period of daily activity. The Helgerud group found that feeding suppressed and fasting stimulated ACAT activity. The enzyme LCAT is thought to promote cholesterol mobilization from peripheral tissue to the liver[131c] and, when LCAT is deficient, hypercholesterolemia is likely to be present.[132] Takatori et al.[133] reported that *trans* fatty acids fed to rats suppressed LCAT activity. In this way, *trans* fatty acids might be presumed to be involved in increasing cholesterol levels. However, Carolyn E. Moore et al.[134] found that free and total serum cholesterol levels were decreased in rats fed *trans* fatty acids. They observed a decreased LCAT activity but speculated that this decrease "may have been related to a reduced amount of substrate (free cholesterol)." Michihiro Sugano et al.[135] subsequently confirmed the finding of Moore et al. that cholesterol absorption was markedly decreased and rapidly excreted in the feces of rats fed a *trans*-fat diet compared with those fed a *cis*-fat diet. This beneficial finding may partially offset the negatives sometimes associated with *trans* fatty acids.

Dietary cholesterol has been a subject of research for about three-quarters of a century. Regrettably, animal experiments do not always elucidate the actions of cholesterol in humans. As Ancel Keys[136] has pointed out, the rabbit and various birds are ultrasensitive to cholesterol, while the rat, dog and cat are insensitive. Man's reactions to cholesterol may fall somewhere between sensitive and insensitive animal models.

The optimal value of blood cholesterol is debatable. Hirotsuga Ueshima et al.[137] reported in *Preventive Medicine* that strokes, among groups studied in Japan, seemed to increase at serum cholesterol levels under 160 mg. %. Several articles in the same issue of *Preventive Medicine* objected to details in the Ueshima study and stressed that there is no data from the U.S. to provide a basis for determining a lowest safe level of total cholesterol.[*] It was, however, suggested that 180-200 mg. % may be optimal for most persons. M. F. Oliver[139] quoted and agreed with this statement of W. B. Kannel and T. Gordon[140] that appeared in an earlier issue of *Lancet,* "Serum cholesterol is not a strong risk factor for coronary heart disease." Oliver suggested we define "raised cholesterol" as being in excess of one standard deviation over the mean of the population being studied. He also suggested we not overestimate the importance of lowering serum cholesterol in those with levels already below the median.[**]

Albert B. Lowenfels[141] has speculated, on the other hand, that *decreased* serum cholesterol may be linked with *increased* cholesterol excretion. Since cholesterol and its degradation products are implicated in the pathogenesis of colon cancer, it becomes reasonable that a low level of serum cholesterol, while being heart-protective, could increase the risk of colon cancer. Others maintain, however, that lower serum cholesterol levels might be caused by cancer.[142] Of course, both positions could be correct. Supporting the former position, Geoffrey Rose et al.[143] found a negative correlation within populations between blood cholesterol and colon cancer. Some persons with lower levels of blood cholesterol may form more bile salts, perhaps in part because more polyunsaturated fat is being consumed (instead of saturated fat and cholesterol). Carcinogen-forming bacteria, feeding on the increased quantity of these bile salts, could add to the risk of colon cancer. (We will consider the possible relationship between cholesterol and cancer a little later in this section.) In spite of the debate as to optimal levels of serum cholesterol, the preponderance of opinion is that the health of

---

[**] The work of Harold D. Chope and Lester Breslow,[138] done about 30 years ago, seems to be generally ignored. They reported that the mortality of persons under 70 years of age was unaffected by blood cholesterol levels. For those 70 or older, the higher the cholesterol, the lower the mortality.

[*] Decreasing even excessively elevated cholesterol levels by means of drugs may be questionable. In the Lipid Research Clinics Coronary Prevention Trial,[156,157] the incidence of coronary heart deaths at seven years was 8.6% in the placebo group and 7.0% in the cholestyramine resin-treated group. There was no significant difference in total deaths between the two groups because the suicide rate was much higher among those treated with the drug.

most persons would be benefited if their cholesterol levels were lowered.

Ancel Keys[136] has developed an equation showing how the change (Δ) in blood cholesterol (B.C.) can be predicted in terms of the change (Δ) in the dietary intake of saturated fat(S), polyunsaturated fat (P) and cholesterol (C). The formula is: ΔB.C. = 1.3 (2ΔS - ΔP) + 1.5 ($\sqrt{C_o}$ - $\sqrt{C_c}$). In this formula, ΔB.C. is the predicted change in total blood cholesterol given in terms of ΔS, the percent change in calories due to saturated fat; ΔP, the percent change in calories due to polyunsaturated fat; $\sqrt{C_o}$, the square root of the original consumption of dietary cholesterol (C_o) expressed in milligrams per 1,000 calories of diet; and $\sqrt{C_c}$, the square root of the current intake of dietary cholesterol expressed in milligrams per 1,000 calories of diet.[*] If you were to *reduce* your consumption of saturated fat from 15% total calories to 5%, then ΔS in the formula would be the difference between 15 and 5 or 10. If you were to increase your consumption of polyunsaturated fat from 5% to 10%, then ΔP would be 10 - 5 or 5. Finally, suppose your original consumption of cholesterol (C_o) were 800 mg./day on a total intake of 2,000 calories/day, i.e., 400 mg./1,000 calories. Suppose further that your cholesterol intake were reduced to 200 mg./day on the same total calorie intake of 2,000, i.e., to 100 mg./1,000 calories for your current cholesterol consumption (C_c). Substituting the values into the equation, ΔB.C. = 1.3 (2 X 10 - 5) + 1.5 ($\sqrt{400}$ - $\sqrt{100}$) = 19.5 + 1.5 (20-10) = 19.5 + 15 = 34.5 mg./dl.

This formula is applicable only after the dietary changes have been in effect for a month or two. Furthermore, it may not accurately predict the blood cholesterol change for any particular individual. Donald J. McNamara[144] has stated that a given individual may absorb as little as 20% or as much as 85% of the

---

[*] In this and in other of his formulas Keys makes no provision for the possibility that various polyunsaturated fatty acids may not be equally effective in lowering blood cholesterol. A 1986 study by Paul J. Nestel[143a] indicates that omega-3 oils (the marine oils) may be more effective than the omega-6 oils for this purpose.

cholesterol in his/her diet. Furthermore, this is, as he says, "only one variable in terms of the individualized responses to dietary lipids." The amount of fiber in the diet may, for example, have considerable effect. Then too, a recent study by Suk Y. Oh and Lorraine T. Miller[144a] shows there is great difference between hyper- and hypo-responders in the effect on plasma cholesterol of eating eggs. The Keys' equation is of use primarily in connection with population groups. However, we can learn some interesting things through examining it. First, a given percentage *decline* in saturated fat is twice as important as the same percentage *increase* in polyunsaturated fatty acids (pufas). The relative unimportance of the cholesterol consumption is shown by the square roots in the formula. Obviously, the biggest changes in blood cholesterol can be effected through reducing saturated fat consumption. However, it is probably best to work on all three factors. In any dietary efforts to lower blood cholesterol, keep in mind, however, that it may be more healthful to achieve a better saturated to polyunsaturated fat ratio through *reducing* an unnatural factor in the diet (excessive saturated fat) than by *increasing* another unnatural factor (excessive polyunsaturated fat).

I speculate that a dangerous practice related to dietary cholesterol may be to consume a very low cholesterol diet for a few days and then change to a high cholesterol intake for several days. I speculate that during the period of low cholesterol intake the body will increase its endogenous production of cholesterol to compensate for the low dietary level. Then, if one begins a period of high cholesterol consumption there may be a lag before the body reduces its endogenous cholesterol production and this is the time cholesterol may be laid down in the arteries. I speculate that continually consuming large amounts of cholesterol might be safer than cyclically varying between a high and a low and back to a high cholesterol diet.

Reducing saturated dietary fat generally means a shift away from animal products in favor of vegetables where the fat is polyunsaturated. However, Paul J. Nestel et al.[145] reported that when cattle were fed supplements of vegetable oil in their diets the ratio between polyunsaturated fatty acids to saturated fatty acids increased ten times. When five men and one woman were fed this meat in their diet, the reduction in their plasma cholesterol was "highly significant in five of the six subjects." David H. Blankenhorn[146] cites studies showing that polyunsaturated marine or vegetable fatty acids can be introduced into poultry and pork with little or no increase in feeding cost. If, while awaiting the general availability of such animal products, we increasingly substitute fish and other seafood* for standard animal foods, it will help reduce plasma cholesterol. (The mechanism by which this occurs, as suggested by Santhirasegaram Balasubramaniam et al.,[147a] is probably through an increase in the transfer of cholesterol into bile.) Daan Kromhout et al.,[148] after a 20-year study in the town of Zutphen, the Netherlands, reported an inverse dose-response relationship between fish consumption and death from coronary heart disease. Mortality from coronary heart disease was more than 50% lower among those who consumed at least 30 grams (about one ounce) of fish per day than among those who did not eat fish. They concluded that eating as little as two fish dishes per week may be of preventive value. Ocean fish (particularly the fatty, cold-water varieties) may be especially beneficial since they contain more eicosapentenoic and docosahexanoic acids than do the fresh-water species.[149] (However, the presence of larger amounts of these long-chain polyunsaturated fatty acids means that they will be more subject to oxidation than fresh water varieties. Furthermore, Stein E. Vollset et al.[149a] noted no relationship between   fish   consumption   and   20-year   mortality

---

* Judith Krzynowek[146a] relates that cholesterol values in seafood have been historically overstated by the precipitation method. The gas-liquid chromatograph now in use gives much lower, more accurate values. Nobuko Iritani et al.[147] showed that oysters and clams, historically reported to be high in cholesterol, *lowered* plasma cholesterol levels in rats. By the way, M. Sugano et al.[147b] reported that when male rats were fed a diet containing 5% chitosan (a polymer of glucosamine—an aminosugar—prepared from the chitin of sea crabs) their plasma cholesterol dropped 25% to 30%. J. J. Nagyvary et al.[147c] also found that chitosan had superior cholesterol-lowering capability in rats.

from coronary heart disease in a study in Norway involving 17,000 respondents to a postal dietary survey. The Vollset cohort had a high average fish intake and an older age composition. Vollset and his colleagues noted that, in a Lutheran Brotherhood study in the U.S. of 14,000 symptom-free men having a low average level of fish consumption, there was also no evidence of an inverse association between coronary mortality and dietary fish. A study by J. David Curb et al.[149b] of Japanese men in Hawaii similarly found no statistically significant relationship between fish consumption and coronary heart disease. The seeming contradictions between these three studies and the Kromhout results await resolution. Nevertheless, Richard B. Shekelle et al.,[149c] in restudying the results of their famous Western Electric Study, concluded that this study supports the Kromhout findings.

Several studies, including one by William S. Harris et al.,[149ca] one by D. Roger Illingworth et al.[149cb] (from the same laboratory as Harris et al.) and one by L. A. Simons et al.[149cc] have shown that dietary fish oils may, by inhibiting the synthesis of VLDL triglyceride, be especially active in reducing plasma triglyceride levels. Beverly E. Phillipson et al.[149cd] reported marked decreases in levels of cholesterol and of triglyceride (as much as 45% and 79%, respectively) in hypertriglyceridemic patients put on a diet high in fish oils. They also found that a vegetable oil diet had much less effect. Triglyceride is carried not only by the VLDL but also by the chylomicrons, a lipoprotein produced in the intestinal mucosa from dietary fat.[149cg] Levels of triglyceride have been reported by G. Schonfeld et al.[149ce] and by Ikuo Nishigaki et al.[149cf] to be significantly higher in diabetics. This suggests the possibility that modest amounts of dietary fish might be of value in managing disease. E. Schimke et al.[149ch] have, in fact, reported that cod-liver oil fed to diabetics resulted in tendencies to normalize both hypo- and hyper-aggregability of platelets. Surprisingly, however, they found no influence on the levels of triglycerides. D. Roger Illingworth et al.[149cb] state that in normal humans virtually all the apoprotein B in LDL is derived from the intervascular catabolism of VLDL. Therefore, they maintain, "the rate of synthesis of LDL can be mediated either by a lower rate of VLDL production or by a reduction in the proportion of VLDL apo B converted to LDL (i.e., an increased rate of removal of VLDL remnants)." Dietary fish obviously may be valuable. Consumption of fish and/or of eicosapentenoic acid capsules, however, may compromise vitamin E status and, conceivably, may therefore sometimes be harmful to the cardiovascular system. Simin N. Meydani et al.[149d] cite the work of C. G. Mackenzie et al.[149e] showing that concurrently supplementing fish or fish oils with vitamin E may not eliminate the problem. More research as to the value of dietary fish, cod-liver oil and eicosapentenoic acid is obviously needed. Meanwhile, let the doctrine of the golden mean dictate your dietary policy.

Many suggestions for reducing excessive serum cholesterol will be found in other chapters of this book. However, *Nutrition Reviews* [150] reported that D. Kromhout,[151] as another part of the Zutphen study, showed that body weight was "the most important determinant of serum cholesterol."

A reduction in total blood cholesterol may be useful, but such a reduction will not necessarily effect as beneficial a change in HDL-cholesterol. The HDL-cholesterol (HDL-C) is the cholesterol that is attached to high-density lipoproteins (HDL) and it is generally believed to be beneficial if this value increases.* It is also believed to be beneficial if LDL-cholesterol (LDL-C), the cholesterol attached to low-density lipoproteins (LDL), decreases. The low-density lipoproteins (LDL) are secreted by the liver as very-low-density lipoproteins (VLDL) which transport triglycerides and small amounts of cholesterol. Some of the VLDL travel to fatty tissues where the triglycerides are removed.[152] VLDL are heterogeneous in size and composition including lipolyzed particles

---

* The anti-atherosclerotic action of HDL was originally suggested over one-third of a century ago by Barr et al.,[151a] but the idea remained relatively ignored in clinical practice until about a decade ago.

(remnants), some of which form intermediate-density lipoproteins (IDL) that are eventually converted to LDL.[153] Other VLDL remnant particles are removed by LDL receptors on the liver cells and degraded. Those VLDL particles not converted to IDL and those escaping this degradation form LDL,* which is then supplied with cholesterol by body tissues, especially by the adrenal gland.[152] Thus, the amount of LDL and LDL-cholesterol is controlled by the liver's LDL receptors.

Michael Brown and Joseph Goldstein of the University of Texas Southwestern Medical School at Dallas were awarded the 1985 Nobel Prize for Physiology or Medicine for work involving operation of the LDL receptor. Approximately one person in 500 has a defective LDL receptor gene and so their cells are deficient in removing LDL-C from the bloodstream. [154a-c] Therefore, they have a greater risk of atherosclerosis and heart attacks. Those with two such defective genes often die of heart attacks before they reach adulthood.[154a]

Cholesterol is carried in the bloodstream by LDL to various organs, including the adrenal gland and the ovary, where it is converted to steroid hormones such as cortisol and estradiol.[155] Cholesterol is also the precursor of progesterone, testosterone, aldosterone and vitamin D. Accumulation of free cholesterol (that which has not been converted for body purposes) reduces the cell's ability to make its own cholesterol by turning off the body's synthesis of the enzyme *HMG-CoA reductase* that acts as a catalyst for cholesterol production.[155,155a]**

---

* Vitzchak Oschry et al.[154] hold, in opposition to majority opinion, that in hypertriglyceridemic subjects not all VLDL can be metabolized to LDL.

** Students of chronobiology will be interested in knowing that this enzyme undergoes a diurnal periodicity in the hepatocytes. Olafur G. Björnsson et al.[155b] have covered their discovery in an interesting paper that you may wish to obtain through your librarian. A key step in the biosynthesis of cholesterol is the reduction of 3-hydroxy-3-methylglutaryl (HMG)-CoA to mevalonate (a precursor in the biosynthesis of cholesterol) and this reaction is catalyzed by HMG-CoA reductase. A potent inhibitor of HMG-CoA reductase called *compactin* (also known as ML-236B) was discovered by Akira Endo et al.[155c,d] in the culture broth of the fungus *Penicilium citrinum*.

Leaving our emphasis on LDL-related phenomena, let's note that HDL carries cholesterol to the liver for transformation into bile acids which are used for digestive processes in the intestines. Therefore, HDL is believed to be protective against atherosclerosis. Many studies support this view, including the massive ten-year study sponsored by the National Heart, Lung and Blood Institute.[156-158] Risk is believed to increase when the LDL-C level exceeds 100 mg./100 ml., and for values above 150 mg./100 ml. risk is much greater.[159] It is generally considered wise to attempt to achieve not only a lower LDL-C, but a higher HDL-C/LDL-C ratio. However, Schlierf et al.[160] stress that: "Although there is consistent evidence that a high HDL cholesterol level is indicative of a low risk of coronary heart disease in industrialized populations, evidence is inconclusive that manipulation of HDL leads to an alteration of risks." R. F. Heller[160a] goes even further when he suggests that: "The associations between lipoproteins and both coronary heart disease (CHD) and cancer may be spurious, and enzyme induction may be causally related to all the features of the pattern of correlations." He goes on to say, "The apparent protection against CHD given by low total cholesterol and high HDL-cholesterol levels may be related to low level of clotting factors." I think, nevertheless, that we should assume, until proved to the contrary, that nondrug manipulation of HDL and HDL-C to higher levels and LDL and LDL-C to lower levels is generally beneficial from a heart-health standpoint.

Fiona C. Ballantyne et al.[161] have summarized much of what is known about HDL and LDL. The major component of HDL is apolipoprotein B (apo B).* HDL consists of two main

---

* The protein constituents of lipoproteins are called apoproteins or apolipoproteins. Among the apolipoproteins that have been studied are A-II, A-IV, B, B-48, B-100, C-I, C-II, E-2, E-3 and E-4.[162,163] The principal form of apo B is synthesized in the liver and is called B-100![164] The apo B form of intestinal origin is known as B-48 and is predominant in chylomicrons but is not found in normal LDL.[164] Many of these various apolipoproteins are composed of subfractions. In the case of circulating apo A-I forms, about 79% of A-I is A-I$_4$, about 6% of A-I consists of A-I$_5$ and A-I$_6$, while less than 2% consists of A-I$_2$ and A-I$_3$.[163]

subfractions, HDL$_2$ and HDL$_3$.** The major component of LDL is LDL$_2$ and there are two minor components, LDL$_1$ and LDL$_3$. Each of these subfractions may itself be heterogeneous, e.g., HDL$_2$ has been found to consist of two subfractions, HDL$_{2a}$ and HDL$_{2b}$. It is believed that a high level of HDL$_2$ may be most associated with lowering heart risk, just as it is suspected that an increased LDL$_2$ level may be most associated with increased heart risk.[161] Women have higher levels of HDL$_2$ and are less prone to coronary heart disease than are men.[161] Athletes, such as weightlifters, who take androgens have even lower levels of HDL$_2$ than other men.)[161a] The possible contribution of low HDL$_3$ to heart risk should, however, not be discounted. (Even early work by J. W. Gofman et al.[166] showed that both HDL$_2$ and HDL$_3$ were decreased in subjects at most risk of coronary heart disease, while the LDL subfractions were increased. The Gofman study was published in 1966 but attracted very little attention at the time.)

The levels of apolipoprotein B (or simply apoprotein B), the major apoprotein of LDL, and apolipoprotein A-I and A-II, the apolipoproteins of HDL, provide additional prognostic information in estimating a patient's risk of coronary artery disease (CAD). James J. Maciejko et al.[167] concluded that, "Apolipoprotein A-I by itself is more useful than HDL cholesterol for identifying patients with CAD." Peter O. Kwiterovich and Allan D. Sniderman[168] confirmed that apo A-I levels, like HDL-cholesterol levels, are associated with a lower prevalence of CAD, while the levels of

---

Apolipoprotein A-I is a potent activator of the LCAT enzyme in the serum.[163a] Apo C-I (a constituent, along with apo C-III, of the very-low-density lipoproteins) and apo C-II also activate LCAT to a lesser degree.[163a] Apo C-II also activates the enzyme lipoprotein lipase.[163a] Plasma apolipoprotein A-II has been found, by Puchois et al.,[163b] to be greatly elevated (45% above normal) in alcoholics and is thus a biochemical indicator of alcohol abuse.

** Another component, HDL$_4$, has recently been identified by R. J. Deckelbaum et al.[165] HDL$_4$ contains apo A-I and apo A-II. Body position at the time of, or shortly before, blood withdrawal significantly influences cholesterol and apolipoprotein levels. When patient is prone, blood becomes dilute; when patient stands, it becomes concentrated, thus altering lipid levels. (*American Family Physician* (1986) 34, no. 3: 296).

apolipoprotein B, like LDL levels, are associated with increased CAD.* Recent studies, as J. Scott et al.[169] observe, have found a stronger negative correlation between apo A-II and both prevalent myocardial infarction[170] and peripheral vascular disease[171] than between either HDL-cholesterol or apo A-I concentration and those diseases. Scott and his associates cite other studies indicating that apo A-II seems to be a cofactor for two enzymes involved in lipoprotein metabolism—lecithin: cholesterol acyl transferase (LCAT)[172]** and hepatic endothelial lipase.[173]

The reasons for low HDL and high LDL concentrations being associated with a risk of atherosclerosis have not been fully elucidated. We have already noted LDL is the principal carrier of cholesterol that is transported to and is taken up by cells. Plasma LDL is a precursor of the lipids and proteins that are deposited in the intima of the arteries which is associated with atherosclerosis. On the other hand, HDL carries free cholesterol that has been removed from tissues. It is possible that HDL may also function by inhibiting the uptake of LDL by the cells.[174] A beneficial action of HDL and perhaps especially of HDL 2 probably involves its ability to scavenge cholesterol from cells of the arterial wall.[174] (A synthetic HDL-like complex has been developed and preliminary work shows it to be effective *in vitro* in removing lipids from smooth muscle cells cultured from atherosclerotic plaques of human aorta.)[174]

Achieving increased HDL and HDL-C while simultaneously decreasing LDL and LDL-C can be accomplished in several ways. For one, the HDL-C/LDL-C ratio (and also any prevalent hypertriglyceridemia) will be improved by increasing consumption of eicosapentenoic acid (EPA) as found in fish

---

* M. F. Reardon et al.[168a] have reported that the severity of atherosclerosis in men is strongly related to LDL-C and apolipoprotein B concentrations. However, in women it is related to triglyceride concentrations in plasma IDL (intermediate-density lipoproteins) and LDL and to the cholesterol and apolipoprotein concentrations in IDL. Thus, the status of the IDL takes on greater importance for women.

** Subsequently, Armin Steinmetz and Gerd Utermann[72a] reported that both apo A-I and apo A-IV also activate LCAT.

oils.[175-178] (We will be discussing EPA further in Chapter 4 in connection with cod-liver oil.) A second way to favorably influence the HDL-C/LDL-C ratio is simply to consume a diet low in total fat, low in saturated fat, low in cholesterol and moderate (not high) in polyunsaturated fat.[179] Richard S. Cooper et al.[179] suggested that a ratio of about 1 between saturated and polyunsaturated fats may be optimal. A third way of beneficially raising the HDL-C/LDL-C ratio is to increase consumption of oleic acid, a monounsaturated fatty acid whose most common source is olive oil. A report by Fred H. Mattson[180] showed that olive oil reduces LDL-C but has no effect on HDL-C.

Among the other ways to increase the HDL-C/LDL-C ratio is through moderate consumption of alcohol.[181,182] Joanne E. Cluette et al.[182] reported that monkeys fed ethanol had significantly greater HDL nonesterified cholesterol, with about 60% of the HDL being represented by the HDL 3 subfraction.* Aerobic exercise also beneficially affects the HDL-C/LDL-C ratio.[183,184] Interestingly, Naruhiko Nagao et al.[184] reported that athletic training requiring vigorous activity seemed to cause an increase in both HDL-C and apo A-I and a decrease in the cholesterol/HDL-C ratio. They found that especially the apo A-I value tended to increase in proportion to the amount of training. Another way to beneficially affect the relevant parameters is by eating a vegetarian diet.** Cooper et al.,[179] and independently Paul J. Nestel,[185] showed that a vegetarian diet significantly reduced the levels of total cholesterol and LDL-C while only modestly decreasing the beneficial HDL-C. The changes resulted in an increase in the HDL-C/LDL-C ratio. More recently, Masarei et al.[186] found that the decrease in HDL-C was primarily in the HDL2-C fraction. Frank M. Sacks et al.[187] also reported that vegetarians had much lower levels of LDL, but they found,

---

* In recent research among 535 men attending a health-screening center in Australia, J. K. Allen and M. A. Adena[182a] found that in these persons the division of cholesterol among its fractions was "apparently independent of both alcohol consumption and cholesterol synthesis."

** Garlic may be an important factor in lowering cholesterol. E. Ernst et al.[184a] have reported the effect and have cited other studies with similar results.

contrary to Cooper et al.,[179] Nestel[185] and John R. L. Masarei et al.,[186] that the vegetarians also had slightly but significantly higher levels of the beneficial HDL-C.* The Sacks' group also observed that the vegetarians had lower levels of triglyceride and VLDL that carries most of the triglyceride in the plasma. Excessive coffee drinking may, however, upset some of the benefits of an otherwise good diet. Paul T. Williams et al.[188] reported that, in men, apo B and LDL-cholesterol were unrelated to intake of coffee up to 2-3 cups/day but positively associated with intake above 2-3 cups/day. (Women were not studied.) Earlier, D. S. Thelle et al.,[189] as part of the Tromso heart study, had reported that coffee raises serum cholesterol. Almost simultaneous with the Williams work, Olav Helge Forde et al.,[190] also as part of the Tromso heart study, found that cholesterol concentrations dropped significantly in men with hypercholesterolemia who abstained from coffee drinking. (Again, women were not studied.)

To help put the HDL/LDL and HDL-C/LDL-C ratios in proper prospective, however, we should note that high values for HDL and HDL-C may not be an unmixed blessing. Dietary fat is usually associated with the incidence of both coronary heart disease (CHD) and colon cancer. HDL and HDL-C, on the other hand, while *inversely* related to the incidence of CHD, may be *directly* related to the incidence of cancer. While HDL and HDL-C are heart-protective, they may work against cancer protection. Perhaps it is a case of HDL and HDL-C protecting so well against heart disease that what is left to cause death is simply other causes, among which is cancer. Ancel Keys[191] has stated that there was no significant difference in the HDL-C levels of the dead of all causes and the survivors and between heart disease survivors and those who died of heart disease. The only

---

* Subsequently, Frank M. Sacks et al.[187a] reported that lactovegetarians had 24% higher LDL-C levels and 7% higher HDL-C levels than strict vegetarians. They concluded that ingesting fatty dairy products raises the LDL-C level on a percentage basis about three times as fast as it raises the HDL-C level.

significant difference in HDL-C levels continued to be in those who died of cancer.

It is widely known, as we noted earlier, that cholesterol serves useful body functions, although it is seldom suggested that cholesterol, at any dosage, might be beneficial in preventing atherosclerosis. In an interesting example of the *reverse effect,* the work of Russell L. Holman,[192] done some 40 years ago, showed that experimental arterial lesions in rabbits were *prevented* by cholesterol. Dr. Holman suggested that cholesterol may be primarily protective and only secondarily alterative. It is surprising that this research has been neglected for these 40 years.*

We noted earlier that low serum cholesterol may be associated with an increased cancer death rate. The Framingham Heart Study has shown an inverse relationship between naturally occurring serum cholesterol levels and cancer risk for men (but not for women).[192a] The same finding that lower cholesterol levels are associated with higher cancer mortality has been observed among the men participating in the Puerto Rico Heart Study and in the Honolulu Heart Study.[192a] This inverse relation agrees with other epidemiological evidence showing (in references cited by Victor Herbert)[193] that low serum cholesterol seems to be associated with increased risk of cancer. The International Collaborative Group[194] investigated the circulating cholesterol level and ten-year cancer mortality in 61,567 men aged 40 to 69 years from 11 population studies in 8 countries. They reported that: "Those dying of cancer within one year of cholesterol determination had mean cholesterol levels 24 to 25 mg./dL lower on the average than the rest of the men. For years 2 through 5 and 6 through 10, the inverse association diminished markedly, with differences in mean cholesterol levels of only 4 to 5 mg./dL and 2 mg./dL, respectively." They concluded that: "These findings are

---

* Perhaps it is not really surprising. Holman's finding could be in error as most scientists learning of the results would quickly conclude. *Reverse effects* are neither expected nor looked for. When they occur, they are sometimes interpreted as being errors. Yet, if cholesterol at some dosages might protect against atherosclerosis, it would be worth replicating the experiment on the chance that Holman was correct.

consistent with the hypothesis that lower cholesterol levels in cancer decedents are due to the effect of undetected disease on cholesterol levels." Manning Feinleib[195] has, on the other hand, recently reviewed the epidemiological evidence for a possible relationship between hypocholesterolemia and cancer and concluded that the data does not support a cause-and-effect relationship. Furthermore, in regard to cholesterol consumption, Feinleib states, "The data from dietary studies, both at the group level and at individual levels, indicate that, if anything, higher intakes of cholesterol appear to be related to cancer rather than lower levels." In this connection, we should note David F. Horrobin[196] says that the more malignant the tumor, the higher may be its cholesterol content. He states that in patients with breast or brain cancer the serum cholesterol levels may be very elevated. He warns that although in terminal cancer, because of cachexia, serum levels may fall, they should not obscure the importance of the early rise.

One reason for the state of confusion could be that cholesterol may sometimes be more dangerous, sometimes less dangerous. Smith[197] has made the point that, like other unsaturated lipids, cholesterol can be affected by free radical processes just as can polyunsaturated fatty acids and their esters. Many of the studies concerning cholesterol that have been done for the past three-quarters of a century have failed to consider this fact and have used oxidized cholesterol rather than cholesterol itself. Thus, it may be that cholesterol may have improperly received some of the blame that should have been given instead to oxidized cholesterol. C. B. Taylor et al.[198] suggested that all studies on the induction of atherosclerosis by feeding cholesterol may have contained oxidized sterols that were atherogenic, whereas if cholesterol itself had been used it might not have been atherogenic.

What can we do to minimize our intake of oxidized cholesterol? First, we can make sure that all foods containing cholesterol are stored in well-sealed containers and refrigerated. In addition, it might be wise to reduce consumption of dried milk or dried egg products (egg noodles being an example) that contain oxidized sterols.[197,197a] In this case, macaroni (which is egg-free) might be a healthful substitute. Leland L. Smith[197] gives other examples of foods having oxidized sterols, even including baker's yeast which contains cholesta-3,5-dien-7-one, and brewer's yeast which contains ergosterol 5∝, 8∝−peroxide, cerevisterol and 5∝, 8∝−ergosta-6,22-diene-3 beta, 5,8-triol. (Sometimes health faddists state that one should not buy products where the list of ingredients contains names of unpronounceable chemicals. The three chemicals just named, even if they were not forms of oxidized sterols, would seem to easily qualify brewer's yeast for removal from their shopping lists.)

(continued from page 228)

Butter, which contains about 40% unsaturated fats, but is usually thought of as being saturated, may be a healthful source of fat. However, this issue is hotly debated and the curious reader is referred to the arguments of the antibutter side represented by R. W. D. Turner[199] and the rebuttal by the probutter side represented by J. A. L. Gorringe.[200] M. J. Hill[201] reported that animals, while on a low-fiber diet, showed an increased fecal bile acid concentration as dietary fat was increased. However, on a high-fiber, high-fat diet, fecal bile acid increased when the fat was sunflower oil but not when the fat was butter. Fecal bile acid is a probable negative as far as colon cancer is concerned, so Hill's results[202] are a "plus" for butter.* On the other hand, bile acids in the colon inhibit absorption

---

* Based on rat experiments, fiber, fed as wheat bran, develops greater acidity of intestinal contents. This acidification inhibits degradation of acid into carcinogens. (A *reverse effect* could be operating. See pages 33-35 for contrary studies.) Paradoxically, while fiber may protect the colon, it could promote cancer in the stomach since the effect on gastric contents is opposite, i.e., it makes the stomach less acid. Perhaps this explains the very low incidence of colorectal cancer among the Japanese (who eat a relatively unrefined, high-fiber diet) and their high incidence of stomach cancer.[203] Further confusion regarding fiber comes out of a study of W. Haenszel et al.[204] who, in working with Hawaiian Japanese, found that colorectal cancer is correlated, not only with meat consumption, but with the frequency of legume intake. Legumes are rich in fiber, so perhaps it is not just fiber, but cereal fiber that protects. (A subsequent 38-country epidemiological study by Gail E. McKeown-Eyssen and Elizabeth Bright-See [205] supports the idea that cereal fiber is the only fiber whose consumption is negatively

of both sodium (which may sometimes be good to inhibit) and water, thus having a laxative effect.[206]

The various negative aspects of eating only unsaturated fats might logically be expected to result in a decrease in longevity. Denham Harman[207] reported on an experiment with male rats that demonstrated this effect. Harman fed various groups of rats either lard, olive oil, corn oil or safflower oil at levels of 5%, 10% and 20% of their respective diets. The mean life span of animals was longer when fat was at a level of 5% or 10% than when it represented 20% of their diet. Among the groups fed the 20% fat diet, those fed the lard (primarily saturated fat) had considerably longer mean life spans (but not longer maximum life spans) than the other groups. Harman also called attention to the work of R. J. Morin, who found that when mice were given either 15% safflower oil or 15% coconut oil (which is very saturated) in their diet, the mean life span of the safflower oil group was 8.7% less than that of the coconut oil group. More recently, Miroslav Ledvina and Milena Hodanova[211] fed one group of female rats a diet supplemented with sunflower oil and another with sunflower oil plus alpha tocopherol for their entire life spans. The mean life span of the tocopherol and sunflower oil group was 704 days; that of the sunflower oil without vitamin E group, 620 days; and that of a control group, 690 days. The results, although favoring use of vitamin E when polyunsaturated fat was fed, were not considered to be statistically significant.

Harman[207] also reported on another experiment, this one with female rats, regarding the effect of various fats on death due to cancer. Those groups fed the lower amount (5% of diet) of various types of fats developed far less cancer than those fed fats at the 15% or 20% levels. However, among the rats fed fats at the 20% level,

---

associated with colon cancer.) Although dietary fiber generally speeds up transit time of chyme through the intestines, Barbara Olds Schneeman[204a] has reported that fibers such as guar gum and pectin delay the "rate of progress to more distal regions of the gut." This, as Schneeman notes, could contribute to the reduction in food intake associated with their ingestion. I wonder, however, if the slowed transit time of guar gum and pectin might make nonexistent the beneficial reduction in colon cancer that is associated with the ingestion of other fibers.

those given the more saturated diet (lard and olive oil) developed less cancer through the age of 16 months than those given the polyunsaturated fat. Harman did not report on the number in each group that eventually developed cancer, but the maximum life spans of animals in the various groups were approximately equal, thus making me wonder if cancer might have simply been delayed but not avoided. Harman's data shows that the olive oil group, through the age of 16 months, developed less cancer than did the lard group. He does not comment on this, but this fact also seems surprising since olive oil is less saturated than lard (but, of course, is much more saturated than corn or safflower oil).* Obviously, I have some

---

* A recent study by C. B. Wood et al.[207a] showed that, among 60 patients with malignancies, the ratio of stearic (a saturated acid) to oleic acid in their erythrocyte cell membranes was consistently lower than among healthy controls or controls with other diseases; i.e., in contrast with Harman's study, the use of oleic acid is probably more dangerous from a cancer standpoint than is the use of saturated fat. Furthermore, J. Booyens and L. Maguire[207b] suggest that oleic acid, and not the essential fatty acids, could be responsible for the tumorigenicity that has been reported. Earlier, Booyens et al.[90d] had reported that oleic acid enhanced the proliferation of osteogenic sarcoma cells in culture. Epidemiological data may, however, tend to exonerate oleic acid. The diets of Greece and of Italy contain large amounts of oleic acid in the form of olive oil. In the year 1964 the standardized death rates for these countries and for the U.S. in regard to cardiovascular problems and from neoplasms were given by Preston et al.[207c] as follows:

Country		Standardized Cardiovascular	Death Rates Neoplasms	Ratio of Stand. Death Rates (Cardiovascular/Neoplasms)
Greece	- males	.00104	.00083	1.25
	- females	.00090	.00054	1.67
Italy	- males	.00192	.00099	1.94
	- females	.00138	.00069	2.00
U.S.A.	- males	.00270	.00092	2.93
	- females	.00153	.00070	2.19

For both males and females (but especially for males) the relative death rates from cardiovascular causes were considerably lower in Greece and Italy than in the U.S. At the same time, the standardized neoplasm death rates for the U.S. were about the same as those of Greece and Italy. Let's keep in mind, however, that death rates are determined by many factors and that consumption of oleic acid might be merely associated rather than causally related. The data suggest, nevertheless, that oleic acid might be beneficial from a cardiovascular standpoint and that it does not seem to add to human cancer mortality.

problems with this experiment but concur with one of Harman's conclusions: "Although the rat tumor incidence appears to increase with increasing unsaturation of dietary fat, the differences are not statistically significant."

Harman[208] also reported that when mammary carcinogenesis in mice was brought on by the carcinogen 7,12-dimethylbenz-alpha-anthracene (DMBA), tumor incidence was greater when the dietary fat was corn oil in contrast to the tumor occurrence in those fed the saturated coconut oil. Lipid peroxidation of the corn oil was an apparent causal factor as shown by the fact that, 179 days after DMBA was administered, tumor incidence was just 40% in the mice fed corn oil with 20 mg. of vitamin E, while 73.6% of those fed corn oil with only 5 mg. of vitamin E developed tumors. Charles F. Aylsworth et al.[209] confirming that high levels of polyunsaturated fat promote DMBA-induced mammary tumorigenesis, reported that the mode of action seems to be through inhibition of intercellular communication. Their observations are important since they provide evidence that "unsaturated fatty acids have a direct influence on tumor cell growth rather than acting indirectly through another system (i.e. endocrine system, immune system)." While corn oil might appear to be tumorigenic, a rat study by Eva Kwong et al.,[210] on the contrary, showed that a 20% corn oil diet caused tumors to regress. (However, tumors continued to grow in rats fed diets containing free fatty acids from corn oil.) They concluded that something in corn oil was associated with tumor regression. (These results and conclusion are contrary to not only the work of Denham Harman[208] and Charles F. Aylsworth et al.,[209] but that of Selenskas et al.[126c] reported earlier.)

Mary G. Enig et al.[122] has found interesting correlations between dietary fat intake and cancer mortality over a 60-year period. In reviewing the extensive literature, Enig et al. reported that many studies show significant positive correlations between cancer mortality and both total fat and vegetable fat,* but no correlations or

---

* Peanut oil and corn oil (and other peanut and corn products) may pose an additional threat in the form of aflatoxin. Thomas H. Jukes[212] has cited an FDA spokesman who, on

negative correlations for animal fat. After being criticized by several scientists and reviewing the relevant studies, Enig et al.[122a] retracted the "clean bill of health" they had erroneously given animal fat as a cause of cancer. They modified their position to state that all dietary fat components should be further studied as possible cancer-causing agents. Dietary fat seems to be a promoter rather than an initiator of cancer, but the mechanisms of its action are unknown.[122b,c]

Excessive fat, and especially polyunsaturated fat, appears to also have a negative effect on the central nervous system. Denham Harman et al.[214] discovered that the number of errors rats made in running a maze increased with the degree of unsaturated fat in their diet. Those fed 5% fat did better than those fed 20%. Among those fed 20% lard or 20% safflower oil, the lard group showed much better ability to run the maze. However, when each of a group of rats was fed 20 mg. of vitamin E in addition to a 20% safflower oil diet, their ability to run the maze was almost as good as that of the lard-fed group. In this particular experiment, there was no significant difference in life span among the various groups so Harman theorizes that the negative effect of polyunsaturated fats (unless protected by additional vitamin E) may be greater on the central nervous system than on the rest of the body.

With a diet whose fat content consists almost entirely of the polyunsaturated variety there is also a danger that gallstones may develop. Alan F. Hofmann et al.[215] reported on studies showing that an excessive intake of unsaturated fats can lead to bile lithogenicity (gallstones). Paradoxically, and exemplifying the *reverse effect,* even though gallstones consist primarily of solid cholesterol, reducing the cholesterol intake too severely actually encourages their formation.[216] Then, a little later, George W. Melchior et al.[217] observed that safflower oil caused gallstones to develop in monkeys, but coconut

---

November 14, 1977, estimated that 66 lifetime cancers per 100,000 persons could develop from aflatoxin contaminated peanut and corn products. Aflatoxin problems do not arise only from improper storage conditions. A study by E. B. Lillehoj et al.[213] found that amounts of aflatoxin B₁ in corn, before harvest, ranged from 1 to 430 parts/billion.

oil apparently had a protective influence due, they speculated, to the latter's slower turnover rate in the bile acid pool.*

It seems apparent, then, that too great a consumption of unsaturated fats can be detrimental to health. However, if vitamin E is present to prevent rancidity, the unsaturated fats, consumed in modest amounts, are not dangerous. On the contrary, as we have seen in this chapter, they are essential for the body's production of prostaglandins which, in turn, are needed to assure health.

In studying the various animal experiments one should keep in mind that most of them involve ingestion of uncooked fat, whereas humans often consume cooked fat. The pyrolysis of fat produces a complex mixture of aldehydes, ketones, unsaturated aliphatic compounds and other chemicals, most of which remain unstudied in biological systems.[218a] Among these compounds are possible carcinogens and some could act synergistically. On the other hand, I speculate that these carcinogens at some dosages, and under some states of synergism, might exhibit *reverse effects* and be cancer-protective. (Some studies show no relation between fat and cancer.[219] Could *reverse effects* be masking reality?)

As important as both unsaturated and saturated fats are to health, it seems probable that most of us in the United States consume too great a quantity of total fat.** As we age, our intestinal absorption of linoleic acid may increase if an experiment with rats is applicable to humans. D. Hollander et al.[220] found that the ability of rats to absorb linoleic acid as they aged increased 5-fold both in the jejunum and in

---

* Persons with healthy gall bladders are likely to have a high phospholipid-cholesterol ratio in their bile, according to Dr. Ronald K. Thompkins of Ohio State University. One could take supplemental lecithin to increase the phospholipid-cholesterol ratio. However, I am concerned with the healthfulness of some lecithin products and tell of these concerns in Chapter 5 in connection with choline. (Gallstones, which are solidified cholesterol, are likely to form when there is not sufficient bile acid to keep the cholesterol suspended. Studies by Dr. Leslie J. Schoenfield et al.[218] showed, by the way, that giving chenodeoxycholic acid—a naturally occurring bile acid—dissolved gallstones in some patients in from six months to two years, although the procedure is not without risk.)

** Reduction in fat intake can, however, be overdone. William Fears et al.[219a] have cited the work of R. A. Frisch,[219b] who has shown that menarche begins when the body achieves a certain percent of body fat. Women who are "under-fat" because of *anorexia nervosa* or because of excessive exercising may have amenorrhea and reproduction difficulties.

the ileum. As we age, it might be important to restrict fatty acid consumption if our ability to absorb it increases.

Too much fat in the diet is detrimental to health and longevity. It can lead to an excess of fat in the bloodstream where it coats the red blood cells and causes them to stack together like a roll of coins, called the *rouleau formation*. In regard to cancer, dietary fat seems to act, as we noted earlier, at the promotional stage of carcinogenesis rather than as an initiating agent.[122b,c,221] Dietary fat has been shown, in experiments with female rats, to raise the level of serum prolactin and may thereby promote growth of mammary tumors.[222*] Administering an antiprolactin drug eliminated the tumor-promoting effect of the high-fat diet, whereas giving an antiestrogen drug was only partially effective.[224] It seems probable that dietary fat promotes mammary cancer through its action in raising the concentration of both prolactin and of estrogen. Dietary fat may promote colon cancer, on the other hand, according to H. L. Newmark et al.[225] by increasing the levels of ionized fatty acids and bile acids in the contents of the colon.[**]

P. Stevens et al.[226] point out that evidence from hunting and gathering communities of East Africa supports the theory that both animal and plant foods of neolithic man were low in fat but relatively rich in essential fatty acids. Thus, they maintain that advice to reduce total fat but relatively to increase essential fatty acids in the diet is not a recommendation for a "change in diet" but a move to return to the original human food structure.

S. Boyd Eaton and Melvin Konner[227] have made detailed estimates of the dietary components of paleolithic man. They point out that today's domesticated animals are fatter than their wild ancestors because of their steady food supply and their reduced physical activity. Furthermore, modern breeding and feeding procedures have further increased the fat content to satisfy man's

---

* Prolactin inhibits tumor growth when administered early but enhances growth of tumors when given late. D. F. Horrobin[223] supplies a rationale for this finding.

** H. L. Newmark et al.[225] suggested that the risk of colon cancer may also depend on the dietary levels of phosphorus and calcium. They have proposed that increasing the calcium content of the diet and/or decreasing the phosphorus content might be preventative.

desire for tender meat. Eaton and Konner cite a study by H. O. Ledger[228] showing that the mean carcass fat of 15 different species of free-living African herbivores of today averages 3.9%. This contrasts with a fat content of 24%, 30% or even more in domesticated animals bred and raised for meat tenderness. [227] Furthermore, there is not only less fat in wild animals but its composition is different than that of domesticated species. Eaton and Konner cite a study of M. A. Crawford[229] and another by C. K. W. Wo and H. H. Draper[230] that reported the fat of wild game has five times as much polyunsaturated fat. Additionally, a study by M. A. Crawford et al.[231] and one by J. Dyerberg et al.,[232] both of which were cited by Eaton and Konner, showed that the fat of wild animals contains about 4% eicosapentenoic acid compared to negligible amounts in domestic beef. (Modern man's only noteworthy dietary sources for this valuable nutrient are fatty, cold-water fish and fish oils such as cod-liver oil.) Interestingly, Eaton and Konner maintain that the amount of cholesterol in the diet of primitive man was about the same as that of modern man since the amount of cholesterol in meat, according to R. M. Feeley et al.,[233] is unaffected by fat content. This helps support cholesterol's relative unimportance to our health (as shown by the formula of Ancel Keys[136] cited earlier).

Whereas, the ratio of polyunsaturated-to-saturated fat in the current American diet is about .44,[227] and the U.S. Select Committee on Nutrition and Human Needs[234] recommends a ratio of 1.0, the late paleolithic diet may have been more like 1.41.[227] If there is merit to returning to a more primitive diet, a decrease in the consumption of red meats with their man-manipulated fat content and an increase in our intake of vegetables, poultry (for its polyunsaturated fat) and fish (for its eicosapentenoic acid) must be prime considerations.

There may be danger, however, in increasing our absolute intake of polyunsaturated fat. The nutrition committee of the American Heart Association points out that no large population has consumed polyunsaturated fats for many years with demonstrated safety, and high-fat diets may lead to weight gain. Furthermore, polyunsaturated fats may not only increase the risk of gallstones in some persons, but they are cocarcinogenic in laboratory animals and they can alter cell membranes.[235] On the other hand, a study by Constance Kies, cited in *Medical World News*,[235a] suggests that a low-fat, high-fiber diet might increase the risk of bone disease by decreasing the amount of calcium absorbed by the body.

In thinking about polyunsaturated fats we should, however, resist the temptation to consider the various polyunsaturated fatty acids as being equivalent. Their effects on platelet aggregation and on thrombosis may be very dissimilar and even opposite. I think a reasonable objective is to reduce total fat consumption, greatly reduce saturated fat intake and slightly increase one's relative (but not necessarily one's absolute) intake of *cis*-linoleic acid and of gamma-linolenic acid while reducing use of the *trans* fatty acids.

A Note About Aspirin

It has long been established that aspirin (acetylsalicylic acid) inhibits prostaglandin synthesis. Prostaglandin E2 is a pyrogen (i.e., a fever-inducing agent) and when the body experiences infections it reacts by causing a fever to help fight that infection.[236] Aspirin, by inhibiting prostaglandin synthesis (via the cyclo-oxygenase pathway)[237-239] reduces the fever.* Considerable research has been concerned with this action of aspirin, but those interested in medical

---

* The body combats infection by increasing the rate at which metabolic functions occur—and this leads to fever. It is true that excessive fever may cause brain damage (although swabbing the forehead with a damp cloth at room temperature may keep the head temperature at a safe level). Elsewhere in the body fever serves a valuable function that we all too often negate with antipyretics. Those interested in studying the benefits of fever are referred to *International Symposium on Fever* edited by James M. Lipton,[240] to *Fever—Its Biology, Evolution and Function* by Mathew J. Kluger,[241] to several studies[241a-c] cited by Gordon W. Duff and Scott K. Durum[241d] and to the work of Simon.[242] Duff and Durum[241d] cite the work of K. A. Smith et al.[241e] showing that the mitogenic action of the lymphokine interleukin-1 on T cells is probably mediated by the lymphocyte product interleukin-2. Harvey B. Simon[242] suggests that endogenous pyrogen is identical with interleukin-1, a mononuclear cell product that enhances the function of lymphocytes. Duff and Durum[241d] reported on *in vitro* work showing that, "The T-cell proliferative response to interleukin-1 (and to the lymphokine, interleukin-2) was greatly increased at 39°C compared to 37°C." They continued by saying, "These findings suggest that, if similar events occur *in vivo*, fever may have important immunoregulatory significance and call into question the current indiscriminate use of antipyretic agents." They pointed out, however, that "antipyretic drugs may be useful

history will find the definitive early studies in three articles appearing in the same issue of *Nature New Biology*.[243-245] This work helped J. R. Vane win a Nobel Prize in 1982. Since the major substrate of the cyclo-oxygenase enzyme is arachidonic acid,[246] the amount present to follow the lipoxygenase pathway to the leukotrienes is probably increased by consuming aspirin.**

Aspirin also affects the production of other prostaglandins that are unrelated to fever and can thus upset the entire body. For example, consider just one side effect of aspirin ingestion—bleeding and ulceration of the gastrointestinal tract. This effect (more common in women than in men) is probably caused by aspirin's reducing the synthesis of prostaglandins that increase the resistance of the gastric mucosa to the acid environment.[249] This mechanism also suggests the vital part played by vitamin E and the polyunsaturated fatty acids in the prevention of ulcers since they encourage the manufacture of the protective prostaglandins. (Based on a rat experiment by A. A. van Kolfschoten et al.,[250] it appears that BHT may also protect the stomach against injury from aspirin without affecting its pharmacological activity.)

---

in auto-immune diseases where the immune response is detrimental to the host." Using cell cultures, Vincenzo Rossi et al.[242a] have found that interleukin-1 induced secretion of prostacyclin in the endothelial and smooth muscle cells of the vascular walls. This discovery may exemplify another advantage of fever if interleukin-1 is the endogenous pyrogen. The discovery is also likely to lead to new strategies in antithrombic therapy. To the extent that aspirin may negate the effect of interleukin-1, that action would seem to work against aspirin's antithrombic properties.

** It seems puzzling why aspirin should be so effective in combating inflammation since, by its blocking of cyclo-oxygenase but not of lipoxygenase, it fosters the metabolic pathway by which arachidonic acid forms very active flammagens.[247] (William F. Stenson and Charles W. Parker,[247a] however, cite Siegel et al. as having shown with *in vitro* studies, that both aspirin and indomethacin, in high doses, block the lipoxygenase pathway in platelets and neutrophils.) Gerald Weissman[248] speculates that NSAID—nonsteroidal anti-inflammatory drugs (e.g., aspirin, indomethacin, piroxicam and ibuprofen)—can induce the neutrophil to form metabolites which act as endogenous inhibitors of inflammation. Of course, aspirin and the other NSAID are far from perfect antiflammagens. Indomethacin, which inhibits only the cyclo-oxygenase pathway, did not stop formation of the flammagen 12-HETE.[249] However, the drug BW75SC, which inhibits both cyclo-oxygenase and lipoxygenase pathways, acted as an effective antiflammagen.[249] A subsequent study by M. Fletcher-Cieutat et al.[249a] yielded results suggesting that aspirin may indirectly suppress production of lipoxygenase products by enhancing the lipoxygenase-inhibitory effects of 15-HETE.

J. G. Collier and R. J. Flower[251] discovered that, in experiments with 4 men aged 22 to 29, aspirin (in dosages of 600 mg., 4 times daily over a period of a week) caused a fall in concentration of both E and F type prostaglandins in their semen. (They did not measure changes in other types of prostaglandins present in the semen.) These researchers pointed out that oligospermic men (men with low sperm count) have abnormally low concentrations of seminal prostaglandins. A. K. Didolkar et al.,[252] in experiments with rats, also concluded that aspirin impairs spermatogenesis. Men who are trying out for fatherhood should obviously avoid aspirin. It should be apparent, however, that I am not recommending taking of aspirin as a birth control technique.

H. U. Comberg et al.[253] reported that F. ten Hoor and H. M. Van de Graaf found aspirin completely prevented the hypotensive action of elevated dietary linoleic acid. We might note also that the excessive use of aspirin can cause a rapid and irregular pulse, edema, asthma, albuminuria, tinnitus, deafness, allergy and interaction with other drugs.[254,255] Amy L. Daniels and Gladys J. Everson[255a] showed, a half-century ago, that aspirin promotes excretion of ascorbic acid in the urine. H. S. Loh and C. W. M. Wilson[255b] more recently have found that the drug can cause ascorbic acid depletion in normal persons. It has also been reported that aspirin poisoning causes the death of 200 persons annually.

An interesting experiment by G. B. West[256] demonstrated that aspirin was far more toxic in rats fed a high carbohydrate diet than it was in rats fed large amounts of protein. A deficiency in magnesium greatly increased the toxicity, especially in pregnant animals (Figure 10). Daily doses equivalent to three 5-grain tablets four times a day in humans resulted in many dead fetuses in animals fed the high carbohydrate diet. Gastric ulceration in nonpregnant rats was very severe on the high-carbohydrate diet. It is dangerous to extrapolate results of animal experiments to man, but perhaps in humans also (and especially during pregnancy) aspirin may be more dangerous to those on a high-carbohydrate diet, particularly if they are deficient in magnesium.

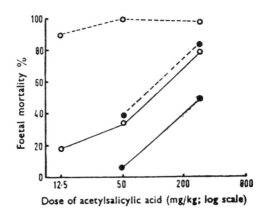

Figure 10. Toxicity of aspirin in pregnant rats fed a high protein diet (•-•) or a high carbohydrate diet (o-o). The effects of magnesium deficiency are shown by the broken lines. Note that magnesium deficiency and the high carbohydrate diet markedly increase the toxicity. Reproduced from G. B. West, *Jrl. Pharm. Pharmacol.* (1964) 16: 788-793, with permission of the publisher.

Aspirin also suppresses interferon's induction of the enzyme indoleamine 2,3-dioxygenase.[257] However, aspirin does not seem to affect interferon's induction of 2,5-oligoadenylate synthetase and protein kinase[257] which are believed to mediate antiviral activity.[258] Since aspirin does not seem to affect the synthesis of these latter two enzymes, it is (at least for this reason) not countermanded for use in treating colds.

In the attempt to reduce the toxic effects of aspirin, some physicians[259] recommend taking aspirin and acetaminophen at the same time so as to limit the intake of each drug to "safe" levels. Other physicians[260] fear that if aspirin were to be used with acetaminophen it would increase acetaminophen's hepatoxic potential and also work toward depletion of glutathione. The depletion of glutathione would be likely to occur even if the drugs were given alternatively instead of together.[260]

Those, then, are some of the negative effects of aspirin. On the other hand, many benefits may derive from aspirin ingestion.

Ryunosuke Kumashiro et al.[261] have found that low-dose aspirin is effective in preventing stress-induced ulcers in rats. (In a related study, A. Robert[262] reported that intestinal ulcers formed in rats following treatment with indomethacin and flufenamic acid due, apparently, to depletion in body tissues of endogenous prostaglandins.) *In vitro* animal studies have shown aspirin to effectively inhibit sorbitol and fructose formation in diabetic lenses and to also inhibit the enzyme aldose reductase. Thus, there could be beneficial implications for inhibiting formation of cataracts. Edward Cotlier et al.[263] have, in fact, favorably reported on cataract retardant effects of aspirin administered to diabetic and nondiabetic patients. Even cancer may be favorably affected by aspirin. James J. Kolenick et al.[264] found that aspirin inhibited formation of pulmonary metastases in mice. Gabriel Gasic et al.[265] also favorably reported on aspirin's effect in reducing metastases in cancerous mice. Metastasis is reduced by thrombocytopenia (a condition in which there is a decrease in the number of platelets)[266] Gasic suggests that metastasis may be produced via platelet aggregation by tumor cells.[265] Thus, aspirin in inhibiting such aggregation, might be of value in cancer therapy.*

However, perhaps the most beneficial aspects of aspirin are its anodynous and anti-inflammatory effects and its power to inhibit platelet aggregation. A tremendous, worldwide research effort is now underway to determine the optimum level of aspirin in protecting against atherosclerosis, heart attacks and stroke.[274-294] One study[293] showed that the benefits of aspirin in preventing stroke may be limited to men. The finding has not been explained and it seems likely that future studies will show that aspirin may also reduce the incidence of stroke in women. Aspirin inhibits cyclo-oxygenase

---

* There are other platelet deaggregators that may find clinical application in the inhibition of cancer metastasis.[267-272] Kailash C. Agarwal and Robert E. Parks [273] reported that forskolin, derived from the roots of an Indian plant, *Coleus forskohlii,* is one such possible anticancer tool. When administered intraperitoneally to mice it inhibited tumor colonization in the lungs by more than 70%. In addition, Hans-Inge Peterson [273a] reported that two transplanted rat tumors (a fibrosarcoma and a hepatoma) were significantly reduced by not only aspirin but by two other prostaglandin inhibitors, indomethacin and diclofenac-sodium.

acetylation,[*] as we have noted, and thus beneficially suppresses formation of thromboxane that causes platelet aggregation. The problem is that aspirin also detrimentally suppresses vascular prostacyclin production which would otherwise inhibit platelet aggregation. From the great number of experiments, it looks as if a very low dosage of aspirin (say 20 mg. per day) will suppress thromboxane yet have very little effect on vascular prostacyclin.[**]

A single dose of only 50 mg. of aspirin has been found by two groups of investigators[296,297] to inhibit vascular prostacyclin formation. Patrignani et al.[298] have reported, however, that a daily dose of just 20 mg. of aspirin inhibited the formation of thromboxane without altering that of prostacyclin. (Astonishingly, H. Sinzinger et al.[299] discovered that long-term daily administration of just 1 mg. of aspirin modified platelet behavior.) To help put such a dosage in perspective, keep in mind that the recommended daily maximum dosage of aspirin (for any reason) is generally given as 4,000 mg.[300,301] Don R. Swanson[302] has recently reviewed the status of this work in considerable depth. The clinical effectiveness of aspirin and other manipulators of the arachidonic acid-thromboxane A2 pathway has also been reviewed by J. R. A. Mitchell.[303***] A study by H. C. S. Wallenburg et al.[303b] indicates that low-dose aspirin, through suppressing production of thromboxane A2, may restore prostacyclin/thromboxane balance in pregnancy. This could work to prevent pregnancy-induced hypertension and pre-eclampsia.

A possible reason for the *reverse effect* that exists when aspirin is used to deaggregate platelets relates to its metabolite, salicylate.[304] Salicylate given to rats blocks the inhibitory effect of aspirin on

---

[*] Aspirin can also influence platelet function in ways other than via cyclo-oxygenase inhibition.[295]

[**] Margareta Thorngren et al.[286,287] reported that a fish diet with its content of eicosapentenoic acid (discussed earlier and covered more completely in Chapter 4) acts by a different mechanism to inhibit platelet aggregation. Thus, such a diet might be useful in conjunction with aspirin therapy.

[***] For a while, it was fashionable for physicians to prescribe Persantine ® in addition to aspirin in the attempt to achieve a lower incidence of cerebral or retinal infarction or death. An extensive trial showed that the results of "aspirin only" administration and of the combined therapy were essentially identical.[303a]

vascular cyclo-oxygenase and the concomitant formation of thromboxanes A2 and B 2.[305-307] Therefore, as more aspirin is taken, the salicylate builds up and it then reverses aspirin's deaggregating effect.[304,308] The blocking effect of salicylate on vascular cyclo-oxygenase is greater than the effect on platelet cyclo-oxygenase.[304] E. Dejana et al.[306] found that the optimal ratio of salicylate:aspirin needed to completely inhibit the effect of aspirin on vascular walls was 5:1, whereas a 10:1 ratio completely inhibited the aspirin effect on platelet cyclo-oxygenase activity. Thus, it may be useful to employ appropriate amounts of salicylate in conjunction with aspirin therapy.

Some studies have reported aspirin to cause a greater prolongation of bleeding time (and therefore show more deaggregating power) in men than in women.[308] The reason seems to be that the blood salicylate level is much higher (about 50% higher) in women than in men.[308] When the results of the various studies are in, I believe the favored therapy for facilitating platelet deaggregation (and thus aiding in prevention of repeated strokes and heart attacks) will be very small amounts of aspirin,* perhaps combined with somewhat larger amounts of salicylate.

---

* Studies of postmyocardial infarction patients by E. Walter et al.[309] suggest that long-term aspirin doses of 1.5 gram/day led to increased blood pressures after six months. It seems apparent that aspirin therapies of the future designed to prevent repeated strokes and heart attacks will employ much smaller aspirin intakes than those used by Walter and his coworkers.

Hypothesis:
A *Reverse Effect* Involving Aspirin and Cancer Metastases Will Be Discovered.

We have seen that the work of James J. Kolenick et al.[264] and of Gabriel Gasic et al.[265] showed aspirin inhibits formation of metastases in cancerous mice. We also observed that the *in vitro* research of Duff and Duran[241d] found that the T-cell proliferative response to interleukin-2 was increased at 39° C (i.e., under fever conditions) compared to 37° C. Recently, Steven A. Rosenberg et al.,[310] Beverly Merz,[311] Michael T. Lotze et al.[312] and Charles G. Moertel,[313] as well as subsequent studies published in the *New England Jrl. of Medicine* of April 9, 1987, reported that metastatic cancer was favorably treatable with interleukin-2. Interleukin-2 not only activates helper and cytotoxic T-cells but also that special kind of lymphocyte, the natural killer cell.

Putting these facts in juxtaposition suggests that aspirin, through its fever-lowering power, will tend to inhibit the T-cell proliferative response to interleukin-2, thereby reducing the T-cell's cancer combatting potential and thus cancer metastases might be promoted. But the studies of Kolenick and of Gasic indicate, to the contrary, that aspirin can reduce the formation of metastases. We can therefore speculate that at some dosage aspirin's power to lower fever and thereby to reduce the action of the T-cell proliferative response (i.e., aspirin's possible tendency to *increase* metastases) will be overcome by aspirin's power to *reduce* metastases. At that dosage level there should occur a *reverse effect* in aspirin's influence on metastases. Determining dosage levels at which *reverse effects* occur, not only with aspirin but with various other drugs in different disease states, could be important in optimizing therapies.

"There are more things in heaven
and earth, Horatio,
Than are dreamt of in your
philosophy."
— William Shakespeare, *Hamlet*,
Act 1, Scene 5

"Disagreement among those seeking
the truth is a blessing greater than
the agreement of the assured."
— Kenneth L. Patton

"Scepticism in regard to present
methods and ideas can lead to
progress. Scepticism can also result
in a refusal to accept the new, the
great, the untried."
— Walter A. Heiby, *Live Your Life*
(New York: Harper and Row,
1966)

CHAPTER 4

Vitamins A, D and K—Potential Anticancer Agents

Vitamins A. D, K and E, being fat-soluble, tend to accumulate in the body as long as there is sufficient fat present. In this way they are unlike the water-soluble vitamins, the B complex and C, which tend to leave the body rather rapidly.

Vitamin A

Technically, vitamin A (also known as *retinol*) is sometimes called vitamin A_1 because of the existence of a related substance, A_2 (also known as *dehydroretinol*), having a slightly different chemical formula—$C_{20}H_{27}OH$ for A_2 instead of $C_{20}H_{29}OH$ for A_1. Vitamin A_2 is found in the liver oil of fresh-water fish, is slightly less active in mammals than vitamin A_1, but performs similar functions. When we talk about vitamin A we are referring to the A_1 variety. Both forms of the vitamin exist in alcohol (retinol), aldehyde and acid forms. The natural aldehyde form is called *retinaldehyde* and was formerly known as *vitamin A aldehyde, retinal* or *retinene*. The acid form is called *retinoic acid* and it exists in both *cis* and *trans* acid isomeric forms.

Vitamin A activity has been measured in international units (I.U.). However, with the advent of so many forms, there is an increasing tendency to use "retinol equivalents" (R.E.) to measure activity. One R.E. is equal to 5 I.U. Thus, the RDA for men is 5,000 I.U. or 1,000 R.E.; that for women is 4,000 I.U. or 800 R.E.

The conversion of carotenes (and also of cryptoxanthin, the yellow pigment of corn) to retinaldehyde and then to retinol takes place primarily in the intestinal mucosa. (A very small amount of the retinaldehyde formed from the carotene is oxidized to retinoic acid.) The efficiency of the absorption and the utilization of the various forms of vitamin A depend on many factors, including the amount of fat in the diet, method of food preparation, completeness of digestion and the availability of vitamin E and thyroxine. It has been estimated that about one-sixth of the vitamin A precursors will be converted, on average, in the healthy person. In those with gastroenteritis, diabetes or an underactive thyroid the conversion may be especially inefficient or nonexistent.

Retinol (either that synthesized from carotene or absorbed from dietary fish oil) is esterified again with long-chain, mainly saturated fatty acids (such as palmitic acid), incorporated into lymph chylomicrons, transported to the blood and then the liver. In the liver, vitamin A is stored in the parenchymal cells as retinyl esters, mainly retinyl palmitate. After hydrolysis of the retinyl esters, the free retinol is conjugated with a retinol-binding protein (made by the liver) and then travels from the liver via the plasma to various parts of the body.

Excessive consumption of vitamin A tends to damage the hepatic cells in which it is stored. Furthermore, retinoic acid, although not stored in the liver, may also be toxic if, under prescription, large quantities are consumed. Synthetic derivatives of retinoic acid called retinoids—some of which have vitamin A activity—are not stored in the liver and may be far less toxic than retinol, retinyl esters or retinoic acid. About 1,500 retinoids have thus far been synthesized according to Gary L. Peck,[1] and soon there may be thousands. The search for vitamin A analogues revolves around the development of congeners that have high vitamin A activity with low toxicity and the discovery of their varying effects on body processes. Recent research has concentrated on finding synthetic retinoids which display greater antitumor activity but less toxicity. For example, the synthetic analogue *retinyl methyl ether* has a high tissue specificity for the mammary gland and a lower toxicity than the natural retinyl acetate. Synthetics can be modified to affect their degree of water or of fat solubility. The fat-soluble forms travel to fatty (e.g., mammary) tissue while the water-soluble forms go to the bladder.

While retinol circulates in the body via a retinol-binding protein (RBP), retinoic acid circulates, instead, bound to serum albumin. It is speculated by S. Smith and D. Goodman[1a] that toxicity occurs when retinol is presented to the membranes in a form other than RBP. After RBP and the retinoic acid bound to serum albumin have arrived at the membranes, there are at least two intracellular binding proteins that transmit retinol and retinoic acid, respectively, *within* the cells. The RBP and the serum albumin are left at the cell wall to recirculate and then to repeat their performance in bringing these forms of vitamin A to the cell wall. David E. Ong and Frank Chytil[2,3] and J. Ganguly et al.[4] report that the cellular retinol-binding protein (CRBP) has been found in all tissues (of adult animals) with the exception of skeletal muscles and heart. The cellular retinoic acid-binding protein (CRABP), although present in the eye, brain, testis, ovary and uterus (of adult animals), is absent in heart muscle, small intestine, kidney, liver, lung, gastrocnemius muscle, serum and spleen. The presence of both proteins in an organ suggests that both retinol and retinoic acid have functions in that organ. In the rat fetus, CRABP occurs much more widely than it does after birth, a fact that suggests retinoic acid may have an important role in embryogenesis.

Recently, other vitamin A-binding proteins have been discovered and David E. Ong[4a] has provided a review. Cellular retinal-binding protein (CRALBP) and interstitial or interphotoreceptor retinol-binding protein (IRBP) are unique to the retina. (High levels of CRBP and CRABP are also present in the retina.) Another substance, cellular retinol-binding protein type II (CRBP[II]) seems to be restricted to the epithelial cell layer of the villi of the small intestine and is probably involved in retinol absorption. Still other carrier proteins for vitamin A are likely to be discovered in the future.

The various forms of vitamin A are not always interchangeable. Retinoic acid can be substituted for retinol in the chemical reactions involving general growth, epithelial differentiation and tumor control. Retinoic acid cannot, however, completely substitute for retinol in processes relating to vision and to reproduction. Animals given retinoic acid as their only source of vitamin A are, therefore, blind and sterile but otherwise in a good state of health.[5] Retinoic acid and retinol differ in other actions. As we observed in Chapter 2, W. J. Pudelkiewicz et al.[6] reported that high levels of vitamin A acetate depressed the tissue levels of vitamin E in chicks. However, John G. Bieri et al.[7] related that rats fed a low level of retinoic acid had much lower plasma tocopherol levels than those fed retinol. Later, John G. Bieri and Teresa J. Tolliver[8] reported retinoic acid caused twice as much tocopherol to be excreted in the feces. Addition of .2% taurocholic acid (a bile acid) reversed this inhibition of tocopherol absorption.

While retinol is absorbed through the lymphatic system and then travels via the blood to the liver, retinoic acid is not absorbed in this way. Instead, after being formed from the oxidation of retinaldehyde (from beta-carotene cleavage) in the intestines, it is transported through the portal circulation. (Not only the intestines, but other tissues such as the liver and kidney can also form retinoic acid.) Then it is transported in the plasma bound to serum albumin in a manner similar to other long-chain free fatty acids and is excreted through the bile. Retinoic acid is rapidly metabolized and it soon becomes relatively unavailable for body processes. These facts help account for the different actions of retinol and retinoic acid.

Vitamin A in Physiology and Therapy

Vitamin A is responsible to a large degree for the appearance of the skin. When there is a shortage of vitamin A, a condition of rough, dry skin called *hyperkeratosis* may develop. Shortage of this vitamin can also cause dry hair, dandruff and broken fingernails. Vitamin A is reported to be a factor in eliminating blackheads and whiteheads and in helping to cure psoriasis.

Vitamin A has also been widely reported to aid in the treatment of acne. However, a finding by the Southeast Scotland Faculty of the College of General Practitioners[9] failed to validate this therapy. Carefully controlled studies failed to show vitamin A to be effective in curing acne, but results suggested that deterioration was lessened by use of the treatment. In spite of this negative notice, Samuel Ayers, Jr. and Richard Mihan[10] reported good results when vitamin E was used with vitamin A. They stated that they successfully treated over 100 cases of acne as well as other skin problems with daily administration of 100,000 I.U. of vitamin A and 1,600 I.U. of vitamin E. Kligman et al.[10a] have also reported good results in using retinol to treat acne, but only when the daily dosages were in the 300,000-500,000 range. (Such dosages can, of course, be dangerous and should be used only when prescribed by a physician.)

Do not confuse "vitamin A activity" with vitamin A. As I have indicated, many studies suggest that the vitamin itself, unless used in enormous dosages, does not appear to be of much value in treating acne. However, the retinoic acid derivative 13-*cis* retinoic acid or isotretinoin (trade name *Accutane®*) is being reported on very favorably for the treatment of cystic acne in *The Lancet, Dermatologica, Muenchener Medizinishe Wochenschrift* and in other journals. Isotretinoin is reported to be useful also in treating generalized pustular psoriasis,[10b] cancer and oral leukoplakia.[10c, 11] On the other hand, there have been reports that children whose mothers took Accutane® during pregnancy were born with nervous system defects, brain damage, congenital heart disease, etc.[11a-c] Then too, 13-*cis* retinoic acid and other retinoids fed to experimental animals have been found to raise the level of serum triglycerides.[12] Isotretinoin is reported to have also caused symptoms of depression, including crying spells, malaise and forgetfulness.[13] The *Physicians' Desk Reference*[14] gives other side effects and states that 90% of the users develop cheilitis (inflammation of the lips) and about 40% experience conjunctivitis. Several recent reviews also provide warnings concerning its use.[14a-d*] In 1986, muscle damage was added to the list of consequences.[14da*]

The blindness that afflicts thousands of children in Indonesia each year is apparently related to vitamin A deficiency. At one time it had been reported that this problem, instead of being due to a vitamin A deficiency, is often caused by a lack of protein. For vitamin A to circulate in the blood and be available to the cells there must also be protein circulating in the blood. However, Alfred Sommer et al.[15] reported large numbers of Indonesian children free of the protein-deficiency disease kwaskiorkor showed deficiencies of vitamin A. Mortality increased, almost linearly, with severity of xerophthalmia. Mild vitamin A deficiency was directly associated with 16% of all deaths of children aged from one to six years. V. Reddy et al.[15a] and K. Vijayaraghavan et al.[15b] similarly found that in malnourished children with vitamin A deficiency, particularly those at risk of developing keratomalacia, vitamin A was the main limiting factor.

George Wald discovered how rhodopsin, opsin and retinene (an oxidized form of retinol) undergo molecular changes in the photoreceptive cells of the retina when influenced by light. Because of this discovery, Wald shared the 1967 Nobel Prize for Physiology or Medicine with Haldan Keffer Hartline and Ragner Granit. Retinol, in the form of retinene, is essential for this reaction. As we noted earlier, other forms of vitamin A will not do the job. Therefore, a lack of sufficient retinol may be the cause of night blindness—difficulty in adapting to either darkness or to bright lights.

---

* A related retinoid, etretinate, that is also used for skin disorders, may be even more dangerous. W. Grote et al.[14e] tell about a severely malformed fetus conceived four months after terminating maternal etretinate treatment. C. Vahlquist et al.[14f] compare the effects of isotretinoin and etretinate with special attention to their effects on serum lipoproteins. Recently, Susan Bershad et al.[14g] and Pochi[14b] also have reported that isotretinoin and etretinate increase levels of triglycerides and of LDL-cholesterol in both men and women and, therefore, could possibly be heart-threatening. Furthermore, John J. DiGiovanna et al.[14i] reported tendon and ligament calcification as another effect.

A therapy of vitamin A and E supplementation is reported beneficial in patients having the typical ocular and systemic symptoms of abetalipoproteinemia, a disease due to almost complete absence of betalipoproteins.[16] This, as do many other reports, indicates a synergistic action between vitamins A and E.

Vitamin A is useful in reducing one's susceptibility to sties, chalazions and other eye infections. Vitamin A is also of value in maintaining the health of mucous membranes in the nose, throat and lungs because it is vital in the formation of mucopolysaccharides which are required for epithelial membranes to remain healthy. Therefore, vitamin A is an important factor in combating the effects of air pollution. It is also useful, through its action on the immune system, for avoiding colds and other respiratory diseases such as tuberculosis and lung cancer. It can prove valuable in combating nasopharyngitis with its resultant postnasal drip. Vitamin A offers good protection against colds and other infections, not only by influencing the immune system, but by its lubricating action on the mucous membranes of the mouth, nose and bronchial tubes.

Let us note, parenthetically, that one's susceptibility (S) to developing a cold or any other infectious disease is directly related to the virulence (V) of the invading organisms and is inversely related to one's resistance (R). In other words, your chances of coming down with an infectious disease is given by the equation $S = V \div R$. If one's resistance is high then, no matter what the virulence, it will be virtually impossible to show cold symptoms (the ratio of $V \div R$ being very small). The germ theory of disease has overemphasized the importance of germs (V) in the occurrence of disease. Killing germs by means of drugs—including large amounts of vitamin A which are being used as a drug—still leaves unchanged one of the "causes," the body's underlying condition. Opponents of the germ theory have, on the other hand, overstressed the importance of the body's preexisting state (R) that permits or inhibits the invasion and multiplication of germs and downplayed consideration of the virulence factor. It's yet another case where neither polarized viewpoint is completely correct. That causation of disease is multifactorial is well illustrated by the fact that an organism, human or otherwise, can be colonized by bacteria and not be ill. Furthermore, in matters of human health and disease, the psychological variables may often take precedence over more "physical" components.

Vitamin A has beneficial effects on the immune response and they probably relate, at least in part, to its favorable influence on the thymus gland. This gland, lying high in the chest, is relatively large in infants and in children but is much smaller in adults. Its importance in adults may have been underestimated.[16a] The thymus gland enters into the immunological processes that fight disease and infection. Dr. Eli Seifter et al.[16b] have found that vitamin A can increase the size of the thymus gland in mice and thus increase ability to fight infection. They also reported that vitamin A partially prevented thymic involution due to stress.* R. R. Watson[16c] found that a high retinol intake beneficially increased T-lymphocyte mitogenesis in mice, but at even higher intakes of retinol there was a *reverse effect* and T-cell mitogenesis was inhibited. (Does this argue that use of very high doses of retinol in cancer therapy may be contraindicated?)

Another mechanism by which vitamin A may act in stimulating the immune system is through an effect on the body's production of gamma globulins. At any rate, M. D. Appleton et al.,[17] in experiments on rats, concluded that vitamin A plays a role in the biosynthesis of gamma globulins, many of which have known antibody activity.

The influence of vitamin A injections on the immunological response of mice was studied by M. Jurin and I. F. Tannock.[18] Daily vitamin A injections for five days before and after the mice were sensitized with sheep red blood cells occasioned a large production of antibodies. Furthermore, when vitamin A was injected into female mice with male skin grafts the mean rejection time of the grafts was reduced. (This suggests to me the possibility that a vitamin A *deficiency* might be useful in improving the prognosis in human

---

* Research by Allan L. Goldstein[16c,d] indicates that thymosin, a hormone secreted by the thymus gland, decreases rapidly with age. Although thymosin injections may prove to be of use in prolonging life and in increasing immunity to diseases, one must not conclude that oral supplements of thymus gland can be of any value. (Proteins, including bottled glandular proteins, break up into peptides and then into amino acids during digestion and thus lose their original identity and properties.)

organ transplanting.) Benjamin E. Cohen and L. Kelman Cohen,[19] also as a result of mice experiments, concluded that vitamin A exerts a powerful adjuvant-like stimulatory effect on the immune response. They also reported that, when given concomitantly with corticosteroids, vitamin A prevents the usual steroid-induced immunosuppression.

Another related experiment showing the effect of vitamin A against infectious agents is also interesting. Benjamin E. Cohen and Ronald J. Elin[20] reported that they treated mice with four consecutive daily injections of 3,000 I.U. of vitamin A palmitate (an enormous amount for a mouse) and then challenged them with either a gram-negative or a gram-positive bacterium or a fungus *(Candida albicans)*. Mice treated with vitamin A showed a significant decrease in mortality compared with control animals. The vitamin A did not, however, affect *in vitro* growth of the challenge organisms. The scientists concluded that vitamin A induces nonspecific resistance to infection in mice.

Vitamin A and Cancer

Smokers, who engage in self-induced polluting, should perhaps take vitamin A (along with ascorbic acid) supplements to help reduce the probability that they will get lung cancer. An important experiment was conducted some years ago by Dr. Umberto Saffiotti, et al.[21] and the findings were reported at the Ninth International Cancer Congress in Tokyo in October, 1966. The scientists subjected the lungs of a group of 53 hamsters to benzo(a)pyrene, one of the main cancer-causing chemicals in cigarettes. Thirteen cases of squamous metaplasia developed in the bronchus or the trachea of these 53 animals. Then, to a similar group of 46 animals, they gave large dosages of vitamin A palmitate and, after one week, exposed them to benzo(a)pyrene. The vitamin A acted favorably on their lungs and, of the 46 animals, only one developed a microscopic squamous tumor in a bronchus and one developed a patch of squamous metaplasia in the trachea.

Other experiments of Saffiotti[22] also showed an inhibition of carcinogenesis by vitamin A for the induction of squamous cell papillomas in the forestomach. Even earlier, Elizabeth W. Chu and

Richard A. Malmgren[23] had found analogous effects of vitamin A palmitate in inhibiting carcinogenesis induced by either benzo(a)pyrene or DMBA in the gastrointestinal tract and the cervix of hamsters.

Vitamin A also seems to protect against cervical dysplasia and carcinoma. Seymour L. Romney et al.[25] reported that women with a low intake of vitamin A (under 3,450 I.U. daily) are 2.76 times as likely to have severe cervical dysplasia or carcinoma *in situ* than women with a higher intake. (They discovered that women with below-normal intake of either beta carotene or vitamin C were even more at risk.) Arnold Bernstein and Beth Harris[25a] found that women with cervical intraepithelial neoplasia showed statistically lower levels of serum vitamin A. We should, however, not conclude that one or more vitamin deficiencies cause cancer, but simply that they may be causal factors in a complex etiology.

Other studies have shown that tumor growth elsewhere in the body is also inhibited by massive dosages of vitamin A. However, since vitamin A is generally stored in the liver, it seems probable that in some cases it might not reach the desired site, i.e., the cancerous tissue, in adequate amounts (and this is why the retinoids may be so very important).

Vitamin A, in the form of retinyl acetate, especially when administered with selenium in the form of sodium selenite, has been found by Clement Ip and Margot M. Ip[25b] to effectively suppress mammary tumorigenesis induced in rats by 7, 12-dimethylbenz(a)anthracene (DMBA). Rats were divided into four groups: (1) the control group whose diet included .3 mg. selenium and 8 mg. of vitamin A palmitate; (2) the control diet plus 4 mg./kg. diet of selenium as sodium selenite; (3) the control diet plus 250 mg./kg. diet of retinyl acetate; and (4) the control diet plus 4 mg./kg. of selenium and 250 mg./kg. of retinyl acetate. The additional selenium and/or retinyl acetate was given starting two weeks before administering DMBA. The final tumor yields (compared to the control group) were reduced to 51% with selenium alone, to 36% with retinyl acetate alone and to just 8% with selenium plus retinyl acetate (Figure 1).

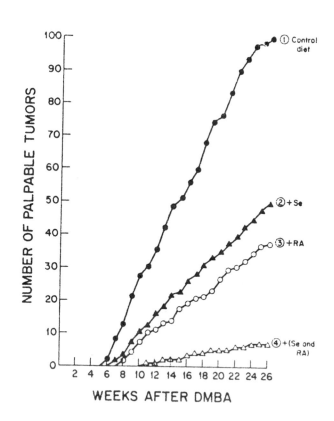

Figure 1. Effect of Se and/or RA supplementation in the diet
on the appearance of palpable mammary tumors in rats given a
total dose of 15 mg. of DMBA. Reproduced from Clement Ip
and Margot M. Ip., *Carcinogenesis* (1981) 2, no. 9: 915-918,
with permission of the publisher.

Vitamin A acetate (retinyl acetate) has been known for many
years to be very effective in preventing breast cancer induced in
animals by carcinogens such as N-methyl-N-nitrosourea (NMU).
The result of Moon et al.[26] making use of retinyl acetate to reduce the
number of mammary tumors induced by NMU is shown in Figure 2.

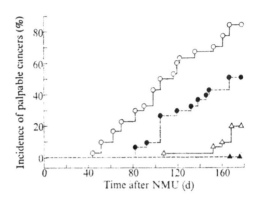

Figure 2. Effect of retinyl acetate on the time of appearance of palpable mammary cancers which were confirmed histologically at necropsy. Rats were placed on retinyl acetate or placebo diet 3 days after the second i.v. injection of either 5.0 mg. or 1.25 mg. NMU per 100 g. body weight. The rats were palpated for mammary tumors twice weekly for the duration of the experiment. Treatments were: o, high dose NMU, placebo diet; ●, high dose NMU, retinyl acetate diet; white triangle, low dose NMU, placebo diet; black triangle, low dose NMU, retinyl acetate diet. Reproduced from R. C. Moon and C. J. Grubbs, *Nature* (1977) 267:620 by permission of the publisher and of the authors.

In large dosages retinyl acetate is, however, very toxic. In fact, Clifford W. Welsh et al.[27] reported that massive feeding of retinyl acetate (82 mg./kg. ration) to estrone- and progesterone-treated mice resulted in a substantial increase in mammary carcinomas. It is another example of the *reverse effect.* At any rate, a new retinoid, *N-(4-hydroxyphenyl)-all trans-retinamide,* was observed by Richard C. Moon et al.[28] to be effective in preventing breast cancer in experimental animals and yet is far less toxic than retinyl acetate. The efficacy and safety of a retinoid in a rat may or may not be related to its action in women. Clinical trials of a long-term nature are needed to get the answer. Those especially interested in problems of breast cancer will find the binding of various retinoids to human breast cancer cells discussed by Andre Lacroix and Marc E. Lippman.[29]

The mechanism involved in vitamin A's action in fighting cancer appears (at least in some cases) to involve the DNA and the incorporation into the DNA of the nucleoside *thymidine*. Hisako Ueda et al.[30] discovered that the degree of *inhibition* of cell proliferation of human mammary carcinoma cells *in vitro* by the retinoids paralleled their capacity to inhibit thymidine incorporation. (Retinoic acid was especially active in inhibiting cell proliferation and thymidine incorporation.) Ueda concludes that this action suggests that the suppression of DNA synthesis is the primary cause of restriction of cell growth, but one is left wondering if normal cells might also be detrimentally affected.

Various retinoids have been found effective *in vitro* against human melanoma cells. Reuben Lotan[31] reported on the ability of retinoic acid to inhibit cells derived from six human melanomas (and four breast carcinomas). Frank L. Meyskens, Jr. and Sydney E. Salmon[32] published the *in vitro* results of using retinoids on metastatic melanoma cells. They stated that their data (in one case showing 80% inhibition) provided support for a clinical trial of selected retinoids in micrometastatic and advanced melanoma. Another report of the *in vitro* inhibiting effects of various retinoids on melanoma cells was published by Frank L. Meyskens, Jr. and Bryan B. Fuller.[33]

Retinoids have been used successfully in treating many types of cancer. Retinoids may also be useful in controlling precancerous conditions. J. Gouveia et al.[34] reported on a study of 70 volunteers who had at least 15 packet-years of smoking experiences (number of packets smoked per day multiplied by the number of years of cigarette smoking) and underwent bronchial biopsy. Of these, a group treated with a retinoid, etretinate, showed far less metaplasia than those not so treated.

The use of retinoids and their potential is reviewed by Beverly A. Pawson et al.[35] in an article entitled "Retinoids at the Threshold: Their Biological Significance and Therapeutic Potential." However, W. Bollag[35a] issues these words of warning: "The promising results achieved with certain premalignant and malignant changes are accompanied by a series of side-effects in skin, mucous membranes, muscles, joints, and bones, as well as changes in serum lipids and hepatic function and teratogenicity. These limit the usefulness of the present retinoids." Furthermore, Saxon Graham[36] points out that retinoids may sometimes increase the risk of prostate cancer, Hodgkin's disease and leukemia.

Vitamin A has also proved useful in potentiating the effect of chemotherapy. The anticancer drug BCNU is effective against murine (mouse) L1210 leukemia, and Martin H. Cohen[36a] reported that optimal results were achieved when vitamin A was given along with caffeine six hours before the BCNU (Figure 3). Dr. Cohen also discovered the interesting fact that coffee given 15-30 minutes after the BCNU further increased the value of the drug. In a related study, Shigetoshi Hosaka et al.[36b] found that the development of hepatic tumors induced in mice by 2-acetylaminofluorene was significantly suppressed in both size and number by giving them a solution of .2% caffeine as their drinking water without use of chemotherapeutic drugs and without use of vitamin A other than that normally present in their diet.*

Based on investigations by Dennert and Lotan, Reuben Lotan[37a] has presented some interesting cytotoxic effects of retinoic acid spleen cells cultured with myeloma cells. Figure 4 shows that, depending on the concentration of the myeloma cells, the cytotoxic effect was greatest at a concentration of retinoic acid between 10^{-8} M and 10^{-6} M, then a *reverse effect* set in with lessening cytotoxicity. The dosage limits set by the experimental protocol were such that a possible negative cytotoxicity (i.e., a cancer-promoting effect) could not have been discovered. In further regard to experimental protocol, one might wish that separate cell cultures had been used for each

---

* Lee W. Wattenberg[37] has reported that green (unroasted) coffee beans inhibited mammary neoplasia induced in the rat from administration of 7, 12-dimethylbenz(a)anthracene. The anticancer action is believed to result from an increased glutathione S-transferase activity caused by the kahweol palmitate and cafestol palmitate in the green coffee beans. Wattenberg notes that foods contain many inhibitors of carcinogenesis, including phenols, indoles, aromatic isothiocyanates, methylated flavones, coumarins, plant sterols, selenium salts, protease inhibitors, ascorbic acid, tocopherols, retinol and carotenes. However, Wattenberg cautions that "the fact that a compound exerts an inhibitory effect against carcinogenesis in an experimental system does not necessarily mean that overall it will be beneficial to the host."

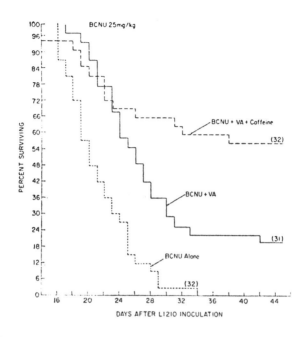

Figure 3. Enhancement of the antitumor effect of 25 mg./kg. BCNU by vitamin A and vitamin A plus caffeine. Reproduced from Martin H. Cohen, *Jrl. of the National Cancer Institute* (1972) 48: 927-932.

different dosage rather than simply adding an increased dosage to the same culture. (The time intervals, necessarily lengthened by the additive procedure, might have been a factor in the results.)

Many of the effects of vitamin A and its analogues have been reviewed by Reuben Lotan.[37a] Although we have just noted that Lotan reported retinoic acid can inhibit cancer cells, he[37b] also found that it can stimulate, *in vitro,* the growth of murine (mouse) melanoma cells.   Later, Samuel Baron et al.[38] demonstrated that trans-retinoic acid can enhance tumor growth in mice.

Retinoic acid can stimulate *in vitro* embryonal carcinoma cell differentiation[38a-c] and in other ways may mediate carcinogenesis.[38d,e]

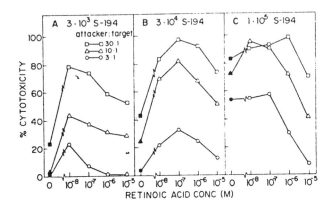

Figure 4. Stimulation of cell-mediated cytotoxicity by retinoic acid. C57BL/6 spleen cells were cultured with nonproliferating BALB/c myeloma S194 cells (added at the numbers indicated at the top of each panel) in the presence of various retinoic acid concentrations. After five days the cytotoxic activity generated in the spleen cells was assayed. Reproduced from Reuben Lotan, *Biochimica et Biophysica Acta* (1980) 605: 33-91, by permission of the publisher, Elsevier Biomedical Press.

Propagation of eukaryotic cells depends on growth factors such as the epidermal growth factor (EGF) which can stimulate proliferation of epidermal and fibroblastic cells.[38f] Retinoids can enhance binding of EGF to its receptor and thus could promote carcinogenesis. [38f] (Edward W. Schroder and Paul H. Black[42] have written an article with the ominous title "Retinoids: Tumor Preventers or Tumor Enhancers.") If, in addition to activating receptors, there are blocking receptors (as postulated in Chapter 1), then retinoids, by acting on them, could inhibit cancer. Thus, the action of the retinoids in promoting or inhibiting is explainable in terms of the *reverse effect*. Lawrence Levine and Kazuo Ohuchi[38d] say, "We suggest that the use of vitamin A and some of its analogues to prevent chemical carcinogenesis is premature; they may enhance, not inhibit tumor formation." And that is a thought that is presented throughout this book. Vitamins and minerals may act to benefit or to harm. Nutrition must become a science of *reverse effects* and principles must be stated in terms of dose-response relationships.

Vitamin A can also act as a cocarcinogen under certain experimental conditions. It accelerates development of malignancies in animals treated with the carcinogens DMBA and Rous sarcoma virus.[39,40] Furthermore, David M. Smith et al.[41] reported that among hamsters given the carcinogen benzo(a)pyrene along with hematite, those fed 2,400 mcg. retinal acetate per week had a significantly higher incidence of respiratory tract tumors than those given 100 mcg. per week. In related experiments with MNNG, a colon carcinogen, T. Narisawa et al.[41a] found that rats *deficient* in vitamin A developed significantly fewer colon tumors than rats fed normal amounts of vitamin A.* Other animal experiments have shown that vitamin A compounds can sometimes enhance and sometimes inhibit the growth of chemically induced malignant growths.[42] Some tumors may be vitamin A dependent just as other tumors may be steroid-hormone dependent.[41b]

Vitamin A alcohol can also act as a cocarcinogen. This substance and perhaps all other cocarcinogens, as pointed out by David Gaudin et al.,[43] inhibit the DNA repair process. Gaudin and his group state that inhibitors of the DNA repair process may find use in the field of cancer therapy. This is specifically true of vitamin A alcohol. It can act as a cocarcinogen or it can enhance the antileukemic effect of the chemotherapeutic agent *bis-chloroethylnitrosourea*. Gaudin et al. suggest that the antitumor effect and the cocarcinogenic effect may be explainable by the same phenomenon, namely the inhibition of DNA repair. This action of vitamin A alcohol is thus another example of a substance working to either cause or to cure a disease in a dose-responsive *reverse effect*. In addition, H. J. Juhl et al.[44] have reported that different retinoids induce sister-chromatid exchanges (SCEs). These are exchanges in replicating or in newly-replicated DNA strands that occur between homologous sites on two (sister)

---

* Narisawa and his associates observed that animals fed the vitamin A-deficient diet consumed less calories than did the control animals. Thus, the observed effects could have been due, not to vitamin A deficiency per se but to calorie restriction. It is often difficult to accurately determine a cause for a given effect.

chromatids of one chromosome. Since SCEs are generally induced by carcinogens, it may be postulated that the retinoids, while at some dosages effectively fighting cancer, may at other concentrations induce cancer. If true, they would be illustrating the *reverse effect*.

On the other hand, retinol can sometimes inhibit the formation of SCEs. S. Qin et al.[45] found that retinol inhibited SCEs and chromosome aberration induced by four indirect carcinogens. Nevertheless, retinol had an enhancing effect on chromosome aberration induced by benz(a)pyrene and DMBA. Qin and his associates speculated that retinol exerts its anticarcinogenic effects by inhibiting forms of the cytochrome P-450 isoenzymes required for activation of precarcinogens. (The generally beneficial actions of the P-450 microsomal enzyme system of the liver were discussed in Chapter 2 and will be covered again in Chapter 6.)

In Chapter 2 we noted the report of A. Lopez[23a] regarding the concentration of vitamin E in the serum levels of lung cancer patients, other hospitalized patients and in free-living controls. Lopez also reported that the serum of lung cancer patients showed just 57 mcg.% beta carotene and 46 mcg.% vitamin A compared with, respectively, 96 mcg.% and 54 mcg.% of other hospitalized patients and 122 mcg.% and 63 mcg.% of free-living controls. The data suggests a possible interrelationship between beta carotene and vitamin A (and also between vitamins C and E) and the incidence of lung cancer. S. Atukorala et al.[24] reported that serum vitamin A concentrations in lung cancer patients were significantly lower than those in patients of similar age with either nonmalignant lung or nonlung diseases. The levels of vitamin A in the lung cancer patients, but not in the controls, were significantly correlated with serum concentrations of retinol-binding protein (RBP) and zinc. Low levels of zinc might reduce the synthesis of RBP and thus mobilization of vitamin A from the liver and in this way a zinc deficiency could be a cancer threat. The recent work of Miroslav Malkovsky et al.[24a] suggests that the anticancer action of vitamin A (or at least of the vitamin A acetate which they studied) is mediated through an immunological process.

It is interesting to note that an epidemiological study by Jeremy D. Kark et al.[45a] of 3,102 individuals in Evans County, Georgia, showed that, compared to controls, persons who eventually developed cancer had significantly lower mean serum retinol levels at least 12 months before the diagnosis of cancer. (A subsequent study of Evans County data by Izchak Peleg et al.[45aa] failed to confirm, however, the strong dose-response relationship between baseline retinol levels and subsequent cancer.) H. B. Stähelin[45b] found that subjects with low vitamin A levels were at risk for stomach cancer but did not find the correlation extended to other cancer sites. (They reported, however, above-average vitamin A levels in heart disease, perhaps because vitamin A levels correlate strongly with total serum cholesterol. Stroke victims, despite low serum cholesterol, also had higher than average levels of vitamin A.) At any rate, it seems apparent that the serum levels of vitamin A may be inversely related to the probability of getting cancer—although it is, of course, possible that this is not a causal but a concomitant relationship. Anyway, some evidence suggests that massive supplements of vitamin A or of beta carotene will do little to increase levels of serum retinol except in cases of serious serum retinol deficiency.[45c]

However, extensive literature[46] shows that vitamin A and especially its precursor beta carotene have roles in the prevention of cancer. (Beta carotene and the other carotenoids that are synthesized by plants protect the plants from free radicals formed during photosynthesis.[46a] Perhaps this protective action against free radicals is also the agent in human cancer prevention.) One example of such research is a 19-year study of middle-aged men that was conducted by Richard B. Shekelle et al.[47] Lung cancer developed in 14 of 488 men who had a low-carotene diet but in only 2 of another group of 488 that ate a high-carotene diet. An interesting conclusion (that will have to be verified or denied by future studies) was that vitamin A from noncarotene (i.e., nonvegetable) sources such as liver, dairy products and egg yolks, was *not* protective. Protection came from a high consumption of carotene in the form of vegetables. Of course, it seems possible to me that it was not just the carotene that may have provided the protection, but perhaps the high-fiber content of the vegetables that speeded up intestinal transit time and thus reduced self-toxic action.[*] At any rate, a related experiment by Curtis Mettlin et al.[49b] dealing with white male patients with lung cancer came to a similar conclusion. Mettlin found that there was a reduced relative risk of lung cancer occurring, especially among heavy smokers, in those having a high amount of vitamin A precursors in their diet (particularly in the form of carrots and milk). Research by E. Bjelke[50] and a follow-up study by Gunnar Kvale et al.[51] resulted in similar findings. They also stressed the strong negative correlation between lung cancer incidence and the presence of carrots and milk in the diet. Takeshi Hirayana,[52] in a 10-year follow-up study of 122,261 men aged 40 years and above, similarly found that diets containing a large amount of green and yellow vegetables helped protect against prostate cancer.[**] Abraham M. Y. Nomura et al.,[52b] in studying serum specimens of 6,800 men of Japanese ancestry in Hawaii from 1971 to 1975, recently reported that the odds of their developing lung cancer were significantly less among those who, years earlier, had high levels of serum beta carotene. A high dietary level of retinol or of other retinoids was found by Carlo La Vecchia et al.[52c] to be inversely and strongly related to the risk of cervical cancer. Beta carotene, and not vitamin A per se, seems to be the anticancer factor.

The intestinal enzyme called carotenoid dioxygenase cleaves the beta-carotene molecule to form vitamin A. Richard G. Cutler[52d] suggests that tissue levels of beta carotene might be *inversely* related

---

[*] Leonard E. Gerber and John W. Erdman, Jr.[48] reported that beta carotene was far more effective in increasing wound strength than an equivalent amount of retinol given as retinyl acetate. There may be other yet-to-be-discovered benefits in carrots and other food sources of carotenes and carotenoids as compared with a vitamin A pill. For example, the carotenoids canthaxanthin and phytoene, *which have no vitamin A activity*, were effective in reducing tumors in mice.[49] Abscisic acid, another of the carotenoids, has been shown by R. W. Shearer[49a] to be a potent preventer of azodye-induced liver carcinogenesis in the rat. (Abscisic acid is found in seed coats, ripe fruit and mature leaves and is the hormone responsible for keeping seeds and buds dormant.)

[**] On the contrary, a study by Martin Y. Heshmat et al.,[52a] involving a dietary interview of 181 black prostate cancer patients, concluded that increased amounts of vitamin A during the age period 30-49 years enhanced the risk of prostatic cancer. Heshmat et al. noted that increased vitamin A would require additional retinol-binding protein for its transport which, in turn, would require additional zinc for its synthesis in the liver. Heshmat et al. speculated that this chronic lowering of zinc available for prostatic tissue might eventually promote the development of cancer.

to levels of carotenoid dioxygenase (while the body's vitamin A levels would, of course, be *directly* related to the levels of the enzyme). I speculate that supplementary use of vitamin A (by acting in accordance with Le Chatelier's principle) might suppress the body's conversion of beta carotene to vitamin A, thus increasing body levels of the valuable beta carotene.* Furthermore, I suggest that this sparing action of vitamin A on beta carotene, rather than the vitamin itself, may be the reason vitamin A is sometimes beneficially associated with reduced cancer risk.

Beta carotene is among the most effective substances known for quenching the excitation energy of singlet oxygen and also for trapping certain organic free radicals.[53,53a]** Beta carotene was reported by John Rhodes[53c] to have potentiated human interferon *in vitro* (whereas retinoic acid and retinol inhibited the stimulatory action of interferon on monocyte membrane function). Either the quenching of free radicals or the effect on monocyte membranes could help account for beta carotene's anticancer power.*** One should, however, resist the temptation to quickly conclude that, just because food sources containing vitamin A or its precursors may offer some cancer protection, the same results might be achieved through pill consumption. In this connection it is interesting to note that the carotenoid canthaxanthine, which is without pro-vitamin A activity, has antitumorigenic action.[53e] You get it when you eat carrots but not when you take a pill.

Furthermore, Jules Duchesne[54] presents a thought-provoking view of cancer and of vitamin A therapy. Duchesne says, "...cancer

---

* Le Chatelier's law states that if the equilibrium of a system is disturbed by a change in one or more of the determining factors (e.g., an increase in retinol) the system tends to adjust itself to a new equilibrium by counteracting as far as possible the effects of the change (e.g., an inhibition of the conversion of beta carotene to retinol).

** At high pressures, such as exist in hyperbaric oxygen treatment, beta carotene shows a *reverse effect* and becomes a pro-oxidant. (Vitamin E, on the contrary, at high pressure continues to act as an antioxidant.)[53b]

*** Giuseppe Rettura et al.[53d] found that beta carotene (90 mg./kg. diet fed to female rats following intragastric administration of the carcinogen DMBA) showed decreased tumor incidence in a time-dependent way. Rats fed beta carotene starting three weeks after DMBA instillation was begun developed far fewer tumors than groups whose feeding of beta carotene was begun later.

is not, as is thought, a disease but is actually, at the cellular level, a natural process of anti-ageing." Duchesne holds that there is an inherent contradiction in the use of vitamin A in cancer therapy. He continues: "Indeed, while substances like retinoids, such as vitamin A, oppose cancer growth by generating free radicals, it must be stressed that the latter are factors which, at the same time, accelerate ageing because they have the fundamental property of progressively eroding DNA. This means that one is caught between two opposing tendencies, so that one must opt for the most appropriate dosage of vitamin A, i.e., the best suited to obtain the maximum effect on the cancer and minimum action on senescence."

A recent study by Walter C. Willett et al.[54a] casts doubt on the hypotheses relating intake or serum levels of vitamin A to reduced risk of cancer. The Willett group measured retinol, retinol-binding protein (RBP), vitamin E and total carotenoids in 1973 in the serum of 111 subjects who were free of cancer at the time but were diagnosed as having cancer during the subsequent five years. These data were compared with those in 210 controls, matched for age, sex, race and time of blood collection, who remained free of cancer. Mean levels of retinol, RBP and carotenoids were similar for cases and controls (although vitamin E levels were somewhat lower in subjects who later developed cancer). Astonishingly, the retinol levels in 18 subjects who subsequently developed lung cancer were actually higher than in their matched controls. Gina Kolata,[54b] in what strikes me as being an overly pessimistic view of the possible role vitamin A might play in cancer prevention, quotes Willett as saying, "There is no basis for proposing that vitamin A protects against human cancer and there is almost zero evidence to justify taking vitamin A." It takes more than one study to upset a large mass of research suggesting that vitamin A and the carotenoids are cancer antagonists. Nevertheless, Willett's study is disturbing.

Whether or not vitamin A per se is effective in preventing cancer, it seems likely that beta carotene is of value. A randomized trial of beta carotene involving more than 20,000 male physicians over 40 years of age is now underway.[54c-e] Half the group, chosen at random, will receive 50 mg. of beta carotene daily; the other half will receive an inert placebo, but none will know which they are taking. In about five years the effects on cancer incidence should begin to be published.* In the meanwhile, a high-vegetable diet and beta carotene in supplement form are available for those who prefer to guess that favorable anticancer activity will be reported.

Uses of Vitamin A in Other Therapies

Let's leave the subject of cancer and consider the implications of vitamin A deficiency in the etiology of arthritis. Roger J. Williams reports on a study by T. Benedek[55] showing that vitamin A was below normal in the blood of 52 out of 58 rheumatoid arthritis patients. Vitamin A stimulates the adrenal gland to produce cortisone and it also helps maintain the synovial membrane, thus giving us two possible reasons for its favorable effect on the joints. Constance E. Brinckerhoff[56] reported that, in rat experiments, 3-cis-retinoic acid significantly reduced inflammation associated with adjuvant arthritis, an experimentally induced arthritis in rats that resembles human rheumatoid arthritis. Retinoic acid inhibits collagenase and production of prostaglandin E by rheumatoid synovial cells[56a] and thus may be useful in treating rheumatoid arthritis. Pilot studies are now in work testing retinoids in the treatment of psoriatic arthritis. If successful, controlled trials using retinoid in treatment of rheumatoid arthritis are likely to follow.

Dr. Isobel Jennings,[57] states that, although no research has indicated that a vitamin A deficiency might cause diabetes, it is likely that its deficiency might exacerbate the condition. A diabetic person tends to be short of zinc, and, as will be discussed later in this chapter, a zinc deficiency is likely to lead to problems in mobilizing "A" from the liver for use elsewhere in the body. Thus, a deficiency in vitamin A would be exacerbated by a shortage of zinc.

---

* I speculate that all the participating doctors in the study, since they know its purpose, might consciously or unconsciously tend to increase their consumption of vegetables over the next five years. Thus, both the beta carotene and the placebo group might show a reduced cancer incidence relative to nonparticipating doctors. Even the protocol of a carefully controlled double-blind study may have flaws that could be impossible to prevent. (How many participants do you suppose there would be if they were simply asked to take for a five-year period either an unknown substance or a placebo?)

Vitamin A is valuable in treating ulcers and is, in fact, important in ameliorating the effects of many types of stress. Vitamin A helps maintain the health of the mucous cells and thus aids in protecting the tissues of the stomach from the effects of excess acid. Not only ulcers, but other types of wounds may be amenable to vitamin A treatment. Rat studies[57a] have indicated that 13,000 I.U. of vitamin A (far more than that suggested by the National Research Council to support growth, reproduction and longevity of normal rats), accelerates wound healing. The extra vitamin A promotes early inflammatory reaction to wounding and increases the influx of macrophages to the site of the wound. Impaired wound healing is one of the complications of cortisone therapy. Topical vitamin A is reported to restore corticoid-retarded healing toward normal.[58,59]

Vitamin A helps prevent premature aging because it acts beneficially on cell walls. There is also a good probability that vitamin A, contrary to the statement of Duchesne,[54] can add to longevity. Interesting experiments with rats, conducted by Dr. Henry C. Sherman et al.[60] of Columbia University, have shown that their life spans can be increased significantly by giving them vitamin A. The Sherman group reported that rats fed modestly increased amounts of vitamin A lived approximately 10% longer than controls. Perhaps Sherman's results might be explainable in terms of vitamin A's beneficial effect on cell walls, although he did not draw that conclusion.

Sex and Reproduction

Vitamin A is important in maintaining the health of the sex glands and also in the production of male and female hormones. Dr. Isobel W. Jennings[57] cites experiments with male rats deprived of vitamin A. In these rats an absence of testosterone and degeneration in the germinal epithelium of the testes was noted. Other rats, similarly deprived of vitamin A but injected with testosterone, showed no degeneration of the testes. Analogous, but somewhat less dramatic results were observed in female rats. (Dr. Roger J. Williams[61] reports that "rats require about twenty times as much vitamin A for maximum reproduction as they need merely to maintain passable health and normal vision.") A recent study by Unni et al.[61a] found that the function of

Sertoli cells of the rat testes was decreased by withholding vitamin A (although supplementing with retinoic acid). When retinyl acetate was administered their function improved and there was an attendant increase in the number of spermatogonia in mitosis.

A study by David H. Van Thiel et al.[62] showed vitamin A (retinol) requires alcohol dehydrogenase to convert it to *retinal* that is essential for spermatogenesis.* Alcohol dehydrogenase is the enzyme needed to metabolize alcohol and so the reason chronic alcoholics are often infertile may be because this enzyme is not available for the retinol-to-retinal conversion.** Experiments have shown that bulls suffering degeneration of the seminiferous tubules of their testes regained full fertility when given vitamin A. Dr. Jennings warns, however, that excessive doses of vitamin A can be more damaging than a deficiency in the effect on the germinal epithelium of the testes. More recent studies relating vitamin A to reproduction have been reported by H. F. S. Huang and W. C. Hembree,[64] by M. R. S. Rao et al.[65] and by Rina Singer et al.[66] Singer reported that vitamin A was present at almost twice the amount in seminal fluid of highly fertile men compared with that of oligospermic men.

Studies by B. Ahluwalia et al.[67] have shown that zinc increases vitamin A uptake by the seminiferous tubules of rat testes and this may, of course, apply to men also. (They also concluded that vitamin A is bound to what was then an unknown protein—now called the retinol-binding protein.) Thus, large amounts of vitamin A are made effectively even larger, and possibly sometimes more dangerous, by megadoses of zinc. Furthermore, Jonathan Cohen and S. Burt Wolbach[68] have reported that intensification of testicular hemorrhaging in rats caused by hypervitaminosis A occurs by

---

* Noel W. Solomons[63] suggests that zinc may be a factor in the type of alcohol dehydrogenase that converts retinol to retinal and, if this conversion is impeded, night blindness could result.

** To add to the problem of alcohol-vitamin A interaction, Charles S. Lieber[63a] has cited the work of M. A. Leo et al.[63b] showing that alcoholics commonly have low vitamin A levels in their livers. Such depletion might contribute to the liver lesions associated with alcoholism.

simultaneously administering vitamin E. It should be noted that the Cohen and Wolbach experiments, like some of the others, used dosage levels of vitamin A in the range of 100-250 I.U. per gram of body weight, which is equivalent to 700,000 or more units daily for a 70 kg. (150 lb.) person. They used vitamin E in dosages of 10 mg. to 100 mg. per 50 grams of body weight, which is equivalent to 14,000-140,000 mg. for a 70 kg. person. Remember the *theory of the reverse effect* and don't let the results of using these huge dosages frighten you if you are supplementing vitamins A and E in moderation.

J. Cecil Smith, Jr. et al.[69] have reported that zinc is, in fact, required to maintain normal concentrations of vitamin A in plasma. They indicated that cases of depressed vitamin A therapy may respond to zinc supplementation. This group[70] also presented data showing that zinc-deficient rats had only 55%-60% of the liver levels of retinol-binding protein (RBP) compared to controls. Furthermore, the plasma RBP level of the zinc-deficient rats was only 14 mcg./ml. compared to a value of 50 in control rats fed a zinc-sufficient diet. When it is realized that retinol is the main form of vitamin A in plasma and that it circulates bound to a specific transport protein, RBP, the necessity of adequate zinc is emphasized.

The endocrine aspects of vitamin A that we considered earlier in regard to fertility may have application to the control of drinking in alcoholics. An interesting study by F. S. Messiha[70a] has shown the effect of vitamin A oral administration on voluntary intake of alcohol in rats. Female, but not male, rats showed a statistically significant reduction in voluntary intake of ethanol by vitamin A treatment of 500 mg./kg. daily for five days. It is believed this aversion to drinking resulting from vitamin A intake is related to the vitamin's antiestrogenic property. Messiha suggests that vitamin A with zinc may be useful in reducing voluntary alcohol consumption, particularly in the female alcoholic.

In setting the RDA for vitamin A, the National Academy of Sciences took no cognizance of a possible seasonal variation in our requirements. J. Glover et al.[71] reported that concentrations of retinal-binding protein (RBP) concentrations in the plasma of ewes and of castrated rams varied seasonally. Plasma RBP concentrations were minimal (20-30 mcg./ml.) during the summer but in late August and September they rose dramatically to peak values (80-100 mcg./ml.). These elevated values of three times the minimal values were maintained through the breeding season and then declined. They also reported equally dramatic changes in plasma RBP values with maximums in males corresponding with the breeding period and in females with the egg-laying period. Is it possible that corresponding variations in human plasma RBP might exist as an atavistic carryover of a period when human sexuality may have been seasonally cyclic?

Absorption of Vitamin A

If you are planning to take vitamin A supplements, you should know that not all forms are equally absorbable by the body. Studies by J. M. Lewis et al.[82] with normal children and adults have shown a great absorption superiority of aqueous vitamin A compared with the oily product. Increased storage also results from ingestion of the aqueous product (but, if one is overdosing, the aqueous product might be more dangerous). The Lewis group also reported that in persons with conditions affecting fat absorption (cystic fibrosis of the pancreas and obstructive jaundice) vitamin A dispersed in an aqueous vehicle brought excellent rises in the blood concentration of the vitamin in contrast to a flat absorption curve when an oil preparation was used. More recently, intestinal absorption tests made by Warren J. Warwick et al.[83] of cystic fibrosis patients confirmed that vitamin A alcohol in oil-water emulsion is the form absorbed best. Worst was A palmitate in oil and intermediate was "A" alcohol in oil and "A" palmitate in emulsion. Warwick et al. also observed that, since the number of stools per day is an inverse indicator of retention time, absorption of fat-soluble vitamins is always abnormal when one has four or more stools per day. The Greek principle of the golden mean is applicable even to defecation!

In Chapter 2 we saw that the absorption of Vitamin E is inhibited in the presence of polyunsaturated fatty acids and observed that this fact is at variance with popular belief. Daniel Hollander[84] has reported that the absorption of the other fat-soluble vitamins (A, D and K) is also inhibited by the polyunsaturated fatty acids. Ideally, one should not use supplements of vitamins A, D, E or K following a meal which includes salad dressing that contains polyunsaturated fat.

Many studies have reported that prolonged dietary restriction in animals increases longevity. A 1986 study by Daniel Hollander et al.[84a] showed that when the diet was restricted in female mice their absorption of vitamin A increased. In light of the work of Henry C. Sherman,[60] reported earlier, showing that vitamin A-supplemented rats lived 10% longer than controls, it is interesting to speculate that the increased longevity of diet-restricted animals may be due, at least partially, to increased absorption of vitamin A. An excessive intake of vitamin A, on the other hand, can cause problems and perhaps dieting humans should be especially wary of supplementation.

A number of studies have shown that large, nonphysiological concentrations of vitamin A cause free retinol (not bound to its carrier, RRP) to labilize membranes, which results in leakage of enzymes.[72] In at least one disease, viral hepatitis, excessive amounts of supplemental vitamin A could be especially threatening. Retinol-binding protein (RBP) is produced in the hepatocytes and this protein, as you will recall, combines with retinol for release from the liver. In hepatitis, levels of RBP are reduced and thus vitamin A may circulate in the body as free retinol, which is far more toxic than retinol bound to RBP.[73,74] Therefore, we see that there is at least one disease (and more may be discovered) where excessive vitamin A could be especially dangerous. Be wary of using megadoses!

An excess of vitamin A has also been known to cause such symptoms as loss of hair, sore lips, bruising, nose bleeds, increased intracranial pressure, painful joints and depression of thyroid activity, although the symptoms are reported to disappear when the vitamin is no longer taken. Excessive intake of vitamin A can also produce mental disturbances, nausea and vomiting, hemorrhages and fatigue, as well as skin disturbances and bone deformities. Both an excess and a deficiency are reported to be a cause of edema. A huge excess can lead to loss of calcium from the bones and resulting bone fragility. Vitamin A supplements (even if only 5,000 units) may be dangerous for patients undergoing chronic renal dialysis.[74a] Pregnant women, especially, will want to avoid an excess of vitamin A. It can cross the placental barrier and, in large dosages, can cause fetal damage such as cleft palate, eye damage, syndactyly (webbing of two or more fingers or toes) and deformities of the brain and skull such as exencephaly and hydrocephaly. The teratogenic action, according to J. W. Millen and D. H. M. Woolam,[75] is potentiated by cortisone and diminished by insulin.

In studying neural-tube defects in the curly-tail mouse, it has been learned that the genetic predisposition for vitamin A to be teratogenic is passed from generation to generation through the mother.[75a] A similar genetic phenomenon may apply to humans. It has already been reported that the risk of having a child with neural-tube defects is increased for sisters (but not for brothers) of mothers of children with such defects. The risk is not increased for relatives of fathers of such children.

Millen and Woolam also have shown, in experiments with rats, that large amounts of the vitamin B complex reduce the toxicity of vitamin A and, if the same effect occurs in humans, this could be useful information when large amounts of vitamin A are required for a specific purpose. Rat studies have also shown that vitamins A and D reduce each other's toxicity. Other studies, with rats and chicks, indicate that vitamin E partially counteracts vitamin A toxicity.[76] Alcohol, on the other hand, may potentiate vitamin A toxicity if experiments on rats are applicable to humans. Marie Anna Leo et al.[77] reported that when ethanol and vitamin A were fed to rats severe liver lesions occurred. Excessive amounts of vitamin A could, perhaps, be especially dangerous to alcoholics.[77a]

The various prescribed forms of vitamin A are also not without danger, but here, at least, you will be taking them under a doctor's direction. Gary L. Peck[78] warns that retinoids are potentially teratogenic. Therefore, fertile, sexually active women who do not use birth control should probably not use retinoids at the present time. Your physician should know the dangers and be able to guide you.

All interactions of vitamin A with drugs are not necessarily bad. An interesting experiment with rats suggests that vitamin A may protect against gastric ulceration induced by large dosages of aspirin. G. Rettura et al.[78a] found that a group of 10 rats given 100 mg. of aspirin in addition to their commercial chow over a period of 7 days developed a total of 17 ulcers. Another group of 10 rats given, in addition, 250 mg. of vitamin A palmitate developed a total of just 5 ulcers and a third group of 10 rats given 1 mg. of vitamin A had a total of only 3 ulcers (Table 1). Note, in the table, the possible *reverse effect* at a level of 100 mg. of vitamin A. This level of vitamin A produced a total of 19 ulcers in groups of 10 rats compared to a total of 17 in another group given no vitamin A. (As is typical, the researchers did not comment on this phenomenon.)

Your use of supplemental vitamin A should be discussed with your doctor if you are undergoing tests. For example, vitamin A can increase (or give false positive indications for) cholesterol, SGOT, prothrombin time and sedimentation rate and can reduce (or give false negative indications for) the erythrocyte count and/or hemoglobin and the leucocyte count.[79,79a] Furthermore, tests for bilirubin, alkaline phosphatase and aspartate amino-transferase may all show falsely elevated values in those taking supplements of vitamin A.[80] Then too, there may be interactions between vitamin A and cholestryramine and between vitamin A and neomycin.[81] Taking vitamin A should be avoided during extended tetracycline treatment because the combination can cause pressure within the skull attended by severe headaches, nausea and visual disturbances.[81a] Such facts illustrate the importance of your physician knowing what vitamins and minerals you may be taking.

Good food sources for beta carotene and the other less-productive provitamin A carotenoids (which the body converts partially, but not always very efficiently, to vitamin A) are green and yellow vegetables (except corn and yams).* Some examples are

---

* Some carotene enters the circulation and when large amounts are ingested carotenemia occurs and is characterized by a yellow pigmentation of the skin. This condition can be

carrots, turnip greens, dandelion greens, parsley, kale, spinach, watercress, apricots, canteloupes and papaya. Other good sources for vitamin A are beef and pork liver, milk, butter, egg yolk and, best of all, fish-liver oils.

S. R. Ames[81b] found that rats fed a diet deficient in vitamin E developed low vitamin A blood levels even when administered vitamin A by mouth or by injection. The vitamin A levels became normal when vitamin E was restored to the diet. Such a finding, though of considerable interest, must not be extrapolated in our minds to apply to large dosages of vitamins A and E. If you supplement your diet with vitamin E, recall that this vitamin, although widely reported to have a sparing effect on vitamin A, may actually displace some of the vitamin A, thus reducing its effectiveness. However, Walter C. Willett et al.[81c] reported that, over a 16-week period, a daily supplement of 800 I.U. of alpha tocopherol caused only an insignificant reduction in plasma retinol and plasma carotenoids. Interestingly, a daily supplement of 25,000 I.U. of retinyl palmitate did not appreciably affect blood levels of plasma retinol, alpha tocopherol or carotenoid. On the other hand, when M. Frigg and J. Broz[81d] injected chicks intravenously with a huge dose of vitamin A (that would correspond with many millions I.U. in a human) and more modest levels (0, 50, 100 or 150 mg./kg.) of vitamin E, tocopherol levels in the plasma were modestly reduced. Such massive dosages were used that it seems safe, for all practical purposes, to ignore this study since the work of Willett found no such effect at modest levels of vitamin A supplementation.

Also arguing against a detrimental vitamin A and E interaction, Samuel Ayers, Jr.[81e,f] has reported excellent results in treating patients with various skin diseases (Darier's disease, pityriasis rubra pilaris, ichthyosis and acne vulgaris) using simultaneous administration of vitamins A and E. He prescribes 50,000 I.U. of

---

distinguished from jaundice by the absence of yellow pigmentation in the sclera of the eye. Kemman et al[81aa] have associated carotenemia with anovulation and amenorrhea. D. V. Vakil et al.[81ab] have reviewed many of the other relevant studies. A variant of carotenemia called lycopenemia, caused by excessive consumption of tomatoes, has been reported by Peter Reich et al.[81ac]

Table 1

Rx	BW change	Thymus, mg.	Adrenal, mg.	Deaths	Rats w ulcer	Tot. ulcers
Water	+45	422±24	63.2±2.0	0/10	0 (0%)	0
Vit. A	+49	508±9	63.8±3.3	0/10	0 (0%)	0
Aspirin, 100 mg.	+19	268±20	72.5±1.2	4/10	6/6 (100%)	17
Asp. + 100 µg. vit. A	+23	379±26	65.1±1.5	1/10	6/9 (67%)	19
Asp. + 250 µg. vit. A	+32	483±30	70.1±0.8	0/10	2/10 (20%)	5
Asp. + 1 mg. vit. A	+35	507±27	67.6±1.3	0/10	2/10 (20%)	3

Thus, 250 µg. (750 I.U.) vit. A protects against 100 mg. aspirin (LD_{40}). If rat data apply to man, each aspirin (325 mg.) should contain 800 µg. vit. A, and 12 tablets (60 grains; 9,750 µg. vit. A) would equal approximately 29,000 I.U. vit. A. A dose of 24 tablets/d (maximum recommended) would equal approximately 60,000 I.U. vit. A, still below acute toxicity for humans. Taken from G. Rettura et al., Jrl. of the American College of Nutrition (1984) 3, no. 3: 291-292 (abstract no. 162), with permission of the publisher, Alan R. Liss, Inc.

vitamin A twice daily and 400 I.U. vitamin E, two to four times daily (certainly large amounts), with smaller maintenance doses after the condition has been controlled.

The literature relating to hypervitaminosis A in teenagers or in adults has generally involved daily ingestion of vitamin A in amounts of 100,000 I.U. or more. However, William A. Farris[85] reported symptoms of hypervitaminosis A in a 16-year-old boy who had taken just 50,000 I.U. of vitamin A daily for 2 1/2 years. Victor Herbert[86] also reported on several other cases where relatively low levels of supplementary vitamin A caused problems. An issue of *Nutrition Reviews* [86a] cited still other cases. *Toxic individuality,** my term for individual variation in toxic effects, may vary over a wide range.

Older persons may be in even more danger of hypervitaminosis A than are 16-year-olds, judging from absorption experiments with rats. It is often wrong to extrapolate results of animal experiments to human application but, nevertheless, Daniel Hollander[84] reported that young (1.5-month-old) rats absorbed 24.8% of vitamin A, while older rats (39 months of age) absorbed 37.3%—about a 50% increase.** As we age it could be even more important to be wary of megadoses of vitamin A!

Even more modest supplementation of vitamin A could conceivably represent a threat to health. A disturbing study by Freudenheim et al.[86b] suggests that for women taking calcium supplements increased intakes of vitamin A may be associated with a decreased mineral content in the bones. This was a dietary study in which the subjects were asked to complete two dietary records each month over a four-year period, which generated a total of 7,353 usable records. Studies of dietary habits are difficult to administer and subject to the vagaries of memory. Nevertheless, is it possible that excessive vitamin A supplementation might be a factor in causing osteoporosis?

---

* "Toxic individuality" is the mirror image of Roger Williams' term "biological individuality" which is so often invoked to justify a more-is-better attitude.

** By the way, he also reported that the young rats absorbed 14% of cholesterol that was given them, while old rats absorbed 38%—over twice as much. Again, we can't extrapolate to humans, but could dietary cholesterol represent a greater threat as we age?

Vitamin D—the Prohormone that is Still Called a "Vitamin"

So-called vitamin D is probably without biological activity. It is, however, converted in the liver and kidney to metabolites which have biological activity as steroid hormones. The body's provitamin D (which I will call "vitamin D" as does everyone else) comes from two sources: production in the skin and absorption in the intestine.

Vitamin D, like vitamin A, is fat-soluble. It controls calcium homeostasis and regulates growth and development of bone. Interestingly, Johnnie L. Underwood and Hector F. De Luca[86c] have shown that vitamin D is not necessary for, and does not stimulate directly, bone growth and mineralization. They discovered that vitamin D acts to foster bone growth and mineralization indirectly by elevating plasma calcium and phosphorus levels.

Through facilitating calcium absorption by the intestinal mucosa, vitamin D works to prevent rickets in children and the corresponding disease, osteomalacia in adults. Its mode of action may be through its metabolite $1,25(OH)_2D_3$ to form a calcium-binding protein in the epithelial cells of the ileum where calcium transport takes place. Another hypothesis is that the effect of vitamin D is to alter the lipid composition of the membrane and hence membrane permeability.[86d] Vitamin D also encourages absorption of phosphate, which is needed not only for forming bone and creatine phosphate for muscle action, but to produce the body's energy source, adenosine triphosphate (ATP).

There are 3 well-known forms of vitamin D called D_2, D_3 and D_4, although about 20 more varieties are known to exist. The substance originally called D_1 was found to be part of D_2. Ergosterol, a vegetable substance which occurs in yeast, molds and ergot, when acted upon by ultraviolet light, is converted into vitamin D_2. Vitamin D_2 is also known as calciferol, ergocalciferol or viosterol. The animal variety of vitamin D (especially prevalent in fish-liver oils) is called vitamin D_3[*] and is also known as cholecalciferol or calciol. Vitamin D_3 is also the form produced in the skin through the action of sunlight upon 7-dehydrocholesterol[**]   (one of the valuable chemicals the body makes from cholesterol). A provitamin D_3 is first formed which is then converted thermally to D_3.[87b-f,88] A third variety, vitamin D_4, of vegetable origin, is formed by irradiating a derivative of ergosterol. It is of far less importance than D_2 and D_3.

Cholecalciferol is converted in the liver to the prohormone $25(OH)D_3$,[***] which is also called 25-hydroxycholecalciferol, calcifediol or calcidiol and is generally thought to be inert biologically at physiological concentrations. However, this is obviously not true since low concentrations of $25(OH)D_3$ stimulate production of prolactin and growth hormone. High concentrations (10^{-6} to 10^{-5} M) of $25(OH)D_3$ show a *reverse effect* and inhibit such production.[88c] Low serum $25(OH)D_3$ levels have been reported in patients with a variety of liver disorders.[89,89a] Limited quantities of $25(OH)D_3$ are produced by healthy persons to avoid vitamin D intoxication from solar exposure. Nevertheless, the concentration of $25(OH)D_3$ in blood plasma is 5 to 10 times more than that in any other tissue.[89b]

---

[*] Although I call vitamin D_3 the "animal variety," it has been found in the calcinogenic plant, *Solanum malacoxylon* in the form of 1,25-dihydroxyvitamin D_3.[87,87a] A principle with activity similar to that of 1,25-dehydroxycholecalciferol has also been found in *Cestrum diurnum* (the day-blooming jessamine). Ricardo L. Boland[87a] has reported that vitamin D_3 sterols have also been discovered in *Solanum torvum, Solanum verbascifolium, Trisetum flavescens, Dactylis glomerata* and *Medicago sativa*. Such discoveries emphasize how inappropriate it is to call vitamin D_3 the "animal variety."

[**] It is believed that in northern latitudes there has been an evolutionarily effective selection for white skins that allows increased photoactivation of 7-dehydrocholesterol into vitamin D. In southern latitudes a selection for black skins prevents up to 95% of the ultraviolet from reaching the deeper layers of the skin where vitamin D is produced. Thus, the dangers of rickets in northern latitudes and of vitamin D toxicity in the southern latitudes are reduced.[87b] While sunlight and other sources of ultraviolet light are forming the precursor of vitamin D, they are also creating the carcinogen cholesterol-$5\alpha,6\alpha$-epoxide.[88ba-bc] Interestingly, Homer S. Black and Jarvis T. Chan [88bc] reported that a combination of dietary antioxidants (1.2% ascorbic acid, .5% BHT, .2% dl-α tocopherol and .1% reduced glutathione) inhibited the formation of cholesterol-5 $\alpha,6\alpha$-epoxide and reduced the number and severity of ultraviolet light-induced squamous cell carcinomas in the skin of mice.

[***] Small amounts of $25(OH)D_3$ are made *in vitro* by several types of phagocytic cells and converted into three metabolites, probably a lactone derivative of $25(OH)D_3$, 24,25 $(OH)_2D_3$ and a novel, unknown compound that is not 1,25$(OH)_2D_3$.[88a,b]

The prohormone 25(OH)D₃ then travels to the kidneys where the hormone 1,25(OH)₂D₃, known as calcitriol, is formed. Norman H. Bell et al.[90] have presented evidence that 1,25(OH)₂D₃ then, in a feedback mechanism, inhibits hepatic production of 25(OH)D₃. Although, until recently, it was widely accepted that 1,25(OH)₂D₃ is produced only in the kidneys, it has been discovered that this hormone is also made in the placenta[95] and, in addition, can be produced by cultured human bone biopsy cells, by cultured human osteosarcoma cells, by embryonic chick calvarial cells,[90a-c] and by abnormal lymphoid tissues in patients with lymphomas.[90ca] In patients with sarcoidosis, neither kidneys nor parathyroid hormone seem to be needed to produce 1,25(OH)₂D.[90d-h] Even human melanoma cells, when incubated with 25(OH)D₃, produced 1,25(OH)₂D₃—found almost entirely inside the cells—and 24,25(OH)₂D₃ which was distributed evenly between cells and the medium.[90i]

The various vitamin D metabolites travel via the serum vitamin D-binding protein—now shown to be identical with human G c protein.[91] This protein in humans and in animals has a similar, but not identical, structure. Further evidence that it is a hormonal rather than a nutrient-type transport system was provided by R. Bouillon and H. Van Baelen.[92] (The current knowledge about vitamin D-binding protein has been reviewed by John G. Haddad, Jr.)[93] When the 25(OH)D₃ arrives in the kidney, it is converted (under the control of the parathyroid hormone, the renal tubular intracellular phosphate, the plasma calcium and the enzyme 1-alpha-hydroxylase along with minor factors including prolactin, growth hormone, insulin and estrogens) to the hormonal form, 1,25(OH)₂D₃, also called 1,25-dihydroxycholecalciferol, or 1∝25(OH)₂D₃ or calcitriol.[94,94a] This is the hormone that catalyzes calcium and phosphate transport from the lumen of the gut to the bloodstream.* The classic sites of vitamin D

---

* Problems of calcium transport (and of changes in bone mineralization) experienced by older persons are often related to problems of vitamin D metabolism. The problem is often not one of insufficient sunlight or insufficient dietary vitamin D so much as it may be inefficient conversion in the kidneys to the active metabolite. A study of K. S. Tsai et al.[91a] of 10 normal premenopausal women, 8 normal postmenopausal women, 10 elderly women and 8 elderly women with hip fractures showed that 25(OH)D did   not

action are the intestines, bone and the kidneys, but many additional target tissues[**] have recently been identified.[94b,c] Another metabolite, 24,25-dihydroxycholecalciferol, or 24,25(OH)$_2$D, is also a physiologically common form of vitamin D and it too is made in the kidney. In healthy persons on a normal diet the ratio of 25(OH)D to 24,25(OH)$_2$D to 1,25(OH)$_2$D will be approximately 1000:100:1.[96] In a recent review, Anthony W. Norman et al.[94b] have cited much support for the concept that 24,25(OH)$_2$D plays a vital role in many biological responses, probably working in concert with 1,25(OH)$_2$D.[94b][***]

Some believe, incidentally, that alternative metabolites of 25(OH)D—24,25 dihydroxycholecalciferol and 25,26 dihydroxycholecalciferol, which is also made in the kidney—or even 25(OH)D itself, may play a role in bone mineralization in addition to (or instead of) 1,25(OH)$_2$D.[****] The majority view seems to be, however, that the 1,25(OH)$_2$D form alone is required for bone mineralization.[97,97a] W. G. Goodman et al.[97b] have recently reported that 24,25(OH)$_2$D$_3$ seems to promote maturation and mineralization of osteoid. However, they were "unable to ascribe to this compound a bone-specific effect on either osteoid maturation or mineralization independent of changes in the concentration of calcium in serum induced during repletion of this metabolite of vitamin D."

---

decrease with age, but serum 1,25(OH)$_2$D was lower in the elderly groups. They concluded that the inability of the aging kidney to synthesize 1,25(OH)$_2$D could contribute to the pathogenesis of osteoporosis. The work of B. Riis et al.[91b] suggests, however, that 1,25(OH)$_2$D is not the only vitamin D metabolite responsible for calcium absorption in the gut.

[**] One such site is the pancreas where Norman et al.[94d] have shown that a vitamin D deficiency inhibits production of insulin.

[***] D. F. Guillard-Cumming et al.[94ba] have subsequently reported that serum values of 24,25(OH)$_2$D$_3$ and the ratio of 24,25(OH)$_2$D$_3$ to 25(OH)D are significantly lower in patients having Paget's disease of the bone. Perhaps this finding will lead to a therapy for the disease. Specifically, I speculate that the 25-fluoro analogs of vitamin D—24,24-F$_2$-1,25(OH)$_2$D$_3$—might be useful (references 497-497d of Chapter 7).

[****] Generally, body quantities of D$_3$ and D$_2$ compounds are not distinguished but are simply referred to as 25(OH)D or 1,25(OH)$_2$D, etc. This practice is likely to change in light of the recent discovery by L. Tjellesen et al.[96a] that vitamins D$_2$ and D$_3$ are metabolized in different ways in man.

Nevertheless, as noted earlier, there is considerable evidence that 24,25(OH)$_2$D may often work in concert with 1,25(OH)$_2$D.[94c,97c-e] When it comes to chickens and the hatchability of eggs, they do work synergistically. A. W. Norman[97f] has reported that when 1,25(OH)$_2$D is the sole vitamin D source to hens they lay fertile eggs, but the majority fail to hatch. When administered with 24,25(OH)$_2$D the eggs hatch normally. In any event, 1,25(OH)$_2$D acts with the parathyroid hormone to mobilize calcium in addition to its role in bone mineralization.

Vitamin D, as 1,25(OH)$_2$D$_3$, stimulates calcium transport primarily in the duodenum while promoting phosphate absorption mainly in the jejunum (at least in rats and chickens).[97g] The action of vitamin D, in facilitating the transport of calcium, seems to involve a two-step process.[97h] When 1,25-dihydroxyvitamin D$_3$ is injected into a rat's veins, the first response of the small intestine's calcium transport mechanism (as shown by alkaline phosphatase activity) reaches a maximum at 6 hours and then declines until it is effectively gone at 12 hours (Figure 5). The second response begins at about the 12th hour and reaches a maximum about the 24th hour. (This is not a *reverse effect*. Time is involved. Furthermore, it is not a single action but the effect of two different responses.)

Both vitamin D$_3$ from food or made in the skin, or the synthetic precursor D$_2$, undergo the same metabolic conversions to form 25(OH)D$_3$ or 25(OH)D$_2$ and 1,25(OH)$_2$D$_3$ or 1,25(OH)$_2$D$_2$. Both the D$_3$ and D$_2$ forms are equally effective in the rat and probably in humans.[98] The widespread stories about the superiority of D$_3$ are true for chicks and New World monkeys, but probably not for man. I suspect that the stories are based on nothing more than the "religion" that holds all things that are "natural" (say D$_3$) to be superior to all things that are "synthetic" (say D$_2$). The fact that there exists a synthetic D$_3$ and the fact that a small amount of perfectly natural D$_2$ may be present in fish-liver oils would seem to somewhat upset the "natural" versus "unnatural" line of reasoning. Interestingly, the analog 1 alpha-OH-D$_2$ appears to be less toxic in rats than is the corresponding D$_3$ form, possibly because of a lessened ability to mobilize calcium from bone.[95]

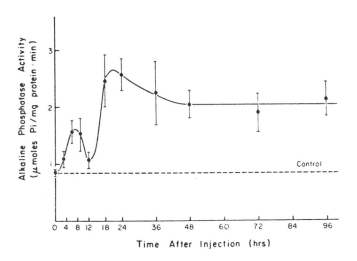

Figure 5. Time course of intestinal alkaline phosphatase activity following a single intrajugular injection of 500 pmol of 1,25(OH)₂D₃. Each point represents the mean ± SEM of at least five animals. Reproduced from Bernard P. Halloran and Hector F. DeLuca, *Archives of Biochemistry and Biophysics* (1981), 208, no. 2: 472-486, by permission of the publisher, Academic Press, and of the authors.

Vitamin D in Physiology and in Therapy

Because vitamin D is so important in calcium and phosphorus absorption, it is vital to the growth of bones, mending of broken bones and the prevention of osteoporosis, osteomalacia and backaches. Vitamin D also encourages the development of strong white teeth, jaws large enough so teeth will not be crowded and the prevention of tooth decay and periodontitis. Modest amounts given daily to children will prevent rickets, but relatively high dosages are required to successfully treat this disease.*

Vitamin D seems to have immunoregulatory properties. William F. C. Rigby et al.[99] reported that 1,25(OH)₂D₃ is a potent *in*

---

* History tells us about the ancient Britons who, in treating a child for rickets, went through a ritual in which the child was passed through a cleft in an ash tree. However, the ritual was performed *only in the presence of full sunlight* (thus providing, of course, vitamin D). Beware of judging all "superstitious acts" as being worthless.

vitro inhibitor of phytohemagglutinin-induced lymphocyte blast formation. Jacques M. Lemire et al.[99a] demonstrated that 1,25(OH)$_2$D$_3$ is a potent inhibitor of immunoglobulin (Ig) production by human peripheral blood mononuclear cells *in vitro*. Lemire et al. reported that, of all other vitamin D metabolites examined, only 24,25(OH$_2$)D$_3$ at a concentration of 10^{-7} M had a similar inhibitory effect. They suggested this action is mediated through vitamin D's "antiproliferative effect" on Ig-producing B cells and/or helper T cells.

Vitamin D is important in the health of the skin and may be useful for the treatment of psoriasis.[99b] It may be of value in treating tetany as well as for problems associated with malfunction of the parathyroid gland. Vitamin D has been found to stimulate the ovaries and is said to sometimes increase the sex drive in both men and women. A. M. Reed and his collaborators[100] noted an occasional increase in libido as well as sexual capacity of both sexes and an improvement in the rhythm of the menses in a few cases where very large doses of vitamin D were taken.

Adelle Davis[101] recommended that menstrual discomfort would be eased if prior to and during menstruation women would take daily 5,000 units of vitamin D and 9 tablets, each containing 250 mg. of calcium and 125 mg. of magnesium. However, like other popular nutrition writers, Adelle Davis was often too enthusiastic about excessive use of vitamins. Here, she is recommending what could well be a dangerous amount of vitamin D.

Let's consider briefly at this point some of the modern advances in vitamin D therapies. Both 25(OH)D$_3$ and 1,25(OH)$_2$D$_3$ are available as prescription products. In addition, a number of other synthetic vitamin D compounds have been developed and, of these, dihydrotachysterol is especially interesting. This compound is used in treating persons with hypoparathyroidism. Vitamin D functions, not only to increase absorption of calcium from the gastrointestinal tract and to put minerals in the bones, but to facilitate resorption of calcium and phosphate from the bones as needed. However, dihydrotachysterol is far more efficient than vitamin D for this purpose because it can be converted to dihydroxycholecalciferol—also known as 1,25-dihydroxyvitamin D$_3$ or 1,25(OH)$_2$D$_3$—by the kidneys without being limited by the liver's normal controlling mechanism. Synthetic 1,25-dihydroxyvitamin D$_3$ has been used by J. C. Gallagher et al.[102] for the treatment of patients with postmenopausal osteoporosis. The Gallagher group reported completely eliminating a negative calcium balance in their patients. By increasing the calcium absorption, use of supplemental calcium by such patients can be reduced. Another snythetic analog, 1-alpha hydroxyvitamin D$_3$, has been used successfully to treat hypocalcemia and hypomagnesemia due to malabsorption resulting from small bowel resection.[102a] Subsequently, David M. Slovik et al.[102b] reported that 1,25(OH)$_2$D was deficient in elderly osteoporotic patients. Then, J. C. Gallagher et al.[103] found that treating postmenopausal women with 1,25-dihydroxyvitamin D$_3$ resulted in significant increases in trabecular bone volume. They were unwilling, however, to draw conclusions about the long-term efficacy of 1,25(OH)$_2$D$_3$ therapy for postmenopausal osteoporosis. This condition will be discussed further in the calcium section of Chapter 7.

Vitamin D seems to be a factor in cancer prevention—at least of colon cancer. Cedric Garland et al.,[103a] noting that mortality rates from colon cancer in the U.S. are highest in populations exposed to the least amounts of sunlight, decided to study dietary vitamin D as a possible factor in its etiology. A 19-year prospective study in men by Garland et al. showed that the risk of colorectal cancer was inversely correlated with dietary vitamin D and calcium. In the quartiles of a combined index of dietary vitamin D and calcium from lowest to highest, the observed risks of colorectal cancer were 38.9, 24.5, 22.5 and 14.3 per 1,000 population.

Vitamin D may also eventually find application in cancer therapy. Chisato Miyaura et al.[103b] have shown that 1,25(OH)$_2$D$_3$ can induce human myeloid leukemia cells to differentiate into mature myeloid cells. It can also, according to Yoskio Honma et al.,[103c] prolong the survival time of mice inoculated with murine leukemia cells. M. R. Haussler et al.,[103d] in studying human promyelocytic leukemia cells, found that they contain some 4,000 receptors for 1,25(OH)$_2$D per cell. Subsequently, R. J. Majeska and G. A. Rodan[103e] found that 1,25(OH)$_2$D$_3$ exhibits complicated effects on cultured rat osteosarcoma cells. At low concentrations, the hormone inhibits cell proliferation but shows a *reverse effect* at higher concentrations by increasing cell numbers. Robert U. Simpson et al.[103f] presented data suggesting that 1,25(OH)$_2$D$_3$ receptors exist on both myelocytic and lymphocytic leukemia cells. They found that the presence of these receptors qualitatively predicted the efficacy of 1,25(OH)$_2$D$_3$ to inhibit cell proliferation. H. C. Freake et al.,[103g] at about the same time, arrived at a similar conclusion.

K. Colston et al.[103h] discovered that human melanoma cells have high-affinity receptors for 1,25(OH)$_2$D$_3$. *In vitro* studies using vitamin D with human melanoma showed a dose-related increase in cell doubling time.[103i] R. J. Frampton et al.[103j] subsequently found that the vitamin D metabolites, 1,24,25(OH)$_2$D$_3$ and 1,25,26(OH)$_2$D$_3$ inhibit *in vitro* proliferation of human melanoma cells. This may be a quite important discovery since both these components have less biological activity than 1,25(OH)$_2$D$_3$ and so they may find use in anticancer therapy.

J. A. Eisman et al.,[103k] in examining 168 human breast cancers, found 1,25(OH)$_2$D$_3$ receptors in 53%. They demonstrated (as shown in Figure 6) good inhibition *in vitro* of T47D human breast cancer cells with 1,25(OH)$_2$D$_3$ at a concentration of .1 nM and much better inhibition at 1.0 nM. (Studies were not carried out at other concentrations that might, conceivably, have shown a *reverse effect*.) A great future probably lies ahead for the use of vitamin D in cancer therapy!

Vitamin D congeners (e.g., *calcifediol, dihydrotachysterol, alfacalcidol* and *calcitriol*) are much less toxic than standard vitamins D$_2$ and D$_3$ and show great therapeutic promise. They show particular promise in treatment of osteodystrophy and of hypoparathyroidism, as well as in other disorders not helped by the standard forms of vitamin D.[104] Many other clinical applications of the various vitamin D compounds are discussed by H. F. DeLuca[105] and by J. A. Kanis.[106] Possible uses for newly discovered forms of vitamin D such as calcitronic acid, cholecalcitroic acid, 25-hydroxyvitamin D$_3$-

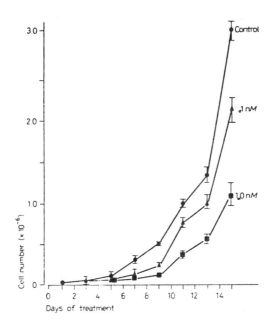

Figure 6. Inhibition of replication of T47D human breast-cancer cells by 1,25(OH)₂D₃. The T47D cells were incubated in a medium containing 0.07 μM insulin (control) and insulin with 0.1 or 1.0 nM 1,25(OH)₂D₃. Cell numbers were determined every second day. There was a dose-dependent inhibition of cell replication apparent after about five days. Interestingly, the effect of 1,25(OH)₂D₃ was dependent on the effect of insulin. Reproduced from J. A. Eisman et al. in *Modulation and Mediation of Cancer by Vitamins,* ed. F. L. Meyskens and K. N. Prasad (Basel, Switzerland: S. Karger AG, 1983) pp. 282-286, with permission of the publisher.

26, 23-lactone and 1,25-dihydroxyvitamin D₃-26,23-lactone remain to be developed. [95,107-107b] Many other vitamin D metabolites (as well as some postulated to exist, but not yet discovered) are shown in charts constructed by A. W. Norman et al.[94b] and by Helen L. Henry and A. W. Norman, [107c] but possible therapeutic uses for most of these are yet to be suggested. However, two vitamin D compounds incorporating fluoride will be discussed in the fluorine section of Chapter 7 in connection with osteoporosis therapies. Russell W.

Chesney,[96] by way of warning, reminds physicians that vitamin D intoxication can occur after the use of any form of vitamin D. He warns that when intoxication occurs, "...most patients are poisoned since physicians expect a rapid rise in serum calcium after giving vitamin D2 and D3 and continue to increase the dose, not recognizing the fact that these compounds may require several weeks to act." Nevertheless, physicians are generally aware that all forms of vitamin D, its metabolites and its analogues must be used cautiously, with monitoring of the serum calcium levels to avoid toxicity.

Antivitamin D compounds could also be therapeutically useful.* Hector F. DeLuca briefly discusses antivitamin D compounds which might be potentially valuable for treating hypercalcemia, but he observes that the search is still on for an effective antivitamin D compound.[108] His patent[108a] contains much additional information on antivitamin D compounds.

Is Vitamin D Supplementation Required?

Vitamin D is unique in that it is made by the body when ultraviolet light (from the sun) impinges on the skin. Much of the vitamin D is washed off, however, even in cold water unless adequate time is allowed for absorption to occur through the skin. However, the ability of human skin to synthesize vitamin D through use of sunlight decreases with age according to M. F. Holick and J. MacLaughlin.[109] This diminishing ability to make vitamin D is probably an important factor in vitamin D-deficiency bone disease that often affects the elderly. I think it also argues in favor of vitamin D supplementation by older persons, perhaps especially by women (who tend to be more affected by bone loss than men). As we age we tend to have increasing difficulty in producing 25(OH)D in the liver.[110] This decline of 25(OH)D in normal women is shown in Figure 7. In addition to the difficulty older persons have in making as much vitamin D as they did when they were younger, the dietary intake of vitamin D

---

* Vitamins (and drugs) have two parts—one structural which permits them to bind to their respective receptors and the other which is responsible for the biological activity. An antagonist lacks the biological activity but has the necessary structure to bind to the receptor. Thus, the antagonist jams the receptor so the vitamin (or drug) cannot operate.

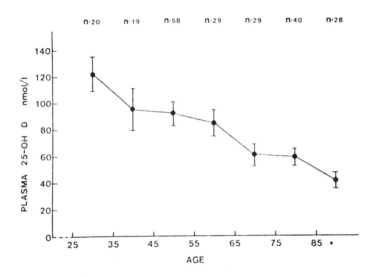

Figure 7. Plasma 25-hydroxyvitamin D concentrations (mean ± s.e.) in normal women in the age range 20-96 years (1 nmol/1=0.4 ng/ml). Reproduced from M. R. Baker et al., *Age and Ageing* (1980) 9: 249-252, with permission of the publisher, Bailliere Tindall, and of the authors.

tends to decrease with age, the ability to metabolize vitamin D in both the liver and the kidney may decline and even absorption of the vitamin from the gut may be impaired.[110] Most of these factors would seem to favor supplementation as one ages.

The dietary absorption of calcium also declines with age according to J. R. Bullamore et al.[110a] and this decline is related to many vitamin D actions. However, the presumption that the activity of the enzyme 1-alpha-hydroxylase, that is used to convert 25(OH)D to 1,25(OH)$_2$D in the liver, diminishes with age may be false. At any rate, aging, according to D. V. Havlir et al.,[110b] does not diminish 1-alpha-hydroxylase activity in the rat. If dietary intake of vitamin D and production of 25(OH)D decline with age (and they seem to do so), then there will, of course, be less of the active metabolite 1,25(OH)$_2$D even if 1-alpha-hydroxylase activity is unimpaired. However, whether or not the activity of this enzyme is impaired in men, it probably declines in menopausal women. Indirect evidence suggests that estrogen deficiency detrimentally affects the activity of this enzyme in women.[110c]

Sunlight generally accounts for considerably more of the body's vitamin D content than do dietary sources. The synthesis of vitamin D from the skin's pool of 7-dehydrocholesterol is rapid but limited, most of the production occurring during the first 2 1/2 minutes of exposure to ultraviolet light. Significant production of vitamin D also occurs only during the first few of a series of successive exposures.[110d] These results argue in favor of very limited exposure to sunlight (as do the negative remarks I made about excessive sunlight earlier in connection with vitamin E). The passive therapy of gardening or of a walk in the sun is health preserving. But avoid the wrinkle-making, leathery-skin-producing toasting ritual that is all too common on the beaches of the world.

D. E. M. Lawson et al.[111] reported that, even in subjects given a vitamin D supplement 20 times that generally present in the British diet, the plasma concentrations of $25(OH)D_3$ were only within the range reached by the British people during the summer. This fact would, it seems, argue in favor of either dietary supplementation or ultraviolet treatments for the British during the winter. It also suggests to me that the RDA of Americans ought to be subject to modification in terms of exposure to the sun or possibly to other sources of ultraviolet radiation.* The elderly should especially be wary of having too little of the active vitamin D metabolite in their plasma. John L. Omdahl et al.[114] reported that, in their study, plasma $25(OH)D_3$ was significantly lower in the elderly than in younger subjects. They noted a nadir in January and a zenith in September with women consistently showing lower $25(OH)D_3$ values regardless of seasonal influence. They also found that plasma alkaline phosphatase, an index of bone loss, was inversely related to the $25(OH)D_3$ values. The Omdahl group observed that healthy elderly

---

* R. M. Neer et al.[112] reported that "Vita-Lite" lamps of the Duro-Test Corp. significantly increased efficiency of intestinal calcium absorption in persons who received no ultraviolet light from the sun. M. S. Devgun et al.,[113] however, observed that such lamps caused no increase in 25(OH)D levels of patients exposed to them.

men supplementing with 400 I.U. daily had normal plasma alkaline phosphatase levels, but women taking 400 I.U. daily maintained elevated alkaline phosphatase levels. They suggested that elderly women may require more than 400 I.U. of vitamin D supplementation. Omdahl et al. ended their report with a recommendation that elderly Americans either consider use of vitamin D supplements and/or obtain increased sunlight exposure (but note Lawson's research, also cited above, that shows brief exposure to the sun may suffice). Comments by Ross P. Holmes and Fred A. Kummerow disputing some of the Omdahl conclusions and a reply by John L. Omdahl and Philip J. Garry and another reply by A. Michael Parfitt appeared in the *American Journal of Clinical Nutrition.*[115]

Then too, Daniel Hollander and Hella Tarnawski[115a] recently reported normal absorption of vitamin D_3 in aging animals. If this finding is also true of humans, then it seems possible that malabsorption of vitamin D_3 could be ruled out as a cause of bone disease among older persons. Perhaps even more disquieting is another recent report by Claus Christiansen and Paul Rodbro[115b] that serum levels of vitamin D metabolites 25(OH)D and 1,25(OH)₂D and 24,25(OH)₂D did not differ significantly between younger and older postmenopausal women.* They concluded that 1,25(OH)₂D is "unlikely to be significant in the development or treatment of a majority of women with postmenopausal osteoporosis." However, B. E. Christopher Nordin et al.[115d] reported, more recently, that feeding elderly women 15,000 I.U. of vitamin D_2 weekly resulted in significantly raised levels of 25(OH)D and reduced rate of cortical bone loss. (It seems apparent that endogenous 1,25(OH)₂D was also increased, although this was not covered in the study.)

---

* This finding, however, as far as 25(OH)D is concerned, contradicts the study of M. R. Baker et al.[110] cited earlier and whose findings were shown in Figure 7. The serum levels determined by Christiansen and Rodbro may also be subject to question. Assessment of serum 1,25(OH)₂D levels must be done over time periods when body weight is stable. The serum level of this hormone is reported to vary directly with body weight and colonic intake.[115c] Thus, a patient fasting without knowledge of his physician might easily mislead the doctor into giving an incorrect evaluation of the level of this metabolite.

Recent studies[116,117] show that vitamin D produced by the skin has longer lasting physiological effects than dietary vitamin D. The human liver synthesizes 25(OH)D, as we have explained, and then later, after vitamin D has served its physiological functions, the liver inactivates vitamin D to a polar metabolite of 1,25 dihydroxyvitamin D for excretion in the bile. The vitamin D formed in the skin diffuses gradually into the blood so the liver's uptake and conversion to 25(OH)D occurs more slowly than a similar amount of vitamin D derived from the diet.

Excellent food sources for vitamin D are fish-liver oils,* especially halibut oil which contains far more vitamin D than does cod-liver oil. Vitamin D is also found in milk,** butter and the yolk of eggs (especially in the summer if the cows and chickens have been out in the sunshine). It is also found in fish, in chicken and in beef and pork liver. However, several studies suggest, as we have noted, that the body generally makes more vitamin D from sunlight than it takes in from a normal diet.[110,111]

Many vitamin D supplements are combined with calcium or bone meal in spite of the fact that it has been known for more than a half century (since 1932) that vitamin D can lose its potency when this is done.[118] Tetsuya Takahashi and R. Yamamoto[119] found that vitamin D_2 is rapidly isomerized to isocalciferol and isotachysterol in powders prepared with dibasic calcium phosphate. They also reported that mixtures of vitamin D_2 and ascorbic acid, folic acid, thiamin or pyridoxine caused a similar reaction. If you're going to take vitamin D supplements you'll probably want to use those containing just this vitamin or combined with vitamin A, while avoiding combinations with other vitamins or minerals. I am less concerned, however, about the possible nonefficaciousness of vitamin D combination pills than I am about the occasional presence of a fishy smell. If a pill smells of fish oil we can suspect the presence of rancidity due to health-sapping peroxides. If one is going to supplement, I think it

---

* Although fish-liver oils are strong sources of vitamin D, only traces occur in the livers of man and the other mammals.[116]

** Yogurt, unless it has been vitamin enriched, will be devoid of vitamin D since it is destroyed by the fermentation process[117a]

best to use encapsulated vitamin D, not just because there is no calcium or other nutrients with which it might interact, but because it is protected from the negative effects of oxygen.

Should one take vitamin D supplements? Supplemental vitamin D may be important during the period of accelerated growth preceding sexual maturation. At any rate, Joseph A. Johnston[119a] states that it is likely that the need for vitamin D is related, not to body size, but to variations in the increase in body length. For a younger person, but one beyond adolescence, supplementation is probably unnecessary if he or she is getting adequate exposure to sunlight and eating foods rich in vitamin D. For older persons, however, depending on the vitamin D content of their diet, supplementation may be of value. (Persons with lactose intolerance who must forego dairy products also may tend to be deficient in vitamin D unless they regularly expose their skin to the sun or take a supplement.) According to A. Michael Parfitt et al.,[120] the best estimate for a safe daily intake of vitamin D for older persons is not the RDA of 200 to 400 I.U.,* but 600 to 800 I.U. However, these scientists report that, in one study,[122] a daily dose of 2,000 I.U. produced hypercalcemia in 2 of 63 elderly persons. They speculate that the margin of safety between an effective and a dangerous dose may be less than it is in younger persons. Furthermore, Fred A. Kummerow[123] has estimated that our vitamin D intake from food is 2,435 I.U. per day, most of which has been added to these foods by man under the doctrine of "enrichment." If he is correct, some of us may already be getting too much vitamin D even if we take none in pill form! Ross P. Holmes and Fred A. Kummerow[123a] present, in fact, a strong case for curtailing—preferably abolishing—fortification of foods with vitamin D. They say, "populations at risk could be monitored closely and counseled to prevent vitamin D deficiency." On the other hand, R. Bouillon[123b] of Belgium maintains that "vitamin D deficiency is much more endemic than previously recognized." (In that connection he cites the clinical usefulness of measuring serum 25(OH)D to detect any deficiency or excess.)

---

* The RDA varies from 200 I.U. to 400 I.U. depending on sex and age, with 200 I.U. extra recommended for pregnant or lactating women.[121]

Obviously, the debate about vitamin D is lively! It may be that some of us are already getting too much vitamin D and that others of us are deficient.* Each of us must learn to read our own body like a book and help our nutritionists and physicians decide such questions as to whether or not we should use a particular supplement.

Dangers of Excessive Vitamin D

Symptoms associated with an excess of vitamin D are nausea, headaches, fatigue, lack of appetite, cramps, depression of brain function, kidney damage, diarrhea and dizziness. But some of these conditions are also symptomatic of other disorders. Excess of vitamin D has caused loss of hair, joint pains, bone pain, headache, enlarged liver and spleen, increased intracranial pressure, high blood pressure, kidney failure and death. Large amounts of vitamin D can lead to hypercalcemia (an excess of calcium in the blood, having been drained from the bones)[122,123d] and a subsequent laying down of calcium in the soft tissue. Hypercalcemia may, in turn, be a risk factor in the formation of kidney stones. In pregnancy, vitamin D can cross the placental barrier and, in large doses, can give the fetus hypercalcemia and mental retardation. Then too, even mild excesses of vitamin D_3 have caused arteriosclerosis in monkeys according to Peng Shi-Kaung et al.[124] A daily intake of just 500 I.U. was enough to cause problems, although a monkey is considerably smaller than a person. (One should not, however, conclude that effects are always proportional to body size. Metabolic effects of the same dosage per kg. of body weight may be quite different in different species.) Many other studies suggest that excessive vitamin D is implicated in the onset of arteriosclerosis. (It is, however, often difficult to sort out prime causes from concomitant phenomena and contributing influences. Suppose that the prime cause of arteriosclerosis and atherosclerosis is shown to be scarring resulting from a bombardment of the arterial wall by free radicals. If this should prove to be the case, then we ought to fight the cause and be less

---

* Iris Robertson et al.[123c] suggest that high-fiber diets may lead to wastage of vitamin D and its metabolites derived from sunlight and thus cause rickets or osteomalacia.

concerned with the body's action of patching the abrasions with cholesterol and calcium, facilitated by vitamin D.)

In a related area, a study concerning ischemic heart disease in Great Britain showed a strong correlation between vitamin D intake and mortality rates.[125] Vitamin D is known to enhance lead absorption and this fact was put forth as a possible explanation of the association. Other studies[130] have shown that vitamin D can increase the absorption of cadmium, strontium, lead and nickel, all of which are potentially toxic and possibly even carcinogenic.

A disturbing rat study of over a half century ago by Robert F. Light et al.[125a] showed that a large overdosage of vitamin D, just insufficient to produce toxic symptoms in the first and second generations, given over a long period, produced "striking pathological changes" in the third and fourth generations. Could vitamin D overdosage leave us without detrimental effects while setting up the possibility of harm in future generations? For that matter, it has already been about two generations that vitamin D supplementation of our foods has been at what might be, for some persons, excessive levels.

To suggest the possible dangers of holding simplistic views of vitamin D metabolism, note that in hypoparathyroidism $25(OH)D_3$ is normal but $1,25(OH)_2D_3$ is low; in primary hyperparathyroidism $25(OH)D_3$ is normal but $1,25(OH)_2D_3$ is high; in both Type I and Type II vitamin D-resistant rickets $25(OH)D_3$ is normal but in Type I $1,25(OH)_2D_3$ is low and in Type II it is high; and in postmenopausal osteoporosis $25(OH)D_3$ is normal but $1,25(OH)_2D_3$ is low.[126]*

---

* There is evidence that estrogen therapy can restore the levels of $1,25(OH)_2D_3$.[127] However, G. Finn Jensen et al.[128] reported that $1,25(OH)_2D_3$, administered in clinically acceptable doses, is without value in the treatment of postmenopausal osteoporosis and may actually be detrimental. They also reported that estrogen, alone or in combination with calcium, results in a significant increase in bone mineral content. Parathyroid hormone (PTH) supplementation may also be of little help in osteoporosis. R. Neer et al.[128a] infused synthetic human PTH intravenously for 24 hours. The result was an increase in $1,25(OH)_2D$ in controls but not in osteoporotic patients. More recently, K. S. Tsai et al.[128b] concluded that an impaired ability of the aging kidney to synthesize $1,25(OH)_2D$ could be a factor in the decreased ability to absorb calcium and in the development of osteoporosis. The work of G. Finn Jensen et al.[128] suggests that another factor or factors may be at work. In addition to calcium, fluoride and $1,25(OH)_2D$, could injections of $24,25(OH)_2D$ be helpful? J. Reeve et al.[128c] found that $24,25(OH)_2D$, administered over a

Supplementation with vitamin D will generally increase the levels of $25(OH)D_3$—possibly resulting in hypercalcemia due to both increased intestinal absorption and bone resorption—while conceivably leaving the levels of the other vitamin D metabolites unchanged. Large doses of vitamin A (50,000 to 100,000 I.U. daily) may also work to induce hypercalcemia by exacerbating bone resorption.[129] Obviously, supplementation, except under the guidance of a physician, might be a dangerous undertaking. We don't want to overdose on vitamin D, but, on the other hand, a minority of persons may be deficient. Among the groups that may be at risk of deficiency are the very young and the very old, invalids, dark-skinned persons living in northern latitudes, others receiving very little sunlight and those who avoid dairy products.

If you are under a doctor's care and he is conducting tests, be sure to tell him if you are using supplements of vitamin D. A large intake of this vitamin can give false positive or elevated readings in the albumin test and the nonprotein nitrogen (NPN) test for abnormal renal function.[79] It may also be responsible for false negative or decreased values of alkaline phosphatase.[79] If your source of vitamin D is a large amount of cod-liver oil, it could result in a false positive or elevated values in the protein-bound iodine test for abnormal thyroid function.[79] The Sulkowitch test for urine calcium may also be spuriously elevated if the patient has taken vitamin D.[131] On the other hand, drugs your physician may have prescribed could inhibit vitamin D and perhaps your doctor will suggest an increase in your intake.** Cortisol, for example, antagonizes the action of vitamin D and reduces absorption of calcium from the intestines.[132] In addition, there may be interactions between vitamin D and cholestyramine, glutethimide[81] and the anticonvulsants. Furthermore, cathartics, through increasing peristalsis and by causing damage to the intestinal wall, can inhibit vitamin D absorption. It is essential that your doctor

---

six-month period to five patients with osteoporosis, was not beneficial. However, I have not yet seen any reports that it has been tested in conjunction with supplementary calcium, fluoride and $1,25(OH)_2D$.

** A vitamin D deficiency in rats has been shown by Carla Bazzani et al.[131a] to increase the basal pain threshold and the analgesic effects of morphine. However, tolerance to morphine developed faster in vitamin D-deficient rats.

know not only about medications you may be using, but also about supplements (or cathartics) you may be taking!

Let's close our discussion of vitamin D with an interesting vitamin-drug *reverse effect*. It has been known for some time that phenytoin (Dilantin®) accelerates metabolism of vitamin D and causes a loss of calcium.[132a] It has been recently reported by Marielle Gascon-Barre et al.[132b] that, based on data from just one patient, plasma concentrations of $1,25(OH)_2D$ were relatively independent of the dose of phenytoin administered, but this was not true of $25(OH)D$. As shown in Figure 8, the plasma concentrations of $25(OH)D$ were increased by low phenytoin concentrations, but then underwent a *reverse effect* by declining as the phenytoin dosage increased and/or as the length of time of exposure to the drug increased. It seems likely that many dose-response *reverse effects* of drug-vitamin interactions will eventually be discovered—and many are likely to have therapeutic implications.

Cod-Liver Oil

Since cod-liver oil is a common source of vitamin D (and also of vitamin A), let's say a few words about this product. Cod-liver oil is not only a strong source of these vitamins but it has also been found to contain eicosapentenoic acid (EPA) which we met in Chapter 3. Eicosapentenoic acid is a precursor of the thromboxane TxA_3 and the prostacyclin PGI_3.[133b-e]* *In vitro* studies have shown that thromboxane TxA_3 does not aggregate platelets[133g,h] the way thromboxane TxA_2 does or, at worst, TxA_3 aggregates platelets only weakly[133i] while PGI_3 is as antiaggregatory as PGI_2.[133h,j,k] The discovery by Sven Fischer and Peter C. Weber[133m] that PGI_3 is formed *in vivo* in man after he consumes eicosapentenoic acid and that dietary EPA does not inhibit *in vivo* formation of PGI_2 from arachidonic acid is

---

* It is unsaturated EPA (not saturated EPA) that beneficially increases bleeding times. A study by N. A. Begent et al.[133f] showed that the bleeding time of small mesenteric arteries of rats fed unsaturated EPA showed significant increases after four to seven weeks compared to those fed hydrogenated (saturated) EPA.

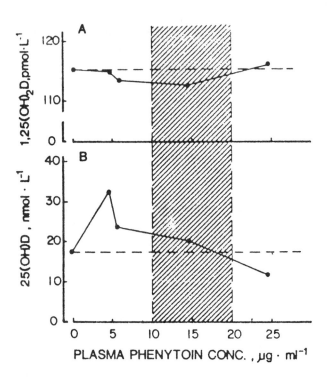

Figure 8. Relationships between the plasma 1,25(OH)₂D (A) and 25(OH)D (B) concentrations and the plasma phenytoin concentrations. The patient also received primidone (300 mg./day), which gave rise to an average plasma phenobartibal concentration of 5 m g./ml. at all phenytoin concentrations. The hatched zone represents the usual therapeutic range of phenytoin. Graph reproduced from Marielle Gascon-Barre et al., *Jrl. of the Amer. College of Nutrition* (1984) 3: 45-50, with permission of the publisher, Alan R. Liss, Inc. The graph illustrates an interesting vitamin-drug *reverse effect* as discussed in the text.

important support for the thesis that EPA reduces the risk of coronary heart disease. Briefly, it is theorized that TxA₃ is less thrombogenic than TxA₂ (which we met in Chapter 3), while

PGI₃ may be as antithrombotic as PGI₂ (which we also met in Chapter 3). It is even speculated that EPA may competitively inhibit the conversion of arachidonic acid to TxA₂ in the platelets.[133n] The increased bleeding tendency and the rarity of heart disease among Greenland Eskimos is at least partly explainable by the large amounts of EPA present in their diet.[133,133a]

A possible benefit of fish oils may be their modification of plasma levels of the very low- and low-density lipoproteins. William S. Harris and William E. Connor,[134] commenting on the Eskimo diet, reported that eicosapentenoic and docosahexenoic acids present in fish oils significantly decreased the very low-density lipoprotein and low-density lipoprotein plasma levels but left the levels of high-density lipoproteins unchanged. Subsequently, they [134b] observed that human subjects fed a salmon-oil diet (40% calories as fat and 50 mg. of cholesterol) for four weeks showed average declines in cholesterol levels from 188 to 160 mg./dl. and in triglycerides from 77 to 48. The LDL and VDL cholesterol levels changed from 128 to 108 and from 13 to 8, respectively. As before, there was no change in the HDL-cholesterol levels. For comparison, a vegetable-oil diet caused similar declines in cholesterol but left triglyceride levels unchanged. T. A. B. Sanders et al.[134c] found that feeding cod-liver oil to healthy male volunteers resulted in a significantly lengthened bleeding time after three weeks. Bleeding time returned to presupplementation value five weeks after withdrawal of the supplement.

R. Saynor et al.,[134d,e] studying the effect of omega-3 fatty acids in patients with cardiovascular disease, reported highly significant declines in serum-triglyceride concentrations and in total cholesterol. HDL-cholesterol increased significantly, suggesting, as Sanders[134c] observes, that omega-3 fatty acids may convey long-term benefits in delaying atherosclerosis and reducing the probability of thrombosis. Bonnie H. Weiner et al.[134f] reported, in late 1986, significantly less atherosclerosis in swine fed cod liver oil.

However, D. B. Jones and T. M. E. Davies[135] caution about concluding that the consumption of EPA is without possible problems. They warn that its excessive use can reduce the platelet count by 15%, which could, in turn, be expected to produce fewer platelet interactions and a reduction in the release of beta-thromboglobulin.* They also list several other fatty acids in fish oil that influence platelet behavior, so we cannot even be sure that only EPA is causing the observed effects. G. Hornstra et al.[135ac] point out that the (n-3) fatty acids (of which eicosapentenoic acid as well as alpha-linolenic acid are examples) cause changes in cardiac lipids in animals that lead to cardiac necrosis.** Furthermore, although cod-liver oil has a distinct antithrombic effect in rats,[136a] arterial blood pressure has been reported to be significantly increased by feeding them cod-liver oil.[136b]

However, man apparently has a more favorable reaction and such findings stress how important it is to choose the proper animal for an experiment if the phenomena could be species-specific. (Caution must always be observed when drawing conclusions for man from animal experiments.) Reinhard Lorenz et al.,[136c] feeding healthy 22–24-year-old male volunteers with a cod-liver oil supplement of 40 ml./day, observed that systolic blood pressure tended to decline. Cod-liver oil taken by humans apparently does not raise blood pressure as it does in rats. Earlier, T. A. B. Sanders et al.[134c] had also reported a reduction of blood pressure in human volunteers given cod-liver oil.

Then too, J. Z. Mortensen et al.[136d] carried out a double-blind crossover study with 20 healthy males, aged 25 to 40 years, who were given 4 g./day of n-3 or n-6 polyunsaturated fatty acids derived from fish and vegetable sources respectively for 4 weeks, separated by 4 weeks without dietary supplementation. They found that with the n-3 fish-oil supplement blood pressure, plasma total lipids, triglycerides and very low-density lipoprotein (VLDL) fell significantly, whereas plasma antithrombin III rose and bleeding time

---

* C. R. M. Hay, A. P. Durber and R. Saynor[135a] reported that platelet count was considerably lowered after 6 weeks on an EPA supplement. However, R. Saynor and D. Verel[135ab] found that the count remained depressed for only about 6 months and that by 12 months had returned to the pre-oil level.

** Horrendous physiological effects occurred when H. M. Sinclair[135b,136] made a 100-day self-study of the effects of ingesting a diet containing only marine animal foods and water. Such a study does not, of course, condemn a diet containing fish oil or cod-liver oil. It simply points out the merit of a balanced diet.

also increased significantly.* Paul J. Nestel et al.,[136e] in a related study using five normal persons and two with hypertriglyceridemia, also reported that VLDL was lowered "profoundly" with fish-oil supplementation, while the effect on LDL was inconsistent. B. E. Woodcock et al.,[136f] in studying patients with peripheral arterial disease, found that fish-oil supplementation significantly lowered blood viscosity and plasma triglyceride concentration, while plasma cholesterol and HDL remained unchanged. P. Singer et al.[136g,h] recently reported on the effects of dietary supplementation with two cans of mackerel daily for two weeks in 15 normotensive volunteers, 14 patients with mild hypertension and 8 patients with type IV and V hyperlipoproteinemia. The normotensives showed markedly lower systolic and diastolic blood pressures at the end of the period on the mackerel diet, whereas in hypertensive and hyperlipemic subjects only the systolic pressure was significantly decreased. (A similar experiment as part of the same study, but using herring instead, resulted in only minor blood pressure changes.)

An interesting possibility is that fish oils may have application in the treatment of autoimmune diseases. Dwight R. Robinson et al.[136i] reported that marine lipids, as menhaden oil, "markedly reduce the severity of glomerulonephritis and its associated mortality in inbred strains of mice developing autoimmune disease, a model for human systemic lupus erythematosis." Many other examples of the benefits of eating fish and/or use of marine oils in moderation were given in Chapter 3.

In spite of the many benefits of marine oils such as cod-liver oil, I suggest that you not consume them to excess. Experiments on animals by Erik Agduhr and Nils Stenström[137] were reported in their book with the frightening title, *The Appearance of the Electrocardiogram in Heart Lesions Produced by Cod-Liver Oil.* The animals suffered toxical changes, notably in the heart, but in many

---

* More recently, Heinz Juan and Wolfgang Sametz[136da] showed that dihomogamma-linolenic acid (DGLA) stimulates EPA to further increase the release of antiaggregatory trienoic prostaglandins.

other organs as well.* K. L. Blaxter et al.[138] reported that calves given cod-liver oil developed muscular dystrophy. The researchers concluded that the disease was not caused by hypervitaminosis A or D (a logical possibility since cod-liver oil is rich in these vitamins), but rather that it was due to the oil's content of polyunsaturated fatty acids. It is also interesting to note that when scientists desire to produce muscular dystrophy in rabbits for experimental purposes, they do so by feeding the animals cod-liver oil. The cod-liver oil's mode of action is to produce a vitamin E deficiency which, in turn, causes muscular dystrophy. Lesions of the skeletal muscles occur not only in rabbits and in calves, as noted above, but in guinea pigs, rats, goats and sheep that have been fed cod-liver oil.[138a] It is not just cod-liver oil, however, that may cause problems. Simin N. Meydani et al.[138b] warn that other types of fish oil and fish itself, if eaten in excess, may adversely affect vitamin E status. As vitamin E declines, serum levels of lipid peroxide will rise. Yoshiki Kobatake et al.[139] reported that when rats were fed either eicosapentenoic acid (EPA) or docosahexanoic acid (DHA), serum lipid peroxide levels were elevated more in animals fed DHA than in those fed EPA.

Many of these detrimental effects may be due not to the cod-liver oil and other fish oils themselves and to the inevitable peroxides they create, but to additional peroxides caused through careless processing. A book by F. Peckel Möller[140] relates the difficulty of keeping cod-liver oil from turning rancid. The book was published in 1895, so perhaps there is now greater appreciation for the fact that the oil must go from the fresh liver of the cod to an airtight bottle very rapidly to minimize rancidity. The marine oils may now be safer since the dangers of peroxidation are more widely known. However, I wonder if the oil is kept under hermetic seal throughout the processing and whether the air has been removed from the space at the top of the bottle and replaced with nitrogen to minimize formation of free radical intermediates and semistable peroxides. I also wonder about the

---

* We noted earlier Nestel et al.[136e] reported that a diet rich in fish oil beneficially decreased the triglyceride-transporting very low-density lipoprotein. However, the fish-oil diet detrimentally decreased the high-density lipoprotein (HDL) lipids and the A₁ apoprotein.

possible carcinogenicity of the reagents used to remove "impurities" leaving, perhaps, more-dangerous remnants.

Even if cod-liver oil or other marine oils were completely free of peroxides, would they remain unaffected by peroxidation after entering the body? Denham Harman[134a,139a] cautions that the use of supplemental marine oils, with their eicosapentenoic and docosahexenoic acids, may increase the peroxidizability of the serum lipoproteins and might even increase the chance of senile dementia. Docosahexenoic acid is taken up by the brain and concentrated in the phospholipids of neurons in the perikaryon and in the synaptic area.[139a] Harmon views this as a threat if peroxidation is not controlled. It seems to me his opposition to supplemental fish oils hinges not so much on whether they are detrimental per se, but on whether their peroxidation can be minimized. Consuming additional amounts of vitamins A and E, selenium and other antioxidants might permit us to enjoy the benefits of marine oils (especially platelet deaggregation) while keeping their peroxidation to a tolerable minimum.

Acrolein, a cross-linkage agent used in tanning, is formed to the extent of .7-1.5% in cod-liver oil when it is exposed to air oxidation![139b] Cross-linking of collagen as noted in Chapter 2 is a pro-aging phenomenon.

Then too, G. R. Mizuno et al.[141] reported on the volatile amines (ethylenediamine and 1,4-butanediamine) present in menhaden oil that may combine with nitrite to form carcinogenic nitrosamines. It may be possible that cod-liver oil presents a similar problem. On the other hand, Rashida A. Karmali et al.[141a] found that marine oil reduced the rate of growth of tumors transplanted into rats. They speculated that the inhibitory effect of the eicosapentenoic and docosahexenoic acids on the tumors may be linked partially to the fact that they depress arachidonic acid metabolism.

Nevertheless, I suspect a *reverse effect* might operate under some dosages to foster rather than inhibit tumor formation if eicosapentenoic and docosahexenoic acids tend to suppress the immune system. Vicki E. Kelly et al.[141b] reported that when mice bred to be a model of fulminant systemic lupus erythematosus were given a dietary supplement of 20% menhaden fish oil, their lupus was suppressed. Since lupus is an autoimmune disease, this action indicates that the immune system of these animals was suppressed by the menhaden oil with its large content of eicosapentenoic acid. In other research, Richard N. Podell [141c] did a 12-week, double-blind study of the effects of eicosapentenoic acid on 37 patients with another autoimmune disease, rheumatoid arthritis. The experimental group who ate a diet low in animal fat, high in vegetable oil and each day took 10 capsules of Max EPA® (a source of eicosapentenoic and docosahexenoic acids) experienced a reduction in morning stiffness and a decrease in the number of tender joints. Thus, eicosapentenoic and docosahexenoic acids, through inhibition of the immune system, may play a role in treating autoimmune diseases. At the same time, it also alerts us to the possibility that, in suppressing the immune system, cancer and other diseases might be fostered. Until dose-response relationships and possible *reverse effects* can be worked out for various diseases, it behooves laymen to avoid experimentation.

Fish oils, like other nutritional entities, obviously have their positives and their negatives. The concerns I have expressed, however, refer primarily to overuse of the concentrated fish oils, not to the fish from which they are derived. Cod and other fish oils are valuable foods, but I think it best to get these oils indirectly by eating fish. I prefer the high-fat, cold-water,* high-calorie fish such as salmon, lake (not brook) trout,** mackerel and whitefish. I think it is better to eat lesser amounts of the low-fat, low-calorie fish such as cod, catfish, snapper, halibut and brook trout. These are also, of course, healthful foods but are less-concentrated sources of eicosapentenoic acid. N. Chetty and B. A. Bradlow[141d] suggest that daily consumption of 200–400 grams of fish (1/2–1 lb.—a rather large amount) might be optimal to inhibit platelet aggregation. As an alternative, they speculate that 1 to 4 grams of EPA daily might be

---

* A benefit of cold-water fish (low arachidonic acid) was noted in Chapter 3. EPA differences vary with EPA content of algae eaten by the fish or eaten lower down the food chain.[141ca] Farm-fed fish have virtually no EPA.

** The expressed preference for lake trout is made only in consideration of oil content. Lake trout may sometimes have contaminants not present in brook trout.

useful, but they stress that optimal amounts of EPA are yet to be determined.

Salmon, the usual commercial source of omega-3 fatty acids, is high in the food chain and therefore might contain industrial pollutants such as PCBs. (If you are considering taking omega-3 capsules, ask your supplier to get an analysis from the manufacturer.) Mackerel, being lower in the food chain, might be a safer source but is not generally used.Nevertheless, both—like other fish oils—contain the natural toxin cetoleic acid.[141da]

Vitamin K—for Blood Clotting and for Possible Use in Combating Cancer

This fat-soluble vitamin is used by the liver to manufacture prothrombin which, in turn, is converted by various activators into thrombin which aids in blood clotting. (The thrombin changes fibrinogen in the blood to fibrin that forms the clot.) This propensity of vitamin K for coagulating blood is what led to its name. It was named vitamin K for *Koagulation* (as it is spelled in Denmark) by the Danish scientist, Henrik Dam, who discovered it in 1929, isolated it in pure form in 1939 and later shared a Nobel Prize with the American scientist, Edward A. Doisy, who synthesized it.

There are several fat-soluble varieties of vitamin K and it also occurs in water-soluble form. The oil-soluble forms are vitamin K_1, now known as *phylloquinone,* which is found in vegetables, and vitamin K_2, now called *menaquinone-7,* which is synthesized by bacteria. There are many other forms of vitamin K_2 homologues. The synthetic, water-soluble vitamin K_3 is now often called *menadione.* Vitamin K is incorporated in the chylomicrons present in the blood and is also present in lymph. A new class of vitamin K-dependent proteins which bind calcium has been discovered and recently reviewed by James J. Corrigan.[141e]

Bleeding areas under the skin (purpura)—black and blue marks—may be a sign of vitamin K deficiency (or of a shortage of vitamins C and P). Vitamin K can be useful in controlling excessive menstrual flow and in treating strokes or other types of hemorrhaging, but only when such hemorrhaging is due to a deficiency of prothrombin or of coagulation proteins known as *factor VII, factor IX or factor X*. (This vitamin does not check bleeding in the normal individual.) Many possible modes of action for vitamin K have been proposed, but it is now speculated that the vitamin regulates the synthesis of vitamin K-dependent coagulation proteins in the ribosomes.[141f]* At pharmacological concentrations vitamin K possesses anti-inflammatory action, including usefulness in rheumatoid arthritis.[142] Vitamin K is useful for body functions, but can it sometimes cause cancer?

V. Egilsson[142a] hypothesizes that malignancy may be caused by disturbed vitamin K physiology of the cells and that cancer might sometimes be caused by vitamin K. P. Hilgard[142b] agrees and points out that a diet-induced vitamin K deficiency is effective in inhibiting tumor growth and tumor dissemination. Furthermore, coumarin and its derivatives[142c] are vitamin K antagonists that are found in the tonka bean (sometimes prescribed by herbalists) and in powerful antimetastatic drugs. Either vitamin K excess or vitamin K deficiency may be causes of cancer or useful cancer therapy.

In spite of Egilsson's views[142a] that vitamin K might cause cancer, the work of Kedar N. Prasad et al.[142d] suggests that vitamin K3 may be a potentially useful anticancer agent. Prasad et al.[142d] reported that vitamin K3 (and to a lesser degree K1) inhibited cultures of mouse neuroblastoma, melanoma and glioma cells. In a serum-free medium but with vitamin K3, glioma cells did not grow at all and the other two types of cells showed 2-3 fold higher sensitivity to vitamin K3 than they did if cultured in a serum-free medium. R. T. Chlebowski et al.[143] determined that both vitamins K1 and K3 are cytotoxic *in vitro* against L1210 murine leukemia cells. They found that warfarin, whose anticoagulant effect antagonizes vitamin K's coagulatory propensity, can be used with vitamin K to achieve a synergistic anticancer effect (Figure 9). Roman T. Chlebowski et

---

* Geoffrey J. Blackwell et al.[142] have reported that vitamin K's ability to cause aggregation of human platelets seems to involve an interference with the mobilization and/or utilization of calcium ions. Vitamin K's aggregation power can be overcome by increasing the levels of extracellular calcium ions.

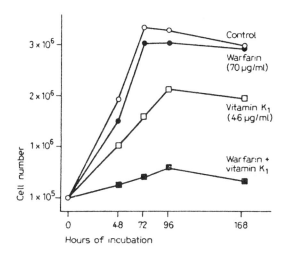

Figure 9. Effect of warfarin and/or vitamin K_1 on growth of L1210 leukemic cells. Cells at an initial concentration of 1×10^5/ml. were exposed continuously to the indicated concentration of drug, and cell count was made at the indicated time intervals. Cultures were maintained at 37.5°C in an atmosphere containing 5% CO_2 and 95% air. Reproduced from R. T. Chlebowski et al., in *Modulation and Mediation of Cancer by Vitamins*, ed. F. L. Meyskens and K. N. Prasad (Basel, Switzerland: S. Karger AG, 1983), pp. 276-281, with permission of the publisher.

Note: These are not *reverse effects* since the x-axis shows time, not dosage.

al.[143a] have recently provided a review of vitamin K in the treatment of cancer. Perhaps vitamin K may hold potential for human cancer therapy if we can discover and then eliminate those serum factors that might thwart its action. If vitamin K can both cause and cure cancer, it would be another example of the *reverse effect* and the importance of dose-response relationships.

Vitamin K may be of value in the treatment of some cases of coronary thrombosis and in serious cases of nose bleeding, as well as when symptoms include bloody vomit or bloody stool. Vitamin K is an aid to the proper functioning of the liver, heart, kidney and the adrenal glands. In cases of hypertension, vitamin K (along with vitamins C and P) may be of help in preventing or stopping hemorrhages in the eye. A study by A. C. Casey and E. G. Bliznakov[144] showed that vitamin K increased phagocytic activity in rats. However, John I. Gallin et al.[145] reported that high concentrations of vitamin K3 inhibited phagocytosis of human neutrophils. Therefore, this is perhaps another example of the *reverse effect*.

A therapy, introduced by R. L. Merkel,[146] for treating nausea and vomiting of pregnancy consists of simultaneous administration of 5 mg. of vitamin K and 25 mg. of vitamin C. Jonathan V. Wright[147] states that addition of vitamin B6 makes the therapy even better.

Normal body requirements for vitamin K are probably less than 1 mg. daily and are provided by food. Good sources for this vitamin are alfalfa,* spinach, broccoli, lettuce, turnip greens, cabbage, cauliflower, algae, pork, beef liver and beef kidney. A very strong source is green tea. Vitamin K is also manufactured in the intestinal tract when there are thriving colonies of acidophilus bacteria. The absorption of phylloquinone and the various menaquinones is facilitated by bile and pancreatic juices. Thus, disorders such as obstructive jaundice or bile fistula, which reduce absorption of vitamin K from the bowel, may lead to a vitamin K deficiency. Malabsorption syndromes caused by sprue, pellagra, bowel shunts, regional ileitis or ulcerative colitis can also produce a vitamin K deficiency. Aspirin and sulfa drugs destroy the body's stores of the vitamin. (Interestingly, however, an increased analgesic effect is reported to occur when salicylates or opiates are concomitantly administered with vitamin K.)[148] Vitamins A and/or E, in large amounts, will also antagonize the action of vitamin K.[148a]

---

* Possible problems could result from the excessive ingestion of alfalfa, its seeds and its sprouts. Discussion of such problems belongs not here but rather in an herb book. Let's just note for now that several studies report monkeys fed alfalfa seeds or sprouts in large quantities (40% of their diet) develop systemic lupus erythematosus.[147a] Then too, among four groups of rats fed either bran, cellulose, pectin or alfalfa at 15 g./100 g. diet, detrimental mucosal changes of the jejunum and colon were most severe in those fed alfalfa.[147b] Bran showed the least detrimental changes, then cellulose and then pectin.

A Note About Mineral Oil

Mineral oil, often used as a laxative, should never be allowed to enter the body. It hinders the body's assimilation of calcium and phosphorus. Furthermore, it absorbs the fat-soluble vitamins A, D, E and K in the intestines. It should never be recommended for treating constipation. Mineral oil, and liquid parafin which is also used as a laxative, can cause rectal leakage.[149] They are even suspected of increasing the risk of gastrointestinal cancer.[149] The carcinogenicity of many mineral oil fractions has, in fact, been reported by J. W. Cook et al.[150]

Another place the evil of mineral oil shows up is in cold creams. It is reported that their use can rob the skin of estrogen, adrenal hormones and, of course, vitamins A, D, E and K. Women should avoid creams containing mineral oil. Use, instead, those having a base of avocado oil, bone marrow or some other vegetable or animal fat.

More Dangers

Dangers of fish oils and of EPA, cited *passim* on pages 317-321 and elsewhere, are discussed further on the following page.

Possible Dangers of Simultaneously Administering Aspirin and Fish Oils

Aspirin and fish oils, as we have seen in Chapters 3 and 4, work through prostaglandin chemistry. Many of their benefits relate to thinning of the blood. The benefits are apparent but the dangers may be more subtle.

Hans Olaf Bang and Jorn Dyerberg[151] reported that, although Greenland Eskimos consume very little fish, they have a large intake of eicosapentenoic acid that derives from eating of whale and seals. Interestingly, the widely-held belief that the Greenland Eskimos have a low incidence of heart problems may be false. Claudi Galli cites M.C. Ehrström[152] as reporting that coronary heart disease in this population is quite common. (Greenland Eskimos also have nearly a 2-fold higher incidence of stroke than do their Danish counterparts.)[153] Attempting to draw dietary heart-health conclusions for fish eating, non-Eskimos from data relating to non-fish eating Eskimos who may have heart disease could be fraught with error.

Bang and Dyerberg[151] reported that "in four Greenland Eskimos with the longest bleeding time this measurement was repeated 24 hours after the intake of 1.5 grams acetylsalicylic acid." They found the bleeding times of the four Eskimos were shortened (rather than being lengthened as would normally be the case in non-takers of EPA). Thus the combination of aspirin and eicosapentenoic acid can result in a *reverse effect*.

George L. Royer et al.[154] relate that aspirin, and to a lesser extent ibuprofen (Motrin®), increase the values of serum glutamic oxaloacetic transaminase (SGOT), serum glutamic pyruvic transaminase (SGPT) and stool guaiac. Is it possible that fish oils (and other platelet deaggregators) might also detrimentally modify some of these same parameters? What other dangers may exist in the consumption of fish oils, especially if complicated by simultaneously taking aspirin, tetracycline, quinidine, quinine, heparin, protamine sulphate, warfarin (Coumadin®) or other anticoagulant, antiaggregating drugs, vitamins and foods?

"What a man sees depends both upon what he looks at and also upon what his previous visual-conceptual experience has taught him to see."
— Thomas S. Kuhn, *The Structure of Scientific Revolutions* (Chicago: The University of Chicago Press, 1962)

"The most beautiful thing we can experience is the mysterious. It is the source of all true art and science. He to whom this emotion is a stranger, who can no longer pause to wonder and stand rapt in awe, is as good as dead."
— Albert Einstein

CHAPTER 5

The Remarkable Vitamin B Complex and the Dangers of Excess

Originally, this group of water-soluble vitamins was thought to be just one vitamin—vitamin B. Subsequent research has identified a series of vitamins. These various vitamins are grouped as a complex because they are usually found together in plant and animal tissues and the function of any one of them depends, in general, on the presence of one or more of the others. All of the B vitamins are vital to mental and physical well-being, and it is important to caution against taking one or two of them alone since this could cause deficiencies in the others. Those curious about the many ways in which the various B vitamins interact with each other are referred to an article by H. E. Sauberlich.[1]

The B vitamins do their extensive work through the formation of *coenzymes,* nonprotein substances associated with the activation of enzymes. The purely protein part, which is the principal constituent of an enzyme, is called the *apoenzyme* which, along with the coenzyme, forms the complete enzyme or *holoenzyme.* In performing body functions, the apoenzyme absorbs the substance on which it is to act (the substrate) but cannot complete the reaction until the coenzyme arrives. After the reaction is completed both the apoenzyme and the coenzyme are free to act again on another substrate molecule. The B vitamins in forming many types of coenzymes provide essential functions in keeping the body youthful throughout a long lifetime.

The performance of these functions is, however, limited to the ability of the body's cells to make apoenzyme. Thus, extra vitamins beyond body requirements may form superfluous coenzyme that cannot find apoenzyme with which to bind. Therefore, not only are the vitamins wasted, but the materials and energy used to make the coenzyme and then the energy to break it down for subsequent excretion are also wasted. Fatigue could be an undesirable result.

Often one hears that there is no limit to the healthful intake of the various B vitamins since they are water-soluble and will, presumably, simply be excreted if present to excess. We saw earlier that it is possible to take too much of vitamins A, D, E and F (and will later see that vitamin C can also be overconsumed). Similarly, it seems reasonable that taking large amounts of the B complex may create body stresses (while perhaps chelating out essential minerals) as the body must work to excrete the excess. It even seems plausible that, in some cases, an excess might produce a *reverse effect.* I think one should be cautious about consumption of megadoses unless he or she is attempting to meet a specific therapeutic need. Another possible exception to the golden mean might be where there is evidence that a particular vitamin in large dosage may have beneficial longevity effects (e.g., the animal experiments with pantothenic acid we will tell about later in this chapter). *Orthomolecular nutrition,* a term introduced by Dr. Linus Pauling, insofar as it refers to "correct molecules" (whatever that may mean in practical application) is, of course, fine. However, if the word "orthomolecular" is taken to mean "more is better," the concept is dangerous. Resist the temptation, whether in regard to exercise, sex, working, relaxing, eating or taking any kind of food supplements, to conclude that if "some is good, more is better." The ancient Greek principle of the *golden mean* applies in many, many areas.

H. Baker and O. Frank[2] reported that colon adenocarcinoma removed by surgery, as well as the uninvaded adjacent tissue, showed above-normal amounts of many B vitamins—although a below-normal amount of vitamin B_{12}. As has been said, "The significance of a fact is measured by the capacity of the observer." It is possible—although I think unlikely—that the body in the case of some cancers could be using B vitamins to fight the tumor as part of a defense mechanism. More often the cancer, like healthy tissue, is being nourished by the vitamins. Many studies have shown that, in treating cancer, vitamin antagonists, rather than vitamin therapy, might in some cases be therapeutic. (Many such examples will be cited on the pages that follow.) One also wonders if an excess of some of the B vitamins might have helped cause or have exacerbated some cancerous conditions. So, when taking B vitamins as well as other nutrients, let's apply the golden mean. *More* is not necessarily *better*. On the other hand, Herman Baker et al.[3] reported that, unlike colon tumor, metastatic liver adenocarcinoma from the colon primary tumor contained far less (up to as much as 28 times less) of many of the B vitamins than normal liver tissue. Obviously, we have much to learn about the role vitamins play in either fostering or inhibiting various cancers.

If you are taking megadoses of any of the B vitamins and are being treated by a physician, be sure he knows of your vitamin consumption. Megadoses of these vitamins are incompatible with many drugs.[4] Then too, the B complex increases prothrombin time and may cause hemorrhage with anticoagulants. If drugs have been prescribed for you, be sure your physician knows the effects of various vitamins (B complex or others) that you may be taking. To optimize his treatment of any condition he must know which drugs are interfered with (so he can perhaps recommend you stop taking the vitamins) and those which are potentiated (so he can perhaps cut his recommended dosage of the drugs).

Let's make one other observation before getting into the specifics of the B vitamins. It is widely reported that the B vitamins made by the *Lactobacillus acidophilus* bacteria in the intestines represent a useable source of supply. This is far more questionable than many authors would lead one to believe. The vitamins are certainly produced by the intestinal flora, but, since it seems likely that the vast majority are simply excreted, this is an unreliable source. Let us now consider, in turn, each of the known B vitamins and several associated nonvitamins, including B_{15} and B_{17}.

Vitamin B_1

Vitamin B_1 is the chemical *thiamin chloride,* commonly known as just *thiamin.* In England and on the Continent it is known as *aneurine* (meaning a preventer of nervous disease). Thiamin is often thought of as "the nerve vitamin" (which is implied in the name aneurine) but pantothenic acid, vitamin B_{12}, calcium, magnesium, lecithin and many other nutrients could also earn a related appellation. Three micrograms of vitamin B_1 are equal to one International Unit (i.e., 1 mg. is equivalent to 333 I.U.).

The loss of vitamin B_1 in cooking of vegetables may range from 25% to 50%. Canning is even more B_1-destructive, not because of the higher temperature involved as is often stated, but simply because vitamin B_1 is highly soluble in water and the water is often discarded (but not in commercial canning in which cooking is done in the can).

Vitamin B_1 is readily absorbed by the body, but the body cannot store it for more than a few days and much is lost through perspiration. When this vitamin is absent carbohydrates are not properly utilized; pyruvic acid accumulates, causing a deficiency of oxygen (hypoxia). Severe deficiency of thiamin can lead to the ancient disease beriberi which is marked by inflammatory or degenerative changes involving the nerves, digestive system and heart. In the western world, thiamin-deficiency heart disease is often associated with alcoholism. Neurological abnormalities such as peripheral neuropathy, myelopathy (a disorder of the spinal cord or the bone marrow), cerebellar signs and Wernecke's encephalopathy also are often present.[4a] In the latter disease, ophthalmoplegia (paralysis of the eye muscles) and nystagmus (involuntary oscillation of the eyeballs) may be seen.[4a] Cerebellar ataxia (muscular incoordination due to disease of the cerebellum) often occurs and memory function may be impaired.[4a] In the Wernecke-Korsakoff syndrome (which only a few alcoholics develop and these are mostly Caucasian rather than Black) there seems to be a specific abnormality of thiamin-binding to the enzyme trans-ketolase.[4b]

R. Prasad et al.[5] reported that a B_1 deficiency in rats resulted not only in a decrease in the uptake of calcium and zinc but an increase of the toxic metal cadmium. Thiamin (and also vitamin B_{12}) is reported to be useful in treating amblyopia, an impairment of the field of vision and ability to focus that results from overindulgence in alcohol and/or tobacco. Thiamin has also been reported beneficial in the correction of defective chemotaxis in the Shwachman-Diamond syndrome[5a] (a rare disease affecting exocrine pancreatic function).[5a]

Thiamin-responsive inborn errors of metabolism have been recently discussed by M. Duran and S. K. Wadman.[5b] Inherited disorders in which thiamin supplementation may have a beneficial effect are maple sugar disease (an inborn error affecting the degradation of the branched chain amino acids leucine, isoleucine and valine), lactic acidemia and the syndrome of megaloblastic anemia with sensorineural deafness and diabetes mellitus.[5b]

Pyruvic acid may accumulate from carbohydrate metabolism if there is not sufficient thiamin. When thiamin is present, however, it combines with the pyruvic acid to form the coenzyme, *cocarboxylase,* also known as *thiamin pyrophosphate (TPP)* which is needed to digest carbohydrates. If, on the other hand, pyruvic acid is allowed to accumulate, nervous irritation may result. TPP also acts as an enzyme in reactions producing ribose, the vital pentose (five-carbon atom) sugar needed to produce ribonucleic acid (RNA) that is used by the cell for the formation of proteins.

Dr. Ruth Flinn Harrell[6] has reported on using vitamin B_1 to improve learning ability. Dr. Harrell conducted a 6-week study involving children at the Presbyterian Orphans Home at Lynchburg, Virginia. The 104 children ranged from 9 to 19 years of age. Half were given a vitamin B1 pill daily; the children in the other half were given a placebo. The half that received the vitamin B1 gained about one-fourth more in learning ability than the group given placebos. It is possible that the diet of these children was originally deficient in vitamin B1. Thus, the learning ability of those given B1 was, perhaps, merely brought up to just normal. At any rate, we should not assume that vitamin B1 will improve the learning ability of anyone whose diet is already adequate in this vitamin.

In another study[6a] Dr. Harrell and her associates found that the intelligence of children at the ages of 3 or 4 years was significantly higher if mothers received vitamin supplements during the latter part of pregnancy. The children of 612 women of Norfolk, Virginia, were studied and it was found that the intelligence of the children was greatest when the mothers received a supplement of thiamin, riboflavin, niacinamide and iron but less so for those receiving only thiamin or only ascorbic acid. However, let vitamin-supplement enthusiasts note this quotation from the Harrell report: "No significant differences were demonstrated in a similar study among Kentucky mountain women, where the usual and unsupplemented diet was found to be more nearly adequate than that used in the Norfolk homes."

Harrell et al.[6b] subsequently administered not only supplementary thiamin but a broad spectrum of other vitamins and minerals to mentally retarded children. They reported significant increases in the children's I.Q. ratings. However, George Ellman et al.,[6c] attempting to replicate the study, found no significant effects. Caislin Weathers[6d] and also Forrest C. Bennett et al.[6e] found no significant effects in Down's syndrome patients given the same supplement. Three studies against one suggest that we must not assume vitamins or minerals given in amounts exceeding those needed to correct for deficiencies will be effective in increasing learning ability.

More recently, in 1985, Jay Chanowitz et al.[7] pointed out that at least one possibly significant factor in the design of the Harrell et al. study not replicated in the other studies was the concomitant administration of thyroid by the Harrell group. Therefore, Chanowitz and his associates administered the identical supplement used by

Harrell and her associates (including 150 mcg. per day of levothyroxin) to a group of institutionalized mentally retarded adults. No significant I.Q. improvements were observed.

A deficiency of thiamin impairs collagen synthesis and lowers the activity of lysyl oxidase (the enzyme that catalyzes collagen cross-linking which is a basic step in the formation of mature collagen of normal tensile strength).[7a] Such a lack of thiamin will, therefore, result in diminished breaking strength of a wound. However, the fact that a thiamin deficiency implies poor wound healing does not mean that a megadose given to a thiamin-adequate patient will result in wound healing superior to what would be achieved by simple thiamin adequacy.

The blood level of thiamin may be related to the probability that one may develop glaucoma. Edward A. Asregadoo[7b] reported that, in a sample of 38 patients with glaucoma and 12 controls, the patients had a significantly lower thiamin blood level than the controls. Poor thiamin absorption was also prevalent among the glaucomatous patients. (A deficiency of thiamin in patients with glaucoma does not necessarily imply causation. The deficiency and the disease might be caused by a common factor.) Asregadoo also reported that ascorbic acid blood levels (that have sometimes been associated with glaucoma) were not statistically different in patients and in controls.

Thiamin may be useful in treating depression. Some types of depression involve increased monoamine oxidase (MAO) activity and MAO inhibitors are often used to reduce the MAO levels. Donald J. Connor[7c,12] has reported that thiamin tends to decrease MAO activity in persons whose depression is associated with raised MAO levels. *
In a double-blind study of 21 college male students with a history of

---

* If thiamin is, in fact, an MAO inhibitor then, if it is consumed as a supplement, there exists the possibility of adverse effects resulting from consumption of cheddar, camembert, gruyere, stilton and some other cheeses, beer, red wine, pickled herring, chicken livers, yeast extract and other foods containing tyramine. Tyramine is ordinarily metabolized through the action of the monoamine oxidases. However, when the MAO are inhibited, tyramine, a potent vasopressor, acts in the blood vessels to produce severe hypertension and such other symptoms as stiff neck, nausea, vomiting, headache, palpitations and, rarely, death.[7d] Gary D. Tollefson[7e] cites studies showing that MAO activity seems to be positively correlated with age and may be higher in women, peaking at the time of ovulation. Lower MAO activity may occur during alcoholic intoxication and in amphetamine users. Higher MAO activity may occur during alcohol withdrawal.

mental illness or attempted suicide, he found that large oral doses of B_1 (400 mg./day) over a short period of just three days can affect MAO enzyme activity. As we will note shortly, there is doubt that thiamin can be efficiently absorbed by most persons at dosages anywhere near this level, but depressed persons could, conceivably, be an exception. At any rate, Connor reported there was a drop in MAO activity in all but one patient and his rise in MAO activity was slight. Connor concludes with suggestions for further research regarding the possible effects on MAO activity of the rest of the vitamin B complex and of other vitamins.

Thiamin may have immunotherapeutic potential. A. Theron et al.[7f] injected 50 mg. of thiamin intramuscularly in adult volunteers and examined effects on neutrophil functions and mitogen-induced lymphocyte transformation. Thiamin caused stimulation of neutrophil motility *in vitro* and *in vivo* and increased lymphocyte transformation *in vivo*. Theron et al. speculate that the probable mechanism of these effects involves protection of these functions due to oxidizable groups in the thiamin molecule competing with similar groups on neutrophil and lymphocyte membranes for toxic oxidative products of the peroxidase/H_2O_2/ halide system. (We will consider this system further in Chapter 9.) Both the *in vivo* stimulation of neutrophil motility and lymphocyte transformation to mitogens suggest that supplementary thiamin might play a beneficial role in the immune system.

Thiamin discourages bees from stinging, according to Dr. Harry Mueller of Harvard and chairman of the insect allergy committee of the American Academy of Allergy. Dr. Mueller reported that about 70% of adults will be protected on any day they take 100 mg. of thiamin (50 mg. for children). According to Dr. Mueller, the vitamin is excreted in perspiration and its odor repels the bees. It has also been reported that taking 100 mg. of vitamin B_1 30 minutes before being exposed to mosquitoes will sometimes discourage them from stinging. I have, however, experimented with taking far more than 100 mg. of this vitamin every day for an extended period (and also large amounts of vitamins B_6 and C that are sometimes recommended for this purpose), but the mosquitoes still stung. My experience is borne out by a study of Walter G. Strauss et al.[8] in which numerous chemicals were studied for possible use as systemic mosquito repellents in man. Vitamins B1 and B6 (and all other substances tested) were found to be ineffective. (Vitamin C was not tested.) I speculate that if any of these vitamins repels mosquitoes it means they are being excreted via the skin, perhaps suggesting the kidneys are being overtaxed.

Sources of thiamin are brewer's yeast, wheat germ, bran, whole grain cereals (all but about 10% of the vitamin is removed when cereals are refined), potatoes, legumes, leafy greens, nuts, peanuts, pork, beef heart, liver, milk, yogurt and egg yolk. Excessive consumption of sugar or of alcohol tends to drain the body reserves of thiamin since it is used in the metabolism of these products. Consumption of thiamin is reported[8a] to reduce the desire for sweet-tasting foods, but we must resist the temptation to conclude that a fact that may be true for thiamin-short persons will be true for those who are thiamin-sufficient. Antithiamin factors have been found in a large number of foods, including the mung bean, rice bran, mustard seed, flax seed, blackberries, blueberries, beets, brussels sprouts and red cabbage.[9] Those eating large amounts of such foods or drinking excessive amounts of tea* might find supplementation to be of value.

F. Tenconi et al.,[9b] after referencing several additional studies showing that thiamin is poorly absorbed by the oral route, discuss the merits of a novel B1 derivative, benzoyloxymethylthiamin. With oral administration of this derivative to healthy volunteers, the plasma levels of B1 attained significantly higher values than possible using thiamin itself. The blood levels of B1 also remained at high levels eight hours after treatment, whereas the blood levels of B1 in those given thiamin returned to basal values within four hours. The usual way to achieve high B1 blood levels is via parenteral administration of thiamin. Tenconi et al., after doing toxicity studies with mice,

---

* Pintip Ruenwongsa and Supakorn Pattanavibag[9a] reported that when thiamin-deficient rats were given tea instead of drinking water for 20 weeks the conversion of pyruvate to acetylcholine was reduced by 35%. However, no neurological symptoms were observed. The decreased synthesis of acetylcholine was ascribed to a reduction in pyruvate dehydrogenase activity.

concluded that human oral administration of the new derivative is safer than giving thiamin parenterally.

Dangers of Excessive Thiamin

Taking excessive amounts of thiamin may be dangerous. A great excess of thiamin is reported to result in a deficiency of manganese since that element is needed for thiamin's metabolism. It is further contended that, unless excessive thiamin is balanced by taking supplemental manganese, sexual lassitude and possibly sterility may result. K. C. Hayes and D. Mark Hegsted,[9c] however, have reported that no more than 5 mg. of thiamin can be absorbed from an oral dose.* If true, the 50 mg. and 100 mg. or more often seen in pills appears not only to be wasteful, but perhaps involves, it seems to me, a possible body stress to effect its disposal. M. W. J. Older and J. W. T. Dickerson[10] state that the well-nourished, healthy human body contains about 25 mg. of vitamin B1 and that it has no means of storing any excess taken in the diet. This adds support to the idea that excess thiamin consumption is, among other possible negatives, a waste of money.

Thiamin plays a role in nerve excitation by potentiating the various effects of acetylcholine.[11] Thiamin is concentrated in the myelin sheath of nerves and this is where acetylcholine synthesis occurs. Therefore, vitamin B1 is often recommended for nerve problems. Joseph R. DiPalma and David M. Ritchie[13] have, however, issued this warning: "Effects of excess thiamin on the nervous system include: nervousness, convulsions, headaches, weakness, trembling and neuromuscular paralysis. Reports of thiamin toxicity on the cardiovascular system include rapid pulse, anaphylactic shock, peripheral vasodilatation, cardiac arrhythmias

---

* The Donald J. Connor[7c] study, cited earlier, where 400 mg. of vitamin B1 reduced MAO activity, seems to prove that high dosages can be absorbed. It is now known that thiamin is absorbed by two processes—the one a transport mechanism similar to that used in sodium transmission and another involving intracellular phyosphorylation in the intestinal mucosa. These processes for thiamin transport, as well as mechanisms for transporting other vitamins, have been discussed by R. C. Rose.[9d] Rose comments that, "The earliest view that water-soluble vitamins are absorbed in the intestine by simple diffusion has been modified as a result of more recent studies that indicate specific transport and metabolic processes for each of the nutrients."

and edema." Some of these symptoms might be the result of a thiamine-caused deficiency of magnesium. Yoshinori Itokawa et al.[14] point out that since the thiamine-dependent enzymes (pyruvate dehydrogenase, alpha-ketoglutarate dehydrogenase and transketolase) require magnesium, it is possible that excess thiamin could lead to magnesium deficiency. It is also reported not only to have a diuretic effect but also to be constipative.[15] Parenteral administration of thiamin hydrochloride has reportedly caused anaphylactic shock.[15a] Parenteral injection of the vitamin B complex, in sensitive persons, may cause urticaria (a skin eruption), angioedema (another skin problem) and contact dermatitis[15a] Serum thiamin levels of SIDS infants are often very high, perhaps because of excessive absorption.[15b]

If you are under a physician's care, be sure to tell him if you are taking thiamin (or any other vitamin or mineral). In some cases the thiamin might interact with drugs he may have prescribed. M. Soukop and K. C. Calman[16] reported that cancer patients on fluorouracil therapy were found to be thiamin-deficient. When the thiamin was replaced there was a rapid progression of the tumors. We often hear the advice that drugs will cause vitamin deficiencies (that's true) and that we should take vitamin supplements to compensate. (That could be false.)

Vitamin B₂

Vitamin B2, also known as *riboflavin* and formerly known as *vitamin G,* is called *lactoflavine* in Europe because of its abundance in milk. Vitamin B2 has also been called "the youth vitamin" (although all vitamins are really youth vitamins) because it is essential for a beautiful, healthy, wrinkle-free skin. Riboflavin is also required for healthy hair and nails. Riboflavin and folic acid are said to be the vitamins most deficient in the diet of many Americans.

The many functions of riboflavin relate primarily to two coenzymes, *riboflavin monophosphate* and *flavin adenine dinucleotide.* These coenzymes are attached to the *flavoproteins*—important enzymes that act as catalysts in oxidation-reduction reactions. Many of these flavoproteins contain iron, molybdenum or another metal, a fact which helps demonstrate the important interrelationships between minerals and vitamins.

Ordinary cooking (boiling) does not destroy vitamin B_2 (as it does B_1) but the vitamin is leached out of vegetables by hot water. Thus, if the "pot liquor" is thrown away, much of the riboflavin will go with it.* Although boiling does not cause significant loss of this vitamin, roasting and frying can result in losses of 30% to 60%. Storing of foods also causes them to lose some of their B_2 content. A large amount of riboflavin is lost in milk when it is irradiated to create vitamin D.

The need for riboflavin is probably roughly in proportion to the amount of protein being eaten.[16a] Riboflavin is especially required during growth, pregnancy, lactation and wound healing.[16a] A syndrome for riboflavin deficiencies in humans is generally characterized by angular stomatitis (fissures at the angles of the mouth), glossitis (inflammation of the tongue), seborrheic dermatitis about the nose and scrotum and by vascularization of the cornea.[16a] Riboflavin deficiency is not characterized by neurologic abnormalities or by change in attitude, activity or appetite which often appear when thiamin is deficient.[16a]

Animal experiments[17] have implicated a riboflavin deficiency as a cause of cataracts. However, Harold W. Skalka and Joseph T. Prchal[18] found no association, in humans, between riboflavin deficiency and early cataract formation. Older cataract patients did, on the other hand, have more deficiency of vitamin B_2, while older patients with clean lenses showed no such deficiency. The scientists concluded, nevertheless, that the degree of riboflavin deficiency generally encountered is not cataractogenic.

On the other hand, it seems possible that riboflavin may exert a *reverse effect,* i.e., excessive amounts might lead to the formation of cataracts. Riboflavin present in the epithelium of the lens and in the aqueous humor is a photosensitive entity which helps foster the production of superoxide. Large amounts of ascorbic acid generally protect the epithelial membranes in the lens against superoxide-

---

* Pot liquor may also contain nitrates and nitrosamines, so throwing it away could be the best policy.

caused damage.[19] Conversely, if the level of riboflavin is high, while that of ascorbic acid is low, superoxide may be formed in excess of amounts controllable by the available superoxide dismutase. The cation pump activity of the lens might therefore be damaged with cataracts a possible result.

A lack of vitamin B_2 may be a cause of *Ménièré's syndrome,* a disorder of the labyrinth of the ear which leads to recurrent attacks of dizziness, tinnitus (ringing of the ears) and deafness which is often accompanied by nausea and vomiting. Dr. M. Atkinson[20] has successfully used vitamins B_2 and B_3 to treat patients with this problem, although others have employed, in addition, vitamin B_6, pantothenic acid and other members of the B complex.

Vitamin B_2 enters into the synthesis of catalase, an enzyme that is important as an antioxidant and therefore, perhaps, as a cancer preventative. Yogurt contains a substance or substances that inhibit tumor progression, but it is not known if vitamin B_2 is responsible. Nevertheless, G. V. Reddy et al.[21] observed a 28% inhibition of tumor growth in yogurt-fed mice. F. J. Lemonier et al.[22] reported that riboflavin reduced the incidence of hepatoma in animals given aflatoxin. Richard S. Rivlin[23] also discovered that a deficiency of riboflavin enhanced tumor development in rats when they ingested azo dyes. Rivlin noted, however, that Morris and Robertson and also later researchers had found that a *lack* of riboflavin in the diet of rats inhibited tumor growth. Subsequently, M. Lane and F. E. Smith[24] showed that a riboflavin deficiency has an antitumor effect in man. They reported that such a deficiency may be of value in treating lymphomas and polycythemia vera. Rivlin[25] again reviewed the riboflavin-cancer connection in 1973. Among other things, he pointed out that riboflavin inhibits the body's uptake of the folic acid antagonist, methotrexate, and this could work against the effectiveness of cancer therapies involving suppression of folic acid. Riboflavin deficiency in the rat also greatly increases the rate at which prostaglandins E_2 and F are synthesized [25a] and this may relate to the favorable anticancer action. When a deficiency of a substance such as riboflavin works to either enhance or inhibit cancer, obviously more research is needed, and also, perhaps, recognition of dose-related *reverse effects*.

Vitamin B_2 (along with vitamin B_1, choline and inositol) is important in assuring that the liver will maintain a proper balance between androgenic and estrogenic hormones. The liver regulates the balance between the two and if the regulation is not completely effective, a woman may produce too much testosterone and become hirsute, develop male-type balding, a deeper voice, acne, an enlarged clitoris, amenorrhea and increased muscular strength. Similarly, a man may produce too much estrogen and develop feminine characteristics such as enlargement of the breasts (gynecomastia), decrease in size of the testes and loss of sex drive. The liver may fail to keep the hormone production in proper balance if there is a deficiency of any of the four members of the B complex mentioned above.

Recently, it has been reported that exercise increases the riboflavin requirements of young women. (Men were not studied.) Belko et al.[25b] determined the amount of riboflavin required for an erythrocyte glutathione reductase activity coefficient of 1.25 during both exercise and no-exercise periods. They concluded that exercise increased vitamin B_2 requirements in healthy young women and that the RDA is inadequate to achieve biochemical normality.

An interesting experiment might be interpreted as throwing additional doubt on the adequacy of the RDA of riboflavin which, depending on age and sex, is about 1.5 mg. per day. Ernest Beutler[26] reported on an experiment using nine volunteers, five of whom had a daily riboflavin intake averaging above the RDA of 1.5 mg. and four having lower intake levels. In each case he measured the activity of red blood cell glutathione reductase which requires the riboflavin-containing enzyme (flavin adenine dinucleotide) for its activity. Beutler found that the activity of glutathione reductase was strongly stimulated by giving these persons 5 mg. of riboflavin daily for eight days. The stimulation was greatest in those originally most deficient in vitamin B_2, but the stimulation was observed even in those subjects originally having a daily dietary intake of riboflavin exceeding 2 to 3 mg. An increase in red cell concentration of flavin adenine dinucleotide could also be detected in most cases, especially when the dietary intake of riboflavin had previously been less than 1.5 mg. per day. The conclusion was drawn that even individuals eating a normal diet that met the RDA requirement for riboflavin received insufficient amounts of this vitamin to maintain saturation of red cell glutathione reductase.[*] Riboflavin deficiency and glutathione reductase deficiency have been associated with hypoplastic anemia, so it is important that we realize the typical dietary intake of riboflavin may sometimes be inadequate. The study would seem to offer a case for the need of supplementary riboflavin. However, supplementary riboflavin may not be efficiently absorbed. Although classed as a water-soluble vitamin (as are other members of the B complex), riboflavin has low solubility in water (1 gram in 3,000-15,000 ml.).[27b] A new liquid vehicle (Aqua-Biosorb)[**] is reported to make vitamin B_2 (and also vitamins A and E) more bioavailable.[27c] Nevertheless, just because one rightly (perhaps) concludes that the National Academy of Sciences recommended dietary allowance for riboflavin is set too low, does not imply it should be exceeded many-fold. An overdose is reported to cause itching and parasthesia (a tingling or burning sensation of the skin). Always be cautious about excessive supplementation.

If you take supplemental vitamin B_2 and are undergoing tests, be sure to tell your physician. Excessive B_2 can lead to false positive indications of bilirubin (on the Icterus Index) and can also make unreliable the diagnex blue test (for impaired gastric function and free hydrochloric acid).[27,27a] In addition, Solomon Garb[27] cautions that large doses of riboflavin can spuriously elevate urine catecholamine levels.

Liver and other organ meats and brewer's yeast are fine sources for riboflavin. Other good sources are fish roe, wheat germ, wheat and rice bran, soybeans, navy beans, eggplant, green leafy

---

[*] It may, however, not be beneficial to stimulate glutathione reductase beyond that provided by the RDA value of riboflavin. Furthermore, excess riboflavin might undesirably change other enzyme systems.

[**] Trademark of R. P. Scherer (Australia) Pty. Ltd., patent pending.

vegetables, avocados, yogurt, eggs, milk, cheese, broccoli, mushrooms, peanuts and nuts.

Vitamin B₃

Vitamin B₃ exists as niacin (also known as nicotinic acid) and was formerly called vitamin P-P (for pellagra preventative). The amide, nicotinamide (niacinamide) is another form of the vitamin and is much more soluble in water than is the acid. Vitamin B₃ is not destroyed by cooking or canning.

Many of the functions of vitamin B₃ which we will cover hinge primarily on two coenzymes called pyridine nucleotides, of which it is the primary constituent. These pyridine nucleotides are called *nicotinamide adenine dinucleotide (NAD)* and the similar compound, but with an extra phosphate, is known as *nicotinamide adenine dinucleotide phosphate (NADP)*. These coenzymes are essential to oxidation-reduction reactions required for the health of all tissue cells and operate by catalyzing the action of enzymes called *dehydrogenases*. One of these compounds, *lactic-dehydrogenase,* oxidizes lactic acid to pyruvic acid but only if NAD is present. (Earlier, we noted that thiamin is required to further process pyruvic acid.) Obviously, vitamin B₃ must be made available in sufficient quantity to permit these chemical reactions to occur.

A severe niacin deficiency is likely to cause the disease pellagra (meaning "rough skin"). Relatively recently, in 1920, Wilson and then Goldberger speculated the disease was due to the poor biological value of the protein in corn.[27d] (Corn is now known to be deficient in the amino acid trytophan, which is converted in the body to niacin.)

Pellagra is often characterized by diarrhea, vomiting and dysphagia (difficulty in swallowing).[27d] Mental symptoms such as irritability, headaches, sleeplessness and loss of memory generally occur early in untreated cases.[27d] Later, if still untreated, psychosis with delerium and catatonia may be present.[27d]

Vitamin B₃ (along with folic acid and vitamin A) is believed to be involved in the complicated chemical transformation that converts cholesterol into the sex hormones. Furthermore, Isobel W. Jennings[142] says: "Nicotinamide co-enzymes are known to be required for the oxidation of testosterone to androstenedione in the liver and kidney. This reaction is one link in the chain leading to the synthesis of the oestrogens. Deficiency, therefore, may be expected to result in lowered oestrogen production."

B3, according to Dr. Abram Hoffer, is useful in treating varicose veins. Vitamin B3, in the form of niacinamide, is also sometimes reported to be useful in treating diarrhea. It is also reported to be helpful in treating hypogeusia, a deficiency in ability to taste. (This condition, which is often helped by taking vitamin A and zinc, is discussed more fully in Chapter 7 in connection with that mineral.)

Vitamin B3 has been employed in the treatment of schizophrenia with improvement, in some cases, reported to have occurred within 24 to 48 hours. Schizophrenia, according to "orthomolecular therapists," results from the body's inability to convert tryptophan into niacin. (The theory is that niacin is required to neutralize a product of the adrenal glands that is called *adrenochrome* which in excess was formerly thought to lead to schizophrenia. According to William M. Petrie and Thomas A. Ban,[27e] the theory has been abandoned.) The primary symptom of the illness is dysfunction of sensory perception, attended by detrimental changes in thought, mood and behavior. Since the illness reportedly responds to treatment with vitamin B3, suggesting therefore that it is of metabolic origin, Dr. Bella Kowalson has recommended it be renamed "metabolic dysperception." According to a report of the Department of Health, Education and Welfare (now known as the Department of Health and Human Services), it is the leading illness in the United States of persons under 39 years of age.

Drs. A. Hoffer and Humphrey Osmond have worked in this field for some 25 years. They employ massive doses of niacin ranging from daily amounts of 1 gram to as much as 30 grams in advanced cases and generally match it with an equal amount of ascorbic acid. The following nutrients are also sometimes used: vitamins B6, B12, A, D, E and L-glutamine.

In treating schizophrenia, Drs. Hoffer and Osmond have found that niacinamide does not work as well as niacin and may actually induce depression. Flushing and cutaneous vasodilation often follows ingestion of niacin, probably due to the release of prostaglandins.[28-30a] Work by Brita Eklund et al.[30b] offers support for this theory and suggests that the prostaglandins being increased in the vascular wall are PGE_2 and probably PGI_2 and other cyclo-oxygenated products. Concomitantly, histamine is released from the mast cells. It is reported that this flushing can be reduced through taking ascorbic acid along with vitamins B_1 and B_6 or by ingesting aspirin and antihistamines.* (Cyproheptadine and Periactin® are sometimes prescribed by doctors to reduce the flushing, but this use of drugs to control a vitamin seems especially weird to me.) The flushing can also be reduced if the niacin is taken with meals or with large amounts of water, milk or other liquids. Gunnar Aberg and Nils Svedmyr[31] have published interesting full-color thermographic pictures of a man's torso before and after niacin ingestion. After taking a total of about 450 thermograms of 10 male volunteers, they concluded that temperature increases generally began in the face and later spread to the neck, shoulders and arms. Temperature increases in the face were often of short duration and, in many volunteers, face temperatures decreased below those at the start of the experiment.

In regard to the use of niacin and niacinamide in treating mental problems, many health-minded persons may be astonished to learn that "orthomolecular" psychiatrists also use drugs such as phenothiazines and, when this treatment fails, employ electroconvulsive therapy. Furthermore, although "orthomolecular" physicians claim that niacin reduces the amounts of phenothiazines required, the opposite is probably true and B_3 also increases hospitalization time. A study by T. A. Ban[32] reported that patients on phenothiazine and a placebo spent 67 days in the hospital as compared to 90 days for those on phenothiazine plus niacin and 88 days for those on phenothiazine plus niacinamide. In another study, patients on chlorpromazine and a placebo spent 211 days in the

---

* Dose-response relationships between aspirin and niacin-induced flushing are discussed by Jonathan K. Wilkin et al.[30]

hospital as compared to 214 days for those on chlorpromazine plus niacin and 353 days (more than 50% longer) for those on chlorpromazine plus niacinamide. With these results, why would vitamin B3 be prescribed for such patients? Several articles by various authors representing both the pro and con sides of orthomolecular treatment will be found in a book edited by George Serban.[33]

Vitamin B3 has been used successfully by Dr. A. Moncrieff[34] in treating angina pectoris.* Then too, niacin has been reported to increase the ratio of high-density lipoproteins (HDL) to low-density lipoproteins (LDL) in the blood, which is generally considered to be beneficial for protecting the arteries and the heart. (We must, however, always be wary of too quickly drawing conclusions. Could it be that the niacin is simply driving the LDL into the intima of the arteries where it could do damage? The Coronary Drug Project Research Group[35] reported that niacin, although lowering serum lipids, did *not* provide heart protection or affect total mortality data.)** Niacin continues to be studied, however, for its LDL-lowering effect. John P. Kane et al.[36] reported that, in conjunction with the bile acid sequestrant colestipol, niacin shows promise as a treatment of patients at high risk from elevated levels of LDL.

The work of J. Ferreira-Marques[37] with 150 patients indicates that vitamin B3 has an antipruritic (anti-itching) action. He employed a dose of 200 mg. of nicotinamide five times a day. Another valuable use for vitamin B3 is to increase the mobility of the joints, according to Dr. William Kaufman.[38] Dr. Kaufman found that massive dosages of niacinamide improved the joint mobility of many patients, although he reported that some received no benefit. He also observed

---

* The report should, however, not be taken too seriously. Only three patients were involved, the report was merely in the form of a letter and Dr. Moncrieff says the observations were "outside my usual therapeutic scope."

** A trial by M. F. Oliver et al.[35a] of the drug clofibrate resulted in significant *decreases* in fatal and nonfatal myocardial infarcts in men compared to those given a placebo. However, deaths of men from all causes were significantly *higher* in the clofibrate group. Whether in regard to niacin, to clofibrate or other test substances, studies must not be limited to an investigation of one aspect of health while ignoring other aspects of health.

that when niacinamide therapy was discontinued, joint mobility declined to what it had been before treatment started.

Niacin has been used for decades in the treatment of pellagra and is a "cure-all" for its symptoms, including that of photosensitivity. Walter B. Shelley and E. Dorinda Shelley[38a] suggest it be considered for any photosensitivity state of obscure nature. Vitamin B3 is also reportedly useful in ameliorating the effects of a "bad trip" on LSD. This treatment is well known by LSD devotees among the drug subculture and has received wide notice in the underground newspapers. Robert A. Wilson[39] relates that about 4 grams of vitamin B3 and an elapsed time of 15 to 45 minutes are required to quiet the effects of a bad trip.

Niacin and niacinamide, although both are forms of vitamin B3, are not completely interchangeable. Whereas niacin dilates the blood vessels, niacinamide does not. This is sometimes considered an advantage in favor of niacinamide (although large dosages can cause nausea) since niacin may, as has been indicated, produce an undesirable reddening (flushing) and itching of the skin and a feeling of excessive warmth. However, where dilation of the blood vessels is desired or in any other applications involving stimulation of the circulation such as treatment of cold feet, acne, hearing difficulties or migraine headaches, niacin, rather than niacinamide, would be preferred.

We noted earlier that niacin causes the release of histamine from the mast cells. At the same time, the niacin stimulates the mast cells to release heparin, a factor in the production of lipoprotein lipase which reduces the level of cholesterol and triglycerides in the blood. (This release of heparin and also niacin's stimulation of prostacyclin formation and the resulting vasodilatory effect, as well as its antiaggregatory action on platelets, may be beneficial in preventing and treating arteriosclerosis and high blood pressure resulting therefrom. However, in a study cited earlier,[35] use of niacin showed neither an increase nor a decrease in mortality of heart patients.)* Heparin also helps blood maintain its normal clotting action. In addition, heparin prevents the red blood cells from clustering

---

* Over the short term, however, niacin may raise the blood pressure.

together by reinforcing their negative electrical charges (thereby causing them to repel one another). When cells cluster together in a roll—sometimes called the *rouleaux formation* because they resemble a roll of coins—only the outside cells will experience an efficient oxygen interchange as the blood passes through the capillaries of the lungs. Incidentally, negative ion generators are reported to also put a negative charge on red blood cells, thus obviating the clumping effect.

Niacin may also affect sleep habits. In some cases it may cause insomnia. On the other hand, Dr. Hoffer says that for the past ten years, during which time he has taken three grams of niacin daily, he has required only six hours of sleep nightly. Dr. Hoffer believes that the declustering effect of niacin on the red blood cells is the reason. When the clumps of red cells are broken up, the additional surface means that their ability to carry not only oxygen but other nutrients as well is greatly increased. Furthermore, the single cells can travel through the tiniest capillaries throughout the body, including those of the brain. Thus, less sleep is required because the blood is operating more efficiently to refresh the body. Such a finding, since it involves just one individual, must, of course, be considered to be merely anecdotal. (We must all learn to distinguish between such "facts" and findings resulting from properly controlled studies.) The declustering effect of niacin may also bring on an increase in one's energy level throughout the day. Then too, niacin taken by those who have had a stroke might permit the red blood cells to carry more oxygen to various organs, including that portion of the brain damaged by the stroke so it may be able to operate more efficiently. Many of the actions of niacin and of its derivatives have been reviewed by W. Hotz.[39a]

If you decide to use niacin (as contrasted with niacinamide), you may be interested in this point made by Gay Gaer Luce.[40] She relates that the skin's reaction to histamine follows a circadian (daily) rhythm, peaking early in the evening when corticosteroids from the adrenal gland are at their lowest levels. Ms. Luce also tells of antihistamine drugs whose effects are also subject to a circadian rhythm. In one experiment, a morning dose, taken at 7 A.M., was less effective but lasted about 17 hours. A similar dose taken at 7 P.M. was more effective but lasted only a few hours. The new science of *chronopharmacology* could greatly influence the time of day for which various vitamins, minerals and medicines will be prescribed.

If you desire to take niacin (in fairly high amounts) rather than niacinamide, but are one of those for whom the flush is intolerable, it might seem logical to consider using timed-release tablets, although elsewhere in this book I tell of my generally negative attitude toward all timed-release products. Specifically, Norman A. Christensen et al.[41] reported that patients experienced greater frequency and severity of side effects with timed-release niacin than with plain niacin. By the way, when niacin is taken in large dosages (e.g., four grams daily, at the rate of one gram four times a day, as is sometimes used in treating schizophrenia) the flushing phenomenon no longer occurs after 24 to 36 hours. Dr. David Hawkins explains[42] that on low dosages of niacin the flush will continue indefinitely, but high dosages "wash out" the histamine from the mast cells so that sufficient histamine will no longer be released to cause further flushing. Hawkins' term "wash out" may represent a too-innocuous view of reality. Once the histamine and the heparin (that have been released through the action of niacin) have been used up in metabolic processes, will there be sufficient new quantities formed to meet body needs? As we noted earlier, niacin, although lowering serum lipid levels and increasing the HDL/LDL ratio did not provide heart protection and did not affect total mortality data.[35] If lowering serum lipids and raising the HDL/LDL ratio is beneficial to longevity, niacin must have *increased* the death rate due to factors (including arrythmia)[35] unrelated to serum lipids.

Adverse Effects of Excessive Vitamin B₃

Dr. Hawkins relates that his patients have taken 20 to 40 grams of niacin daily for prolonged periods with no adverse effect. However, Hawkins warns that niacin is contraindicated for those with peptic ulcer, hypertension, diabetes or gout. (Niacin can sometimes, but rarely, cause an increase in uric acid, an intolerance for sugar that simulates diabetes, and ulcers of the gastrointestinal tract.) If you have a serious   health   problem   it   is   essential   to   check with your physician before starting any type of megavitamin therapy. Unless one is under a doctor's care, I would be especially wary of taking so much niacin that all of the histamine is released from the mast cells. Histamine has functions in the body and should be present to perform those functions. Histamine stimulates visceral muscles, dilates capillaries and stimulates salivary, pancreatic and gastric secretions. It is also thought to be a neurotransmitter. On the other hand, according to Carl C. Pfeiffer,[42a] who is echoed by Durk Pearson and Sandy Shaw[42b,c] and by Saul Kent,[42d] excessive histamine may lead to premature ejaculation* in the male and rapid orgasm in the female. However, they hold that a deficiency of histamine may make ejaculation impossible in the male and orgasm impossible in the female. I have not been able to discover the biochemical rationale for this line of reasoning and believe that its scientific status is something less than fact. Furthermore, if the presence or absence of histamine were a factor in timing the male and female orgasms, various antihistamines including vitamin C (which reduces histamine) ought to be a factor in orgasmic response. As far as I know, this has not been reported. One should learn to distinguish between a concomitant effect and causation. The fact that histamine may sometimes be released during orgasm (the reddening of the torso of both men and women called "the sexual flush" by Masters and Johnson) does not prove that niacin facilitates orgasm. One might, instead, argue that if niacin has already released the histamine from the mast cells, it will no longer be there to promote orgasm.** Nevertheless, the concomitant blood vessel dilation

---

* "Premature" ejaculation may be defined as ejaculation before both partners want it and a man's "long-staying," within reason, is appreciated by many women. However, such "long-staying" may not be healthful. The occurrence of benign prostatic hypertrophy is correlated with habitually expending more than ten minutes to complete one act of sexual intercourse.[43]

** Le Chatelier's law, which we met in Chapter 4, would suggest that the presence of released histamine might actually inhibit orgasm. Le Chatelier's law states that if the equilibrium of a system is disturbed by a change in one or more of the determining factors (e.g., an increase in histamine) the system tends to adjust itself to a new equilibrium by counteracting as far as possible the effect of the change (e.g., an inhibition of orgasm).

(especially if it occurs in the penis) might have favorable sexual implications.

It should be obvious that I think niacin (or niacinamide) in megadosages (amounts several times the RDA), even in the absence of the contraindications mentioned earlier, may be dangerous. A literature review of the side effects and toxicity of niacin is provided by Loren R. Mosher.[44] Victor Herbert[45] states that liver damage, dermatoses, elevated serum glucose, elevated serum uric acid, elevated serum enzymes and peptic ulcer are all possible consequences of taking excessive amounts of niacin or niacinamide. James C. Woodard[45a] found, in studies with rats, that large amounts of nicotinamide produce renal cortical necrosis. The stress of methylating similar amounts of nicotinamide allowed the formation of hydrocephalus and other congenital abnormalities in litters from females receiving choline, methionine and vitamin B12 (all good sources of methyl groups). Other toxic effects of niacin and niacinamide have been recently reviewed by Leslie Alhadeff et al.[45b]

Pregnant women with diabetes and taking tolbutamide may wish to discuss with their physicians the possible dangers of also taking nicotinamide. Morris Smithberg[46] reported that treatment of pregnant mice with tolbutamide plus nicotinamide produced a significant increase in defective fetuses compared to treatment with tolbutamide alone.

There is an additional danger in taking excessive amounts of vitamin B3, at least if taken in the form of nicotinamide. Nicotinamide can potentiate the tumorigenicity of certain agents. R. Schoental[47] reports that rats pretreated with injected nicotinamide show an increased tumor incidence after being exposed to streptozotocin, heliotrine and diethylinitrosamine. Furthermore, 6-AN, a drug that shows potent antitumor activity against mammary adenocarcinoma in mice is made powerless by nicotinamide.[48]

If you are taking supplemental amounts of niacin and are undergoing tests, be sure to tell your physician. Above-normal amounts of niacin can give excessive or false positive indications for glucose tolerance (the differential diagnosis), uric acid, diagnex blue test (for impaired gastric function), glucose (Benedict's test) and urine catecholamines.[27]

Niacin can be made in the body out of tryptophan, an essential amino acid available in high-grade protein, but vitamin B 6 must also be present. The generally accepted equivalence is that 60 mg. of tryptophan converts to 1 mg. of niacin. In pregnancy the ratio could be nearer 30:1. Neither relationship may be valid when the diet contains only limited amounts of tryptophan.[48a]

Liver, brewer's yeast and bran are outstanding sources for vitamin B 3. Good sources are other meats, chicken, fish, milk, peanuts, nuts, whole grain products, rice polishings, mushrooms, peas, molasses and whole grain products.* Coffee is not a good source but, interestingly, the coffee bean contains trigonelline which, during roasting, is converted to niacin. A cup of coffee provides 1 to 2 mg. of niacin.[48c]

Vitamin B₆

Vitamin B 6 exists as three natural vitamers: pyridoxine (the alcohol), pyridoxal (the aldehyde) and pyridoxamine (the amine). Pyridoxine hydrochloride is a commonly available synthetic form. Two of the related natural phosphorus compounds, pyridoxal phosphate and pyridoxamine phosphate, enter into the amino acid reactions called *transamination* and *decarboxylation.* In transamination, an amino group (NH_2) is shifted from a donor amino acid to an acceptor acid to form a new amino acid. This makes it possible to build amino acids from acids that are devoid of nitrogen. In decarboxylation, on the other hand, carbon dioxide is removed from an amino acid. This process is required in the formation of some hormones. Pyridoxal phosphate also acts as a catalyst in

---

* Much of the niacin in some grains is reported to be in the form of nicotinyl esters which are not available to humans.[48b] When the staple cereal is relatively low in tryptophan (such as corn or millet) a nutritional deficiency disease, pellagra, may result. However, in making tortillas, Mexicans traditionally steep the grain overnight in lime water which hydrolyzes the nicotinyl esters and makes the niacin available. Pellagra is much less common in Mexico than in other corn-eating populations, such as those of South Africa.[48b]

removing sulfhydryl groups (mercapto SH groups) from amino acids containing sulphur. Approximately 50 reactions requiring pyridoxal phosphate have thus far been discovered and many of the uses of B 6 which we will describe relate to these reactions.

Much of the research has used the terms pyridoxine and vitamin B6 as synonyms. B. Shane and E. E. Snell[48d] have shown that pyridoxine is not convertible to pyridoxal by mammalian tissues. Thus, vitamin B supplements containing only pyridoxine may not be useful when pyridoxal is specifically required. Furthermore, I suspect some of the experimental results that appear to be in conflict may be due to the fact that different forms of vitamin B 6 were being administered.

Vitamin B6 contributes to the prevention and cure of pellagra. A deficiency can cause whiteheads on the face and can also result in acne. A shortage of vitamin B 6 can cause a rare type of anemia in which the red blood cells are too small (rather than the usual iron-deficiency type) in persons susceptible because of a defective hereditary factor. A deficiency of vitamin B 6 can also lead to an increase of urea in the blood, cracks around the eyes and edges of the mouth, cramps in the arms and legs, diarrhea and early-morning nausea (especially in pregnant women or those on the Pill).

A vitamin B6 deficiency can produce irritability, insomnia and mental depression. Pyridoxal phosphate is required in the synthesis of serotonin from tryptophan so a B6 deficiency (as could occur in the premenstrual period) might readily cause these symptoms. A. D. G. Gunn[48e] has reviewed the many trials using B6 to alleviate the premenstrual syndrome and most of them have shown beneficial effects. Gunn tells of an ongoing multi-center, double-blind trial involving 1,000 women in the United Kingdom in which either 100 mg. of pyridoxine or a placebo is being administered daily. He reports that preliminary results look encouraging for use of vitamin B6 in combating premenstrual syndrome. A confusing note is engendered, however, by Carolyn D. Richie and Ratree Singkamani[48f] who reported, in 1986, that the pyridoxine status, as measured by plasma levels of pyridoxal 5'-phosphate, is not altered in women with premenstrual syndrome. They concluded that pyridoxine deficiency is therefore unlikely to contribute to the occurrence of this syndrome. (The possible role of B6 in alleviating the premenstrual syndrome may relate to its role in the GLA-to-DGLA-to-PGE1 conversion as discussed in Chapter 3. If so, the status of a woman's Δ 6-desaturase enzyme, as also covered in Chapter 3, may determine whether or not B6 could be helpful.) On the other hand, Karen Schuster et al.[49] reported that there was no relationship between vitamin B6 status and the incidence or degree of morning sickness in pregnant women.

A study by David A. Bender and Lena Totoe [49a] has shown that an intraperitoneal injection of a solution containing 2 mg. of pyridoxine chloride given to rats resulted in an inhibition of hepatic metabolism of tryptophan attended by a huge uptake of this amino acid by the brain. The rats weighed 180-200 grams, so this dosage would correspond with an injected dose of 700 mg. in a 70 kg. person. This is a large dose, but perhaps not greatly in excess of amounts sometimes used clinically for treatment of depression (and premenstrual syndrome). The rats injected with B6 showed reduced exploration and curiosity which might be accounted for by the increased amount of the neurotransmitter 5-hydroxytryptamine which was found to be present. Bender and Totoe suggested that B6 may inhibit the enzyme tryptophan oxidase and thus enhance the antidepressant action of tryptophan.

A deficiency of vitamin B6 can cause convulsions in persons of all ages, including cerebral seizures which occur in some mental cases and in older persons.* It is likely that a need for greater amounts of certain vitamins, in this case of vitamin B6, may be inherited. If other children in the family were subject to convulsions, the obstetrician should be told since he or she may wish to give the infant vitamin B6 before symptoms develop. A controlled trial, however, failed to show B6 supplementation protects children from recurrent febrile convulsions.[50] It is sometimes stated that convulsions due to vitamin B6

---

* The seizures and neurologic damage resulting from a B6 deficiency seem to be caused by defective binding of pyridoxal 5'phosphate to the apoenzyme glutamate decarboxylase.[49b,c] The lack of this enzyme leads to a deficiency of gamma-aminobutyric acid (GABA) which is an inhibitory neurotransmitter in the central nervous system.[49b,c]

deficiency can occur in the fetus and may even lead to abortion or stillbirth unless the pregnant woman is given the vitamin. These symptoms related to vitamin B6 deficiency may be due, at least in part, to a magnesium shortage. Many studies by Guy E. Abraham et al[51] and by others support the postulate that B6 aids the transport of magnesium across cell membranes. However, as far as B6 preventing seizures is concerned, current evidence suggests that its anticonvulsant efficaciousness is limited to very specific conditions[52] Nevertheless, A. Bankier et al.[52a] maintain that the physician should consider the diagnosis of pyridoxine-dependent seizures in any infant with intractible epilepsy regardless of the pattern of seizures or response to anticonvulsants. Interestingly, M. Ebadi et al.[52b] reported that, while a deficiency of vitamin B6 can cause seizures, larger amounts of pyridoxal phosphate (but not other forms of vitamin B6), injected into rats, produced epileptic seizures. This gives us yet another example of the *reverse effect*. However, it seems likely that other forms of the vitamin also show *reverse effects*. Joseph R. DiPalma and David M. Ritchie[52c] have pointed out that "pyridoxine causes convulsive disorders due both to an excess of the vitamin or to a deficiency state."

J. S. Kroll[52ca] also warns about use of pyridoxine supplementation for a convulsing neonate. He cautions that there is risk of profound sedation even to the point of ventilation being needed. Kroll suggests that physicians using B6 for a convulsing neonate have full resuscitation facilities close at hand.

Herbert Schaumberg et al.[52d,e] reported on seven patients who developed ataxia and severe nervous-system dysfunction while taking two grams or more of B6 daily. All improved after withdrawal. Two grams of B6 is, of course, huge and should not frighten us into avoiding modest supplementation. Let's observe, however, that quantities far less than two grams daily might be dangerous if consumed for extended periods and perhaps might be especially dangerous for alcoholics. (Henry M. Middleton III et al.,[87] in experiments with rats, reported that the mucosal uptake of pyridoxine was greatly increased by the presence of high ethanol concentration.) Nevertheless, in an extended study of 630 women taking 80-200 mg.

of vitamin B6 daily for premenstrual syndrome, M. G. Brush and Marta Perry[87a] reported "only minimal side-effects were noted and certainly no neuropathy was seen."

If insufficient vitamin B6 is present in the body the amino acid tryptophan is not converted into niacin but produces xanthurenic acid instead. The xanthurenic acid may damage the pancreas and lead to diabetes. A lack of pyridoxine can make one susceptible to respiratory infections and sore throat (because of an attendant deficiency of antibodies). On the other hand, increased quantities of the vitamin may stimulate production of antibodies and thus be of help in fighting infections such as the common cold. Vitamin B6's mode of action in this regard is through its beneficial action on the thymus gland in its production of T-lymphocytes. By the way, a vitamin B6 deficiency in pregnant rats is reported to reduce the size of the thymus not only in the mother but also in her fetuses.[53] Rat experiments by S. C. Cunnane et al.[53a] have shown that pyridoxine deficiency leads to decreased thymus fat weight. However, plasma, liver and thymus phospholipid levels of linoleic and gamma-linolenic acids were increased when pyridoxine was deficient. These results support reports (as related in Chapter 3) that vitamin B6 is needed for both linoleic desaturation and gamma-linolenic acid elongation and thus for formation of prostaglandin E1.

There are many other applications for vitamin B6. Craig G. Burkhart[54] reports on the benefits of pyridoxine in treating *herpes gestationis* (a vesicular or bullous skin eruption occurring during pregnancy). M. A. Packham and S. C.-T. Lam[55] suggest that, since vitamin B6 inhibits platelet aggregation and fibrin formation, it could be a useful antithrombotic agent. U. N. Das[56] notes that pyridoxine is required for normal activity of the enzyme delta-6-desaturase which mediates the conversion of *cis*-linoleic acid to gamma-linolenic acid, the precursor of the prostaglandin PGE1. Thus, according to Das, the antithrombic action of vitamin B6 is related to its ability to enhance formation of the PGE1 prostaglandin.* A derivative of vitamin B6 (pyridoxal 5'-phosphate) is probably an antithrombic agent which

---

* Further evidence supporting the possibility that vitamin B6 may be an antithrombotic agent is given in a *Lancet* editorial.[56a]

not only inhibits platelet aggregation but also prolongs clotting time.[56b,58a] Many other properties of vitamin B6 may be due to its influence on prostaglandin synthesis.

A deficiency of pyridoxine may be the primary cause of atherosclerosis according to Kilmer McCully, M.D., Professor of Pathology at the Harvard Medical School.[56c,d] He postulated that the original lesion is caused by homocysteine, which is formed from the amino acid methionine when B6 is absent. The homocysteine creates free radicals that can destroy healthy cells, thus creating a lesion. (P. H. Proctor and J. E. McGinness[56e] more recently reported that these free radicals consist of superoxide that is formed as homocysteine is oxidized to homocystine.) Once the lesion has developed, cholesterol, triglycerides, calcium and other chemicals form around it to produce the atheroma. When B6 is present, on the other hand, the homocysteine is converted to the harmless substance, *cystathionine*. Under this theory it is the shortage of vitamin B6 and/or excess of methionine (found in animal protein) rather than the presence of cholesterol or triglycerides, that is the causal factor in this disease. However, Phyllis A. Cohen et al.[56f] reached a contrary conclusion. In experiments with rats, the Cohen group found that in animals fed B6 there was no tendency to produce cystathionine. Nevertheless, Edward J. Calabrese[57] has recently reviewed extensive evidence for the support of the homocysteine theory of atherosclerosis. In cases of homocystinuria that are not helped by B6 therapy, David E. L. Wilcken et al.[57a] and L. A. Smolin et al.[57b] reported betaine may succeed in lowering plasma homocysteine levels with resulting clinical improvement.* Homocystinuria is just

---

* Homocystinuria is a condition that can be secondary to defects in conversion of homocysteine either to cystathionine or methionine.[57d] I. Yoshida et al. [57e] have reported that supplementary pyridoxal phosphate (administered initially at 500 mg./day and then gradually increased to 1,000 mg./day) resulted in liver injury to a patient with homocystinuria. J. V. Murphy et al.[57d] found that three schizophrenic patients with homocystinuria caused by difficulty in converting homocysteine to methionine improved "dramatically" with folic acid therapy. Lars E. Brattström et al.[57f] reported finding that "folic acid, administered to nonfolate-deficient normal men and women, almost invariably and significantly reduces the plasma concentrations of homocysteine, measured as homocysteine-cysteine mixed disulphide, both in the fasting state and after a methionine load." They speculated that homocysteinemia might contribute to

one of several B6-responsive genetic conditions. Others are B6-responsive anemia, xanthurenic aciduria, cystathionuria, hyperoxaluria and gyrate atrophy of choroid and retina.[49b]

Vitamin B6 is sometimes used in the treatment of Parkinson's disease. It is especially important, however, that those being treated with levodopa for parkinsonism follow their physician's instructions regarding B6. He will likely instruct such patients to limit their intake of pyridoxine to the RDA of 2 mg. (which could mean restriction of fortified breakfast cereals). However, if the patient also has certain other diseases or is taking drugs which have rendered him B6 deficient, or if levodopa is being administered with the dopa decarboxylase inhibitor, *carbidopa,* the physician may prescribe supplementary B6. Follow his advice!

G. LeLord et al.[58] have found vitamin B6 to be valuable in treating autism in children. The LeLord group gave large amounts of the vitamin (along with magnesium because large amounts of B6 might otherwise increase irritability). Of 44 children, 15 exhibited moderate clinical improvement with worsening on termination of the trial. Benefits of B6 in the treatment of autistic children seem to relate to an improved turnover of dopamine and a reduction of excessive levels of urinary homovanillic acid (the main metabolite of dopamine).[58d,e]**

Women taking contraceptive pills may be deficient in vitamin B6. The Pill is believed to compete with the vitamin for binding sites on the apoenzyme. A. L. Luhby et al.[58b] have estimated that 80% of the women taking the Pill for six months or longer show an abnormal tryptophan metabolism. They found that metabolism of tryptophan became normal when these women took a 2 mg. B6 supplement daily. There is an increased risk of thrombosis and embolism in women taking oral contraceptive hormones.[58c] There is also potential

---

postmenopausal arteriosclerosis and osteoporosis. They also speculated that, if this proves to be the case, use of folic acid might be prophylactic.

** Kenneth L. Davis et al.[58f] recently reported that concentrations of plasma homovanillic acid before treatment of schizophrenic patients is highly correlated with the severity of the illness. I wonder if B6 therapy would reduce the levels of homovanillic acid in this condition as it does in autism.

risk of accelerated atherosclerosis among Pill users in accordance with the homocysteine theory discussed earlier.[58c]

Vitamin B6 (along with other members of the B complex, inositol and choline) is a lipotropic factor, i.e., it helps control fats in the body. The presence of vitamin B6 and of these other vitamins aids the liver in disposing of excessive amounts of estrogen since this hormone is a fatty substance. (Such control is important since estrogen may be a causative factor in cancer.) If you are a woman on the Pill, be sure you are getting adequate amounts of the entire vitamin B complex, especially vitamins B6, B12, inositol, choline and folic acid (and also vitamins C and E). Observe, however, my use of the words "adequate amounts." The study by Phyllis A. Cohen et al.,[56f] to which I recently referred, showed that rats fed a high-pyridoxine diet (500 mg. per kilogram diet) gained 20% in mean body weight and 40% in mean liver weight. When the rats were put on a pyridoxine-deficient diet, fat was mobilized and their weight was reduced. This is just another example of the benefits of moderation and dangers of excess. Beware of megadoses of this or any other vitamin or mineral!

There are other applications for vitamin B6. Some persons experience a sensitivity to monosodium glutamate (MSG) that is sometimes referred to as the "Chinese restaurant syndrome." K. Folkers et al.[59] found that many (but not all) persons experiencing MSG sensitivity were helped by taking 50 mg. of pyridoxine daily. They reported a concomitant increase in the erythrocyte glutamate-oxalacetate transaminase activity, a deficiency of which may be the cause of the problem. Folkers et al.[59a] have more recently reported that those sensitive to monosodium glutamate are likely to have a low basal specific activity of aspartate transaminase. In a study of 155 students who did not take B6 they found 27 with a low activity of this enzyme. When these 27 were given 12.5 mg./kg. body weight of monosodium glutamate, 12 showed symptoms of the "Chinese restaurant syndrome." In double-blind trials these 12 responders were given 50 mg. of pyridoxine daily or a placebo for 12 weeks and then given glutamate as before. After decoding, it was found that nine had received the B6 and three the placebo. After treatment with

B6, eight of the nine showed no sensitivity to glutamate, but all three given the placebo evinced symptoms of a glutamate reaction as they had before.

There are yet other uses for vitamin B6. Pyridoxine in combination with thiamin and magnesium oxide is often beneficial in treating hyperoxaluria in adults and children. Among various favorable reports is one from Russia where V. Revusova et al.[59b] found that 60 mg. (but not 20 mg.) daily of pyridoxine reduced calcium-oxalate nephrolithiasis. (The treatment, however, can sometimes be complicated by resulting pyridoxine poisoning.)[59c] Dr. A. W. Schreiner has shown that topical applications of vitamin B6 may be useful in correcting some skin conditions. I think the mechanism whereby skin health is improved may involve pyridoxal phosphate—a conversion product of B6—acting as a catalyst in the formation of niacin from tryptophan. Thus, it seems to me that it could be the niacin that is causing the good effects. Vitamin B6 is also reported to be useful in relieving hemorrhoids and pruritis (itching). A popular writer (John M. Ellis, M.D.) reported B6 to be useful in aiding finger flexibility and the pain of arthritic hands, but this has been denied by other investigators. Dr. Ellis and others [60-63] have, however, published several papers regarding the often-beneficial effect of B6 on the carpal tunnel syndrome which involves wrist pain and other symptoms. Alan Gaby and J. V. Wright[64] found that, in treating over 50 cases of carpal tunnel syndrome with pyridoxine, symptoms disappeared permanently in nearly every case. S. Pilar[65] has reported that pyridoxine is useful in treating the carpal tunnel syndrome in pregnancy and is safe for use during this period.

Both the pyridoxal and pyridoxal phosphate forms of vitamin B6 have been shown to inhibit sickling of erythrocytes *in vitro*.[66] Subsequently, Clayton L. Natta and Robert D. Reynolds[66a] found that plasma concentrations of pyridoxal phosphate were significantly lower in sickle cell patients than in controls. Oral supplementation of 50 mg. pyridoxine twice daily increased plasma and erythrocyte levels of pyridoxine phosphate and there was a slight but not significant rise in red cell number, hemoglobin and hematocrit. One patient experienced reduction in frequency and duration of painful crises.

As mentioned earlier, riboflavin in large dosages has the reputation of reducing the desire for sugar. Vitamin B6 also is reported to have this property, probably because it is a cofactor in the enzyme *glycogen phosphorylase* which mobilizes the conversion of liver-stored glycogen to glucose. Quantities of glucose in the blood would probably tend to diminish one's interest in consuming sugar.

According to G. Delitala et al.,[67] supplemental pyridoxine in the amount of 300 mg. daily can stimulate a beneficial increase in peak levels of growth hormone (somatostatin).* The growth hormone, produced by the pituitary gland, stimulates muscle growth, helps activate the immune system and helps to burn fat and is thus a factor in weight control. Thus, stimulation of the growth factor is valuable, but Delitala also reported that vitamin B6, in amounts of 300 mg. daily, causes a decrease in plasma prolactin, which could have negative implications for lactating women. G. Delitala et al.[69] also reported that 300 mg. of daily pyridoxine caused a significant decrease in serum thyrotropin in six patients with primary hypothyroidism, so this also could be a detrimental effect.

The growth hormone stimulation by pyridoxine which we have just noted can be further stimulated by exercise. Costanzo Morietti et al.[70] reported that six young, healthy subjects given 600 mg. of pyridoxine via saline infusion and then exercised showed two to

---

* A. Isidori et al.[67a] have reported that oral administration of 1,200 mg. of 1-lysine and 1,200 mg. of 1-arginine increased the growth hormone, a fact widely popularized by Durk Pearson and Sandy Shaw.[67b] T. J. Merimee et al.,[68] however, found that much greater amounts of lysine and arginine were required. They reported that the minimum effective arginine load needed to cause growth hormone release was 1/6 gram per pound of body weight in men and 1/2 gram per pound of body weight in women, which are, of course, gigantic dosages. Kikuo Kasai et al.[68a] reported that intravenous infusions of 12 grams of glycine resulted in an increase in serum levels of growth hormone. Excesses of one or a few amino acids can, however, sometimes lead to an undesirable increase in uric acid and other adverse effects.[68b] Furthermore, according to Roman J. Kutsky,[68c] growth hormone increases the capacity to form tumors. Creutzfeldt-Jakob disease may be another consequence of supplementary growth hormone.[68d,e] In Chapter 1 we noted other problems associated with growth hormone supplements (reference 107f of that chapter). The National Health Institutes suspended distribution of the hormone pending further evaluation of its safety[68f] but later the FDA approved a genetically engineered product.[68g] New cautions were cited in 1987 by Regelson.[68h] Interestingly, Mitchell E. Geffner et al.[68i] reported, in 1986, that growth is not necessarily dependent on growth hormone.

three times as much plasma growth hormone as did controls given only the saline infusion. The infusions were given before, during an eight-minute maximum workload on a bicycle, and during the recovery phase. Exercise alone greatly increased the amount of growth hormone. Pyridoxine without exercise also increased the growth hormone but was far less effective than exercise alone, which was, in turn, less effective than combined pyridoxine and exercise.* Other growth factors exist,[71a, b] many of which were discovered by Rita Levi-Montalcini and Stanley Cohen, 1986 Nobel laureates.

Supplemental vitamin B6 may also have a beneficial effect on the muscles. In experiments with rats, John H. Richardson and Marsha Chenman[72] reported that vitamin B6, given daily, increased muscle contraction time and increased the time before onset of fatigue. Between the growth hormone effect and this fatigue-fighting property, it would seem that supplemental B6 might find application in athletic training.

Some of the applications for B6 which we have mentioned may hinge on its apparent ability to aid the transport of magnesium and zinc (and perhaps of other minerals) across cell membranes. Guy E. Abraham et al.[73] reported that 100 mg. of vitamin B6 given twice a day to premenopausal subjects resulted in increased magnesium levels in plasma and in red blood cells. Lee and Leklem,[73a] however, in a study with premenopausal and postmenopausal women, found no evidence that vitamin B6 influences the levels of plasma and red blood cell magnesium.

Nevertheless, the effect of vitamin B 6 in fostering zinc absorption has been reported by many investigators. The action of this vitamin on zinc is not simply the fostering of its uptake as most references would lead one to believe. In actuality, vitamin B6 shows a *biphasic reverse effect* on zinc uptake; at least it does so in rats. R. Prasad et al.[74] have reported that, in rats, a B6 deficiency results in a significant *increase* in zinc absorption. Thus, a normal B6 intake reverses the high-zinc absorption of the B6-deficiency state (by resulting in *diminished* zinc absorption) just as a high intake of B6 reverses the normal B6-state by again resulting in an *increase* in zinc   absorption.

---

* T. Tolis et al.[71] found 200 mg B6/day did not change growth hormone levels.[133]

Prasad et al. also reported that a B6 deficiency resulted in increased absorption of calcium and also of the toxic metal cadmium. The literature is thus far silent as to whether these metals (and perhaps others also) exhibit *biphasic reverse effects* under the influence of different B6 dosages. Obviously, nutrition must become a science of dose-response relationships.

Adverse Effects of Excessive B6; Possible Benefits of a Deficiency

If, for any reason, you are using or are planning to use B6 supplements and are under a doctor's care, be sure to discuss your supplementation program with him. In some cases he may applaud your use of supplements. For example, the drugs hydralazine, isoniazid and penicillamine interact with B6 to cause an increased excretion of the vitamin-drug complex. Peripheral neuropathy may result if the supplies of B6 become deficient. If your physician is doing blood tests it may be especially important for him to know if you are supplementing with vitamin B6 since it can cause elevation in the level of serum glutamic oxaloacetic transaminase (SGOT). Solomon Garb[27] states that it is not clear if this elevation in SGOT is an artifact or is caused by slight liver damage.

Although I have given bad notice to a condition of pyridoxine deficiency, such a deficiency might be of value in treating certain cancers, and if you have cancer perhaps your physician might desire to *restrict* your intake of this vitamin. Fred Rosen et al.[75] tell about experiments by F. Bishoff et al., by B. E. Kline et al. and by others who fed a pyridoxine antagonist, 4-deoxypyridoxine, to tumorous animals who were already on low-pyridoxine diets. The result was a favorable combating of the tumors. Tumors, like normal tissue, need vitamins and minerals for their growth, so it should not surprise us that withholding one or more nutrients might result in tumor shrinkage. In other work, M. L. Littman et al.[75a] found that supplementary vitamin B6, in the form of pyridoxamine dehydrochloride, accelerated growth of ascitic Sarcoma 180 in mice and shortened their life span.

Experiments by at least three independent groups of scientists using the anticancer drug KTS on tumorous rats have shown the drug to be more efficient when the animals were fed a B6-deficient diet.[76] In this connection it is interesting to note that, not vitamin B6, but vitamin B6 antagonists (vinyl and ethynyl analogues of pyridoxal) are active inhibitors of mouse mammary carcinoma and in some cases the inhibition may be reversed by pyridoxine.[77] It is an amazing display of *reverse effects* among vitamin B6, B6 antagonists and cancer.

George P. Tryfiates et al.[78] reported on a related study. Rats were fed a pyridoxine-deficient diet and others were fed, respectively, supplements of various amounts of the vitamin. After 25 days on the various diets, the rats were injected with hepatoma cells and then were killed 16 days later. Both animal growth and tumor growth paralleled the level of dietary pyridoxine. The growth of the tumors was inhibited at low levels of vitamin B6 but grew rapidly at high levels of the vitamin. I think it would be of value to repeat this experiment with middle-aged rats who are beyond their period of rapid growth. In such animals, would a pyridoxine deficiency cause tumors to stop growing while causing no worse than tolerable harm to the rest of their bodies? Such an experiment might be suggestive for guidance in human cancer therapy. Let's note, however, that just because a pyridoxine deficiency may be valuable in unusual cases is no indication we should diminish our concern about having sufficient amounts of this vitamin to meet our needs.

In fact, if you are tempted to assume that vitamin B6 should always be restricted in cancer therapy, let me abort that conclusion. Dennis M. DiSorbo and Gerald Litwack[79] reported that *in vitro* experiments showed pyridoxine retarded growth and eventually killed rat hepatoma cells. They concluded that their findings suggest the potential use of vitamin B6 as an antineoplastic agent. More recently, Dennis M. DiSorbo, this time working with Larry Nathanson,[79a] reported that growth of a culture of human melanoma cells was severely inhibited when pyridoxal was added to the culture medium. Subsequently, DiSorbo et al. [79aa] discovered that vitamin B6 can inhibit growth of B16 melanoma cells, not only *in vitro* but also *in vivo,* in mice. The DiSorbo group also reported that preliminary results with human patients indicate that topical applications of pyridoxal cream "can significantly retard the growth of locally recurrent malignant melanoma."[*]

In what I think of as being a related study, J. Dozi-Vassiliades et al.[79b] found that pyridoxine hydrochloride enhanced sister-chromatid exchange (SCE) rates in cultured normal human lymphocytes. (You will recall we met the phenomenon of SCE in Chapter 4 in connection with retinoids. SCE are exchanges in replicating or newly-replicated DNA strands that occur between homologous sites on two, sister, chromatids of one chromosome.) No increase in SCE frequency was found when lymphocytes were treated with pyridoxal-5-phosphate or 4-pyridoxic acid to which vitamin B6 is finally converted. The *theory of the reverse effect* suggests the possibility that a substance that enhances the SCE rate might be a cancer fighter. It is to such substances that oncologists should, I believe, direct their attention.

Nursing mothers should ask their obstetricians about the advisability of restricting B6 intake. According to the work of G. Delitala,[67] which we recently noted, and also according to the *Drug Interaction Index* [80] pyridoxine may suppress the normally elevated prolactin hormone levels which stimulate the production of breast milk. Pyridoxine is, in fact, sometimes used purposely to suppress lactation. D. Scaglione and A. Vecchione[81] reported that lactation was suppressed in 89.3% of 1,592 women treated daily with 600 mg. of pyridoxine. Obviously, large amounts of vitamin B6 have a powerful drug action and should be used only with great respect for the possible consequences. Although G. Delitala had reported that a 300 mg. daily dose of B6 decreases plasma prolactin, G. Tolis et al.[82] found no such effect. The Tolis group, giving 200 mg. of B6 to normals and 400 mg. to patients with galactorrhea-amenorrhea (and having increased prolactin levels), found after two months of B6 therapy there was no decrease in prolactin, no decrease in the flow of

---

[*] After this was written, Larry Nathanson[79c] announced that vitamin B6, topically applied as pyridoxal, may combat melanoma. His team applied a cream of 50% pyridoxal on the lesions of two men, aged 63 and 70, 4 times a day. Fifty percent necrosis and regression occurred after 14 days. Nathanson said, "This is the first demonstration, to our knowledge, of the antitumor effects of pyridoxal in established human malignancies."

milk and no resumption of menses. If these various reports are equally believable, it would seem to require a daily intake of more than 400 mg. to suppress lactation. Don't you suppose other hormone effects (some perhaps undesirable) might be occurring in both men and women taking excessive B6?

One hormone that might be affected is Vitamin D. Fumio Shimura et al.[83] have reported that pyridoxal 5-phosphate has an inhibitory effect on the $1,25(OH)_2D_3$ receptor system *in vitro.* If this effect occurs *in vivo,* vitamin B6 may regulate responses to $1,25(OH_2)D_3$ in the intestines, perhaps for the better (at modest dosages) and perhaps for the worse (at excessive dosages). Thus, this could eventually be shown to be another *reverse effect.*

Those who decide to greatly increase their intake of vitamin B6 above that of the other vitamins may find it necessary to take additional amounts of vitamin B2. Vitamin B6 tends to combine with B2 and the resulting shortage of riboflavin may cause irritation of the eyes. Then too, numerous studies[84] indicate that excessive pyridoxine enhances the toxicity of cadmium in rats. Furthermore, beware of megadoses of vitamin B6 since, according to Victor Herbert,[85] it can cause liver disease.

Good sources for vitamin B6 are fish, liver, other organ meats, other meats, whole grain cereals, wheat germ, bran, brown rice, rice polishings, cabbage, beets, royal jelly, peanuts, pecans, seeds (especially sunflower), legumes, avocados, potatoes, yams, bananas, vegetable oils, milk, egg yolk, crude cane (but not beet) molasses and brewer's yeast. Flaxseed is reported to contain an antipyridoxine factor, a peptide called linatine.[86] However, few persons other than those frequenting health-food stores eat flaxseed, and the latter are probably taking B6 supplements.

Vitamin B12

This vitamin was discovered in 1948 in England by Dr. E. Lester Smith and, independently, in America by E. L. Rickes and his associates, who isolated it from liver. As long ago as 1926, Minot and Murphy had discovered that liver contains a factor that is effective in curing pernicious anemia, but not until 1948 was the substance isolated. The substance is, of course, vitamin B12 and its very complicated structure was determined by Dorothy Mary Crowfoot Hodgkin. For her discovery she was awarded the Nobel Prize in Chemistry in 1964. The red color of vitamin B12 is due to its cobalt content.

Vitamin B12 belongs to a group of compounds called corrinoids—most of which have vitamin B12 activity. Cobalt is at the center of most of these molecules* and it may be attached to a cyanide (CN) group, in which case the compound is called *cyanocobalamin,* or to a hydroxyl (OH) group, which then is termed *hydroxocobalamin.*[89,89a] The various cobalamins are very sensitive to light. Hydroxocobalamin, to cite just one example, is the photolysis product of cyanocobalamin.[89b]

Vitamin B12 functions through coenzymes such as *adenosinecobalamin* (thought, by the way, to be the form vitamin B12 generally takes in foods) or *methylcobalamin.* In fostering the formation of nucleic acids, the mode of action of the B12 coenzyme is probably that of a carrier for formyl and hydroxy-methyl groups which are required to produce purines and pyrimidines—nucleotides needed to synthesize nucleic acids. A B12 coenzyme also enters, along with pantothenic acid, into the so-called *isomerism reactions* whereby carbon units are rearranged within a compound (as is required in forming some amino acids such as aspartic acid). Coenzyme B12 is also involved in the formation and transfer of labile methyl groups as will be described in connection with choline.

Along with folic acid, vitamin B12 promotes formation of blood corpuscles. A shortage of either of these B vitamins can cause amenorrhea and even pernicious anemia. Shortages of vitamin B12 may be due to an interference with its absorption that could be caused by various drugs, including contraceptive pills. B12 may also help combat fatigue, nervous irritability, mental depression, insomnia and

---

* Cobalt-free corrinoids have been isolated from phototropic bacteria and used to synthesize corrinoids which contain copper, rhodium, zinc or iron instead of cobalt as a central atom.[88,88a]

lack of balance. Dwight Landis Evans et al.[89c] suggest that a B 12 deficiency may show up as psychiatric manifestations long before anemia or spinal cord disease occur. (H. Baker et al.[89d] have examined the vitamin content of normal brain segments and reported that the thalamus is especially rich in B 12.) Recently, Martin G. Cole and Jaroslav F. Prchal[90] reported that serum B 12 levels were much lower in 20 subjects aged 65 or over with Alzheimer-type dementia than in 20 age-matched subjects with non-Alzheimer-type dementia and 20 age-matched subjects with no dementia.

Along with B6 and folic acid, vitamin B 12 is required for the synthesis of the nucleic acids, DNA and RNA. Vitamin B 12 is anecdotally reported to be useful in treating asthma, hives, seborrhea, psoriasis, eczema and facial neuralgia. Vitamin B 12 has also been reported useful in treating sudden deafness (if treated promptly), glaucoma, osteoporosis, multiple sclerosis, diabetes, amblyopia (loss of vision due to tobacco poisoning), herpes zoster (shingles), hepatitis, arthritis and shoulder bursitis. Along with the rest of the vitamin B complex, vitamin B 12 is said to be beneficial to the health of the scalp and the hair. Through its action in stimulating the bile, it reportedly helps control the cholesterol level of the blood. Many of these effects are, however, based on purely anecdotal evidence.

Vitamin B 12 is an important constituent of semen and is also found in the uterus. Vitamin B 12 has been found to improve the fertility of sperm used for artificial insemination of cattle.[90a] Dr. Alan A Watson[90b] has reported B12 to be deficient in azoospermic human semen (Figure 1). Ralph Carmel and Gerald S. Bernstein[90c] recently reported that, in man, seminal plasma is the most concentrated source of transcobalamin II (a B 12 transporting agent). Their work suggests that the seminal vesicles are a principal source.[*]

A. Hanck and H. Weiser[90e] reported that vitamin B 12 (injected or oral), and its combination with vitamins B 1 and B 6, and, separately, vitamins K and C inhibited inflammation in paws of rats where

---

[*] Serum levels of transcobalamin II, and also of cobalamin and cobalumin-binding capacity, are higher in women, while serum levels of transcobalamin III are higher in men.[90d]

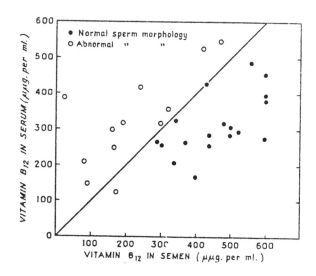

Figure 1. Levels of vitamin B₁₂ in semen as a function of the amount of the vitamin in serum. Note that normal sperm morphology is related to the presence of large amounts of B₁₂ in the semen. Reproduced from Alan A. Watson, *Lancet* (Sept. 29, 1962): 644, with permission of the publisher.

inflammation had been induced. Large dosages were used (e.g., 5 to 20 mg. of B₁ and of B₆ per kg. of body weight, equivalent to 300-1,400 mg. in man—a dangerous amount, at least as far as B₆ is concerned). They compared the result to that achieved through use of phenylbutazone. Perhaps periodontal problems, including gingival inflammation, might also be ameliorated through use of these B vitamins, but at the high dosages used by Hanck and Weiser it could be quite hazardous.

Vitamin B₁₂ sometimes may be an important factor in combating fatigue. Dr. F. R. Ellisard and Dr. S. Nasser,[91] working at Kingston and Long Grove Hospitals in Great Britain, gave massive injections of vitamin B₁₂ (10,000 mcg. weekly) to patients who had unexplained feelings of fatigue. They experienced an improvement and a feeling of well-being. A control group of patients given a placebo instead of vitamin B₁₂ showed no improvement until they, too, were given B12; then they reported similarly favorable results. One should not, however, make the assumption that there is a close relationship between injection of vitamin or other nutrient and its oral intake. Especially in the case of B12, very little that is taken by mouth may find its way past the gastrointestinal tract. Even the use of B12 injections may be of doubtful value for combating fatigue in the absence of anemia in spite of the report of Ellisard and Nasser. Tin-May-Than et al.[92] reported on a double-blind study in which subjects *free of anemia* were given either a 1 mg. cyanocobalamin or a placebo injection three times a week for six weeks. There was no significant difference between the two groups, thus suggesting that B12 injections be confined to treating those with anemia.

Intramuscular injections of vitamin B12 (in the hydroxocobalamin form known as B12b) have been valuable in treating some cases of senile dementia. When successful, it may be because those individuals had not been absorbing B12 properly, perhaps due to a deficiency of the "intrinsic factor."

The intrinsic factor is a mucoprotein produced by the hydrochloric-acid-producing parietal cells in the stomach that is important for the absorption of B12 (although a small amount of B12 can cross the intestinal barrier without the intrinsic factor being present). Some individuals do not produce the intrinsic factor and they must either receive their B12 by injection or be given B12 by mouth along with dried stomach tissue, calcium and magnesium. Then the B12 will pass through the ileum just as if the naturally produced intrinsic factor were there to act as a carrier. Besides the intrinsic factor, other vitamin B12-binding proteins exist and have been the subject of recent reviews by Elizabeth Jacob et al.,[93] as well as by Herzlich and Herbert.[93a] R binders (cobalophilins) that bind cobalamin are found in almost all body secretions. Of these, salivary R binder binds far more than the bile R binder which, in turn, is far more effective than are the pancreatic R binders.[93a] Vitamin B12 is transported via receptors in the ileum of the small intestines by means of transcobalamin II (TCII).[93b] The B12-TCII complex circulates in the body primarily bound to transcobalamin I, a glycoprotein related to gastric R binder.[93b]

The existence of a pancreatic intrinsic factor for vitamin B_{12} known to be one of the R binders) had been sought for more than 50 years. W. Veeger et al.[94] found that when pancreatic enzymes were given B_{12} absorption was sometimes improved. It is now known that pancreatic enzymes may also play a role in releasing food-bound cobalamin.[93a] Thus, those with intestinal malabsorption problems may sometimes experience a B_{12} deficiency.

Even though a B_{12} deficiency is quite rare, J. T. Henderson et al.[95] have found that even those showing poor absorption of vitamin B_{12} in the fasting state generally absorb it when food is given. Those ingesting excessive alcohol on a daily basis may, however, be an exception. Victor Herbert[96] states that alcoholics may have damaged the endoplasmic reticulum of the ileal epithelial cells. As a result, absorption of vitamin B_{12} may be subnormal.

Sources of Vitamin B_{12} and Possible Deficiency Problems

Vitamin B_{12} comes almost exclusively from animal protein such as liver, other meats, fish, milk, yogurt, cheese and eggs. The yeast *Candida utilis* is a concentrated source of cobalamin and, according to J. Michael Poston and Brian A. Hemmings,[97] "warrants serious consideration as a dietary supplement." Perhaps it will, in due course, become commercially available. Eggs, although containing B_{12}, may, nevertheless, inhibit its absorption. Alfred Doscherholmen[98] has reported that eggs contain inhibiting factors not only for iron and biotin, as has been known for a long time, but also for vitamin B_{12}.

The vitamin is made in the human colon but little or none is absorbed.[99] Vegetarians may find, however, that B_{12}-producing bacteria in the nodules of some legumes, in seaweeds and turnip greens, as well as in fermented soybean foods such as tempeh may be sources of this vitamin.[100] Anyway, although B_{12} is water-soluble, it can be stored for an extended period in the liver. Even if the liver's stores were to be depleted, the body would efficiently reabsorb the B_{12} excreted by the bile into the intestines in the absence of any intestinal malabsorption problem. It is reported that vegetarians are especially good at developing this ability to recycle vitamin B_{12} instead of losing much of it via the urine, as is typical of meat eaters.

Nevertheless, Allen Dong and Stephen C. Scott[101] observed that vegetarians who did not supplement with B 12 or multiple vitamin tablets had serum B 12 levels below normal. They found that 92% of the vegans (total vegetarians), 64% of the lactovegetarians, 47% of the lacto-ovovegetarians and 20% of the semivegetarians had serum B 12 levels below normal. It seems safest to get this vitamin from animal sources (such as liver, other meats, fish, milk, yogurt, cheese and eggs) or in the form of a pill.

Fiber itself (especially pectin), so prominent in the vegetarian diet, may also threaten body supplies of vitamin B 12. R. W. Cullen and S. M. Oace [102] have reported that pectin-fed rats excreted greater amounts of B 12 than did rats fed either a fiber-free diet or diets containing up to 50% cellulose.

Breast milk of vegetarian mothers may be deficient in vitamin B 12 according to scientists at the University of California Medical Center in San Diego. Breastfeeding is highly beneficial to infants (as well as to the mothers) and it is certainly difficult to find anything negative to say about it.* Vegetarian mothers should supplement their diets with vitamin B 12 so their breast milk will then be baby's ideal food.

We have pointed out that a B 12 deficiency may exist in those having inadequate intrinsic factor (or factors if we count the pancreatic R binder as well as the gastric variety), in alcoholics and in those consuming virtually no animal protein. Women taking oral contraceptives may be deficient in B 12.[104a] Those taking some other drugs may also become B 12 deficient. Colchicine may damage the intestinal wall and thus cause inefficient body take-up of B 12; cholestyramine may inhibit functions of the intrinsic factor; neomycin may both damage the intestinal wall and interfere with the function of the intrinsic factor; para-aminosalicylic acid may cause decreased absorption of the vitamin; and potassium chloride may decrease the pH of the illeum and thus inhibit absorption of B 12.

---

* There is a negative, however, for preterm infants. Preterm infants grow more rapidly on artificial formula than they do on banked breast milk.[103] The anti-infective and immunological properties of breast milk are, by the way, severely impaired by pasteurization.[104]

There is yet another class of individuals who may be short of B12. Victor Herbert[105] relates that an increased requirement for B12 (and also for folic acid) may occur in any body condition that increases the body's metabolic rate. Examples are those with hyperthyroidism, those showing increased hematopoiesis (blood formation) or those having a fever. Pregnant women may find that the fetus may wipe out their stores of B12. Then too, persons with certain cancers (such as those of lymphoproliferative tissues) may find the cancer depletes body supplies of B12. I suspect, however, that some of these conditions could be examples of the body's protective mechanism rather than an indication to use a supplement.

Perhaps even those megadosing with vitamin C may be deficient in vitamin B12. D. V. Frost et al.,[105a] well over 30 years ago, cited studies by Frost et al.[105b] and by N. R. Trenner et al.[105c] showing that vitamin B12 is destroyed by vitamin C. E. M. Stapert et al.[106] reported (about 30 years ago) that ascorbic acid in the presence of copper destroys vitamin B12. A. J. Rosenberg[107] reported that cupric ion alone had no effect on cyanocobalamin, while ascorbic acid, without cupric ion, had some but little destructive effect. However, ascorbic acid, or dehydroascorbic acid, and cupric ion together effectively destroyed B12. About the same time, Hastings H. Hutchins et al.[107a] found that cyanide-free B12 analogs in ascorbic acid solutions were far less stable than cyanocobalamin. Many years later, Victor Herbert also reported that ascorbic acid may destroy B12. (These various experiments were performed *in vitro,* and thus the results may not be applicable *in vivo.*) If it is ever demonstrated that *in vivo* ascorbic acid is antagonistic to the cyanocobalamin type of vitamin B12, one could simply take it with meals and ascorbic acid between meals. However, orthomolecular therapies employing massive dosages of ascorbic acid have been used frequently and there have been no reported signs of anemia that should occur if supplies of vitamin B12 were inadequate. Those interested in exploring the possibility that B12 is destroyed by vitamin C are referred to articles by Victor Herbert[108,109] and a rebuttal by Harold L. Newmark, et al.[100] Dr. Herbert[111] reports, however, that the B12 is protected against destruction if it is in the form of cyanocobalamin (as Hutchins et al.[107a] had determined some 30 years earlier). Perhaps Herbert and Newmark are talking about different B12s. In fact, Martin Marcus[112] recalls that H. P. C. Hogenkamp[112a] pointed out that, of the various forms of B12, only aquocobalamin seems to be affected by vitamin C. (Aquocobalamin is a very minor constituent of food—the methyl, hydroxy and adenosyl cobalamins being more common.)[112] Finally, Marcus[112] states that it was the heat used in Dr. Herbert's experiments, not the vitamin C, that destroyed the B12. The argument that began with the work of Frost et al.[105b] and Trenner et al.[105c] in 1950, well before Herbert got interested, goes on. Herbert[112b] maintains the position that ascorbic acid destroys vitamin B12 and continues to castigate those with an opposing view.* He is probably correct *in vitro,* but is he correct *in vivo?* Shirley Ekvall et al.[112d] reported that when 40 children with myelomeningocele (a kind of spina bifida) were given 1.65 grams of supplementary ascorbic acid, there was no sign of a vitamin B12 deficiency. They consider it very improbable that megadoses of ascorbic acid could induce a B12 deficiency in man. John D. Hines,[112e] basing his opinion on 90 subjects taking over 500 mg. of ascorbic acid daily, believes that 2% to 3% of persons megadosing on "C" will ultimately develop a B12 deficiency. On the other hand, Mary Ann Sestili,[112f] after reviewing the various B12 studies, states that destruction of cobalamins other than aquocobalamin by vitamin C is very unlikely as long as they are not exposed to light.

Vitamin B12 Analogues

Bacterial overgrowth in the small intestines can result in production of vitamin B12 analogues (cobamides).[113] Haruki Kondo et al.,[113a,b] J. Fred Kolhouse and Robert H. Allen,[113c] J. Fred Kolhouse et al.,[113d] and Mitchell Binder et al,[113e] among others, have made extensive studies of B12 analogues. In patients with bacterial overgrowth problems, unabsorbable cobamides tend to be produced in static areas of the intestinal tract and they can interfere with B12 absorption. Of four patients with intestinal bacterial overgrowth, two

---

* Herbert[112c] maintains, however, that moderate amounts of iron in the diet will reduce the damaging effects of ascorbic acid on vitamin B12.

had low B 12 levels, two had small bowel diverticulosis and two had partial intestinal obstruction.[113] Three of the four had anaerobic organisms in their gut.[113] B. Mackler and V. Herbert et al.[113f] have suggested that, even in normally healthy persons, the primary source of B12 analogues in human tissues may be enteric bacteria.

A study by Victor Herbert et al.[114] maintains that many multivitamin products contain spurious, possibly dangerous analogues of vitamin B 12. In support of Dr. Herbert's contention, Nina V. Myasishcheva et al.,[115] using *in vitro* experiments, showed methylcobalamin analogues interfere with the synthesis of cobalamin enzymes in human lymphocytes. It may be some time before the problems are resolved. Meanwhile, it might be wise to avoid vitamin supplements containing vitamin B12. However, even declining to take such pills will not allow us to completely avoid B12 analogues. These analogues have been found in large amounts in human serum and in the human liver, red cells and brain. Herbert[114] credits R. H. Allen [115a] as having postulated that they may derive from eating animals raised on feed supplemented with vitamins and minerals. Herbert and his colleagues[114] have shown that nutrients capable of damaging the B 12 molecule and converting it to analogues include thiamin, nicotinamide, vitamins C and E, copper and iron. It seems reasonable to me to presume that such damage might take place not only in the bodies of meat-producing animals but in humans, perhaps especially those supplementing their diet with B 12 and the above-mentioned nutrients. Another possibly dangerous source of B12 analogues is that currently popular "health food," spirulina (a blue-green algae of the family *Oscillatoriaceae*). Spirulina is advertised to contain large amounts of vitamin B12, but Victor Herbert and George Drivas[116] have found that more than 80% of what appears to be B12 is really analogues of the vitamin that have no B 12 activity for humans. Some of these analogues could actually be antagonists of B12 and might be harmful. On the other hand, Herbert et al.[116a] recently reported that B12-analogue levels similar to those of Americans have been found in Kalahari desert bushmen who take no supplements. Another recent study by Herbert et al.[116b] has identified enteric bacteria as a major if not the main source of B12 analogues. The fact that supplements contain these analogues would seem to be relatively irrelevant. Furthermore, is it possible that, during the eons these compounds have been present in the human gut, the body may have developed a use for them?

Possible Dangers of Excessive B₁₂

In treating pernicious anemia, B₁₂ is often injected on a regular basis and in such cases hypersensitivity to B₁₂ can sometimes develop. C. N. Ugwu and F. J. Gibbins[117] report on one case of hypersensitivity developing after several years of treatment. They stress that it is important for physicians to be aware of this "rare but potentially lethal reaction." A. Dupre et al.[118] have observed that injected B₁₂ can induce acne. By the way, when B₁₂ is injected it should be given by the intramuscular or deep subcutaneous route rather than intravenously. Robert S. Hillman[119] discovered that intravenous injection of B₁₂ can result in transitory exanthema (a skin eruption) and anaphylaxis. Vitamin B₁₂ injections may be very overprescribed. David A. Knapp et al.[119a] maintain that vitamin B₁₂ was "prescribed/administered unappropriately some 8 million times in 1980-1981."

Vitamin B₁₂ may sometimes work against the attempt to cure cancer. A. D. Ostryanina[120] has reported that vitamin B₁₂ increases the activity of four carcinogens in experimental animals. L. A. Poirier et al.[121] found a B₁₂-adequate diet accelerated liver cancer in rats that had been given carcinogens. With a B₁₂-deficient diet, on the other hand, the hepatomas grew much less rapidly.

Similarly, in an *in vivo* study relating the effects of protein, vitamin B₁₂ and aflatoxins on the rat liver, Punya Temcharoen et al.[121a] found that, although aflatoxin combined with a low-protein diet had toxic and carcinogenic effects, there was no toxic effect on the liver in rats fed aflatoxin and a high-protein diet. However, hepatoma and hyperplastic modules were found in rats fed aflatoxin, a high-protein diet plus vitamin B₁₂.

Another upsetting possibility is that excessive B₁₂ may be very detrimental not just to animals but also to men and women who have cancer. Ralph Carmel and Leopoldo Eisenberg,[122] in a study of 139 patients with nonhematologic malignancy, concluded that a high serum level of vitamin B12 usually implied a poor prognosis. In their study, mean survival for such patients was just one month, whereas the survival time for all other patients in the study was four months. J. C. Linnell and D. M. Mathews[122a] reported that patients with primary hepatoma have methylcobalamin levels in tissues, including the brain and liver, from 3 to 25 times normal levels. Linnell[89a] speculates that methylcobalamin may promote tumor growth just as lack of it inhibits such growth.

Nitrous oxide, the anesthetic, can interfere with B12 metabolism which leads to an impairment of *de novo* thymidine synthesis.* This inhibition of thymidine synthesis, in turn, has been found by A. C. M. Kroes et al.[122c] to reduce *in vitro* proliferation of rat leukemia cells. Yasuhiko Kano et al.[122d] demonstrated similar effects on human cell lines which suggests nitrous oxide, through its depressing effect on B12 metabolism, might inhibit certain tumors *in vivo.* Such findings provide additional warnings that supplemental B12 might be detrimental to the cancer patient just as a deficiency of this vitamin might be therapeutic. The cancer patient may need less of vitamin B12 and perhaps less of other vitamins also rather than the megadoses that are sometimes recommended. (On the other hand, until appropriate studies are done we can't rule out the possibility that at very high doses of B12 there could be a *reverse effect* with B12 becoming a cancer antagonist. Supporting this possibility, a study by Norio Shimizu et al.[122e] reported that intraperitoneal administration of methylcobalamin suppressed proliferation of MH134 tumor in mice and increased their longevity.)

Pantothenic Acid

This vitamin, which was at one time known as vitamin B5, was discovered by Roger J. Williams. The role of pantothenic acid

---

* Detrimental effects of the anesthetic nitrous oxide have been known for many years. As recent as 1986, nitrous oxide was still causing neurological damage and death. Robert F. Schilling,[122b] after reporting on two such deaths, postulated that "nitrous oxide anesthesia may precipitate neurologic disease in people with unrecognized deficiency of vitamin B12."

(pantothenate) in body chemistry involves coenzyme A, a complicated compound containing this vitamin. Under the influence of coenzyme A, pyruvic acid (which was formed from glucose by a process called *glycolysis*) is converted to *acetyl coenzyme A*. This coenzyme is required by the adrenal glands for the conversion of acetic acid to cholesterol and other sterols. Acetyl coenzyme A is also required (along with choline) for the production of acetylcholine, so important for nerve transmission. Fritz Albert Lipmann discovered coenzyme A and its significance in the intermediary metabolism, and for this he shared the Nobel Prize in Medicine or Physiology in 1953 with Hans Adolph Krebs, who developed the Krebs cycle.

Acetyl coenzyme A is essential for numerous reactions required for building of many complicated compounds that are produced during the Krebs cycle and the coenzyme A portion of acetyl coenzyme A is released to make more acetyl coenzyme A from pyruvic acid. The acetyl part becomes part of the citric acid molecule that is involved in this cycle and is eventually degraded to carbon dioxide and hydrogen atoms. In the Krebs cycle, oxaloacetic acid, produced from the metabolism of fats, carbohydrates and proteins, is oxidized to carbon dioxide and water.

The Krebs cycle is also known as the *citric acid cycle* or the *tricarboxylic acid cycle* since citric acid and the other tricarboxylic acids are formed in the process. This cycle starts and ends—after many chemical conversions—with oxaloacetic acid and it continues again and again.

Hydrogen atoms are given off at various stages of the Krebs cycle. These hydrogen atoms are oxidized to water by a series of enzymes in a process called the *electron-transport system* and this is the main way in which the cell produces ATP to supply the energy needed for the various reactions of body chemistry. This process is called *oxidative phosphorylation*.

The Krebs cycle, and the subsequent oxidation of hydrogen atoms to form water via the electron-transport system, is the common pathway for converting foods to energy. The mitochondria, where these reactions occur, are often called the "powerhouses" of the cell.

The ATP created in the electron-transport system supplies the energy to run the various processes of the body. Each mole[*] of ATP provides the body with 8,000 calories[**] of energy in being transformed into adenosine diphosphate (ADP). Each mole of ADP will, in turn, supply another 8,000 calories on being converted to adenosine monophosphate (AMP). Engines are never 100% efficient and the body is no exception. About 50% of the food energy is used for body processes; the rest goes into heat. The AMP and the ADP may be converted back again to ATP as food is oxidized to supply the energy to make the transformations.

By now we should have a great appreciation for pantothenic acid, which through coenzyme A, the Krebs cycle and the electron-transport system gives rise to the all-important ATP. Since pantothenic acid is essential to the energy-producing process, adequate amounts of this vitamin are required to combat fatigue and help assure youthful longevity.[***] (Thiamin, niacin and riboflavin are also involved in the working of the Krebs cycle, so to help fight fatigue one must have an adequate amount of all the B vitamins.)

Pantothenic acid is reported to be useful for maintaining a youthful appearance, including proficiency in reversing that sign of aging, skin wrinkling, and in delaying the graying of the hair as well as loss of hair.[****] Stress shows up in may diverse ways. Pantothenic acid will probably not grow hair; it may, however, help overcome the stress patterns sometimes associated with hair loss. Pantothenic acid is reported to be useful in overcoming the effects of many kinds of stress. Rats fed this vitamin exhibited significantly improved exercise tolerance and resistance to radiation-induced injury.[123a,b] Humans taking 10 grams/day of pantothenic acid showed

---

[*] A mole is a weight in grams numerically equal to the molecular weight.

[**] These are small calories. The food calorie is 1,000 times as large.

[***] D. Branca et al,[122f] reported that pantethine (the disulfide form of pantetheine, which is the B-aminoethanethiol ester of pantothenic acid) induced a significant increase in coenzyme A in both perfused liver and liver homogenate while pantothenic acid did not. They suggest this compound may therefore have some physiological significance. This may be the kind of research on which vitamin purveyors could build a "story."

[****] Pantothenic acid may or may not delay graying of hair in humans, but it does have this ability in rats and the action is potentiated by zinc.[123]

increased ability to withstand cold-water stress as shown by blood chemistry values.[123b] Christopher Nice et al.[123c] reported on a study by R. G. Early and B. Carlson[123d] that concluded 30 mg. of pantothenic acid daily delayed the onset of fatigue in exercising humans. Christopher Nice et al.,[123c] however, in a controlled study of 18 highly trained distance runners exercised to exhaustion on a treadmill found no effects in supplementing one gram/day of pantothenic acid. Nevertheless, D. Litoff, et al.,[123e] in a double-blind crossover study, reported that 7 highly trained distance runners, after bicycling for 40 minutes or until exhaustion, had mean lactate values of 5.1 mEq./1. on placebo compared to 4.25 mEq./1. when taking 2 grams/day of pantothenic acid. This represents a 16.7% decrease of lactate while taking pantothenic acid. The Litoff group also found that while the athletes were on pantothenic acid there was an 8.4% decrease in oxygen consumption.

Fatigue, headaches, personality changes, abdominal problems, numbness and tingling of the extremities and loss of antibody production are symptoms that may be the result of a pantothenic acid deficiency, and their cure can be effected by the use of this vitamin if that was the cause of the problem. This is, of course, the key to the truth or falsity of so much anecdotal evidence. Any of a multitude of problems can be corrected by a vitamin or a mineral IF (and that is a big IF) the cause of the problem was a shortage of that particular nutrient.

Pantothenic acid is vital for the proper operation of the thyroid gland. It is also required for proper functioning of the adrenal glands which, when not operating efficiently, can bring on mental depression, excessively low blood pressure and reduced secretion of hydrochloric acid by the stomach which, in turn, may lead to anemia. Pantothenic acid is an important factor in digestion and also in the absorption of food through the intestines.

Pantothenic acid is needed for production of cortisone, one of the hormones secreted by the adrenal glands that is used to prepare the body to meet a stress. Synthetic cortisone has been found effective in treating arthritis, thus indicating that the body's own production of cortisone may be deficient. Use of the amino acid cysteine in conjunction with pantothenic acid is reported to improve results with arthritic patients.

Pantothenic acid appears to be useful in wound healing and therefore supplementation may be of value after operations. J. F. Grenier et al.[123f] reported on the effects of pantothenic acid supplementation in wound-healing experiments using rabbits. Such post-operative supplementation improves healing of aponeurosis tissue (a fibrous or membranous sheet for attaching or enclosing muscles) without affecting skin healing. (Aponeurosis is a more collagenic tissue than is skin.) Histological examinations showed a significant increase in the number of fibroblasts which synthesize collagen fibers. The investigators found that pantothenic acid not only accelerates healing, but also improves the quality of the scar. They also noted that, although vitamin C and zinc are known to be beneficial in wound healing, many other nutrients may be of additional value and it will be up to future research to find them. Subsequent work by Marc Aprahamian et al.,[124] also with rabbits, showed that daily ingestions of 20 mg./kg. body weight of pantothenic acid significantly increased aponeurosis strength and otherwise suggested that supplements of this vitamin induced an accelerating effect on the normal healing process.

Pantothenic acid (because it stimulates production of cortisone) has also been found effective in combating allergies such as hay fever. Tendencies toward allergies that run in families may simply be an indication of a hereditary requirement for much larger than normal amounts of pantothenic acid. Even a mild deficiency in pantothenic acid will affect the immune system* by causing a reduction in the numbers of white blood cells and antibodies resulting in the prevalence of infections (such as sore throat). Increased quantities of pantothenic acid may be helpful in fighting infections, including the common cold.

---

* Over 30 years ago, Ashton L. Welsh[124a] reported that massive amounts of pantothenic acid combined with vitamin E were used successfully in treating 67 patients having lupus erythematosus. Since lupus is known to be an autoimmune disease, this suggests that massive amounts of pantothenic acid (and/or vitamin E) may show a *reverse effect* by depressing the immune system.

Gout is a disease in which uric acid accumulates instead of being converted, as it normally is, into urea and ammonia. When pantothenic acid is lacking, this beneficial conversion is not made. The fact that gout tends to run in families may indicate a hereditary need for unusually large quantities of this vitamin. Anecdotal evidence exists for beneficial use of pantothenic acid, not only for gouty arthritis, but also for osteo and rheumatoid arthritis. A study by the General Practitioner Research Group[124b] showed possible (almost statistically significant) improvement in rheumatoid arthritis but no benefit in osteoarthritis.

Pantothenic acid appears to serve a vital function during reproduction.[125] Dr. Roger J. Williams suggests that it is possible that many stillbirths, premature births, malformed babies and mentally retarded babies may be due to the lack, during pregnancy, of pantothenic acid. The richest natural sources for this vitamin, royal jelly[*] and codfish caviar, are both closely linked with reproduction. It seems likely that human beings, during reproduction, require unusually high amounts of pantothenic acid.

Pantothenic acid may be a prolongevity factor. Thomas S. Gardner[126] found that royal jelly, already noted to be a concentrated source of pantothenic acid, increased the life span of fruit flies by 16.5% Using just calcium pantothenate added to their drinking water, the average life span increase was an impressive 27.8%.[**] This work was followed, about ten years later, by a related study using mice.

Roger J. Williams[128] tells of an experiment with mice in which pantothenic acid (in the form of .3 mg. of pantothenate per day) was found to increase their mean life span by about 20%. However, in checking the original research he did with Richard B. Pelton,[129] I find that I have a problem with the experiment's protocol. Pelton and

---

[*] Royal jelly contains testosterone (11-12 ng./g. for native royal jelly and 31-36 ng./g. for the lyophilized variety).[125a] The many anecdotes telling of increases in libido following ingestion of royal jelly thus have a rationale. Above-normal testosterone levels may, however, pose a threat if an undiagnosed prostatic carcinoma should exist.

[**] When Gardner[127] fed fruit flies biotin, pyridoxine and sodium yeast nucleate (Fleischmann Yeast) in addition to pantothenate, their life span increased by a remarkable 46.6%.

Williams grouped the mice six or seven to a cage. As we saw in the introduction, when this is done the stronger, more aggressive animals tend to get enough food to survive while the rest may sicken from starvation. Thus the experiment could really have been a study in aggressive behavior rather than one involving the (possibly incidental) consumption of pantothenic acid. The experiment was done a quarter of a century ago; perhaps it will be repeated some day using individually caged mice. If the finding that pantothenic acid increases the life span of mice is confirmed and if that finding is applicable to human beings, this vitamin could be an important contribution to the project of increasing longevity.

Sources of Pantothenic Acid

Pantothenic acid is found widely in foods. (In fact, the very name of this vitamin, given it by Williams, comes from the Greek word meaning "everywhere.") One of the finest sources for this vitamin, as we have noted, is royal jelly, the substance that converts a worker bee into a queen and perhaps helps the queen to live much longer than the workers. Good sources, in addition to royal jelly, are brewer's yeast, liver, egg yolk, kidneys, other meats, salmon, milk, molasses, peanuts, soybeans, seeds, whole grains, bran, rice polishings, wheat germ, mushrooms, alfalfa, sweet potatoes, zucchini, squash, cabbage, corn, peas and broccoli. Pantothenic acid is also available as a supplement in the form of calcium pantothenate.

Roger J. Williams[130] makes the interesting point that general vitamin supplements are usually woefully short of pantothenic acid. Williams notes that human milk contains 18 times as much pantothenic acid as thiamin, which suggests that infants, at least, require far more pantothenic acid than thiamin. He notes also that human muscle, the most abundant tissue in our bodies, contains 11 times as much pantothenic acid as thiamin.

Apparent Safety of Excessive Pantothenic Acid

The literature does not seem to mention any problems deriving from excessive intake of pantothenic acid. It is interesting to note, however, that mammary carcinoma is reported to be depressed in rats when pantothenic acid is deficient.[131] On the other hand, in animal experiments using the antitumor agent semicarbazone, pantothenic acid (and thiamin) beneficially increased the antitumor activity of semicarbazone.[132]

Folic Acid

Folic acid has an impressive collection of synonyms, among which are vitamin M, folacin, pteroylpolyglutamic acid and pteroylmonoglutamic acid. Folinic acid is a variant form having the same effect as folic acid. The term folate is sometimes used synonymously for any of these names. Folic acid deficiency is reported to be the most common vitamin deficiency throughout the world.[132a] Certain groups—alcoholics, pregnant women* and the elderly—may be especially deficient in this vitamin. In a study among elderly persons residing in their own homes, L. Elsborg et al.[133a] found the average folate intake was only one-third of the RDA. (Low as this figure is, it assumes the total folate of food is absorbable, which may not be the case.)

The mucosa of the duodenum and jejunum produce the enzyme conjugase (or folic deconjugase) which splits polyglutamic folic acid to form monoglutamic folic acid. Inside the mucosal cell, monoglutamic folate is reduced by tetrahydrofolic acid to form the physiologically active form of folic acid. Folic acid is then released from the mucosal cells of the upper intestinal tract into the portal circulation.[133b]

When folic acid is assimilated it is converted to tetrahydrofolic acid and then, in turn, into several coenzymes. The main function of these coenzymes, which are found throughout the body, but primarily in the liver, is probably to produce nucleotides needed to synthesize nucleic acids. The folic acid coenzymes are also required, along with coenzymes of other vitamins, to construct certain amino acids needed to build protein and also for the metabolism of most, if

---

* Folic acid is the only vitamin whose requirement doubles during pregnancy.[133]

not all, amino acids. Various coenzymes of folic acid also supply carbon and hydrogen for synthesizing labile methyl groups, thus adding to those supplied by choline as well as by betaine and methionine. (The body's use of labile methyl groups will be discussed further in connection with choline.)

Folic acid is essential for building red blood corpuscles. It helps promote good appetite and increases the stomach's production of hydrochloric acid (thus aiding digestion and iron absorption). Folic acid is a factor in the body's manufacturing of prostaglandins and helps the liver in performing its function. It aids in the treatment of anemia (including sickle cell anemia).[133ba]

Folic acid has a potpourri of uses in body chemistry. A deficiency of folic acid may detrimentally affect the immune system and cause chronic candidiasis.[133c] A folic acid deficiency is also implicated in mental disease. At any rate, when pregnant rats were deprived of folic acid their offspring were intellectually inferior. Then too, patients with senile dementia generally have folic acid (and ascorbic acid) concentrations below the normal range and M. J. Bober[133d] suggests this may apply to many other mentally ill older persons. Related to this suggestion is the possibility that folic acid may be of value in treating schizophrenia.[134] In addition, E. H. Reynolds and G. Stramentinoli,[134a] both in their own research and in cited references, show that a deficiency of folic acid is associated with depression.

Dr. Carl C. Pfeiffer[135] states that, in the female having low amounts of histamine, folic acid can be used to elevate the histamine level in the blood and tissues and may thus provide easier orgasm. I have indicated earlier, however, in connection with niacin, that I know of no rationale to support the validity of the histamine-orgasm hypothesis. (A cold increases the histamine level in the blood, but I know of no data to suggest that colds increase sexuality or orgasmic capacity.)

The diet of the expectant mother is usually deficient in folic acid. Since experiments with pregnant mice have shown that folic acid deficiency can lead to malformed offspring, and, since there is a likely parallel with human pregnancy, expectant mothers should probably supplement their diet with this nutrient. In fact, at least one type of birth defect in human babies seems to be related to a folic acid deficiency. K. M. Laurence et al.[136] of the Welsh National School of Medicine in Cardiff conducted a controlled double-blind trial to prevent a recurrence of a neural-tube defect in babies of women who had one child with such a defect.[*] Sixty women were given 4 mg. of folic acid daily before and early in their pregnancy, while 51 were given a placebo treatment as a control. Among the controls, six babies were born with a neural-tube defect. Among those receiving folic acid, there were no babies showing such a defect. G. M. Stirrat[137] expresses uncertainty, however, that folate alone or in combination with other vitamins is effective for this purpose. Nevertheless, in another study,[138] this one involving almost 1,000 mothers with a history of previous offspring having a neural-tube defect, recurrence rates were just .7% for 454 fully supplemented mothers and 4.7% for 519 unsupplemented mothers. Supplements were given before conception occurred and included not only folic acid but also other vitamins and minerals. Elwood,[138a] however, reviewing the use of vitamins in the attempt to prevent neural-tube defects, expresses concern over their safety.

Bolo O. A. Osifo et al.[138b] have reported that serum folic acid levels were higher in febrile pediatric patients and higher yet in those that were convulsing. They also found that the folic acid content of the cerebrospinal fluid was slightly lower but not significantly different in convulsing children. (This finding supports the previously known fact that there is an efficient blood-brain barrier for folate. The folate level of the cerebrospinal fluid being slightly lower during convulsion may relate to the discovery of O. R. Hommes and E. A. M. T. Obbens [138c] that the blood-brain barrier for folate can be damaged in the rat by heat applied to the brain and that this induces seizures.) Additionally, the O s i f o   g r o u p   r e p o r t e d   t h a t   s e r u m

---

[*] When the fetus is only a few weeks old, the neural plate folds to form the neural tube, which is the foundation for the brain, the spinal cord and the rest of the central nervous system. Normally, the neural tube closes at an embryonic age of about four weeks. Anencephaly (absence of cerebrum, of cerebellum and of the flat bones of the skull), spina bifida (defect in the closure of the vertebral canal) or encephalocele (hernia of the brain through an opening in the cranium) can occur if the neural tube fails to close.[136a]

cobalamin levels had a definite decrease in febrile convulsion. These facts (higher serum folic acid and lower vitamin B 12) during febrile convulsion may be subtle examples of body wisdom that we will understand in the future. Certainly, for now, it would be premature to attempt clinical modification in the serum levels of these vitamins with the objective of molifying febrile convulsion.

Studies of Richard R. Streiff,[139] reported in the *Journal of the American Medical Association,* have shown that women taking oral contraceptives tend to be deficient in folic acid. Streiff found that the bone marrow of some women on the Pill showed evidence of megaloblastic anemia, which is a condition associated with a serious lack of folic acid. He reported that monoglutamic folate does not seem to be affected by the Pill, but absorption of polyglutamic folate was reduced by about 50% in volunteers taking oral contraceptives. Others[140] have reported that the Pill inhibits the absorptive enzymes which are essential for the body to absorb this vitamin from food and cause an increased synthesis of folate-binding macroglobulin. However, Streiff found that women taking oral contraceptives could absorb folic acid in the form of a dietary supplement. It seems apparent that women on the Pill should supplement their diet with folic acid. It is especially important that any folic acid deficiency be rectified before the occurrence of pregnancy to protect the fetus from possible damage. Interestingly, D. W. Dawson[140a] presents evidence suggesting the possibility that a folate deficiency may be a factor in causing infertility.

Folic acid supplementation may be of value in periodontal health. Richard I. Vogel et al.[141] reported that such supplementation may increase the resistance of the gingiva to local irritants and thus lead to a reduction in inflammation. They also reported that a folic acid rinse caused a large absorption of the vitamin by the gingival tissues. In a double-blind study, those rinsing with a folic acid solution showed a significant decrease in inflammation compared to that shown by the placebo group. In a related study, Angela R. C. Pack[141a] also found that a solution of 5 mg. folate per 5 ml. of water used as a mouthwash improved gingival health. She concluded that the action seems to be through local rather than systemic influence.

Folic acid (along with niacin and vitamin A) is believed to be essential in carrying out the complicated chemical transformation whereby the body converts cholesterol to androgens and estrogens. Therefore, it is interesting to speculate on the possibility that women taking dosages of this vitamin might note an enlargement of their breasts. Furthermore, according to Isobel W. Jennings,[142] folic acid increases the androgenic action of testosterone.

Richard F. Branda and John W. Eaton[141b] reported that *in vitro* experiments involving human plasma exposed to simulated strong sunlight caused a 30% to 50% loss of folate within 60 minutes. Furthermore, light-skinned persons exposed to ultraviolet light as dermatological treatments have subnormal folate concentrations. Branda and Eaton have speculated that dark skins are prevalent in populations exposed to intense sunlight as a protection against folate depletion (as well as protection for vitamin E and riboflavin, which are also light sensitive).

Blood deficiencies associated with maturation-failure anemia can be corrected by taking folic acid. However, vitamin B_{12} must be taken at the same time or the spinal cord will degenerate. This phenomenon has led to a law of questionable merit. In the United States it is illegal for any supplement to be sold without prescription if it contains more than the RDA value of .4 mg. of folic acid. (The supplement may contain .8 mg. if it is labeled "for pregnant or lactating women." Even prescription dosages are now limited by the FDA to 1.0 mg. per tablet.) Does this indicate that folic acid is a toxic substance? It definitely does not! This law is in effect, not because folic acid supplementation might be dangerous, but simply because it might interfere with a diagnosis of vitamin B_{12} deficiency. If such a B_{12} deficiency were allowed to persist it could result in a degeneration of the spinal cord. The law was designed to protect those who do not eat animal foods supplying vitamin B_{12}. Why not, instead, warn vegetarians to supplement their diet with a B_{12} pill? Under this line of logic, why does the government not limit the amount of vitamin C that can be put in a pill since it interferes with the test for occult blood in the stool? Other examples of vitamins and minerals affecting laboratory tests are cited throughout this book.

Drug-Folate Interactions

There is a negative aspect to folic acid supplementation that should be noted. The folic acid content of cancer cells is unusually high, so if one has cancer or has had a cancerous tumor removed it may be wise to limit one's folic acid intake. In fact, experiments using antagonists such as methotrexate that tend to keep folic acid from functioning (by blocking the synthesis of the coenzyme tetrahydrofolate) [142 a-c] have been successful in treating cancers.* (On the other hand, methotrexate can display a *reverse effect* and, while being used to treat psoriasis, can *cause* cancer.)[143, 143a] The toxic effects of methotrexate are, in turn, often controlled by *calcium leucovorin,* the calcium salt of folic acid. If cancer should be present in a state of arrested development the extra folic acid might be very dangerous indeed if it should stimulate the cancer cells to more-rapid growth. It would be ironic (horrible might be a more appropriate word) if, in the attempt to improve nutrition, we ended up stimulating some cancer cells.

Folic acid may, however, help protect cancer-free persons against chromosome breakage. A modest amount of folic acid decreases the number of chromosome breaks in cells in culture mediums.[143b-e] In a 1986 study of spontaneous chromosome aberrations, human lymphocytes were cultured by Xin-Zhi Li et al.[143d] with and without folic acid. Chromosome breaks were seen less frequently in the culture containing folic acid. Grant R. Sutherland[143e] had shown earlier that folic acid not only inhibits expression of heritable fragile sites on human chromosomes but that methotrexate increases expression of those sites. (Induction of chromosome breaks in cancer cells by methotrexate is probably the mechanism by which this drug works in cancer therapy and the reason folic acid may negate the therapy.)

---

* We saw earlier that the anesthetic nitrous oxide can suppress vitamin B_2 metabolism and thereby act to inhibit some cancers in animals.[122b] Nitrous oxide also impairs folate metabolism. Yashuhiko Kano et al.[142d] and Kroes et al.[122c] have speculated that nitrous oxide alone or in combination with methionine or methotrexate might be of value for human cancer treatment. In some cases when methotrexate is ineffective in treating cancers, other antifolates have proved effective![142e-h]

There is a group for which supplementary folic acid could act as a cancer preventative. Folate taken by women using oral contraceptives may reduce the risk of cervical cancer. William A. Check[144] reported on the work of Charles E. Butterworth demonstrating that young women with mild to moderate cervical dysplasia showed improvement in the condition after taking 10 mg. of folate orally each day for three months. (There is no evidence that oral contraceptives increase the risk of cervical cancer of women in general, but they may hasten the progression of cervical dysplasia to carcinoma.) Based on their own research and that of S. Wassertheil-Smoller et al., Charles E. Butterworth and Denise Norris[145] conclude that deficiencies of both folic acid and of vitamin C are involved in the pathogenesis of cervical dysplasia. But remember, if you already have either detected or undetected cancer, folic acid supplementation might be harmful.

We noted earlier that the Pill can reduce the body's level of folic acid. A shortage of folic acid can also be caused by ingestion of various other drugs that tend to inhibit its absorption from food. One of these drugs is dilantin, which is prescribed for epileptics.* One might presume that when dilantin is used, taking a folic acid supplement might be advisable. Not necessarily so; folic acid is reported to sometimes throw an epileptic into convulsions. Could this be the body's way of telling the epileptic to refrain from taking supplementary folic acid? On the other hand, a study by T. del Ser Quijano et al.[145b] observed that serum folic acid levels were significantly lower in chronic epileptic outpatients and the lowest folic acid levels were found in those with the most severe psychological disturbances. How to handle folic acid deficiency in those with epilepsy is obviously problematical.

Not only dilantin but various other drugs can cause vitamin deficiencies. However, is it possible that this phenomenon is

---

* I am citing the generally held opinion that dilantin reduces the intestinal absorption of folate. E. W. Nelson et al.[145a] found that, in studying 11 subjects, dilantin had no such effect.

sometimes an example of "body wisdom,"* as it may be in the dilantin-folate reaction? How often in vitamin-drug interactions might supplementing with additional vitamins be just as deleterious as it could be in the dilantin-folate case?

In any event, if you are using a folic acid supplement and are under a doctor's care, be sure to tell him what you are doing. We have already mentioned the possible negatives in the use of folic acid by the cancer patient or by a patient on methotrexate therapy. Other drugs may also interact with folic acid. Various anticonvulsive drugs, cholestyramine, pyrimethamine, salicylates, sulphasalazine, triamterene and trimethoprim all decrease folic acid absorption or inhibit its functions.[140] Aspirin in therapeutic doses can also contribute to low folic acid levels.[145c] If any of these drugs have been prescribed, your physician may in some cases suggest an increase in folate supplementation.

Be cautious about using folic acid to excess. It is true that Alfred Zettner et al.[146] reported that large oral doses of 25 to 1,000 mg. given daily for a limited time in treating four hyperuricemic men gave no evidence of toxic effects. However, Joseph R. DiPalma and David M. Ritchie[147] found, to the contrary, that a large intake of folic acid can lead to renal cell hypertrophy. They noted that, in animal experiments, large doses of folic acid have caused an "increase in DNA synthesis and total protein content along with hypertrophy and hyperplasia of the kidney epithelial cells." Other possible toxicities of folic acid are controversial but include mental changes, sleep disturbances, gastrointestinal upset, malaise, irritability and excitability in normal volunteers.[147] Richard Hunter et al.[147a] orally administered 15 mg. of folic acid daily to men and women volunteers but abandoned the study "after 1 month of a projected 3-month period because of unexpected development of increasingly disturbing toxic effects in the majority." On the contrary, Lajla Hellström[147b] gave 15 mg. of folic acid or placebo daily to healthy volunteers in a double-blind randomized trial and reported that psychic reactions in

---

* The teleological argument of "body wisdom" seems, to me, to be valid and a logical derivative of the evolutionary process.

the two groups did not differ. Nevertheless, two studies, one with rats by P. C. Wilson et al.[147c] and another with men by D. B. Milne et al.,[147d] found that even modest levels of folic acid can depress zinc assimilation.* A study by Mukunda Mukherjee et al.[147f] showed that high plasma folate or low zinc levels in pregnant women were associated with fetal distress. Carl C. Pfeiffer[147g] warns that "folic acid in oral doses greater than 5 mg. per day is apt to produce muscle restlessness, myoclonic (muscle) jerking, and occasionally seizures (convulsions)." Glucose markedly increases the absorption of folic acid[147g] and will tend to make large dosages become huge dosages.

Sources of Folic Acid

Folic acid is manufactured by the intestinal bacteria. However, animal studies suggest that folic acid is absorbed primarily in the first third of the small intestines rather than in the colon where it is made. Excellent food sources for folic acid are black-eyed peas, liver, yeast, wheat germ, bran, dry beans (lentils, limas, navy), asparagus, spinach and other green leafy vegetables. (The vitamin's name derives from the word *foliage* since it was first isolated from the foliage-like leaves of spinach.) If allowed to stand at room temperature, however, vegetables lose much of their folic acid. The metabolism of vitamin B 12 and of folic acid are interlocked, the higher intake of one demanding commensurate increases in the other. One consuming excessive amounts of alcohol is, by the way, apt to be deficient in both these vitamins. (Beer drinkers are an exception,[147h] a fact that is probably related to the high content of folic acid in brewer's yeast.)

Para-aminobenzoic Acid

This tongue twister is called PABA for short. It was at one time mistakenly thought to be a vitamin.

---

* On the contrary, a study published in 1986 by L. Wada et al.[147e] showed that, in both the human and the rat, there was no adverse effect of folic acid on zinc absorption. In fact, the serum level when folic acid was given with zinc was higher, but not significantly higher, than the serum level resulting from zinc administered alone.

PABA may be a factor in delaying the onset of gray hair and has been reported to occasionally help gray hair to regain its natural color. Many investigators, however, have been unable to confirm this. C. J. D. Zarafonetis,[148] as reported by Franklin Bicknell and Frederick Prescott, succeeded in darkening gray hair when massive doses of PABA (6 to 48 grams daily) were given for long periods. Bicknell and Prescott do not rule out the possibility that PABA may have been acting, in this case, as an internal hair dye rather than as a vitamin. They warn against the continual ingestion of excessive PABA since it can cause leukopenia (a condition in which the number of leukocytes circulating in the blood is abnormally low).

PABA reputedly aids, as does pantothenic acid, the action of the adrenal glands in their production of cortisone and can, therefore, presumably be helpful in treating arthritis. It is said to act in some men, but only rarely in women, as an aphrodisiac, but I have seen no studies to support this statement. PABA (and also folic acid which contains PABA as part of its molecular structure) may be useful to postmenopausal women. In interacting with whatever estrogen production still exists, the PABA supposedly contributes to skin health. Krehl[148a] cites the work of Zarafonetis showing some value for PABA in treating lupus erythematosus, scleroderma and dermatitis herpetiformis. However, Krehl cautions that "toxic hepatitis, drug fever and nausea and vomiting may occasionally result from PABA, and much more careful work must be done before any serious recommendation can be made for its use in dermatological conditions."

In Chapter 2 I reported on the successful use of vitamin E to treat Peyronie's disease (which involves a bending in the penis that makes intercourse painful, if not impossible). Else Kierkegaard and Birgit Nielson[148b] reported success in treating such patients with vitamin E plus a large amount (12 grams daily in 3 divided doses) of the potassium salt of PABA, potassium para-aminobenzoate (KPAB). This same chemical has been used by Meyers[148c] (along with reserpine) in treating scleroderma with considerable relief of symptoms, healing of ulcers and increased joint mobility. Meyers stated that the good results were probably due more to the KPAB rather than to the reserpine.

PABA must not be taken if you are using the sulfonamides.[148d] The chemical composition of PABA and sulfa are similar. Harmful bacteria are "fooled into thinking" sulfa is PABA (which they normally eat) so they consume it and die. The presence of too much PABA would dilute the effect of the sulfa.

Applying an ointment containing PABA has proved effective in alleviating the effects of sunburn. PABA is said to form a chemical bond with the keratin layer. Therefore, it is considered best to apply the ointment about 45 minutes before going out in the sun. The PABA will then have sufficient time to build up a shield in the keratin layer that should protect one for several hours. However, P. J. Osgood et al.,[148e] using *in vitro* studies with a mouse lymphoma cell line, have reported that dermal binding with PABA may enhance a photocarcinogenic effect and so this product cannot be recommended. Osgood et al. emphasized, however, that their results do not necessarily predict a response of human skin to the presence of PABA during exposure to ultraviolet light.

A popular writer of a few years ago, Adelle Davis, recommended PABA ointment for treating unpigmented areas (vitiligo) of the skin. Like much of her other "information," this seems to be erroneous. Regarding PABA's presumed value in treating vitiligo, Franklin Bicknell and Frederick Prescott[149] say that "further investigations have failed to substantiate this."

PABA is reported to act as an antioxidant to scavenge those methyl and acetyl free radicals that would otherwise damage cells, and thus it may be an anti-aging factor. There is, by the way, a questionable rejuvenation technique which is related to PABA. The Rumanian rejuvenative therapy of Dr. Ana Aslan is based on giving the patients injections of procaine combined with potentiating ingredients, a combination which she calls Gerovital H$_3$. An oral version known as KH$_3$ is sold widely throughout Europe and a similar formulation, GH$_3$, is sold in the United States. In the body, procaine* breaks down into PABA and diethylaminoethanol (DEAE), which participates in the synthesis of choline and acetylcholine and which is related to DMAE (that will be discussed in Chapter 9). Before this transformation takes place, the procaine is said to have a direct beneficial effect on the central nervous system. It is conceivable that procaine finds its way to brain areas that may not be significantly permeated by procaine's breakdown products, PABA and DEAE, and is converted to these end products when those destinations are reached. (This theory is reminiscent of the well-known fact that DOPA penetrates the brain barrier and is then converted to dopamine, whereas dopamine itself will not cross that barrier.) Benjamin S. Frank, M.D., and Philip Miele[150] state that this breakdown of procaine leads to the creation of purines.

Many beneficial effects of GH₃ therapy are reported by some patients, for example, alleviation of arthritic symptoms and recoloration of hair. The mechanism of GH₃ therapy may involve a reactivation of the endocrine glands, especially of the pituitary and the adrenals. Procaine is reported to sometimes increase male potency, possibly because, unlike other MAO inhibitors, it is said to allow serotonin and norepinephrine to coexist. Most of the statements about GH₃ therapy are purely anecdotal; studies, when they exist, are often contradictory. Zung et al.[150a] found Gerovital to be efficacious in treating depression and indicated that it seemed to provide additional benefits. On the other hand, Edwin J. Olsen et al.[150b] and Israel Zwerling et al.[150c] reported negatively. A very thorough review by Adrian Ostfeld et al.,[150d] based on 285 articles and books describing the treatment of more than 100,000 patients over a period of 25 years, concluded that except for a possible antidepressant effect there is no convincing evidence of effectiveness.

Good sources for PABA are brewer's yeast, liver, milk, wheat bran, wheat germ, whole grain cereals, seeds, nuts, green leafy vegetables and molasses. In conclusion, let's note that supplemental use of PABA (orally or dermally or injected as procaine) is highly

---

* Procaine can be checked in the *Physicians' Desk Reference* under the brand name Novocain®. (There are many contraindications to the use of procaine.)

questionable, especially if your doctor is planning tests. (It falsifies the chymex pancreatic test.)[150e] The recommendation of several popular "nutrition" writers to take in excess of 1,000 mg. daily is unethical. Its safety has not been proved. Those with skin sensitivity and those who have had previous bouts with melanoma might be especially wary about excessive use of PABA.

Inositol

Inositol is sometimes called myoinositol to distinguish it from eight other stereoisomers. Like choline, inositol is usually found in only insignificant quantities in vitamin supplements. Inositol appears to be produced by the body in sufficient quantity to meet normal needs and thus it is no longer generally considered to be a vitamin.

Inositol is found in the body in the form of phosphatidylinositol in the phospholipids of cell membranes and in plasma lipoproteins. Inositol is a lipotropic substance, i.e., it plays a role in the metabolism of fats. Large amounts are present in heart muscle and brain and skeletal muscle, making it likely that it may serve functions in these tissues.[150f] Various investigators have, in fact, shown that inositol is synthesized from glucose in many tissues, including peripheral nerve, the lens of the eye, the kidney cortex and the intestinal mucosa.[151]

Inositol deficiency in animals causes an accumulation of triglycerides in the liver and intestinal lipodystrophy (a disturbance of fat metabolism, also called Whipple's disease, characterized by infiltration of the intestinal wall and lymphatics by glycoprotein-filled macrophages).[151a] Inositol metabolism has been found to be altered in human diabetics.[151a] Douglas A. Greene et al.[151b] reported that impairment of sciatic nerve conduction velocity in diabetics was associated with a decrease in free inositol compared with that present in the nerves of nondiabetics fed the same diet despite similar plasma levels in both groups. In rats, K. R. W. Gillon and J. N. Hawthorne[151c] discovered that inositol injected intraperitoneally restored nerve conduction velocity to normal. David A. Simmons et al.[151d] reported on observations that suggest impaired inositol concentrations in peripheral nerve may derange the processes regulating turnover of phosphatidylinositol. This condition, in turn, may contribute to the development of diabetic polyneuropathy. Such findings have led to interest in the possibility of modifying dietary intake of inositol for the prevention and treatment of disease.

Cathryn E. Stokes et al.[151e] have reported that inositol is concentrated in human anterior temporal cortex. This is the area thought to be associated with current memory, a problem with the aging human brain. Stokes et al. found that the inositol concentration in this area fell steadily with age until, at age 90, it was only about one-half that at age 20.

Ghafoorunissa[152] has reported that semen is the richest source of free inositol. Rat studies have suggested that inositol, after being synthesized from blood glucose, is secreted in the rat epididymis and that the secretory process is controlled by androgens.[152a] However, its presence in the male sex organs (females were not studied) is not altered by inositol deficiency, nor can oral inositol reach these organs in significant quantity. Thus, although it may be an important factor in sexual performance, it would appear that supplementary intake for this purpose is a waste of money.

Many pesticides contain lindane which is known to destroy inositol. There is evidence also that caffeine can destroy inositol. Sources for inositol include wheat germ, oatmeal, blackstrap molasses, lecithin, brewer's yeast, grapefruit, oranges, peaches, raisins, cantaloupe, peas, lima beans, cabbage, peanuts, nuts, sesame seeds, beef heart, beef brain and liver. Cereals contain inositol in the form of the hexaphosphate, *pytic acid*. It is partially available to the body through the action of the enzyme *phytase* which is found in the intestinal mucosa. Large amounts of inositol are present in human milk and so it may be a desirable additive in infant formulas.

Choline

Choline, like inositol, is a lipotropic substance. It is a constituent of plasmalogens, which are abundant in the mitochondria of the cells, and of sphingomyelin which is found in the brain. Many of the functions of choline relate to its being a source of labile methyl groups (CH₃). Methyl groups are commonly found in organic compounds, but they are generally fixed and not detachable. When a methyl group is detachable and can be transferred to another compound it is called *labile* and the process of transferring it is known as *transmethylation*. The process is employed by the body to construct many valuable substances. Choline, in providing labile methyl groups, therefore performs a desirable function. As a matter of fact, choline itself is formed in the liver by methyl groups combining with beta-hydroethylamine, which is itself produced in the body from methionine, assisted by folic acid and vitamin B₁₂. (Taking exogenous choline thus conserves body stores of methionine for other purposes such as building protein, removing lead from the body and destroying free radicals.) Betaine, the oxidative product of choline, may also serve as an important methylating agent when normal methylating pathways are impaired through ingestion of drugs such as alcohol or because of nutritional imbalances.[152b]

Choline is required to move digested fats from the liver to other parts of the body. A deficiency of choline produces liver and kidney disorders in rats. Administering choline to treat human liver disorders such as fatty liver and cirrhosis has, however, produced inconsistent results.[153]

Although choline is involved in the digestion of fats, perhaps even more important is its role, along with *acetyl coenzyme A* (which we met when we discussed pantothenic acid and the Krebs cycle) and the enzyme *choline acetyltransferase,* in producing acetylcholine. Acetylcholine is one of the neurotransmitters essential for the transmission of impulses along the nerves.* How acetylcholine is released by neural impulses and thus causes muscles

---

* In addition to acetylcholine, which acts at what are called *cholinergic-type synapses,* there are other neurotransmitters that operate at other types of synapses. Some of these other excitatory transmitters are *norepinephrine, dopamine* and *serotonin.* Possible excitatory transmitters, as given by Arthur C. Guyton,[154] are *L-glutamate* and *L-aspartate.* Inhibitory transmitters such as *gamma aminobutyric acid (GABA)* and *glycine* exist and *taurine* and *alanine* are suspected of acting as such. Many other neurotransmitters have been recently discovered.

to contract was discovered by Sir Bernard Katz. For this discovery he shared the Nobel Prize for Medicine or Physiology in 1970 with Ulf von Euler and Julius Axelrod. (Von Euler and Axelrod were cited for their work with another neurotransmitter, noradrenaline, also called norepinephrine.)

Acetylcholine fires neurons, probably because it increases the neuron's permeability, thus permitting positively-charged sodium ions to enter. The firing of the primary neuron across the synapse (the gap between a primary and a secondary neuron) stimulates the secondary neuron. After the secondary neuron is stimulated, acetylcholinesterase quickly inactivates the acetylcholine so the secondary neuron may rest prior to its next stimulation. The stimulation and refractory cycle happens many times per second and is facilitated by the presence of calcium ions but inhibited by the presence of magnesium ions. When such impulses arrive at a neuromuscular junction, muscles are activated. * However, in *myasthenia gravis* there is difficulty in transmitting nerve impulses to muscle fibers. It has been postulated that myasthenia gravis may be an autoimmune disease where the individual has developed antibodies against his own muscles, causing them to be damaged by those antibodies. Treatment generally involves inhibition (usually by a drug such as neostigmine or physostigmine) of the production of cholinesterase so the acetylcholine can build up enough, it is hoped, to result in activation of the muscle fiber.

---

* Among the body's muscles is, of course, the heart muscle and, based on animal experiments, one must consider the possibility of *reverse effects*. I. A. Boyd and C. L. Pathak[154a] have published concentration-response curves of the action of acetylcholine on perfused frog hearts. The first peak in the concentration-response curve occurred at 10^{-11} g./ml. in three hearts, at 10^{-13} g./ml. in seven hearts, at 10^{-15} g./ml. in two hearts and at 10^{-17} in one heart. A *reverse effect* occurred at 10^{-9} g./ml. in seven hearts and at 10^{-11} g./ml. in six hearts. Although these response curves show variation from heart to heart, on average there was increasing inhibition of the heart rate to a first peak as the concentration of acetylcholine rose to about 10^{-13} g./ml. This was followed by a *reverse effect* and declining inhibition as acetylcholine concentration continued to increase to about 10^{-9} g./ml. and then heart-rate inhibition finally reversed again and rose to cardiac arrest at an acetylcholine concentration of 10^{-7} g./ml. The great individual variation shown here in the concentrations at which *reverse effects* occurred in frog hearts warns us that possible *reverse effects* in human hearts could also take place at widely varying levels of acetylcholine.

Underactivity of cholinergic mechanisms (i.e., the mechanisms to produce acetylcholine) has been implicated in many diseases. Thus far, however, tardive dyskinesia (an iatrogenic side effect caused by use of neuroleptics in the management of psychotic illness) seems to be the only disorder whose symptoms have been reliably reduced by choline or lecithin.[154b,c]* However, different ranges of doses or durations of treatment may yet yield results in other diseases related to impaired cholinergic neurotransmission.[155] Successful use of choline and of lecithin in treating mania[156]** and ataxias[157] has been reported. Nevertheless, a recent report by Jan Volavka et al.[157a] that choline can be increased in plasma without any appreciable effect on EEG throws doubt on choline's ability to significantly affect cholinergic transmission.

Raymond Levy[158] wrote of the possible therapeutic value of choline in Alzheimer's senile dementia and calls it "probably the first rational approach to the treatment of this condition." Later, Levy[159] suggested judgment as to choline's efficacy in treating Alzheimer's dementia be withheld pending outcome of current trials. Paz Chuaqui and Raymond Levy[160] reported on the plasma levels of 12 patients participating in a double-blind trial of lecithin (a choline precursor) in senile or presenile Alzheimer's dementia. Choline levels show a decline after one or two months, often followed by a subsequent rise. The authors stated that all previous trials of lecithin in dementia have lasted between three weeks and three months, so it is possible that patients were assessed when plasma choline was at its lowest level. The relationship between the peak level of choline in the plasma and cognitive performance had been described in one study but then failed to be replicated in subsequent studies. Nevertheless, Chuaqui and Levy seem to imply that if choline can be maintained at a satisfactory level, the prognosis for Alzheimer's dementia may be improved. More recently, George A. Vroulis et al.[160a] used a double-blind crossover trial of piracetam plus lecithin (with 53%

---

* Lecithin was discovered in the latter half of the 19th century by Felix Hoppe-Seyler.[154d] In 1877 he founded the journal, *Hoppe-Seyler's Zeitschrift für Physiologische Chemie*. Many of the articles in this world-renowned publication are in English.

** Choline might potentiate the effects of lithium in treating manic patients.[156a]

phosphatidylcholine) to treat five Alzheimer's patients. They reported substantial memory improvement in three patients.

Erythrocyte choline levels have been reported by Bruce L. Miller et al.[160aa] and by other groups to be elevated in a subset of patients with Alzheimer's disease. This does not, however, suggest that choline may be detrimental to them. On the contrary, Miller and his associates noted that E. F. Domino et al.[160ab] reported patients with high baseline erythrocyte choline levels may respond better to treatment with oral lecithin than those with low levels. I speculate that these facts suggest erythrocytes may sometimes be detrimentally harboring choline rather than permitting it to engage in the formation of acetylcholine.

Choline, in large amounts, may act as a memory improver. Studies by N. Sitaram et al.[160b,c] showed that when healthy volunteers, aged 21 to 29, were given 10 grams of choline chloride, their ability to recall unrelated words was significantly increased. Stimulated production of acetylcholine, and its beneficial effect on neurotransmission, probably accounts for choline's reportedly good effect on memory. On the other hand, Kenneth L. Davis et al.[160d] reported that normal subjects given large amounts of choline chloride (4 grams, four times a day for a daily total of 16 grams) in a double-blind trial, showed no effects in either short-term or long-term memory. They suggest, however, that the effects of lower dosages of choline on long-term memory should be studied.*

---

* Edith L. Cohen and Richard J. Wurtman[160e] reported that free-choline concentrations in the blood serum and brain of the rat vary with dietary choline consumption. However, as noted earlier, Jan Volavka et al.,[157a] using psychiatric patients, found that choline can be increased in plasma and red blood cells by 300% or 400% without any effect on the EEG. They suggested this indicates choline in peripheral blood has no effect on central cholinergic transmission. If this study is replicated with nonpyschiatric patients, it would seem to throw doubt on the ability of dietary choline to aid not only memory but any other mental phenomena such as tardive dyskinesia or Alzheimer's disease. However, the work of Volavka, and any subsequent replication, needs to be reconciled with the earlier research of Dean R. Haubrich and A. Barbara Pflueger.[160f] They found, by measuring the concentration of dopamine's metabolite, homovanillic acid, in the rat brain, that oral administration of either choline or physostigmine stimulated the brain's metabolism of dopamine. Their studies indicated that choline augments central cholinergic function and suggested that the mechanism involves stimulation of the role of synthesis and release of acetylcholine.

Experiments cited by Dr. Roger J. Williams[161] showed that rats deprived of choline developed cancer. But, as Dr. Williams notes, "From these experiments, it cannot be concluded that choline is the only nutrient to be watched in connection with cancer prevention. It is not that simple. In these particular rats, choline may have been a limiting factor, but in other animals or human beings some other nutrient or nutrients might play a comparable role." This is a very important point. The most vital nutrients for any particular person are the ones in which he or she may be deficient.

Tomiko Ageta et al. [161a] have found choline in human semen but not in other human body fluids that were examined (saliva, vaginal fluid, blood, serum, urine and breast milk). The significance of the finding remains to be elucidated.

An increased choline requirement has been shown to exist in rats fed ethyl alcohol.[162] Alcohol alone fed to monkeys to the extent of 40%-50% of their calorie requirements did *not* result in cirrhosis or any other liver disease when the diet was complete. Alcohol did, however, induce cirrhosis when fed to rats in combination with a lipotrope-deficient diet that was not by itself cirrhogenic.[163] Regrettably, other experiments with subhuman primates have shown that chronic use of alcohol—even when consumed with an adequate diet—can lead to hepatitis and cirrhosis. [163a-c] It seems conclusive that, contrary to the widespread belief, an adequate diet will not prevent development of cirrhosis in alcoholics.

The liver and also the brain (as has been learned recently) can synthesize lecithin by methylation of phosphatidylethanolamine using phosphatidylethanolamine-N-methyltransferase (PeMT).[163d] The synthesis is dependent on the concentration of magnesium ions and on the pH. An *in vitro* study by Steven H. Zeisel et al.[163d] has shown that when the caudate lobe of calf liver is incubated in the presence of magnesium, formation increases with pH and reaches a maximum at 8.5 pH and then shows a *reverse effect* and declines. Without magnesium being present, lecithin production increases to a pH level of 7.5 but then shows a *reverse effect* at increasing levels of pH (Figure 2). Many other physiological phenomena occur with

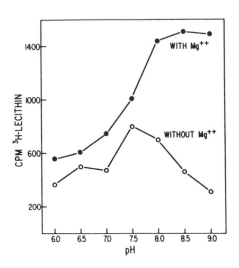

Figure 2. pH and magnesium dependence of PeMT. Reproduced from Steven H. Zeisel et al., *Nutrition and the Brain,* ed. A. Barbeau, J. H. Growden and R. J. Wurtman (New York: Raven Press, 1979) pp. 47-55, with permission of the publisher, Raven Press.

increasing efficiency until a pH level of 7 to 7.5 is achieved—i.e., the level present in the body—and then their efficiency generally declines.

All forms of choline, including that found in B complex pills or in lecithin, should be avoided in cases of parkinsonism, unless one's doctor indicates otherwise. Generally, in treating this disease, the attempt is made to block the action of acetylcholine rather than to encourage its formation.

If you are under a doctor's care and also decide, for whatever reason, to supplement your diet with choline (or lecithin) be sure your doctor knows. Lynn Wecker et al.[164] reported on studies with rats and mice that indicated dietary choline reduces the side effects and lethality of many drugs. (The microsomes of the cells are very active drug metabolizers and their major lipid is phosphatidylcholine.)[163e] Smokers might find it interesting to know that choline-supplemented chow greatly reduced nicotine toxicity in rats (but whether or not there is a human application has not yet been reported). These results suggest that choline can dramatically affect the detrimental action of some drugs and I think it could also conceivably reduce the beneficial action of the same or other drugs. Choline does, in fact, attenuate the analgesic effect of morphine in rats.[165] Perhaps this undesirable attenuation of a desirable effect could also occur in humans who have been prescribed morphine.

Food sources for choline include lecithin, brewer's yeast, liver and other organ meats, fish, egg yolk, milk, fruits, leafy green vegetables, wax beans, snap beans, soybeans, cabbage, peas, seeds, wheat germ and molasses.* Lecithin, for use as an emulsifier, is added to processed foods: about .3% in chocolate, .1% to .5% in margarine, up to 2% in bread dough and cake batter and .5% in ice cream.[165a] Large amounts of choline are present in foods, so it is doubtful that supplementation will generally serve a useful purpose except perhaps when excessive amounts of alcohol are consumed. Furthermore, the body can synthesize choline by using the labile methyl group of the amino acid methionine. It was, in fact, this reaction that led Du Vigneaud to develop the concept of transmethylation reactions. Since choline is made by the body and no cofactor for enzymatic action is known to contain choline, it is not generally considered to be a vitamin.

However, if you're going to take additional choline, you may wish to know that choline in tablets is generally in the form of *choline chloride, choline bitartrate* or *choline dihydrogen citrate,* which must be converted to phosphatidylcholine (a precursor of acetylcholine) by the body.** Thus, it is more efficient to take choline in the form of phosphatidylcholine, which is available in lecithin, so the body does not have to use up nutrients and energy to make the

---

* On the other hand, the edible portions of many plants inhibit cholinesterase activity. (We met acetylcholinesterase—one of the cholinesterases—earlier in explaining how acetylcholine functions at the synaptic knobs in facilitating neurotransmission.) Among these plants are broccoli, beets, asparagus, eggplant, potatoes, turnips, radishes, celery, carrots, horseradishes, oranges and apples. Raspberry leaves, white clover, yellow jessamine and boxwood, often recommended by herbalists, also inhibit such activity.[166]

** A rat study by A. A. Odutuga and A. J. Ogunleye[166a] showed that phosphatidylcholine was increased in vitamin E deficiency.

conversion. Richard J. Wurtman et al.[166b] have, in fact, reported that lecithin is considerably more effective in raising human serum choline levels than equivalent amounts of choline. However, the widely touted reason for using lecithin supplementation, namely to reduce cholesterol levels, is in doubt. Margaret Cobb et al.[167] fed healthy human volunteers 7.5 grams of lecithin three times daily for a four-week period. They found no evidence of a reduction in blood cholesterol nor did they find a change in the lipids of the bile.* On the other hand, lecithin is reported by Marian T. Childs et al.[168] to beneficially increase HDL levels in humans. It also beneficially lowers LDL levels, but does not do so as effectively as does corn oil.

If one is going to employ lecithin supplementation, it should be done thoughtfully. Lecithin is generally processed with hexane and some remnants may remain. Then too, commercial lecithin contains considerable amounts of linoleic acid which may form peroxides even if protected by encapsulation since oxygen can diffuse through the capsule. Powdered lecithin should probably be vacuum sealed or packed with nitrogen and kept under refrigeration. Furthermore, high intakes of lecithin or choline may produce gastrointestinal distress, anorexia, depression and disturbance of the cholinergic-dopaminergic-serotoninergic balance.[168f]

Biotin

Biotin, formerly known as vitamin H, is associated with a healthy skin and is a factor in the metabolism of protein and fat .

---

* Carlos Krumdieck and C. E. Butterworth[168a] noted that J. R. Murphy[168b] showed not all lecithins serve equally well as substrates for the lecithin: cholesterol acyltransferase (LCAT) enzyme, the main catalyst for cholesterol esterification. Krumdieck and Butterworth also reported that the polyunsaturated lecithin from soybeans has been found by C. W. M. Adams et al.[168c,d] to accelerate the resorption of cholesterol much more effectively than the relatively saturated lecithin from eggs. The soybean lecithin was much more effective in preventing cholesterol-induced atheroma in the rabbit. A study by Madelyn J. Hirsch et al.[168e] showed that lecithin consumption also lowered serum cholesterol concentration in healthy volunteers, although it increased serum triglyceride levels. It will be interesting to observe whether the study of Hirsch et al. or that of Cobb et al. is replicated by further research. (Follow such future research by making use of *Citation Abstracts* as discussed in the introduction.)

Biotin's primary mode of action is through enzymes in association with the amino acid lysine. One related role of biotin is to act in carboxylation reactions where, as discussed in connection with vitamin B6, carbon dioxide is transferred from an enzyme to other compounds. Biotin is a cofactor of a number of enzymes called *carboxylases* which are needed to catalyze carboxylation, and it has been suggested that defective intestinal absorption of biotin can result in multiple carboxylase deficiency.[169] The carboxylase of acetyl coenzyme A is vital in the working of the Krebs cycle which we discussed earlier in this chapter in connection with pantothenic acid. Many of the properties of biotin relate to this function or to its use in the synthesis of fatty acids, its role in the production of energy from glucose or the part it plays in the formation of nucleic acid, glycogen and some of the amino acids.

Some persons with inherited disorders of biotin-dependent carboxylases may be helped by huge supplementary intake of this vitamin.[169a] There are two major forms of these inherited disorders. There may be a primary enzyme deficiency in the activity of biotin holocarboxylase synthetase, the enzyme that attaches biotin to various apocarboxylases forming holoenzyme.[169a] The second major disorder relates to a deficiency in the enzyme biotinidase. This enzyme catalyzes the cleavage of biotin from biocytin or biotinyl peptides.[4b,169a-c] B. Wolf et al.[169a] state that all children with a biotinidase deficiency have improved clinically after being given oral biotin.

A shortage of biotin is variously (often anecdotally) reported to cause cancers to grow more rapidly and to induce fatigue, sleepiness, loss of appetite, high cholesterol levels in the blood, heart trouble, muscular pain, dry scaly skin, skin infections, loss of hair, sores on the tongue, nervousness, mental depression and insomnia. Isobel W. Jennings[142] reports that,"in biotin-deficient rats, deficiency of male sex hormones causes degeneration of testes with delayed spermatogenesis and abnormal spermatocytes."

Biotin is a cofactor of an enzyme used by the body to manufacture the amino acid arginine. When arginine is in short

supply the sex drive of both men and women decreases and, at least
in mice, the thymus gland is adversely affected. When the thymus is
affected then, generally, the immune system will also be affected.
Morton J. Cowan et al.[170] reported on three siblings with deficiencies
in several carboxylases which depend on the cofactor biotin, thus
suggesting inherited defects in biotin metabolism. Although two of
the children died, 10 mg. of oral biotin daily corrected the
Candida dermatitis, corneal ulceration and alopecia in the third.
Many studies show that biotin, vitamins B_6 and B_{12} and other
members of the B complex are needed in optimal amounts for a well-
functioning immune system.

I know of no research that relates biotin to human fertility.
However, P. H. Brooks et al.[171] reported that sows whose feed was
supplemented with biotin produced more live piglets than did
controls. Also, the remating interval was significantly reduced on
average from 15.31 days to 6.23 days. Just because biotin may make
sows sexy and/or fertile is no reason to expect a similar action in men
and women. However, as we noted above, biotin is related to the
body's production of arginine which may have sexual implications.

Biotin may also be of value in combating the graying of hair.
Both biotin and pantothenic acid deficiency result in graying of the
fur of black mice,[172] but whether or not the phenomenon occurs in
the hair of humans remains to be demonstrated. Perhaps even more
important for hair care in men is biotin's reported propensity to
metabolize excess dihydrotestosterone to products that will not inhibit
hair growth. It is said to also aid the process of moving cystine
molecules into the hair shaft, thus facilitating protein synthesis and
hair growth. A biotin-responsive immunodeficiency associated with
alopecia was reported by Brendan M. Charles et al.[173] Nevertheless,
the role of biotin in hair health is at best controversial.

We have noted the many postulated causes of sudden infant
death syndrome (SIDS) and will be discussing the problem further in
the next chapter. A deficiency of biotin is implicated as a possible
cause. A. R. Johnson et al.[174] reported that the livers of infants dying
of SIDS were significantly lower in biotin than livers of infants of
similar age who died of explicable causes.

The Vitamin B Complex

Biotin is produced by the intestinal bacteria, but this production can be adversely affected by sulfa drugs. Excellent food sources are royal jelly and torula yeast. (Torula is far superior to brewer's yeast as a source for biotin, but this is not, in my opinion, a sufficient reason for preferring torula over brewer's yeast.) Good food sources for biotin are liver, brewer's yeast, wheat germ, egg yolk, corn, unpolished rice, peanuts, nuts, soybeans, lima beans, peas, cauliflower, mushrooms, cane molasses and milk.

Many nutritionists believe that one should avoid eating raw egg white. Not only can raw eggs present a possible source of salmonella poisoning, but they contain avidin (also called avid-albumin) which combines with biotin and makes it unavailable to the body. Franklin Bicknell and Frederick Prescott[175] report that the avidin in the white of one raw egg will combine with approximately 20 micrograms (mcg.) of biotin. However, Bicknell and Prescott also cite the work of I. I. Kaplan[176] who reported about his treatment of a group of ten cancer patients. Dr. Kaplan maintained each of them on a diet low in biotin through their eating the whites of 36 to 42 eggs daily. No beneficial effect on the disease was noted, but it was considered that the general condition of the patients was markedly improved and they showed no biotin deficiency.* On the contrary, studies cited by Jean-Pierre Bonjour[176b] indicate that "egg-white injury" can occur when there is an excessive intake of raw eggs.

Anyone who would rather not take the risk of salmonella poisoning or of losing biotin through eating raw eggs, might prefer to poach or boil them. The biotin-binding propensity of the egg white is, however, largely offset by the biotin contained in the yolk (about 12 micrograms). In fact, when Kogl and Toennis, in 1936, first isolated a crystalline substance and named it biotin, it was egg yolk that they used as their raw material. Anyway, an experiment with rats conducted by Ruth Okey[177] suggests that excess biotin is beneficially reduced by avidin. This research indicated (as had earlier studies by G. Gavin and E. W. McHenry) that biotin may lead to deposition of

---

* Many years later, in 1985, R. P. Bhullar and K. Dakshinamurti [176a] reported that HeLa cells cultured in a biotin-deficient medium showed a reduced rate of protein synthesis. It should not astonish us that cancer cells, like other cells, require vitamins to function.

excess dietary cholesterol in the liver. There was even some indication that avidin may help remove excess cholesterol deposits from the liver, but if avidin is used up combining with biotin it will not be available to remove cholesterol. This then is yet another example of the thesis that vitamin overdose may be dangerous. The fact that Vincent du Vigneaud[*] reported, in 1947, that biotin showed a procarcinogenic effect with butter-yellow (a carcinogen that is no longer used to color butter or margarine) also emphasizes that one should generally avoid megadoses. As far as I know, studies of biotin's possible procarcinogenic effects with other carcinogenic hydrocarbons have not yet been made. Until they are, go easy on excessive use of this vitamin.

"Vitamin B₁₅"—Pangamic Acid

Substances called "vitamin B_{15}" have, for many years, been used in Russia, in Germany and in other countries and often called *pangamic acid* or *calcium pangamate*. "B_{15}" is not, however, a vitamin. A *vitamin* is defined by Victor Herbert, M.D., as an "organic chemical compound which is neither carbohydrate, fat, nor protein; which is necessary for normal human metabolism; which the body does not make itself in adequate amounts to sustain normality, so lack of which produces a specific vitamin deficiency disease (such as beriberi, pellagra, rickets, or scurvy), and provision of which corrects that deficiency." The body does not become diseased when we withhold the various substances called "B_{15}" and so "B_{15}" is obviously not a vitamin.

Most of the remarkable reports about so-called "vitamin B_{15}" are based on Russian research and, regrettably, we are not sure just what formula they have been using. It now turns out that most extant literature is hopelessly obsolete. The 8th edition of *The Merck Index* states that diisopropylamine dichloroacetate, sodium gluconate and glycine are ingredients of pangamic acid. The 9th edition of *The*

---

[*] Du Vigneaud was awarded the Nobel Prize in Chemistry in 1955 for work on pituitary hormones.

Merck Index gives the structure of pangamic acid as *D-gluconic* acid 6-bis(1-methylethyl) amino acetate. The 10th edition[177a] states there is no clear chemical identity for pangamic acid and products sold under this name vary considerably in composition. In spite of its lack of status as a vitamin, I will continue to use the phrase "vitamin B 15" as a shorthand expression for talking about substances said to have "B 15 activity."

There are three major forms of "vitamin B15." The one patented by Ernst Krebs, Jr. [177b] combines calcium with d-glucono-dimethyl aminoacetic acid but is not commercially available. The "B15" that was commercially available until recently supposedly had as its main ingredient N,N-dimethylglycine (known simply as DMG). Victor Herbert, M.D.[178] states, however, that DMG products do not appear to be dimethylglycine but methylglycine hydrochloride, which is of different composition and reactivity. Another commercial form combines calcium or sodium compounds with diisopropylamine dichloroacetate and is known as DIPA for short. Dichloroacetate has been found to be mutagenic and, therefore, probably carcinogenic.[179,179a] Furthermore, DMG is a tertiary amine that has been found to react with sodium nitrite in amounts simulating salivary and gastric nitrites to produce the carcinogenic substance nitrososarcosine and the more dangerous dimethylnitrosamine.[180,180a]

One of the reported benefits of "vitamin B15" is to supply methyl groups. (You will recall that we discussed transmethylation earlier in this chapter in connection with choline.) Dr. Roger Kendall of Food Science and Da Vinci Laboratories (who manufactured the DMG form of "B15" and now markets DMG as a solo supplement) states that the DIPA form, although containing many methyl groups does not act as well as the DMG type as a methyl donor, i.e., the methyl groups are not "labile." In fact, Victor Herbert,[181] relates that the DIPA type sometimes *worsens* methyl depletion and creates kidney problems in rats. Furthermore, Dr. Herbert states that, contrary to the statement of Dr. Kendall, the DMG type does not have labile methyl groups either. Transmethylation is absolutely vital to life for creating essential substances including adrenaline, creatine and phosphocreatine (the latter two being important in connection with the operation of the muscles). Transmethylation is also required for detoxifying poisons. The body continually excretes methyl groups and so they must be replaced. We noted earlier that choline is a methyl donor, but it would appear that the nonvitamin "B15" is not. Furthermore, Woodward,[45a] based on rat studies, reported that N,N-dimethylglycine actually has an antimethyl action.

The oxygen-sparing effects of "B15" have been reported by several observers. If true, this would be important for athletes, of course, but announced effects of "B15" in reducing the buildup of lactic acid, if true, would be perhaps of even greater importance. An article by L. Barnes[182] reported on a study by Thomas V. Pipes of the Institute of Human Fitness, Escondido, California. Dr. Pipes did a one-week double-blind comparison of 5 mg. daily DMG with a placebo in 12 male college track athletes. His subjects ran to exhaustion on a treadmill both before and after the test week with each athlete training normally during the test week. Dr. Pipes found that the DMG group showed a 23.6% increase in time to exhaustion.

However, Robert N. Girandola et al.,[183] reporting on a study of subjects orally ingesting six .40 gram tablets of calcium gluconate and N,N-dimethylglycine (a former, popular formula for "B15"), reached a contrary conclusion. During acute, submaximal exercise, these subjects, when compared with controls, showed no difference in oxygen kinetics during exercise or recovery, heart rates and resting or exercise blood lactates. The scientists concluded that the "pangamic-acid" resulted in no metabolic or circulatory advantages. D. G. Black and A. A. Sucec[183a] similarly found no measurable effect on aerobic endurance in a controlled study of 18 physically active men upon daily administration of six 50 mg. tablets containing DMG and calcium gluconate.

More recently, M. Harpaz et al.,[183b] in a double-blind, placebo-controlled crossover study, observed the effects of 200 mg./day of N,N-dimethylglycine on 20 active males doing aerobic exercise. After 21 days of treatment with "B15" there was no apparent advantage to the use of this nonvitamin in either submaximal or maximal performance.

In related research, G. Lynis Dohm et al.[184] studied the effect of various pangamic acid preparations on the endurance of exercised rats. None of the substances affected time to reach exhaustion by treadmill running, nor physiological parameters relating to liver or muscle function, nor the urinary excretion of creatinine. Another study by Michael E. Gray and Larry M. Titlow[184a] similarly concluded that orally administering six 50 mg. tablets of pangamic acid (Gluconic 15) daily to track athletes produced no significant changes in short-term maximal treadmill performance.

"Vitamin B15" has been used in treating atherosclerosis, skin problems, emphysema, eczema, mental retardation, alcoholism, asthma, arthritis, diabetes, chronic hepatitis and cirrhosis of the liver. Bernard Rimland, Ph.D., Director of the Institute for Behavior Research located in San Diego, California, has reported "vitamin B15" to be of value in treating speech defects as well as for use with retarded, autistic and emotionally disturbed children. I suspect that most of these results achieved through use of "B15" were figments of the imagination. However, a controlled study relating to immune response has shown "B15" to be beneficial. Charles D. Graber et al.[185] have reported on the immune-response-modifying properties of DMG in humans. The Graber group found a four-fold increase in antibody response to pneumonococcal vaccine in those receiving DMG orally as compared with controls. Other than the generally discredited Russian experiments, this would seem to be one of a very few studies supporting any "B15" or B15 component.

Do not allow anything I have said to encourage you to use the nonvitamin "B15" or whatever replacements follow its commercial demise. (Currently one answer to the possibly pending death of "vitamin B15" is the marketing of DMG without any other ingredients.) I have pointed out earlier that the DMG type of "B15" (and of course DMG itself) is reported to encourage formation of nitrosamines which are carcinogenic. I also pointed out that the still-available DIPA type, although banned for sale by the FDA, is mutagenic (and probably carcinogenic) and also that it may reduce (rather than increase) the methyl groups available for body chemistry. Furthermore, P. W. Stacpoole et al.[186] state that dichloroacetate causes hind limb paralysis, degeneration of testes and vacuolation of myelinated tracts of the cerebrum in rats and dogs. Dogs show ocular lesions and a man developed polyneuropathy. Then too, Dr. Victor Herbert[181] concludes that the massive "evidence" for the beneficial effects of "pangamic acid" is largely anecdotal and that there is a dearth of controlled studies. Let's remind the "vitamin" sellers of the ancient Hippocratic dictum: *Above all, do no harm.* Do not sell us cancer and other illnesses under the guise of "nutrition"!

"Vitamin B₁₇"—Laetrile

Amygdalin (or laetrile with a small letter "l") has been reported to be an effective control for cancer. "Laetrile" (with a capital "L") is a trademark for a substance patented by E. T. Krebs and E. T. Krebs, Jr.[187] which they claimed to have synthesized. (Amygdalin is the chemical D-mandelonitrile-beta-D-glucosido-6-beta-D-glucoside, while laetrile has the formula 1-mandelonitrile-beta-glucuronic acid. Each, however, has several alternate chemical names.)[187a] More recently, Laetrile was synthesized by a group of scientists[188] working at Johns Hopkins University and with the U.S. Food and Drug Administration. Interestingly, they found this substance, and also amygdalin, to be mutagenic on the Ames test. Since mutagenicity strongly suggests carcinogenicity, this is, indeed, a challenging twist of events. However, the *reverse effect* might, conceivably, be applicable to defend the possibility that laetrile (in different dosages) could be an agent acting both as a cure and as a cause of cancer. Laetrile is not a vitamin, but I will continue to use the term "vitamin B₁₇" (with quotation marks) given it by the Krebs.

Amygdalin was so-named by Robiquet and Boutron Charlard who, in 1830, first isolated it from bitter almond. (It was synthesized by Campbell and Haworth in 1924.) A related cyanide-containing glucoside, named *linamarin,* was isolated by Jorissen and Hairs in 1891. A few years later, Dustan and Henry isolated the cyanophoric glucosides *lotusin* and *dhurrin* and rediscovered linamarin, which they named *phaseolunatin.* The cyanide-based prussic acid is present in about 50 orders of higher plants. Among the glucosides that have been isolated, in addition to those already named, are sambunigrin, prulaurasin, prunasin, vicianin, corynocarpin, taxiphyllin, manihotoxin, lotaustralin, acacipetalin, triglochinin and gynocardin. These various plant-derived sources of prussic acid, other than amygdalin, seem to have been largely ignored in cancer research. (Scientists desiring to explore the cancer-controlling possibilities of naturally occurring cyanophoric glucosides other than amygdalin could begin their studies with *Cyanogenesis in Plants* by Muriel Elaine Robinson.[189] This article is extensively referenced with about 75 citations. Scientists may also find the chapter by Eric E. Conn[190] with 31 citations in *Toxicants Occurring Naturally in Foods,* to be of considerable interest.)

"Vitamin B17" is found in apricot kernels, as well as in the kernels of most other fruits, especially quince, peaches, plums, cherries, apples and nectarines. Ernst T. Krebs, Jr.[191] says: "When civilized man eats less than the whole fruit, for example by discarding the seed or kernel, he experiences a specific and total deficiency not only in oils and proteins but in minerals and such vitamins as vitamin B17 (nitriloside) which is found only in the seed, not in the flesh of the fruit. By discarding the seed or kernel, man experiences a specific and total deficiency of vitamin B17 so far as that fruit is concerned. Let me remind you that were man by circumstances limited to no source of food but apricots, peaches, plums, cherries and the like and ate only their fruit without their seeds he would in a short time develop a fatal deficiency in proteins and fats, not to mention vitamins. He would die from this deficiency just as the white rats (in an experiment performed by Dr. Roger Williams) died from the deficiency produced by eating only the starch of wheat without the seed germ and bran. But if he ate the seeds or kernels with the fruit flesh, he would get proteins, fats and other nutrients essential to health." What Krebs fails to say is that such a person might eventually die from cyanide poisoning.

Cranberries, crabapples, red and black raspberries, blackberries, blueberries, loganberries, boysenberries, huckleberries and gooseberries, alfalfa tops, beet tops, macadamia nuts, bitter (but not the ordinary) almonds, navy beans, broad beans, garden peas and most other legumes are also rich in "vitamin B17." Apple seeds contain quite a bit of this "vitamin." Millet and buckwheat are especially rich in "vitamin B17." Sprouted seeds contain much greater quantities than do the corresponding plants when mature.

John Beard, Ph.D., of the University of Edinburgh, many years ago in 1902, developed the trophoblastic theory of cancer. Since then the theory has been expanded by Dr. Ernst T. Krebs, Sr., Ernst T. Krebs, Jr., Dr. Howard Beard (no relation) and by doctors in various countries (primarily, until recently, outside of the United States). The trophoblastic theory states that a certain type of cell produced in the pregnant female is similar to the type of cell that becomes a cancer cell. Occurring in the pregnant female, such a cell is perfectly normal. But when such a cell occurs in a nonpregnant female or in a male, it is a pathological occurrence and cancer may result. These cells, with their possibly dangerous consequences, are stimulated by the presence of estrogen but are, on the other hand, supposedly controlled in healthy persons by a proteolytic enzyme called chymotrypsin. (Proteolytic enzymes are chemicals that hydrolyze protein—i.e., along with water, they convert protein into proteoses, then into peptones, then into peptides and, finally into amino acids. The process is called *proteolysis*.) However, chymotrypsin exists primarily in the pancreas (surrounded while it remains there by an inhibitor so the organ will not be digested) and in the alkaline pH of the intestines where it digests polypeptides.

A modest number of intact protein molecules will pass from the gastrointestinal tract into the bloodstream. Specifically, J. L. Ambrus et al.[192] and S. Avakian[193] showed that trypsin and chymotrypsin are absorbed into the bloodstream from the intestinal tract of humans. However, if any considerable amount of proteolytic enzymes circulated in the bloodstream, good tissue, as well as cancerous tissue, would be digested. This fact would seem to me to undermine the trophoblastic theory.* However, the theory continues to be

---

* Inhibitors of trypsin and chymotrypsin, found in seeds of corn and soybeans, have been shown to also inhibit tumor promotion and to arrest emphysema.[194] Protease inhibitors in seeds of rice, beans and corn inhibit breast, colon and skin cancers in animal experiments.[194a] However, this could simply exemplify the *reverse effect* rather

promulgated by those advocating the use of laetrile.** For the same reason it seems to me irrelevant to take proteolytic enzymes by mouth to either fight cancer or to prevent its occurrence. Yet this practice is often prescribed by "metabolic therapists" as part of a regime for treating the cancer patient and by some nutritionists as a preventive measure.

Ernst T. Krebs, Jr., in working with chymotrypsin, found that it did not seem to be able to control cancer that had already started. Therefore, he felt that the search for a cancer-control agent would have to continue. Krebs's long-continuing search that was to end in the development of the reputed anticancer factor laetrile is told in a fascinating manner in the book, *Laetrile—Control for Cancer,* by Glenn D. Kittler.[195] (To give balance, however, to Kittler's excessive enthusiasm, read *Nutrition Cultism: Facts and Fiction* by Victor Herbert[196] or Dr. Herbert's article entitled *Laetrile, The Cult of Cyanide.*)[197]

Krebs reported that enzymes called beta glucosidases accumulate in large quantities near cancer cells. He maintains that these enzymes exist throughout the body but are supposed to be present in much larger concentrations near cancerous areas.*** After extensive work, Krebs reportedly developed, from apricot seeds, a nitriloside compound, *lae*vomandeloni*trile*-beta-glucuronide, i.e., "Laetrile." It is presumed that the beta glucosidases that are present in the

---

than condemn the trophoblast theory. Nevertheless, the mechanism by which trypsin inhibitors fight cancer probably relates to their property of blocking neutrophil production of superoxide.[194b] (We will consider superoxide in Chapter 9.)

** Furthermore, this error has encouraged the use of low-protein diets in treating cancer under the theory that chymotrypsin should be saved for killing trophoblasts rather than being used up in digesting protein. But animal protein, including meat and dairy products, is needed to supply adequate amounts of iron, calcium and possibly also of vitamin B_{12} or the cancer patient must receive supplements to meet deficiencies in these nutrients. (However, we noted earlier in this chapter that B_{12} may more often be associated with the *cause* rather than with the *cure* of cancer.) Then too, eating a diet consisting mainly of fruits and vegetables could leave the cancer patient short of an adequate caloric intake, which might exacerbate a possibly already-emaciated condition.

*** Irving J. Lerner[198] states that beta glucosidase does not exist *in vivo.* Thus, an injected dose of laetrile is probably excreted intact in the urine without any significant metabolic consequences. Food does contain beta glucosidase, however, so oral laetrile is not always so innocuous.

cancerous area act on laetrile, releasing its cyanide component and also a chemical called benzaldehyde, both of which act, according to trophoblastic theory, to kill the cancer cells. Neither the cyanide nor the benzaldehyde injures normal cells, according to this theory, since those cells contain an enzyme *rhodanese* which renders these chemicals innocuous and the cyanide is excreted in the urine as thiocyanate.* That's the theory, but what are the facts? D. M. Greenberg[199b] shows that the area of the cancer cell contains neither more beta glucosidase nor less rhodanese. Furthermore, Victor Herbert[197] cites several references for the fact that cyanide is not immediately detoxified to thiocyanate by rhodanese. Finally, says Dr. Herbert,[197] human cancer cells do *not* release cyanide from laetrile—and so the fundamental tenet of the trophoblastic theory is false.

Cyanide poisoning from the eating of foods does exist. A thought-provoking book, *Toxic Constituents of Plant Foodstuffs*, edited by Irvin E. Liener[200] is an excellent place to begin your investigations of this subject and should prove to be intriguing. Certain grasses, pulses, root crops and fruit kernels containing cyanogenetic glucosides can be life threatening. Evidence suggests that the isothiocyanate in millet may be responsible for endemic goiter that occurs in 51% of the population in a province of western Sudan.[201]

At least six different cyanogenetic glucosides have been identified in edible plants: amygdalin, prunasin, dhurrin, sambunigrin, lotaustralin and linamarin. Amygdalin (often confused with laetrile) and prunasin are found in the bitter almond and in the kernel of fruits of the Rosaceae family. Dhurrin is found in sorghum and in other grasses. Sambunigrin is present in the elderberry. Lotaustralin and

---

* Thiocyanate may not be as innocuous as supporters of the trophoblastic theory would like you to believe. It is a goitrogenic agent. It has been reported [199] that in eastern Nigeria, where an unfermented form of cassava (containing a cyanogenetic glucoside) is a principal item in the diet, goiter is very common. I. B. Umoh et al. [199a] have implicated thiamin deficiency as a factor in tropical ataxic neuropathy in persons eating large amounts of cassava and cassava derivatives that contain the nitriloside limarin. Perhaps those taking laetrile might also be more likely to be poisoned if they are deficient in thiamin.

linamarin are found in pulses (the edible seeds of leguminous plants such as peas and beans), in flaxseed and in cassava. Foods containing these cyanide compounds that are generally consumed by humans, as reported by Dr. Liener, are: cassava, sweet potato and yam; maize and millet; bamboo and sugar cane; peas and beans—especially lima or butter bean; kernels of almond, lemon, lime, apple, pear, cherry, apricot and plum (including the prune). In early years of the 20th century a species of lima beans was responsible for poisoning of humans and of animals in Europe. Bitter almonds have also caused death, and oil of bitter almonds was, at one time, a not uncommon means of committing suicide. Poisonings from cassava have been reported periodically for hundreds of years. In light of such reported poisonings from cyanide-containing foods, should we not ask just how completely rhodanese protects normal cells? A meal where many of these foods might be consumed at the same time is probably unsafe.

Cyanide's usual mode of action is that of a respiratory inhibitor, its site of action being the enzyme *cytochrome oxidase*. A Keith Brewer,[202] states that cyanide also enhances the uptake of potassium by the cancer cell, thus raising its pH (and cancer cells are reported to die in a few hours when their pH reaches 8.5 or higher). * By the way, Max Gerson, M.D., whose unorthodox cancer therapy of a generation ago stressed consumption of foods containing potassium, would be pleased to know a rationale now exists for a conclusion he arrived at through clinical experience. If Dr. Brewer's work is valid it would seem that potassium, rather than laetrile, is the more vital component of "laetrile therapy" (although that does not imply the therapy is safe). Perhaps the nomenclature will be changed to "high-pH therapy" and laetrile simply relegated to the position of

---

* They also are reported to die at a pH of 6 or under, as occurs in hyperthermia therapy. Any deviation from a pH of 7 to 7.1 in either normal or cancerous cells leads to death of the cell.[202a] Cancer cells lose their ability to control their pH and are thus more readily destroyed than are normal cells by pH manipulative techniques.[202b] M. Von Ardenne[202a] explains that aerobic glycolysis of cancer cells (discovered by Warburg over a half-century ago) makes it possible to induce a useful element of selectivity between cancerous and normal tissue by increasing the acidity of the cancerous tissue. This is achieved through raising the blood glucose concentration.

potentiating the cell membrane to allow potassium to enter. * By the way, cyanide, entirely apart from its possible role in treating cancer, may be of some value to the body. R. D. Montgomery[203] has suggested that trace amounts of cyanide may benefit the body by acting as a brake in cellular oxidative processes.

Although enthusiasts have concentrated their attention on laetrile's cyanide fraction, they have paid little attention to its benzaldehyde component. Fig fruit has been used in folk medicine throughout the world as an anticancer agent. M. Kochi et al.[203a] found that fig extracts suppressed Ehrlich carcinoma in mice. Then, Setsuo Takeuchi et al.[204] reported that the active carcinostatic agent in fig is benzaldehyde. They also reported success in preventing papilloma in mice by oral induction of benzaldehyde combined with beta-cyclodextrin. More importantly, they announced that oral ingestion of enteric-coated benzaldehyde and beta-cyclodextrin tablets were effective in treating human cancer patients with adenocarcinoma and squamous cell carcinoma. Furthermore, they discovered that this benzaldehyde product was more effective against human malignant tumors than against experimental tumors in mice. In related work, Kochi et al.[204a] treated 90 patients having inoperable carcinoma in terminal states and 12 patients in serious condition with benzaldehyde in the form of beta-cyclodextrin benzaldehyde orally and rectally at a daily dose of 10 mg./kg. in four doses. They reported that "19 patients responded partially (>50% regression)." In two subsequent studies, Pettersen et al. reported that the effect of benzaldehyde on human cervical cancer cells involved a reduced rate of protein synthesis[204b] and that above a concentration of 6.4 mM there was a marked decrease in survival of these cells..[204c] Akoko Ishida et al.,[204d] in related work, found that the cytotoxic effect of

---

* Since potassium is the main cation in cancer tissue regardless of diet, [202b] might it, instead, be better to attempt inhibiting the cancer cells' uptake of this element? Cancer cells contain only miniscule amounts of calcium compared to normal cells. [202b] If they could, somehow, be forced to take up more calcium and less potassium, would their growth be inhibited? Some success in fighting cancer has been achieved by fostering the absorption of rubidium and cesium by cancer cells since these elements transport only water into the cells, whereas potassium carries glucose in addition to water. [202b] This phenomenon is discussed further in Chapter 7.

either benzaldehyde or hyperthermia on HeLa cells was enhanced when both were used together. To strike a negative note, however, Raymond Taetle and Stephen B. Howell,[204e] while reporting benzaldehyde inhibited certain leukemia cells, concluded that benzaldehyde "lacks significant activity against most human tumors tested."

Laetrile has been used for cancer control in Mexico and in other countries. (However, the often-heard statement that laetrile is legal and freely prescribed in many countries is apparently false.) Laetrile is used intravenously at levels of about three to nine grams per day. Laetrile is not considered, even by enthusiasts, to be especially effective in brain tumor, severe metastasis of the liver, nor for the fast-growing cancers. However, the vast majority of tumors are of the slow-growing type that laetrile enthusiasts hold to be amenable to laetrile therapy. Lung cancer is reported to be quite responsive to laetrile because (they say) when laetrile is injected it is carried by the blood to the right heart, lungs, then through the left heart before its effect is reduced by the action of the liver and kidneys. In light of a study by Dr. Mathew M. Ames et al.,[205] it seems ridiculous to expect *injected* laetrile to be effective for anything. Although laetrile or amygdalin by mouth may be highly dangerous, Dr. Ames et al. have reported that parenteral administration, even of massive doses, is ineffective for either benefit or harm. When injected, close to 100% of the unchanged laetrile or amygdalin molecules are recovered in the urine. Studies have shown that many samples of laetrile are contaminated, and so I think its capacity for harm, even when injected, should not be ignored.*

Enthusiastic supporters of laetrile and amygdalin believe that cancer is preventable if one's diet contains adequate "vitamin B 17" just as scurvy is prevented if the diet contains an adequate amount of

---

* Most amygdalin pills and injectables are produced in Mexico without adequate quality control. John Jee et al.[206] reported that the percentage of amygdalin per tablet varied from a high of 57.3% to a ridiculous low of .4% of the labeled contents. Five tablets tested were below 10% of the amounts shown on the labels. The average of five groups of injectables ranged from 46% to 55% of the labeled amounts. The laetrile injectables were heavily contaminated by amygdalinamide, amygdalin acid and 2-propanol. Examples of contaminated laetrile products that contained the subpotent D epimer of amygdalin have been discussed by J. Paul Davignon.[206a]

ascorbic acid. Ernst Krebs, Jr. believes that the daily diet of early man may have contained as much as 50 mg. of the so-called "vitamin B17" as contrasted with the diet of modern man, which may not contain that much in a year.

In Hunza, located in the northern part of Pakistan, where the inhabitants are said (hearsay) to eat a great number of apricot kernels and thus ingest large amounts of vitamin B17, there is reported to be virtually no cancer (possibly also hearsay). Victor Herbert, M.D.[197] states that cancer *does* exist in Hunza. Nevertheless, if the incidence of cancer is relatively low it would be especially noteworthy since many of the Hunzakuts are said to live to ages well in excess of 100 years, and so Hunza's longevity statistics may belie the oft-stated doctrine that cancer is a disease of old age. (Their life-style is, however, probably a more significant determinant of longevity than any food they may eat.) Ernest Krebs, Jr. has reported that the Taos Pueblo Indians of New Mexico, who have a low incidence of cancer, drink a concoction made of ground kernels of cherries, peaches and apricots, all of which are concentrated sources for "vitamin B17." Eskimos also, according to Krebs, before being exposed to the white man's diet, seldom, if ever, contracted cancer. Here the reason seems to be, according to Krebs, the large amounts of caribou meat in their diet. The caribou eats arrow grass which contains a large amount of "B17." The Eskimo often eats the contents of the caribou's stomach as sort of an hors d'oeuvre and thus gets enough "B17" to provide protection against cancer. Such facts, Krebs argues, strongly favor the thesis that cancer, like scurvy, rickets, beriberi, pernicious anemia and pelagra is a metabolic disease amenable, as are these other diseases, to prevention and treatment by factors normal to the diet. Scurvy is preventable or curable with limes (ascorbic acid), rickets with fish bones (vitamin D), beriberi with rice polish (vitamin B1), pernicious anemia with liver (vitamin B12 and folic acid), pelagra with vitamin B3 and cancer is presumed preventable with "vitamin B17." It should be obvious, however, that a combination of many other factors might be cited to account for the relative absence of cancer among the Hunzacuts and the Eskimos.

Contrary to this statement by Krebs, the *Federal Register*[207] argues that there is a complete lack of correlation between a high-nitriloside diet and a low cancer incidence. The *Federal Register* points out that some cancers that are rare or absent in North America and Western Europe occur in populations having high levels of nitriloside in their diets.

Furthermore, to put Krebs's statement in perspective, consider this comment of David M. Greenberg.[208] Dr. Greenberg says: "The claim that the betacyanogenic glycosides represent a new hitherto unrecognized water soluble vitamin (vitamin B17) is refuted by the following facts: (1) no evidence has ever been adduced that laetriles are essential nutritional components. (2) laetriles have never been shown to promote any physiological process vital to the continued existence of any living organism.* (3) no specific disease has been associated with a lack of laetrile in any animal. Since experimental animals (mice, rats, guinea pigs) have been maintained in good health over a number of generations on synthetic diets of pure chemical components, but containing no laetriles, it is evident that lack of this material is not associated with any disease."

Kanematsu Sugiura, at Sloan-Kettering Cancer Center, has done research on mice to determine the effects of amygdalin on spontaneous mammary tumors. Kanematsu Sugiura[211] is quoted as saying, "The results clearly show that amygdalin significantly inhibits the appearance of lung metastases in mice bearing spontaneous mammary tumors and increases significantly the inhibition of the growth of the primary tumors over the appearance of inhibition in the untreated animals." Subsequent experiments have not substantiated Sugiura's earlier enthusiasm. C. Chester Stock et al.[211a] reported that "all independently conducted experiments of 3 independent observers and the carefully controlled blind experiments in which Sugiura participated have failed to confirm Sugiura's initial results." Then later, in 1977, so-called "dramatic results" using

---

* This may not be completely true. It is reported [209,210] that amygdalin (like catalase and superoxide dismutase) will beneficially scavenge hydroxyl radicals. These studies, however, bear no apparent relationship to the question of whether or not amygdalin has any therapeutic efficiency in treating cancer.

amygdalin on mammary tumors in mice were announced by Harold
W. Manner, Ph.D.[211b] formerly of the Biology Department of Loyola
University in Chicago.

What were Manner's techniques and what were his "dramatic
results"? Instead of using just amygdalin in treating their
experimental group of 84 mice, Manner's group also used massive
doses of vitamin A and, every other day, they injected each tumor
with a group of enzymes (Wobe-mugos® from Germany). Manner
reported that after six to eight days an ulceration appeared at the
tumor site and within the ulceration was a pus-like fluid. This fluid,
containing dead malignant cells, was aspirated before the second and
subsequent enzyme injections. Twenty-one tumorous mice in a
control group were injected instead with a physiological saline
solution. The amygdalin, vitamin A and the Wobe-mugos® enzymes
were, of course, withheld from the control group.

Manner reported that, "Among the 84 experimental mice, 75
underwent complete remission of the primary tumors. This
represented 89.3 per cent. The remaining 9 mice showed partial
remission, or 10.7 per cent." In the control group that received no
treatment all the tumors continued to grow, endangering the lives of
the animals. Please note, however, that the results refer to primary
tumors, not to metastases. It should also be observed that since
Manner killed the mice promptly after analyzing the tumors for
regression, his reported 89% success ratio—remarkable as it may
appear to be at first glance—actually is below surgery's 100%
success record in treating human breast tumors. (When a woman's
breast tumor is removed she is not sacrificed to make the 100%
record a reality.) Only if Manner had kept the mice alive and
subsequently observed for possible cancer recurrences at the same
site or at metastasized locations, could his animal research be
legitimately compared with orthodox therapies. Victor Herbert, M.D.
has suggested that Manner should have used the term "digestion"
instead of "remission" since that is what the enzymes did to the
tumors. (By the way, proteolytic enzymes injected into *any* tissue
will dissolve it and at the same time, relates Dr. Herbert, may cause
fatal anaphylaxis.) Then too, was not the aspiration procedure

tantamount to performing surgery? In addition, the mice should not only have been analyzed for tumors but for possible therapy-induced damage to major organs, especially the kidneys.

To establish a human treatment protocol based on the research thus far done seems premature. With the many defects in Manner's experimental protocol and the negative results of the numerous other laetrile experiments, it seems pointless to further waste the time of qualified scientists who should, instead, be doing useful research. If Manner's work is replicated, however, it should be by an independent laboratory using double-blind studies with the results, including analyses of the animals' organs, being published in a scientific journal. Furthermore, I would hope that any such experiment would be modified so that the animals, after treatment, could be kept alive (the way human cancer patients are) to await development of possible metastases or other problems. It must be remembered that human cancer patients may have tumors removed by surgery or shrunk by chemotherapy and yet die later because of metastases or because of pneumonia contracted due to a weakened immune system.

The federally sponsored tests of laetrile therapy—in which special diets of fresh fruits, vegetables, whole grains and little meat were used—showed, as the results were published in May, 1981, that laetrile was ineffective in controlling human cancers. One-third of the patients participating had received no prior treatment with anticancer drugs, most patients were in generally good condition and none were disabled, so it would appear that the protocol for the experiment was good. However, advocates of "metabolic therapy" are dissatisfied with the experiment's protocol since the immunological system was, they say, not adequately stimulated with sufficient vitamin A or thymus and other glandular tissues, the amount of vitamin C given was too small and no proteolytic enzymes were given. It is, therefore, unlikely that the cause of laetrile will be put to rest as a result of this study. Some of the laetrile people who have the most to lose if these results hold up are even claiming that only patients "considered hopeless by modern medicine" were used. Ernst Krebs, Jr.[212] is quoted as saying, "These people were dying patients. They had received every other modalities (sic), and every other modality failed." Obviously, Krebs's information as to the experiment's protocol is at variance with that presented in *Science*.[213] Those desiring to study this clinical trial more deeply are referred to an article by Charles G. Moertel et al.[214] and subsequent correspondence.[215]

Although the effectiveness of laetrile continues to be debated, it is claimed by laetrile proponents (but not reported in the medical literature) that laetrile is often effective in reducing the pain that is generally present in those with advanced cancer. However, this seems difficult to understand in terms of the work of Dr. Mathew M. Ames, reported earlier, that parenteral administration of laetrile results in no action at all and that the laetrile ends up unchanged in the urine. If pain reduction occurs, it is most likely due to the cyanide content. K. M. Birch and F. Schütz[216] found that cyanate fed to animals caused sedation before it produced seizures and death.

The reported-to-be-successful experiments using amygdalin or laetrile with rats have employed large daily dosages of 400 mg. to 2 g. per kg. of body weight. When it is realized that it reportedly takes about 68 apricot seeds to equal just one gram of laetrile, it is apparent that apricot kernels can, at best, be thought of only as a preventative rather than as a cure or control once cancer has started in a human being. To eat that many kernels each day might be dangerous, although individuals have consumed that many and lived to tell their story. However, such large quantities cannot be recommended; they might, in some cases, prove to be dangerous and perhaps even fatal. Apricot kernels have caused the death of children in Australia. This was reported in *The Poison Plants of New South Wales* by E. Hurst.[217] Another reference of interest entitled "Cyanide Poisoning from Apricot Seeds among Children in Central Turkey" was written by James W. Sayre, M.D. and Sukru Kaymakcalan.[218] By the way, if apricot kernels are swallowed without adequate mastication they are reported to be relatively safe (and also, of course, ineffective) and they will show up as chunks in the feces. If the kernels are chewed well or ground in a blender the cyanide in the kernel becomes more effective (and more dangerous).

The dangers of eating apricot kernels, and also the oral ingestion of laetrile tablets, can be exacerbated if vitamin C is taken at the same time. Vitamin C encourages release of cyanide from amygdalin and laetrile, and so the likelihood of cyanide poisoning with its accompanying hypotension, vomiting and diarrhea is increased.[219,219a,220] Tapan K. Basu[220a] has reported that vitamin C also reduces the availability of cysteine which is required in the detoxification of cyanide to form thiocyanate prior to exretion in the urine (Figures 3 and 4).

Cyanogenetic glucosides (laetriles) have been considered to be poisonous since antiquity. The "penalty of the peach" (execution using prussic acid) is mentioned in an Egyptian papyrus preserved in the Louvre; and ancient Romans used laetriles to commit suicide.[221] In modern times the poisonings continue. Victor Herbert[197] cites many cases, including one reported in the May 10, 1977, issue of the *Thousand Oaks (California) News Chronicle*. This newspaper carried a story about the author of the *Little Cyanide Cookbook,* June DeSpain, who was hospitalized and almost died from acute cyanide poisoning after eating 25 apricot kernels. Additional reports of laetrile's poisonous nature can be found elsewhere.[222] Dr. Herbert cites the possible danger of laetriles in producing goiter, encephalopathy, demyelination and cataracts and, based on rat experiments, also discusses the possibility that they could be teratogenic. *The Merck Index* gives a much more extensive list of cyanide toxicity symptoms.

Kenneth B. Liegner et al.[223] have suggested that agranulocytosis (a decrease in the number of granulocytic leukocytes in the peripheral blood) may result from use of laetrile. Then too, laetrile toxicity studies in dogs by Eric S. Schmidt et al.[224] are both interesting and frightening. Symptoms included vomiting, involuntary defecation and urination, respiratory problems including hyperventilation and gasping, difficulty in seeing and hearing, motor ataxia, inability to stand and coma. The Schmidt article also cites studies (human and animal) which can be interpreted as indicating that, in cases of

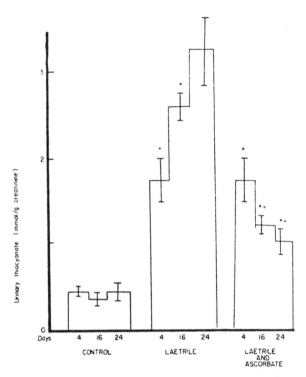

Figure 3. Effect of megadoses of ascorbic acid on the urinary levels of thiocyanate in guinea pigs treated with laetrile. Each bar represents SEM ± with at least 10 animals. Reproduced from Tapan K. Basu, *Canadian Jrl. of Physiology and Pharmacology* (1983) 61: 1426-1430, with permission of the publisher.

advanced cancer, laetrile may shorten rather than lengthen life. Kathleen T. Braico et l.[225] report on how laetrile caused the death of a child. Some individuals who have a diminished capacity to detoxify cyanide to thiocyanate, either because of a genetic predisposition or because of a diet low in sulphur amino acids, may be at increased risk.[226] Clearly, there is great possibility for harm for those who

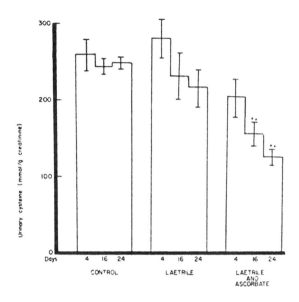

Figure 4. Effect of megadoses of ascorbic acid on the urinary levels of cysteine in guinea pigs treated with laetrile. Each bar represents SEM ± with at least 10 animals. Reproduced from Tapan K. Basu, *Canadian Jrl. of Physiology and Pharmacology* (1983) 61: 1426-1430, with permission of the publisher.

believe G. E. Griffin's statement (which appears in his book *World Without Cancer*), "Laetrile is even less toxic than sugar."

I hope I have convinced you that any possible value in laetrile is currently offset by its many negatives. However, if you are consuming amygdalin and are taking Benedict's glucose test for impaired carbohydrate metabolism, be sure to tell your physician. Use of amygdalin may lead to increased or false positive values in this test.

The ultimate irony to the story of laetrile is that it may eventually be proved to *cause* cancer. Earlier, we reported that the Johns Hopkins group found Krebs's type of "Laetrile" to be mutagenic (and therefore probably carcinogenic). Calvin C. Willhite[227] reported that laetrile administered orally to pregnant hamsters caused skeletal malformations in the offspring.* Intravenous laetrile caused no teratogenic effects. Animals are not people, but the results of this research in orally administered laetrile may, at first glance, be alarming. Furthermore, Victor Herbert[197] lists five other lines of evidence for the concept that laetrile may cause cancer and he cites the associated references. The interested reader is encouraged to order this article through his or her local library. However, the fact of laetrile's mutagenicity (and thus possible carcinogenicity), in light of the *reverse effect,* suggests that at different concentrations laetrile might also cure cancer. The *reverse effect* must, however, never be used except to suggest possibilities. Controlled clinical and laboratory studies must provide the answers, and so far laetrile's power to combat cancer has not been demonstrated.

Cyanide poisoning includes many undesirable effects. Donald R. Harkness, M.D. and Sandra Roth[228] cite such symptoms as sedation, seizures, cataracts, weight loss, weakness and death. Now, if cancer is to be added to such a list it would seem that laetrile is far more dangerous than is generally believed. Laetrile is reported to be a one-billion-dollar-per-year industry. Thus, there obviously exist those who have a sufficient financial stake in laetrile to whip up public enthusiasm in spite of the fact that their position has become untenable.

To absolutely assure that I will be castigated by both prolaetrile and antilaetrile forces, let me say this: I see no animal or clinical evidence that suggests laetrile to be effective against cancer. However, since laetrile has mutagenic properties, I believe at some dosages, depending on the species, it will *cause* cancer; at other dosages it will be ineffective for either causing or curing cancer; and at still other dosages it may work to *cure* cancer. It is possible that some of the presumed cures involving laetrile may have employed dosages that were within what may be a very small "therapeutic window." No animal or clinical study has yet been done that was designed to discover laetrile's possible dose-responsive *reverse effects* and a conceivably-existent therapeutic window. When such

---

* Subsequently, Patricia Doherty et al.[227a] showed that cyanide is teratogenic in hamsters.

studies are done it could be a great day for laetrile. Such studies might also encourage the habitual establishment of experimental protocols designed to discover cancer-fighting *reverse effects* in many other mutagenic (and possibly cancer-causing) substances. Furthermore, such laetrile studies could move up the time when the experimental protocols of other animal and clinical studies will be consistently designed to facilitate discovery of *reverse effects* rather than to mask their existence. However, the studies should be done by the laetrile proponents and should be scrutinized by the non-proponents of laetrile.

Some More Nonvitamins of the B Complex

Other factors also associated with the B complex have been discovered but they are no longer considered to be vitamins. Carnitine (formerly called B$_T$)* may be required as a vitamin by neonates prior to their developing the system for its synthesis.[229] Adults who normally synthesize carnitine from lysine and methionine through a series of biological transformations involving iron and vitamins B$_3$, B$_6$ and C may also sometimes be short of this nutrient. Carnitine is required to metabolize fatty acids and,like other factors the body normally synthesizes (such as arginine and histidine), it may sometimes be produced in only marginal amounts.[229] Cereals, fruits and vegetables contain little or no carnitine. The word carnitine is derived from *carn,* meaning *of an animal.* Tempeh, however, which is often eaten by vegetarians, contains carnitine derived from the mold used in the fermentation process.[230]

Carnitine is important for operation of the muscles, including those of the heart. If persons who avoid meat because its fat may be bad for their cardiovascular system are also among those individuals who synthesize carnitine very inefficiently, they may be endangering their hearts. Carnitine promotes cardiovascular health not only through facilitating heart-muscle action, but by dilating blood

---

* The T of B$_T$ stands for *Tenebrio.* Many years ago (in 1952) carnitine was discovered to be a growth factor for the meal worm, *Tenebrio molitor.*[228a]

vessels, by raising HDL-cholesterol levels in the blood and by reducing triglyceride levels.[230a] Those who desire to pursue carnitine and its chemistry should read the paperback book *Carnitine: The Vitamin BT Phenomenon* by Brian Leibovitz [230a] and check out its numerous references.

Carnitine, in its L form may be of value in connection with a weight loss program and with aerobic activity.[230a] Robert E. Keith,[230b] writing in 1986, notes, however, that to save money it is sometimes used in the DL form. Keith suggests that, since the D-isomer may inhibit the valuable L-isomer, it may be best to avoid the DL form.

Supplementary carnitine might conceivably be of value in increasing the fertility of men. Infertile men have been found by a number of investigators, including Nongnuj Tanphaichitr[230c] and J. C. Soufir et al.,[231] to have much lower levels of carnitine in their seminal fluid. In both fertile and infertile men, carnitine levels in the semen increases with abstinence. The semen concentration of carnitine and of the enzyme carnitine acetyltransferase depends on an effect of testosterone [228a] The motility of ejaculated sperm (an index to fetilizing capacity) is correlated with their content of acetylcarnitine.[228a,230c]

In a 1986 review, Peggy R. Borum and Sandra G. Bennett [232] presented evidence for the essentiality of carnitine. They made the point that supplementary carnitine may be especially needed not only by preterm infants but by children with various forms of organic aciduria, by dialysis patients, by patients being treated with drugs such as valproic acid and by patients undergoing metabolic stresses such as trauma, sepsis and organ failure. The Borum and Bennett review called my attention to the research of D. Rudman et al.[233] who reported that a carnitine *deficiency* is associated with liver cirrhosis while R. K. Fuller and C. L. Hoppel [234] found that *excessive* carnitine is associated with this disease. These facts suggest the possible presence of a *reverse effect*.

As we will consider later in Chapter 9, it may be possible to use carnitine as a carrier for derivatives of BHT, tocopherols and other antioxidants. If they could be carried into the inner membrane of the mitochondria it might lead to greatly increased longevity.

Among other factors associated with the B complex that no longer have status as vitamins are lipoic acid (or thioctic acid), B 4 (an undetermined factor in wheat germ, grass, yeast and liver), adenylic acid, B10 and B11 (a folic acid-like factor affecting chicks), orotic acid (sometimes called B13)* and B 14 (a crystalline factor isolated from human urine). These factors have, at best, doubtful status as vitamins or perhaps even have assured status as nonvitamins.

---

* The whey portion of soured milk contains sizable amounts of orotic acid. Orotic acid is reported to be a precursor in the biosynthesis of the nucleic acids in the cytoplasm of cell nuclei.

The   "Niacin Effect"

On pages 345 and 348 we noted that niacin beneficially lowered serum lipid levels and increased the HDL/LDL ratio. If the Coronary Drug Project Research Group[35] that conducted this study had stopped after making these discoveries they might have concluded that niacin was an aid to heart health. However, they went further and found that longevity was not increased and heart health was not improved, at least one reason being that cardiac arrhythmia tended to occur.

Scientists, in setting experimental protocols and in subsequently drawing conclusions from their studies, should guard against being misled by what I call the "niacin effect." Beneficial results may sometimes be obvious but negative developments may be far more subtle.

"Read every day something no one
else is reading. Think every day
something no one else is thinking.
It is bad for the mind to be always
a part of a unanimity."
— Christopher Morley

"Men are wise in proportion not to
their experience but to their
capacity for experience."
— George Bernard Shaw

"A problem is a chrysalis that
awaits its butterfly. When its time
has come, the solution will emerge.
Never believe the chrysalis will
fail in its destiny. Never believe a
problem will remain, for long,
unsolved."
— Walter A. Heiby, *Live Your
Life* (New York: Harper and Row,
1966)

CHAPTER 6

Vitamin C—Problem
Solver or Problem *Causer*?

The great Arab traveler, Ibn Batuta, visited China about 60 years
after Nicolo Polo, his brother Maffeo and the former's son Marco.
Ibn Batuta[1] tells us that in the large ships of ancient China (which
carried a crew of 300 and a large number of passengers besides the
occupants of 60 private cabins) vegetables, grown on board in pots,
were eaten as a prevention against scurvy. This accounts for the long
voyages undertaken by the Chinese at a time the crews of European
ships suffered from this disease. Then, in the 16th century, the
English admiral, Sir Richard Hawkins, made the discovery that
consumption of citrus fruits would prevent scurvy. Unfortunately,
the idea fell into disuse at the time of his death in 1622. Over a
century later, in 1753, Dr. James Lind published a treatise on scurvy
in which he told of his controlled experiments. He demonstrated that

this is a diet-deficiency disease and that citrus fruits would prevent and cure it. Albert Szent-Györgyi von Nagyrapolt, destined to win the Nobel Prize, isolated a chemical from ox adrenal glands and called it *hexuronic acid*. A few years later, having evidence of its antiscorbutic properties and that it was in fact identical with the factor being called vitamin C, he suggested the name *ascorbic acid*. Some other names that have been used for compounds with vitamin C activity are l-ascorbic acid, l-xyloascorbic acid and l-threo-hex-2-enoic acid gamma lactone.[1a]

The appellation, "beauty and youth vitamin" that is sometimes used for vitamin C may be suggestive, but it is subject to the same comment that was made in connection with some of the other vitamins. Vitamin C contributes greatly to the firmness of the tissues through its work in building collagen (as we will discuss a bit later). It tends to minimize bruising caused by capillary breakage and the red blotches that are often seen in the skin of older persons. However, vitamin C should not be stressed unduly as a beauty and youth vitamin. The body needs not only vitamin C but a complete array of other nutrients to assure beauty and youthfulness.

Vitamin C may function in metabolizing carbohydrates or proteins or both. If it does so it is probably because it can act as a hydrogen carrier (similar to the way hemoglobin acts as a giver and receiver of oxygen). Vitamin C, like the constituents of the B complex, is water-soluble. Dehydroascorbic acid is a stereoisomer of l-ascorbic acid having virtually no antiscorbutic activity. Another stereoisomer, erythorbic acid (which is also called d-isoascorbic acid or d-araboascorbic acid), has antiscorbutic power equal to that of ascorbic acid,[2] although earlier studies erroneously reported it to have only a weak antiscorbutic effect. Erythorbic acid also has good antioxidant activity and is widely used as a food preservative. It has shown good ability to prevent nitrosamine formation from nitrates in bacon and other cured meats. A third stereoisomer of l-ascorbic acid, l-araboascorbic acid, is without any antiscorbutic activity. A somewhat oil-soluble form of the vitamin, ascorbyl palmitate, which is, incidentally, very soluble in alcohol, is also a valuable nutrient. It will be discussed later in this chapter and again in Chapter 9.

Is Ascorbic Acid a "Vitamin"?

Some believe that the term "vitamin C" may be an unfortunate one. The implication is that vitamins are required by the body in only minute amounts. This is, perhaps, not true of vitamin C and therefore the terms "ascorbic acid," "ascorbate" or "ascorbyl palmitate" could be semantically superior. It is true that ascorbic acid or the ascorbates in minute amounts will banish the grosser aspects of scurvy but, according to some, a subclinical scurvy will still exist unless one consumes amounts of "vitamin C" beyond those usually associated with a vitamin.

Irwin Stone[3,3a] maintains that "vitamin C" is not a true mammalian vitamin but rather a liver metabolite that in most animals, other than man, is produced by the body. Dr. Stone has made the point, in personal correspondence with me, that: "Scurvy is the only potentially fatal human genetic disease that Medicine treats so casually, prescribing 1% or less of the daily ascorbate needed for its full correction! It is this chronic lack of correction which induces the present high incidence and morbidity of cancer, heart and vascular diseases, the collagen diseases, kidney disease and many others." Stone considers scurvy to be just the more apparent aspect of what he calls hypoascorbemia (i.e., low ascorbic acid) consisting of all examples of both clinical and subclinical scurvy. Stone terms hypoascorbemia "our most widespread disease." The disease will be corrected, according to Dr. Stone, only after we stop thinking of ascorbic acid as being a vitamin and begin to think in terms of medical genetics.

Why medical genetics? The human body (unlike that of most of the lower animals) cannot synthesize ascorbic acid because of a genetic fault which has caused an absence of an enzyme, L-gulonolactone oxidase, in the human liver, and so it is presumed that large amounts should be consumed. Irwin Stone speculates[3] that the mutation occurred in an ancestor of man (in the Primate Suborder Anthropoidea) during the late Cretaceous or early Paleocene periods about 60 million years ago (or about 25 million years ago according to Chatterjee).[3b] Plants and many animals produce ascorbic acid from glucose.* The invertebrates, insects and fishes do not make it. [3b] The amphibians and reptiles and birds of lower order produce ascorbic acid in the kidneys, while most mammals and birds of higher order make it in the liver.[3b] S. Shah and N. Nath[3c] recently reported that the goat synthesizes ascorbic acid not only in the liver but also in the prostate gland. (This discovery, they say, "not only establishes animal prostate as an alternative site for ascorbic acid biogenesis but also indicates the exciting possibility of ascorbic acid playing certain important but specific role in male reproductive events.") The primates, including man, are generally incapable of producing ascorbic acid. Chatterjee[3b] speculates that the emergence of the ability to synthesize ascorbic acid that arose with the amphibians suggests that somehow a greater need for the vitamin was linked to the move from the oceans to the land.

Other mammals besides man that are also unable to manufacture their own ascorbic acid are guinea pigs, the apes, most monkeys and an Indian fruit-eating bat.** They, like man, must, therefore, get ascorbic acid from their food. According to Stone, early man probably obtained, in most cases, adequate amounts of ascorbic acid from his diet. However, after the discovery of fire and cooking, man no longer consumed as much as he needed. Whereas raw meat and raw fish were good sources of this vitamin, much of it was lost in the cooking process. Similarly, as man began to cook vegetables and fruits he lost additional sources of ascorbic acid. The resulting hypoascorbemia or a chronic "sub-clinical" scurvy condition of early man (particularly of those who had emigrated from the tropics where fruits were more plentiful) may have been a factor in his limited longevity. Dr. Stone states that hypoascorbemia, being caused by an enzyme dysfunction, is similar in etiology to other genetic diseases brought on by the absence of an enzyme, e.g., phenylketonuria,

---

* Dr. Stone[4] states that "...it is the ascorbate ion that is physiologically active and at the pH of living tissue it is not present in the acid form." Following Stone's lead, however, I will use the terms *ascorbic acid, ascorbate* and *vitamin C* interchangeably.

** When young ascorbutic guinea pigs are injected intramuscularly with L-gulonolactone oxidase they synthesize vitamin C.[5]

galactosemia and alkaptonuria. Modern man, through consumption of fresh fruits and vegetables is in a better position, but he is still woefully lacking in adequate amounts of ascorbic acid. "It is my judgement," says Stone, "that for full health man should ingest the same large quantities of ascorbate that he would otherwise be producing in his own liver, had this mutation not occurred." It seems to me, on the other hand, that it is probable that man may have evolved in such a way that he requires somewhat less ascorbic acid.

Edward J. Calabrese[6] presents, in fact, the interesting thought that man's loss of the ability to synthesize ascorbic acid may have increased his chances of survival in a malaria-infested environment. Later in this chapter we will discuss how individuals with a G-6-PD enzyme deficiency are sensitive to ascorbic acid-induced hemolysis. Calabrese speculates that, in an area where malaria was common, a G-6-PD deficiency could be lifesaving, but only if the body content of ascorbic acid were concomitantly reduced. Thus, he says, a reduction in the ability to synthesize ascorbic acid was a trait that helped the survival of early man.

Stone[7] has published data (Table 1) which indicate the milligrams of ascorbate produced in the livers of selected mammals for each 70 kilograms of body weight (70 kilograms being the approximate weight of a man).

The table's data indicate that man, if he synthesized vitamin C as does a rat, would produce 1.8 grams to 4.9 grams of ascorbic acid daily in an unstressed condition and up to 15.2 grams under stress. However, problems are involved in drawing conclusions based on vitamin production in animals. It has been pointed out[8a] that animals producing endogenous ascorbic levels at high rates also oxidize it very rapidly and so maintain plasma levels of less than 1 mg. per deciliter comparable to those present in humans consuming 60 to 100 mg. per day. Then too, we know that ruminants absorb large quantities of the B vitamins from their intestinal tract, whereas human beings may absorb only minor amounts. Setting up a table showing such large absorption in ruminants and minor absorption in humans might lead, following Dr. Stone's line of reasoning, to the conclusion that man needs far greater amounts of the B vitamins from food

Table I

Mammal	Ascorbate Produced (Mg.)
Rat, unstressed	1,800 [*]
Rat, unstressed	4,900 [*]
Rat, stressed	15,200
Mouse	19,250
Rabbit	15,820
Goat	13,300
Dog	2,800 [**]
Cat	2,800 [**]
Human	0

or supplementary sources than may, in fact, be the case. At any rate, drawing conclusions about humans from animal data is always a risky venture. It seems even more risky to take a normal condition in animals (i.e., to make vitamin C) and a normal condition in humans (i.e., to *not* make vitamin C) and then to conclude that the human condition is detrimental while the animal condition is not. Evolutionary theory might, if anything, suggest just the opposite. In fact, Y. Kagawa et al.[9,10] report that man does not metabolize ascorbic acid in the same way as ascorbate-synthesizing animals do. In the latter, dehydroascorbic acid is irreversibly converted to 2,3-diketo-l-gulonate having no vitamin C activity, but this reaction occurs only at a low rate in man. Instead, dehydroascorbic acid in man is reduced to ascorbate, which thus is a conserving mechanism. Emil Ginter[11] points out also that man, unlike ascorbate-synthesizing animals, does not oxidize ascorbate to carbon dioxide. Thus, Stone's extrapolation from ascorbate-

---

[*] Interestingly, a rat mutant unable to synthesize vitamin C has recently been bred for experimental purposes.[a]

[**] I. B. Chatterjee et al.[8] report that the dog and cat produce only about one-eighth the ascorbic acid produced by the rat, facts at odds with Stone's data.

synthesizing animals to man is not tenable.

Then too, Robert B. Rucker and Michael A. Dubick[12] hold that if humans synthesized ascorbic acid at rates similar to other animals they would probably do so in the amount of 50 to 400 mg./day. They argue that the high estimates of Stone, Pauling and others are overestimates based on extrapolations from synthetic rates *in vitro* without consideration of actual concentrations of ascorbic acid precursors *in vivo*.

In further regard to evolution, Miriam Rosin et al.[12a] have suggested the possibility that man may have evolved mechanisms to protect himself from exogenous vitamin C. If such mechanisms exist they may very well be adequate to protect man against vitamin C found in food, but can they protect against megadoses in the form of pills?

To complicate matters further, Muge Cummings[13] presents interesting information suggesting that some persons may manufacture vitamin C in their bodies. Cummings points out that if the absence or inactivity of the enzyme l-gulonolactone oxidase is a simple recessive genetic trait, then mutations will result in the ability to synthesize vitamin C. The idea of endogenous "C" manufactured by humans was suggested earlier by the work of E. M. Baker et al.[14] who showed that d-glucuronolactone is converted to ascorbic acid in the human body. The idea of endogenous "C" production was also promoted by Roger J. Williams and Gary Deason[15] but, surprisingly, these reports seem to have remained dormant in the archives of science.

Speaking of the "archives of science," a study conducted more than 30 years ago suggests that humans can sometimes synthesize vitamin C. Kalyan Bagchi[16] reported that lactating women apparently synthesized vitamin C. A group of 25 healthy, lactating Bengali women whose ascorbic acid intake (40-50 mg. daily) was either less than recommended or borderline, secreted 40-50 mg. in their milk in addition to some in their urine. Thus, their outgo of vitamin C was apparently greater than their intake, while they showed no signs of scurvy. R. Rajalakshmi et al.[17] reported on their own study and discuss many other studies suggesting endogenous vitamin C production may occur during pregnancy and during lactation. Then, two years later, they[18] presented evidence for the synthesis of ascorbic acid in the human placenta.

Dr. Linus Pauling[19] speculates that the human requirements of ascorbic acid are between 3,000 and 9,000 grams per day. Obviously, these figures of Dr. Pauling, and those cited by Dr. Stone, are in excess of the consumption levels of most persons.

Some have argued that taking large amounts of ascorbic acid is a waste of money since the excess will simply be excreted. However, Dr. Pauling has pointed out what he calls the fallaciousness of this reasoning. He maintains that a steady state is set up in the body such that the ascorbate in the blood is proportional to the ascorbic acid or ascorbate consumption. The amount of ascorbic acid excreted in the urine will be reduced, and the concentration in the blood increased, if the daily supplement is divided into at least four dosages and taken throughout the day.

Prominent among those associated with administering massive amounts of vitamin C in the treatment of various conditions are F. R. Klenner[19a] and Robert F. Cathcart, III.[19b] Cathcart, by "titrating to bowel tolerance," determines the amount of vitamin C that causes diarrhea in a given patient and then prescribes a dosage just below that amount.

Does Vitamin C Help Prevent Colds? Effects on the Immune System

When the body is under stress the ascorbic acid or ascorbate intake should, according to Dr. Stone's theory, be increased up to the amount the liver would manufacture if the enzyme were not missing. Irwin Stone recommends, for example, that 1,500 to 2,000 mg. of ascorbic acid be taken at the first symptom of a cold. According to Dr. Stone, this should be followed within 20 to 30 minutes with a similar dose and then one more 20 to 30 minutes later. Additional doses should be taken if there are further symptoms of a cold.

The Merck Manual (13th edition)[20] reports that there is a reduced duration of disability due to colds among persons taking as much as eight grams of ascorbic acid on the first day of the disease. This volume comments, however, that such persons could be transmitters of the disease since, while their feeling of well-being is enhanced, their virus-shedding is not reduced. Then, in the current (14th) edition[20a] they have dropped the former report and simply state, "Ascorbic acid or high doses of citrus juices are popular, mostly on lay recommendation; no adequate scientific data confirm any benefit."

Thomas C. Chalmers[21] studied many of the trials that were made to determine the effect of vitamin C on colds. He observed that "in all nine of the randomized or double blind studies, patients treated with ascorbic acid prophylactically tended to have less severe symptoms than those who received placebo." More recently, Alan B. Carr et al.[22] studied self-reported cold data for 95 pairs of identical twins who took part in a double-blind study of vitamin C tablets. The treatment group received one gram of ascorbic acid per day for 100 days and each corresponding identical twin received a placebo well matched in taste and appearance but having lactose substituted for the ascorbic acid. There was only a modest difference between the groups, but the average duration of colds in the "C"-treated group was shortened by 19%.

We noted earlier that d-isoascorbic acid (as contrasted with l-ascorbic acid) has very weak antiscorbutic power. However, a study by K. Mary Clegg and Jennifer M. MacDonald[23] suggests it may have power to prevent colds. They reported that, in a survey of double-blind design, three groups of approximately 70 student volunteers took either one gram l-ascorbic acid, one gram d-isoascorbic acid or placebo tablets every day for 15 weeks. The group taking the d-isoascorbic acid had 34% fewer colds than the other two groups. The investigators point out that A. Murata et al.[24] had reported that studies with bacteriophages have shown both l-ascorbic acid and d-isoascorbic acid have virucidial activity. *

---

* Murata[24a] subsequently reported that vitamin C *in vitro* inactivates many kinds of viruses.

However, since l-ascorbic acid, in their study, failed to show power against colds, Clegg and MacDonald seem to feel that the importance of the beneficial results using d-isoascorbic acid is somehow diminished.

Many studies have concluded that vitamin C is efficacious in alleviating symptoms of a cold. To cite one such study, N. Subramanian et al.[25,8] found that ascorbic acid renders histamine biologically inactive through rupturing its imidazole ring and breaking the histamine down to hydantoin, acetic acid and aspartic acid. Figure 1 shows the decrease in histamine in the presence of ascorbic acid and the concurrent oxidation of the latter. By the way, optimizing the blood's content of histamine could be important even in those not suffering symptoms of a cold. C. Alan B. Clemetson[26] reported that, when the ascorbic acid level of human blood plasma falls below 1 mg./100 ml., the whole blood histamine level increases exponentially as the ascorbic acid level decreases. Orally administered ascorbic acid (one gram daily for three days) to 11 volunteers resulted in a reduction in the blood histamine level in every instance. What amount of ascorbic acid intake results in a low enough histamine level (or too low a level) for optimal health? No one knows, but it could be above (or below) the RDA recommendation.* By the way, the *in vitro* experiment by Natarajan Subramanian et al.[25] cited above showed that when copper was present along with ascorbic acid the histamine was destroyed much more efficiently.** Perhaps copper should be included in the various cold-fighting remedies. Vitamin C depresses intestinal absorption of copper,[26d] however, and thus they probably should not be taken

---

* Histamine stimulates visceral muscles, dilates capillaries and stimulates salivary, pancreatic and gastric secretions.[26a] Could excessive intake of vitamin C reduce histamine to the point that body functions (including production of stomach acid) might be inhibited?

** The formation of hydrogen peroxide plays a vital role in this reaction. Itarv Yamamoto and Hitoshi Ohmori[26b] found that when additional hydrogen peroxide is added to the ascorbate-copper system, histamine breakdown is accelerated. (Lawrence R. De Chatelet et al.[26c] had noted earlier that the bactericidal activity of ascorbate was greatly enhanced by the addition of copper and hydrogen peroxide, although neither of the additives alone nor in combination showed any such activity.)

together.[*] Rat studies[27] have shown that, although ascorbic acid depresses intestinal uptake of copper, it has little or no effect on copper excretion. Subsequently, a study was made by Elizabeth B. Finley and Florian L. Cerklewski[27a] of the copper status of young adult men. Using self-selected diets, each took a 500 mg. ascorbic acid supplement with every meal (1,500 mg./day) for 64 days. Copper status was analyzed periodically beginning with the 28th day. Serum ceruloplasmin was significantly reduced throughout the supplementation period. Serum copper was also reduced but not significantly. However, after the supplementation period there *was* a significant increase in serum copper. Although the observed effects of copper reduction were within physiologically normal ranges, ascorbic acid was confirmed as a copper antagonist for men as had earlier been shown to be the case with laboratory animals.

Many other studies have concluded, on the other hand, that vitamin C is ineffective in cold prevention or treatment. Since vitamin C acts as an antihistamine, it would seem likely to be useful for that type of cold (stuffy, runny nose) where histamine overproduction is an important factor in contributing to the unpleasant symptoms. However, where the cold symptoms are more general it seems likely that using vitamin C would be of little benefit. (I do not think, however, that we can rule out the possibility that histamine—in spite of the attending unpleasant symptoms—may be performing a protective or curative function.)

B. K. Nandi et al.[28] and I. B. Chatterjee et al.[8] point out that the antihistaminic property of ascorbic acid differs from that of antihistaminic drugs. Ascorbic acid, as we have seen, ruptures the imidazole ring, making histamine biologically inactive. Antihistamines, on the other hand, bind to receptor sites of the cell membrane, protecting the cell from histamine action. Macrobiotics

---

[*] Much itchiness is reportedly caused by histamine, and itchiness undergoes a circadian rhythm, generally peaking during the hours of sleep. It seems to me that, to the extent vitamin C inactivates histamine and to the extent that the itchiness is histamine-related, vitamin C taken at bedtime might solve the problem. Supplementary copper, taken earlier in the day so its absorption is not adversely affected by the ascorbic acid, might also sometimes prove helpful.

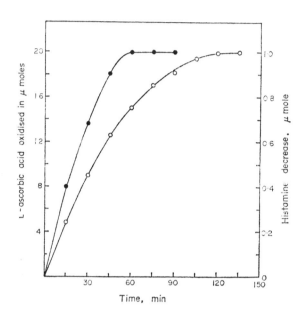

Figure 1. Oxidation of l-ascorbic acid and biotransformation of histamine. •-•, oxidation of l-ascorbic acid; o-o, decrease of histamine. Reproduced from N. Subramanian et al., *Biochem. Pharmacol.* (1975) 22: 1671-1673, with permission of the publisher, Pergamon Press, Ltd.

enthusiasts may, incidentally, be interested to learn that Nandi et al.,[28] in performing their histamine experiments on rats, used whole cereal diets (wheat, rice and corn), without supplementation of other dietary ingredients, to induce the stress that led to the production of histamine. (This diet is, in fact, now commonly used to induce scurvy in laboratory animals.)* At any rate, valuable as this destruction of excessive histamine may be, it is not without possible problems. Will vitamin C destroy only excessive histamine or will it also destroy histamine needed for body functions?

---

* Cereal in the diet of an omnivore (such as man) would, however, not be expected to act as it does in the diet of a carnivore (such as the rat).

R. Hume and Elspeth Weyers[29] have shown that there is a significant fall in the ascorbic acid levels in human leucocytes within 24 hours of the onset of a cold. Levels return to normal on the cessation of symptoms. Their results also suggested that the leucocyte levels of ascorbic acid could be increased by taking supplemental vitamin C. C. W. M. Wilson[30] has reported that, upon supplementation, the uptake of ascorbic acid by the leucocytes is greater in females than in males. Moreover, the effects occurred predominantly with what Wilson terms the toxic variety of colds (attended by sore throat, headache and fever). Colds with catarrhal symptoms (cold in head, cough, nasal obstruction and nasal discharge) showed, instead, ascorbic acid moving out of the leucocytes and into the plasma.* There is as yet no evidence that these physiological effects bear any relationship to the amelioration of cold symptoms. The drop in ascorbic acid levels in leucocytes occurs in cases of myocardial infarction, with the immune depression of pregnancy, aging and corticosteroid treatment and may be just a response to stress. It is, in fact, now being seriously questioned whether leucocyte ascorbic acid is reliable for use in estimating body pool size of ascorbic acid. Anita J. Thomas et al.[30b] reported that leucocyte ascorbic acid levels failed to identify six of seven elderly patients shown to be deficient on an oral vitamin C saturation test.

Vitamin C, as has been suggested, may be useful in reducing cold symptoms where the symptoms are primarily due to the presence of histamine. It is not known whether vitamin C has any antiviral power that would help fight colds, although, as we saw earlier, it does show *in vitro* antiviral activity.[24,24a] At any rate, vitamin C seems powerless to destroy bacteria. An experiment by Prakash G. Shilotri and K. Seetharam Bhat[31] demonstrated the effect of ascorbic acid on leucocyte function and bactericidal action. For 15

---

* An earlier study by C. W. M. Wilson[30a] (before he discovered that different types of colds are attended by different ascorbic acid uptake action in the leucocytes) involved use of aspirin. Wilson showed that aspirin inhibited the uptake of ascorbic acid by leucocytes but, during colds, this phenomenon was completely reversed and, under the influence of aspirin, leucocytes actively absorbed ascorbic acid. Curiously, it took three weeks for the increased uptake to decline to normal after recovery from the last cold symptom. These actions could provide a rationale for the frequent prescription of aspirin to relieve the toxic symptoms of colds.

days normal human subjects were given 200 mg. of ascorbic acid daily and for the following two weeks they were given 2 g. daily. The scientists found that daily intakes of 200 mg. had no effect on the ability of leucocytes to kill bacteria. Furthermore, intakes of 2 g. of vitamin C daily significantly *reduced* the leucocyte's bactericidal activity (Figure 2). (This suggests that the immune system may be depressed at high levels of ascorbic acid.) Then, four weeks after withdrawal of ascorbic acid supplementation, bactericidal activity returned to normal.* By the way, Bani Basu et al.[33] reported that the uptake of dehydroascorbic acid by leucocytes *in vitro* is much higher than that of ascorbic acid.

Ascorbic acid will also move into erythrocytes, *in vivo,* but nowhere near as readily as it moves into leucocytes. Ralph Golden and Frederick Sargent III[34] showed that insulin promotes this transport of ascorbic acid into both erythrocytes and leucocytes. Then, 21 years later, G. N. Schrauzer and W. J. Rhead[35] reported that persons taking gram amounts of vitamin C daily for extended periods show signs of a systematic conditioning. This conditioning is characterized by lower plasma and erythrocyte levels of ascorbic acid and a higher level of ascorbic acid excretion in the morning urine compared with those levels in controls who took large amounts of vitamin C for a shorter period. Still more recently, J. Ludvigsson et al.[36] reported that women taking vitamin C showed increased serum levels of "C" but they found no change in leucocyte levels of the vitamin. Some of these reports are obviously contradictory and suggest that more research needs to be done.

Support for the hypothesis that colds are ameliorated by supplemental vitamin C is suggested by the possible effect of this vitamin on interferon production. The ability of ascorbic acid (and also sodium salicylate and caffeine) to alter the serum level of interferon in mice was investigated by William F. Geber et al.[37]

---

* Those who like to more deeply understand phenomena are referred to "The Effects of Ascorbic Acid on Bactericidal Mechanisms of Neutrophils" by Charles E. McCall et al.[32] This article relates that ascorbic acid inhibits the hydrogen peroxide-myeloperoxidase-halide reactions which are implicated in the bactericidal activity of phagocytic neutrophils.

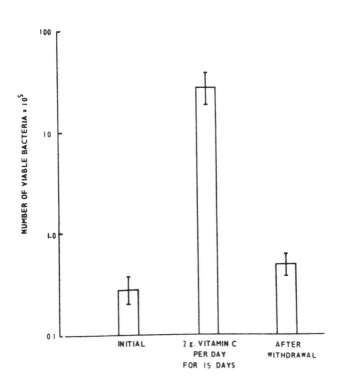

Figure 2. A profile of bactericidal activity of leukocytes before, during supplementation of 2 grams of vitamin C daily for 15 days and after withdrawal of vitamin C. Reproduced from Prakash G. Shilotri and K. Seetharam Bhat, *Amer. Jrl. of Clinical Nutrition* (July, 1977) 30: 1077-1081, with permission of the publisher.

Ascorbic acid at 666 mg./kg. (a huge amount, beyond the range of most megadosing humans) increased the interferon production in the mice. This amount of ascorbic acid showed a much larger interferon response than did caffeine at 100 mg./kg. (another huge dosage) but much less than sodium salicylate at the rather high dosage of 100 mg./kg. (At the still higher dosage of 300 mg./kg., sodium salicylate showed a *reverse effect* and interferon production decreased.) The levels of all three "drugs" used in this study were so beyond typical physiological range that they offer little guidance as to what might occur at more nominal dosages.

In a related study, Benjamin V. Siegel[38] found that ascorbic acid added to cultures of certain mouse cells after stimulation with polyinosinic acid-polycytidylic acid increased the synthesis of interferon.* He had earlier reported[39] increased interferon production in mice fed a diet containing vitamin C after stimulation with a virus. Then, Helen Dahl and Miklos Degre[40] related that ascorbic acid enhanced interferon levels in human embryo skin and lung fibroblasts induced by a virus. However, ascorbic acid did not increase interferon levels in lung fibroblasts induced by a different virus. Thus, it remains to be reported what, if any, effect vitamin C may have on interferon production stimulated by cold viruses. In fact, Dahl and Degre conclude that "the minor benefits of questionable validity are not worth the potential risk, however small that might be."

In more recent work, it has been shown that vitamin C has the ability to increase the production of prostaglandin E2 (PGE2). B. V. Siegel and Jane I. Morton[40a] reported that, when ascorbate was added to macrophage cultures derived from bone marrow of mice, PGE2 production increased 90%-100%. They suggested this may explain vitamin C's failure to augment the activity of natural killer cells even though interferon production is enhanced.

Even though vitamin C may actually inhibit the ability of white cells to destroy bacteria, as reported earlier,[31] a number of studies suggest that "C" may have some beneficial effects on the immune system. E. M. S. Gatner and R. Anderson[44] reported that the neutrophils from tuberculosis patients which showed impaired directed motility (chemotaxis) had that defect corrected *in vitro* when treated with ascorbate. R. Anderson[45] reported, in a related study, that calcium and sodium ascorbate stimulated the chemotactic responsiveness of neutrophils from patients with lepromatus leprosy.

---

* This word is often used in the singular form, although the interferons are a family of at least 16 different proteins and glycoproteins. All have the ability to protect cultured cells against infection by viruses. In addition, they have many other biological regulatory functions, including cellular proliferation, morphology, differentiation, enzyme induction and antigen function in the immune response.[38a]

(Surendra N. Sinha et al.[46] subsequently reported that blood ascorbic acid levels were reduced in lepromatus as well as in tuberculoid leprosy patients. They suggested that ascorbic acid supplementation might have a beneficial effect on leprosy patients and aid in the healing of trophic ulcers.)

Murata and Morishige[47] found that surgical patients who receive blood transfusions can be partially protected against serum hepatitis by taking vitamin C. (F. P. Mc Ginn and Judith C. Hamilton[48] have expressed concern that ascorbic acid deficiencies in stored blood may contribute to the healing problems of patients requiring blood transfusion.) In another study, A. Rebora et al.[49] reported that ascorbic acid administered to two children with inordinate susceptibility to skin infections due to defective bacterial killing power of their neutrophils was effective in suppressing infectious recurrences. In a separate study, A. Rebora et al.[50] stated that ascorbic acid was effective in improving chemotaxis and bacterial-killing power of the neutrophils in three other patients.

Assessment of a number of studies regarding ascorbate and immunity was made by W. R. Thomas and P. G. Holt.[51] They concluded that the data suggests an important role for "C" in the immune function but that there is no evidence that megadoses are justified. Then too, R. Anderson and Annette Theron[52] made the point that defective neutrophil motility is implicated in many diseases, including rheumatoid arthritis, diabetes mellitus, measles, bacterial infection, influenza, herpes, warts and allergies. They observed that while certain antibiotics and other drugs may impair neutrophil activity, calcium and sodium ascorbate have been useful in their own studies, as in the research of others, in working to improve neutrophil function.

To add to the possible benefits for vitamin C, W. Prinz et al.[53] have reported that ascorbic acid has another positive effect on the human immune defense system. Male university students given one gram of vitamin C daily for 75 days showed a statistically significant increase in the serum levels of IgA, IgM and C-3 complement. (C-3 complement increases the rate of mobilization of leukocytes and the rate of phagocytosis of foreign cells.) Thus, this research suggests that vitamin C beneficially affects this process. To contradict these favorable results, R. Anderson et al.,[54] in studying the effects of ascorbate on human volunteers, concluded that ascorbate at levels of two to three grams daily showed that serum levels of IgG, IgA, IgM, C-3 and C4 were unaltered. They did, however, find that certain functions of neutrophils and lymphocytes were benefitted. Thus, the group of studies reported in this and in the preceding paragraphs must as a whole be rated as giving a small plus to the idea that supplemental "C" may be beneficial in combating colds.

Then too, *Lancet*[55] notes that various investigators have reported (and we also noted earlier) that subnormal levels of polymorphonuclear-leucocyte ascorbate generally exist in the immune depression of pregnancy, in aging and during corticosteroid treatment. Thus, a deficiency of "C" is shown to be detrimental, but it certainly does not prove that an excess is beneficial. Furthermore, after an extensive review of the literature, W. R. Thomas and P. G. Holt[51] make the point that the high concentration of ascorbate and dehydroascorbate in leucocytes and their rapid expenditure during infection and phagocytosis suggests vitamin C functions in the immune process. More studies are obviously called for to delineate the role of vitamin C in the immune process.

In studying the effect of ascorbic acid on immunity, R. H. Yonemoto[55a] gave one group of volunteers 1,000 mg. of ascorbic acid (AA) for 7 days and gave a second group 3,000 mg. for 14 days. Both groups showed heightened lymphocyte blastogenesis. Then, in what I suspect might be evidence of a *reverse effect,* he reported: "Curiously, 1 day following cessation of the 14-day AA ingestion period, the response of the 3 g AA group was significantly less than the placebo and the 1 g group."

Sometimes, as my interpretation of Yonemoto's finding suggests, vitamin C could act against immunity. In some cases, vitamin C may even encourage the growth of detrimental yeast infections. W. Byron Smith et al.[56] have reported that *in vitro* experiments show ascorbic acid inhibits intracellular killing of *Candida albicans* (formerly called *Monilia albicans*). Since candidiasis is a common complaint, this may be distressing news to many vitamin C enthusiasts. However, the investigators note that they are "unaware of an increased incidence of fungal infections in subjects ingesting massive quantities of l-ascorbic acid." On the other hand, some ascorbic acid may be useful in controlling *Candida.* Iancu Gontzea[57] reported that guinea pigs fed a diet with supplemental "C" showed diminished phagocytic activity of their leucocytes to *Candida* as their vitamin C intake was reduced. More recently, Thomas J. Rogers et al.[57a] found that, although guinea pigs receiving only small amounts of ascorbic acid were susceptible to *Candida* infections, megadose levels of "C" did not seem to influence resistance to this microorganism. (Apparently they did not study the possibility that growth of *Candida* might have been enhanced at high levels of ascorbic acid.) Thus, there is agreement that modest amounts of ascorbic acid are useful in protecting against *Candida,* but a possible disagreement as to whether a *reverse effect* occurs at high levels of the vitamin.* But, even if a *reverse effect* exists in the action of vitamin C on *Candida* that does not necessarily mean there could be a *reverse effect* in treating colds. It would, however, be ironic, wouldn't it, if modest dosages of "C" worked to treat a cold but large doses exacerbated its symptoms? There is no proof of such a phenomenon but the concept of the *reverse effect,* applicable to so much "C"-phenomena, alerts us to its possible existence also in the therapy of colds. Perhaps a study of dosage levels used in the various trials of vitamin C relative to colds, in full cognizance of a possible *reverse effect,* might yield interesting results!

Is it worth taking a possible risk of dangerous side effects (as will be reported later) to use megadoses of "C" in the attempt to alleviate the effects of a cold? If one's typical cold tends to involve

---

* The incidence of *Candida* infection has risen steadily in recent years as the widespread use of antibiotics has weakened our immune systems. Nystatin is a currently popular drug for controlling *Candida,* but Jan Kabelik[57c] found garlic extract to be more effective *in vitro.* A. Tynecka and Z. Gos[57d] also reported *Candida albicans* sensitive to garlic juice. Gary S. Moore and Robin D. Atkins[57e] also determined that garlic extract was a strong inhibitor of *Candida.* A study by Judith A. Appleton and Michael R. Tansey[57f], however, as well as another by Tynecka and Gos,[57g] reported variable results using garlic against *Candida.* A recent review by Moses A. Adetumbi and Benjamin H. S. Lau[57h] covers the use of garlic as an antibiotic.

just a stuffy, runny nose—the kind of cold that some studies have indicated is most helped by "C"—one may decide to answer "yes." If, on the other hand, a person's colds tend to involve fever, sore throat, headaches, i.e., more general symptoms that seem less amenable to palliation, his answer might appropriately be "no." Even though vitamin C supplementation may be of some value in combating a cold, it is not necessarily wise to use the vitamin as a preventive aid. Perhaps it is healthful to reduce excess histamine produced by a cold or by other forms of stress. However, under normal conditions is it healthful to destroy histamine (which serves valuable body functions, possibly including that of a neurotransmitter) through use of vitamin C?

Cold Fighting and the Bioflavonoids; Their Possible Mutagenicity

Those fighting colds often take various bioflavonoids in addition to vitamin C. At least one flavonoid, quercetin, is effective against some viruses, and it is possible that it might also reduce the infectivity of cold viruses. An *in vitro* study by T. N. Kaul et al.[57i] concluded that the flavonoid quercetin exerts inhibitory effects on the infectivity of herpes simplex virus type 1, polio virus type 1, parainfluenza virus type 3 and respiratory syncytial virus. The flavonoids naringin and hesperidin had no discernible effect on the infectivity of any virus.

However, using the Ames salmonella test, many bioflavonoids have been reported to be mutagenic, e.g., quercetin, quercitrin, quercitin, rhamnetin, galangin, tamarixetin, morin, myricetin, kaempferol, fisetin and rutin, and therefore they should probably not be consumed to excess.[58,59,59a-c] We should not fear the bioflavonoids, however, since animal experiments have shown that they do not seem to cause cancer. Aeschbacher et al.[59d] fed mice quercetin (one of the most powerful mutagenic flavonols *in vitro*) at concentrations 1,000 times greater than the estimated daily human intake of all flavonoids (50 mg.) with no detectable mutagenic effect. Many other studies, cited by Hans-Ulrich Aeschbacher,[59d] and more recent research by G. S. Stoewsand et al.[59e] and C. C. Willhite[59f] concluded that quercetin is also not carcinogenic and/or teratogenic in mice, rats and hamsters.*

On the other hand, interesting possibilities exist in the use of quercitin in hyperthermia treatment for cancer. This treatment is more effective at an acidic pH and Jae Ho Kim et al.[60d] have shown that quercitin, by decreasing the amount of lactate in cancer cells, lowers their pH. We should note, nevertheless, according to C. Sirtori et al.[61] that mutagenic or carcinogenic agents are also factors that tend to accelerate the advent of senility. R. E. Hughes and H. K. Wilson[62] have also reported that flavonoids, possibly by chelating trace elements, can inhibit a large number of enzymes. However, Hughes and Wilson also point out, on the plus side, that flavonoids depress the breakdown of ascorbic acid into metabolites that could be an important factor in the mutagenesis theory of aging. (The flavonoids, by binding copper, reduce the destructive effect of this metal on vitamin C.)[60a]** Ingestion of flavonoids is most likely another example of the merit of moderation in all things.

By the way, vitamins labeled as being derived from rose hips or acerola cherry generally contain only small amounts of vitamin C from such sources and hence have very small, probably completely safe, amounts of bioflavonoids. Such products are supplemented to a large degree with synthetically produced ascorbic acid to bring them up to the labeled potency. Vitamin P activity (and "vitamin P" is not

---

* The theory of the *reverse effect* suggests that if a substance is a mutagen and possible cancer-promoter, we should ask if it ever reverses and becomes a cancer-fighter. Lee W. Wattenberg and J. Lionel Leong[60] reported that three flavones (quercetin pentamethyl ether, beta naphthoflavone and rutin) inhibited skin tumor formation in mice initiated by benzo(a)pyrene. The first two flavonoids, but not rutin, were effective in inhibiting pulmonary adenoma in mice. Use of betanaphthoflavone was especially effective, resulting in almost 100% inhibition. Joachim Kühnau[60a] and K. Morita et al.[60b] have also reported that flavonoid-containing foods and flavonoids themselves have antimutagenic and tumor-inhibitory effects (i.e., they show a *reverse effect*). Kühnau[60a] says: "There is reasonable evidence that the cytostatic and anti-carcinogenic activity of food flavonoids, which distinguishes these compounds from all other nutrients, is a fundamental phenomenon which warrants in itself the conclusion that flavonoids must be looked upon as 'semi-essential' food elements." Ito et al.[60c] also suggest flavones of vegetables (and glutathione in the case of onions) may suppress chemically-induced cancer.

** On the other hand, if a hair analysis suggests one may be already low in copper, the bioflavonoids might exacerbate the deficiency.

generally considered to be a vitamin) is displayed by at least 40 substances. Among the substances that show vitamin P activity are rutin (derived from buckwheat), hesperidin (found in most citrus fruits, especially in the white of orange peel), quercitrin or quercitron (from the bark of the quercitron oak tree and found also in grapefruit), naringin (from grapefruit), epicatechin and unidentified factors in lemon peel. (Tangerine peel contains a poisonous flavone, *tangeretin,* which makes it unusable as a bioflavonoid source. It should probably not be used in marmalade.)

Rutin and the other bioflavonoids are effective in decreasing capillary fragility.[62a*] It has even been reported that the bioflavonoids have been found useful in relieving hot flashes during menopause.[62b] In addition, Faith B. Davis et al.[63a] found, using an *in vitro* technique, that quercetin stimulated Ca^{2+}-ATPase at low concentrations, but in high amounts showed a *reverse effect* and inhibited this enzyme. (Then too, using rat experiments, J. P. Tayayre and H. Lauressergues[65] have reported that oral administration of the bioflavonoids with vitamin C has been useful in combating inflammation. (Huge dosages were used—far beyond those taken by megadosing humans. In addition, the rats made their own ascorbic acid.)

Then too, S. D. Varma, et al.[64] tell that the flavonoids probably help prevent the onset of diabetic and galactosemic cataracts, at least in animals. In a follow-up study, Varma et al.[64a] found that the flavonoid quercitrin decreased the accumulation of sorbitol in the lenses of diabetic animals. Through quercitrin's inhibition of the enzyme aldose reductase (which affects sorbitol production), the onset of cataract was effectively delayed. The flavonoids act as antioxidants primarily because of the phenolic hydroxyl groups they contain.[66]

---

* Those who bruise easily and develop the black and blue marks of *purpura* may wish to consider taking extra bioflavonoids to strengthen their capillaries. (Incidentally, those black and blue marks, that may turn yellow, green and brown, provide optical evidence of the conversion of hemoglobin to yellow bilirubin which is further oxidized to green biliverdin and to other bile pigments.) However, Walter H. Lewis and Memory P. F. Elvin-Lewis[63] relate that hesperidin, quercitrin and rutin are vasopressor agents (i.e., they may increase blood pressure) and thus one wonders about the wisdom of using vitamin P for treating or for avoiding strokes.

Even though the bioflavonoids are efficacious in these various applications, Dr. Pauling and others have questioned their usefulness in fighting a cold. However, Doctor Z. Zloch[67] of Charles University, Pilzen, Czechoslovakia, has done research that may tend to support the value of the bioflavonoids when used in conjunction with ascorbic acid. Robert S. Goodhart[67] states that Dr. Zloch "...has reported that treatment of vitamin C-deficient, long term 'factor P'-deficient guinea pigs with both bioflavonoids (quercetrin or epicatechin) and ascorbic acid showed a significantly favorable influence of the bioflavonoids as compared with results obtained with treatment with ascorbic acid alone. According to Zloch, there was a more rapid restitution of the body weight and decrease in the proportion of ascorbic acid present in the liver, kidney and adrenals as dehydroascorbic acid, a manifestation, perhaps, of an antioxidant effect of the flavonoids. Reported also were a decrease in serum cholesterol and an increase in serum albumin, as compared to findings in animals treated with ascorbic acid alone."

Subsequent findings suggest that the bioflavonoid quercetin can alleviate cold symptoms by inhibiting the release of histamine. Elliott Middleton, Jr. et al.[67a] reported that quercetin "markedly inhibited antigen-induced, calcium-independent basophil activation in the 1st stage of histamine release and was also inhibitory in the antigen-independent, calcium-dependent 2nd stage." Quercetin inhibited histamine release at concentrations of 5 to 50mM (80% to 100% inhibition at 50 mM). They reported, however, that rutin (the 3-0-rhamnosylglucoside of quercetin) lacked inhibitory activity.

It seems likely that many of us would benefit from an increased consumption of bioflavonoids in spite of their possible mutagenicity, providing we can risk a possible increase in blood pressure. Very small amounts are found in most supplements. It is reported that the edible portion of an orange contains 16 times as much bioflavonoids as ascorbic acid. In juice form, the ratio is greatly altered since most of the bioflavonoids are in the pulp that is generally rejected, but, even in the case of juice, there is about twice as much bioflavonoids as ascorbic acid. One might conclude that we need far more bioflavonoids than ascorbic acid. The reasoning is, I believe, fallacious.

The progenitors of man, according to Dr. Stone, met most of their ascorbic acid requirements, not through diet, but as a conversion product of glucose. Thus, their bioflavonoid needs, like ours, were not necessarily related to the relative concentrations found in their diet.

If, in spite of what I have said, you are still a big "C" enthusiast, it may be especially important to consume extra amounts of ascorbic acid during the season of highest sunspot activity—September to October and February to March. L. Peter Cogan[68] presents evidence that increased positive ionization in the air caused by the additional sunspot activity has some very negative effects on the body. Positive ionization is reported to affect the body's acid-alkaline balance and to decrease the ability of blood plasma to combine with carbon dioxide. Since the presence of carbon dioxide stimulates the respiratory center, the low carbon dioxide causes a reduction in both the intake and the consumption of oxygen. Mr. Cogan points out that inadequate oxygen intake causes the body to produce an insufficient amount of heat. The resulting thermal imbalance is an invitation for cold viruses to attack. During the two periods a year of maximum sunspot activity it may be especially important to consume an adequate amount of ascorbic acid. It seems to me, however, that the 11-year sunspot cycle would be so overpowering as to dwarf this twice-a-year effect.[*]

Use of vitamin C and the bioflavonoids for fighting colds is compatible with one view of biological processes. However, there is another way of looking at the human organism and at the phenomenon of the cold. Some healers would prefer to simply let a cold run its course and might argue that the vitamin C is merely suppressing the symptoms.

At any rate, whether or not vitamins are used in fighting a cold, one should seek the cold's underlying causes. Man may get sick through his own actions and inactions rather than from just the

---

[*] L. Peter Cogan[68] and R. E. Hope-Simpson[68a] discuss the 11-year sunspot cycle in relation to the incidence of influenza. (Interestingly, this disease, or rather group of diseases, is named because epidemics were formerly attributed to the influence of the stars—and the sun is, of course, a star.)

environment. It should, moreover, be kept in mind that it is far easier to *avoid* a cold (by getting sufficient sleep, exercise and relaxation, by eating regularly, by having regular and frequent bowel movements, by having an adequate intake of vitamins and minerals and by minimizing stressful conditions such as smoking or exposure to cold temperatures or to cold germs) than it is to cure a cold.

Let me repeat an earlier question before we leave the subject of cold fighting: Could it be that excessive amounts of vitamin C might work against the cold-curing process? Is it possible that some studies examining the effects of vitamin C on the course of colds have used such high dosages of "C" as to negate any possible therapeutic benefit because of the occurrence of a *reverse effect*?

Dosages and Uses of Vitamin C

There are widely varying opinions as to what constitutes an optimal intake of vitamin C. Dr. Irwin Stone, perhaps the first person to regularly use massive doses of ascorbic acid, took 3,000 mg. to 5,000 mg. daily for some 40 years beginning in the 1940s. During periods of great stress (in one case a serious auto accident) he increased his daily intake to 30 or 40 grams. Dr. Frederick R. Klenner took 20,000 mg. per day for many years and prescribed far higher levels for patients with individual problems. Dr. Abram Hoffer, about whom we have written in connection with vitamin B₃ and schizophrenia, has given patients as much as 90 grams of ascorbic acid daily without, he reports, any sign of toxicity. Those desiring to study the pros and cons of vitamin C in treating schizophrenia can refer to articles in the *American Journal of Psychiatry*[69] in which Dr. Linus Pauling takes the "pro" side and three other researchers take the "con" side.

There has been considerable speculation about vitamin C's possible ability to favorably influence mental alertness and efficiency. Such speculations have been based on vitamin C's ability to raise the intercellular concentrations of cyclic adenosine monophosphate (cAMP). Kristine Adams,[70] however, reported that no differences in psychomotor performance were found in a double-blind crossover trial involving a group of 20 young men when plasma vitamin C levels were high (16.28 ± 3.75 mg./l.) and when they were low (6.5 ± 3.88 mg./l.). There were no significant differences found in an hour-long auditory vigilance test for alertness, a digit-symbol substitution test for short-term memory and a memory-for-digits test for measuring immediate memory. Dr. Adams also found no significant difference in subjectively rated sleep quality, alertness, concentration or mood. She observed, however, that her work does not rule out the possibility of subtle deleterious effects in psychomotor performance or mood, particularly at vitamin C levels lower than those existing in her subjects. Nevertheless, a study exists that is even less favorable to vitamin C. David Benton[71] found that large doses of "C" produce disruption of psychological functioning, resulting in decreased reaction times and decreased psychomotor coordination. On the other hand, G. J. Naylor[72] reported vitamin C to be of value in treating manic and depressed patients. An experiment involving a two-day double-blind, placebo-controlled crossover trial of a single three-gram dose of ascorbic acid was carried out in a group of 11 manic and 12 depressed patients. Naylor observed that the severity ratings during the ascorbic acid-treated day were significantly lower than those of the placebo-treated day.

Ascorbates or ascorbic acid (especially when taken with calcium) may be useful in relieving allergic conditions such as hives, hay fever and sinus infections (as noted earlier). It is popularly believed that ascorbic acid is often able to relieve those suffering from asthma and from hay fever. However, recent research by Dr. Bryant R. Fortner et al.[73] at the Fitzsimons Army Medical Center in Aurora, Colorado, has indicated that daily doses of four grams of ascorbic acid do nothing to suppress allergic reactions to ragweed or june grass. These scientists expressed doubt as to vitamin C's ability to ameliorate any allergic response. In a subsequent study, Stanislaus Ting et al.[74] gave 20 subjects with mild asthma a short course of megadose treatment (500 mg. four times daily for three days and 1 g. prior to spirometric evaluation). Ting found no benefits of vitamin C against bronconstriction but remained open to the possibility of improvement over a period of time.

We have already noted the ability of vitamin C to act as an antihistamine and thus it may have applications in treating asthma. E. Zuskin et al.[75] reported that ascorbic acid inhibited histamine-induced airway constriction in humans. It is now known, as pointed out in Chapter 3, that prostaglandins are involved in both the onset of asthma and in its control. The research of L. Puglisi et al.[76] suggests that the therapeutic effect of ascorbic acid in human bronchial asthma may be related not only to its control of histamine, but to an effect on prostaglandin synthesis. In further work, C. Brink et al.[76a] presented evidence suggesting that ascorbic acid beneficially modulates cyclo-oxygenase activity, thus leading to a reduction of airway responsiveness to histamine.

Supplemental ascorbate may also help prevent liver damage that could be caused by some drugs. For example, Richard J. Hargreaves et al.,[77] in an experiment with mice, reported that ascorbic acid protected against liver damage caused by acetaminophen. In another experiment with mice, R. G. Busnel and A. G. Lehmann[78] observed that injection of high doses of vitamin C (500 mg. per kg. weight—i.e., equivalent to about 35,000 mg. in a 150 lb. person) prevented any swimming impairment due to ethyl alcohol.

Then too, H. Sprince et al.,[79] in surveying the literature, reported that ascorbic acid has a protective action against at least seven toxicants associated with heavy drinking and heavy smoking. These toxicants are ethanol, acetaldehyde, nicotine, carbon monoxide, N-nitroso compounds, cadmium and polynuclear hydrocarbons.

The drinking of alcohol greatly reduces the plasma ascorbic acid concentration. It has been stated by E. M. Baker et al.[80] and by N. Krasner et al.[81] that the clearance of alcohol from the blood is proportional to the ascorbic acid concentration of the leucocytes. The Krasner group suggested that the activity of alcohol dehydrogenase, the enzyme employed by the body in alcohol's metabolism, may vary with the concentration of ascorbic acid. If so, "sobering up" should be hastened by taking additional "C." A study by Herbert Sprince et al.[81a] showed that ascorbic acid provides protection against acetaldehyde, a toxicant associated with the drinking of alcohol (and with the smoking of cigarettes). Interestingly, R. G. Busnel and A. G. Lehmann[81b] found that swimming impairment in mice due to alcohol consumption was prevented by high doses of ascorbic acid. The alcohol-induced intoxication, when not obviated by vitamin C, lasted beyond the elimination of alcohol from the blood, suggesting that a metabolite (perhaps acetaldehyde), rather than alcohol itself, may have been responsible for the swimming impairment. Then too, findings reported by Virginia Fazio et al.[82] suggest that alcohol may reduce the availability of ascorbic acid from food and predispose to a vitamin C deficiency. Earlier, M. O'Keane et al.[83] had shown that subclinical scurvy is common in alcoholics.

Smoking also detrimentally affects the leucocyte ascorbic acid concentration according to C. J. Schorah et al.[84] In the Schorah study, smokers were found to have an increased number of circulating white cells (which is a typical body reaction to invading chemicals or organisms). Nevertheless, the total ascorbic acid in the leucocytes was less than that in the leucocytes of nonsmokers. In the 1960s we heard statements to the effect that one cigarette destroyed 25 mg. of vitamin C in the body—an idea first published by W. S. McCormick[84a] in 1952. Such claims had no quantitative support,* but the definitive study by Omer Pelletier,[84b] as well as other studies cited by Pelletier, firmly established the negative effects of smoking on the body stores of "C." O. S. Hoefel[84c] recently summarized a number of related studies and concluded that vitamin C supplements help protect against some of the effects of smoking. In his own research he found greater differences in the ascorbic acid levels between smokers and nonsmokers when the smokers were also heavy users of alcohol. A study by Herbert Sprince et al.[85] indicates that the function of supplementing "C" seems to involve protection of the body against acetaldehyde toxicity that results from smoking and drinking.

---

* If each cigarette destroyed 25 mg. of vitamin C, smokers who did not take supplements would rapidly develop scurvy. They do not. Smoking is deadly, of course, but it has only a modest propensity to destroy "C."

Vitamin C should perhaps sometimes be recommended to drug addicts who desire to kick their habit. Valentine Free and Pat Sanders[85a,b] and also Alfred F. Libby and Irwin Stone[85c] have published studies showing that ascorbic acid is beneficial in drug-addiction therapy. Suppression of withdrawal symptoms and of the psychological "high" of narcotic addicts (as well as the suppression of pain in cancer patients) seems to be due to ascorbate's destruction of opioid receptors.[85d] Robert E. Willette et al.[85d] reported that inhibition of analgesia in mice was dose-dependent, had a rapid onset (two hours) and long duration (48 hours). Ascorbate in oral doses over 8 mg./kg. also protected against lethal doses of morphine. Destruction of receptors reached a maximum at 10^{-3}M or about 100 mg. of ascorbate per kg. of body weight (i.e., equivalent to 7 g. daily in a 70 kg. person).* Then a *reverse effect* set in at higher ascorbate concentrations with receptor destruction decreasing. Animal experiments can do no more than suggest the possibility of similar phenomena in humans. However, the *reverse effect* displayed in the analgesia experiments of Willette et al. suggests to me the possibility that human cancer patients treated with ascorbate might be given such high doses that pain could be increased over that which would have existed if they had been given lower dosages.

Ascorbic acid, in some cases, will not only act to prevent toxicity, but also will act to detoxify poisonous agents. It has been reported to play a role in nullifying the toxicity of saccharin and other artificial sweeteners or an excess of vitamins A and D (which we noted earlier can be toxic). It is also useful in reducing the effects of various poisons such as fluorine, cadmium, benzene and carbon tetrachloride. Vitamin C's detoxifying property involves its influence on the action of liver enzymes.[86] As a result of *in vitro* studies with guinea pigs, V. G. Zannoni et al.[86a] speculated that lipid peroxidation is detrimental to drug metabolism and vitamin C might be working as an antioxidant to reduce lipid peroxidation, thereby improving drug metabolism. They reported, however, that "the rate of lipid

---

* Since rats make endogenous vitamin C, the equivalent in a 70 kg. human would be greatly in excess of 7 g.

peroxidation was, in fact, somewhat lower in microsomes deficient in the vitamin." Vitamin C was exhibiting greater antioxidant power at the lower concentrations. Judith L. Sutton et al.,[87,87a] in further experiments with guinea pigs, reported that both a very low (scorbutic) level and a very high level of 300 mg./day (equivalent to five grams per day for man) affect the liver concentration of cytochrome P-450 and cytochrome b_5, as well as the activities of various other drug-metabolizing enzymes.[*] Francis J. Peterson et al.[87d] similarly reported that long-term consumption by guinea pigs of massive amounts of ascorbic acid (2 to 86 g. per kg. diet) for nine months significantly depressed hepatic P-450 and the liver's metabolizing enzyme activities. Separately, addition of ascorbic acid (100 mM) *in vitro* to guinea pig microsomes significantly increased oxygen consumption, but this was partially reversed by adding superoxide dismutase and/or catalase. Peterson and his colleagues concluded that excess ascorbic acid inhibits drug metabolism by mechanisms involving the generation of oxygen free radicals.[**] E. Ginter et al.[87f] subsequently reported on several different *reverse effects* involving high and low levels of ascorbic acid with cytochrome P-450, triglycerides and cholesterol. Since a normal level of "C" reverses a low level in its effect on the cytochromes and a high level of "C" reverses the effect of a normal level of "C" on

---

[*] The action of the cytochrome P-450 family of hemoprotein isoenzymes is not always favorable. The work of Qin et al., as discussed in Chapter 4, showed that retinol may exert its anticarcinogenic effects by inhibiting some of the P-450 enzymes required to activate precarcinogens (reference 45 of Chapter 4). I speculate that the partial suppression of cancer by theophylline (in tea)[87b] or by caffeine[87c] may relate to an inhibition of one or more of the P-450 enzymes.

[**] Samuel Schvartsman et al.[87e] did a rat study relating to the effects of paraquat, the herbicide used to kill various weeds, including marijuana plants. When paraquat-fed rats were treated with ascorbic acid (or better yet with ascorbic acid plus riboflavin) their survival rate was significantly increased over those fed just paraquat. Superoxide and other toxic types of oxygen are produced by paraquat.[87ca, ea] It seems to me that if ascorbic acid, in the Schvartsman study, is protecting against paraquat by inhibiting the generation of free radicals, we have a *reverse effect* compared to that of the Peterson study where ascorbic acid aided the generation of free radicals. In experiments with mice, Ron Kohen and Mordechai Chevion[87ea] showed that iron increased the toxicity of paraquat. They found that the iron chelator desferrioxamine increased the survival of mice poisoned with paraquat. (They did not suggest it, but it seems likely that the role of ascorbic acid in reducing paraquat toxicity may involve its effect in chelating iron.)

cytochromes, we have an example of a *biphasic reverse effect*. This effect suggests again the virtue of moderation in vitamin consumption. Vitamin C may also be of value in reducing the hazards associated with nitrosatable drugs and foods (i.e., those capable of being converted into nitroso compounds such as nitrosamines). More will be said about this later in connection with vitamin C and cancer.

Many nutrients other than vitamin C, as well as many drugs, affect the microsomal enzyme system and the way it handles drugs and poisons. Kamala Krishnaswamy[87g] has cited studies by C. S. Catz et al.,[87h] by G. C. Becking[87i] and by V. G. Zannoni and P. H. Sato[87j] showing that not only vitamin C deficiency, but also riboflavin and tocopherol deficiencies can decrease enzyme activities participating in various reactions. Other research by G. C. Becking,[87k] as cited by Krishnaswamy, has demonstrated that a vitamin A deficiency affects the mixed function oxidase system, examples of such effects being a reduction in hepatic N-hydroxylase and N-demethylase activities. On the other hand, Krishnaswamy cites a study by A. G. Wade et al.[87l] showing that thiamin deficiency can enhance the metabolism of heptachlor and aniline. Attallah Kappas et al.[87m] reported that a low-carbohydrate, high-protein diet decreased the half-life of antipyrine from 16.2 hours to 9.5 hours and increased the half-life of theophylline from 5.2 hours to 7.6 hours. They also cited studies showing that cigarette smoking increased the *in vivo* metabolism in man not only of nicotine but also of phenacetin and theophylline. In another study, Kappas et al.[87n] found that mean plasma half-lives of antipyrine and theophylline were each decreased 22% after healthy volunteers were fed a diet containing charcoal-broiled beef. They also cited animal studies[87p,q] showing that feeding of charcoal-broiled beef stimulated the oxidative metabolism of phenacetin as well as of benzo(a)pyrene. Krishnaswamy[87g] cited studies by T. C. Campbell and J. R. Hayes,[87r] as well as by J. C. Son-Lucero et al.,[87s] showing that deficiencies of magnesium, iron, potassium, zinc, calcium, copper and iodine can result in altered drug metabolism through their effects on the microsomal enzyme system. Campbell and Hayes[87r] have extensively reviewed many additional studies relating to the role of nutrition in the drug-metabolizing enzyme system, while A. Douglas Bender,[87t] as well as D. J. Smithard and M. J. S. Langman,[87u] have reviewed the pharmacologic effects of nutrients and drugs as a function of aging.

Vitamin C for Other Uses in Healing

A lack of ascorbate may be a factor in backaches. Dr. James Greenwood, Jr.[88] has stated that in many cases when patients with disc lesions were given 500 to 1,000 mg. of ascorbic acid daily, their back pains disappeared. Vitamin C is, in fact, recommended for relief of bone pain in various diseases. M. Smethurst et al.[89] and T. K. Basu et al.[89a] reported that ascorbic acid, used either alone or (better) in conjunction with calcitonin, gave good relief of bone pain to those having Paget's disease.

A primary function of ascorbic acid is to act in the formation of hydroxyproline, which is a constituent of collagen. Collagen is a major component of connective tissue, which is the stiff, jelly-like material that acts like a cement in holding together all the cells of the body. Collagen is strictly protein in nature and vitamin C is not one of collagen's components, but collagen cannot be synthesized without the vitamin. Calcium and vitamin A are also needed in the formation of collagen but, like vitamin C, act merely as catalysts and do not enter into collagen's structure.

Some contend that ascorbic acid should be employed immediately as first-aid treatment for accident victims and should also be used before and after surgery. Way back in 1942, Dr. G. Ungar[89b] published the results of some guinea pig experiments. Using anesthetized animals, Dr. Ungar dropped weights on them from different heights. Weights dropped from heights that would kill 100% of the animals resulted, instead, in 100% survival if the animals were injected shortly after the trauma with ascorbic acid equivalent to seven grams in a 150 lb. person. Accidents and surgery introduce severe stress, and vitamin C is reputed to be useful in combating stress.

John A. Wolfer et al.[90] reported that a deficiency of vitamin C was a detrimental factor in wound healing. They stated that human subjects on prolonged ascorbic acid depletion show about 50% diminution in tensile strength of healing wounds. Such depletion delays development of tensile strength from three to five days up to the fourteenth postoperative day.[90] The essential function for vitamin C in wound healing seems to be that it catalyzes the hydroxylation of proline and lysine during synthesis of collagen.[90a]

William W. Coon,[91] in studying 150 surgical patients, stated that 200 mg. of vitamin C daily was sufficient for saturation or near-saturation of tissues. He concluded, "the requirement for ascorbic acid in the usual patient undergoing a major operation is probably not much greater than that expected in a comparable sample of the normal population." In yet another study, one involving 63 surgical patients, Thomas T. Irvin and Dilip K. Chattopadhyay[92] reported that surgery was followed by an increase in ascorbic acid requirements. There was an average of 42% reduction in circulating leukocyte ascorbic acid levels on the third postoperative day. Although the investigators concluded that their work suggests a need for increased vitamin C in surgical patients, they stated it is unlikely the postoperative changes in leucocyte ascorbic acid have pathological significance in wound repair.

Others are far more enthusiastic about the use of vitamin C in healing. T. V. Taylor et al.[93] stated that his findings suggest vitamin C as being valuable in accelerating the healing of pressure sores (bed sores). More recently, W. M. Ringsdorf, Jr. and E. Cheraskin[94] reported on many aspects of vitamin C in fostering wound healing. They concluded that, in subjects judged not to be deficient in vitamin C, wound healing was greatly accelerated when they administered to those subjects daily doses of 500 to 3,000 mg. of the vitamin, i.e., roughly 8 to 50 times the RDA of 60 mg. Their subjects were recovering from surgery, other injuries, decubital ulcers and leg ulcers due to hemolytic anemia. In a study based on many cases where ascorbic acid was employed topically, orally and parenterally in the treatment of burns, David H. Klasson[94a] gave good notice to use of the vitamin. He concluded that ascorbic acid relieves the pain of minor burns, hastens the healing period and aids in combating the accumulation of toxic protein metabolites.

Hyperbaric oxygen therapy is sometimes employed in the treatment of a number of diseases. Such therapy could involve the danger of oxygen toxicity and it is occasionally suggested that, since vitamin C can act as an antioxidant, it may offer protection. S. S. Epstein and Y. Bishop[185a] did, in fact, do studies that supported this thesis. However, Robert A. Roth and Lizabeth A. Dotzlaf[185b] later decided that 1.5 g./kg. ascorbic acid provided no protection against pulmonary oxygen toxicity when rats were exposed to oxygen at a pressure of one atmosphere.

Vitamin C, Pregnancy and Crib Death

One sometimes reads that it is important for women to take large quantities of ascorbic acid during pregnancy. C. Alan B. Clemetson[96] speculates that ascorbic acid deficiency (which can lead to histamine intoxication) might predispose to *abruptio-placentae* (premature separation of the placenta prior to delivery of the infant). Possibly its incidence and that of megaloblastic anemia of pregnancy might be reduced with vitamin C supplementation. However, Victor D. Herbert[97] states that where the mother is taking excess vitamin C the fetus may develop (as has the mother) catabolic machinery for handling the excess. The fetus born with this catabolic machinery for destroying excess "C" may develop *rebound scurvy* if he or she now eats a normal diet.* Pregnant women should seek opinions from their obstetricians if they plan to take ascorbic acid in large quantities. Pregnant women may wish to call the attention of their obstetricians to an article in *The Canadian Medical Association Journal* in which W. A. Cochrane, M.D.[98] reported on observations in children, as well as in animals, suggesting that an ascorbic acid dependency in

---

* Adults who have been taking massive dosages of "C" but who wish to cut down, should do so gradually, perhaps by 10% or 20% daily, to avoid the possibility of developing rebound scurvy, a condition which is, however, far less serious in adults than it may be in infants. Adults may, however, experience such symptoms of scurvy as bleeding gums, loosening of the teeth, muscular pain and skin roughening.

the young may be induced by exposure to the vitamin *in utero.* (The same article notes that excessive vitamin D intake by mothers sensitive to vitamin D may cause mental retardation in the offspring.) Pregnant women taking vitamin C may also wish to call their physician's attention to a study by E. P. Samborskaya and T. D. Ferdman[99,99a] which reported that 16 or 20 pregnant women developed menstrual-type bleeding within three days of taking six grams of ascorbic acid per day.

A deficiency in ascorbic acid has been widely reported in the lay press to be a factor in "crib death" or "sudden infant death syndrome." Dr. Archie Kalokerinos has reported good success through use of "C" in eliminating crib death among Australian aborigines. However, the Australian College of Pediatrics could find no scientific basis for the claims.[100]

Vitamin C and Cholesterol

According to Dr. Constance Spittle,[101,102] ascorbic acid breaks down triglycerides and mobilizes cholesterol out of the arteries and sends it to the liver, where it is converted into bile acids and subsequently excreted. She reported that, while cholesterol of young healthy persons declined after they had been given vitamin C, it rose in those with coronary artery disease. She attributed this to mobilization of arterial cholesterol. Then too, E. Ginter et al.[103] reported that 15 g. of pectin and 450 mg. of ascorbic acid fed to mildly hypercholesterolemic patients dropped their total cholesterol levels far more than did pectin alone.* Their levels of high density

---

* Increasing the intake of dietary fiber may reduce plasma cholesterol and this could sometimes be beneficial. Wheat bran, contrary to popular belief, does not seem to be of value for this purpose, but fibers in fruits and vegetables are effective. George V. Vahouny[104] reported that pectins, guar gum and oat bran (but not wheat bran) are effective for lowering plasma lipids, particularly plasma cholesterol. Thomas et al. [104a] speculate that increased bile acid excretion may have been due to stimulation of the mechanism for steroid excretion in the rat. On the other hand, Irma H. Ullrich et al.[105] stated that a high-fiber diet, compared with a high-carbohydrate, low-fiber diet, provided no additional short-term cholesterol-lowering effect over that derived from a diet equally high in carbohydrate and starch but low in fiber. R. E. Hughes[105a] has cited several studies

lipoproteins remained unchanged; thus the ratio of HDL to LDL increased. On the contrary, C. J. Bates et al.[106] reported a strong positive correlation between vitamin C status and plasma HDL cholesterol in men, but *the correlation was not observed for women*. On the other hand, a study by Virginia E. Peterson et al.[107] showed no such drop in cholesterol levels. The Peterson group fed nine hypercholesterolemic persons four grams of ascorbic acid daily for two months. There was no significant change in plasma cholesterol or triglyceride levels. They also reported no significant change in triglyceride concentrations of the major lipoprotein classes, but their data shows small, possibly unfavorable, declines in HDL and small, but possibly unfavorable, increases in the LDL fraction.

Gregory E. Johnson and S. Scott Obenshain[108] in a follow-up study reported that vitamin C given male volunteers at levels of one gram daily showed no effect on serum cholesterol, HDL, LDL or triglycerides. Then too, Abdur R. Khan and Frank A. Seedarnee[109] reported that 13 normal young female volunteers given one gram of vitamin C daily for four weeks showed no effect on the cholesterol content of HDL, LDL or VLDL. Similarly, V. D. Joshi et al. [110] found that ascorbic acid has no effect on total cholesterol and HDL-cholesterol in normal young persons. Thus, the studies of Gregory E. Johnson, of Abdur R. Khan and of V. D. Joshi with normal women and men agree with the study of Virginia E. Peterson using hypercholesterolemic persons, each indicating that vitamin C shows no effect on plasma cholesterol in humans. Interestingly, Khan and Seedarnee suggest that the difference in results of the various studies may be due to a failure of the earlier researchers to take diet and weight of the subjects into account! Later studies by M. L. Burr et

---

showing that increased intake of certain types of dietary fiber (e.g., pectin or guar gum) retards the development of the uterus in young mice, rats and guinea pigs. Hughes, citing a study he did with E. Jones[105b] that involved the life patterns in 46 countries, noted that they had found "a highly significant positive correlation between the reported menarcheal age and the estimated intake of dietary fibre." Hughes went on to state that "correlations with other dietary components for which a monitoring role in menarche has sometimes been claimed, such as fat, protein and energy intake, were significantly weaker." Fiber has value in increasing intestinal transit time (and this is probably very important). Could it be that all those many studies favoring fiber were really favoring some other unknown dietary component present in fiber-containing foods? Fiber has already been discussed in Chapter 3 and will be considered further in Chapter 7.

al.[111] showed ascorbic acid did increase HDL, but the association between them was not strong and Burr et al. suggest it may not have been an example of cause and effect. Recently, in studying mildly hypertensive women, Eunsook T. Koh[111a] reported that, although vitamin C in amounts of 1,000 mg. daily did not change HDL-cholesterol levels, it appeared to reduce significantly VLDL-cholesterol and serum triglycerides. (In addition, ascorbic acid lowered serum sodium levels in 69.5% of his patients. Koh also observed that 64% of his subjects achieved lowered diastolic pressure and 31% experienced lowered systolic pressure.) *   In another recent study, this one of faculty members and students given two grams of vitamin C daily for two months, F. Erden et al.[111ba] reported cholesterol concentrations were decreased and HDL-cholesterol levels were raised significantly. The contradictions shown in some of these experiments strongly suggest that dose-response *reverse effects* are involved. (If not, how could so many competent scientists arrive at such opposite conclusions?) **   Recently, a study by N. Saha and Py Tan,[113a] reminiscent of the earlier work of C. J. Bates et al.,[106] showed that men with a serum ascorbic acid level higher than 1 mg./dl. had a significantly higher level of serum cholesterol than those having lesser serum ascorbate levels. Saha and Tan found no such association of the two parameters in women.

Both dietary extremes of ascorbic acid, in a *biphasic reverse effect,* were shown by David E. Holloway et al.[112] to elevate plasma

---

* Mitsuki Yoshioka et al.[111b] found that in a group of 194 apparently healthy adults (30-39 years of age) from rural Japan, serum ascorbic acid was inversely correlated with systolic and diastolic blood pressure. The association was especially strong with systolic blood pressure. The prevalence of hypertension (140/90 mm. Hg and above) was decreased as the ascorbic acid level increased. The dietary intake of vitamin C was from green vegetables and fruits. Thus, the investigators noted that "serum ascorbic acid may simply reflect the intake of the other important nutrients which influence blood pressure, such as potassium and dietary fiber."

** The season of the year during which a study of vitamin C versus cholesterol is made could account for the discrepancies. Hilary M. Dobson et al.[111c] reported that, in experiments with healthy young men and women, "during the period of May to October, there was no significant difference between the mean cholesterol levels of the groups studied with and without supplements of ascorbic acid. Throughout the period of November to April, however, the group supplemented with ascorbic acid had significantly lower mean cholesterol levels." Dobson et al. found that administering one gram of ascorbic acid daily throughout the year abolished the winter rise in cholesterol levels.

and liver cholesterol in guinea pigs. Then too, S. K. Kamath et al.[113] reported that guinea pigs fed ascorbic acid showed a *reverse effect* (my language) in their serum triglyceride levels. Those fed either .5 mg. or 5 mg. of vitamin C daily had serum triglyceride levels lower than those fed 15 mg., thus demonstrating a *biphasic reverse effect*. The results show that either subscorbutogenic or excessive doses of "C" produce a hypertriglyceridemic condition in guinea pigs and the activity of lipoprotein lipase is believed responsible for the phenomenon.

Whether or not vitamin C is effective in changing blood lipid and cholesterol parameters, we do not know what lipid and cholesterol values are ideal. Even if we knew the "ideal" values for the HDL/LDC ratio, and for total serum cholesterol, vitamin C might not always work toward such ideals. G. W. Evans[114] has shown that ascorbic acid decreases absorption of copper. As we will see in the next chapter, a reduction of copper can increase serum cholesterol and may be heart threatening. It seems likely that, depending on dosages, vitamin C might either decrease or increase cholesterol levels. In a related study, David B. Milne et al.[115] reported that, in monkeys fed high levels of ascorbic acid, serum copper was reduced and serum cholesterol was elevated. S. Kamath et al.[116] reported that serum cholesterol declined in guinea pigs fed modest doses of vitamin C (.5 to 50 mg. per day) but showed a *reverse effect* and rose at higher doses (150 and 300 mg./day). More research in this area is needed but, pending additional data, I think the work of Drs. Evans, Milne and Kamath suggests a danger in megadoses of vitamin C.

So, although the value of ascorbic acid in beneficially affecting cholesterol or lipoproteins is in doubt, it, nevertheless, has a very important function that relates to protection against atherosclerosis. Many studies have shown that vitamin C reduces the incidence of atherosclerosis and the reason probably relates not to an effect on cholesterol but an effect on prostacyclin (PGI$_2$).[117] Johan R. Beetens and Arnold G. Herman[117] have reported that vitamin C enhances the production of 6-oxo-PGF$_{1a}$ by aortic tissue. This prostaglandin is a stable product of prostacyclin. Vitamin C enhances its production probably by protecting the cyclo-oxygenase enzyme. By aiding prostacyclin's platelet deaggregating function, vitamin C offers protection against atherosclerosis.

Vitamin C and Gallstones

Emil Ginter[118] observed that an ascorbate deficiency in guinea pigs often leads to gallstones. Like man, guinea pigs belong, as we have said, to a relatively small group of animals that do not manufacture their own ascorbate. Whether or not the correlation between ascorbate deficiency and gallstone formation will extend to man is yet to be determined.*

Gallstones have been found to consist primarily of cholesterol. The bile produced by the liver and stored in the gallbladder normally carries completely dissolved cholesterol plus bile salts and pigments originating from the breakdown of red blood cells. If the bile could be made more capable of dissolving cholesterol, stones ought to be preventable. Dr. Ginter's studies indicate that increased intake of ascorbic acid (up to normal but not necessarily excessive amounts) leads to an increased amount of bile salts through conversion of cholesterol to cholic acid and its sodium salt, thus avoiding (it is hoped) the formation of gallstones.**

An excess of bile beyond body requirements may, however, not be health-serving, and Bandaru Reddy et al.[120] reported that excessive bile can destroy cells in the villi of the small intestines and also that colon cancer patients have far more bile acids in their colons than do controls. Then too, B. I. Cohen et al.[121] observed that when bile acids were increased in the colon of rats by feeding them cholic acid there was a large increase in colon cancer. It now appears that excessive bile acids are associated not only with colon cancer in rats but with cancer of the colon in humans. The association seems to be especially

---

* It seems to be generally ignored that one should move cautiously in concluding that facts relating to herbivores (such as guinea pigs) apply to omnivores (such as man).

** Recent hamster research by D. Kritchevsky et al.[119] showed dietary pectin promoted regression of gallstones.

true for women and in particular for cancer of the caecum and of the ascending colon. These facts were reported by Dimitrios A. Linos et al.[122] in commenting on the effect of gallbladder surgery. The point was made that gallbladder removal leads to an increase in bile acids and is thus a cancer threat.

Much of the confusion revolving around vitamin C and cholesterol was resolved through the experiments of David E. Holloway and Jerry M. Rivers.[123] Their guinea pigs were fed a cereal-based scorbutic diet and were given intraperitoneal injections of a bile acid, chenodeoxycholic acid, and so the experiment's protocol might be criticizable. Nevertheless, those guinea pigs who were deficient in ascorbic acid, as well as those fed an excess, showed marked inhibition of bile acid synthesis and elevation of cholesterol levels in the plasma and in the liver.* (The bile acid of animals deficient in vitamin C and those fed an excess showed less cholesterol than did controls. This finding might, at first glance, appear to contradict Ginter's results since one might expect a low level of cholesterol in the bile to *protect* against gallstone formation. However, it seems that the importance of an increase in bile salts—that comes with normalizing the intake of vitamin C—overwhelms the influence of the bile's cholesterol increase insofar as gallstone formation is concerned.) Once again, the theory of the *reverse effect* helps us appreciate the reason for confusion surrounding the contradictory experiments involving vitamin C and cholesterol. It is yet another example of the virtue of the principle of the golden mean—moderation in vitamin C intake as well as in all other things.

---

* Holloway and Rivers,[123] in finding that excessive consumption of ascorbic acid leads to marked inhibition in bile acid, called the discovery "most surprising." They reported that virtually all parameters of sterol metabolism, cholesterol 7α-hydroxylase activity, plasma and liver cholesterol, etc., were influenced in a similar manner. *Reverse effects,* although often striking scientists as "surprising," are very common indeed. This study was conducted over a period of seven to nine weeks. When Holloway and Rivers[124] did a similar study in guinea pigs over a period of 21 weeks they found that excessive ascorbic acid no longer inhibited bile acid but actually increased the size of the bile acid pool by 12%. The results of experiments can vary according to the time interval over which the study is conducted! How often is this fact improperly ignored?

Other Applications for "C"

In the strange mix of fact and fancy in scientific as well as in popular literature, ascorbic acid is reported to be useful in treating many physical problems. Ascorbic acid is sometimes prescribed in the treatment of arthritis, bursitis, atherosclerosis, encephalitis, phlebitis, varicose veins, trichinosis, hepatitis, osteoporosis, shingles, hypermenorrhea, postoperative radiation sickness, scarlet fever, tularemia, whooping cough, tuberculosis, multiple sclerosis, prostatitis, meningitis, high blood pressure, influenza, diphtheria, dysentery, measles, chicken pox, virus pneumonia, mumps, pancreatitis, rheumatic fever, kidney infections, acne, prickly heat, canker sores and mononucleosis. K. Jahan et al.[124a] found daily intravenous injections of 1,000 mg. of ascorbic acid to be effective in treating 117 tetanus patients (who had never been immunized against tetanus) when administered in addition to antitetanus serum, sedatives and antibiotics. A study by S. Banic[124b] indicated that, in guinea pigs, even deaths from rabies can be reduced by giving intramuscular injections of 100 mg. per kg. of body weight of vitamin C. G. Petroutsos and Y. Pouliquen[124c] recently confirmed earlier studies that ascorbic acid, administered topically and by subconjunctival injection, is beneficial in treating the alkali-burned human eye.

Vitamin C is said to aid in reducing the viscosity of the synovial fluid which is important to the proper functioning of the joints. Ascorbic acid may reduce the body's lead content (although some research contradicts this) by decreasing the amount of hyaluronidase that, when present, has a negative effect on synovial fluid. E. S. Wilkins and M. G. Wilkins[95] reported that rheumatoid arthritic cells were eradicated *in vitro* when cultured with vitamin C, while normal cells were unaffected. One should always keep in mind, however, that what works *in vitro* may or may not work *in vivo*. However, J. F. Rinehart et al.,[95a] many years earlier, had reported rheumatoid arthritis patients to have low levels of plasma ascorbic acid. Vitamin C (along with vitamin E) may also be useful in treating osteoarthritis.

Edith R. Schwartz[95b] found that guinea pigs having low levels of
vitamin C had large numbers of severely affected sites showing the
classic signs of advanced osteoarthritis. She suggested that diets rich in
vitamin C (and E) might retard the development of osteoarthritis in
humans.

Ascorbic acid has been variously reported as effective[125-128] and
ineffective[128a-c] in treating glaucoma in animals and in humans.* Both
Claus W. Jungeblut[128d-f] and Fred R. Klenner[128g] observed it to be
effective in treating poliomyelitis.** Douglas K. Reilly et al.[128j] found
use of ascorbic acid produced modest improvement in functional
performance in parkinsonism.

Vitamin C has been employed in treating diabetes and is widely
reported to be insulin-sparing. However, Roman J. Kutsky[129] reported
that it acts similarly to alloxan (i.e., as an insulin antagonist). Von W.
Losert et al.[130] observed that, in guinea pigs, the blood glucose, which
is lowered by exogenous insulin, is further decreased by concurrent
administration of high doses of ascorbic acid. They found that, in
humans also, ascorbic acid seemed to increase glucose utilization in
peripheral tissues of the body. This finding, although given wide
publicity, as we have said, seems to be in error. The erroneous
reputation that ascorbate had in seemingly providing an insulin-like
action   was   due,   it   seems,   to   ascorbate's   inhibitory

---

* Such reports suggest the possibility that a dose-response *reverse effect* might be operating.

** The subsequent work of Albert B. Sabin,[128b] using vitamin C given subcutaneously in one
experiment and nasally in another, showed that "vitamin C neither modified the course of the
disease nor prevented paralysis: 80 per cent of the untreated monkeys and 90 per cent of the
treated ones developed paralysis." Sabin continues, "With this data in hand Dr. Jungeblut's
advice was sought and a similar experiment was carried out jointly in his laboratory. In a group
of forty monkeys, among which ten were controls and thirty were treated with varying amounts
of vitamin C, only one monkey, a treated one, escaped paralysis." Sabin concludes, "There is no
apparent explanation for the difference between these results and those reported earlier by
Jungeblut." Earlier, John A. Toomey[128i] had reported that "ingestion by monkeys of massive
doses of vitamins A, B and C did not in any way aid them to ward off the effects of intracerebral
injections of poliomyelitis virus." However, Toomey reported that vitamin D protected monkeys
from poliomyelitis when the virus was subsequently introduced by way of the gastrointestinal
tract. Toomey stated, "It is paradoxical that, though the lack of vitamin D makes monkeys more
susceptible to poliomyelitis, the rise in the morbidity of the disease occurs at the time of year
when human beings theoretically should receive plenty of the antirachitic factor from the
summer sun."

action on gluconeogenesis in liver cells. It is now believed that oxalate—a metabolite of ascorbic acid—causes the inhibition.[131] Vitamin C, then, does not aid insulin-like action but, instead, it now appears that insulin indirectly inhibits the enzyme semidehydroascorbate reductase which is important for regeneration of ascorbate from dehydroascorbic acid.[132] Dehydroascorbic acid causes diabetes when injected into animals and has been found to be present in increased quantities in the blood of persons with diabetes.[132a] C. Alan B. Clemetson[133] has suggested that bioflavonoids be taken with "C" to help prevent its oxidation to dehydroascorbic acid.*

Ascorbic acid reportedly acts as a diuretic and so may be of value in relieving edema. It may also be useful in maintaining body temperature in extremely cold environments. In an extensive study involving soldiers living in a cold environment, Robert Ryer III et al.[134] found no statistically significant differences in performance between those supplemented with 300 mg. of vitamin C (plus various B vitamins) and controls whose diet had not been supplemented. Nevertheless, during exposure to cold while at rest, the supplemented group showed a lesser fall in rectal temperature, and the difference between the two groups was statistically significant.

Like vitamin E, ascorbate may be of value in inhibiting platelet aggregation, which is, in turn, a factor in blood clotting. Constance Spittle,[101] in connection with the cholesterol study which we reviewed earlier, discovered that vitamin C has a powerful antithrombic effect. K. E. Sarji et al.[135] observed that vitamin C produced marked inhibition of platelet aggregation in nonsmoking males. Persons with diabetes mellitus, while having normal plasma levels of vitamin C, generally have significantly lower platelet levels of vitamin C and hyperaggregation of platelets. Sarji discusses some of the implications for those with diabetes. Similarly, "C" may be valuable in reducing the incidence of thrombosis and vascular disease in nondiabetics

---

* Excessive copper is also a factor in this reaction. Ascorbic acid oxidase, a copper-containing enzyme which is found not only in humans but in plants such as cabbage and squash,[133a] catalyzes the oxidation of ascorbic acid to dehydroascorbic acid.

through inhibiting platelet aggregation. E. G. Knox[136] has reported that there is a strong negative correlation between ascorbate consumption and ischemic heart disease and cerebrovascular disease. Furthermore, C. Cordova et al.[137] found that intravenous administration of two grams of ascorbic acid inhibited platelet aggregation in ten healthy volunteers. They also reported, however, that a single oral dose of one gram/day does not clearly affect platelet aggregation in normal subjects. Thus, at normal dosages vitamin C has far less effect on platelet aggregation than does a nominal amount of vitamin E.

Ascorbate is concentrated in the lens of the eye and acts as a defense against superoxide,[138] singlet oxygen[139] and hydroxyl[139a,b] free radicals. Using *in vitro* experiments with rat lenses, Shambhu D. Varma et al.[139d] found that vitamin C protected the ocular lens from free radical damage caused by light in the presence of riboflavin phosphate. The light intensity was similar to that used for reading purposes. Thus, a high concentration of ascorbate in the anterior fluid chamber and the lens might help protect the eye from cataracts.

More recently, in 1986, J. Blondin et al.[139e] examined the effect of dietary vitamin C on lens protein integrity since protein damage, including oxidation and aggregation, is associated with cataractogenesis. When lens homogenates were exposed to ultraviolet light, protease activity in high-vitamin C samples was twice as great as that of low vitamin C samples. Blondin and his associates concluded that the results suggested that vitamin C protects lens structural proteins and proteases against oxidation and may delay cataractogenesis. Earlier, we saw that several studies[64,64a,66] indicated that the flavonoids may also serve a function in inhibiting the formation of cataracts.

Those various studies were done *in vitro* but even more recently, in 1986, J. A. Vinson et al.[140] reported on the effect of ascorbic acid *in vivo* on galactose-induced cataracts in rats. Complete opacification was observed in 69% of the lenses of rats fed 70% dietary galactose for 84 days (the control group). In contrast, only 6% of the lenses were completely opacified in a group fed in addition 1.2 grams of ascorbic acid/liter of drinking water. Furthermore, after 70 days of normal feeding the control group lost just 67% of its opacities while the ascorbic acid group lost 100%. Thus, ascorbic acid was shown effective in both slowing down the progression of galactose cataracts but also in speeding up their regression. One must not conclude, however, that the effect of ascorbic acid on galactose-induced cataracts in rats might have anything more than a remote relationship to any possible influence of ascorbic acid on human cataracts of unknown cause.

Ascorbic acid may protect the retina as well as the lens of the eye. Daniel T. Orgnanisciak et al.[140a] and Zong-Yi Li et al.[140b] (members of the same research team) reported that ascorbate is effective in protecting, or partially protecting, the retina of rats from light damage. It was effective, however, only if administered to the rats prior to light exposure.

Herpes labialis has also been effectively treated with 600 mg. ascorbic acid and 600 mg. of bioflavonoids by G. T. Terezhalmy et al.[141] Healing occurred on average in 4.4 days as contrasted with 9.7 days in controls given a placebo. However, like many other experiments, the protocol of this study may have been less than ideal. The experiment was not double-blind and apparently the researchers themselves did the evaluating of the results. Emotional factors were not considered; blood analyses were not done. Nevertheless, in spite of the shortcomings, the results of the study suggest that vitamin C and the bioflavonoids may be useful in combating cold sores.

Let us cite some more benefits that may accrue from adequate body stores of vitamin C. Ascorbic acid is needed to assure sturdiness of bones, deficiency of this nutrient causing them to break easily. Ascorbic acid is required by the fetus when the teeth are forming or their enamel may be thin and decay problems will be prevalent.

An ascorbic acid deficiency over a period of many years has been implicated in the occurrence of periodontal disease.[141a] Tetsuo Nakamoto and Mark McCroskey[141b] noted that mast cells which are present in gingival tissue may participate in the inflammatory response by liberating histamine. Thus, an ascorbic acid deficiency could be a factor in the development of gingivitis. Supplementary vitamin C may act directly to detoxify the histamine or may change the level of enzymes responsible for histamine metabolism. They suggested that ascorbic levels above the RDA may be required for benefitting gingival tissue which is under a high level of stress from dental plaque.* On the other hand, the value of supplemental amounts of vitamin C to aid periodontal health has been vigorously denied.[141g,h] At any rate, chewable vitamin C tablets could pose a threat to tooth enamel. John L. Giunta[141i,j] and also James L. Dannenberg[142] relate that the ascorbic acid of such tablets may be strong enough to dissolve the enamel. Then too, no matter what type of vitamin C is consumed, if one suddenly terminates megadoses of "C," oral scurvy may occur.[143] If you're going to reduce vitamin consumption, do so gradually.

Dehydroascorbic Acid and the "Morbidity Index"

We mentioned earlier the hypothesized negative effects of dehydroascorbic acid—the oxidized form of ascorbic acid. ** Dr. Irwin Stone speculates that a high ratio of dehydroascorbic acid to ascorbic acid is a cause of, or is at any rate concomitant with, the occurrence of many diseases. The reciprocal of this ratio, called the

---

* In Chapter 2 we saw that vitamin E may also be useful in treating inflammation of the gingiva and oral mucosa (references 143, 144 of that chapter). Interestingly, Tawfik M. A. ElAttar et al.[141c] reported that *in vitro* studies using human gingival tissue showed that testosterone inhibited the cyclo-oxygenase pathway and resulted in lesser amounts of the prostaglandins that are associated with inflammation. Above-normal amounts of testosterone tend to make one sexy and J. P. Gutai et al.[141d] have reported a direct (beneficial) relationship between testosterone and HDL-cholesterol. However, testosterone exacerbates balding and increases the risk of prostate cancer. (Ronald Ross et al.[141e] reported, in 1986, that blacks had just a 15% higher testosterone level but a 100% greater risk of prostatic cancer.) Regarding vitamin C, we have seen that it has a presumably beneficial effect on the immune system. However, it may be questionable, as Roy C. Page and Hubert E. Schroeder [141f] have pointed out in regard to periodontitis, whether the activation of the immune system is protective or destructive. Their interesting book and the relevant references they cite should be consulted if it seems strange that the immune system might work against periodontal health.

** K. Schmidt et al.,[143a] however, speculate that the physiological mode of action of ascorbic acid possibly does not involve oxidation to dehydroascorbic acid.

Morbidity Index, is, according to Stone,[3] a prognostic tool for estimating survival probabilities. Irwin Stone gives values of the Morbidity Index for various diseases (based on the data of B. Chakrabarti, S. Banerjee and J. N. Bhaduri). He gives values of the Index for patients who died, survived or were convalescing from various diseases. For example, those who died from pneumonia had a Morbidity Index of .4; those who survived 1.0 and those who were convalescent 4.5. Normal healthy persons have an average Morbidity Index of 14. That is, the higher the ratio of ascorbic acid to dehydroascorbic acid, the better the prognosis for recovery from each of a long list of diseases. Taking large amounts of ascorbic acid will tend to keep the ratio of ascorbic acid to dehydroascorbic acid at presumably safe levels. Then too, the research of Dr. Zloch, reported earlier in this chapter, indicates that the bioflavonoids will help keep this ratio at high, presumably favorable levels.

On the other hand, the studies of Libuse Stankova et al.[144] suggest that dehydroascorbate may be valuable. They postulate that the reducing capacity of dehydroascorbate may be important for inactivating oxidants and free radicals. Furthermore, as R. E. Hughes[145] has pointed out, the tissues contain reduced glutathione for converting dehydroascorbic acid to ascorbic acid. Then too, the fact that dehydroascorbic acid, but not ascorbic acid, passes the placental barrier from mother to fetus also argues that nature does not consider it to be a poison. (The dehydro-form is converted to ascorbic acid by the fetus.) If, as I pointed out earlier, leucocytes prefer dehydroascorbic acid over ascorbic acid, isn't it possible that "body wisdom" is increasing the so-called Morbidity Index in order to fight the pneumonococci?

Dehydroascorbic acid (DHA) is present in foods, which suggests that man may have developed metabolic uses for it, or at least a means of handling it. And, as we have seen, DHA can be reduced to ascorbic acid. Ron B. H. Wills et al.[145a] found that most fresh fruits and vegetables have less than 10% as much DHA as they have ascorbic acid. Celery was the exception at a level of 41% as much DHA as ascorbic acid. As the produce aged, the amount of DHA, as a proportion of vitamin C, became greater than 50% in celery and cucumber, greater than 25% in potato, cantaloupe and broccoli, between 10% and 20% in brussels sprouts, silver beet, tomato, lemon and orange, but stayed under 5% in banana and parsley. It seems obvious that DHA is natural, although being natural is, of course, not synonymous with being healthful. Nevertheless, it seems likely that Stone's undue concern about the healthfulness of DHA was not warranted.

Furthermore, many investigators have shown that dehydroascorbic acid readily passes the blood-brain barrier, while L. Hammerstrom[146] presented information suggesting that ascorbic acid does not.* In fact, G. R. Martin and Christyna E. Mecca[148] published findings that suggest vitamin C enters various tissues as dehydroascorbic acid that is later converted to ascorbic acid. They speculated that the kidney (and possibly the intestine) may play a role in the distribution of vitamin C by oxidizing it to dehydroascorbic acid which easily penetrates cellular barriers. The more curious reader may wish to learn of the various effects of dehydroascorbic acid on the adrenergic nerve cells in the brain and heart (including an increased release of noradrenaline in both these organs) and its possible influence on various cholinergic mechanisms. If so, read "Pharmacological Properties of Dehydroascorbic Acid and Ascorbic Acid" by Sven Erik Sjöstrand.[149] But let's get back to Stone's *Morbidity Index.* It seems to me that, since dehydroascorbic acid can be readily converted back to ascorbic acid by the body, this whole theory of the *Morbidity Index* is open to serious question.**

---

* Later, however, Reynold Spector and A. V. Lorenzo[147] reported (in the *Amer. Jrl. of Physiology,* vol. 225, pages 757-763, 1973) that in man (and in the rabbit) ascorbic acid enters the brain via the choroid plexus and this system is responsible for the transport of ascorbic acid into the cerebrospinal fluid. Thus, although some of the brain's ascorbic acid originates from the reduction of dehydroascorbic acid which entered via the blood, most ascorbic acid (and other vitamins) enter the brain via the cerebrospinal fluid, thus bypassing the blood-brain barrier. However, Spector and Lorenzo stated that vitamin C, in entering the brain via the choroid plexus, is well controlled by a saturable mechanism so that even the huge plasma levels of "C" that are achievable only by injection would result in a brain-level increase of "C" of less than 10%. These scientists observed that, in light of this fact, it is difficult to see how megavitamin therapy could alter brain function in a patient not markedly deficient in this vitamin.

** Nevertheless, as we have seen, dehydroascorbic acid has many negatives. To cite one more, an elevated hepatic dehydroascorbic acid level in hypercholesterolemic rats is

Vitamin C as an Antioxidant

An important although incompletely understood function of ascorbic acid is that of an antioxidant. Using the electron paramagnetic spin resonance technique, I. Yamazaki et al.[150,151] and, later, Carl Lagercrantz[151a] reported free-radical signals generated by peroxidase with ascorbic acid as the substrate (the substance being acted on). E. M. Baker et al.[152] found that the ascorbate free radical is oxidized in the presence of oxygen to dehydroascorbic acid. Many of the other properties of the ascorbate free radical have been discussed by Benton H. J. Bielski and Helen W. Richter.[139a] Much more recently, Rikuro Sasaki et al.[153,154] reported that they have observed a free radical in human serum at room temperature which they consider to be the ascorbate radical. We have already met free radicals in connection with vitamin E. A more thorough discussion of the role of free radicals will be found in Chapter 9. However, since ascorbate has its own free radical and can act not only as a pro-oxidant but can also act as an antioxidant to quench other free radicals, we will say something more about them at this time.

Free radicals, as you will recall, are chemical entities that have an unpaired electron and, therefore, can sometimes fly about and damage body tissues. However, superoxide radicals, which are generated by the body's membranous NADPH oxidase and possibly by its xanthine-xanthine oxidase system, have both beneficial and detrimental functions. Morimitsu Nishikimi,[138] as we pointed out earlier, has shown that ascorbate can scavenge superoxide. Ascorbic acid, according to B. Leibovitz and B. V. Siegel[155] is only a little less effective in quenching the superoxide anion radical (active in causing peroxidation) than superoxide dismutase. S. Som et al.[155a] later confirmed that the abilities of superoxide dismutase and of ascorbic acid to catalyze the decay of superoxide in animal tissues are similar. Ascorbate is also a scavenger of yet another reactive species, singlet oxygen, as reported earlier![139] We noted too that ascorbate also

---

thought to make the lysosomes fragile (a condition correctable by giving "vitamin P" in the form of quercitin or hesperidin.)[149a]

scavenges hydroxyl radicals.[139a] Then, R. W. Fessenden and N. C. Verma[139b] found that ascorbic acid, in quenching the hydroxyl radical, forms the ascorbate radical. Benton H. J. Bielski and Helen W. Richter[139a] reported that the ascorbate free radical operates in the alkaline pH range. They stated that the ascorbate free radical is a relatively nonreactive species while, in contrast, ascorbate is a good reducing agent and an efficient free-radical scavenger.* Marina Scarpa et al.[155b] have recently found, however, the recycling of vitamin E by ascorbic acid is effective "through the formation of ascorbate radical and its dismutation to ascorbic acid and ascorbate."

It is interesting to note that ascorbic acid may work not only with vitamin E but also with vitamin A (although not necessarily in a related manner). Y. Inada et al.[155c] recently reported a synergism between vitamins A and C as activators of plasminogen formation in cultured endothelial cells. (Plasminogen, occurring in plasma, can be converted to the proteolytic enzyme plasmin which is responsible for slow digestion and lysis of fiber clots.) As we noted in Chapter 2, Hon-Wing Leung et al.[155d] reported that synergistic action occurs between vitamins E and C in the inhibition of peroxidation. However, according to Inada and his coworkers, such synergism between vitamins has never before been reported in regard to cellular functions. They suggest that the combination of vitamins A and C may be effective in preventing thrombosis.

Ascorbic Acid and the *Reverse Effect*

Many years ago, H. Abramson[156] reported that he observed a subnormal oxidation of linolenic acid in almost all tissues of the scorbutic guinea pig, including the brain. Abramson found that the oxidation of fatty acid and of lipids *in vitro* proceeds spontaneously in the presence of oxygen and is catalyzed by ascorbic acid (and by

---

* In the lungs, to cite just one example, ascorbic acid may have an important role to play in extracellular defense against free radicals by acting as an antioxidant.[139a] On the other hand, V. N. R. Kartha and S. Krishnamurthy[39c] reported that ascorbate stimulated

hemoglobin). In other words, they determined that at the lowest levels of vitamin C there exists a pro-oxidant effect with lipid peroxidation proceeding at a very slow rate.

Subsequently, Gottfried Haase and W. L. Dunkley,[156a] doing *in vitro* research, studied the pro-oxidant effects of ascorbic acid (and, separately, of copper) on linoleate. They reported pro-oxidant activity occurred at a concentration as low as $1.8 \times 10^{-6}M$ of ascorbic acid and $1.3 \times 10^{-7}M$ of copper. The pro-oxidant activity increased as the concentrations of ascorbic acid rose up to a maximum at $2 \times 10^{-3}M$. Then they discovered that a *reverse effect* (my language) occurred and pro-oxidant activity declined as the concentration of ascorbic acid was increased further. However, pro-oxidant activity still existed at a $5 \times 10^{-2}M$ concentration of ascorbic acid, the highest that was studied. The researchers found that dehydroascorbic acid also showed pro-oxidant effects, but they were less strong than those of ascorbic acid. The early *in vivo* work of Abramson[156] and the *in vitro* research of Haase and Dunkley[156a] was followed by studies of E. D. Wills,[156b] of Subal Bishayee and A. S. Balasubramanian[156c] and of others.

O. P. Sharma and C. R. Krishna Murti[157] showed that ascorbic acid was a naturally occurring mediator of lipid peroxidation in the rat brain. This finding was consistent with that of A. A. Barber[158] who had reported that lipid peroxidation (as shown by malonaldehyde levels) in incubated liver, brain, testis and kidney tissues of the rat is proportional (at low levels) to their content of ascorbic acid. Then, at higher levels of vitamin C there is a *reverse effect,* i.e., peroxidation decreases as vitamin C begins to act as an antioxidant. E. D. Wills[156b] and also Subal Bishayee and A. S. Balasubramanian[156c] have published graphs showing this *reverse effect.* The graph of the latter is reproduced here as Figure 3.

Using *in vitro* experiments with rat's brain, A. Seregi et al.[159] reported ascorbic acid at the lowest concentrations acted as an antioxidant and at higher, but still low, concentrations induced lipid

---

lipid peroxidation in rat brain tissue *in vitro* at a pH of 5.0. Ascorbic acid has many Jekyll-and-Hyde antioxidant and pro-oxidant actions.

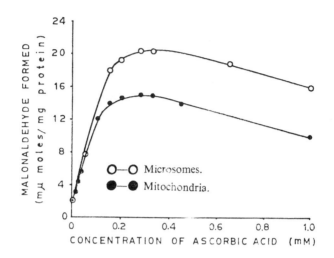

Figure 3. Effect of varying concentrations of ascorbic acid on lipid peroxide formation in mitochondrial and microsomal fractions of rat brain. In a total volume of 0.5 ml. the incubation mixture contained 0.2 M tris-acetate buffer (pH 7.0), 150 mM KCl 0.5 mg. of mitochondrial or microsomal protein and different concentrations of ascorbic acid as indicated. Incubation was for one hour at 37°C. Reproduced from Subal Bishayee and A. S. Balasubramanian, *Jrl. of Neurochemistry* (1971) 18: 909-920, with permission of the International Society for Neurochemistry and the authors. Note the *reverse effect*: the change from increasing to lessening peroxidation—i.e., vitamin C is beginning to show reduced activity as a pro-oxidant prior to assuming an antioxidant role.

peroxidation and the formation of malon aldehyde. * Then, just as the other investigators had discovered, Seregi et al. found that ascorbic acid at a higher physiological concentration inhibited peroxidation of brain microsomes induced by certain agents. They

---

* This action is especially likely to occur in the presence of iron, according to several independent researchers including Athos Ottolenghi.[160] John M. C. Gutteridge et al.[160a] have, in fact, presented evidence suggesting that lipid peroxidation perhaps occurs only when traces of metal ions are present. Other investigators have shown that small amounts of ascorbic acid stimulate peroxide formation in liver mitochondria also.[160b,c]

noted that this is important since the brain is particularly subject to lipid peroxidation. In a similar *in vitro* study, Kovachich and Mishra[159a] recently found that when 1mM ascorbate was incubated with cortical brain slices malonaldehyde was doubled, but at 3mM concentration ascorbic acid acted as an antioxidant and malonaldehyde production was inhibited. When tissue content was maintained at physiological levels, ascorbic acid reduced the formation of malonaldehyde. Somewhat earlier, Ikuo Abe et al.[159b] found, in experiments with the lysosomal fraction of rat liver cells, that incubation, with not only ascorbic acid but also with sodium erythorbate, caused increasing lipid peroxidation and also increasing lysosome labilization between .1 and 1mM of ascorbate and erythorbate. Then, as in the experiments of other investigators, a *reverse effect* set in, with ever-decreasing lipid peroxidation and lysosome labilization occurring between 1 and 10mM.

The effects of ascorbate on lipid peroxidation have also been studied in other tissues. Walter C. Brogan III et al.[160d] reported that in both adrenal and testicular tissues of guinea pigs lipid peroxidation was stimulated *in vitro* by either ascorbate or ferrous ions. Lipid peroxidation increased as the ascorbate concentration rose to 10^{-4}M. At this point a *reverse effect* set in and, as ascorbate concentration continued to rise, lipid peroxidation declined.

Peroxidation of micellar (small colloidal particles of) linoleic acid induced by x-rays is similarly enhanced as low levels of ascorbate increase, but then, at still higher levels of ascorbate, there is a *reverse effect* and peroxidation is inhibited. Albert W. Girotti et al.[160e] found that superoxide dismutase and catalase failed to inhibit ascorbate-enhanced peroxidation, thus suggesting that the effect is not mediated by superoxide or hydrogen peroxide.

Peter J. Hornsby and Joseph F. Crivello,[160f] after citing many of the relevant studies, concluded that:

> The pro-oxidant action of ascorbic acid predominates at low ascorbic acid concentrations in the presence of trace levels of transition-metal ions (free or as certain chelates) that are universal contaminants in in vitro

systems. At the high levels of ascorbic acid present in the cells, in the presence of abundant metal-binding sites, the antioxidant action of ascorbic acid is likely to predominate.

In a related article, E. D. Wills[160g] says:

Firstly, it is quite clear that, in association with iron, the normal function of ascorbate is as a pro-oxidant, producing active oxygen, which is required for the oxidation of proline in peptides to hydroxyproline.[160h] Secondly, experiments carried out *in vitro* clearly show both pro-oxidant and antioxidant effects for the vitamin, depending on the concentration.[156b] It is likely that similar considerations apply *in vivo,* and the precise tissue and intracellular concentrations of ascorbate are likely to be important in determining whether the vitamin acts as a pro- or antioxidant. Furthermore, it is important to appreciate that many of the reactions of lipid peroxidation in the tissue are taking place in a lipid environment and that the water-soluble vitamin C may not always gain ready access to the site of peroxidation. The extent to which vitamin C is primarily a pro- or antioxidant *in vivo* therefore remains an open question.

The studies cited by Hornsby and Crivello[160f] and by E. D. Wills,[160g] as well as those experiments discussed throughout this chapter, suggest that "C" at proper dosage may promote health and longevity. On the other hand, rat experiments have indicated that vitamin C, at high concentrations and under conditions of only marginally adequate vitamin E (50 I.U./kg. diet), can actually *increase* lipid peroxidation.[161] *In vitro* studies, as referenced by Linda H. Chen,[161] have shown that in high dosages vitamin C not only acts as a catalyst of lipid peroxidation but that it can also result in hemolysis (liberation of hemoglobin from red blood cells). Studies by Dr. Chen[161] found, however, that daily dosages of 200 international units of vitamin E per kg. of food eaten can protect rats against these effects. So if you're going to megadose yourself with vitamin C, consider using vitamin E protection.

Vitamin C, Sex and Fertility

Let's consider at this time vitamin C and sex-related effects. Females seem to show a greater utilization of ascorbic acid in response to sexually determined demand of the endocrine glands. H. S. Loh et al.[162] reported that the morning specimen of urine of menstruating women showed a jump in ascorbic acid excretion on the fourteenth day of the cycle. Earlier, H. S. Loh and C. W. M. Wilson[163] had observed (Figure 4) that ascorbic acid excretion in women, during their reproductive years, undergoes a monthly cycle, closely following that of the leutenizing hormone (LH). The only major difference in the cycles of these two compounds generally occurs a few days before ovulation when ascorbic acid briefly declines while the LH continues to climb. The ascorbic acid excretion then changes its direction; both ascorbic acid and LH peak at ovulation and then decline. Note the surge of urinary ascorbic acid (in Figure 4) at ovulation on the fourteenth day of the menstrual cycle as the leutenizing hormone peaks and as basal body temperature also rises close to a peak value. Loh and Wilson also reported that tissue ascorbic acid levels are severely depleted in women after fertilization occurs. The increased metabolic rate at the time of ovulation, as shown by the temperature rise, is considered by Loh and Wilson to mean that the body requires more ascorbic acid. Furthermore, the surge in urinary excretion of ascorbic acid concomitant with ovulation suggests, they say, that it may be used in the ovulatory process. One could just as readily postulate that vitamin C interferes with fertility and that, at ovulation, tissue levels of vitamin C decline so fertilization has a better chance of occurring. M. H. Briggs,[171a,172] as we will discuss soon, presents evidence suggesting that vitamin C may reduce fertility. Masao Igarashi,[163a] however, reported some success in inducing ovulation in

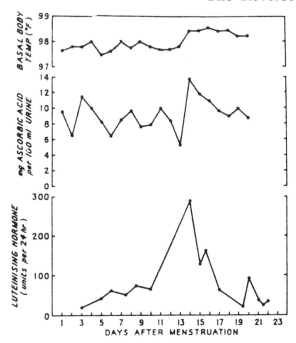

Figure 4. Mean daily values for basal body temperature and
excretion of ascorbic acid in the morning specimen of urine
from five female subjects receiving 500 mg. of ascorbic acid
daily. These values are superimposed on mean values for
excretion of LH in the morning specimen of urine from five
other comparable ovulating subjects. Reproduced from H. S.
Loh et al., *Clinical Pharmacology and Therapeutics* (1974)
16: 390-408 and from H. S. Loh and C. W. M. Wilson,
Lancet (Jan. 16, 1971): 110-112, with permission of the publishers, *Lancet* and C. V. Mosby Company and of Dr. Wilson.

clomiphene-ineffective anovulatory women by administering 400 mg.
of ascorbic acid daily, alone or in combination with clomiphene.
Igarashi cites several studies suggesting, however, that large amounts
of vitamin C may inhibit reproduction. Therefore, further research
could indicate the presence of a *reverse effect*. (A recent report showed
vitamin C enhances release of leutenizing hormone-releasing hormone
in vitro.) [163aa]

The blood of women taking the Pill tends to have a greater concentration of copper in the form of ceruloplasmin, a compound whose presence is generally increased after estrogen is consumed. This is believed to lead, in turn, to the reduced levels of vitamin C that are observed to occur in their plasma, leukocytes and urine.[163b] (Of course, the phenomena could be merely concomitant with the cause of each being another unknown factor.) As noted earlier in this chapter, rat studies have shown that vitamin C depresses intestinal uptake of copper. The copper absorption in women may or may not parallel that of rats. At any rate, additional ascorbic acid is sometimes recommended to Pill-taking women for help in bringing the blood's copper level back to normal.*

Ascorbate is present in large quantities in the interstitial cells of the testes and the ovary. Semen is also reported to contain 10-15 times as much ascorbic acid as is present in whole blood.[165] We should, however, be cautious about assuming that vitamin C may be sexually beneficial. An experiment by P. K. Paul and P. N. Duttagupta [166] shows that vitamin C exerts a beneficial effect on the secreting ability of the male accessory sex glands in the underfed rat. However, in normally fed rats it induces a toxic effect. Then too, Andres Carballeira et al.[167] have reported that *in vitro* experiments with rats' testes have shown that ascorbic acid depresses the conversion of cholesterol into testosterone by the testes. Studies cited by these scientists, and others we will discuss shortly, have shown that vitamin C interferes with cholesterol utilization by the ovaries and adrenals. One must be hesitant about drawing conclusions about people as a result of animal experiments, particularly experiments with rats that make their own vitamin C compared with humans who usually do not. These experiments might, therefore, be worth repeating with guinea pigs who, like humans, do not generally make their own "C." However, insofar as the results of the above-cited experiments could apply to men and women, it would appear that an excess of "C" cannot be considered to be useful in facilitating s e x u a l

---

* While excess dietary ascorbate can induce or exacerbate a copper deficiency, there is a *reverse effect* (at least as far as the brain, spleen and serum are concerned) with low ascorbate levels being associated with copper deficiency.[164]

expression. Then too, there is a report that one gram of vitamin C (but only if taken with vitamin B12) reduced the amount of a man's ejaculate.[168] This was confirmed by G. N. Schrauzer and W. J. Rhead,[169] but must be considered to be merely anecdotal in the absence of controlled studies. N. J. Chinoy and R. P. Buch[170] reported that there is less ascorbic acid in the semen of normospermic (normally fertile) men than in oligospermic (partially infertile) men, and these men, in turn, have less ascorbic acid in their semen than azospermic (completely infertile) men. However, a more recent study by A. Srivastava et al.[170a] showed, contrary to the data of Chinoy and Buch, that the semen of normally fertile men contains considerably more vitamin C than that of azospermic or oligospermic men. Other recent studies by Earl B. Dawson et al.[171] have reported that supplementary intake of 500 mg. of ascorbic acid per day works to halt sperm agglutination, a factor in fertility problems. The Dawson group found that high semen copper levels were associated with sperm agglutination and that vitamin C works to reduce a high copper level. On the other hand, M. H. Briggs[171a] speculates that vitamin C might antagonize the formation of glycoprotein micelles in cervical mucus and thus diminish fertility in women. He [172] gives anecdotal evidence that daily dosages of two grams of ascorbic acid may reduce their fertility.

Adrenal and Sexual Steroidogenesis

Large quantities of ascorbate are also found in the adrenal glands which, in the medulla area, secrete epinephrine (adrenalin) and norepinephrine. The cortex of the adrenal glands secretes the corticosteroids—glucocorticoids (one of which is cortisone), mineralocorticoids (such as aldosterone) and the sex steroids (which supplement quantities produced by the gonads). Considerable amounts of published evidence support the view that vitamin C is involved in the production of these hormones by the adrenal glands. However, A. E. Kitabchi[173] and A. E. Kitabchi and W. C. Duckworth[174] suggest that ascorbic acid may, on the contrary, inhibit steroidogenesis in the adrenal glands.* They speculate that, upon stimulation by ACTH, the adrenals release ascorbic acid before steroidogenesis takes place.** Furthermore, Kitabchi and Duckworth[174] reported that two patients with scurvy showed no adrenal hypofunction and their adrenal steroid secretion remained unchanged with ascorbic acid treatment.

While making *in vitro* studies involving the adrenal cells of rats, Abbas E. Kitabchi et al.[175] found that, when vitamin E was deficient, ascorbic acid concentrations greatly affected ACTH-induced steroidogenesis. This effect was not observed, however, when vitamin E was adequate. They suggested that in a vitamin E-deficient state, steroidogenesis was being affected through an interaction of ascorbic acid with ACTH. Figure 5 shows that, in vitamin E deficiency, inhibition of steroidogenesis increases up to a concentration of about .5mM ascorbate. Then a *reverse effect* sets in with steroidogenesis being less inhibited at higher concentrations of ascorbate. Kitabchi et al.[175] also reported that intraperitoneal injection of vitamin E to the vitamin E-deficient rat abolished the inhibitory effect of ascorbate on ACTH-induced steroidogenesis. The presence of adequate vitamin E also prevented the stimulation of lipid peroxidation by ascorbate (a fact that was confirmed later by Dr. Linda H. Chen[161]). They also found that manganese, cobalt and EDTA were effective in reducing the inhibition by ascorbate of ACTH-induced steroidogenesis.

Evidently, "C" can both promote and inhibit various actions of the adrenals. Using *in vitro* experiments involving incubation of cholesterol with bovine and porcine adrenal glands, Kyutaro Shimizu[176] found that low concentrations of ascorbic acid stimulated

---

* A recent experiment by J. Richardson,[174a] however, found that when stressed mice were given large daily doses of vitamin C they maintained high blood levels of corticosteroids, including glucocorticoid. Since glucocorticoid is known to suppress the immune response, Richardson hypothesized that large doses of vitamin C may reduce the organism's immunity to disease when stress is present. Under the stress of a cold, could vitamin C *reduce* one's cold-fighting and/or cancer-fighting ability?

** Qi-Wen Xie[174b] has reported that S. Bi found acupuncture caused a decrease of adrenal ascorbic acid in rats. I speculate it was simply a case of needle stress stimulating production of ACTH which then proceeded to act in accordance with the speculation of Kitabchi and Duckworth.

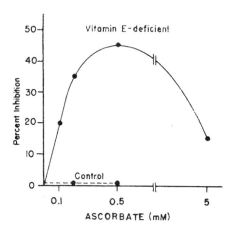

Figure 5. Effect of various concentrations of ascorbate on steroidogenesis induced with 50 microunits of ACTH in isolated adrenal cells of vitamin E-deficient and control rats. Reproduced from Abbas E. Kitabchi et al., *Jrl. of Biological Chemistry* (1973) 248: 835-840, with permission of the copyright owner, The American Society of Biological Chemists, Inc. Note the *reverse effect* that sets in at an ascorbate concentration of about .5mM.

the side-chain cleavage of cholesterol that is involved in steroidogenesis. As the concentration of ascorbate was raised up to about 4mM, the rate of side-chain cleavage of cholesterol, as shown by the presence of isocaproic acid, also increased. Then as the ascorbate was raised further, the side-chain cleavage showed a *reverse effect* by drastically declining and steroidogenesis was inhibited (Figure 6). Ingemar Björkhem et al.[176a] later reported similar results with the maximum rate of cholesterol cleavage occurring between .1 and .5 m mol/l. Then too, Valerie A. Wilbur and Brian L. Walker[177] observed that male guinea pigs fed a vitamin C-deficient diet for three weeks, as might have been expected, showed a lower amount of cholesteryl esters in their adrenals than did a control group. However, another group fed a 100-fold excess

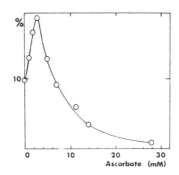

Figure 6. Production of isocaproic acid from cholesterol incubated with porcine adrenal glands and vitamin C. Side-chain cleavage of cholesterol was stimulated up to a concentration of about 4 mM ascorbate and then was inhibited as ascorbate levels increased. (Using bovine adrenal glands, maximum cleavage occurred at about 1 mM.) Reproduced from Kyutaro Shimizu, *Biochimica et Biophysica Acta* (1970) 210: 333-340, with permission of the publisher, Elsevier Biomedical Press and of the author.

of "C" also had a concentration of adrenal cholesteryl esters lower than that of the control group. Small doses and huge doses of "C," in a biphasic effect, each reversed the normal condition of adrenal cholesteryl esters. It is another example of a benefit obtained from a nominal amount of a vitamin and a detrimental condition induced by either a deficiency or by a megadose.

More recently, Willy A. Behrens and Rene Madere [178] found that rats given a high oral intake of ascorbic acid (2% of the diet) showed no significant difference in adrenalin, noradrenalin or dopamine in any tissues analyzed. The authors suggest that some previous reports showing an increase in catecholamines may have involved either higher doses of ascorbic acid or different administration of the doses (i.e., intravenously or intraperitoneally). Then too, as far as the adrenal hormone *cortisol* is concerned, Ingemar Björkhem et al. reported that ascorbic acid cannot be obligatory for any of the different steps in its biosynthesis. Furthermore, they noted that even in advanced scurvy with an increased level of ACTH, plasma cortisol is not reduced but is markedly increased. *Nevertheless,* the fact that the vitamin C concentration in the adrenals exceeds that of any other tissue perhaps suggests that a vital function is being served.* Perhaps ascorbic acid in normal concentrations improves corticoid hormone utilization and prolongs action of these hormones. More research in this area is obviously needed. However, it seems to me the contradictions that are bothering these various groups of scientists are examples of dose-related *reverse effects.*

Ascorbic acid also seems to be a factor in ovarian and testicular steroidogenesis. When the pituitary stimulates the ovaries or interstitial cells of the testes with luteinizing hormone (usually called the interstitial-cell-stimulating hormone in the male) there is a dose-related depletion in the ascorbic acid content of those organs. (The action is similar to the reduction in the ascorbic acid content of the adrenals when they are stimulated by ACTH.) Using *in vitro* experiments with incubated ovarian tissue homogenates of guinea pigs, Stephen J. Pintauro and James G. Bergan[180] reported that ascorbic acid concentration appears to be related to the rate at which pregnenolone is converted to progesterone. The effects are, however, most evident in a very narrow range of ascorbic acid concentrations. At high ascorbic acid concentrations the effect is inhibitory. Here, again, is a *reverse effect* which should warn us that excessive dosages of ascorbic acid may be detrimental. Perhaps high dosages of ascorbic acid may be exhibiting a pro-oxidant action with negative effects on membrane integrity and/or increased lipid peroxidation. In accordance with this speculation, the result may be an inhibition of the interaction of the luteinizing hormone (or ACTH in the case of the adrenals) with the cell membrane, thus reversing the low-dose stimulatory action.

Vitamin C, Exercise and Fatigue

What about the possible effects of vitamin C on exercise and endurance? In studying the physiological response of trained and

---

* But this is not necessarily true. Does plaque on the teeth mean that it serves a vital function? (Actually, it may. See page 702.)

untrained subjects, Bailey et al.[180a] concluded that supplementation of two grams of ascorbic acid had no effect on oxygen uptake during or after exercise. In another study involving 286 male soldiers, George O. Gey[180b] concluded that daily divided doses of 1,000 mg. showed no effect on endurance performance or on the rate, severity or duration of athletic injury. In yet another study of 20 soldiers, carried out under double-blind conditions, Kirchoff[180c] reported that vitamin C had no effect on energy metabolism or on various measurements of circulatory and ventilatory function (pulse rate, blood pressure, oxygen consumption, CO_2 output, etc.)

Nevertheless, others maintain that ascorbic acid is a useful fatigue-fighter. It is possible that vitamin C may increase the content of carnitine in the muscles. (Carnitine is a food factor synthesized in the body from lysine and methionine and was thought at one time to belong to the B complex group of vitamins. It was discussed in Chapter 5.) R. E. Hughes et al.[181] reported that guinea pigs fed low amounts of vitamin C had significantly lower muscle carnitine. They speculate that this could account for the lassitude and fatigue reported to precede scurvy in man. However, we must not fall into the error of believing that, just because a vitamin C deficiency may cause fatigue, a megadose of "C" will bring us super energy. It is a defective form of logic of which vitamin enthusiasts are sometimes guilty. However, H. Howald, B. Segesser and W. F. Körner[182] examined 13 athletes after daily oral administration of placebo over a period of 14 days and again for a similar period after an intake of one gram of vitamin C per day. The performance test was carried out by bicycle ergometry starting at a work load of 30 watts and increasing in 40-watt steps every four minutes until the subjects were exhausted. They found that "vitamin C leads to a more important utilization of free fatty acids as an energy source in the working muscle." Howald and his associates go on to say, "because of its glycogen-sparing effect, both in muscle cells and in liver, this mechanism would have a beneficial effect." The increased availability of fatty acid in the plasma is shown in Figure 7. They also found that, at every level of performance, use of vitamin C resulted in lowered average pulse rates (Figure 8). On the other hand, a negative

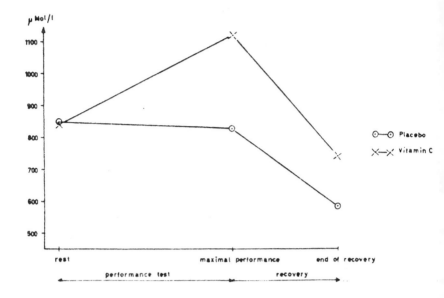

Figure 7. Free fatty acids in plasma. See text. Reproduced
from H. Howald, B. Segesser and W. F. Körner, *Annals of the*
N.Y. *Academy* *of* *Sciences* (1975) 258: 458-464, with
permission of the N.Y. Academy of Sciences and of the
authors.

finding was that vitamin C lowered blood glucose levels (Figure 9).
Howald and his colleagues recommended doses of one gram daily to
achieve beneficial effects in both cardiovascular and metabolic
parameters. On the other hand, R. Buzina and K. Suboticanec[182a]
found that, although increasing plasma vitamin C levels increased
aerobic capacity of young adolescents, the optimal aerobic capacity
was associated with a daily ascorbic acid intake of just 80-100 mg.

Vitamin C could combat fatigue in other ways. Like vitamin E,
ascorbic acid works to detoxify pollutions caused by the environment
and this may help explain the increased energy that is reported to
sometimes occur. Then too, a *diminished* supply of ascorbic acid acts
(like an *increase* in lactic acid does) to reduce alkaline phosphatase
activity and results in less energy being available for

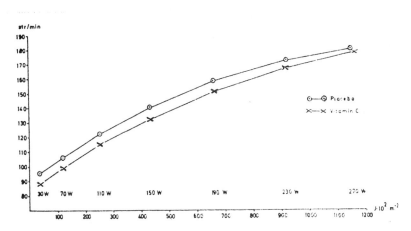

Figure 8. Pulse rate during the performance test. See text. Reproduced from H. Howald, B. Segesser and W. F. Körner, *Annals of the N.Y. Academy of Sciences* (1975) 258: 458-464, with permission of the N.Y. Academy of Sciences and of the authors.

muscle contraction.[183] K. Suboticanec-Buzina et al.[183a] reported that the physical working capacity of adolescent boys is increased as plasma vitamin C rises to a level of .86 mg./dl. and then plateaus. This level is achievable on a daily dietary intake of about 80 mg. of vitamin C. Again, I must caution, however, just because a vitamin C deficiency leads to reduced working capacity and to fatigue is no indication that an excess will be valuable in increasing working capacity or in combating fatigue. Robert E. Keith and Elizabeth Merrill[183b] reported that, four hours after giving 15 healthy males 600 mg. of ascorbic acid, they found no significant differences in maximum grip strength or in muscular endurance. Many of the studies relating athletic performance not only to supplementation of vitamin C but also to supplementation of other vitamins, minerals and foods have been evaluated in a book by Melvin H. Williams.[183c] In general, Williams concludes that further study is required but the present case for supplementation to improve athletic performance is not a strong one.

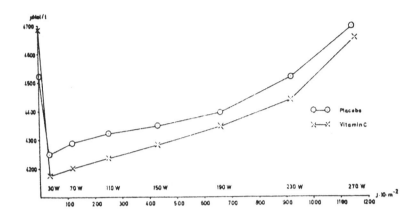

Figure 9. Blood glucose concentrations during the performance
test. See text. Reproduced from H. Howald, B. Segesser and W.
F. Körner, *Annals of the N.Y. Academy of Sciences* (1975)
258: 458-464, with permission of the N.Y. Academy of
Sciences and of the authors.

Furthermore, T. K. Basu[184] has shown that ascorbic acid, in
amounts of three grams daily, reduces body stores of cysteine.*
Cysteine is an essential amino acid that enters into the formation of
ATP energy to run the body. Thus, vitamin C in megadoses could
cause rather than reduce fatigue, which is a *reverse effect*.

Cancer Prevention and Therapy

Many experiments with animals and with humans suggest that
vitamin C may be beneficial in preventing or in treating cancer. This
section will not only tell about these studies but, later, will describe
experiments suggesting that vitamin C may sometimes be detrimental

---

* Dr. Edward Calabrese[185] has pointed out that vitamin C megadoses might be a special
threat to a laetrile patient (and "C" is frequently used in "laetrile therapy") since
cysteine helps protect against the cyanide poisoning that can result from taking laetrile.

in both cancer prevention and in cancer treatment. Does this sound contradictory? It may be just a case of the *reverse effect.*

Studies summarized by Sidney S. Mirvish et al.,[186] and more recent research by J. B. Guttenplan,[186a] show that ascorbic acid can block the nitrosamines,* the carcinogenic chemicals resulting from the consumption of sodium nitrate that is found in sausage. (Meat packers are now adding sodium ascorbate or erythorbate to their products. Ascorbyl palmitate or vitamin E, being oil-based, would probably be more effective and not add to the body's sodium intake.)

An *in vitro* study by E. P. Norkus and W. A. Kuenzig [186b] suggests that "ascorbic acid can block the intragastric formation of mutagenic N-nitroso compounds but that ascorbic acid has no effect on mutagenicity of N-nitroso compounds once they are formed. An *in vivo* study by H. J. O'Connor et al.[186c] that was published in the same issue of *Carcinogenesis* showed, however, that oral vitamin C significantly reduced mutagenic activity and increased intragastric ascorbate levels without altering gastric pH. If you are going to eat cured meat products, take vitamin C during that meal rather than several hours later!

However, whether or not you eat cured meat products, nitrite is introduced into your body via the water you drink.** The analysis of the spring water that I drink shows more than a four-fold increase in the content of nitrate compared to an analysis of the water from the same spring made some 30 years ago.[188] Why? Farming uses nitrate fertilizers which run off soil into streams and can also find their way underground to the sources of spring water. Action of bacteria converts the nitrate to the dangerous nitrite. (To be on the safe side, you may

---

* In connection with the nitrosation of dimethylamine, however, ascorbate does not always work to inhibit formation of nitrosamines. Mirvish et al. reported on experiments showing that ascorbic acid is fairly effective in preventing nitrosation of dimethylamine at a pH of 3 and 4, but at a pH of 2 has little effect, and at a pH of 1 shows a *reverse effect* by *increasing* nitrosation.

** Thomas H. Jukes, Ph.D.[187,187a] states that eating of certain vegetables also introduces nitrate into the body. Lettuce, celery, spinach and beets, according to Dr. Jukes, account for 42% of the nitrates from all food sources. He notes that, while draining cooked vegetables and throwing away the cooking water leads to losses of some vitamins and minerals, it also greatly diminishes their nitrate content. Eating of raw vegetables may increase the nitrate intake of the body, so perhaps it is especially important for raw-food enthusiasts to protect themselves with supplementary ascorbic acid.

wish to take ascorbic acid more frequently so some will always be present in your stomach to work at detoxifying the nitrite that is almost certain to be there.) [188a]*

Nitrosamines are not only present in our foods and in our water but are made endogenously by our bodies. They are also present as volatile pollutants associated with tires and rubber products, leather and automobile fabrics.[180f] A study by Andre E. M. McLean et al.[180g] suggests that persons suddenly switching from a low-protein to a high-protein diet may be under a special threat. A single dose of 15 mg./kg. of dimethylnitrosamine administered to rats who were switched from a low- to a high-protein diet was an effective initiator of liver tumors.

Other experiments also demonstrate that ascorbate inhibits the detrimental action of nitrosamines. Joseph B. Guttenplan[188h] reported that ascorbate inhibited mutagenesis in salmonella that was induced by N-methyl-N-nitrosoguanidine and dimethylnitrosamine. Copper, and to a lesser degree ferric iron, enhanced the inhibition and presumably functioned as catalysts. J. H. Weisburger[189] has provided a recent review of the part played by N-nitroso compounds in gastric and esophageal cancer and the preventive role of vitamin C.

Continuing in the matter of cancer prevention, C. L. Leuchtenberger et al.[189a] found that ascorbic acid and l-cysteine reduced the carcinogenic effect of tobacco and marijuana smoke in cultured hamster lungs. Humans are not hamsters, but would it not seem good preventative action for tobacco and pot smokers (and those frequently exposed to smoke) to take vitamin C and perhaps cysteine also?

---

* Often the advice is given to take vitamin C, in divided doses, several times during the day. Except from the standpoint of possibly protecting the stomach from nitrosamines, this would seem unnecessary since, according to Anders Kallner et al.,[188b] only 3% of the body's pool of vitamin C is lost per day. Jean T. Snook et al.,[188c] in a related study, found that taking 240 mg. of ascorbic acid every fourth day was essentially equivalent to taking 60 mg. daily. On the other hand, if megadoses of "C" are ingested, they will be absorbed more efficiently if the dose is divided. D. Hornig et al.[188d] found that while 75% of a single daily oral dose of one gram of ascorbic acid was absorbed, the absorption was reduced to 44% of a two-gram dose, to 39% of a three-gram dose, to 28% of a four-gram dose and to just 20% of a five-gram dose. By the way, about 30 mg./day of vitamin C is secreted into the stomach—an interesting exampie of "body wisdom."[188e]

In regard to cancer therapy, as contrasted with cancer prevention, it is speculated that vitamin C may kill tumor cells through the creation of intracellular hydrogen peroxide.[189b] Normal cells control the transport of vitamin C so that no more is absorbed than is needed for cells to function. The fact that some tumors in experimental animals accumulate above-normal amounts of "C" suggests that cancer cells may sometimes lose homeostatic control for this vitamin.[189c,190] Therefore, some cancer cells may die through taking up "C" and through its intracellular production of hydrogen peroxide. The efficiency of "C" in combating a given type of cancer might vary directly with that particular cancer tissue's loss of homeostatic control over the entrance of "C." This would explain the apparent failures and apparent successes of "C" in inhibiting cancer.

In relatively early work relating vitamin C to cancer control, K. Yamafuji et al.[190a] reported on its use to inhibit growth of sarcoma-180 in mice. Ascorbic acid, dehydroascorbic acid and 2, 3 diketogulonic acids were each active in inhibiting the growths, and the inhibition was enhanced by the presence of cupric ions. More recently, Kedar N. Prasad et al.[190b] observed that 99% of cultured mouse neuroblastoma cells and rat glioma cells were destroyed by various agents after they had been potentiated. (Vitamin C did not potentiate the effect of all agents. In fact, it *reduced* the cytotoxic effect of methotrexate, probably because vitamin C can inactivate certain drugs.) Curiously, sodium D-ascorbate—having the mirror-image structure of sodium L-ascorbate and without vitamin C activity—was also effective in potentiating some of the growth inhibitors. Among the other *in vitro* experiments, ascorbate has produced a cytotoxic effect against Ehrlich ascitic carcinoma cells [190c] and on proliferating murine (mouse) ATP C+ cells.[190d] F. S. Liotti et al.[190d] reported that ascorbic acid *enhanced* multiplication of ATP C+ cells at low dosage (10 mg./ml.), but *inhibited* multiplication at high dosages (30 mg./ml. and up). They similarly reported that dehydroascorbic acid *enhanced* multiplication at low dosage (10 mg./ml. and 30 mg./ml.), but inhibited it at high dosages (60 mg./ml. to 960 mg./ml.). If such a *reverse effect* occurs not just *in vitro* in animal cancer cells, but *in vivo* in human cancers, what dosage of vitamin C might enhance proliferation and what dosage might inhibit it?

Vitamin C is reported by N. Bishun et al.[191,191a] to affect cell proliferation and DNA synthesis in two tumor cell lines, called Hep2 and KB. The investigators reported that the ratio of dead to live cells of each type increased with increasing concentrations of ascorbic acid (Figure 10). They failed to report, however, (but one of their graphs clearly shows) that the two highest concentrations in the case of the Hep2 cells and the four highest concentrations in the case of the KB cells show a *reverse effect*. At these higher concentrations there was less effective killing of the cells. It is just another example of scientists ignoring the existence of a *reverse effect*, even though their own data clearly indicate its presence.

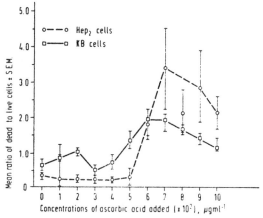

Figure 10. Effect of various concentrations of ascorbic acid on the ratio of dead to live cells in two cell lines. Reproduced from N. Bishun et al., *Oncology* (1978) 35: 160-162, with permission of the publisher, S. Karger AG, Basel. Note the *reverse effect* that occurs at higher concentrations of ascorbic acid. More is not always better!

William F. Benedict et al.[193] have reported that ascorbic acid at low, noncytotoxic concentration, inhibited morphological transformation of mouse embryo cells after exposure to the carcinogen 3-methyl cholanthrene (MCA) for 24 hours. Moreover, the treatment often resulted in a reversion to normal cells. Following a subsequent study, Benedict et al.[193a] suggested that ascorbic acid was effective in suppressing the progression of cancer in mouse embryo cells "only prior to a stage where an initiated cell achieves the capacity to grow in semisolid medium and to produce tumors in immunosuppressed animals."

Earlier, in connection with folic acid, I mentioned vitamin C as a factor involved in the pathogenesis of cervical dysplasia, a cell change that sometimes leads to cancer of the cervix. Sylvia Wassertheil-Smoller et al.[193b] have reported that, while sexual activity and young age at first intercourse are associated with high risk of cervical dysplasia, so is a vitamin C daily intake below 88 mg. The investigators reported that 68% of U.S. women in their reproductive years have a vitamin C intake below 88 mg. In a subsequent case-control study by Seymour L. Romney et al.[193d] of 80 women who had sought a Papanicolaou test, the 46 who had either one or two consecutive suspicious smears in a 12-month period had significantly lower (36 versus 75 mg./dl.) plasma vitamin C concentrations than the 36 controls. It may be important for women at high risk of cervical dysplasia to assure that their vitamin C intake is well above the RDA of 60 mg.*

---

* Nitrosamines have been found in vaginal secretions of women with trichomoniasis.[193c] Not only is prompt medical treatment of trichomoniasis important, additional "C" for such women might be useful to reduce the risk of nitrosamine-induced cancer.

Another phase of cancer prevention may relate to the effect of ascorbic acid on rectal polyps. Jerome L. DeCosse et al.[194] reported on using vitamin C to treat rectal polyps of five patients with family polyposis. Three grams of ascorbic acid were given orally as one gram timed-release capsules, three times a day. During a 4 to 13 month study, rectal polyps disappeared in two, regressed partially in two and increased in one. In another study of three additional patients, one had a reduction in rectal polyps and two were unaffected. Rectal polyposis is a premalignant disease that may lead to colon cancer but, since such polyps are subject to long-term cyclic variation, it may be difficult to ascribe their regression to the use of vitamin C. (The fact that timed-release vitamin C was used also makes this study questionable. As will be seen shortly, it is doubtful just how much of timed-release "C" enters the body.) Nevertheless, in an experiment with mice challenged with the carcinogen dimethylhydrazine (DMH), those given oral vitamin C developed less than one-half the number of colorectal tumors that occurred in the controls.[195] To the extent that vitamin C may be a beneficial factor in polyp treatments, the action probably hinges on its antioxidant power to control intestinal bacteria and fecal steroid metabolism. A more recent study by Frank E. Jones et al.[195a] showed that ascorbic acid had no effect on the incidence or density of large bowel tumors induced in mice by DMH. However, ascorbic acid acted synergistically with BHA to more effectively reduce tumor incidence than when BHA was used alone.

M. Eymard Poydock et al.[196] have also reported on research suggesting the possible value of vitamin C in treating cancer. The mitotic activity of Sarcoma 37, Krebs-2 and Ehrlich carcinomas transplanted into mice was inhibited after injection with a mixture of ascorbic acid, calcium ascorbate and vitamin B12 without apparent toxic effects. (The mixture consisted of 340 mg./kg. of body weight ascorbate and 20 mg./kg. of vitamin B12.) When vitamin C or B12 was administered alone there was no apparent effect on mitosis or on the morphology of the cells. The ascites fluid from the mice treated with the vitamin mixture showed few tumor cells and these were in various stages of disintegration. The experimenters also reported an increase in lymphocytes, monocytes and neutrophils. Later, no tumor cells could be found and monocytes and macrophages were abundant. It has been suggested that the cytocidal action of the ascorbate against the tumors may be due either to the intracellular generation of hydrogen peroxide and/or to an enhancement of the immune system. In another study, large amounts of vitamin C orally administered to rats with benzo(a)pyrene-induced tumors were found by G. Kallistratos et al.[196a] to beneficially affect the animals' survival (Figure 11).

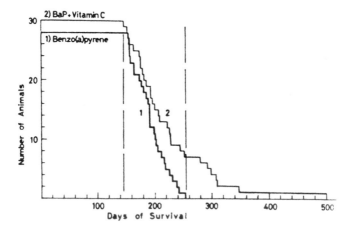

Figure 11. Mortality curve of Wistar rats treated with either a single subcutaneous injection of 10 mg. benzo(a)pyrene or with a 10 mg. benzo(a)pyrene injection plus a simultaneous oral administration of vitamin C. Reproduced from G. Kallistratos et al., *Naturwissenschaften* (1984) 71: 160-161, with permission of the publisher, Springer-Verlag.

Studies by J. U. Schlegel et al.[196b] have shown that ascorbic acid protects against the induction of bladder tumors in mice. However, Mark S. Soloway et al.,[196c] in their experiments, failed to confirm this. A protective effect against skin cancer, however, may be more real. I. A. Sadek and N. Abdelmegid[197] reported that toads injected daily for eight weeks with 10 mg./kg. body weight (equivalent to only about 700 mg. in man) showed inhibition of skin papillomas that had been induced by painting the skin with the carcinogen DMBA. In other experiments by Wolcott B. Dunham et al., [197a] the incidence of dermal malignant lesions induced in mice by ultraviolet light were reported to be decreased with high statistical significance by adding ascorbic acid to the diet. Then too, David G. Morrison et al.[197b] reported that injections of ascorbic acid or retinyl palmitate (but especially both injected together) significantly inhibited pulmonary neoplasms in mice exposed to fiberglass dust.

Some years ago, L. Benade et al.[198] found that ascorbate is highly toxic to Ehrlich ascites carcinoma cells *in vitro*. They also observed that the toxicity is greatly increased by concomitant administration of 3-amino-1,2,4,-triazole (ATA), although ATA alone is virtually without effect. The cytocidal action of ascorbate, as noted earlier, is believed due to its fostering of the intracellular generation of toxic hydrogen peroxide that is produced when ascorbic acid is oxidized by the cells. ATA is believed to act by inhibiting the enzyme catalase, thus decreasing the ability of the cancer cells to detoxify the hydrogen peroxide.

Richard F. Wagner et al.,[198a] in a review entitled "Nutrition and Melanoma," analyze a number of studies showing that vitamin C is effective against melanoma. They cite the work of S. Bram et al.,[198b] who found that vitamin C was selectively toxic *in vitro* to both mouse and human melanoma cells. Copper added to the ascorbate resulted in a two- to five-fold increase in toxicity to melanoma.* P. G. Parsons and L. E. Morrison[198d] subsequently reported that ascorbate induces DNA breaks in human melanoma cells. Wagner et al. also reported on the work of J. M. Varga and L. Airoldi [198e] showing that mice pretreated with hemicalcium ascorbate in their drinking water experienced a delayed appearance of melanoma and the three-month survival rate was increased by 12%-50%. Varga and Airoldi speculated that, since hemicalcium ascorbate had no direct toxicity to melanoma cells *in vitro*, the beneficial action was probably due to an increase in host resistance.

---

* A study by G. L. Fisher et al.[198c] found, however, that persistently high levels of serum copper were associated with a poor prognosis in patients with melanoma.

Vitamin C has also been found to potentiate the action of the anticancer drug BCNU in inhibiting leukemia in mice. Carleen Moore et al.[198f] found that mice inoculated intracerebrally with leukemic cells died in 10 days. BCNU (25 mg./kg./day) administered intraperitoneally once or twice a day increased the life spans of the mice by 73% and 123% respectively. Vitamin C (250 mg./kg./day) given as 125 mg./kg. twice a day increased the life spans only slightly. When both vitamin C and BCNU were administered together once or twice a day, however, the life spans were increased 104% and 237% respectively.

Research has also shown that vitamin C can induce immunity against some cancers in mice. Frances E. Knock et al.[199] have reported that ascorbic acid, like selected sulfhydral inhibitors, promotes significant immunological response in Ehrlich ascites tumors and still stronger response in S-180 tumors. Ehrlich or S-180 ascites cells were incubated in their own ascitic fluid and sodium ascorbate. The treated cells were then injected intraperitoneally in mice. The mice received two booster shots at seven-day intervals and then seven days later were challenged with untreated ascites cells (several times the normally fatal dose). Increasing numbers of survivors were taken as an indication of partial or complete immunity to the fatal cancer dose. Effective doses of sodium ascorbate corresponded to just 12 grams in a 60 kilogram patient. Cancer cells are rich in microvilli compared with normal cells, and the ability of vitamin C to cause blebbing (blistering) and a reduction of these microvilli is held to be responsible for the immunity.

Wolcott B. Dunham et al.,[199a] at the Linus Pauling Institute of Science and Medicine, studied the effect of vitamin C on large malignant skin tumors (squamous cell carcinomas) and other lesions in mice intermittently exposed to ultraviolet light. They reported that, "A pronounced effect of vitamin C in decreasing the incidence and delaying the onset of the malignant lesions was observed with high statistical significance."

In another study from the Linus Pauling Institute of Science and Medicine, Linus Pauling et al.[199b] reported on the effect on the incidence of spontaneous mammary tumors of different amounts of

L-ascorbic acid contained in the food of mice. Striking delays in the appearance of mammary tumors were observed between control groups and groups fed .076% or greater amounts of ascorbic acid (by weight) in the diet. A tabulation published as part of the study shows that, at the age of 114 weeks when the experiment was terminated, those mice given large amounts of vitamin C (4.2%-8.3% of the diet by weight) survived in much greater numbers than either the controls or those administered lesser amounts of the vitamin.

Vitamin C may also be valuable as part of an otherwise orthodox treatment of cancer. An extensive study on the effect of ascorbate in treatment of cancer was done by Ewan Cameron and Linus Pauling.[200] In a clinical test, 100 terminal cancer patients were given supplemental vitamin C (usually 10 grams daily by intravenous infusion for about 10 days and orally thereafter) as part of their therapy. Their progress was compared with 1,000 similar patients treated identically but who received no supplemental vitamin C. The mean survival time of the ascorbate-treated patients was over 4.2 times as great (more than 210 days) as for the controls (50 days). Deaths occurred for about 90% of the ascorbate-treated patients at one-third the rate of the controls. The other 10% had a much greater survival time, averaging over 20 times that of the control group. It might seem obvious from this study that ascorbate can be effectively used in the treatment of cancer.* However, the fact that Cameron and Pauling used nonrandomized subjects suggests that their conclusions may be questionable.[200a] Nevertheless, a study by Robert H. Yonemoto et al.[201] showed that *in vitro* human lymphocyte blastogenesis was increased by oral ingestion of 5 grams of ascorbic acid daily and increased further by ingestion of 10 grams. The researchers stated that, since *in vitro* lymphocyte reactivity

---

* In Chapter 4 we saw that coffee administered to animals with vitamin A was more effective in controlling cancer than vitamin A given alone. (Reference 36a of Chapter 4.) Perhaps, similarly, caffeine administered with vitamin C could be a more effective antitumor therapy than vitamin C alone. Animal studies at various dosages (not simply a test under the "more is better" doctrine) might be a valuable prelude to possible clinical use. (One of the "unorthodox" treatments of cancer in current use employs coffee enemas.)

correlates well with the prognosis of cancer patients, ascorbic acid may be valuable in the restoring of immunological competence in such patients.

A more recent experiment, however, seems to contradict the findings of Cameron and Pauling and the suggestive results of Yonemoto. E. I. Creagan et al.[202] of the Mayo Clinic found that, in a double-blind controlled experiment using placebos and involving 60 paired cancer patients, there was no benefit from giving 10 grams of ascorbic acid daily. Nevertheless, Michael Jaffey[203] argues that there is a strong probability that vitamin C approximately doubled the survival time of patients in the Cameron and Pauling trial and that an alternative interpretation of the Mayo Clinic trial could also lead to the conclusion that vitamin C is of value in cancer therapy. Jaffey says: "Despite a speculative element because based only on the condensed, published data, these conclusions have sufficient possibility of validity as to call for full further investigation. The conclusions on method are that the broad, inductive approach may have potential value when the randomized method cannot be used; that it also may facilitate, to the public's benefit, the release of probably valuable, inexpensive, non-toxic treatments pending decisive proof; and that a greater return on the research dollar might result from a formal acceptance of the probabilistic element in scientific proof."

Subsequently, Charles G. Moertel et al.[203a] of the Mayo Clinic did a randomized, double-blind comparison of the use of high-dose vitamin C (10 grams daily) or placebo in 100 patients with advanced colorectal cancer who had no prior chemotherapy. They reported that none showed objective improvement. Scientists do not, however, consider negative results in adenocarcinoma of the colon, one of the most resistant cancers to any kind of therapy, to indicate the general ineffectiveness of that therapy against other neoplasms.[203b] However, as Robert E. Wittes[203b] pointed out, Cameron and Pauling[200] had suggested that vitamin C had a strong, beneficial effect in this disease.

In his 1986 book, Pauling[203c] accuses Moertel of misrepresenting in pretending that the protocol of Moertel's study replicated that of Cameron and Pauling. Dr. Pauling says: "The Moertel paper and a spokesman[203b] for the National Cancer Institute who commented on it both suppressed the fact that the vitamin C patients were not receiving vitamin C when they died and had not received any for a long time (median 10.5 months). They announced vigorously that this study showed finally and definitely that vitamin C had no value against advanced cancer and recommended that no more studies of vitamin C be made. Their results provided no basis whatever for this conclusion, because in fact their patients died only after being deprived of the vitamin C. To the extent that their study showed anything, it is that cancer patients should not stop taking their large doses of vitamin C." Pauling and Cameron[203d] stated in a press release, "It is likely that some of the Mayo Clinic patients died as a result of the rebound effect when their high-dose vitamin C was taken away from them." Pauling and Moertel[203e] have recently debated the proposition: "Megadoses of Vitamin C are Valuable in the Treatment of Cancer."

The Moertel study, with appropriate modifications suggested by Pauling, should now be replicated with other cancers. Regrettably, Cameron and Pauling may have sent Moertel down a dead-end clinical alley. Perhaps cells associated with colorectal cancer act like normal cells in the sense they inhibit entrance of ascorbic acid. If vitamin C cannot enter the cancer cell it cannot produce the hydrogen peroxide needed to kill that cell. A study should now be done on cancers (such as melanomas) where the cells might allow vitamin C to enter.* To think of cancer as a single disease may not only be semantically incorrect but curatively unproductive.

There will be more human studies, however, and they will not use just vitamin C alone but use it for possible synergistic effects in drug therapies. Remember, Carleen Moore et al[198f] found vitamin C used alone to treat leukemia in mice showed little effect. When used

---

* We noted earlier that Parsons and Morrison[198d] reported that ascorbate induces breaks in the DNA of human melanoma cells. On the other hand, G. Meadows and R. Abdallah[203f] reported, in 1986, on an *in vivo* study involving the effect of vitamin C on the spontaneous metastasis of B16-BL6 melanoma in mice. They concluded that "ascorbate lacks direct antimetastic activity on B16-BL6 melanoma." A clinical trial of vitamin C and human melanoma patients would obviously be out of order unless the work of Meadows and Abdallah is contradicted by a similar study with mice, rats, guinea pigs or primates.

synergistically with the drug BCNU there was, however, a dramatic increase in longevity of 237%! Similar success stories using vitamin C in human cancer therapies seem likely to eventuate. Nevertheless, even if vitamin C, under some circumstances, can be used to effectively *treat* cancer, it might, as we will discuss later in this chapter, also be a *cause* of cancer.

Possible Dangers of Excessive Vitamin C

In spite of my enthusiasm for the health-yielding benefits of adequate amounts of vitamin C, I believe that ascorbic acid may, in some cases, present dangers concerning which many nutritionists, scientists, physicians and laymen remain unaware. We have already noted possible problems of excess vitamin C taken while pregnant. We have also seen that excessive vitamin C can reduce bactericidal activity of leucocytes, that it may promote yeast infections and that it may destroy body stores of cysteine. Vitamin C may also sometimes, by depressing absorption of copper from the intestines, reduce available amounts of various copper-based enzymes, including superoxide dismutase. The action of vitamin C in reducing copper assimilation may also, as we related earlier, upset the zinc/copper ratio and thus detrimentally affect blood cholesterol. Ascorbic acid increases the body's absorption of iron and it facilitates production of hemoglobin. As a note of caution, however, vitamin C supplementation for patients having an iron overload (e.g., in cases of thalassemia) may be dangerous.[204]* Then too, the iron-based enzyme *catalase* is inhibited, according to Charles W. M. Orr,[205] by ascorbate alone but is more rapidly inhibited when copper is also present. The inhibition by

---

* Ascorbic acid, however, is generally at a low level in iron-overloaded patients probably because it is degraded by iron.[204a] Supplementing vitamin C in iron-overloaded patients, as mentioned on page 164 and as will be discussed further in chapter 7, is generally contraindicated. It is just such contraindications that sometimes make therapy difficult. B. Halliwell and J. M. C. Gutteridge[204b] have reported that feeding iron-overloaded patients ascorbic acid, in the absence of desferrioxamine, has sometimes caused death. They speculate it is because the iron and ascorbic acid combination increases lipid peroxidation and generates hydroxyl radicals.

ascorbate is also exacerbated in the presence of either iron (surprisingly, since catalase contains iron) or of EDTA (*ethylene diamine tetraacetic acid,* which is also called *edetic acid*). In a 1986 study, Allan J. Davison et al.[205a] speculate that a free radical semidehydroascorbate is the damaging species. As another negative, we will see in Chapter 8 that vitamin C may increase tissue levels of the poisonous minerals, mercury and lead.

Earlier we saw how ascorbic acid, especially in the presence of copper, deactivates histamine. Acetylcholinesterase, a group of enzymes found in blood and in various tissues that catalyze hydrolysis of acetylcholine, is also inactivated by ascorbic acid in the presence of copper. Eilat Shinar et al.[205b] have elucidated the role of ascorbate in reducing the cupric complex to the cuprous state. Ascorbate produces hydrogen peroxide and then hydroxyl radicals which inactivate the acetylcholinesterase. The residual enzymatic activity decreases as the cuprous ion concentrations rise up to about 10^{-5}M. A *reverse effect* then sets in and residual enzymatic activity increases with a further rise in copper concentration (Figure 12). Ascorbic acid and copper obviously play an important role in the biological damage caused by the resulting hydroxyl ions.

M. E. Briggs et al.[206] have expressed concern about the possibility of oxalate-based kidney stones forming in some persons taking megadoses of "C".* (Vitamin C increases the amount of oxalate in the urine, but the possibility of stones forming seems to be fairly remote. However, I wonder about the advisability of taking large amounts of "C" along with eating oxalate-containing foods such as spinach, rhubarb, strawberries, beets, cabbage, chocolate and cocoa. I also wonder about the wisdom of taking supplemental "C" along with foods such as gelatin which contain large amounts of glycine, an amino acid that forms oxalate.) Adverse effects of excessive "C" such as nausea, abdominal cramps and diarrhea are more frequently

---

* A study by Karl-Heinz Schmidt et al.[206a] showed, however, that when healthy men took 10 grams of ascorbic acid daily the change in urinary oxalate was low and was similar to the change that can result from consuming normal diets. Howard Posner[206b] has supported the idea that ascorbate represents little danger of oxalate formation, while R. Swartz[207] has taken the opposing view. Charles J. McAllister et al.[207a] cite oxalate-induced problems in a patient with renal insufficiency who was given an intravenous infusion of vitamin C.

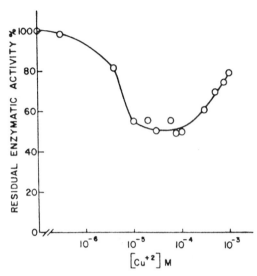

Figure 12. Effect of copper on the initial rate of inactivation of acetylcholine esterase in the presence of 2 mM ascorbate. The initial rate of inactivation was based on the loss in enzymatic activity after five minutes of incubation. Reproduced from Eilat Shinar et al., *Jrl. of Biological Chemistry* (1983) 258, no. 24: 14778-14783, with permission. Note the *reverse effect* at a cuprous ion concentration between 10^{-5} and 10^{-4} M.

reported. Menstrual bleeding in pregnant women has also been observed. In the previous chapter we noted the possible destruction of vitamin B_{12} by excessive "C" and the fact that "C" increases cyanide toxicity. Excessive "C" can, according to P. Malathi and J. Ganguly,[207b] decrease ubiquinone production concentration in the liver of vitamin-A deficient rats. Furthermore, megadoses of vitamin C may diminish body stores of minerals such as sodium, magnesium and potassium as they are coexcreted in the urine. Not only will excessive ascorbic acid have this undesirable effect on these minerals, but several groups of scientists, including Yuk-Chow Ng et al.[207c] have found that vitamin C inhibits endogenous Na+,K+ATPase in isolated cells (but not in intact cells). Svoboda and Mosinger[207d] reported Na+,K+ATPase inhibition increased as vitamin C rose to 10^{-4}M but then a *reverse effect* set in and, at higher levels, enzyme inhibition declined.

A possible, though probably remote, danger of megadose "C" is that it might tend to demineralize bone. Diane L. Bray and George M. Briggs[207e] fed 14-day-old guinea pigs a diet of 8.7% ascorbic acid for six weeks, while control animals were fed .2% ascorbic acid. The 8.7% group had decreased bone density. The levels of ascorbic acid used were, of course, huge, and humans do not always react as do animals. Nevertheless, could these results suggest a possible threat to the bones of humans megadosing on "C"? The growing bones of children might be the most threatened, but even in such cases I presume the possible danger may be remote.

M. H. Briggs,[208] who was the first to report that women taking the Pill had lowered levels of ascorbic acid in their leucocytes and platelets, more recently concluded[209] that megadose "C" may increase the risk of cardiovascular disease in Pill users. Briggs reported that "C" plus the Pill leads to increased production of an estrogen, ethinyl estradiol. He concludes that the overall effect of the megadose "C" is to convert a low-estrogen pill into a high-dose pill.

Even consuming vitamin C concomitantly with bananas might not be completely safe for all persons. Ascorbic acid is a cofactor in the hydroxylation of dopamine which leads, in turn, to the synthesis of the neurotransmitter norepinephrine.[209a] John W. Dunne et al.[210] reported that bananas, a rich source of biogenic amines, when consumed with amounts of ascorbic acid frequently used in the attempt to prevent colds, can increase the body's content of sulphate-conjugated dopamine (Figure 13). On the other hand, bananas and placebo raised the levels of norepinephrine sulphate more than they were raised by bananas eaten with ascorbic acid (Figure 14). Dunne et al. observed no negative effects when normal male subjects consumed vitamin C with bananas, but speculated on the possibility that hypertensive or older age groups might be affected. Dunne did not suggest it, but I wonder if the extra dopamine and norepinephrine present in the plasma might affect brain levels of these catecholamines to the extent

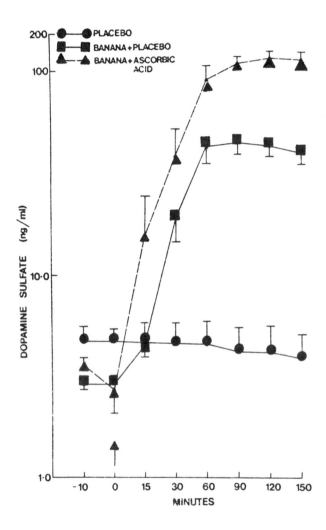

Figure 13. Effect of eating bananas (arrow) on plasma dopamine sulfate concentration after treatment with ascorbic or matched placebo in normal males (n=6). Placebo was administered in the control study but the banana was omitted. All values are mean ± SEM. Reproduced from John W. Dunne et al., *Life Sciences* (1983) 33: 1511-1517, with permission of the authors and of the publisher, Pergamon Press, Ltd.

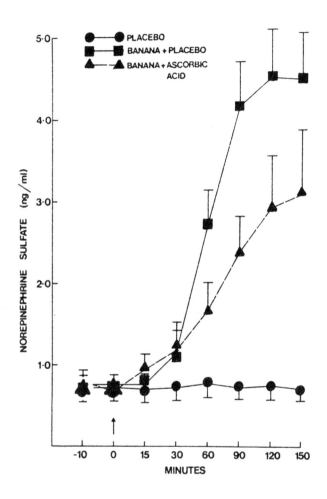

Figure 14. Effect of eating bananas (arrow) on plasma norepinephrine sulfate concentration after treatment with ascorbic acid or matched placebo in normal males (n=6). Placebo was administered in the control study but the banana was omitted. All values are mean ± SEM. Reproduced from John W. Dunne et al., *Life Sciences* (1983) 33: 1511-1517, with permission of the authors and of the publisher, Pergamon Press, Ltd.

they might be sexually stimulating. If so, banana sales might soar!

In addition to all those possible threats to health, in some cases large dosages of vitamin C may be detrimental to persons (especially black males) who have erythrocytes with a glucose-6-phosphate dehydrogenase (G-6-PD) deficiency. Thienchai Udomrath et al.[211] reported that 12.3% of black men studied were so affected. Orientals, male Serphardic Jews and other males of Mediterranean origin may also show this G-6-PD deficiency. Such affected persons who use large amounts of vitamin C can develop intravascular hemolysis followed by hemolytic anemia and there has been at least one death. Udomrath and his associates suggested that persons who might be deficient in the G-6-PD enzyme be tested for such a deficiency before consuming massive amounts of vitamin C.* Additionally, there may be even more serious problems with this vitamin.

Could Vitamin C Sometimes be a Factor in CAUSING Cancer?

There is suggestive evidence that vitamin C in megadoses might cause cancer. Dr. Vernon C. Bode[213] stated that ascorbate "degrades DNA even at very low concentrations." Then too, Dr. H. F. Stich et al.[214] and also Hirohisa Omura et al.[215] reported, on the basis of *in vitro* experiments, that vitamin C, especially in the presence of copper, has a mutagenic effect. The mutagenicity, as shown by the Ames test, occurs, however, over only a narrow range of concentrations of the ascorbate-copper mixture.** Iron has also

---

* In G-6-PD deficiency there could also be a problem with dehydroascorbic-acid metabolism. S. Basu et al.[212] have reported that dehydroascorbic-acid reduction in human erythrocytes is accomplished through the action of reduced glutathione. This reduction depends not only on glutathione reductase but also on G-6-PD.

** As a therapeutic application of the *reverse effect* (my example, of course), Eiji Kimoto et al.[216] reported that large doses of ascorbate together with copper: glycylglycylhistidine complex significantly prolonged the life span of mice inoculated with Ehrlich tumor cells. Rationale for the action, it seems to me, involves the DNA of the cancer cells being damaged concomitantly with that of the normal cells. Although their normal cells also died, the mice continued to replace these through normal body processes and thus the cancers were overcome.

been shown to potentiate the mutagenic effect of ascorbate. Stich et al.[214] point out also that their *in vitro* data may not necessarily apply to man because of man's lack of free copper or iron ions within the cell which is, of course, the site of action in DNA splitting. (E. P. Norkus et al.[215a] subsequently reported that ascorbic acid does not have intrinsic mutagenicity, evaluated in a modified Ames bacterial system, if deionized water is used.) In continuing this ascorbic acid research, Dr. Stich[217] showed, with *in vitro* experiments, that manganese enhanced the frequency of DNA aberrations but produced less inhibition of mitosis. The mitosis-inhibiting and chromosome-damaging actions of ascorbate appear to be due to the formation of hydrogen peroxide whose production is enhanced by copper, iron and manganese. Dr. Stich found that catalase virtually abolished both mitosis-inhibiting and chromosome-damaging action of ascorbate because it neutralized hydrogen peroxide. Research of Miriam P. Rosin et al.[218] also suggests that the mutagenic metabolites of ascorbate probably involve peroxide radicals since catalase prevented mutagenesis and toxicity. H. F. Stich et al.[219] also found, by means of *in vitro* tests, that commercially available vitamin C pills can damage chromosomes. Stich called the chromosome aberrations "relatively severe" and reported that they ranged up to 42%. He stressed, however, that this does not permit the conclusion that a similar effect occurs in man.

Here is another related negative effect. With *in vitro* experiments, vitamin C has caused a phenomenon known as *sister-chromatid exchanges* (SCEs) in ovary cells of Chinese hamsters according to W. Donald MacRae and H. F. Stich.[220] SCEs (which we met in Chapter 4 in connection with retinoids) are exchanges in replicating or in newly replicated DNA strands that occur between homologous sites on two (sister) chromatids of one chromosome.* These exchanges are known to be induced by a broad range of mutagenic and carcinogenic agents.

---

* Harlow K. Fischman et al.[220a] recently reported that the level of SCE in six female Alzheimer's disease patients was significantly greater than in controls. Is it possible that vitamin C (through producing SCE) could be a cause of Alzheimer's disease? The work of G. Speit et al.,[222] which we will promptly review, seems to indicate (except for a single 2,000/kg. dosage) that vitamin

The fact that vitamin C causes SCEs adds support to the idea that it may be mutagenic and/or carcinogenic.

Using *in vitro* experiments, S. M. Galloway and R. B. Painter[221] observed that ascorbate not only caused an increase in sister-chromatid exchanges in Chinese hamster ovary cells (as we noted had been reported by MacRae and Stich) but also in human lymphocytes. They also found that ascorbate caused a dose-dependent inhibition of DNA synthesis in He La cancer cells. The authors pointed out that the reported effect of vitamin C prolonging the lifetime of terminal cancer patients may result from its DNA-damaging ability since cancer cells have very little catalese to inhibit the effects of the hydrogen peroxide that is produced because of the ascorbate. They say, "...ascorbate may act beneficially to kill cells of cancer patients but detrimentally to cause mutations and perhaps even cancer in persons with normal life expectations."

Keep in mind that these SCE experiments were *in vitro*. In contrast, G. Speit et al.[222] reported that *in vivo* experiments did not lead to an induction of sister-chromatid exchanges in the bone marrow of Chinese hamsters. The test doses ranged from 200 to 10,000 mg./kg. body weight (i.e., between 14,000 and 700,000 mg. in a 70 kg. human) and were administered orally as well as by intraperitoneal injection. In the case of the earlier *in vitro* tests, the SCEs are believed to have been induced by the activity of peroxides and radicals formed by the oxidation of the ascorbate. Catalase, as well as sulfhydryl compounds such as cysteine and glutathione, by virtue of their reducing capacity, are believed responsible for the antimutagenic effect of the *in vivo* experiments. By the way, one dosage level (2,000/kg. body weight, orally administered) yielded a significant increase in the incidence of SCEs which the scientists dismissed because neither lower nor higher dosages produced SCEs. (It is, therefore, at least remotely possible that vitamin C at a certain dosage may produce *in vivo* SCE

C does not cause SCE *in vivo*. Anyway, even if we could prove vitamin C at a certain dosage causes SCE *in vivo*, that wouldn't prove that such SCE could lead to Alzheimer's disease. Concomitancy of events is far more common than etiological linkage of those events. *Ability to cause does not prove causation.*

exchanges.) The scientists concluded that "the actual mutagenic danger to man does not appear to be as great as findings on ascorbate *in vitro* might lead one to suspect." These studies warn us to draw only tentative conclusions from *in vitro* tests until they are duplicated *in vivo* since the body has many defense mechanisms that could negate test-tube results. Interestingly, in June, 1986, G. Krishna et al.[222a] reported that a huge dosage of ascorbic acid (6.68 g./kg. body wt.) acted as an anti-SCE agent both *in vitro* and *in vivo* in mice when SCEs were induced by cyclophosphamide and mitomycin C. Furthermore, Yoshihide Suwa et al.[223] have found that ascorbic acid *reduces* the *in vitro* mutagenicity of coffee as analyzed by the Ames test. Nutrition abounds with confusing phenomena that may often be examples of unrecognized *reverse effects.* Nevertheless, in experiments with mice and rats, J. Fielding Douglas and James Huff[223a] found that feeding them enormous amounts of l-ascorbic acid (0, 25,000 or 50,000 ppm., i.e., at 0, 2.5% or 5% in the diet) there were no observed differences in neoplasms between treated and control groups.

In experiments with tumorous guinea pigs, J. A. Migliozzi[224] reported that tumor regression occurred in 55% of the animals receiving .3 mg./kg. per day of ascorbic acid. Animals given 10 mg./kg. per day showed tumor inhibition but no regression. Tumors in animals given 1 g./kg. per day (equivalent to about 70 grams in a 150 lb. person) grew with no sign of regression, thus reversing the effect at lower dosage. People are not guinea pigs, but one wonders about the megadoses of vitamin C in amounts approximating 70 grams daily that are employed by some clinicians.

At least four studies by C. H. Park and his associates[224a-d] have shown that l-ascorbic acid affects growth of human leukemic colony-forming cells *in vitro.* The cells of about 50% of patients with acute nonlymphocytic leukemia were affected, the growth of leukemic cells of 33% being enhanced by ascorbic acid while the growth of leukemic cells of 17% was inhibited. In a separate experiment, the cells of one patient were divided into groups. Enhancement of leukemic colony growth increased as ascorbic acid concentrations rose. A maximum in colony growth occurred at an ascorbic acid concentration of .3 mM, then showed a *reverse effect* as enhancement declined at higher levels of ascorbic acid, but did not show inhibition at any level. It would seem that *in vitro* tests should be made of a leukemic patient before deciding to use vitamin C supplementation.[*] If this were done, vitamin C supplementation could, perhaps, be useful in treating the 17% that might be amenable to such therapy. In the absence of such tests, vitamin C should probably not be given to leukemic patients.

Another possible negative influence of vitamin C in regard to cancer is that it has been found by Toni Huwyler et al.[224f] to inhibit human natural killer (NK) cell activity. NK cells are able to lyse certain types of tumor cells and they are also possibly involved in surveillance mechanisms against neoplasia. Whether or not a *reverse effect* may exist at a different dosage and thus might act to foster NK cell activity has not been determined.

Ascorbate may not be carcinogenic itself, but, in the presence of the mutagen N-hydroxy-2-acetylaminofluorene, it has been shown by H. A. J. Schut et al.[225] to increase that chemical's mutagenicity.[**] In another study, S. Banic[227] found that vitamin C promoted the induction of sarcomas in guinea pigs by methylcholanthrene. S. S. Mirvish et al.[228] reported that ascorbate seemed to promote the induction of forestomach tumors in rats fed morpholine and nitrite, but at the same time reduced the occurrence of liver and lung tumors in the same animals! Other interesting phenomena were discovered by D. J. Korpatnick and H. F. Stich,[229] who observed that mice who were force-fed by esophageal intubation sodium ascorbate (in amounts equivalent to 1.4-7.0 grams in a 70 kilogram person) and

---

[*] We noted that Carleen Moore et al.[198f] found that vitamin C used alone to treat leukemia in mice showed little effect. However, up to 70% increase in survival of mice bearing P388 lymphocytic leukemia when treated with hydroxocobalamin (vitamin B12) and sodium ascorbate or with just dehydroascorbate has been reported recently by Herbert F. Pierson et al.[224e] The results of their study may suggest modifications in the experimental treatment of human leukemia. (A subtle *reverse effect* involving the vitamin B12 component may exist since, as we saw in Chapter 5, B12 may sometimes work to promote cancer.)

[**] Interestingly, Saeko Sakai et al.[226] reported that vitamin E and BHT *inhibited* the mutagenic action of this chemical, whereas vitamin C increased its dangers two- or three-fold.

the carcinogen MNNG showed enhanced DNA fragmentation compared to mice fed MNNG alone. However, they reported that ascorbate alone fed to mice will not fragment DNA. On the other hand, when ascorbate and MNNG were incubated at 37°C for 30 minutes before force-feeding, the ascorbate caused a *reverse effect* and the mixture produced *less* DNA fragmentation than had MNNG alone. The studies by and cited by Miriam P. Rosin et al. [230] also indicate the pro and con complexities of the interactions between carcinogens and vitamins such as ascorbic acid. Nutritional studies yield many surprising *reverse effects!**

Subsequently, Sigmund A. Weltzman and Thomas P. Stossel [231] reported that phagocytic leukocytes from normal humans can produce mutations in bacteria. Formation of such endogenous mutagenic products of an inflammatory response, while inhibited by vitamin E, sulfhydral compounds, superoxide dismutase, catalase, mannitol and benzoate, is increased by vitamin C. On the other hand, a study by David E. Amacher and Simone C. Paillet[232] suggested that ascorbate has a very narrow mutagenic range. They concluded that, although their experiments confirmed that sodium ascorbate and ascorbic acid can be toxic, the genotoxic hazards associated with them are minimal. Furthermore, Dr. R. J. Shamberger et al. [233] have shown that vitamin C protects against chromosomal damage induced by several carcinogens. In light of these somewhat conflicting studies and the considerable body of research cited earlier which points to vitamin C being beneficial for cancer prevention and therapy, studies of interactions between carcinogens and nutrients such as "C" should be given a high priority. Such studies should be made by scientists aware of the importance of dose-response relationships between carcinogens and nutrients and with full cognizance of the possibility of *monophasic, biphasic, triphasic* (or even *polyphasic) reverse effects.* Scientists should be alert to the

---

* Shyh-Horng Chiou[230a] subsequently confirmed that ascorbic acid in combination with metal ions had very high DNA-scission activity. Recently, in a study with the subtitle "A New Strategy for Cancer Chemotherapy," Nathan A. Berger et al. [230b] (writing not in regard to vitamin C but to the drugs tiazofurin and selenazofurin) called for "designing chemotherapy combinations...to synergistically potentiate the effects of DNA strand-disrupting agents." Ascorbic acid seems to be such an agent.

possibility that seemingly contradictory experimental results at different dosages may be examples of a polyphasic *reverse effect*. Tomorrow's knowledge of nutritional-physiological interactions is apt to be elucidated in dose-response tables rather than in simple statements.

Let's also remain aware that a given nutrient, say vitamin C, can operate through different mechanisms. Certain tumor cells accumulate larger amounts of vitamin C during megadose therapy than their normal counterparts and it is theorized, as noted earlier, that cells could die by a mechanism involving the production of hydrogen peroxide.[234] Other cancer cells and normal cells would be less affected by this mechanism, but might be subject to DNA modification as also suggested earlier. Making use of known mutagens such as ascorbic acid and applying the principle of the *reverse effect,* could, after appropriate animal tests, lead to successful human cancer therapies.

Vitamin C could be especially dangerous if taken with tryptophan pills that many use as a sleep aid. Hisayuki Kanamori et al[235] have shown, using *in vitro* experiments, that vitamin C and tryptophan[*] in a phosphate buffer produced several reaction products, two of which were mutagenic. These compounds were indoles (as might have been expected since tryptophan was their progenitor). Indoles, which are present in the Brassica family of vegetables (cauliflower, cabbage and brussels sprouts), seem to *protect* against cancer, so if they are also a possible *cause* of cancer at a different dosage we would once again have an example of the theory of the *reverse effect*. Various indoles could, of course, have different properties and those in vegetables are not necessarily the same as those found in the Kanamori study.

As I have stressed, the theory of the *reverse effect* suggests that many nutrients (and drugs) may have Jekyll-and-Hyde functions in disease-health applications. Furthermore, only if a substance has the potential for harm is it apt to have, at a different dosage, the potential for prevention and cure. From the large number of studies we have

---

[*] Tryptophan, even without vitamin C, was reported by Samuel M. Cohen et al.[235a] to promote urinary bladder carcinogenesis in rats. Fatty liver also may occur.[235b]

reviewed, vitamin C would seem to qualify as one of the Jekyll-and-Hyde nutrients.

Food Sources and Supplements

Some food sources for vitamin C are red and green peppers, parsley, black currants, horseradish, kohlrabi, collards, spinach, garlic, broccoli, brussels sprouts, citrus fruits and their juices, black raspberries, strawberries, cantaloupe, honeydew melon and tomatoes. Cooked fruits and vegetables contain, in general, about one-half as much vitamin C as the raw specimens. Those getting their vitamin C only from food may experience a seasonal variation in its availability. During winter and spring the vitamin C intake is likely to be low due to the increased expense (and thus a lower intake) of fresh fruit and vegetables and to the consumption of old potatoes which have less of the vitamin at this time of the year.[236]

A wild fruit, *Terminalia ferdinandiana,* found in Australia, has 50 times the concentration of vitamin C in oranges.[237] It is a food of Australian aboriginals and is reported to taste like gooseberries. Other concentrated food sources of the vitamin are the sea buckthorn *(Hippophae rhamnoides),* ambla or emblic *(Emblica officinales),* rose hips *(Rosa canina),* * dattock fruit *(Detarium senegalense)* and acerola or Barbados cherry *(Malphighia punicifolia).* [237] O. O. Keshinro[237aa] reported that iyeye or Spanish yellow plum *(Spondias mombin),* indian fruit *(Termindia cartapa),* oro bush mango *(Cordyla pinnata),* obiedun *(Cola millennii),* cashew fruit *(Anacardium occidentale)* and guava *(Psidium guajava),* among other fruits he listed, have especially high amounts of vitamin C.

S. Boyd Eaton and Melvin Konner[237b] have calculated that the mean ascorbic acid content of 27 vegetables eaten by recent hunters-gatherers is 26.8 mg./100 gm. Using this estimate, the amount of daily vitamin C in the diet of paleolithic man would have been about

---

* Interestingly, the concentration of vitamin C in rose hips varies widely from species to species. D. S. Rathore[237a] reported that while *Rosa multiflora* contained just 68 mg./100 g., *Rosa santicana* was found to have 2,584 mg./100 g.

392 mg. (The calculation of Eaton and Konner excludes the *Terminalia ferdinandiana* eaten by Australian aboriginals which would make the estimate much higher.) This amount of vitamin C intake is probably seldom achieved today except by vegetarians or those who supplement. Obviously, it is greatly in excess of the RDA.

Foods containing vitamin C and the vitamin itself can have a great effect on the absorption of nonheme iron (but not of heme iron) and this is especially noteworthy when other absorption promoters (such as meat and fish) are not present. However, contrary to the findings of earlier investigators, James D. Cook and Elaine Monsen[238] suggested that "animal tissue and ascorbic acid enhance iron absorption by the same mechanism." Leif Hallberg and Lena Rossander[239] reported on the effect of ascorbic acid on iron absorption from various meals. Despite only a 3-fold variation in the content of nonheme iron in the meals, there was a 7-fold difference in absorption of nonheme iron (.13 to .98 mg.) and a 20-fold variation in percentage absorption (2.2% to 45%). Thus, vegetarians may find it especially valuable to either include foods rich in vitamin C with all their meals or to supplement with pills. There are many subtleties to food iron absorption, some of which we will consider in the next chapter.

Some of these statements and conclusions do not, however, seem to apply in cases of vitamin E deficiency. Linda H. Chen and Richard R. Thacker[239a] reported that vitamin C supplementation significantly lowered the total iron level of vitamin E-deficient rats. Interesting as these results are, they are probably not relevant to humans who, unlike the rat, do not generally make their own vitamin C. They suggest to me, however, the possibility that large amounts of "C" (analogous perhaps to any amount of supplementary "C" in an animal that makes it endogenously) might show a *reverse effect* by inhibiting iron absorption in a vitamin E-deficient state. (This is, however, only "armchair chemistry" and requires experimental confirmation or denial.)

We have already noted that vitamin C supplementation may be dangerous in patients having an iron overload. In the case of such patients it is very important to control the vitamin C intake, and physicians managing such patients will give appropriate warnings. However, when such patients are administered desferrioxamine via subcutaneous injection, urinary iron is invariably increased by giving large doses of ascorbate.[240] Ascorbate can promote iron *absorption* but, when desferrioxamine is given it promotes iron excretion.

Regardless of the vitamin C content of the diet, it may be useful to take ascorbic acid supplements if tissue saturation is to be achieved. It has been claimed that ascorbic acid tablets degrade during normal storage. S. H. Rubin et al.[241] have reported, however, that ascorbic acid tablets retain 95% of their potency over a period of five years. The minor degradation to dehydroascorbic acid is of no concern. As we noted earlier, dehydroascorbic acid was at one time alleged to have diabetogenic activity because of an experiment involving massive, intravenous, even lethal injections into rats.[133] In spite of this and regardless of Stone's negative views, the biological utility of dehydroascorbic acid is well established.

Vitamin C is available under the label "mixed ascorbates." In the selenium section of Chapter 7 I report on a study regarding the possible nonexistence of selenium-ascorbate in a product labeled to contain it. I wonder if it is not reasonable to also question the commercial reality of some of the other "ascorbates" which to my knowledge have not been studied.

It is financially important and perhaps also health-wise important that any vitamin C or other supplement you take be assimilated by the body. If you carefully study your feces you may sometimes find intact or partially digested pills. Most vitamin pills should probably be taken after meals when the higher levels of stomach acid will help dissolve them. (As noted earlier, I think vitamin E is an exception to this rule.) The importance of pills being digested is borne out by a case reported by R. E. Vickery.[242] Vickery reported a woman had taken massive dosages of vitamin C tablets that caused an obstruction at the ileocecal valve. During surgery, multiple, hard, rock-like objects varying in size from large marbles to aspirin were found in the ileum, with the larger ones occluding the ileocecal valve. I suspect the woman may have been taking the tablets between meals (perhaps every hour to fight a cold) and thus did not have adequate stomach acid levels to aid in their digestion. This is, however, pure speculation on my part.

What about timed-release forms of vitamin C? E. Stewart Allen[243] observed that timed-release vitamin C capsules (Ascorbicap® brand) were very effective. Allen found that blood level and urine excretion measurements of 15 medical students, ages 21 to 29, showed optimal availability of vitamin C over a 12-hour period for a timed-release 500 mg. capsule compared with either a single 500 mg. dose or three 157 mg. doses given at 4-hour intervals.

A more recent study by Susanne Yung et al.[244] reached a less favorable conclusion regarding timed-release capsules. Yung et al. compared the efficiency of different forms of ascorbic acid absorption in humans. The intravenous dose was 85% recovered in the urine as ascorbic acid and its major metabolites. In contrast, just 30% was recovered from the solution and tablets forms. A considerably smaller fraction, about 14%, was recovered from the timed-release capsule. The timed-release capsule was less than one-half as efficient as a standard tablet. (The relatively small amount of ascorbic acid metabolites recovered in the case of the timed-release capsule shows that most of the vitamin went out of the body via the feces without entering into metabolic processes.)

I hope additional studies will be forthcoming to see if the dismal results of the Yung group or the very favorable earlier results of Allen are more typical of timed-release products whether they be of vitamins or of minerals. Until the studies are done and favorably reported in scientific journals, one should avoid timed-release products. Anyway, as far as vitamin C is concerned, studies by J. T. L. Nicholson and F. W. Chornock[245] and J. S. Stewart and C. C. Booth[246] showed that it is absorbed mainly in the proximal part of the small intestine (the upper region near the stomach). Thus, some timed-release pills may break up after they have passed this point and be relatively worthless. If absorption is primarily at one particular part of the intestines, why would one desire any vitamin C to be released later? I speculate, however, that timed-release "C" might protect the colon against bile acid oxidation.

Small amounts of vitamin C are absorbed via the buccal mucosa (in the cheeks) and the mucous glands at the base of the tongue. * The amount absorbed will be increased if powdered vitamin C is dissolved in water and allowed to stay in the mouth awhile before swallowing. Rate of passage of vitamin C through the buccal mucosal cells into the blood is generally greater in males because they usually have lower ascorbic acid concentrations in their buccal cells and in their blood. Buccal uptake of vitamin C is pH-dependent and increases as time of retention of the solution in the mouth is lengthened. When the solution was retained in the mouth for five minutes, males absorbed 82% and females 71% of ascorbic acid solution at pH 3.4; at pH 6.0 males absorbed 49% and females 44%. When the solution was retained in the mouth for just one minute, absorption was only one-third to one-fifth as great.[247] Ascorbic acid, with its lower pH, should be absorbed much better in the mouth than ascorbates. Absorption is also increased by the presence of sodium, calcium or glucose, but fructose has little effect.[247a]** A prominent commercial product of powdered ascorbates and also vitamin C chewable tablets are sweetened with fructose.

Some powdered vitamin C is effervescent. Thomas N. Imfeld [248] cites a study by C. M. Schweizer et al.[248a] reporting on the possible erosive action of effervescent vitamin C tablets. Imfeld shows a photograph illustrating complete loss of buccal enamel due to the prolonged misuse of vitamin C-containing effervescent tablets to the point that the patient's amalgam restorations had become loose.

Vitamin C may be taken not only by mouth, but physicians may administer it parenterally (subcutaneously, intramuscularly or intravenously). In this case, sodium ascorbate or sterile, isotonic solutions phosphate-buffered to about 6.8 pH, are generally used.

---

* Buccal administration can sometimes be very efficient. M. D. D. Bell et al.[246a] reported that the bioavailability of morphine was 40%-50% greater after buccal than after intramuscular administration. They also reported that when the drug was given via the buccal route the adverse effects were generally less than when the drug was given intramuscularly.

** Glucose, while aiding intestinal absorption of ascorbic acid, inhibits its entrance into human granulocytes. (Fructose does not inhibit assimilation of vitamin C by granulocytes.)[247b]

Since ascorbic acid is water-soluble (except for the oil-soluble form, ascorbyl palmitate) it can be stored by the body in only limited amounts (e.g., in the adrenal glands). The need for ascorbic acid varies tremendously in accordance with age, habits (such as smoking and drinking), stress and drug intake, including aspirin.

If you are going to take megadoses of "C," in spite of what you are reading, then to reduce the possibility of either an upset stomach or diarrhea, it may be advisable to swallow the ascorbic acid with food. If problems still occur, change your brand as the condition may be exacerbated by the filler that is used. Other possibilities to avoid stomach upset or diarrhea are to gradually build up to the desired dosage over a period of time or, instead of taking ascorbic acid, switch to the nonacidic forms such as sodium ascorbate (unless you are on a sodium-restricted diet), calcium ascorbate or ascorbyl palmitate. (Nicotinamide ascorbate, used by veterinarians as an analgesic, is, as far as I know, not readily available for human consumption. I wonder if it has been tried as an aspirin substitute. Being a compound formed by two vitamins—vitamin B3 and ascorbic acid—it would seem likely to be relatively safe.)

Some persons who experience allergic reactions to corn may find vitamin C upsetting since it was probably manufactured from this grain. Switching to a product made from the acerola (barbados) cherry of the West Indies or the plum-like fruit of the South American camu-camu bush may solve the problem providing the bulk of the pill's vitamin C content comes from the product indicated on the label rather than, as well it might, from corn instead.

Some persons have tried taking ascorbyl palmitate powder dissolved in fruit juice. (Regrettably, it is not very soluble in water or juices, but is very soluble in alcohol.) Ascorbyl palmitate has been shown to potentiate *in vitro* the effect of vitamin E in greatly reducing the amount of peroxides and free radicals[248b] and if it also works this way in the body it may qualify as an antiaging, prolongevity factor. J. C. Bauernfeind[248ba] has reported that ascorbyl palmitate has fairly good solubility not only in alcohol (at 25°C) but also in a phospholipid-tocopherol premix formulation (an example of such a commercial preparation being Ronoxan A). Ascorbyl palmitate has very limited solubility, however, in vegetable oils. The antioxidant effectiveness of ascorbyl palmitate in vegetable oils is believed due to its strong synergistic action with the tocopherols contained in such oils.

What about the safety of ascorbyl palmitate? O. Garth Fitzhugh and Arthur A. Nelson[248c] reported that when rats were fed l-ascorbyl palmitate or d-isoascorbyl palmitate for nine months in concentrations of 2% and 5% of the diet, only the 5% levels were toxic. The *Kirk-Othmer Encyclopedia of Chemical Technology,* 2nd edition,[249] states that, although ascorbyl palmitate is not shown in the list of acceptable antioxidants for the United States, it is shown as accepted in foods by Canada at a level of .2%. This is the same as Canada's acceptable level for the tocopherols (vitamin E). The 3rd edition[250] of this work shows no U.S. level for ascorbyl palmitate but states that it is suitable for use in food products. The *Code of Federal Regulations*[251] states that ascorbyl palmitate is generally recognized as safe when used in accordance with good manufacturing practices. However, just because a chemical may be safe as a food preservative does not mean we can safely "go overboard" on big dosages. If large dosages of ascorbic acid are viewed as being dangerous, then that attitude must be even more emphasized when it comes to the relatively untested form of vitamin C—ascorbyl palmitate.

Don't Take Megadoses of Vitamin C!

Vitamin C may hold possibilities for giving us increased health and perhaps increased longevity because of its role as an antioxidant. However, a study by J. E. W. Davies et al.[252] in which 1% of the diet of guinea pigs was ascorbic acid showed that such massive dosages do *not* prolong survival of guinea pigs.*   On the contrary,

---

* Harold R. Massie et al.[252a] found that 1% ascorbic acid (1,430 mg./kg. body weight—i.e., about 100 grams for a 70 kilogram person) in the drinking water of mice increased their average life span by 8.6% or 20.4%, depending on how the data were interpreted. There was, however, no increase in maximum life span. Since mice make their own vitamin C, a dosage such as given in this study must be viewed as being huge.

massive doses *shortened* their life span. Davies et al. point out, however, that "C" in nominal dosages may operate to increase the life span because of its antioxidant effect. Moreover, based on another guinea pig experiment, there seems to be a *reverse effect* in the antioxidant power of ascorbic acid when it is used in great excess. L. H. Chen and M. L. Chang [161,253] reported that high levels of vitamin C supplementation of 10 mg./100 g. of body weight per day (equivalent to about 7 grams daily in a 150 lb. person) lowered tissue antioxidant potential when vitamin E was marginally adequate. The hemolytic and peroxidizing effect of even higher "C" levels (equivalent to 20 grams daily in a 150 lb. person) was, however, counteracted by increasing the level of vitamin E.* Lydi Sterrenberg et al.[253a] similarly concluded that "vitamin E determines whether the pro-oxidant activity of vitamin C is expressed." The Sterrenberg group found that the sensitivity of the microsomal membranes to ferrous ion/ascorbic acid-induced lipid peroxidation is highly dependent on the vitamin E content of those membranes.

J. C. Bauernfeind[248ba] noted G. Kelly and B. M. Watts[255a] have speculated that a copper-ascorbic acid complex may be responsible for the pro-oxidant effect of ascorbic acid in aqueous animal-fat systems that are low in tocopherols. Kelly and Watts,[255a] as well as B. M. Watts and M. Faulkner,[255b] found that this pro-oxidant effect could be eliminated through use of sequestering or chelating agents.

E. D. Wells[256] reported that magnesium and inorganic iron increase the rate of ascorbate-induced peroxidation while calcium and most heavy-metal ions inhibit it. O. P. Sharma and C. R. Krishna Murti[257] speculated that the free radicals liberated by ascorbic acid are probably involved in the oxidation of unsaturated fatty acids and this now seems to be well established.

---

* L. H. Chen and M. L. Chang [161,254] have reported that adequate, but normal, vitamin C supplementation in guinea pigs increased the plasma vitamin E level to improve tissue antioxidant status. They speculate that vitamin C at modest levels may favor the glutathione peroxidase system for removal of peroxide in a way additive with vitamin E. A more recent study by Linda H. Chen and Richard R. Thacker[255] showed that rats given high amounts of supplementary "C" had significantly lower plasma levels of vitamin E and also lower levels of reduced glutathione in their erythrocytes. These studies ought to warn the high-C enthusiasts to increase their vitamin E intake if it doesn't succeed in scaring them into reducing their use of excessive "C."

Ascorbic acid, as it oxidizes, produces the superoxide free radical but, as we will see in Chapter 9, superoxide has both negative and beneficial effects.[258] Rolando F. Del Maestro[259] has reported that, in *in vitro* experiments, ascorbic acid can sometimes degrade hyaluronic acid. The action is dependent on both the concentration of ascorbic acid and on the presence of metal (probably iron) contamination. Sometimes, as we have seen, ascorbic acid acts as a pro-oxidant and, under different conditions, as an antioxidant.

Another interesting vitamin C experiment with guinea pigs was conducted by B. K. Nandi et al.[260] of the University College of Science, Calcutta, India. This group found that maximum growth was achieved at a dosage of ascorbic acid corresponding to a daily intake of 700 mg. by a 150 lb. (70 kg.) person. Greater quantities of vitamin C up to 10 times that amount neither increased nor decreased their growth rate (but, of course, health relates to far more than rate of growth).

Human beings are not guinea pigs and certainly they are even further removed biologically from fruit flies. However, antioxidant effects might have some similarities. H. R. Massie et al.[260a] reported that when *Drosophila melanogaster* were fed ascorbic acid in their water their longevity was reduced.* Interestingly, however, Table 2 shows that survival of those given .10M ascorbic acid was closer to that of controls than groups given either .01M or .05M. This suggests to me the possibility of a *reverse effect* if the experiment were carried out at higher concentrations of vitamin C. Perhaps life spans would be increased at higher concentrations. (On the other hand, the 20% survival datum at the 10M concentration is likely just a statistical variation and survival rates might therefore decrease further at higher concentrations.) When scientists are not cognizant that *reverse effects* might conceivably occur, they are unlikely to construct an experiment's protocol in such a way as to make such a

---

* I expressed concern earlier about the reliability of experiments when animals are housed more than one per cage. Obviously, my concern extends to studies using fruit flies where the more aggressive may live longer simply because they can more effectively compete for the food and/or the water.

Vitamin C—Problem *Solver* or *Causer?* 533

Table 2

Compound	80% survival	Median survival (days)	20% survival	% change from control median
Control	35	46	55	
0·01 M ascorbic acid	33	42	52	−8·7
0·05 M ascorbic acid	33	43	48	−6·5
0·10 M ascorbic acid	35	44	50	−4·3

Median survival times of *D. melanogaster* (Ore-R Males) maintained as adults on medium containing varying molar concentrations of ascorbic acid. Medium tubes were changed twice daily except on weekends when flies were placed on control medium. Reproduced from H. R. Massie et al., *Experimental Gerontology* (1976) 11: 37-41, by permission.

discovery possible. At any rate, Figure 15 shows the detrimental effects of .05M ascorbic acid on the life span of fruit flies.

If you are using vitamin C in megadoses and are undergoing physical tests, be sure your doctor knows of your vitamin consumption. (Conversely, physicians who faithfully question patients about any medication they may be taking must learn to ask also about their patient's vitamin and mineral consumption.) Howard B. Stein et al.[261] have reported that megadoses of vitamin C can greatly increase uric acid levels in the urine (possibly interfering with a correct diagnosis of gout).* Megadoses can lead to decreased or false negative indications with the benzidine or guaiac tests for occult blood.[263] Megadoses of vitamin C can also falsely show increased serum glucose levels (Benedict's test), which might result in an incorrect diagnosis of diabetes in a normal subject. On the other hand, megadoses of "C" can falsely show decreased glucose levels with the test using combistix and with the test using the oxidase method. (The hexokinase method for testing levels of serum glucose is, however, reported to be unaffected by the presence of excessive amounts of antioxidants such as vitamin C.) Furthermore, ascorbate may interfere with the measurements

---

* On the contrary, William E. Mitch et al.[262] reported that 4 to 12 grams of ascorbic acid, taken in divided doses, had no effect on serum uric acid or uric acid excretion by the kidneys in normal subjects when measured by the phosphotungstate reduction technique. When subjects ingest large amounts of ascorbic acid and their uric acid is measured by a nonspecific method, then it will be falsely reported as having increased. Mitch et al. suggest, however, that in subjects with gout or hyperuricosuria, ascorbic acid may cause a true increase in the renal clearance of uric acid.

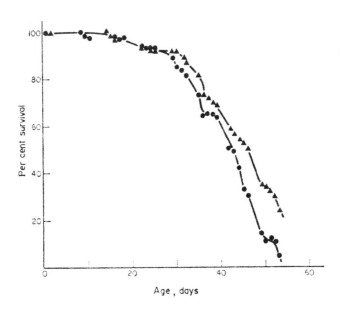

Figure 15. Survival of Oregon-R *Drosophila melano-gaster* males at 25°C expressed as percent surviving after emergence versus time in days. Triangles represent the water control and circles 0.05M ascorbic acid. One hundred flies were used for each group and the medium was changed twice daily. Reproduced from H. R. Massie et al., *Experimental Gerontology* (1976) **11:** 37-41, by permission.

of glucose neonatal cerebrospinal fluid, important in the differential diagnosis of meningitis.[265a] Then too, vitamin C can cause spuriously high levels in the test for serum creatinine.[264] Vitamin C is also reported to sometimes suppress the results of tests for serum bilirubin, aminotransferases, lactate dehydrogenase, 17-hydroxycorticosteroids and urobilingen.[265] Ascorbic acid can also lead to false negative indications for cholesterol, hemoglobin and porphobilinogen.[265b] Ascorbic acid can, on the other hand, produce false positive readings for catecholamines, serum glutamic oxaloacetic acid transaminase (SGOT) and 17-ketosteroids.[265b]

Megadoses of vitamin C should, perhaps, not be taken concurrently with aspirin. Grace Y. Lo and Frank Konishi[266] reported that rats fed aspirin and vitamin C (which was the daily equivalent of about 40 grams in humans) developed more gastric lesions than those consuming only aspirin. The dose was huge, besides which the rat makes additional "C" endogenously. Still, if you are taking vitamin C at the 2-, 5- or 10-gram (or higher) level you may want to add this to the long list of "cautions." At any rate, C. W. M. Wilson[266a] reported that when 600 mg. aspirin was taken with 500 mg. vitamin C the uptake of vitamin C by the leukocytes was completely arrested. This inhibition occurred even when doses of vitamin C as great as 2,000 mg. were taken. High doses of "C" can raise aspirin levels in the blood and lead to salicylism and such symptoms as tinnitus (ringing in the ear), deafness, dizziness, nausea, restlessness, delirium, rapid breathing and burning sensations.[266b] Johansson and Akesson recently reported that "at low ascorbic acid intake, acetylsalicylic acid (3 grams per day) increased urinary ascorbic acid, but at high ascorbic acid intake (1 gram per day) acetylsalicylic acid decreased urinary ascorbic acid." They speculate that the former effect may reflect decreased protein binding and tissue uptake of ascorbic acid by acetylsalicylic acid, while at high amounts of ascorbic acid the *reverse effect* (my language) was probably due to an inhibited absorption of ascorbic acid.

Vitamin C can affect the action of many other drugs and some of these interactions were given earlier in this chapter. A study by Francis J. Peterson et al.[267] suggested that long-term, excessive ascorbic acid consumption (in guinea pigs) may inhibit drug metabolism. When the animals were fed for nine months 86 grams of ascorbic acid per kilogram of food (about equal to 86 grams daily for a human) they showed much lower levels of liver cytochrome P-450.* They also demonstrated much poorer ability to metabolize drugs such as p-nitroanisole, aminopyrine and aniline. The scientists

---

* David B. Milne and Stanley T. Omaye[268] reported that guinea pigs fed a vitamin C-deficient diet showed a 48.2% drop in cytochrome P-450. It's another example of a *biphasic reverse effect* since nominal amounts of "C" reverse the action of both a deficiency and an excess. It is also another example of the merit of moderation.

speculated that long-term massive levels of vitamin C can be detrimental to the hepatic mono-oxygenase system because of mechanisms involving the generation of oxygen free radicals. Virtually no one takes 86 grams of vitamin C daily for long periods, but could lesser amounts affect drug metabolism in humans? If you are taking supplemental vitamin C and you are prescribed drugs, let your physician decide if you should decrease (or increase) your "C" intake.

Megadoses of vitamin C, as we have seen, can either interfere with or can potentiate various drug therapies. "Orthomolecular physicians" who employ large amounts of "C" should be aware that "C" is incompatible with therapies using certain drugs.[269] Such physicians must realize that vitamin C can interfere with the action of antipyrine and atropine by increasing their excretion.[269a] On the other hand, vitamin C potentiates the action of quinidine, quinine, primidone, barbiturates, amphetamines and sulfonamides by decreasing their excretion.[269a,b] Vitamin C shortens the prothrombin time in animals receiving coumarin anticoagulants, and George Rosenthal[270] cites a case in which this held true in a human. Recently, George V. Rebec et al.[270a] reported that ascorbic acid "may be effective in potentiating the clinical response of haloperidol and related antipsychotic drugs." If any of these drugs has been prescribed for you, be sure your physician knows the drug-related effects of vitamin C so that he can advise you accordingly.

The Body Pool of Ascorbic Acid and the RDA

Much speculation has appeared in the literature in regard to the probable body-pool size of ascorbic acid in man. Isotope studies have postulated 1,500 mg. as the maximum body-pool size. Anders Kallner et al.[271] concluded that a daily intake of 100 mg. ascorbic acid would be appropriate to maintain the body pool. By the way, Dr. Kallner's two colleagues on this study were associated with F. Hoffman-LaRoche & Co., the world's largest manufacturer of vitamin C, so it would seem that they certainly had no bias toward understating optimal vitamin C consumption.

However, Emil Ginter[272,273] points out that some of the body's vitamin C may be metabolically inert and he favors a value of approximately 5,000 mg. for the ideal body-pool size of ascorbic acid. Ginter[273] says: "If we presume fractional ascorbate turnover, even in the presence of such a high pool, to be 3% in 24 h, then to keep the ascorbate pool at the maximum size, the daily input of ascorbate into the pool would have to be 150 mg. If we take into account the partial degradation of ascorbate in the gastrointestinal tract, the incomplete absorption of single large doses of vitamin C and the fact that part of the absorbed ascorbate is excreted in the urine without ever reaching the tissues, then the daily dose of vitamin C needed to ensure maximum steady-state levels in the tissue is probably one order higher than the official recommended dietary allowances and one order lower than the doses used in megatherapy. It should be emphasized that this is only a rough estimate because there are at least three ascorbate compartments, each with a different turnover rate, in the human body. In addition, we must take into account the considerable individual variability existing in man." Earlier, I cited William W. Coon[91] as stating that 200 mg. of daily vitamin C was enough to achieve saturation. Jerry A. Tillotson and Richard J. O'Connor,[274] however, like Ginter, concluded from studying the ascorbic acid (AA) pool size in the monkey, that "the potential, function and contribution of all the AA compartments may have been overlooked." Thus, the possibility exists that saturation is not achieved at daily intakes of 150 mg. (Ginter) or 200 mg. (Coon). However, in the absence of a histamine-related or collagen-related problem, there is no good current evidence that higher levels are generally useful. Nevertheless, we saw earlier that research by S. Boyd Eaton and Melvin Konner,[237b] averaging figures from several studies of recent hunter-gatherers, indicated that the diet of paleolithic man may have contained about 392 mg. of vitamin C per day. If the concept of the RDA had existed in those times the value for vitamin C would likely have been set, based on dietary intake, at a level far higher than the present 60 mg.

Tissue ascorbic acid saturation levels are higher in young guinea pigs than in old guinea pigs. J. E. W. Davies et al.[275] found that the liver, adrenals, spleen and brain of old animals had lower saturation levels of ascorbic acid than the corresponding tissue of young animals. Davis et al. noted that this supports an earlier suggestion by Rh. S. Williams and R. E. Hughes[276] that ascorbic acid retention may be a function of the metabolic activity of the tissue. If this finding is applicable to humans it would argue that older persons may need less ascorbic acid than younger persons.

We have seen that ascorbic acid (AA) can show a *reverse effect* by functioning as an antioxidant or as a pro-oxidant. H. Peter Roeser[204a] observes that "at low concentrations of AA (less than 0.08 mM), lipid peroxidation of microsomes or tissue homogenates is greatly enhanced, both in the presence and absence of iron." Then he goes on to state, "When AA is administered in megadose quantities (1 g/day in humans or 1.5g/kg. of diet in animals), the dominant effect also appears to be pro-oxidant." Based on the evidence presented in this chapter, daily megadoses in the 3- to 10-gram range, which are sometimes recommended, appear to be dangerous.

The Lingual Test for Vitamin C

The proposal to test body stores of vitamin C by timing the decoloration of a drop of dye solution placed on the tongue is believed to have been made first by T. Giza and J. Weclawowizc[277] in Poland in 1960. E. Cheraskin and W.M. Ringsdorf, Jr. have been prominent proponents of this test.[278-280] It now seems, howver, that the test is without validity. A well-controlled study by P.J. Leggott et al.,[281] as discussed in the October, 1986 issue of *Nutrition Reviews,* [282] concluded lingual vitamin C test values and salivary vitamin C levels are not related to changes in vitamin C intake and are not consistent with plasma or leukocyte concentrations of vitamin C. The non-validity of this test could affect many conclusions. The study by K.E. Sarji[135] (page 475), for example, used the test to judge vitamin-C levels.

"We might perhaps agree that the history of science is a history of errors, for it is the nature of the scientific process that one error be replaced by a new error. Nevertheless in this process of replacing one error with another (or one truth with another), scientific thought proceeds. There is no such thing as a final statement about ultimate truth. The difference really is whether an error is productive or sterile. The history of science is the history not only of fertile error but also of fertile truth."
— Erich Fromm, from *Dialogue with Erich Fromm* by Richard I. Evans (New York: Harper and Row, 1966)

"Normally we do not so much look at things as overlook them."
— Alan W. Watts, *The Joyous Cosmology* (New York: Pantheon Books, 1962)

CHAPTER 7

Minerals for High Vitality—Threatening if Oversupplemented

Minerals are vital to neuromuscular transmission, act as enzyme cofactors and in other ways play important roles in promoting health and longevity. The body's requirement for minerals is just as great as its need for vitamins. Overdosages of minerals can, however, be just as threatening as overdosages of vitamins. Many of the metals influence each other's absorption and we will be calling attention to some of these interactions. Charles H. Hill and Gennard Matrone[1] have presented support for their hypothesis that elements whose physical and chemical properties are similar will act antagonistically to each other. Now, let us consider, in turn, the various mineral requirements of the body.

Calcium

The parathyroids are four tiny glands at each end of the lobes of the thyroid gland. They secrete a hormone, parathormone, which regulates the calcium concentration in the blood and tissues. It is generally agreed that the parathyroid hormone, parathormone (PTH), mediated by vitamin D, acts directly on bone and maintains serum calcium levels by taking the element from bone.* PTH secretion is stimulated when calcium assimilation is decreased either because of insufficient intake of calcium-containing foods and supplements or because of malabsorption. Serum PTH also increases with aging in normal and in osteoporotic subjects, perhaps as a reaction to deficient renal secretion of 1,25(OH)$_2$D brought on by age-related decreases in kidney function (i.e., the PTH is attempting to "push" the kidney to hydroxylate more 25-OH-D to 1,25(OH)$_2$D). However, contrary to what one might suspect, at a given age the PTH often (but not always) will be lower in those with osteoporosis. (Obviously, PTH is affecting more than bone resorption; the mechanisms are incompletely understood.) A group at the Mayo Clinic has confirmed that osteoporosis is inhibited by estrogen because it makes bone less sensitive to the parathyroid hormone.

A hormone, *calcitonin,* secreted by the thyroid gland and thus sometimes called *thyrocalcitonin,* reduces the calcium ion concentration in the blood by inhibiting bone resorption (and increasing bone formation) and thus works opposite to the parathyroid hormone.** However, the calcitonin mechanism is weak and the calcium level in the extracellular fluid is almost entirely set by the parathyroid gland. Nevertheless, studies by Hugh McA. Taggart

---

* Bone resorption is a process by which the body's immediate needs for calcium and other minerals may be met. Osteoporosis occurs when bone resorption chronically exceeds bone formation.

** As will be seen later, Guy E. Abraham[195] holds that magnesium stimulates production of calcitonin while suppressing the parathyroid hormone.

et al.[1a] suggest that calcitonin deficiency may be involved in postmenopausal osteoporosis. The level of calcitonin is generally greater in men than in women and decreases with age in both sexes,[2] which may help account for the fact that osteoporosis tends to occur as we age and that it affects women more than men. Seizo Yoshikawa and his associates[3] have found that when calcitonin is administered with calcium supplements it can increase bone in elderly osteoporosis patients.* Several calcitonin preparations—including human, salmon and eel—are available for clinical use. A recent study by Robert D. Tiegs et al.[3b] concluded, however, that "postmenopausal osteoporosis is not associated with, and does not result from calcitonin deficiency. On the contrary, excessive skeletal calcium release may stimulate calcitonin secretion in patients with the disorder."

Parathormone and calcitonin are concerned primarily with the control of the calcium free ion concentration in plasma. It is these free calcium ions that are the most important component of the much larger supply of total body calcium. Not only is calcium present in bone and tissue but, in the plasma itself, much of the calcium (about 55%) is bound to albumin and to other protein and is therefore not freely diffusible. The plasma also contains diffusible but non-ionized calcium, although only the ionized calcium is physiologically active.[3c]**

Calcium, a vital element, is not generally present in sufficient quantities in foods to meet the needs of all persons. There is probably no other vital element that is in shorter supply in the typical

---

* Calcitonin is used not only in the treatment of postmenopausal osteoporosis but also for Paget's disease and hypercalcemia.[3a] Calcitonin also acts as an analgesic and it can, in addition, potentiate morphine analgesia.[3aa]

** More tests are generally performed on total calcium since measurement of just the ionized calcium is more difficult.[3c] Physicians might be wise to specify "ionized calcium" when ordering tests. A high level of ionized calcium in the blood is associated with low blood pressure. Total circulating calcium has been found to be unrelated to blood pressure in some studies and, in other studies, to be associated directly with blood pressure.[3d] Graham A. MacGregor[3e] stresses the importance of also measuring ionized calcium levels in conjunction with serum pH because overbreathing causes an alkalosis and could reduce ionized calcium levels. Intracellular levels of free calcium ions are also important. The journal Cell Calcium,[3f] in mid-1985, devoted an entire issue of 14 chapters to the "Measurements of Cell Calcium."

American, high-phosphorus, high-protein diet. (Nevertheless, as we will see later, it is simplistic to believe that protein and phosphorus always depress the calcium balance. Protein detrimentally affects the calcium balance only at low intakes of calcium and phosphorus concomitant with a high intake of protein.)

At any rate, calcium present in foods or taken as supplements may not always be adequately absorbed in the presence of fiber or of competing minerals. W. P. T. James et al.[3g] have pointed out that calcium is absorbed not only in the small intestines but also in the colon and that the role of each could be approximately equal. In fact, from their experimental results they concluded that calcium absorption from a high-fiber diet could depend largely on the absorptive ability of the colon. I speculate it is possible that a colon overloaded with mucus (a condition perhaps correctable with colonic therapy) might therefore be a factor in the etiology of osteoporosis.[*]

Many cellular functions are regulated by the intracellular concentration of calcium. Calmodulin is a low molecular weight protein involved in this regulation through an interaction with various enzyme systems.[4] Among the uses of calmodulin is that of a sexual function. It stimulates the pathway to testosterone by facilitating transport of cholesterol to mitochondria. Calmodulin may also be involved in the response of the Leydig cells of the testes to the leutenizing hormone.[5] A review of this multifunctional regulator of cellular functions was written by Wai Yiu Cheung[6] and is titled "Calmodulin: An Overview."

Calcium controls endocytosis and exocytosis (the intake and output of substances through cell membranes). It also functions in

---

[*] Most of the absorption by the colon takes place in the proximal half, while the distal portion serves primarily for storage.[3h] Excessive mucus will not only inhibit absorption of calcium but also that of other nutrients. ((Sodium, chloride, vitamins B₁, B₂, B₁₂ and K are absorbed in the colon.)[3h] The fact that absorption occurs high in the colon suggests a reason colon therapy may be superior to the enema. Although removal of excessive mucus may often be a valuable benefit of colonic therapy, can it be overdone? Mucus protects the underlying mucosa from enzymatic and mechanical injury and also, perhaps, from pathogenic organisms.[3i] Gross et al.[3j] propose that another valuable function of the mucus layers of the respiratory tract and of the gastrointestinal system is the scavenging of highly reactive, oxygen-derived entities that might otherwise damage the underlying mucosa. Removing excessive mucus may often be health serving, but we must remember the golden mean.

the metabolism of glycogen, the storage form of glucose. Calcium plays a role in steroidogenesis, in insulin release and in taste and olfaction mechanisms.[7]

Calcium exhibits an interesting *reverse effect* in the activity of the enzyme adenyl cyclase, which catalyzes the formation of cyclic AMP (cyclic adenosine monophosphate) from ATP (adenosine triphosphate). Laurence S. Bradham et al.[8] reported that, although calcium ions are required to activate this enzyme, a larger amount, showing a *reverse effect,* blocks its action. More, as in so many other examples, is *not* better.

Calcium is needed for clotting of the blood and for regulating the beat of the heart. Studies by Richard D. Estensen et al.[9] indicate that calcium (as well as magnesium) plays a role in human peripheral blood neutrophil function. Calcium can relieve the itching of hives as well as pruritis due to other organic or psychogenic causes. A number of studies, begun in 1966 by G. M. Grodsky and L. L. Bennett and cited by S. L. Howell,[10] have shown that calcium is an essential factor for secreting insulin. Calcium also plays a role in stimulating the release of acetylcholine at the neuro-muscular junction.* A deficiency of calcium can lead to muscle cramps ("Charley horses"),** abdominal pain, nervousness, irritability and heart palpitations. Calcium ions play an important role in sustained exercise by coupling actin and myosin and increasing the contractility of heart and skeletal muscles.[10a]*** Calcium reduces sensitivity to pain and some find that it acts as an effective headache remedy. Calcium also helps protect the body against lead poisoning (an ever-present problem because of

---

* Contrary to the action of calcium, this release of acetylcholine is inhibited by sodium, magnesium and manganese ions, as well as by the poisons lead and mercury.[11]

** Mats Hammar et al.[12] reported that oral calcium gave good clinical improvement in pregnant women with leg cramps. The total serum calcium concentration increased but the ionized serum calcium concentration was unchanged.

*** J. M. Lopes et al.[10b] reported that caffeine beneficially acts before and after the onset of fatigue by operating on the sarcoplasmic reticulum of muscle tissue, increasing calcium permeability and making the calcium readily available for muscle contraction. Although caffeine may increase physical (and mental) functioning on a short-run basis, prolonged ingestion showed a *reverse effect* by decreasing the capacity of mice to perform continuous work (i.e., swimming to exhaustion).[10c] While coffee drinking by adults may temporarily increase their "pep," coffee consumed by "hyperkinetic" children may calm them down![10d]

automobile exhausts, industrial pollution and smoking of tobacco).

Another important use of calcium involves the chemical serotonin. Serotonin is manufactured in various parts of the body, including the nerve cells of the brain. It is produced from the amino acid tryptophan, but only if calcium is present. Serotonin, and its subsequent conversion to melatonin, is required for normal sleep. (During waking hours the brain's serotonin is neutralized by enkaphalins with very little serotonin being converted to melatonin. Near the end of our wake period melatonin production increases and we become sleepy.) Serotonin is also required for other functions such as constriction and dilation of blood vessels, contractions of the intestinal tract, production of adrenal hormones and for controlling the acidity and the volume of gastric juice. And so the importance of serotonin (and of tryptophan from which it is made), and of calcium which must be present for the synthesis of serotonin to occur, is evident.

Calcium, along with ascorbic acid, is a factor in the strength of collagen that constitutes the body's connective tissue. Calcium is essential for maintaining the health of the capillaries. Without sufficient calcium they become fragile, break and cause hemorrhages.

A lack of calcium may be a contributing factor, along with other mineral deficiencies, in causing spastic colitis. A calcium deficiency may be a source of colic in a baby. The lack of calcium can cause children to hold their breath when frustrated, even to the extent of becoming unconscious. Its lack in sufficient supply can be a cause of fragile teeth. It has been suggested that, in plentiful supply, calcium can act to tighten loose teeth and repair bone damage caused by pyorrhea. However, H. Rottka et al.[13] reported that human periodontal disease is apparently not improved by oral calcium supplementation of 1,000 to 2,000 mg. daily—at least not when supplementation is given over a period of only 9 to 12 months. Nevertheless, this study used calcium supplementation alone rather than in conjunction with vitamins C and D, fluoride and estrogen and so one cannot conclude that calcium plus these other factors would similarly be without beneficial effect.

Calcium joins with phosphorus, magnesium, iron, vitamin D and other nutrients in forming bones and teeth. About 99% of the calcium in our bodies is found in the bones and teeth and the remaining 1% circulates in the body fluids and tissues. Calcium and phosphorus are used to form hydroxyapatite, a calcium-phosphate compound in the bone, in the approximate ratio of two to one. Vitamin D, in the form of $1,25(OH)_2D_3$ (known as calcitriol), helps control the process which is further promoted by the presence of vitamin A, the B complex and C, magnesium and lactose (milk sugar). Phosphorus is generally plentiful in foods, but you may find it desirable to supplement your diet with calcium and possibly even with vitamin D from fish-liver oils if you are elderly and especially if you are a woman.

There is a relation between calcium and the menstrual cycle, the blood calcium dropping steadily in the period prior to menstruation. During menstruation, and for several days before its onset, women may wish to take more calcium and magnesium in the attempt to reduce headaches, insomnia, nervousness and mental depression. A popular writer of nutritional faddism (Adelle Davis) recommended that one or two calcium tablets per hour be taken for relief of menstrual cramps. On the contrary, treating symptoms, as we are suggesting here, may be simplistic. Just because certain minerals tend to be at low levels in the blood during the time of menstruation does not prove that the body requires supplementation. It is questionable whether we should try to smooth out the body's monthly mineral rhythms.

Let's point out another calcium-related rhythm—this one having a daily rather than a monthly cycle. In rats, and therefore perhaps in man, the efficiency of calcium transport from the intestines into the blood varies with the time of day. Jerzy Wrobel[14] has reported that in rats there was a diurnal rhythm in calcium-transport efficiency that rose during the night.* The rhythm persisted even in fasted rats and was maintained even under conditions of constant illumination. Earlier, J. Wrobel and G. Nagel[16] had reported that the periodicity of this rhythm could, however, be shifted not only by the light-dark cycle but by the time of food presentation. In fact, they state that the time of food intake was the more important synchronizer of the calcium-transport cycle. It seems conceivable to me, however, that the rhythm, since it also persists in fasted rats, may be determined at least partially by a rhythmicity of the parathyroid gland. Rats are nocturnal animals, so I suspect that calcium transport in man in a fasting state might peak during daytime hours. Hun Ki Min et al.[17] found that calcium (and also magnesium) excretion via the urine peaks in the early morning with a maximal fall in the evening. (Peak excretion of sodium and potassium occur late in the morning. Phosphorus excretion, they report, is almost exactly 180° out of phase with calcium and magnesium excretion.)

In related research, Horace M. Perry III et al.[17a] have reported that studies of M. Markowitz et al.[17b] and of W. Jubiz et al.[17c] showed a diurnal variation of ionized calcium in young men that is unrelated to dietary intake, serum phosphate or serum albumin concentrations.

A different diurnal variation of serum calcium and phosphorus recently has been discovered to occur in postmenopausal women. Horace M. Perry III et al.,[17a] early in 1986, reported that the hourly means of ionized calcium and phosphorus demonstrate a significant diurnal variation with similar apogee, nadir and periodicity. The effect of meals on the serum concentration of calcium and phosphate ions is shown by a sinusoidal increase of each during the mid-morning. However, there is a downturn hours before the evening meal which Perry and his associates suggest demonstrates that the diurnal variation is related to intrinsic rather than extrinsic causes.

---

* Subsequently, Wrobel[15] reported that the diurnal fluctuation in calcium transport became established when rats were about six weeks of age. Younger rats, 23 days old, showed very little diurnal fluctuation. He also reported a shift in phase of the rhythm when rats adapted, from the 14th day of life, to a reversed light-dark cycle.

Perhaps the calcium-excretion rhythm and the transport rhythms in man can be used to beneficially modify diets. Might it not be possible that concentrating the consumption of high-calcium foods at lunch to maximize calcium entry into the blood would be preferable to the eating of such foods either earlier or later in the day? The idea is, of course, sheer speculation on my part. However, diet planning of the future is almost certain to consider subtleties ignored today. More will be said regarding mineral rhythms of the body later in this chapter when we discuss iron and potassium.

Calcium in the bone and calcium in the blood undergo a continuous interchange—a process called "bone remodeling." In the normal adult bone calcium is completely replaced during the course of about ten years.[17d] In the middle years and beyond, men, but women especially, lose calcium from their bodies at a rate greater than they can replenish it from food. Dietary surveys[18] have shown that men and women, aged 60 and up, generally consume less than one-half the RDA for calcium. Add to this fact the probability that the RDA for calcium itself may be too low and we obviously have a very serious situation. The fact, as I see it, that calcium consumption (especially by women or by elderly men) is generally too low is supported by a study of J. R. Bullamore et al.[19] Using plasma radioactivity measurements after administrating oral calcium isotopes, this group showed that calcium absorption fell with age after about the age of 60 and everyone over 80 that was studied had significant malabsorption. Whether this is due to a decline in gastrointestinal function as one ages or due to a vitamin D deficiency is not known. The fact that the absorption of other minerals does not seem to be greatly affected in the aged suggests that a deficiency in the calcium-binding protein, which is induced by a deficiency of $1,25(OH)_2D_3$, may be the cause.[20] The fact that bone loss with advancing years is especially large in women is shown by the 180,000 to 200,000 hip fractures occurring every year in women over the age of 65. Bone loss is due primarily to lack of calcium in the diet and is exacerbated, in women, by diminishing supplies of estrogen and, in men and women, by decreasing levels of the body's active vitamin D metabolite $1,25(OH)_2D$, by chronic megadoses of vitamin A, by inadequate exercise, by diabetes mellitus, by alcoholic abuse and by smoking. Smoking women show far more bone loss than do nonsmoking women, who in turn experience more bone loss than do obese women, thus making this one of the few points in favor of obesity.[21] Perhaps the additional estrogen associated with obesity and also associated negatively with the incidence of osteoporosis, provides the rationale.

For many people, particularly for women, in the middle years and older, supplementation is essential if they are not to run the risk of osteoporosis (porous, fragile bones, although usually painless) or osteomalacia (softening of the bones, usually accompanied by pain and generally called rheumatism) with possible resultant fracture of the hip. The ability to absorb calcium declines as we age, so a calcium intake adequate to grow our bones may not be enough to maintain them. Robert P. Heaney et al.[22] stresses that if one maximizes bone density at the ages of 30-35, then hip and other bone fractures will be less likely to occur some 40 years later.* William A. Peck[22b] of Washington School of Medicine and chairman of the National Institute of Health Consensus Development Conference on Osteoporosis believes women should obtain 1,000 mg. of calcium daily starting in their 30s or 40s. He maintains that women on estrogen-replacement therapy should also obtain 1,000 mg. daily and postmenopausal women who do not take estrogen should have 1,500 mg. daily.** (The Consensus also stressed the need for vitamin D—but not over 600-800 I.U.

---

* A study by Frances A. Tylavsky[22a] supports Heaney's thesis. Tylavsky found that lifetime calcium intake is a better indicator of bone health than is current calcium intake.

** I think that taking such large amounts of calcium supplements should preferably be done under the direction of a physician who may order measurement of such factors as total body calcium, spinal bone density and bone mineral content of the radius. Such measurements in women, aged 50-79 years, by means of neutron activation analysis and photon absorptiometry were discussed early in 1986 by Stanton H. Cohn et al.[22c] A physician with the know-how to order such tests is also likely to appreciate the dangers of excessive calcium consumption that we will discuss later. (A device intended to monitor bone loss by measuring bones' resistance to vibrations will likely be in use within a few years. It was conceived by Donald Young, a NASA physiologist, and is being developed by Charles Steele, a professor of applied mechanics at Stanford.)[22d]

per day without a physician's guidance.)[22b]*

The hip does not usually break when one falls; more generally the hip breaks and *then* one falls. It is reported that at least 26% of all women over 60 years of age have osteoporosis severe enough to cause vertebral deformity, i.e., a more or less severe version of "dowager's hump."[23] A study by W. A. Wallace,[24] made in Nottingham, England, showed that the incidence of fractures of the proximal femur increased from the year 1971 to 1977 at the rate of approximately 6% per year, but between 1977 and 1981 it rose 10% per year. (Between 1977 and 1981 the elderly population increased by less than 2% per year!) The incidence of hip fractures in women over 75 years of age increased from 8/1,000/year in 1971 to 16/1,000/year in 1981.

The RDA for calcium has been set at 800 mg. per day for men and women (and at 1,200 mg. for adolescents and for pregnant or lactating women). Although not reflected in the RDA, calcium requirements of menopausal women may rise significantly. Robert P. Heaney[25] estimates such requirements at 1,500 mg. per day. Louis V. Avioli[26] not only questions the adequacy of the 800 mg. daily level, but points out that most recent dietary surveys indicate that the average woman 75 years of age or older ingests only 450-500 mg. of calcium per day.** As a result there is, according to R. P. Heaney[27] a bone loss of about 1.5% per year.

Guy E. Abraham[28] disagrees, however, with the idea that a high calcium intake will help prevent osteoporosis.*** He argues that osteoporosis is no more common in those parts of Asia and Africa where the diets are relatively low in calcium (300-500 mg./day). He cites the work of S. Davidson et al. showing that patients with severe

---

* We saw in Chapter 4 that some persons may already be getting vitamin D in excess of these levels just from sunlight and the vitamin D-supplemented foods they eat.

** S. Boyd Eaton and Melvin Konner[26a] have estimated that paleolithic man consumed a diet containing about 1,579 mg. of calcium.

*** L. Nilas et al.[28a] also reported that a calcium intake of 1,000-2,000 grams daily was "ineffective in preventing bone loss in the early menopause." Studies that will be cited later suggest, however, that even calcium alone, without the support of estrogen, phosphorus or vitamin D, may be useful.

osteoporosis given massive doses of calcium showed no improvement in their osteoporosis. Abraham speculates that the calcium went into the soft tissues where it doesn't belong. It seems to me, however, that even though massive amounts of calcium (if taken without the support of estrogen, fluoride and vitamin D) may not help all cases of osteoporosis, that additional calcium might still have proved preventive if taken earlier in life. Nevertheless, if the calcium intake is increased, magnesium consumption should also be stepped up to help send the calcium to the bones rather than into the soft tissues.

Louis V. Avioli maintains that women, especially, have an inadequate calcium intake in the second and third decades of life and that progressive bone loss begins early in the fourth decade. R. P. Heaney et al.,[22] while holding that the RDA is inadequate, states that two-thirds of all U.S. females ingest less than the RDA on any given day and that after age 35 more than 75% of U.S. women have calcium intakes less than the RDA. But, even the minority getting the calcium RDA may be in trouble. R. P. Heaney and R. R. Recker, [28b] in a diet study of 273 estrogen-deprived, nonosteoporotic, middle-aged women, concluded that 55% had insufficient absorption to maintain calcium balance at an intake equal to the 1980 RDA. They concluded further that nearly one-fourth would still be in negative balance at an intake of 1.5 grams/day.

To set an arbitrary level for the RDA without taking cognizance of the body's phosphorus intake; without considering protein consumption; without considering the age-related circulating levels of $1,25(OH)_2D^*$ that is a factor in calcium absorption; without thought

---

* Taking a large amount of supplementary vitamin D is too simplistic to be a good answer to the problem since it will not necessarily be converted to the active metabolite. J. C. Gallagher et al.[29] found that osteoporotic patients and elderly normal subjects had normal levels of 25-OH-D (made in the liver) but significantly lower levels of the active vitamin D metabolite, $1,25(OH)_2D$ (made in the kidney). Thus, this latter conversion to the active vitamin D metabolite is important, along with adequate calcium, to avoid osteoporosis. The conversion may be inhibited by the increased serum phosphate of osteoporotic subjects but, as will be discussed later, this probably does not occur in humans.[111-114] In fact, Hector F. DeLuca[30] states "an important aspect of mineralization of bone is the elevation of plasma phosphorus concentration." Then too, several scientists have reported that phosphate conserves calcium by decreasing calcium excretion in the urine.[31]

as to the age-increasing levels of the serum parathyroid hormone; or without considering the diminishing estrogen levels in the menopausal and postmenopausal woman is just too simplistic for fostering health.* When it is realized, as Avioli says in the above-cited reference, that "there is currently no acceptable mode of therapy that stimulates bone formation" we see how important it is to maintain our calcium intake at acceptable levels. It is possible, however, that this view of Avioli may be a bit too pessimistic. Robert R. Recker et al.[33] reported that calcium carbonate supplementation appeared to reduce bone loss in postmenopausal women. The effect was not as strong as with sex hormone therapy, but they concluded that calcium could be more safely recommended as a preventive measure. Then, C. J. Lee et al.[34] found that, even with a mean age of 70 years, some elderly women can benefit from supplementary calcium and calcium-rich foods to improve bone density. Nevertheless, like so many other areas of health, prevention is preferable to cure.

Based on a study of 58 women with postmenopausal osteoporosis (crush fracture of the spine) compared with 58 normal women, John F. Aloia et al.[34a] found that the osteoporotic group had lower total-body calcium levels and bone mineral content of the radius, had undergone an earlier menopause, smoked cigarettes more and had breastfed less often. They had lower levels of estrone, estradiol and testosterone and reduced levels of 25-hydroxyvitamin D, 24-25 dihydroxyvitamin D and 1,25-dihydroxyvitamin D. To reduce risk of osteoporosis developing, Aloia recommends that smoking be stopped and that an adequate intake of calcium and vitamin D be insured. Furthermore, Aloia maintains that women who have had an early menopause and have low bone mass at the time of

---

* Robert P. Heaney et al.[22] state that after menopause a calcium intake of nearly 500 mg./day is required to produce the same balance effect as moderate doses of estrogen. Anthony Horsman et al.,[31a] in administering ethinyl estradiol to postmenopausal women, found that in amounts below 15 mcg. there was a net loss of bone, but at doses of about 25 mcg. there was a net gain. In the Horsman study no calcium or fluoride supplements were given. Although bone loss is generally a problem of the middle years and beyond, even young female athletes, nonmenstruating because of their strenuous activity, may also be at risk for bone loss.[32] Estrogen deficiency (or possibly an excess of prolactin) may be the cause.

menopause should be offered the choice of medically supervised estrogen and progesterone therapy.

Most of the studies discussed above would seem to make obvious the benefits of supplementary calcium in preventing and perhaps in treating osteoporosis. Even the 1984 National Institutes of Health consensus panel on osteoporosis recommended increased calcium intake.[34b] However, the view that dietary calcium is beneficial in preventing osteoporosis has been objected to by some respected scientists. A mid-1986 article by Gina Kolata[34c] reported that, at a recent meeting of the American Society for Bone and Mineral Research, B. Lawrence Riggs of the Mayo Clinic and independently, C. Christiansen of Golstrup Hospital in Denmark presented studies that failed to show a relationship between calcium intake and osteoporosis. Kolata quotes Richard Mazess of the University of Wisconsin, in regard to large dosages of supplementary calcium, as saying that "there is no evidence of efficacy and the safety has never been evaluated." In addition, Mazess has pointed out that "there is an abundance of data showing that calcium intake in a population is unrelated to bone density." Mazess reportedly calls calcium "the laetrile of osteoporosis."

Non-Bone-Building Uses of Calcium

Calcium may be beneficial to the eye. According to anecdotal reports, calcium may be effective in treating conjunctivitis, photophobia (intolerance of the eye to normally bright light), excessive winking and watering of the eye. K. R. Hightower and V. N. Reddy,[35] on the other hand, reported that increased levels of calcium introduced *in vitro* into lenses of rabbits increased cortical opacity. This was not, however, an *in vivo* experiment with rabbits, but just an *in vitro* experiment with rabbit lenses. It should not frighten us into assuming that calcium is associated with the onset of human cataracts.

In vitro experiments by B. K. Davis[35a] have demonstrated the effect of calcium ions on motility and fertilization of rat eggs by rat spermatozoa. Motility of the sperm increased to a maximum at 1.7 mMCa^{2+} and then showed a *reverse effect* by declining as Ca^{2+} concentration was increased further. Although motility was maximum at 1.7 mM, fertilization rates continued to increase as the calcium ion concentration rose to 3.4 mM (Figure 1). Then as the calcium concentration was further increased, the rate of fertilizing success showed a *reverse effect* by declining. C. Y. Hong et al.[35b] reported that calcium ions stimulate immature human sperm, whereas calcium ions inhibit the motility of ejaculated human sperm. A study by Tu Lin[35c] suggests that steroidogenesis in Leydig cells (the interstitial cells that produce testosterone) is calcium-dependent.

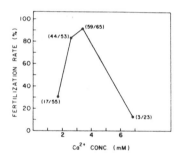

Figure 1. Effect of Ca^{2+} ions on fertilization *in vitro* of rat eggs. The eggs were incubated with epididymal spermatozoa (0.5×10^6 sperm/ml.) in a modified Krebs-Ringer bicarbonate medium containing 10 mg. of albumin/ml. The number of fertilized eggs and the total number are given in parentheses. Graph reproduced from B. K. Davis, *Proc. of the Society for Experimental Biology and Medicine* (1978) 157: 54-56, with permission. Note the *reverse effect* that occurs at a calcium ion concentration of 3.4 mM.

Calcium may also be beneficial in combating muscle fatigue. John H. Richardson et al.,[35d] working with the isolated gastrocnemius muscle of rats, concluded that, beneficial as exercise was, calcium was even more effective in delaying the onset of fatigue.

A severe calcium deficiency can be the cause of very detrimental personality characteristics. Calcium appears to also have a dramatic effect in eliminating symptoms of anxiety neurosis. Persons suffering from anxiety neurosis are apt to have unusually high levels of lactic acid in the blood. (Lactic acid is an end product of the metabolic process known as *glycolysis*.) When sufficient calcium is present it will combine with the lactic acid, thus reducing the probability of anxiety and nervousness being induced for this reason.

This relationship between calcium and blood lactate is demonstrated by the work of two psychiatrists, Ferris Pitts, Jr. and James J. McClure.[36] They noted that four studies in four different countries over a period of 25 years have shown that excessive lactate is produced during standard exercise by patients with anxiety neurosis. In their own research, they injected sodium lactate into anxiety prone patients and a group of controls with the result that it brought on a total of 190 anxiety symptoms among 14 patients with anxiety neurosis and 72 such symptoms among 10 controls. Pitts and McClure, after further experimentation, found that when calcium chloride was injected along with sodium lactate there was a greatly reduced total of 75 symptoms among the patients with anxiety neurosis and a total of just 36 among the controls.

Many persons are fearful that increasing their consumption of calcium may cause it to be deposited in the joints, a characteristic of arthritis. It has, on the contrary, been speculated that when the level of calcium in the bloodstream is too low (rather than too high) the parathyroid hormone stimulates release of calcium from the bones, as we noted earlier, and this is the calcium that may be deposited in the joints to produce arthritis. When calcium consumption is low, a high phosphorus intake (and, remember, health-minded persons using wheat germ, brewer's yeast and lecithin could have an excess of phosphorus) can also activate the parathyroid hormone secretion and thus further aggravate bone loss. Simultaneously, calcium (and also magnesium) may be deposited in the hair, leading to high hair-analysis readings even though the body itself may be deficient in these minerals.

Hair analyses of persons with arthritis generally show large amounts of calcium (along with fairly *high* amounts of magnesium but very low amounts of sodium, potassium and manganese).[37] This situation presumably reflects the condition in other soft tissues. The arthritic individual's problem, however, may be one of calcium usage and it is quite likely that he may actually be short of the mineral.

How Much Calcium is Needed?

One of the factors determining the amount of calcium needed is the intake of acid-forming foods. Protein forms an acid ash, so older persons who are meat eaters may need considerably greater calcium supplementation in order to avoid osteoporosis than vegetarians who are ingesting more alkaline-ash foods.[38] Many studies show that excessive protein consumption increases the urinary excretion of calcium.*

On the other hand, the decrease in the stomach's hydrochloric acid as we grow older might inhibit calcium absorption.** Tablets containing hydrochloric acid or betaine hydrochloride are available. Some persons use, instead, ascorbic acid tablets. The ascorbic acid acts as a substitute for, or rather acts as a reinforcer of, the stomach's hydrochloric acid. Yogurt, kefir and buttermilk are fine sources for calcium in that they also provide lactic acid which helps reinforce the stomach's hydrochloric acid. A lactase deficiency, making milk consumption unpleasant or intolerable, may be another of the many factors in the development of osteoporosis. Consuming yogurt, kefir, buttermilk, acidophilus milk, as well as various cheeses—or using a lactase supplement available at health food suppliers—may be ways for the lactase-deficient individual to get more calcium into his body. Whether one is lactase deficient or not, taking calcium with a glucose polymer might be useful. A number of studies[38c,d] show that intestinal calcium absorption can be increased (by as much as 2-5-fold) in normal subjects and in patients having intestinal obstruction and calcium malabsorption by administering calcium in a liquid formula containing glucose polymer.

---

* Some studies, however, show a compensatory decrease in fecal calcium excretion.[38a]

** A study by George W. Bo-Linn et al.,[38b] however, may cast doubt on the belief that stomach acid is important for calcium absorption. They used cimetidine to depress gastric acid secretion and found the effect on calcium absorption was negligible. These subjects, however, had a mean age of just 28 years which, along with the fact a drug was used, may make the results not applicable as a guide for older persons.

Calcium absorption may be detrimentally affected by alcohol consumption, especially in the confirmed alcoholic with liver cirrhosis. G. W. Hepner et al. [39] state that in cirrhosis the liver does not efficiently hydroxylate vitamin D. Then too, E. L. Krawitt[40,41] reported that animal studies indicate orally ingested alcohol inhibits calcium absorption even when either vitamin D or 25-OH-D3 is given, so it may be that alcohol detrimentally affects final conversion to the active metabolite by the kidney. On the other hand, it is possible that alcohol may interfere with calcium assimilation in ways unrelated to vitamin D. Studies cited by Lindsay H. Allen[42] also confirmed that bone mass is decreased in persons with chronic alcoholism. However, Allen found that both wine and dealcoholized wine actually improved calcium balance in healthy young men. This suggests that the beneficial effect was caused by one or more cogeners in the wine or by stimulation of gastric secretion.

Exercise is another factor in calcium absorption. Unless bones are adequately exercised they will not appreciably absorb calcium even if it is plentiful. Milan Korcok[43] points out that calcium acts to suppress bone resorption while mechanical stress seems to enhance bone formation. He observes that a study by J. F. Aloia et al.[44] showed that postmenopausal women who exercised three times a week *increased* their total body calcium (a measure of bone mass) by 2.6% over a one-year period, while a control group of sedentary women lost 2.4%.

Individuals confined to a bed and lying on their backs for long periods tend to lose calcium. A study of 90 healthy young men by Victor S. Schneider and Janet McDonald[44a] showed that during 5-36 weeks of continuous bed rest calcium balance became negative after two weeks even though the subjects received vitamin D throughout the study. By the end of the first month 200 mg./day was lost and the loss continued up to the 36th week when the study was discontinued. The loss in the calcaneus bone (the heel bone) as a percent of baseline is shown in Figure 2. A related study by G. Donald Whedon[44b] found that bone demineralization occurred primarily in the lower extremities and that the calcium losses were accompanied by sizeable losses of nitrogen which reflected muscle atrophy.

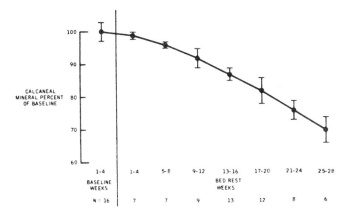

Figure 2. Photon absorptiometry of the calcaneus (heel bone) showing percent mineral loss from ambulatory values during untreated bed rest. Graph reproduced from Victor S. Schneider and Janet McDonald, *Calcified Tissue Int.* (1984) 36: S151-S154, with permission.

Bed exercises will not stop the loss of calcium. Only through standing will the loss be prevented. The theory is that the impact on the spine creates electrical forces that drive calcium into the bones. Orthopedists are, in fact, in some cases implanting electrodes (connected to a low-voltage current source) in fractures that do not properly join. The current attracts calcium ions to the fracture to do the healing. This connection between calcium intake and exercise may be related to the presumed diurnal rhythm reported earlier. During daylight hours exercise is generally greater and could thus be the factor behind the presumed rhythm.

Exercise has a beneficial effect on the HDL-LDL cholesterol ratio and so does calcium. Whereas calcium fed to magnesium-deficient rats was reported by J. J. Vitale et al.[44c] to cause a significant increase in serum cholesterol levels, at higher levels of magnesium there was a *reverse effect* and calcium decreased the levels of serum cholesterol. Alan J. Fleischman et al.[44d] showed that dietary calcium not only decreased serum cholesterol but also serum triglycerides, serum phospholipids and total serum lipids. Earlier, they[44e] had reported results suggesting that the lowering of blood cholesterol is mediated by increased excretion of bile acids. A study of these effects of calcium by Marvin L. Bierenbaum et al.[44f] produced an interesting graph (Figure 3).

Research by Terry L. Bazzarre et al.[44g] determined that total cholesterol decreased significantly for females following yogurt consumption and was lower, but not significantly so, following calcium supplementation. Mean HDL-cholesterol and HDL to total cholesterol ratios for females were significantly higher following yogurt or calcium supplementation. Total cholesterol and HDL-cholesterol were not significantly affected in males—but there were only 5 males studied versus 16 females.

H. Yacowitz et al.,[45] in a 21-day experiment involving the feeding of increased amounts of calcium to 13 men and women, reported a resulting decrease in serum cholesterol. A mean decrease of 14 mg./100 ml. was demonstrated in the serum cholesterol within 96 hours when 2.66 gm. of calcium over the normal daily intake of .71 gm./day was ingested daily.

Calcium not only reduces the level of lipids in the blood, but a rat study by S. Renaud et al.[45a] has indicated that calcium markedly inhibits the effect of saturated fats on platelet functions.* If this effect is also present in man, much of the cardiovascular protection provided by calcium (and by hard water) may be through its action on blood platelets. This effect and those effects described in the previous paragraphs probably bear a relationship to the favorable findings in regard to calcium and blood pressure which we will now review.

Calcium and Blood Pressure

Calcium is a factor in preventing, or at least in delaying, the occurrence of hypertension. Yoshinori Itokawa et al.[46] reported that both body temperature and blood pressure increased in calcium-deficient rats (although blood pressure *decreased* in magnesium-deficient rats). A few years later, S. Ayachi[47] found that calcium

---

* Renaud et al.[45a] found that alcohol exhibited a similarly beneficial action on the clotting activity of platelets, but the effect was lost rapidly as the alcohol disappeared from the blood.

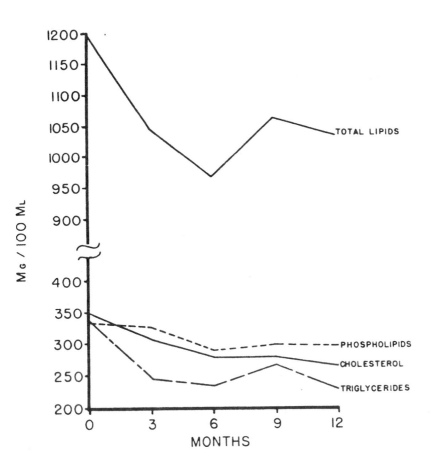

Figure 3. Effect of daily supplementing with 2 grams of calcium carbonate in the diet of 8 men and 3 women, 26 to 61 years of age, who had hypercholesterolemia, hyper-triglyceridemia or mixed hyperlipidemia. Graph reproduced from Marvin L. Bierenbaum et al., *Lipids* (1972) 7, no. 3: 202-206, with permission.

carbonate fed to rats bred to develop high blood pressure significantly delayed (but did not prevent) the advent of hypertension. Then, David A. McCarron et al. [48] reported that inadequate calcium intake may be a previously unrecognized factor in the development of human hypertension.* A group of 46 persons with hypertension had a significantly smaller daily calcium intake than a group of controls (668 mg. versus 886 mg.). Dr. McCarron[50] also reported that another group of hypertensive patients showed low serum concentrations of ionized calcium. Using a data base of the National Center for Health Statistics, McCarron et al.[50a] subsequently analyzed the relation of 17 nutrients to the blood pressure profile of 10,372 Americans from 18 to 74 years of age. Subjects denied a history of hypertension or intentional modification of their diet. The McCarron group found lower calcium intake, as well as lower intake of potassium and of vitamins A and C, distinguished hypertension from normotensive subjects. They found that diets low in sodium were associated with increased blood pressures while high-sodium diets were associated with lower blood pressures. The presence of salt is often associated with high calcium content (as in dairy products) and in some persons increasing calcium intake may be more important than decreasing sodium consumption.

Furthermore, McCarron[51] reported that for any level of urinary sodium, hypertensives excreted more calcium and he suggested that this may indicate parathyroid gland function is increased. McCarron[52] also observed that rats fed a high-calcium diet showed a *decrease* in their blood pressure. McCarron found that rats fed a .50% calcium diet had a systolic blood pressure about 5 points under those fed a .25% calcium diet. Those fed a 4% calcium diet had a systolic pressure on average about 10 points under those fed the .25% calcium diet (Figure 4). In each case the systolic pressure declined with age (as the rats continued on the calcium) rather than increasing as is so typical in most humans eating a normal diet. The amounts of calcium used in this experiment were huge and certainly cannot be used as a guide for human supplementation. Unless this is another example of the *reverse effect,* the experiment does, however, support McCarron's human evidence. Additional support

---

* Unknown, apparently, to the McCarron group was the fact that Herbert G. Langford and Robert L. Watson[49] many years earlier hypothesized that "the prevalence of hypertension is a function directly of net sodium intake but inversely of calcium and potassium intake."

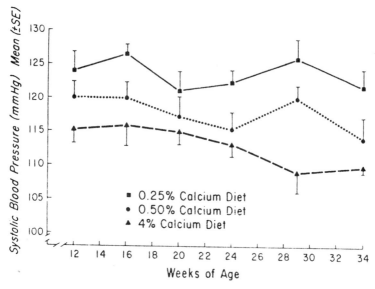

Figure 4. Systolic blood pressure-lowering effect of rats fed high-calcium diets. Graph reproduced from David A. McCarron, *Life Sciences* (1982) 30: 683-689, with permission.

for McCarron's findings is provided by a study conducted by Scott Ackley et al.[53] This group found that, based on a 24-hour dietary recall, considerably less calcium intake from milk was reported by hypertensive than by normotensive men (but not by women). Mario R. Garcia-Palmieri et al.[53a] found an inverse relationship between milk consumption and blood pressure in Puerto Rican men. Recently, McCarron et al.[53b] reported that a supplement of 1,000 mg. of calcium given daily for 8 weeks was effective in reducing hypertension in some but not in all human subjects. In a randomized, double-blind, placebo-controlled crossover study, there was a mean 6.5 mm Hg decrease in standing systolic blood pressure of a group of 32 hypertensives compared with a decrease of only 1.3 mm Hg in a control group of 30 matched normals. In another recent study, Jose M. Belizan et al.[53c] found that healthy young adult volunteers given 1 gram of calcium daily for 27 weeks showed a significant drop in

diastolic blood pressure. The average reduction amounted to 5.6%
for the women and 9% for the men (Figures 5 and 6). A recent
discovery by A. R. Whorton et al.[53d] that calcium helps regulate
prostacyclin synthesis may possibly offer support for McCarron's
and Belizan's findings (but that is my, not Whorton's, suggestion).

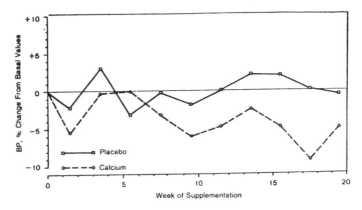

Figure 5. Women's diastolic blood pressure in dorsal position.
Mean percent changes in relation to basal values, by week of
supplementation. In the calcium-supplemented group, effect
stabilized in ninth week of supplementation. Graph reproduced
from Jose M. Belizan et al., *JAMA* (1983) 249, no. 9: 1161-
1165, with permission. Copyright 1983, American Medical
Association.

McCarron is not without his critics. Stanley M. Garn and
Frances A. Larkin[54] criticized his work on several counts. They noted
that the very countries having the lowest calcium intakes have the
lowest incidence of hypertension. Furthermore, epidemiological
studies by Stephen Seely[54a] and by Robert E. Popham et al.[54b]
indicate that countries having the greatest consumption of
unfermented milk proteins tend to have the highest rates of mortality
from ischemic heart disease. (Since cheese does not seem to be
implicated, Popham et al. suggest that a component of lactose,
perhaps galactose, may be the atherogenic factor.) Also contrary to
McCarron, it was reported by Hugo Kesteloot and Joozef Geboers[55]
that, in a survey of 9,321 men, there was a significant

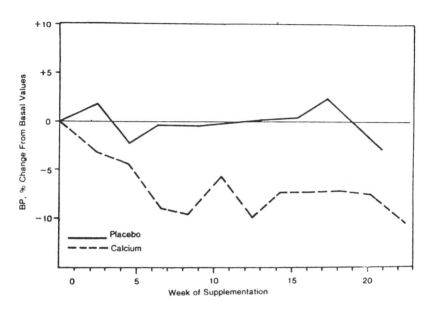

Figure 6. Men's diastolic blood pressure in dorsal position. Mean percent changes in relation to basal values, by week of supplementation. In the calcium-supplemented group, effect stabilized after sixth week of supplementation. In keeping with other reports, the calcium effect on blood pressure seems to be greater in men than it is in women. Graph reproduced from Jose M. Belizan et al., *JAMA* (1983) 249, no. 9: 1161-1165, with permission. Copyright 1983, American Medical Association.

positive correlation between serum calcium and both systolic and diastolic blood pressure. Then too, Harvey W. Gruchow et al.[55a] recently reported that calcium was significantly related to systolic blood pressure only among nonwhite men. (Sodium, phosphorous and alcohol intakes were, however, each related directly and significantly to systolic blood pressure, while potassium was inversely and significantly related to systolic blood pressure.) Earlier, Mordecai P. Blaustein[56] stated that, "a rise in the mean (Ca) 2+ may be the 'final common path' by which most, if not all hypertension is produced." The relationship between calcium and hypertension is obviously a lively topic with a surprising array of contradictory studies. We should note, however, that whether or not calcium works to normalize blood pressure, hypercalcemia may *cause* hypertension.[57]

John H. Laragh and Mark S. Pecker[57a,b] speculate that only hypertensives with low levels of the kidney hormone renin are likely to benefit from increased calcium and/or reduced sodium. They found that high-renin patients had blood pressure *increases* when they took supplementary calcium.* Lawrence M. Resnick, John P. Nicholson and John H. Laragh[57d] maintain that "it is the hypertensive with a low renin, low ionized calcium profile who benefits most by maneuvers increasing serum levels of ionized calcium and/or increasing levels of renin activity, such as is obtained with calcium channel blockade, or oral calcium supplementation. Patients with higher renin activities, who have levels of serum ionized calcium higher than normotensive or other hypertensive individuals, benefit less from calcium-channel blockade and may actually have a pressor response to oral calcium therapy." Several other studies indicate that increased serum calcium may be associated with increased, rather than decreased, hypertension.[55,58,59] Several letters from various scientists disagreeing with McCarron and also McCarron's reply make interesting reading.[60]

A recent study by Paul Erne et al.[59a] reported that intracellular free calcium has been implicated in vascular smooth-muscle contraction and hypertension. The free-calcium concentration in platelets was found to be elevated in a group of 9 patients with borderline hypertension and in a group of 45 with established essential hypertension, but was not elevated in a group of 38 normotensive subjects (Figure 7). Interestingly, many years earlier, Frank F. Vincenzi,[59b] as a result of his studies, suggested that a low intracellular concentration of free calcium ions is necessary for

---

* According to Andreas P. Niarchos and John H. Laragh,[57c] "renin and aldosterone values are at their highest in infancy and decline gradually throughout life in an inverse variance with blood pressure which is at its lowest in infancy. This by itself suggests that the renin system is a blood pressure control system that normally reacts to higher pressures by turning itself off and vice versa."

activity of the Na-K pump.* The seeming contradictions will, most likely, be eventually elucidated in terms of one or more dose-responsive *reverse effects*. (If, contrary to the finding of McCarron, serum calcium is sometimes high in hypertension, "body wisdom" could be acting to normalize blood pressure by providing calcium. I am not suggesting the body works this way, but only suggesting that nutrition is complex.)** If the "anti-McCarron group" is correct, that might explain the beneficial role of calcium antagonists in treating hypertension.***

---

* Paul W. Davis and Frank F. Vincenzi[59c] similarly found that as the calcium ion concentration in erythrocyte membranes increased, Na, K-ATPase was inhibited (Figure 8). They also found that activation (not inhibition) of Ca-ATPase increased as calcium concentration rose, but at a level of about $10^{-3.9}$M showed a *reverse effect* and declined as the calcium level continued to increase. Note that Na, K-ATPase was 35% inhibited at 10^{-5}M Ca, a concentration at which Ca-ATPase is maximally stimulated.

** Nutrition may be complex simply because something is being ignored. The probability is that ionized calcium and non-ionized calcium in the blood work oppositely in regard to hypertension and most of the studies fail to make the distinction. H. G. McKercher et al.,[59d] reported that other physiological studies unrelated to blood pressure also require that a distinction be made between ionized and non-ionized calcium. In their work on the inhibition of placental Ca-ATPase by ethacrynic acid, they found that merely measuring *total* calcium, rather than *ionized* calcium, resulted in artifacts and led to erroneous conclusions.

*** According to William T. Clusin et al.,[61] many of the effects of myocardial ischemia can be attributed to an abnormal increase in intracellular free calcium during diastole. (Details of the calcium channel—a pore in the sarcolemma, the phospholipid bilayer membrane that surrounds cells—and the use of calcium in the interior of the heart and vascular muscle wall are discussed by Kenneth L. Baughman.)[61a] Calcium channel blockers or calcium entry blockers—drugs such as verapamil, D-600, fendiline and diltiazem—interact at the cell surface to impede slow channel transport, the current that carries calcium ions into cells such as those of the heart muscle and interferes with smooth muscle contraction in arterial walls. Thus, these drugs can prevent attacks of angina caused by arterial spasm. Since these drugs are vasodilators, perhaps some of their action (and their use in treating hypertension) is due to this property. Such older drugs as nitroglycerine, morphine, inorganic nitrates and even barbiturates show some calcium antagonism. Calcium blockers interfere with extracellular calcium ions attempting to enter cells, but are reported to have no effect on calcium already present in a bone cell or skeletal muscle cell. Some of the negative aspects of calcium antagonists are given by Jane Kangilaski and Gail McBride,[62] by J. G. Lewis[63] and by Raymond J. Windquist et al.[64] Before you are tempted to conclude that the effectiveness of calcium blockers suggests that we reduce our calcium consumption, note this: D. Lynn Morris[65] observes that clinical experience with the calcium blocker verapamil suggests that calcium reverses its adverse effects! Recent reviews of calcium entry blocking drugs and their mechanisms of action have been provided by David McCall et al.,[65a] by Mattias Schramm and Robertson Towart[65b] and by Dennis W. Schneck.[65c]

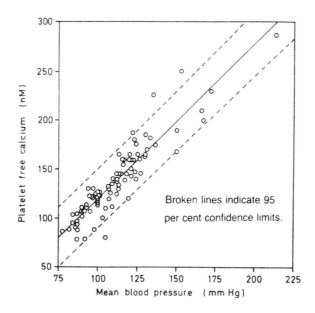

Figure 7. Correlation between mean blood pressure and intracellular free-calcium concentrations in platelets of 38 normotensive subjects, 9 patients with borderline hypertension, and 45 patients with essential hypertension. Reproduced from Paul Erne et al., *New England Jrl. of Medicine* (1984) 310, no. 17: 1084-1088, with permission of *The New England Journal of Medicine*.

It is probably wise to increase the amount of calcium (and potassium) in the diet, but best to do so by giving preference to foods that are, at the same time, low in saturated fats, cholesterol and sodium.

Hard Water Versus Soft Water

Before leaving the subject of calcium we should say a few words about the soft water versus hard water controversy. Henry A. Schroeder[66] published a comprehensive study of the water supplies

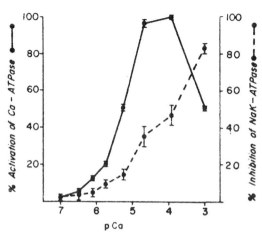

Figure 8. Effect of calcium concentration on Ca-ATPase activation (•—•). Increase is shown up to a pCa value of 3.9 at which a *reverse effect* set in and activation declined. Na, K-ATPase inhibition (•---•) is also shown with no *reverse effect* being in evidence in the concentrations under study. Vertical bars denote two standard errors. Graph reproduced from Paul W. Davis and Frank F. Vincenzi, *Life Sciences* (1971) 10, Part II, 401-406, with permission of Pergamon Press and of the authors.

of many communities throughout the U.S. He found no correlation between water hardness and noncardiovascular disease, but significant correlations for total death rate, cardiovascular mortality and mortality from coronary heart disease. He found that the water's content of magnesium, calcium, bicarbonate, sulfate and dissolved solids, its conductivity, and especially the water's pH, all had significant negative correlations with death rates. The *higher* the values, the *lower* the death rates. Studies by Luciano C. Neri and Helen L. Johansen[66a] and by F. W. Stitt et al.[69] similarly discovered that systolic and diastolic pressures tend to be higher in soft-water areas. Note, in Figure 9, how death rates are related inversely to water calcium. (We should realize, however, that when the water is hard, magnesium and other minerals are likely to be present and one or more of these could contribute to lowering of deaths. On the other hand, Denham Harman[66b] suggests that the higher mortality rate from coronary heart disease in soft-water areas could be due, in part, to *higher* amounts of copper in soft water.)

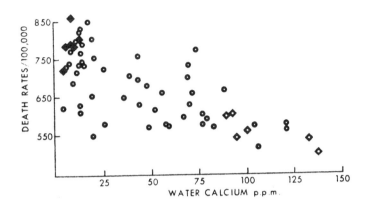

Figure 9. Cardiovascular mortality (1958-64) of males aged 45-64, and water calcium. Graph, modified from F. W. Stitt et al., *Lancet* (Jan. 20, 1973): 122-126, reproduced from Luciano C. Neri and Helen L. Johansen, *Annals of the New York Academy of Sciences* (1978) 304: 203-219, with permission of the authors and of the publisher.

There is, however, a contradictory study that is very interesting. Marvin L. Bierenbaum et al.[67] reported some fascinating statistics involving the water of Kansas City, Kansas, and of Kansas City, Missouri. (The study was criticized by A. Richey Sharrett and Manning Feinleib[67a] and the criticism answered by Bierenbaum.[67b]) In this study the incidence of hypertension among residents of the Kansas side of the river was greater than among those living on the Missouri side even though the water being drunk on the Kansas side was harder and should therefore have been more healthful. However, the hard water contained considerable amounts of cadmium and lower amounts of zinc, factors which presumably may have caused a reversal of the usual rule that hard water is better. However, although cadmium is often considered to be a causal factor in hypertension, cadmium workers, in three studies, have been shown to not have elevated blood pressures.[66a] Nevertheless, there may be a cadmium-hypertension association inasmuch as research cited elsewhere in this book suggests that possibility.

There are two more studies of considerable interest. A Canadian research team headed by L. C. Neri et al.[68] concluded that hard water not only reduced the risk of death from cardiovascular causes, but reduced by a margin of 15% to 30% (depending on geographic area) the risk of death in general. In the matter of blood pressure, F. W. Stitt et al.[69] showed, in a study of the inhabitants of six hard-water and six soft-water towns in England, that blood pressure was greater in soft-water towns. These various studies did not pinpoint the mineral primarily responsible for the good effects of hard water. However, an investigation of water hardness in Ontario, Canada, drinking water by A. A. Allen[70] concluded that protection against sudden death due to ischemic heart disease was due to the water's magnesium component. Mildred Seelig[71] cites many other studies that also now lead to the same favorable conclusion regarding magnesium. A recent study by J. R. Marier and L. C. Neri[71a] found that the percentage of the population with high blood pressure varied inversely with the concentration of magnesium in the drinking water. J. Durlach et al.[71b] have stated that, "only two out of three studies show a reverse correlation between cardiovascular mortality and water hardness. But studies carried out on the water Mg level alone, as opposed to those on water hardness (Ca + Mg) have all shown a reverse correlation between cardiovascular mortality and the Mg level." As we will see later, a study shows that silicon in drinking water may also be beneficial to the heart by inhibiting atherosclerosis. Other research, cited by Earl B. Dawson et al.,[72] links water levels of lithium with lowered annual mortality rates due to atherosclerotic and ischemic heart disease.

These are just a few of the overwhelming number of studies which lead to the general conclusion that hard water is better for the nervous system, for the heart and for the body in general. (George W. Comstock[72a] has reviewed the subject of water hardness in regard to cardiovascular diseases and has cited 149 references.) Hard water contains many valuable trace minerals but its solute consists primarily of calcium and magnesium compounds. If you have a water softener at your house, consider connecting it to only the hot water line. Artificially softened water is deficient in calcium, magnesium and many other minerals. Furthermore, such water may contain sodium, introduced by the softening process. Foods cooked in such water will also have elevated sodium levels.

Food and Supplementary Sources of Calcium

Foods sometimes cited as being good sources of calcium are milk; Swiss, brick, cheddar or Parmesan cheeses; turnip greens; broccoli; almonds; filberts; sunflower seeds; sweet potatoes; green beans; and also salmon and sardines (if one eats the bones). In the case of the turnip greens and broccoli, however, the calcium is tied up as the oxalate and thus may be relatively unavailable. Whatever calcium that exists in spinach, chard, beet greens, sorrel and rhubarb is also in the form of oxalates and so is not very useful to the body.

Dietary lactose (as found in human and in cow's milk and in cheese, but not in soy "milk") facilitates intestinal transport of several minerals including calcium, magnesium, iron, zinc, cobalt and manganese, as well as detrimental metals such as strontium, barium and radium.[73] O. W. Vaughan and L. J. Filer, Jr.[74] point out that other sugars such as glucose, sucrose and fructose have a similar effect when injected, along with calcium chloride, directly into the ligated ileal segment of rats. (Note that this is a benefit of sugar, a substance which generally receives what may be more than its share of polarized condemnation.)*

Although calcium is present in many foods, supplementation may be essential to insure good health, depending on one's age, sex and the presence of calcium antagonists in the diet. Those taking large amounts of ascorbic acid and getting above-average amounts of

---

* Many statements by food faddists in regard to sugar are simply erroneous. For example, Adelle Davis[75] says (without documentation): "The excessive intake of sweets during childhood and adolescence causes facial bones to be underdeveloped and the jaws to remain so small that the teeth are crowded together. Similarly, eating sweets can prevent calcium from being absorbed by an adult." Sugar may be bad for the teeth but not for the reason given by Davis. However, in a 1986 article, A. R. P. Walker[75a] has cited studies by S. M. Garn et al.,[75b] by C. S. Stecksen-Blicks et al.,[75c] by A. R. P. Walker et al.[75d] and by A. S. Richardson et al.[75e] showing that correlations of total sugar intake and snack frequency with caries are sometimes slight, absent or even inverse.

phosphorus (because of high consumption of meats, fish, poultry, eggs, brewer's yeast, wheat germ and lecithin) should be sure that their calcium intake is adequate since phosphorus sometimes increases the body's requirements for calcium. A high-protein intake means that more calcium will be excreted in the urine[76] and this suggests that calcium consumption should probably be increased.

Eating of whole grain cereals rather than refined flour and unpolished rice instead of polished rice is often recommended because of the better mineral content of the unrefined foods. However, June L. Kelsay et al.[77] have reported that dietary intake of calcium, magnesium, iron and silicon were significantly lower on high- rather than on low-fiber diets. They cite references relating to many other studies reaching similar conclusions regarding fiber's inhibiting assimilation of these and other minerals. K. W. Heaton and E. W. Pomare[78] also found that plasma-calcium significantly fell during bran feeding of 14 persons, but there was, beneficially, a significant decline in serum triglycerides. On the other hand, W. van Dokkum et al.[79] reported that, compared with white bread, an increase of dietary fiber through consuming bran in bread increased the mineral intake of calcium, magnesium, iron, zinc and copper, but the fecal excretion of these minerals also increased significantly. As a result, the mineral retention remained almost constant. (Astonishingly, they reported that serum cholesterol *increased* significantly during the coarse-bran-bread diet compared to the white-bread diet.)*

Other research, however, has indicated that phytic acid and phytate (which tend to occur with fiber) may be inhibitors of mineral absorption. One such study was reported by John G. Reinhold et al.[80] Three young men were fed 2.5 grams of phytic acid daily, first

---

* N.-G. Asp[79a] also reported that wheat bran increased total plasma cholesterol and HDL-cholesterol. Many earlier studies have, on the contrary, shown that wheat bran has no effect on plasma cholesterol or triglycerides.[79b] Oat bran, however, lowers cholesterol levels in man.[79c] Guar gum, in the Asp study, significantly lowered plasma cholesterol, while pectin resulted in no significant effect.[79a] A study by R. J. Heine et al.[79d] similarly showed that pectin had no major influence on serum lipid levels. On the other hand, A. Wise and D. J. Gilburt[79e] have cited an earlier study by S. Viola et al.[79f] which reported that 5% dietary pectin reduced the absorption of calcium in rats to two-thirds that of the controls.

as sodium phytate with leavened flat wheat bread for 28 days and then for 32 days as *tanok,* a phytate-rich unleavened wholemeal flat wheat bread. Negative calcium balances persisted after the 60-day period of high-phytate consumption, contrary to what might have been expected from a report by A. R. Walker et al.[81] that the effects of phytate were ameliorated after a few weeks with calcium balances returning to normal. (The Reinhold group found that plasma zinc and serum iron fell after phytate consumption began but, contrary to calcium, later rose.) Whole wheat bread contains a surfeit of minerals, but it is not the amount of mineral in food that is important; the primary consideration is how much of the mineral content enters into body processes. Like so many other health superstitions, the presumed benefits of the whole grains may have been overemphasized and the presumed evils of white flour and polished rice improperly inflated. However, there is more to nutrition than just increasing the assimilation of calcium and other minerals. K. M. Henry and S. K. Kon[82] reported that rats retained supplementary calcium less well when wholemeal bread was eaten than when white bread was consumed. Nevertheless, the wholemeal bread promoted growth better than the white bread and was thus, at least in some ways, nutritionally superior. Obviously, many of the studies are contradictory, but it seems wise to be concerned about the possibility that excessive dietary fiber and excessive phytate may be detrimental to health.

However, the calcium phytate of bran, and of cereals in general, may not be as poor a source of calcium as it is often thought to be. Lindsay H. Allen[83] relates that phytate is digested, through the action of bacteria, to varying degrees in man's lower intestine. The possibility that calcium may be absorbed in the colon might mean that calcium phytate, contrary to general opinion, could provide an assimilable source of this mineral. Even so, many studies cited by David M. Slovik[83a] support the generally held view that fiber and phytate impair calcium absorption. Many of these same studies, as well as others showing that increased fiber induces negative balances of not only calcium but also of magnesium, zinc, iron, phosphorus and copper, have also been reviewed by Joseph T. Judd et al.[83b] In light of this, it may be useful to eat high-fiber foods at a time different from your eating of high-calcium foods (assuming you desire to increase calcium assimilation). Furthermore, if you are using supplementary calcium, magnesium or other minerals, take them well away from a meal containing large amounts of fiber.

Supplementary calcium is available in several forms. The easily assimilable varieties are calcium carbonate (including oyster shell calcium), calcium lactate, calcium gluconate, calcium ascorbate, calcium citrate, amino-acid chelates and calcium orotate (which is, however, more costly). The recovery of heart attack victims may be promoted by orotic acid according to research at the University of New South Wales, Australia.[84] In a study by James L. Robinson and Debra B. Dombrowski,[85] using 29 normal adults taking six grams of orotic acid just once a week, serum urate and cholesterol decreased significantly concomitant with the occurrence of uricosuria (uric acid in the urine). Other reports (some anecdotal) suggest that the orotates may be of value in treating cancer, psoriasis, seborrheic disorders, obesity, multiple sclerosis, retinitis and hepatitis and for controlling cholesterol. Calcium orotate is said to aid also in the body's utilization of other calcium compounds. Sounds good, doesn't it, but there could be a problem. Roberta P. Durschlag and James L. Robinson[85a] found that dietary orotic acid induces severely fatty livers in rats, but other species (including monkeys) showed no hepatic changes. A. Denda et al.[85b] reported that orotic acid not only works as an initiator of carcinogenesis in the rat, but can act as a promoter when 1,2-DMH-2HCl is used as an initiator. Although humans are probably perfectly safe in consuming orotic acid from milk and milk products such as whey, it may be advisable to avoid orotic acid supplementation unless prescribed by a physician who has read the relevant research. Calcium is also available in less easily assimilated forms such as bone meal, dicalcium phosphate and dolomite that require not only vitamin D but a good supply of hydrochloric acid in the stomach for assimilation. The most

economical source is calcium carbonate followed by calcium lactate.[*]
Although calcium gluconate is not very costly, it contains mostly
gluconate and very little calcium. Calcium pantothenate (a source of
pantothenic acid), calcium aspartate and calcium citrate are also usable
forms. Calcium chloride is useful for pickling but too bitter and too
irritating to the stomach for use as a supplement.

As just indicated, calcium carbonate is an economical source of
calcium, but its ingestion could lead to problems. Robert R. Recker[85c]
has reported that calcium absorption from carbonate is impaired in
achlorhydria (low stomach acid) during fasting conditions. Thus, some
persons should avoid taking calcium carbonate except after eating
protein foods (which stimulate the flow of gastric juice). There may be
a problem, however, even if calcium carbonate is taken with protein-
containing meals. Richard Eastell[85d] has reported that "it is unlikely that
there is ever sufficient concentration of hydrogen ions to allow
solubilization of calcium carbonate." (He holds that more reliable
calcium absorption may be obtained from calcium citrate.)[**] There may
be another problem with consuming excessive amounts of calcium
carbonate.

The milk-alkali syndrome was first identified in 1923 and became
more common with the advent of the Sippy antacid regimen for
promoting ulcer healing. It is characterized by hypercalcemia without
hypercalcuria or hypophosphaturia, normal or slightly elevated alkaline
phosphatase, renal insufficiency with azotemia (excessive amounts of
nitrogenous compounds in the blood), mild alkalosis, conjunctivitis and
calcinosis. As Eric S. Orwall[85g] states, the milk-alkali

---

[*] Do not confuse the amount of calcium in a pill with the total size of that pill, e.g., only
between 1/7 and 1/8 of a 10-grain (650mg.) tablet of calcium lactate consists of calcium, the rest
being lactate and water. To make the calculation, you must know the formula for calcium lactate
is $Ca(C_3H_5O_3)_2 \cdot 5H_2O$. Then, recall that the atomic weights of calcium, carbon, hydrogen and
oxygen are, respectively, 40, 12, 1 and 16. Using simple arithmetic, the molecular weight of
calcium lactate turns out to be 308. Solving the equation $40/308 = X/650$, we find that the pill
contains about 84 mg. of calcium.

[**] A study by Michael J. Nicar and Charles Y. C. Pak[85e] similarly concluded that "calcium
citrate provides a more optimum calcium availability than calcium carbonate." However, R. C.
Puche et al.[85f] hypothesize, "hypercalciuria is produced by a modification of tubular physiology
that favors the excretion of citrate, that drags calcium along the tubules." If true, might it not be
inadvisable to take calcium in citrate form?

syndrome continues to occur in persons ingesting large amounts of calcium and absorbable alkali, particularly as calcium carbonate. Will the new "take more calcium" trend lead to a resurgence in the incidence of this syndrome? I think physicians should be alert to this possibility.

Whether or not supplementary calcium should be taken may, among other variables, be a function of the season of the year. O. J. Malm[86] found that better calcium balances are generally achieved between June and December than during the rest of the year. It seems likely that, with a two- or three-month delay factor, this could relate to the increased amount of sunshine and with it the extra vitamin D to foster calcium metabolism. Before you are tempted to conclude, however, that calcium supplements should be taken or increased during the winter, let me point out that body metabolism (for northern hemisphere inhabitants) tends to be slowed down at this time of the year, so less calcium may be needed.

What is the best form of supplementary calcium? Because of its high lead content and possible difficulty in assimilation, it seems very questionable to use bone meal. The Food and Drug Administration[87] found that bone meal tablets averaged 3.6 ppm of lead compared with 5.8 ppm for the powders and they published their analysis of various brands. (I suspect some of the difference may have been due to excipients in the tablets.)* Dicalcium phosphate might be used, but one should ascertain that the dicalcium phosphate is not bone meal or lead may be present in this product as well. Furthermore, Per Rasmussen and Gro Ramsten Wesenberg[88] reported that rats fed bone meal absorbed very little additional calcium from this source. However, the additional calcium that they did absorb apparently was enough to stop the lead of the bone meal from entering their bone tissue. Thus, the lead in bone meal may not be a great threat, but why use a supplement that poses such formidable assimilation problems?

---

* Later in this chapter and in Chapter 8 we will consider possible benefits of minute amounts of arsenic, lead and other "poisons." However, pending possible discovery of low-dose beneficial *reverse effects* of these metals in humans, I would prefer to avoid bone meal and dolomite.

I would also avoid use of dolomite, not only because it may at times be contaminated with lead and other toxic metals, but also because it may be difficult to assimilate. The Food and Drug Administration[87] reported that dolomite samples they tested ranged in lead content between 1 ppm and 8.1 ppm and, as in the case with bone meal, they gave the lead content of various brands. * The *FDA Drug Bulletin*[91] warns that pregnant or lactating women taking bone meal or dolomite to meet their increased calcium needs may have enough lead intake to endanger the fetus or the nursing infant. I suspect that calcium carbonate if derived from oyster shells or clam shells may also sometimes contain lead and other toxic elements because of industrial contamination of coastal waters, although I have seen no studies that indicate this. It might be preferable to use calcium lactate or calcium gluconate.

Adverse Effects

If you are taking supplementary calcium and also undergoing tests, tell your physician. Raised levels of calcium (or reduced levels of potassium) can increase the toxic effects of glycosides while decreased levels of calcium (or raised levels of potassium) can reduce the therapeutic effects.[92] Men with unusually high blood levels of calcium should not use the male hormone enhancers fluoxymesterone or methyltestosterone.[92a] Calcium potentiates the trypanocidal drug action of salicylhydoxamic acid plus glycerol[93] and can also affect the action of other drugs your doctor may have prescribed. Herta Spencer[94] found that use of isoniazide or tetracycline or of diuretics such as furosemide increased urinary calcium, while aluminum-containing antacids not only increased urinary calcium but also increased fecal calcium excretion. On the other hand, taking

---

* H. J. Roberts[89] reported that Bio-Medical Data, West Chicago, Illinois, found in dolomite, parts per million of these toxic elements: aluminum, 187.1; lead, 34.9; nickel, 12.9; arsenic, 24.0; mercury, 11.6; and cadmium, 2.3. Dr. Roberts suggests that physicians having health-conscious patients with unexplained medical disorders ask those patients if they are taking dolomite. Later, Dr. Roberts[90] reported on three additional batches of dolomite as analyzed by Bio-Medical Data. They found ranges of toxic metals as follows: lead, 8 to 13.8 parts per million; arsenic, 6.5 to 8; mercury, 4.7 to 8; aluminum, 42 to 219; tin, 982 to 1,323; antimony, 12.6 to 18.4; barium, 3.9 to 40.5; cadmium, .4 to .54 and nickel, 2.8 to 3.2

supplementary calcium can decrease the antibiotic power of tetracycline,[94a] so if you have been prescribed this drug and are taking supplementary calcium, be sure your doctor knows what you are doing. Significant negative associations between calcium balance and caffeine consumption were reported by Robert P. Heaney and Robert R. Recker,[95] so do you really want that second cup of coffee?* Other drugs, including alcohol (but not wine) can also contribute to calcium loss and thus may intensify loss of bone in aging. Calcium, in excess, can give a false positive reaction on the Diagnex blue test for impaired gastric function. Calcium gluconate (and all other gluconates also) can give a false positive reading on Benedict's glucose test. When your doctor asks you which drugs you are using, in your reply tell him also the vitamins and minerals you are taking.

An excess of calcium, sometimes brought on by taking supplementary vitamin D, can be just as bad as a deficiency.** Robert P. Heaney and Robert R. Recker[96a] have discussed the importance of estimating calcium absorption. They say "an absorption value as high as 0.5 would alert the clinician that calcium supplements were probably not indicated (and might even be contraindicated). By contrast, a value as low as 0.1 would indicate not only that supplements would be required, but that they would probably have to be unusually large." Hunter Heath III and C. Wayne Callaway[96b] point out that, "Hypercalcemia is a common biochemical finding in middle-aged and elderly Western adults that may be worsened by calcium salt ingestion." A laboratory measurement of calcium

---

* More recently, Linda K. Massey and Tracy A. Berg[95a] reported on the effects of caffeine taken by male subjects who had fasted for at least ten hours. When the subjects drank decaffeinated coffee to which 0, 150 or 300 mg. caffeine had been added, their total urinary three-hour excretion of calcium, magnesium, sodium and chloride increased significantly, while zinc, phosphorus, potassium and creatine were not significantly changed. Even more recently, during 1986, James K. Yeh et al.[95b] reported on a relevant study (but it was done with rats rather than with humans). Caffeine was injected subcutaneously each day at either 2.5 mg. or 10 mg./100 g. body weight for two weeks before balance studies began. Urinary excretion of potassium, sodium, inorganic phosphate, magnesium and calcium, but not zinc or copper, was higher in the rats given caffeine. The fecal excretion of zinc and copper was also unaffected by caffeine.

** A number of antivitamin D compounds for potential use in treating hypercalcemia have been synthesized.[96]

absorption should precede a decision to greatly increase calcium supplementation.

Excess calcium can inhibit thyroid activity and can suppress levels of zinc, magnesium* and manganese. In hypercalcemia the nervous system is depressed and central nervous system reflexes become sluggish. The QT interval of the heart beat decreases. Muscles weaken and constipation occurs, probably due to the reduced contractility of the muscular walls in the gastrointestinal tract (an effect opposite to that caused by magnesium and potassium). An excess of calcium can obviously be detrimental to body functions and even modest amounts may be constipating.

A recent study by G. A. Reinhart and D. C. Mahan[96c] showed that, in pigs, calcium: phosphorus ratios above 2.1, with the calcium being excessive but phosphorus adequate, resulted in decreased bone ash and reduced strength of bones. (This suggests to me that, if humans and pigs are similar in regard to calcium: phosphorus ratios relative to bone strength, too much calcium might increase the dangers of osteoporosis—just the opposite of the "take more calcium" edict that is now so popular.) In another pig study, this one by D. D. Hall et al.,[96d] vitamin K appeared to be inactivated in the gut, as shown by greatly increased bleeding times, when excessive amounts of calcium were fed—unless supplemental vitamin K was also given.

There may be yet other problems associated with excessive calcium consumption. B. Fleischhans[97] tells about a doctor(!) who took, for 12 years, 10 to 15 grams of calcium carbonate as an anti-acid drug for his duodenal ulcer. He suffered many symptoms, including disturbed heart action and signs of beginning renal failure. After withdrawal of the drug his condition normalized. That's an extreme situation, of course, but *American Pharmacy* [98] warns that taking more than 2,500 mg. of calcium daily may lead to a rapid deterioration in kidney function. High amounts of supplementary calcium may be especially hazardous to persons   prone   to   develop   calcium   urinary

---

* As stated already, and as will be expanded in the magnesium section, low amounts of magnesium attended by a high intake of calcium may lead to calcium being dumped in the soft tissues.

stones.[98a]*   Oral calcium should also be used with caution when providing mineral supplementation to low-birth-weight infants in order to prevent rickets of prematurity. Geoffrey J. Cleghorn and David I. Tudehope[99] tell of an intestinal obstruction resulting from such neonatal calcium supplementation. Obviously, calcium supplementation can lead to problems. If one greatly increases the calcium intake it is important to also increase the consumption of magnesium. Many of the calcium-magnesium interactions are discussed by Lloyd T. Iseri and James H. French.[99a]

Calcium ions and calmodulin are active in certain fast-growing tumors. W. E. Criss and S. Kakiochi[100] report that in Morris hepatoma cells total calcium is increased three- to five-fold. Dead cells, in general, contain accumulations of calcium.[101,102] H. L. Newmark et al.[102a] and Michael J. Wargovich et al.,[102b] however, have suggested that supplementary dietary calcium may reduce the potential toxicity of dietary fat. They point out animal experiments[102b] have shown that calcium lactate can react with fatty acids and bile acids in the colon to form insoluble calcium soaps that are then excreted. Since fatty acids and bile acids in the feces are thought to be tumor promoters, calcium might—by forming insoluble soaps—work to protect against cancer. At any rate, calcium remains essential to our health and most of us probably need more of this mineral than we are now getting. The problem relates to the improper maintenance of intracellular calcium homeostasis. Better health and increased longevity will result from the eventual resolution of the mysteries of calcium metabolism.

Phosphorus

The work of phosphorus in metabolizing fats, carbohydrates and protein is an important contribution to body chemistry. Phosphorus, in the form of adenosine triphosphate (ATP), is required to assure a

---

* Interestingly, Marielle Gascon-Barre et al[98b] reported that when calcium was restricted in renal stone formers they adapted by showing a highly significant increase in the circulating $1,25(OH)_2D$ concentrations. (It seems reasonable to me that this phenomenon may also occur in those of us who do not form renal stones.)

generous supply of energy and to combat fatigue. The role of phosphorus in forming ADP, creatine phosphate and other chemicals is vital to body chemistry.

Another phosphorus compound, AMP (adenosine 5'-monophosphate), is an intermediate in the release of energy for use by the muscles and perhaps for other types of work done by the cells. Cyclic AMP (adenosine 3', 5'-monophosphate), produced by the action of the enzyme adenyl cyclase and ATP, mediates the actions of a large number of hormones. Much of the work with cyclic AMP was done by Earl W. Sutherland, Jr., for which he was awarded the Nobel Prize for Medicine or Physiology in 1971. C. F. Tam and R. L. Walford [102c] found that older persons as well as younger persons with Down's syndrome have decreased levels of cyclic AMP (cAMP). They speculated that decreased cAMP might be a factor in immune-system dysfunction.

Phosphorus, as phosphates, assists the blood in maintaining the proper acid-base balance. Phosphorus in modest concentrations stimulates the (Na,K)-pump in red blood cells according to Robert W. Mercer and Philip B. Dunham.[103] However, they report that at high concentrations phosphorus exhibits a *reverse effect* and inhibits operation of the pump.

Phosphorus in the form of phosphate radicals plays an essential role at the very heart of the living cell in deoxyribonucleic acid (DNA) and ribonucleic acid (RNA). DNA and RNA consist of large chains of molecules containing not only phosphoric acid but a pentose sugar—Beta-2-deoxy-D-ribose for DNA and Beta-D-ribose for RNA—plus nitrogen bases which are usually purines or pyrimidines. Pioneering work on DNA and RNA has been done and continues to be done by many preeminent scientists. Among these, Arthur Kornberg shared the Nobel Prize for Medicine or Physiology in 1959 with Severo Ochoa. Kornberg discovered an enzyme that promotes the production of DNA while Ochoa discovered the enzyme that promotes production of RNA. James D. Watson, Maurice H. F. Wilkins and Francis H. C. Crick shared the Nobel Prize for Medicine or Physiology in 1962 for determining the structure of DNA. Robert W. Holley, Marshall W. Nirenberg and

Har Gobind Khorana studied the genetic mechanisms of DNA and RNA, for which they shared the Nobel Prize for Medicine or Physiology in 1968. Then, in 1969, Max Delbrück, Alfred Hershey and Salvador Luria shared the Nobel Prize for Medicine or Physiology for research in the genetics of viruses—work so important that, without their results, it is said Watson and Crick could not have discovered the structure of DNA. Relatedly, Odd Hassel and Dereck H. R. Barton were honored with the Nobel Prize for Chemistry the same year (1969) for their research into the shape of molecules, work which also aided the discovery of the structure of DNA. Then, in 1975, Renato Dulbecco, Howard Temin and David Baltimore were awarded the Nobel Prize for Medicine or Physiology for discoveries concerning the interaction between tumor viruses and the DNA and RNA of the cell. In 1978, the discovery and application of enzymes that break DNA into usable pieces for individual study gained the Nobel Prize for Medicine or Physiology for Werner Arber, Daniel Nathans and Hamilton O. Smith. In 1980, Paul Berg, Walter Gilbert and Frederick Sanger were granted the Nobel Prize in Chemistry for their discoveries in nucleic-acid chemistry and for developing ways of finding the order of the individual links in DNA and RNA. Increased knowledge of the vital role of phosphorus, as well as the role of other elements in DNA and RNA, and future controlled manipulation of our genetic constitution, will provide powerful techniques to reduce disease and increase longevity.

Phosphates are components not only of DNA and RNA but also of the phospholipids (such as lecithin) which act as emulsifiers and transporters of fats and fatty acids and increase the permeability of cell membranes. Since phosphorus is an essential component in the body's manufacture of lecithin, it is required for proper nerve and brain function and for sexual vitality.

Phosphorus is needed for building bones and teeth. H. Luoma and T. Nuuja[104] reported that phosphate alone added to a magnesium-deficient cariogenic diet of rats strongly reduced fissure caries. However, phosphate addition, in these magnesium-deficient animals, had undesirable effects such as renal and aortic accumulation of calcium and accumulation of dental calculus. These harmful effects were prevented, however, with the addition of magnesium and fluoride.

Phosphorus performs an important function in the body's use of vitamin B_1. Thiamin may be present in adequate supply but, unless one's body permits phosphorus to efficiently combine with it (by the process called phosphorylating), he or she could show signs of a B_1 deficiency.

Lack of phosphorus can cause retarded growth, rickets, osteomalacia, bone pain, fatigue, nervousness, mental slowness and loss of appetite. A low level of serum phosphorus is also associated with hypertension.[105,106] Hemolysis may occur at very low levels of serum phosphate. Animals fed sufficient quantities of calcium and vitamin D but with almost no phosphorus, have developed rickets. David B. N. Lee and Charles R. Kleeman[107] relate that K. Friedlander and W. G. Rosenthal, as early as 1926, reported improved glucose utilization in diabetic patients by giving intravenous phosphate in the absence of insulin. Lee and Kleeman cite references showing phosphate is a useful addition to treatment of diabetic ketoacidosis. The *large* amount of phosphorus used in forming ATP for supplying energy to propel sperm is suggested by the *low* amount of ATPase present in the sperm of normospermic men and the much greater quantity present in the sperm of infertile men.[107a]

Oral phosphorus mediates a calcium control system for parathyroid hormone secretion resulting in an increase in the amount of the parathyroid hormone present in serum.[108] Changes in parathyroid activity modify, in turn, the manner in which the kidneys handle phosphate. This mechanism presumably accounts for the low level of serum phosphate in hyperparathyroidism and the high serum phosphate of hypoparathyroidism.[109]

A tremendous excess of phosphorus, a condition called *hyperphosphatemia,* may encourage an excessive entry of calcium into the soft tissue cells. A. Hogan[110] reported that 90% of guinea pigs kept on a diet consisting of .8% calcium and .9% phosphorus developed deposits of calcium phosphate. When the amount of dietary phosphorus was reduced to .5% the incidence of deposits was less than 10%. However, the findings of Hogan's guinea pig experiment may not be applicable to humans. In humans, it appears that a high phosphorus intake generally has little effect on the body's calcium balance. J. Jowsey, noting the high-meat diet and relatively low-dairy diet of most Americans, proposed that the resultant low-calcium and high-phosphorus intake was an important factor in causing postmenopausal osteoporosis. This proposal has been widely cited as a fact in many popular nutrition books and articles. (If it were true, would it not also be logical to condemn such high-phosphorus foods as wheat germ, brewer's yeast and lecithin?) However, various studies by Herta Spencer et al. and another study by Robert P. Heaney and Robert R. Recker[111] led Heaney and Recker to conclude that, "the absolute level of phosphorus intake and the calcium-to-phosphorus ratio in the diet are not important factors in determining calcium balance in the osteoporosis-prone subject, at least within the reasonably broad range of these intake variables likely to be encountered in premenopausal women." Modestly high phosphorus intake can, to the contrary, actually aid in the metabolism of calcium. A study by Herta Spencer et al.[112] showed that a high-phosphorus intake had very little effect on intestinal absorption of calcium. Furthermore, the higher phosphorus intake resulted in a significant decrease of urinary calcium (i.e., calcium retention was improved). Other studies have shown that phosphate supplements prevent a negative calcium balance during immobilization, as in bedridden patients.[113] Then too, even in patients with osteoporosis, phosphate is reported to improve the calcium balance![114]

Many other studies support the conclusion that phosphorus, even in excess, generally improves calcium metabolism. When calcium and phosphorus are consumed in goodly amounts, protein also is without significant adverse effect on calcium balance in humans. Sally A. Schuette and Hellen M. Linkswiler[112a] have done a good job of analyzing results of their work and other relevant studies prior to the research of Heaney cited above. Schuette and Linkswiler stress that "it is important to emphasize the diets low in calcium but high in protein and phosphorus consistently have caused slight negative calcium balances.[112f,g,38] Such a dietary condition exists when diets high in protein are consumed unless dairy products, other calcium rich foods or calcium supplements are also consumed." In their own research they noted that when calcium intake was 590 mg., addition of a low protein diet containing 890 mg. phosphorus from meat or from purified proteins and monopotassium phosphate caused a significant increase in urinary calcium, had no effect on apparent calcium absorption and changed calcium balance from positive to negative. In such a case, the popular conception that protein and phosphorus depress calcium balance is true. Remember, however, many studies [111-112g,38,38a] show that generous intakes of calcium, phosphorus and protein—including that found in meat—cause no adverse effect on the calcium balance, except when daily calcium intake is quite high. [112] Although these studies have been done by eminent scientists, the work must be viewed as being simplistic if magnesium intake was ignored. As we have already seen, and as will be discussed again when we consider magnesium, generous amounts of this element are required for healthful interaction of calcium, phosphorus, the parathyroid hormone and calcitonin. [28] Furthermore, in examining the protocol of the various studies, one gets the impression that many of the scientists improperly ignored the distinction between plasma ionized calcium, which is biologically active, and bound calcium, which is inert. [3c]

The typical diet easily supplies enough phosphorus, the primary sources being fish, meat, poultry, navy beans, peas, mushrooms, milk, Swiss and cheddar cheese, egg yolks, peanuts, nuts, wheat germ, bran and whole grains. (Note the absence of fruits and of most vegetables from this list.) Those consuming large amounts of soft drinks may get considerable phosphate from this source. (The May 22, 1986 *Wall Street Journal* reported that, according to the newsletter *Beverage Industry,* soft drinks now surpass water as the most popular U.S. beverage. The average person drank 44.5 gallons of soft drinks in 1985 but just 39.1 gallons of water.)

In spite of the widespread stories regarding mineral loss during the refining of flour, white bread may be superior to whole wheat bread in its effects on minerals present in the digestive tract. Numerous studies support this statement. For example, John G.

Reinhold et al.[115] found that negative balances of calcium, magnesium, zinc and even phosphorus developed after 20 days of eating Bazari (a type of whole wheat) bread. Although Bazari whole wheat bread contains somewhat more zinc and calcium and much more magnesium and phosphorus than white bread, the Reinhold group found the whole wheat bread inferior to the white bread as a source of minerals. Phytate has been shown to be digestible by the rat and presumably man can also digest it, at least to some extent. Presumably, also, in the Reinhold experiment the phosphorus released by the digestion of the phytate formed complexes with the metals and caused them to be excreted in the feces. The literature is replete with studies arriving at a similar conclusion, one regarding the effect of phytate and iron being given a little later in connection with that metal. The health-enthusiast's crusade against white bread could be effectively countered by strong ammunition from the big bakeries. It is possible, however, that phytate is not the culprit and the problem could really arise from the fiber content. A study by Suzanne M. Snedeker et al.[116] showed that subjects lost more iron and copper (but not zinc) via the urine when fed either a high-phosphate or a high-calcium diet. However, plasma iron, zinc, copper and transferrin levels and serum ferritin levels were unaffected by either diet. (Several other studies show, however, that iron utilization is adversely affected when the diet contains large amounts of both phosphorus and calcium.) Thus, phytate and phosphorus may be blamed for an effect being produced mainly by another entity, probably fiber.

The essential consideration for most of us is not that we may be consuming too little phosphorus, but that we make certain, through supplementation, of getting sufficient calcium. On the other hand, vegetarians may have phosphorus levels that are too low. D. A. Isenberg et al.[117] have reported on studies involving 15 vegetarian Asian women volunteers. The quadriceps strength of four of these women was well below normal and all four had abnormally low phosphorus levels. So, although my statement that most Americans (and, in particular, those consuming wheat germ, brewer's yeast and lecithin) may have an adequate or even an excessively high phosphorus level, this is quite obviously not a universal rule. In fact, familial hypophosphatemia is a dominant trait apparently due to poor intestinal absorption and/or poor kidney reabsorption of inorganic phosphate which can result in rickets and dwarfism. In general, however, except for some vegetarians, some alcoholics, persons consuming excessive amounts of aluminum or magnesium hydroxide antacids,[118] and for those with familial hypophosphatemia, the problem is generally not too little phosphorus but too much relative to calcium consumption. It is speculated that overuse of aluminum hydroxide could help cause osteomalacia.[118a] Marion D. Francis et al.[118b] found that phosphorus in the form of orally administered diphosphonates inhibits crystalization of calcium phosphate in vitro and prevents aortic calcification in rats given large amounts of vitamin D₂. The diphosphonate disodium etidronate prevents conversion of calcium phosphate into hyroxyapatite (the basic inorganic constituent of bone) when given in large dosages for long periods. C. J. Preston et al.[118c] reported in 1986, however, that when orally administered to patients with Paget's disease in high dosage (20 mg./kg. daily) for a short period of time it was an effective treatment.

A nondietary source of phosphorus, "strike-anywhere" matches, has caused dermatitis in some persons. A. Chiarenza and C. Gallope[119] reported that the phosphorus sesquisulphide in match heads has caused dermatitis among persons carrying such matches in their pockets. M. C. Steele and F. A. Ive[120] told of recurrent facial eczema in females, even in nonsmokers, due to "strike-anywhere matches." They also noted that sale of such matches is illegal in western Europe.

Iron

Iron is required to form the blood's hemoglobin, which is responsible for carrying oxygen to every cell of the body, and thus iron proves its essentiality to health and longevity. Heme is a red pigment consisting of a ring structure called tetrapyrrole or porphyrin (which contains four subunits called pyrroles) and centered around an atom of iron[120a]* Heme is joined in the bone marrow with the protein globin to form hemoglobin. Each hemoglobin molecule has the capacity to carry four oxygen molecules for use by the tissue cells. Every second about three million red blood cells (erythrocytes) die, break up and the iron returns to the bone marrow to go into the manufacture of fresh hemoglobin for new cells. At the same time, the nonprotein, heme portion of the broken-up hemoglobin is converted into the bile pigment *bilirubin,* which is released into the blood and subsequently secreted by the liver into the bile.

The mucosal (epithelial) cells of the intestinal lining are the sites of iron absorption. Absorption is greatest in the duodenum but occurs in the rest of the small intestines and in the colon. The mucosa are assisted in this function, it is believed, by the protein *gastroferrin,* which is also a normal constituent of gastric juice. Inside the mucosa, iron combines with a beta globulin known as *transferrin.* Transferrin carries iron in the plasma (just as hemoglobin is a carrier of oxygen) to the tissues and to the liver, spleen and other storage areas. Here the ferric form of iron in the transferrin, under the influence of ascorbic acid and the energy supplied by ATP, combines with the protein *apoferritin* to form *ferritin* or a mixture of protein, iron, lipid, sugars, copper and calcium called *hemosiderin.* (The latter is especially likely to form when large amounts of iron are to be deposited. Martin O'Connell et al.[120b] suggested, in 1986, that the conversion of ferritin into hemosiderin in iron overload is biologically advantageous in that it decreases the ability of iron to promote oxygen—radical reactions.) When plasma iron levels become too low, iron is removed from ferritin (and, less easily, from hemosiderin)—possibly assisted by the enzyme xanthine oxidase—and sent via transferrin to wherever the body needs it.** The iron of transferrin is in the *ferric* form in plasma, but it is reduced to the *ferrous* form in the bone marrow

---

* In more primitive species, other metals such as copper or cobalt may take the place of iron.[120a]

** Vitamin A seems to be involved in regulating iron release from the liver. [120c,d] Thus, iron-deficient anemia may be a complication of vitamin A deficiency, as will be discussed shortly.

before being used to form hemoglobin prior to its incorporation into the red blood cells.

Iron not only functions as an integral component of hemoglobin but as a vital element in pigments and enzymes—*cytochromes* and *cytochrome oxidases*—that transfer oxygen within the cells. Later, in Chapter 9, we will meet the important iron-containing enzymes, *catalases* and *peroxidases*. Iron is a component of nearly half the enzymes involved in the energy-producing Krebs cycle that we discussed in Chapter 5 in connection with pantothenic acid.

E. J. Underwood[121] reports that, according to B. Vahlquist, serum iron in men has been found to undergo a diurnal rhythm, being high in the morning and low in the evening. (The rhythm was found to be reversed in night workers. Sleep deprivation also had an effect—that of gradually lowering the serum-iron levels.) James M. Stengle and Arthur L. Schade[122] reported that in a majority of normal human adults the iron-binding capacity of the plasma remained constant. In a minority he found, as had Vahlquist, that the bound-iron level was highest in the morning and lowest in the evening. Giorgio Casale et al.[123] found a circadian rhythm in plasma iron and in total iron-binding capacity (but not in serum ferritin) for older men and women. (The subjects had a mean age of 78 years and had been hospitalized for at least 30 days, so the data may not be applicable to younger, more healthy persons.) The peaks in data for the men generally occurred between 7 AM. and 4 P.M. The women's data generally reached maximum in the afternoon for serum iron and in the evening for total iron-binding capacity, i.e., about four hours after that of the men.(If this diurnal rhythm is present in younger persons and if it ought to be encouraged, then iron-rich foods and supplements should be consumed in the morning or at lunch. If homeostasis in serum iron is preferable, and maybe it would be when sex is on the nighttime agenda, then iron consumption should be encouraged at the evening meal. As I suggest later in this chapter in regard to potassium, I suspect that we should generally encourage diurnal—circadian—body rhythms.) Other studies have been made of the diurnal iron cycle, not all agreeing with the study just discussed. K. Hoyer[124] reported peak iron values in the morning. W. F. Wiltink et al.[125] and Bernard E. Statland et al.[126] independently found the peak to be at about 2P.M. and thus were both in general agreement with the Casale study. On the other hand, Rita Long et al.[127] could find no discernible pattern in serum iron. I think, however, that majority opinion supports the Casale study.

H. S. Lo and C. W. M. Wilson[127a] found, in agreement with the Casale research, that serum iron peaked about 8 A.M. In addition, they discovered that the uptake of ascorbic acid by the leukocytes is enhanced by the presence of ferric iron. Furthermore, Wilson[127b] reported that the diurnal rhythm of plasma iron is synchronized with the rhythm of ascorbic acid, thus optimizing the conditions for maximal absorption of ascorbic acid by the leukocytes.

A deficiency of iron may lead to anemia, which affects women especially and often in some degree throughout half their lives from menarche to menopause, whether because of menstruation or because of the additional iron needs during pregnancy or lactation. M. Staubli[128] reports episodes of pruritus (itching) associated with iron-deficiency anemia in women. Manufacturers of iron tablets would have us believe that supplementary iron is essential for women—which is not true for the majority if they will eat iron-rich foods, take vitamin C and will, as we will relate later, avoid some of the food combinations detrimental to iron assimilation. Some may, however, require supplementation during pregnancy and The Council on Foods and Nutrition of the A.M.A. has stated [129] that many women enter pregnancy with inadequate stores of iron.* A number of nutrition surveys have concluded that a deficiency of vitamin A may contribute to the incidence of

---

* A lead article in the *British Medical Journal,* [130] states that maintenance of hemoglobin concentration at nonpregnant levels does not seem necessary. Furthermore, Stephen S. Entman et al.[130a] report that, among 144 women with toxemia of pregnancy, a striking elevation of serum iron was noted in patients who were most seriously ill. Physicians who are confirmed believers in iron supplementation during pregnancy should read these articles and also one by S. M. Ross et al.[130b]

anemia. Rat experiments have supported this contention since animals deficient in this vitamin often developed anemia and did so even when adequate iron was present. A report of a nutritional survey in Paraguay published by the U.S. Department of Health, Education and Welfare[130c] showed that hemoglobin levels are closely related to plasma levels of vitamin A (Figure 10). Then too, Robert E. Hodges et al.[130d,e] reported that five of eight men developed anemia as a result of experimentally induced vitamin A deficiency.

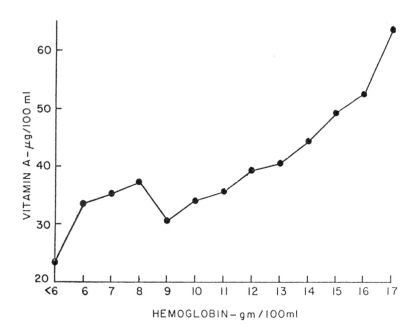

Figure 10. Relationship of serum vitamin A levels to hemoglobin levels from a nutrition survey in Paraguay.

From a knowledge of how ubiquitous is the occurrence of *reverse effects,* one could guess that an excess of vitamin A might also induce anemia. J. M. White[131] has recently reported this phenomenon in a 44-year-old man whose dermatologist had prescribed prednisolone topical steroids and 150,000 I.U. of vitamin A tablets daily. It seems apparent that in the future nutrition facts will be stated in terms of dose-response relationships.

Vitamin E may also be a factor in reducing the problems attending some forms of anemia. The potency of various vitamin E compounds can be measured, as we saw in Chapter 2, by their ability to prevent hemolysis of red blood cells. This suggests the possibility that vitamin E might be used therapeutically to treat hemolytic anemia. O. Giardini et al.[132] treated 26 patients, aged 2-14 years, who had homozygous beta-thalassemia (a disease involving a hereditary defect in hemoglobin synthesis) by administering 300 mg. of alpha-tocopheryl acetate, 10 orally and 16 parenterally, for 15 days. They reported that the vitamin E treatment appeared to effectively reduce the oxidative damage to the red blood cells, principally when administered parenterally perhaps, they speculated, because of poor intestinal absorption of the vitamin in these subjects.

Women who lose large amounts of blood (and, therefore, iron, calcium and other nutrients as well) during menstruation, may develop brittle nails with horizontal ridges which form at the time of the menstrual periods. (Lack of protein, sulphur and vitamin A could, however, also be factors in the formation of horizontal ridges.) A shortage of iron may also cause lack of vitality, poor complexion, bad memory and difficulty in thinking clearly. Iron deficiency in some persons causes them to experience *pica* (the craving for and eating of unnatural substances). Pica may take many forms such as *geophagia* (eating earth) or *pagophagia* (craving for and eating large amounts of ice) or eating of chalk, laundry starch, plaster, tinfoil, paper and even one's own hair (sometimes to such an extreme that it wads in the stomach and may require surgical removal).* Iron deficiency sometimes results in hypothermia when

---

* James A. Halsted,[132a] in reviewing geophagia in man, cites R. S. Lourie et al., [132b] who stated, in 1963, that clay could be purchased in large sacks in southern cities. Lourie noted also that when persons moved north they sometimes had their relatives dig clay from a favorite river bank and mail it to them. Kenneth Redman, [132c] noting that clay in the form of kaolin is a crude drug used to treat diarrhea, dysentery and colitis, shows that

rats are kept at low ambient temperatures. Erick Dillman et al.[133] have reported that the lowered temperature in iron deficiency is due to altered triiodothyronine metabolism. They found that in such cases thyroxine conversion to triiodothyronine is impaired.

Iron deficiency is a factor in impaired immunocompetence according to R. K. Chandra and A. K. Suraya.[134] There is considerable evidence that adequate (but not excessive) iron favorably affects the immune response and reduces susceptibility to infection. The bactericidal action of iron is thought to be related to its ability to catalyze free-radical chain processes.[135] Sufficient iron, but not iron in excess, may be important not only in combating bacterial infections, but in combating yeast-like fungal infections such as candidiasis.** *The Lancet*,[138] citing the work of J. Fletcher et al., observes that "fungal infections of the mouth and vagina are common in patients with iron deficiency, and it is quite possible that merely reflects changes in normal bacterial flora allowing growth of organisms that are normally suppressed." J. Fletcher et al.[139] suggest that insufficient iron may in some way limit production of thymus-dependent lymphocytes. Humbert and Moore cite the work of J. M. Higgs and Wells[139a] who found that of 31 patients with chronic mucotaneous candidiasis, 23 had an iron deficiency. When four patients were treated with iron, three improved, while none of four patients treated with placebo improved.

On the other hand, free iron promotes multiplication of many microbes. Some heme-containing compounds (such as blood or ascitic fluid) also foster bacterial growth.[138] However, iron chelated to body protein is not generally available to the invading organisms. For example, J. J. Bullen et al.[140] have shown that the bacterial-resisting properties of breast milk are due to its high content of

---

its use dates from the time of Christ. Interestingly, Benjamin H. Ershoff and Sol Bernick[132d] found that rats fed a non-heat-processed wheat flour-containing ration were retarded in growth and exhibited pathologic changes in tibias and alveolar bone. A supplement of 1% to 4% clay, however, caused an increase in weight and prevented the pathologic changes. Nevertheless, through a process of cation exchange, clay can inhibit iron absorption (and also, possibly, potassium, mercury and zinc absorption).[132a]

** Unsaturated serum transferrin is an important anticandida factor. It inhibits growth of various microorganisms by binding ferric ions needed for their growth.[136,137]

lactoferrin and transferrin which take up excess iron. Milk's bacteriostatic properties are negated if the iron-binding proteins are saturated with iron.

The golden mean once again comes into play. Iron in moderation, often working through the iron-dependent enzyme myeloperoxidase (of which more in Chapter 9), is infection fighting. In excess, iron may exhibit a reverse, infection-fostering effect. In fact, J. J. Bullen[141] has pointed out that fever lowers the concentration of iron in serum and this favors resistance to infection. (It is obviously not always rewarding to fight a fever or to supplement the diet with iron!)

One of the frightening implications of iron deficiency is its possible association with the development of cancer (at least in rats). Joseph J. Vitale et al.[142] found that rats on an iron-deficient diet developed neoplastic changes in the liver when given the carcinogen dimethylhydrazine. Control rats given either the carcinogen alone or fed on the iron-deficiency diet alone did not develop neoplastic lesions during the period of the study. The high incidence of gastric cancer in Colombia, South America, is attributed by Selwyn A. Breizman et al.[142a] to deficiencies in iron. On the other hand, it is possible that iron in excess may show a *reverse effect* and be a *cause* of cancer. S. H. Kon[142b] notes that uncontrolled iron promotes autoxidation which crosslinks biomolecules and produces destructive activated oxygen. Kon speculates that hydrolyzed iron could be a pathogen that evades control by ferritin and may be a factor in an early stage of preneoplastic carcinogenesis. Furthermore, Raymond J. Bergeron et al.[143] reported that iron at levels comparable to clinical doses for humans (24 mg./kg. body wt.) stimulates growth of L1210 tumor cells in mice. It looks as though too little iron or too much iron may be cancer threatening, thus representing a *biphasic reverse effect*.

Iron supplementation may sometimes be useful to athletes. D. B. Clement and L. L. Sawchuk[143a] present evidence that suggests exercise may impose an iron "cost" on athletes because of erythrocyte destruction, increased elimination of iron and possibly impaired iron absorption. A. Hunding et al.[143b] reported a systemic iron deficiency in 56% of joggers and competition runners, but Edward Colt and Budd Heyman[143c] found only 3 males and 9 females to be iron deficient out of 118 runners and they found only 1 who was anemic. They concluded, nevertheless, that endurance running is associated with an increased risk of iron deficiency and that all runners should have their iron status periodically monitored.

For youthful energy, generous amounts of oxygen under proper control of antioxidants, as we will discuss in Chapter 9, must be delivered by hemoglobin to every cell of the body. Iron is also essential to the sexual function in both men and women because good sex requires rich blood. Although men are less susceptible to energy-sapping anemia and the resultant sexual lassitude, iron is just as important to them in another way. Dr. Edwin W. Hirsch [143d] asks the question: "How do you explain the hardness of the erection?" He then goes on to provide an answer: "Penile tensile strength is not only due to the squeezed-in red blood corpuscles within the firm rubberoid-encased penile erectile bodies, but also to the fact that the hemoglobin or iron atom content of the blood furnishes the requisite element for phallic firmness and hardness." However, if your iron stores are adequate, don't conclude that supplemental iron will make you hyper-sexy. Excessive iron is dangerous, as we have seen and as we will soon discuss further.

Assimilation Problems

Although the body has only a small daily requirement for iron and although far greater than needed quantities are present in the diet, many persons are reported to be iron deficient. Why? Simply because iron is often inefficiently assimilated from food. Good sources for iron are meats (especially organ meats such as liver), oysters, clams, sardines, egg yolk, brewer's yeast, turnip greens, beet tops, peas, parsley, avocados, lettuce, cabbage, red peppers, spinach,* watercress, beans of various types, alfalfa tablets, apricots, peaches, prunes, black cherries, blackberries and other

---

* Astonishingly, according to Darrell R. van Campen and Ross M. Welch,[143e] the oxalate in spinach, while depressing calcium absorption, increases the bioavailability of iron. Supplemental oxalic acid was found to enhance the bioavailability of iron from both spinach and ferric chloride.

berries (and the juices of these various fruits), dates, raisins, nuts, whole grains, bran, wheat germ and black-strap molasses. About half the iron in fish, fowl or meat is *hemoglobin (heme)* iron, the remainder being ferritin and hemosiderin—the *nonheme* iron. About 15% to 30% of the iron in animal protein, but only about 5% of that in vegetables, which is *nonheme* iron, is absorbed by the body. Those consuming a predominantly cereal-based diet—i.e., a macrobiotic diet—may, therefore, be in serious danger of iron deficiency. B. C. Mehta et al.[144] found widespread iron deficiencies among such persons. Long-distance runners may have a need for iron that exceeds the RDA and Michael B. Jacobs et al.[144a] reported an iron-deficiency anemia in a vegetarian runner. The presence of meat enhances the body's absorption of extrinsically added iron and also counteracts a component in vegetables that inhibits the absorption of iron.[145,146] Nevertheless, Bonnie M. Anderson et al.[146a] found that the iron (and zinc) status of Seventh Day Adventist vegetarian women (mean age 52.9 ± 15.3 years) appeared adequate despite their low intake of absorbable iron from flesh foods and their high consumption of fiber and phytate.

If sufficient hydrochloric acid is present in the stomach, nonheme iron will more readily pass through the intestinal wall into the bloodstream. Much anemia is probably caused by insufficient stomach acid and so supplementing the diet with dilute hydrochloric acid (available in pills) may be useful. However, foods such as buttermilk, yogurt, kefir and citrus fruits, all of which contain acids, can provide a boost to the stomach's normal acid supply so that supplementation with hydrochloric acid may not be required.

Ascorbic acid functions in iron metabolism through its ability to reduce ferric to ferrous ions followed by formation of ferrous ascorbate chelates.[146b] Iron is more efficiently absorbed in its ferrous form than in its ferric state. Therefore, nutrients that foster reduction or inhibit oxidation aid in iron assimilation.* Examples of such

---

* To the extent that vitamin C diminishes copper assimilation (as noted in Chapter 6), it could reduce formation of hemoglobin since copper is needed to form it. Take vitamin C with iron but not with copper. (If a large amount of vitamin C is consumed it may interfere with assimilation of copper from food, possibly making it useful to supplement

factors are not only vitamin C, which is especially useful, but also vitamin E. However, ascorbic acid (like hydrochloric acid—as we noted earlier) does not aid the absorption of hemoglobin iron (such as is found in meat). Even the ability of vitamin C to aid the absorption of nonheme iron is reduced when protein is present simply because protein itself, as we have reported earlier, greatly aids in the absorption of the nonheme iron.[147]

Other ways to aid iron absorption are by administering it with the amino acids histidine, lysine, glutamine, glutamic acid and asparigin. Chelating agents, again including vitamin C as well as succinic acid, sugars and sulphur-containing amino acids, are all useful in increasing iron uptake.[148] Many studies, some cited earlier and also those of Luis A. Mejia and Guillermo Arroyave,[149] indicate that adequate amounts of vitamin A are needed for iron metabolism. (On the other hand, Luis A. Mejia et al.[150] found that iron absorption in rats was neither significantly impaired nor augmented by a vitamin A deficiency.) Bile also increases iron absorption. Alcohol slightly increases the amount of iron absorbed. However, some wines (especially red wines) have a high iron content and can greatly increase the amount of iron absorbed.[151] This may seem, to some, a pleasant way to get more iron into the body. However, alcohol depresses the activity of the enzyme *ferrochelatase* which catalyzes the insertion of iron into protoporphyrin to produce heme. Thus, alcohol elevates the level of iron in the blood but inhibits production of hemoglobin.[152]

Iron absorption is inhibited by methionine, proline, serine, phenylalanine, taurocholic acid, tannin (tannic acid), calcium and phosphates (as found in dairy products). Nonheme iron absorption is inhibited by coconut milk.[153] R. J. Dobbs and I. McLean Baird[159] found that whole wheat bread significantly inhibits the absorption of

---

the diet with copper.)[146c] Judith L. Sutton et al.,[146d] in a study regarding the effects of ascorbic acid on the mixed oxidase system in guinea pig livers, speculate on the possibility of what I call the *reverse effect*. They say in regard to vitamin C, "It would be of interest to discover whether at very high intakes of the vitamin, as with deficiency, ascorbic acid causes an increase in caeruloplasmin concentrations, like that which occurs with deficiency, and a shift in the equilibrium of the hepatic iron pool from the ferrous to the ferric form, hence rendering Fe^{2+} less available."

nonheme iron. Dobbs and Baird, as well as those conducting many other studies, have suggested that the absorption of iron is inhibited by phytates. However, Karen S. Simpson et al.[154] reported that, although bran inhibited the absorption of iron in human volunteers, removal of the phytate by endogenous phytase did not alter the inhibiting effect. Thus, it may be that some other factor is responsible for the effects generally blamed on phytate. J. Edward Hunter[155] suggests that the inhibitory component could be fiber. He points out that man should be capable of digesting phytate since the enzyme phytase has been reported to be present in the human small intestine. It is interesting to note that bran (which contains fiber and phytate), when fed to pigs, showed no inhibitory effect on iron absorption.[156] In experiments with rats, S. J. Fairweather-Tait[157] also concluded that wheat bran fiber had no effect on the retention of iron from the diet. Furthermore, Abdullah M. Thannoun et al.[157a] recently reported that iron supplied by fortification in white bread was less available to rats than iron found naturally in whole wheat bread. On the contrary, D. L. McWhinnie and A. J. Mack,[158] in studying young adult volunteers, found, as had R. J. Dobbs and I. McLean Baird,[159] that wheat bran inhibited the bioavailability of iron from the gut. The results of many of these experiments are obviously contradictory and more research is required.

Factors affecting iron absorption are complex indeed. James D. Cook et al.[160] report that soy products inhibit the absorption of nonheme iron. Even so, the iron in soybeans is much better absorbed than the iron in black beans if each is eaten separately, but similar percentages from each source are absorbed when the beans are eaten together.[145] We have noted that iron from animal sources is generally more available to the body, but the iron-rich yolk of egg is usually considered to be an exception. Egg yolk (because of its phosphoprotein called *phosvitin)* will decrease the availability of other iron but, nevertheless, it is a reasonably good iron source. In fact, with rats eating egg yolk along with ascorbic acid, the iron became as available as it is from ferrous sulfate. Thus, contrary to common belief, iron from egg yolk in the presence of vitamin C is, if rat experiments are applicable to humans, as available as iron from meat.[161] Orange juice contains little iron but, because of its vitamin C, if the juice is consumed with other foods (including egg yolk) it will make their nonheme iron far more available.[162] Lard in the diet was found to increase absorption of nonheme (but not heme) iron compared to the same diet with corn oil instead of lard.[163] Oils may actually decrease the iron balance and Wim van Dokkum et al.[164] reported that an increase in linoleic acid from 4 to 16 energy% (at a constant level of fat intake of 42 energy%) caused a decrease in iron balance from 3.3 to 2.3 mg./day.

In a 1986 study, Leif Hallberg et al.[164a] concluded that ascorbic acid was most effective in increasing absorption of iron in foods containing a high content of ligands known to inhibit iron absorption. The effect of ascorbic acid on iron absorption may be related to its ability to reduce ferric to ferrous ions and/or its ability to form soluble iron complexes. Either mechanism would reduce the probability that iron would be bound to ligands such as hydroxyl ions or phosphate ions that would inhibit absorption.

Cauliflower, with its generous amounts of vitamin C, will generally increase the nonheme iron available from a vegetarian meal. Furthermore, vegetarians were found to better utilize iron from a vegetarian diet than were omnivores consuming the same vegetarian diet. Thus, C. Kies and L. McEndree[165] observe that these results support the theory that one's nutritional needs partially determine the absorbability of iron. The environment may also be a factor in iron absorption. Dr. Albert Kruger of the University of California has reported that both positive and negative ions increase the body's assimilation of iron and the production of iron-containing enzymes. (However, in other ways the benefits of negions over posions are substantial.)

Tea, because of the tannic acid, and to a lesser degree coffee (perhaps also because it contains some tannates) will, on the other hand, greatly reduce iron availability.* Timothy A. Morck et al.[166] reported that a cup of coffee reduced iron absorption from a

---

* Hadar Merhav et al.,[165a] studying tea-drinking infants in India, found that 32.6% had microcytic anemia compared to just 3.5% among nontea drinkers. They recommended not giving tea to infants whose main source of iron is milk, grains, vegetables or medicine.

hamburger meal 39% as compared with a 64% decrease with tea. No decrease in iron absorption occurred when coffee was drunk one hour before a meal. However, drinking coffee one hour after a meal resulted in the same iron inhibition as when consumed with the meal. On the other hand, oxalate-containing foods such as spinach and rhubarb that were formerly thought to inhibit iron absorption may, according to recent studies, not have this negative effect. Those desiring to further explore the complexities of iron absorption are referred to an article "Bioavailability of Dietary Iron In Man" by Leif Halberg.[167] At any rate, it seems obvious that we cannot estimate the iron our body is absorbing by simply adding up the iron contents of the foods we are eating.

If you take iron supplements, some nutritionists will tell you that the iron should be organic (e.g., the gluconate, fumarate, lactate or peptonate compounds or an amino-acid chelate) rather than inorganic iron (e.g., ferrous sulphate) since inorganic iron, according to the Drs. Shute, is antagonistic to vitamin E. Then too, inorganic iron, in the presence of vitamin C, is a potent catalyst in the undesirable oxidation of unsaturated fatty acids.[168] Since lipid peroxides are aging factors, this gives us another good reason to prefer organic over inorganic iron. If, however, you do use inorganic iron (and the sulphates are more assimilable than the organic varieties of iron) the Drs. Shute suggest that you take it about 12 hours away from your vitamin E so that neither the iron nor the "E" will be present in the intestinal tract with each other. If iron supplements cause stomach upset, one's "intolerance rate" can sometimes be reduced if those supplements are taken after meals. However, David N. S. Kerr and Stanley Davidson,[169] after doing double-blind testing, concluded that the presumed intolerance to inorganic iron was primarily psychological.

The work of Paul Seligman et al.[170] has shown that absorption of iron from multivitamin/mineral pills can be greatly inhibited by the presence of calcium carbonate and magnesium oxide.* Seligman and

---

* On the other hand, Mary A. O'Neil-Cutting and William H. Crosby[170a] reported, in 1986, that magnesium hydroxide did not significantly reduce iron absorption from

his colleagues also found that iron absorption may be reduced as much as 75% when supplements are taken with meals; They suggest any iron supplement be taken several hours before breakfast or at bedtime.

Adverse Effects

If you are undergoing any tests, tell your physician if you are taking supplemental iron. Iron can cause a false-positive indication on the Diagnex blue test for impaired gastric function. Inorganic iron can cause a false-positive indication on the benzidine and guaiac tests for occult blood. Iron, in the form of ferrous sulphate or ferrous gluconate interferes with the absorption of tetracycline and especially of doxycycline.[171,171a] If these drugs have been prescribed for you, your physician may ask you to refrain from taking supplemental iron, at least in the form of ferrous sulfate. Ananda S. Prasad et al.[171b] reported that women using oral contraceptive agents showed an increase in serum iron and in total iron-binding capacity, but no effect was seen on hemoglobin, hematocrit and erythrocyte count. Erica P. Frassinelli-Gunderson and Sheldon Margen,[171c] in studying iron parameters of 46 women taking the Pill, found that serum ferritin, serum transferrin, serum iron and total iron-binding capacity were significantly increased. However, the red blood cell and hematocrit levels in those using the Pill were lower than normal. The investigators counsel that women using oral contraceptives should avoid supplementary iron.

As we have already mentioned, one of the negative aspects of excessive iron is the possibility that, in ferrous form, it can cause lipid peroxidation. In an *in vitro* experiment with rat-liver liposomal membranes, Manabu Kunimoto et al.[172] reported that ferrous ions in the presence of ascorbic acid induced lipid peroxidation. They reported additionally that neither superoxide dismutase nor catalase had any appreciable influence on the reaction. In a related study, but this one was done *in vivo* with rats, John J. Dougherty et al.[173]

---

an oral supplement. They found that sodium bicarbonate and calcium carbonate significantly inhibited iron absorption, but not if the supplement also contained ascorbic acid. The competitive binding of iron by ascorbic acid, they presumed, allowed uninhibited absorption of the iron.

found that either ferrous chloride or iron-dextran, given by injection, caused lipid peroxidation of dietary fat in the gut. Vitamin E partially protected the rats against lipid peroxidation and did so more effectively than did selenium. Animals deficient in vitamin E are vulnerable to iron toxicity. However, by way of partial protection, Young H. Lee et al.[174] observed that when rats were fed excessive amounts of iron while vitamin E and selenium were limited, catalase activity and also nonselenium glutathione peroxidase activity increased. (Catalase and both selenium glutathione peroxidase and nonselenium glutathione peroxidase work to decrease some of the damage done during lipid peroxidation.)

David K. Melhorn and Samuel Gross[175] found that erythrocyte hydrogen peroxide fragility was abnormally elevated in children with iron deficiency anemia. The fragility of the erythrocytes rose when iron-dextran was administered, supporting the supposition that iron increases red cell lipid peroxidation. (Ferrous iron catalyzes the formation of the hydroxyl radical from superoxide and hydrogen peroxide, a process known as Fenton's reaction [refs. 70 and 71a of Chapter 9]. The hydroxyl radical, in turn, stimulates lipid peroxidation.) Melhorn and Gross found that when the children were given vitamin E with the iron the rise in hydrogen peroxide fragility was prevented (I presume because the vitamin E removed the superoxide which was a factor in producing the lipid peroxidation).

Though the benefits of *adequate* iron are great, perhaps additional words of warning are in order about the negative aspects of *excessive* iron. Copper is essential to assure the proper utilization of iron, so if copper is deficient care must be taken not to overdose on iron. R. G. Kay[176] reports liver-biopsy studies have shown that, concomitant with copper deficiency, there may be excess amounts of iron in the Kupffer cells as well as in the hepatocytes.

Let's observe a way in which copper can help protect against an excess of iron. We noted earlier that ferrous iron can act as a pro-oxidant which is detrimental to body chemistry. The copper compound *ceruloplasmin* is not only an oxidase of various organic compounds but also acts as an oxidase of iron and so is sometimes referred to as "ferroxidase."[176a] It converts reduced (ferrous) to oxidized (ferric) iron, thus preventing iron from acting as an autoxidation catalyst.

Transferrin which, you will recall, transports iron throughout the body, is saturated with iron only in disease. In a diseased state, then, free-radical reactions tend to increase (or depending on one's viewpoint, they increase first and the symptoms of disease follow). At any rate, in cases of excess iron, especially if coexistent with a copper deficiency or a deficiency of other antioxidants—whether or not a diseased state is evident—free-radical reactions, leading to formation of hydroxyl radicals and subsequent lipid peroxidation, are likely to be accelerated and the rate of aging increased. David R. Blake et al.[177] suggests that iron is an exacerbating factor in the inflammation of the synovial membrane in rheumatoid disease as well as in other inflammatory processes. Furthermore, B. Sweder van Asbeck et al.[178] observed a type of meningitis and decreased phagocytosis in a patient with iron overload. We are thus provided for a rationale to avoid supplementary iron unless there is a good reason for using it.

Furthermore, a relatively rare functional disability called hemochromatosis, an inability to screen out unneeded iron, affects a few individuals. The excess iron is stored in the liver, pancreas, testicles, bone marrow and muscles (including the heart). This disability can result in cirrhosis of the liver, diabetes, sterility and heart attack, and so individuals who suffer from this ailment must restrict, rather than increase, their intake of iron.* Except for those having such problems, iron overdosage is usually considered to be rare, although intentional overdosages can result in mental retardation and sometimes in death.[179] However, Jerome L. Sullivan[180] would disagree that iron poisoning is unusual. Dr. Sullivan warns about the cardiotoxicity of excessive stores of iron. He suggests that stored

---

* Although venesection (blood letting) is no longer a general practice, it is valuable in treating hemochromatosis.[178a] Figure 11 illustrates the extended survival of persons so treated. Deferoxamine (desferrioxamine), a complex amine of microbial origin, is also used as an iron chelating compound in treating hemochromatosis. D. R. Blake et al.[178b] reported that at low levels deferoxamine aggravated inflammation in rats. At high levels, however, a *reverse effect* set in and deferoxamine was anti-inflammatory. B. Halliwell and J. M. C. Gutteridge[178c] have speculated on possible explanations of this phenomenon.

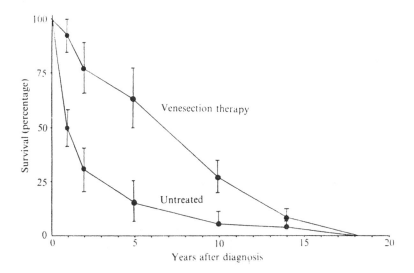

Figure 11. Life-table survival curves after hemochromatosis diagnosis in treated and untreated groups. The vertical lines at each time interval represent ± 1 standard error. Reprinted from Adrian Bomford and Roger Williams, *Quarterly Jrl. of Medicine* (1976) New Series, XLV, 180: 611-623, with permission of Oxford University Press.

iron in normal hearts is a chronic poison, causing arrhythmias and diffuse myocardial fibrosis. Dr. Sullivan maintains that our systems for storing iron evolved under conditions of deficiency. He postulates that the high risk of cardiovascular diseases in affluent societies may result from an inability to adjust to diets rich in iron. Sullivan further postulates that the greater incidence of heart disease among men and among postmenopausal women compared to younger women is due to higher levels of stored iron in the first two groups. For those with an excess of stored iron, vitamin C and/or alcohol may dangerously add to the problem.* A study by L. E. Böttiger and L. A. Carlson[180b] and another by P. C. Elwood et al.[180c]

---

* In cases of accidental poisoning by iron (e.g., if a child swallows ten 200 mg. tablets of ferrous sulphate) magnesium oxide has been recommended as an antidote.[180a]

have shown that hemoglobin in nonanemic healthy persons is directly correlated with serum cholesterol and triglyceride levels.

Then too, although adequate stores of iron are vital to foster the immune response and to ward off infections, high levels of iron favor bacterial and fungal invasions as well as infections such as tuberculosis.[181] The *in vitro* studies with mouse serum done by Ronald J. Elin and Sheldon M. Wolff[182] give support to the idea that excess iron may be detrimental. Elin and Wolff found that excessive iron encouraged growth of *Candida albicans* which cause yeast infections in humans. However, *Lancet*,[138] citing J. M. Higgs et al., states that "patients with chronic mucataneous candidiasis, who have a defect in lymphocyte function, are often helped by iron although they may not be anemic." Earlier in this section we considered the possibility that iron in excess may even be carcinogenic. Again, it's a case of the golden mean and of *reverse effects*. Too great or too little an intake of iron can obviously be very harmful, so you may wish to check your levels periodically with blood and hair analyses.[*]

Magnesium

Most of the body's magnesium is found in the bones, along with calcium and phosphorus. The remainder is located in the soft tissues and in the blood. Magnesium is required as a coenzyme for operation of the sodium pump that transports sodium and potassium ions into and out of the cell. However, Peter W. Flatman and Virgilio L. Lew[189] report that at high concentrations of magnesium, using *in vitro* experiments with giant squid axons, there was a *reverse effect* and the sodium-potassium and sodium-sodium exchange was inhibited.

Magnesium is used in a large number of the body's chemical reactions, including those involving transfer of the phosphate groups

---

[*] A new magnetic device is especially accurate in measuring iron stores. James N. Fordham[182a] relates that in certain hemolytic disorders (such as Cooley's anemia) which require blood transfusions, the iron stores may reach pathological levels and use of a chelator such as deferoxamine may be indicated. This new magnetic tool, using the superconducting quantum-interference device (SQUID), is discussed by Fordham.[182a]

in ATP—so essential for youthful energy! Magnesium is also required to activate the enzymes linking phosphate radicals to glucose in the formation of glycogen and in its subsequent breakdown to glucose in order to supply quick energy. R. K. Rude and F. R. Singer[190] point out that DNA transcription, RNA aggregation and a large number of plasma membrane functions are mediated by optimal amounts of magnesium. Dr. G. K. Eichhorn[191] has concluded that metal ion concentrations, especially of magnesium, may be a factor in aging since DNA replication, transcription and protein synthesis are mediated by metal ions. In addition to its role in DNA replication, magnesium enters into over 70% of the identified enzyme systems. The enzyme *carboxylase,* used in the metabolism of carbohydrates, functions only in the presence of magnesium. Magnesium promotes the efficiency with which amino acids form protein. Therefore, a high-protein diet requires that one consume more magnesium.

Many persons are reported to be somewhat deficient in magnesium. Jessie R. Ashe et al.[183] observed that prenatal diets of nulliparous women (including three graduate and two undergraduate university students, the wife of a university student, a registered nurse, two secretaries and a former elementary schoolteacher) showed a dietary magnesium intake of only 60% of the RDA. As Maurice E. Shils[184] stated, "With increasing ease and frequency of measurement of magnesium in body fluids, it has become obvious that human depletion occurs much more commonly than had been assumed previously." In this regard, Mildred S. Seelig[185] maintains that the published metabolic data indicates the minimal daily requirement for magnesium is above the official RDA of 300 mg. for women and 350 mg. for men and is probably at least 6 mg. per kg. per day. That's about 420 mg. per day for a 70 kg. (approximately 150 lb.) person. Those with a higher than normal calcium intake may have an even higher requirement for magnesium since increased ingestion of calcium increases magnesium loss. Persons consuming diets rich in fiber, such as whole wheat bread, brown rice or oatmeal, may have an even greater need for magnesium and supplementation may be advisable. Others who may be deficient in magnesium include residents of soft-water areas according to T. W. Anderson et al.[186]

Furthermore, I. Szelenyi[187] cites Mildred S. Seelig as believing that certain conditions such as pregnancy or lactation, childhood (especially during periods of rapid growth), postoperative and posttraumatic states (which are associated with higher levels of protein synthesis) require more intake of magnesium. Those with severe shortages are said to have *hypomagnesemia*.

Primary hypomagnesemia, with secondary hypocalcemia, is reported by Ahmad S. Teebi[188] to be not an extremely rare cause of infant tetany. Ahmad speculates that hypomagnesemia, preponderantly a male problem, may be genetic and caused by a rare x-borne allele.

The more common clinical manifestations of magnesium deficiency in adults are categorized by Edmund B. Flink[92] as follows:

1. Neuromuscular manifestations, particularly muscular twitching and tremor of any or all muscles including the tongue, with waxing and waning intensity and often with abrupt onset, are the most common findings. Convulsions occur in severe depletion and are the common signal of trouble in infants and young children.
2. Mental symptoms, which are equally important, include apathy, poor memory, mild to severe delirium (confusion, disorientation, hallucinations, paranoia) and coma.
3. Cardiac manifestations include premature beats, ventricular tachycardia and ventricular fibrillation.

Flink notes that although signs of tetany due to magnesium deficiency may occur in adults, they are not common.

A magnesium deficiency may increase the risk of retinal deterioration in diabetic patients. P. McNair et al.[193] reported that diabetic patients with retinopathy exhibited a definite hypomagnesemia. The magnesium deficiency was most pronounced in those having the severest retinopathy.

Magnesium is an important nutrient for the pituitary gland and for the nerves. Its shortage possibly contributes more than anything else to the great popularity of tranquilizers. When the pituitary gland receives an inadequate supply of magnesium it may fail to function properly in controlling the adrenal glands. (Overactivity of the adrenals can increase the heartbeat and release glucose from the liver which may, on occasion, be important for survival. But, on the other hand, if the adrenals are always hyperactive the condition can lead to inability to cope with life's problems.)

When magnesium is deficient in the extracellular fluid, this condition can lead to a greater release of acetylcholine along with increased muscle excitability that can produce tetany. Although excessive magnesium increases calcium requirements, hypomagnesemia, on the other hand, can bring on a form of hypocalcemia that may persist until the magnesium deficiency has been corrected. When tetany is present in such cases it will not be corrected by administering calcium but is correctable only if magnesium is given.

Another example of magnesium correcting not just hypomagnesemia but also hypocalcemia is its use in the treatment of neonatal convulsions. Many studies cited by G. Stendig-Lindberg and E. Hultman[194] show that hypocalcemia in infants is successfully treated with magnesium rather than with calcium therapy. C. S. Anast et al.[194a] explained this phenomenon by reporting that hypomagnesemia in man can cause the parathyroid gland to become suppressed, which can contribute further to hypocalcemia. Guy E. Abraham[195] cites references for a magnesium suppressional effect on the parathyroid hormone and stimulation of calcitonin secretion. These actions favor the deposition of calcium in the bone rather than in the soft tissues. Furthermore, according to Abraham, magnesium enhances the absorption and retention of calcium, whereas increasing calcium intake tends to suppress absorption of magnesium. Abraham holds that eating a diet low in phosphate and high in magnesium is a more prudent approach to managing osteoporosis than the ingestion of massive amounts of calcium. Abraham also decries the use of calcium blockers when, he says, magnesium can produce the same end result. (Burton M. Altura and Bella T. Altura[95a] state that, "Mg^{2+} appears to be a weak and useful Ca^{2+} antagonist.") Many of the interactions between magnesium and calcium are discussed by Lloyd T. Iseri and James H. French.[99a] Then too, Herbert E. Parker[195b] recently demonstrated other related actions of magnesium. He showed that, in rats, a magnesium deficiency decreased the phosphorus level in bone and blood plasma but increased the calcium content of the kidney, heart, liver, muscles and testes. Dietary magnesium, in Parker's study, affected tissue calcium levels more at normal phosphorus levels than at lower phosphorus levels.

Adequate dietary magnesium plays a significant role in reducing the incidence of cardiovascular disorders. I. Szelenyi[187] cites several references attributing success in the treatment of angina pectoris to use of magnesium salts. Szelenyi also gives six ways in which magnesium opposes the progress of arteriosclerosis:

1. Mg impedes the deposition of Ca in the aortic wall.
2. It lowers elevated serum cholesterol levels.
3. It decreases serum total lipid concentration and, within that scope, also the serum level of triglycerides and beta-lipoproteins.
4. It impedes the "aging" of collagen.
5. It elicits an increase in fibrinolytic activity.
6. It stabilizes blood platelets.

Geoffrey H. Bourne and many other investigators have reported that magnesium has an antihypertensive effect. Robert Whang et al.[196,196a] found hypertensive patients deficient in magnesium required more drugs to maintain their blood pressure than did those with normal magnesium levels. A deficiency of magnesium is reported to lead to constriction of coronary arteries, whereas an adequate supply leads to vasodilatation. T. Dyckner and P. O. Wester[97] reported that 20 patients receiving long-term diuretic treatment for hypertension (and, therefore, perhaps very magnesium deficient) were benefitted by magnesium supplementation.* Supplementation with magnesium aspartate hydrochloride resulted in decreasing their systolic pressure by an average of 12 mm Hg and their diastolic pressure by 8 mm Hg.

However, others, referenced by J. Mendiola, Jr. et al.,[198]report that rat experiments show magnesium slows the heartbeat, while tension is either *increased* or not changed. Still other scientists, including some cited by Mendiola [198] and others cited by Warren Wacker and Bert L. Vallee,[199] have reported that rats, and also humans on magnesium-deficient diets, had a decreased blood pressure. This may be yet another example of the *reverse effect:* a modest intake of magnesium may produce lower blood pressure; large amounts (possibly through inhibiting calcium usage) may lead to increased blood pressure. In attempting to explain magnesium's effect in lowering blood pressure, Hebbel E. Hoff et al.[200] theorize that magnesium's role in the fall of blood pressure may be due to vasodilatation. (They also reported, in experiments with dogs, that magnesium produced a marked rise in skin temperature which persisted for some time.) In corroboration of the speculation of the Hoff group, Altura et al.[200a] reported that magnesium deficiency in rats resulted in reduced capillary, postcapillary and venular blood flow concomitant with reduced terminal arteriolar, precapillary sphincter and venular lumen sizes. Other studies showing magnesium to be effective in reducing hypertension are cited in a more recent issue of *Nutrition Reviews*.[200b] On the contrary, recent research by F. P. Cappuccio et al.[200c] found no fall in blood pressure when 17 unselected patients with mild to moderate essential hypertension were given 15 mmol per day of magnesium as magnesium aspartate. They noted, however, that the period of their study was rather short and therefore cannot be used to draw any definite conclusion about possible long-term effects.

There is yet another way in which adequate magnesium seems to protect the heart. D. Lehr et al.[201] have reported a good correlation in

---

* One must continually resist the conclusion that, just because a supplement aids one who is deficient in a given vitamin or mineral, that supplement will similarly aid those not deficient.

rats between the extent of magnesium loss from the heart and the degree of acute myocardial injury. In fact, Joachim Manthey et al. [202] conclude that a deficiency of magnesium, but *not* of other metals studied, is present in patients with severe coronary heart disease. L. T. Iseri and A. R. Bures [203] maintain that magnesium deficiency may also be the hidden factor in ventricular arrythmias, especially in patients with a strong alcoholic history. Michelle Speich et al. [204] also hold that magnesium depletion may be a cause of arrythmias. In speculating as to why a deficiency of magnesium may influence cardiac arrhythmias, Thomas Dyckner and Per Ola Wester [205] make the following suggestions. Magnesium may exert its influence by:

1. A direct effect;
2. An effect on potassium metabolism; or
3. An effect as a calcium-blocking agent.

They point out that if the effect involves potassium, it may be that a magnesium deficiency interferes with the action of membrane ATPase and thus the pumping of sodium out of the cell and potassium into the cell would be impaired. * Lloyd T. Iseri et al. [206a] have theorized that "magnesium depletion probably interferes with sodium-potassium adenosine triphosphate enzyme activity and causes ionic imbalances and electrical instability of Purkinje's fibres." They continue, "Without obvious magnesium depletion this element in high concentration may still prolong transient inward current, prolong refractory period, increase the membrane potential and control ventricular tachyarrhythmia." In related work, Leon Cohen [207] reported intravenous and intramuscular magnesium sulphate abolished digitalis-toxic arrhythmia in seven patients. The role of magnesium in heart health seems apparent, with only the mode of its action being in doubt.

Joachim Manthey et al. [202] found that patients with severe coronary heart disease (CHD) have lower mean serum magnesium

---

* R. P. C. Bigg and R. Chia [206] discovered that a magnesium deficiency often is present with a potassium deficiency, can also cause it and can prevent correction of the potassium deficiency if potassium supplements are used alone.

levels than those without CHD. R. B. Singh et al[208a] made several other findings relative to cardiovascular disease. They cited their own earlier studies which showed that magnesium deficiency sensitizes the myocardium to the toxic effects of digoxin and other drugs. They observed that, while calcium in the myocardium and in the blood is associated with myocardial hyperexcitability, coronary constriction and ventricular arrhythmias, hypermagnesemia causes dilatation of the coronary artery. They also stated that high intake of vitamin D intensifies damage caused by magnesium deficiency.* Others have also warned that it may be especially dangerous for patients on digitalis to be magnesium deficient and it is recommended that administration of supplemental magnesium be considered for them.[209-211]

Stroke patients have also been reported to often be deficient in magnesium, both in the serum and in the cerebrospinal fluid (CSF). Bella T. Altura and Burton M. Altura[211a] point out that magnesium concentration in the CSF is normally 40% higher than that of the plasma and that cerebral arteries generally have 100% more magnesium than do arteries in other regions of the body. In another study, the Alturas[211b] reported that the amount of calculated free, ionic magnesium in the CSF is estimated to be three times greater than that in the plasma. These facts suggest the vital nature of magnesium for normal operation of the nerves and brain. In yet another study, the Alturas[211c] have pointed out that excess calcium ion uptake in neuronal

---

* On the other hand, according to Robert K. Rude et al.[208] serum concentrations of 1,25(OH)₂D are frequently low in patients with magnesium deficiency. Rude and his coworkers suggested a normal 1,25(OH)₂D level is needed for parathyroid hormone-mediated response to magnesium administration. A low level of 1,25(OH)₂D exacerbates a magnesium deficiency (according to Rude et al.), modest levels of both 1,25(OH)₂D and oral vitamin D are associated with normal magnesium levels and (according to Singh et al.)[208a] a high vitamin D intake reverses the action of normal amounts of vitamin D by once again exacerbating the bad effects of depressed magnesium levels. A *reverse effect* has not really been demonstrated since we are dealing with two different entities, oral vitamin D and serum 1,25(OH)₂D. Even if Singh and his coworkers had made their findings in terms of 1,25(OH)₂D rather than in terms of oral vitamin D, we would not be certain that a *reverse effect* had been demonstrated. Why not? Because the experimental protocol of Singh et al. may not have sufficiently matched that of the Rude group., i.e., the presumed *reverse effect* could have been due to a protocol variable or variables other than that of vitamin D intake. Nevertheless, I think it likely that the presumed *reverse effect* is genuine.

cells is thought to be the prime cause of neuronal death in the brain and that a magnesium deficiency can be an exacerbating factor.

A magnesium deficiency may also be a contributing factor to the incidence of migraine headache. Burton M. Altura[211d] observes that stress, menstruation, pregnancy, alcohol, many diuretics and reserpine, which are all known to provoke migraine, can produce hypomagnesemia. He notes that chocolates and cheeses, which provoke migraine, contain tyramine which, in the presence of low cerebrovascular magnesium, can result in cerebrovasospasm. He points out that there is often a familial tendency to be susceptible to migraine which is consonant with the known fact that magnesium in certain tissues (perhaps including the brain) is under genetic control.

Jerry K. Aikawa[211e] has reported on a study made between 1963 and 1965 by the U.S. Geological Survey and the Heart Disease and Stroke Control Program, U.S. Public Health Service, of two groups of contiguous or nearly contiguous counties of northern Georgia that were known to have much different cardiovascular mortality rates. The garden soil from those counties with the low rate of cardiovascular death contained almost nine times as much magnesium as the soil in the high-rate area.

Writing in 1986, H. Sandvad Rasmussen et al.[211f] reported on a double-blind, randomized, placebo-controlled study of 273 persons suspected of having acute myocardial infarction (AMI). Of 130 patients with proven AMI, 56 received magnesium and 74 received placebo. During the first four weeks after treatment, mortality was 9% in the placebo group and just 7% in the magnesium group. In the magnesium group 21% had arrhythmias that needed treatment compared with 47% in the placebo group.

H. J. Holtmeier and M. Kuhn[212] reported that in Finland, the European country with the highest mortality from coronary heart disease, the average magnesium intake decreased to a third of its original value between 1911 and 1963. Furthermore, they found that in Japan, which has the lowest coronary heart disease mortality rate, the average daily magnesium intake is 560 mg./day which is, of course, far above the RDA set in the U.S. by the National Academy of Sciences. (It is possible that the life-style of the Japanese may require more magnesium than is required by the American life-style, but this seems to me to be only a remote possibility. Holtmeier and Kuhn concluded that due to the environmental changes, technological refinement of food, alteration of food habits and living conditions, an adequate magnesium supply is not assured. They therefore recommended magnesium supplementation for persons not getting an adequate supply of this mineral in their diet.

Holtmeier and Kuhn have considerable company in their doubt about the magnesium adequacy of the typical diet. N. E. Johnson and C. Philipps[213] studied pregnant women in Wisconsin. The magnesium content of their diets was found to range from 103 to 333 mg. with an average value of 204 mg. This contrasts with the RDA for pregnant or lactating women of 450 mg. (which some suspect is also not adequate). Since there seems to be a correlation between birth weight of infants and their mother's supply of magnesium, Johnson and Philipps call for additional studies in this area.

Adequate magnesium may be important as a cancer inhibitor. J. Aleksandrowicz and J. Stachura[214] found confirmation of epidemiological data suggesting a link between magnesium deficiency in the soil and cancer. They also commented on the significance of magnesium deficiency in the pathogenesis of human and animal leukemia. Then too, Jerome M. Blondell[215] has reviewed various lines of evidence that suggest magnesium has an anticarcinogenic effect and concludes that magnesium shows promise as a cancer inhibitor. Its mode of action in working to prevent cancer is thought to lie in enhancing the fidelity of DNA replication. On the contrary, F. M. Parsons and G. A. Young[216] reported that cancer regressed in a group of rats and also in two out of nine human cancer patients when magnesium and potassium *depletion* was induced. More recently, Betty J. Mills et al.[216a] reported that magnesium depletion in rats resulted in a 46% inhibition of tumor growth and they suggested that this could be significant for nutritional management of tumor patients.

Magnesium has been shown to inhibit the formation of both calcium oxalate and calcium phosphate crystals in the urine. Many references supporting the use of magnesium (sometimes along with vitamin B6)* to prevent kidney stones are cited by G. Johansson et al.[217-218a] Research by the Johansson group indicated that urinary excretions of magnesium and calcium in both stone formers and controls were positively correlated. Nevertheless, as subjects showed rising excretion values for both calcium and magnesium, the magnesium/calcium ratio declined. The Johansson group concluded that their clinical experience supports the use of magnesium for the treatment of idiopathic calcium stone formation. An *in vitro* study by P. C. Hallson et al.[219] gives support to the use of magnesium in preventing kidney stones. They induced a magnesium deficiency in normal volunteers by giving cellulose phosphate. The urine of the volunteers was then studied and there was found to be an inverse correlation between magnesium concentration and calcium oxalate crystal formation.

However, Hans Göran Tiselius et al.[220] reported that they found no such favorable results in treating renal stone patients with magnesium oxide. Walther Wunderlich[221] agrees that magnesium is not adequate prophylaxis against the formation of calcium oxalate urinary calculus. He reports that magnesium tends to result in the formation of *larger* crystals.

J. Thomas et al.,[222] attempting to resolve the dispute concerning magnesium's effect in kidney-stone formers, studied the action of various magnesium compounds in the treatment of oxalic lithiasis. The Thomas group experimented with rats and employed chloride, lactate and trisilicate salts of magnesium. They concluded that the anticrystallization action on calcium oxalate was greatest when the trisilicate form of magnesium was used in an amount approximating 300 mg. of magnesium per day.** The scientists stated, however,

---

* Recently, in 1986, J. Eisinger and J. Dagorn[216b] have found that only at high dosages will vitamin B6 help to increase erythrocyte magnesium. They found that dosages of 1 gram or less per day had no effect on intestinal absorption of magnesium and they caution, as have others, about using B6 in dosages that might result in neurological damage. Eisinger and Dagorn left open the possibility that doses of 1 gram or less might have benefits on the levels of leukocyte magnesium.

** Could these results relate to the unsettling fact that the magnesium in magnesium trisilicate is rather unavailable to the body? According to E. G. Huf,[223] only 5% of the

that there were still many failures in clinical treatment. Thus, this use of magnesium to either dissolve or prevent formation of kidney stones may not be as convincing a procedure as popular "health" literature would suggest. Then too, D. A. Levison et al.[224] reported the occurrence of pure silicon dioxide (silica) urinary bladder stones in a patient who had taken magnesium trisilicate three times a day for 40 years for indigestion.

Magnesium sulphate has been used successfully as a tocolytic agent (i.e., one that inhibits premature labor). John P. Elliott,[224a] in a study involving 355 patients with diagnoses of premature labor, found that delivery was delayed in the majority of patients by intravenous administration of magnesium sulphate.

Earlier, in citing some of the manifestations of magnesium deficiency, I included convulsions in infants. A deficiency of magnesium may also be a factor in that mysterious killer of babies—SIDS, Sudden Infant Death Syndrome or, as it is called in Britain, S.U.D., Sudden Unexpected Death in Infancy. We discussed this distressing problem in connection with vitamins C and E and with biotin since lack of these vitamins is thought by some to be a contributing cause. Dr. Joan L. Caddell[225] of the St. Louis University School of Medicine believes, on the other hand, that the culprit may be a critical deficiency of magnesium. Caddell suggests that the mechanism through which magnesium deficiency may act to bring on crib death is the liberation of histamine. We all know from our experience with colds how histamine can cause a swelling and irritation of membranes. Infants can release relatively more histamine than adults and this flood of histamine dilates blood vessels. At the same time, the permeability of capillaries is increased and the blood leaks away from its proper route. Perhaps this is what leads to death. It has also been suggested that the lack of magnesium, leading to excessive histamine, might cause anaphylactic shock. A pregnant woman should make sure that she gets enough of magnesium and manganese since deficiencies of these elements in her diet may be the start of the baby's troubles. After birth, the pediatrician and parents

---

magnesium of magnesium trisilicate is absorbed by the body compared to 21%-25% of the element in the sulphate form.

should make sure the baby continues to receive sufficient quantities of these minerals.

Anesthesia risks are minimized, and postoperative pain is markedly lowered, according to Dr. Josef Lämmle[226] by oral administration of magnesium-potassium salts of aspartic acid. The aspartic salts of magnesium and potassium—now sold by some health food suppliers but formerly available only by prescription under the trade names Spartase, Trophicard and Aspara—are sometimes prescribed by doctors to combat fatigue or sexual lassitude, especially in women. The combination of these salts is also reported to strengthen various muscles (including the heart) and to be effective in counteracting high blood pressure.

Elyett Gueux et al.[226a] reported that, in rats, a magnesium deficiency *increased* plasma triglycerides and free cholesterol levels but *decreased* esterified cholesterol levels. Esterified cholesterol, in turn, is required by the adrenal cortex for the manufacture of the steroids, including cortisol and the sex hormones. Perhaps because of its effect on the adrenal glands, a deficiency of magnesium in rats was reported by M. Santillana et al.[227] to have brought on skin disorders and gray hair. Human prostatic fluid is very rich in magnesium.[227a] Animal experiments have shown that the activity of the enzyme 5-nucleotidase, which is found in human semen, is enhanced by magnesium (but inhibited by fluoride).[227b] Mice experiments by S. Dalterio et al.[227c] have shown that magnesium is required for production of testosterone. Between magnesium ion concentrations of 0 and 5 mM (the upper limit of the range studied) there was a dose-response increase of testosterone production as the magnesium ion concentration rose.

Adverse Effects of Excess

We have already observed some adverse effects attending excessive supplementation of magnesium. Let's now note some other possible negatives. P. Larvor[228] points out that, while calcium stimulates secretion of insulin, vasopressin, catecholamines, FSH, etc., magnesium inhibits many types of cell secretions such as insulin, catecholamines and oxytocin. (Some of these involve *reverse effects*.) Pharmacologic doses of magnesium can have a curare-form action on the neuromuscular junction, presumably through interference with the release of acetylcholine in the motor nerve terminals.[223] These inhibitory effects give us good reasons to not overdo our consumption of magnesium.

In the matter of teeth protection, magnesium may also exhibit a negative action. Popular nutrition writers have been known to make excessive claims for magnesium as a factor in preventing caries. There is undoubtedly an element of truth in their position since magnesium does enter into formation of bones, including the teeth. (F. C. M. Driessens and R. M. H. Verbeeck[228a] theorized that dolomite is formed during the mineralization of tooth enamel.) However, C. Robinson et al.[228b] found that the distribution patterns of magnesium suggest a correlation between magnesium concentration and low density enamel. They make a case for the possibility that magnesium and carbonate-rich enamel near fissures might be a factor in the progress of carious destruction. They also note that S. Thiradilok and F. Feagin[228c] found that magnesium seems to inhibit remineralization. Furthermore, Matti Knuuttila et al.[229] cite many references implicating magnesium in the mineralization of calculus, especially in the formation of Mg-whitlochite. Whitlochite is a form of calcium phosphate which may combine with magnesium (and also with zinc) to form subgingival calculus. Gron et al.[229a] found that the magnesium content of calculus was not only correlated positively with the abundance of whitlochite but negatively with the abundance of octacalcium phosphate. These possibly negative dental effects give us yet another reason to not overdo the intake of magnesium. A caries-enhancement effect of magnesium (in rats) was reported by H. Luoma et al.[230]

Magnesium supplementation is probably also contraindicated, according to Warren E. C. Wacker and Bert L. Vallee,[231] in those with kidney problems. Wacker and Vallee noted that blood pressure is often lowered when magnesium sulphate is administered to patients with glomerular nephritis. Nevertheless, magnesium is probably contraindicated in cases of severe renal disease. In kidney disease the process of urinary excretion is often interfered with and hypermagnesemia may result. Large supplementary amounts of magnesium can also cause diarrhea. John P. Mordes and Warren E. C. Wacker[231a] have written extensively on the dangers of excess magnesium and have cited a total of 471 references.

Although we have cited some negatives to excessive intake of magnesium, hypomagnesemia is probably a far more frequent occurrence. Supplementation may be especially important for those consuming large amounts of alcohol. F. W. Heaton et al.[232] reported that, in a study of four subjects, magnesium excretion rose to 260% of the control value after alcohol ingestion. (Calcium excretion increased 68%, sodium excretion was unchanged and potassium excretion decreased slightly.) The investigators conclude that this excessive excretion of magnesium is the reason hypomagnesemia is so prevalent among chronic alcoholics.

Food Sources and Supplements

Food sources for magnesium are bran, wheat germ, oatmeal, nuts, peanuts, seeds, prunes, figs, chard, kale, lettuce, sorrel, cocoa, beet leaves, kohlrabi, celery, spinach, parsley, brussels sprouts, soybeans, buckwheat, clams, snails, citrus fruits, purple grapes, plums, corn, brown rice, apples and honey.* In some of these foods, however, magnesium may be tied up as phytate or oxalate. The fiber or phytate in the bran of wheat, for example, may inhibit the absorption of magnesium and other minerals (including calcium, iron and zinc) from the intestinal tract, but one need not conclude that wheat bran is to be avoided. It is probably an excellent food; just make sure you get enough magnesium (and other metals) to offset the effect of the fiber or phytate. On the other hand, a disturbing study by George H. Hitchings and Elvira A. Falco[232a] reported that mice fed whole wheat bread were more susceptible to pneumonococcal infection than those fed white bread. In this case an unknown factor in the crude bread was more beneficial to the parasitic organism than to the animal consuming the food. Whole wheat bread seems to be a "health" food for pneumonococci!

---

* Some "nutritional" breads contain the laxative magnesium sulphate (which is also known as Epsom salts). Laxative action might promote weight loss, but it seems at cross-purposes to expect maximum nutritional intake simultaneously with trying to rid the body of the bread's nutrients before they can be absorbed.

The magnesium requirement for men is somewhat higher than it is for women since men excrete more of the element. Sexually active men lose additional amounts in semen—the prostatic component of which is especially rich in this mineral. At one time it was thought that semen components from other glands in the male genital tract were also rich sources of magnesium. R. Eliasson and C. Lindholmer,[232b] however, analyzing split ejaculates, found that the first and second fraction (primarily from the prostate) contained far more magnesium than did later fractions (Figure 12). Interestingly, while acid phosphatase content of the various fractions corresponds with that of magnesium, fructose content does not. Fructose, the fuel that impels sperm, is more concentrated in later ejaculates.[232b]

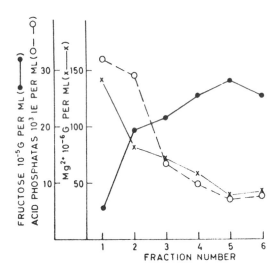

Figure 12. Distribution of magnesium, acid phosphatase and fructose in a split ejaculate. The correlation between magnesium and acid phosphatase indicates that magnesium originates from the prostate gland. Reproduced from R. Eliasson and C. Lindholmer, *Investigative Urology* (1972) 9, no. 4: 286-289, with permission of the publisher, Williams and Wilkens Co., and of the authors.

It is widely held that the magnesium intake should be about one-half that of calcium.* Garry F. Gordon,[232c] however, is concerned that excessive calcium may contribute to arterial calcification. He favors "limited use of calcium supplements, maintaining a 1:1 calcium to magnesium ratio." He goes on to say "a 1:2 calcium to magnesium ratio can be beneficial for short-term treatment." As I have indicated, his is a minority view.

Supplementary magnesium may be taken as dolomite (calcium plus magnesium) but magnesium in this form is not very assimilable and, furthermore, the dolomite may contain excessive lead. If you are going to supplement with magnesium, use instead the more assimilable forms of magnesium oxide, magnesium gluconate, magnesium alginate (which is derived from kelp), magnesium in the form of an amino-acid chelate or perhaps magnesium orotate, but the same reservations stated in regard to calcium orotate would apply.** Furthermore, R. D. Lindeman[233] has reported on studies indicating that physiologic amounts of vitamin D can promote a positive magnesium balance. However, large amounts of vitamin D exhibit a *reverse effect* by increasing urinary magnesium excretion and thus work to create a negative magnesium balance. By the way, although it was at one time believed that calcium and magnesium compete for absorption, it now appears that the intestinal transport of each of

---

* That's a commonly heard idea but it could be simplistic. If magnesium orotate, for example, goes into the body as efficiently as claimed, why wouldn't the "ideal" ratio of magnesium to calcium be lower for those using this form? If calcium orotate but not magnesium orotate were used, why wouldn't the "ideal" ratio be higher? It seems possible, however, that the presumed higher bioavailability of calcium, magnesium and zinc orotates may be fictional. G. Andermann and M. Dietz[232d] found, in a study using female rabbits, that the bioavailabilities of zinc from oral ingestion of zinc sulfate, zinc pantothenate and zinc orotate were virtually the same. Rabbits are not people and zinc orotate may act differently than orotates of calcium or magnesium, but the results suggest that the "orotate story" may be questionable.

** Potassium and magnesium salts of aspartic acid are also available. They have been shown, in several animal experiments, to have a beneficial effect on muscle fatigability. Björn Ahlborg et al.[233b] showed that this effect is demonstrable in humans. They found that by giving each of six young men 1.75 grams of potassium-magnesium-aspartate at six-hour intervals, their capacity for prolonged exercise increased significantly. On the contrary, A. de Haan et al.[233c] found that potassium and magnesium aspartate had no observable effect on short-term intensive muscular activity among human volunteers. Other scientists, cited by de Haan and his associates, have reported 20%-50% increase in human submaximal work load after taking these aspartates.

these ions is largely independent of the other.[233a] Thus, supplements of these minerals can be effective whether they are taken together or separately.

Tell Your Doctor

If you are taking magnesium supplements and are being examined by a physician, be sure to tell him not only about the drugs but also about the vitamins or minerals you may be taking. Magnesium supplements can result in a false-positive indication on the Diagnex blue test for impaired gastric function. Furthermore, the ubiquitous presence of magnesium in so many cathartics and antacids presents a possible threat of hypermagnesemia, and of decreased iron absorption,[234] especially among the elderly who may be overdoing consumption of these drugs.[234a]

In summarizing a study relating magnesium to contraction of vascular smooth muscles and to vascular diseases, Burton M. Altura and Bella T. Altura[234b] said, "...these data are consistent with the hypothesis that [Mg^{2+}] and membrane Mg may exert a regulatory role in vascular reactivity, or peripheral vascular resistance and may have an important functional role in control of Ca uptake, content, and distribution in smooth muscle cells. Certain vascular disease states that are associated with a deficiency (e.g., sudden-death ischemic heart disease, diabetes mellitus, hypertension) or excess (e.g., circulatory shock, renal vascular disorders) in plasma and tissue Mg may be reflections of the direct vascular actions of the lack, or excess of, this metal, respectively." Remember that, while magnesium is probably often undersupplied in the diet and such deficiency can produce dire consequences, an excess can also lead to grave problems.

Zinc

Zinc is a vital mineral needed for many body functions. Definitive studies, however, as reported by Noel W. Solomons,[235] show that many persons do not get the equivalent of the RDA. Solomons says, "The customary intake of zinc does not approach the

RDA level for any adult group. In fact, the mean intake ranged from 46 to 63% of the RDA." Solomons goes on to point out, however, that one need not *absorb* the equivalent of the zinc RDA to maintain growth or health. The important consideration, in addition to the amount of zinc in the diet, is its *biological availability* and we will have more to say on this topic a bit later.

Most of the zinc in the serum is loosely bound to albumin. However, according to Jerry L. Phillips and Parviz Azari,[236] the biologically active complex is zinc-transferrin, not zinc-albumin. We met transferrin in connection with iron, but it is also used to transport not only iron but zinc, cobalt, nickel, copper and manganese. The competitive binding to transferrin accounts for the fact that these metals interfere with each other's absorption. An editorial in the *British Medical Jrl.*[236a] states that a low plasma concentration of zinc is almost certainly due to a change in the concentration of one of the zinc binders—albumin, α_2-macroglobulin, transferrin and amino acids—rather than to a true depletion with a fall in the cell content of zinc.

Zinc is a component of the enzymes carboxypeptidase A and B in pancreatic juice. In this way zinc aids in the metabolism of proteins and facilitates food absorption through the intestines. It is a constituent of many other enzymes and increases the activity of still others. *Carbonic anhydrase,* an enzyme which is involved in the breathing process and present in the gastrointestinal mucosa, the kidneys and in many other areas of the body, contains zinc. It is reported that a low level of zinc in the hair is associated with a deficiency of stomach acid.[237] Zinc contributes to the chemical reactions whereby our bodies synthesize the nucleic acids DNA and RNA. Another valuable property of zinc is that, as a component of *lactate dehydrogenase,* which is important for reactions involving pyruvic and lactic acids, it improves exercise tolerance. John H. Richardson and Pamela D. Drake,[237a] in experiments with the isolated gastrocnemius muscle of rats, reported that oral zinc supplementation resulted in significantly longer fatigue time than was shown by unsupplemented controls. In this regard, Nanaya Tamaki et al.[237b] have shown that, at concentrations lower than .46 mM, zinc is a

more effective activator of the enzyme phosphofructokinase and
therefore of glycolysis than is magnesium. (Glycolysis is the process
of conversion of carbohydrate, in tissues, to pyruvic or lactic acid,
with release of energy.) As the concentration of zinc increases,
phosphofructokinase activity and lactate production continues to
increase, but at .5 mM a *reverse effect* sets in and lactate production
is inhibited (Figure 13). Zinc inhibits the activity of some enzymes,
activates others and then, at different concentrations, may exhibit a
reverse effect by inhibiting those very enzymes it had stimulated.[238]

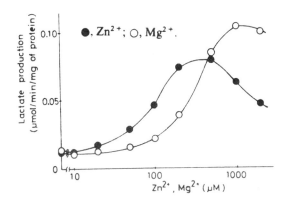

Figure 13. Activation of muscle lactate production by Zn^{2+} or
Mg^{2+}. Reproduced from Nanaya Tamaki et al., *Jrl. of
Nutritional Science and Vitaminology* (1983) 29: 655-662,
with permission of the Center for Academic Publications,
Japan, and of the authors. Note the *reverse effect* as the
concentration of zinc ions increases above 500 µM (.5 mM).
(There appears to also be a *reverse effect* when magnesium
ion concentration exceeds 1,000 µM.)

Drs. William H. Strain and Walter J. Pories[239] point out that
women between menarche and menopause have far higher levels of
zinc (and of other minerals) in their hair than men or premenarchial
girls or postmenopausal women. (M. H. Briggs et al.[240] have
reported, however, that the content of zinc in hair is low in
pregnancy, probably a reflection of the lowered plasma zinc at that

time.) Furthermore, the zinc level in the hair of young men was found, in general, to be lower in summer than in winter, but the small number of persons in the study made the result questionable.[241] K. Michael Hambridge[241a] later confirmed, however, that zinc levels in hair were generally much higher for both boys and girls in February than in September.

Zinc is used in treating various skin problems. A rare congenital defect of zinc absorption, acrodermatitis enteropathica, responds well to zinc therapy.[242] To cite another example, K. C. Verma et al.[243] studied the effect of oral zinc sulphate on patients having acne vulgaris. In a double-blind trial, 29 patients received 60 mg. of zinc sulphate daily and 27 were given a placebo. Of the 29 patients receiving the zinc, 17 (58%) showed significant improvement, while there was no change in the placebo group. Verma reported that the serum vitamin A levels of the treated group rose significantly. (There is, as we noted earlier, a close relationship between zinc and blood levels of vitamin A.)

M. K. Song et al.[243a] have shown that, based on rat experiments, the absorption of zinc and its transport rate is influenced by the amount of arachidonic acid (AA) present. Zinc absorption and transport in rats orally administered .5 mg. of AA decreased but showed a *reverse effect* by increasing when 1.0 mg. or 1.5 mg. of AA was given. Zinc absorption and transport seems to be influenced by AA's modulation of the relative levels of the prostaglandins, PGE_2, $PGF_{2\alpha}$ and PGI_2 in the plasma and small intestine.

As related in Chapter 3, zinc is a factor in the metabolism of linoleic acid. It interacts with delta-6-desaturase to convert linoleic acid to gamma-linolenic acid which, in turn, forms dihomo-gamma-linolenic acid which is partially converted into PGE_1.[244]* In cases of zinc deficiency, the concentration of PGE_1 will generally be quite low. (The concentrations of PGE_2 and $PGF_{2\alpha}$, on the other hand, tend to be significantly higher in the plasma of zinc-deficient rats than in pair-fed controls. Prostacyclin is lower in zinc-deficient rats than in

---

* Copper inhibits Δ6-desaturation of linoleic acid by enhancing oleic acid synthesis and metabolism to eicosatrienoic acid.[245] Lithium also blocks the actions of zinc in fostering formation of prostaglandins.[246]

controls fed *ad libitum*.)[247] Interestingly, evening primrose oil (a natural source of linoleic acid and gamma-linolenic acid) will reverse many biological effects caused by zinc deficiency.* For example, evening primrose oil (but not safflower oil) restored weight of adrenal and thymus glands of rats to near normal after a zinc deficiency had caused them to atrophy. Thus, zinc's effect on the immune system may relate to its beneficial action in forming prostaglandin E_1, a substance especially needed by T-lymphocytes. Prostaglandin E_1 is an antiaggregatory and a vasodilatory agent and this may also explain zinc's beneficial influence in these actions. Therefore, the beneficial action of the essential fatty acids in working to prevent atherosclerosis and hypertension may depend on the availability of adequate zinc.[249] However, the comments to be made later regarding the copper/zinc ratio, and Klevay's opinion that zinc is often overconsumed relative to copper, suggest that we continue to remember the doctrine of moderation. Furthermore, R. F. Borgman et al.[250] reported that high levels of hair zinc (and low levels of hair copper) were related to higher blood pressure in humans.

Drs. Strain and Pories[251] have found that the levels of zinc in the hair and in various body organs of those having atherosclerosis are quite low. Dr. Pories, acting on this information, has treated atherosclerosis successfully by giving zinc supplements. Is zinc deficiency a cause of atherosclerosis? Assuming a cause-and-effect relationship may not be warranted since seemingly causal factors may merely be associated phenomena. However, it has been reported that adequate zinc can lower blood cholesterol levels and that patients with atherosclerosis who are given zinc show improvement even when, in peripheral vascular diseases, the situation is complicated by early gangrene. Philip L. Hooper et al.,[252] on the contrary, point out that rats on a high-zinc diet show an *increase* in serum cholesterol. Furthermore, in a study involving 12 healthy adult men, Hooper et al. found that ingestion of 440 mg. of zinc sulphate per day reduced

---

* Oil containing low amounts of essential fatty acids and high amounts of oleic acid, e.g., olive oil, does not benefit zinc-deficient rats and actually exacerbates skin lesions.[248]

high-density lipoprotein cholesterol (HDL) 25% below baseline values. Since HDL is believed to protect against atherosclerosis, this study indicated that excessive zinc ingestion may be atherogenic in man. (The concept of the *reverse effect* would suggest that the Strain and Pories group and the Hooper group could both be right. Zinc deficiency or zinc excess could cause atherosclerosis.)

Animal research of Dr. L. Klevay[253] has indicated that too great a zinc concentration relative to copper can lead to improper cholesterol handling and heart attacks. Nevertheless, not everyone is agreed as to the existence of a zinc-cholesterol connection. L. Murthy and H. Petering[254] reported that serum cholesterol is inversely related to the level of dietary or serum copper, regardless of the zinc level. Furthermore, Philip L. Hooper and Philip J. Garry[255] present data that indicate even very high zinc/copper ratios (up to 33:1) do not affect lipid metabolism. Other criticisms of Klevay's position have been made by Peter W. F. Fisher and Maurice W. Collins.[256] Nevertheless, a recent study by M. Katya-Katya et al.[256a] of rats supplemented with 200 mg. of zinc/kg. of diet daily for seven months resulted in increased plasma zinc, zinc/copper ratio and cholesterol. All differences were significant after three months (Figure 14). Contrary to the findings of Murthy and Petering[254] cited above, cholesterol levels increased in the Katya-Katya study even though copper was present in what they called adequate amounts. Recent work has also shown that high dosages of zinc (160 mg. daily) lowered the beneficial HDL-cholesterol, whereas low-dose zinc supplementation did not affect lipid or lipoprotein values in either endurance-trained or sedentary men.[256b]

Zinc deficiencies can cause many problems among humans and among animals. Ayhan O. Cavdar[257] reported that mothers of anencephalic babies (those with partial or complete absence of brain) had extreme zinc deficiency in both plasma and red blood cells. It is well known that a deficiency of any of a number of minerals or vitamins can cause teratogenic effects among animals, but here's a surprising note: Lucille S. Hurley and Shyy-Hwa Tao[258,259] found that those teratogenic effects of zinc deficiency were partially eliminated if there was, at the same time, a lack of dietary calcium.

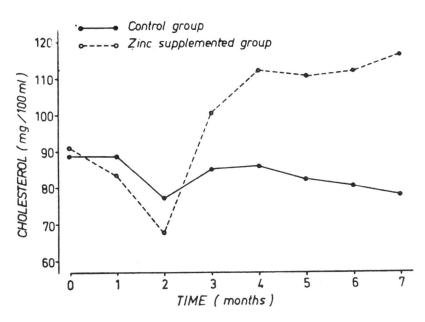

Figure 14. Variation of cholesterol levels in control and zinc-supplemented rats. Graph reproduced from M. Katya-Katya et al., *Nutrition Research* (1984) 4: 633-638, with permission of the publisher, Pergamon Press, and of the authors.

Female rats fed a diet lacking in both zinc and calcium during pregnancy had larger litters, fewer resorptions and fewer malformed fetuses than those fed a diet deficient in just zinc. The latter study showed that the alleviation of the teratogenic effects did not occur in parathyroidectomized rats. This supports the hypothesis that conditions bringing about bone resorption increase the availability of skeletal zinc.

A deficiency of zinc could, perhaps, be a factor in alleviating rheumatoid arthritis. At any rate, Peter A. Simkin[260] fed 220 mg. of zinc sulphate, three times daily, to patients with rheumatoid arthritis. Placebos were given a group of similar patients and both the zinc-supplemented and the placebo patients were instructed to continue with their previous medication. Simkin observed that patients taking zinc sulphate experienced lessened joint swelling, reduced morning stiffness and also fared better in all other clinical parameters than the placebo group.

Zinc interacts with and is related to insulin in ways not completely understood. Using *in vitro* experiments, L. Coulston and P. Dandona[261] reported that zinc strongly stimulates lipogenesis by adipocytes (the major cells in fatty connective tissue). This is similar to the effect of insulin. James M. May and Charles S. Contoreggi[262] discovered that the insulin-like effects of zinc in adipocytes are caused not only by the direct effects of the zinc ion on intracellular metabolism, but also indirectly by effects related to the generation of hydrogen peroxide.

Zinc has been used successfully to treat stomach ulcers. An experiment with rats by C. H. Cho et al.[263] may help explain its beneficial effect. Cho et al. found that intraperitoneal treatment with zinc sulphate reduced gastric secretion and lesions induced by methacholine. Then too, Donald J. Frommer[264] reported that, in a double-blind trial of oral zinc sulphate (660 mg. daily in three 220-mg. doses for three weeks), patients given the zinc sulphate had an ulcer healing rate three times that of patients treated with placebos. Frommer reported that there was no evidence of zinc deficiency in any of the patients and no side effects from the zinc sulphate were noted. Haeger and Lanner, as well as earlier investigators, have reported that oral zinc sulphate also accelerates healing of leg ulcers.[264a] S. L. Wallace et al.[264b] and Carol E. Williamson et al.[264c] suggest that zinc may be useful in treating periodontal and other oral wound healing. It seems likely that these phenomena, like so many other actions of zinc, may relate to its influence on the production of prostaglandins, a topic which we have already considered.

According to a study of Naval Academy students conducted by Adon A. Gordus et al.,[264d] the hair of those earning high grades contained far more zinc, copper and cobalt (and, astonishingly, more aluminum) than did the hair of students of lesser academic accomplishments. On the other hand, one might speculate on the possibility that some persons may have an increased rate of learning because they get rid of excesses of zinc and of the other three minerals by excreting those excesses via their hair.* Under this line of reasoning one would avoid zinc and the other three minerals in order to become a faster learner. This hypothesis illustrates the possibility of opposite lines of reasoning in explaining many types of scientific phenomena. However, similar studies but with rats, made under the direction of Donald Oberleas[264e] at the medical school of Wayne State University in Detroit, support the idea that zinc may increase learning rates. It has been found that zinc-supplemented rats showed improved rates of learning when it came to running mazes.

Nevertheless, there are cases where a high zinc concentration in the hair may be a sign of zinc deficiency elsewhere in the body. Karl E. Bergmann et al.,[265] as well as Karl E. Bergmann and Renate L. Bergmann,[265a] reported that a group of 17 mothers of infants with *spina bifida cystica* generally had much higher hair zinc concentrations (216.2 mcg./g.) compared with controls (81.6 mcg./g.). The hair zinc concentration in the mothers of the diagnosis group increased during pregnancy, whereas it decreased in the control group. It is concluded that mothers of infants with spina bifida have an abnormality of zinc availability. These examples—where high amounts of hair zinc may be associated either with something positive (intelligence) or something negative (spina bifida offspring)—illustrate the perplexity of hair analysis.

Where a nutrient is located in the body is probably of great importance to health. Certainly, this generalization would appear to apply in the case of zinc. Dr. William R. Beisel,[278] scientific advisor to the U.S. Army Medical Research Institute of Infectious Diseases in Frederick, Maryland, says: "It may be that the body readjusts or redistributes its own zinc levels very cleverly. More zinc in the liver may help it to function better, and less zinc in the bloodstream may help the phagocytes function better. Just *where* the zinc is located in the body may be what's important for best defense."

(Continued on page 634)

---

* Perhaps hair zinc may sometimes reflect body stores while hair aluminum reflects excretion. However, as in mothers of *spina bifida* babies (soon to be discussed), it looks as if hair zinc concentrations may also correlate with excretion.

SOME PROBLEMS WITH HAIR ANALYSIS

Hair analysis has many limitations, at least in terms of current technology.[*] In experiments with rats, S. B. Deeming and C. W. Weber[267] found positive correlations between zinc in hair and zinc in bone and testes. However, no correlation was found between zinc in hair and zinc in liver, kidney or blood plasma. Deeming and Weber concluded that, at least for rats, hair zinc is a reflection of dietary intake rather than the state of total-body zinc metabolism. L. M. Klevay[268] reports that he and R. A. Jacob found a positive correlation between copper in the hair and copper in the liver but, like Deeming and Weber, found no similar correlation for zinc. Then too, the work of Bo Bergman and Rune Söremark[269] showed that in adult mice the uptake by the pituitary gland of zinc, administered as zinc benzoate, was considerable, but that zinc given as zinc chloride did not accumulate in this gland. When one learns of a conclusion regarding the body's uptake of a given mineral, that finding should be viewed as one based only on the form of the supplement used in that experiment (e.g., a conclusion for zinc benzoate, but not for zinc chloride). The fact that the uptake of metals varies not only from organ to organ but also varies with the supplement being used, argues that if we are going to supplement our diet with one or more minerals, those minerals ought to be taken in various forms. We do not presently know which tissue concentrations of zinc and of other trace elements correlate well with hair concentrations. Until this is known, the

---

[*] Hair analysis results are not only subject to contamination from the environment but are also subject to the vagaries of the washing procedure employed before using the atomic absorption spectrophotometer. Gary S. Assarian and Donald Oberleas[266] describe the problems and conclude that trace element status through hair analysis is technique-sensitive and therefore may be unreliable. I know from my own unpublished studies using split samples sent to different laboratories just how variable the results can be.

value of hair analysis in estimating mineral needs of the body must remain conjectural.*

It should also be observed that hair analysis can not only be misleading but, even when not misleading, can be subject to misinterpretation. Extremely high levels of zinc or of calcium in the hair may, for example, indicate not an excess but a deficiency elsewhere in the body (as in mothers of spina bifida fetuses). Then too, if hair growth is being inhibited due to disease, average or below-normal amounts of zinc may be incorporated into the hair, but the slower-than-normal hair growth rates may result in high zinc levels. Robert B. Bradford and K. Michael Hambridge[270] reported that this often occurs in the malnutritive disease kwashiorkor. Severe zinc deficiencies are generally accompanied by a loss of hair, but the hair that remains generally shows normal concentrations of zinc.[271] When considering hair analysis, beware of simplistic conclusions!

The racial extraction of the person whose hair is being tested is generally ignored. However, H. Kikkawa et al.[271a] reported that white hair of any race contains more nickel; golden or brown hair of Caucasians contains additional titanium and molybdenum; black hair of Mongolians is rich in copper, cobalt and iron, while the hair of blacks contains more copper and iron.** To the extent this study is valid, it would seem that racial identifications might be desirable before health conclusions are attempted from a hair analysis.

---

* Leukocyte zinc has been suggested as another possible diagnostic tool.[269a] Zinc levels in leukocytes average 25 times higher than in erythrocytes.[269a] Furthermore, leukocytes have a more rapid turnover of zinc than do erythrocytes and should, therefore, be more sensitive to body changes involving zinc.[269a] Low leukocyte-zinc levels, to cite one possible example of diagnostic application, may be predictive of diabetes.[269b] On the other hand, Ananda S. Prasad[269c] has presented data indicating that zinc in neutrophils and the assay of alkaline phosphatase activity in neutrophils may be the best tools for estimating the body's zinc status. (The usual test for diagnosing zinc deficiency is the plasma zinc assay, but Prasad maintains that its results must be evaluated cautiously.)

** On the contrary, M. H. Briggs et al.[271b] reported that Caucasians have more hair copper than blacks. They also found that Asiatics had the highest hair zinc levels while blacks had the lowest.

Another factor that may sometimes be ignored, but perhaps should not, is a variation of hair zinc with the season. I reported earlier that a study[241a] showed hair zinc to be higher (at least in children) in February than in September.

Hair analysis often considers variations due to age and sex but not variations due to weight or height. Philip S. Gentile et al.[272] reported that, in children, relationships between hair zinc concentrations and height, weight and age are linear, positive and statistically significant. In adults there were no statistically significant relationships between height and age, but a negative correlation was found between hair zinc and weight. As far as I know, however, no hair analysis laboratory asks the weight of the person whose hair is being analyzed.

Yet another factor that is ignored in contemporary analysis procedures is hair diameter. In a study related to lead (but probably applicable to other minerals), G. D. Renshaw[273] found great variations in hair lead over a single head due to hair diameter. Mean hair diameters range from 40 to 100 μm. Renshaw reported that minerals are not always uniformly distributed across the diameter of the hair shaft. Whereas zinc was fairly uniformly distributed, the concentration of lead at the surface (highest concentration) to the concentration at the center varied between 2.8 to 1 and 5.1 to 1. Other minerals such as iron and calcium displayed distributions similar to that of lead. I know of no laboratory regularly doing hair analysis that considers hair diameter. I have never seen laboratories caution one to use clean *plastic* scissors when cutting the hair sample to avoid possible metal adulteration from this source. [274] Laboratories universally ask whether or not the hair has been dyed because the dye may contain lead. They ask about the shampoos used since some may contain zinc or selenium. Less often are they concerned about the possible effects of hair-curling solutions or the possible lead content of hair spray. [275] Failure to consider these and the various other factors I have mentioned help keep contemporary hair analysis procedures from attaining the reliability we would like to see.

Even the frequency of washing can be a factor in the amount of trace elements present in the hair. D. Clink[275a] has reported that frequent washers showed significantly lower values of sodium, aluminum, chlorine, titanium, vanadium, arsenic, bromine, iodine, barium and lead; lower but not significantly different contents for manganese, copper, selenium and mercury; and significantly higher values for magnesium and calcium. The effect of shampoos on magnesium and calcium may be due to precipitation of "water hardness minerals" into the hair.[275b]* Those who swim may have elevated hair copper levels if the water has been treated with copper salts to inhibit algae formation.[275b]

As I hinted earlier, the zinc content of the hair may be related to its color. Ewin A. Eads and Charles E. Lambdin[276] observed that darker-colored hair of both sexes had a significantly higher zinc content. Gray hair of both sexes showed a lower zinc/copper ratio than that of corresponding nongraying hair of younger subjects. Other investigators have not, however, been able to confirm this report but provide, instead, many contradictions. Jose G. Dorea and Sueli Essado Pereira[277] cite 22 references relating to hair color and the content of various minerals. Zinc is probably involved in hair pigmentation but so is copper. Perhaps too great an intake of zinc might provide a *reverse effect* through inhibiting copper and its ability to form the enzyme tyrosinase. (Tyrosinase is involved in the production of melanin, which is a factor in hair color.)

There are obviously great problems associated with the interpretation of hair analyses. I think, however, that hair analysis may achieve a better status among medical practitioners when the precautions I have cited are more generally observed. As for now, its status, as discussed by Stephen Barrett,[277a] is at a

---

* Adon A. Gordus et al.[275c] reported that hair washed in zinc- or selenium-containing shampoos (for dandruff control) showed elevated concentrations of the respective mineral. (The same study compared mineral concentrations of contemporary hair with those of hair samples up to 200 years old. High lead and arsenic values were associated with pre-1900 hair samples, perhaps relating to use of those minerals in medicines of the time.)

very low ebb. In reply to Barrett, however, P. J. Barlow et al.[277b] said: "Dismissal of a potentially valuable tool simply because it is misused in some hands seems something of an over-reaction." Letters from William J. Walsh,[277c] from George Hickok[277d] and from Robert S. Waters[277e] favoring hair analysis and a reply from Barrett[277f] appeared in another issue of *JAMA*.

(Continued from page 629)

Zinc deficiency is a factor in a multitude of problems. A shortage of zinc has been reported to occur in persons with varicose leg ulcers and so a cause-and-effect relationship is at least a possibility. Zinc is highly concentrated in the choroid of the eye. Could that be why a shortage of this mineral may be a factor in photophobia (light sensitivity) and conjunctivitis? A deficiency can reportedly cause dental caries and slow healing of wounds, including burns.* (The hair, which normally contains more zinc than any part of the body other than the prostate, spermatozoa and the choroid of the eye, will lose much of its zinc following excessive skin burns.) [280b]

Zinc deficiency can lead to a small thymus gland in zinc-deficient animals. T-cell immunity is detrimentally affected and there may be a low resistance to infections. Zinc deficiency interferes with the T-cell helper function, but in a study by Pamela J. Fraker et al.[281] there was little effect on the B cells for the time periods studied. Perhaps the influence of zinc on the thymus is due to its effect on plasma levels of vitamin A. In any event we know, as reported in Chapter 4, that vitamin A is a factor in the health of the thymus gland. Pamela J. Fraker et al.[282] reported on a relevant experiment. The thymus glands of young adult mice fed a zinc-deficient diet were reduced to one-third normal size and their immune function was greatly impaired. Then, upon supplementation with zinc, the thymus glands were fully reconstructed and the T-cell-dependent antibody-mediated response

---

* The beneficial effect of zinc in wound healing is generally explained by the fact it is a component of various enzymes.[279] However, Milos Chvapil et al.[280] hold that zinc stabilizes lysosomal membranes by a mechanism that is restricted to the membrane's surface. Zinc increaases rate of thrombin-induced fibrin clot formation, thus reducing blood clotting time.[280a] Blood clot occurrence tends to maximize early in the day, leading to increased heart attacks among those doing strenuous morning exercise. (*Healthwise* [Aug., 1987] 10, no. 8: 1; *Physician and Sportsmedicine* [1987] 15, no. 4: 39.) Could this suggest a danger in bedtime zinc supplementation?

was also fully restored. Also, Michael H. N. Golden et al.[283] found that thymic atrophy in malnourished children was reversed by zinc supplementation.

Further support for the possibly-beneficial effect of supplementary zinc relative to the immune response comes from a study conducted by Jean Duchateau et al.[284] Lymphocyte response, however, depended on the starting value of lymphocyte stimulation obtained by administering phytohemagglutinin, i.e., in low responders it was enhanced by oral zinc sulphate, but in high responders it was reduced. The investigators reported that the lymphocyte response does not result from a correction of latent zinc deficiency. They cautioned, furthermore, that their work does not support any clinical conclusion about the benefits of high oral zinc dosages in normal adults. They also pointed out that there is no conclusive evidence that such modified lymphocyte mitogen response could afford any increased resistance to infectious diseases.

Gianni Marone et al.[285] have observed that zinc inhibits *in vitro* histamine release from human basophils induced by several immunologic stimuli. Zinc does not affect the first stage of histamine release but acts to antagonize the action of calcium in the calcium-dependent second stage. The scientists suggested zinc compounds might be considered for treatment of allergies. Furthermore, Jean Duchateau et al.[286] reported on the oral intake of 220 mg. of zinc sulphate by 15 persons over 70 years of age twice daily for one month. Compared with controls, there was a significant improvement of three different immune parameters.

Zinc has also been found effective in inhibiting replication of rhinoviruses, the infectious agents of the common cold. B. D. Korant et al.[287] discovered that zinc displayed antiviral activity in nontoxic concentrations against eight out of nine rhinoviruses.

A study by George A. Eby et al.[287a] suggested zinc gluconate lozenges as a possible treatment for colds. One 23-mg. zinc lozenge or a matched placebo was dissolved in the mouth every two wakeful hours after an initial double dose. They reported that after seven days, 86% of 37 zinc-treated subjects were asymptomatic compared with only 46% of 28 placebo-treated subjects. It seems to me that in only a very immunologically deficient group would 46% have colds after a full week. There were an excessive number of dropouts in this study, a fact that often tends to confuse interpretation of the findings. The scientists themselves expressed reservations as to the validity of their study and called for additional research.

Many other studies indicate that overcoming a zinc deficiency may be useful in promoting the immune response.[288-290] Supplemental zinc is even reported to be useful in treating lepromatous leprosy.[290a] However, in attempting to combat the infectious yeast *Candida albicans* (monilia), David R. Soll et al.[291] reported that using *in vitro* suspensions of the organisms, cells normally formed mycelia in one-half the time it took zinc-starved cells. Interesting as this information may be to the vast numbers of persons suffering periodic *Candida* infections, it seems doubtful to me that the information can be put to use since it is probably just another example of the *reverse effect*. A zinc deficiency is just too dangerous to purposely introduce. Furthermore, according to Ananda Prasad et al.,[292] infection with *Candida albicans* is a frequent complication of zinc deficiency.

Vaginal trichomoniasis may also be effectively treated with zinc. Fred Willmott et al.[293] found that 220 mg. of zinc sulphate twice daily for three weeks successfully treated a woman whose trichomoniasis was recalcitrant to treatment with high dosage metronidazol. He reported that after 15 months of recurrent infection she has now remained free from infection for 4 months. (I wonder if she receives a maintenance dose of zinc. Sometimes preventive measures seem less obvious than therapies.) Incidentally, the sexual organs of men and the male urinary tract contain large amounts of zinc. This is probably effective in reducing the risk of infection after intercourse with a woman infected by *Candida albicans* or *Trichomonas vaginalis.*[294]

Immunodeficiency resulting from gestational zinc deprivation in mice can persist for three generations! Richard S. Beach et al.[295] reported that they fed mice a diet moderately deficient in zinc from day seven of gestation to parturition. Offspring showed decreased immunocompetence through six months of age. Most interestingly, the second and third generation mice, all of which were fed a normal diet, continued to show reduced immune function, although not to the same degree as the first generation. Mice are not people (although in reading research we sometimes act as if they were), but if these results have human applicability, it may be vital that pregnant women receive adequate zinc.[*]

We have seen that zinc plays an important role in the immune function. Does a *reverse effect,* in regard to immunity, however, set in if zinc is overdosed? Yes. Ranjit Kumar Chandra [295a] reported that 11 healthy adult men ingested 150 mg. of elemental zinc twice a day for six weeks. The result was a *reduction* in lymphocyte stimulation response to phytohemagglutinin and also a reduction in chemotaxis and phagocytosis of bacteria by the polymorphonuclear leukocytes. Chandra also observed that high-density lipoprotein decreased significantly and low-density lipoprotein increased slightly. Keep in mind that excessive zinc could have deleterious effects on healthy persons.

Studies by Ananda S. Prasad [296] and others relating to zinc-deficient boys in Egypt (where the phytates in their predominantly cereal-based diet inhibit zinc availability) have clearly demonstrated the importance of zinc for growth and for sexual development. Research by K. Michael Hambridge et al. [297] and by Noel W. Solomons et al. [298] has also found zinc deficiency, as shown by hair analysis, to be related to growth inhibition. However, a study by Phylis B. Moser et al. [299] showed no statistical differences among groups for growth as a function of either dietary zinc intake or hair zinc concentration.

During puberty, boys have an unusually great need for zinc. As the prostate gland, seminal vesicles and testes develop, zinc is drawn to these organs from elsewhere in the body. As a boy masturbates he also loses considerable amounts of zinc. It is quite possible that acne and the lagging of boys behind girls in the matter of height during

---

[*] It is interesting to speculate, however, about the possibility that the baby of a woman who was zinc-supplemented during pregnancy might show a rebound effect if, as a fetus, he became acclimatized to above-normal amounts of zinc. It does happen with vitamin C and may happen with other minerals and vitamins.

puberty may sometimes be due to zinc deficiency because of effects on prostaglandin synthesis (as covered in Chapter 3). Zinc supplements, perhaps along with vitamin B6 which is reported to increase its assimilation, should be considered for use at this time.

Growth of the fetus is reported in a number of studies, including one by John Patrick,[300] to be correlated with maternal leucocyte zinc and with plasma zinc. Patrick measured the rate of growth of the femur length of the fetus using ultrasound and found it to be significantly related to the amount of the mother's zinc.

A study by Harold H. Sandstead et al.,[301] as well as many other studies by Ananda S. Prasad,[302] have shown that zinc is required not only for normal growth but also for sexual maturation. Lucille S. Hurley[303] has reported on the zinc-sexual connection in rats. Zinc-deficient females had abnormal estrous cycles and also showed other effects such as hyperplasia and hyperkeratinization of the esophagus. Their fetuses also showed malformations. Male rats on a zinc-deficient diet of 60 ppm. showed normal growth but testicular atrophy. When the diet included 100 ppm. of zinc, however, growth and testicular morphology were normalized.

Zinc is a constituent of semen—both of the sperms and of the transporting fluid. (Astonishingly, however, Bert L. Vallee[304] has reported that aspermic human semen has the same zinc content as normal sperm.) Furthermore, Dr. Lucy Antoniou, of the Veterans Administration Hospital in Washington, D.C., has demonstrated that zinc seems to be vital to the metabolism of the male hormone, testosterone. Sufficient zinc (as well as every other nutrient) is probably essential for sexuality. Lucy D. Antoniou et al.[304a] studied eight impotent hemodialyzed men. Dialytic administration of zinc (they did not report what kind was used) raised the plasma testosterone level to normal in two patients and improved sexual potency in all. A zinc deficiency can, in fact, lead to gynecomastia, excessive breast development in males. Zinc deficiency may also adversely affect testicular size and so testosterone production may be decreased for this reason.[305] William H. Goldiner et al.[304b] found, however, that in cases of alcohol-induced cirrhosis of the liver, zinc administered as zinc sulphate did not prove to be effective in treating sexual dysfunction.

It has been speculated that the effect of zinc on testosterone may be mediated by the action of gonadotrophins from the pituitary. However, this seems unlikely in light of a report by T. R. Hartoma[306] of a study of men aged 36-60 years. Correlations were studied between serum zinc and serum testosterone, between serum zinc and follicle-stimulating hormone and between serum zinc and luteinizing hormone. A statistically significant positive correlation was found only between serum zinc and serum testosterone. Thus, zinc deficiency evidently operates, not on the pituitary level, but on the testicular level.

Zinc may also play an important role in fertility. T. Riita Hartoma et al.[307] found that, in six out of ten infertile men, serum zinc was below normal. They reported that administering 220 mg. of zinc sulphate three times daily for four to eight weeks significantly raised not only serum zinc but also plasma testosterone and sperm count. Joel L. Marmar et al.[308] reported that 11 men with oligospermia and low semen zinc, after being given zinc sulphate, showed significantly higher mean levels of semen zinc, mean sperm count and mean motility index. Three pregnancies occurred among their wives during the period of treatment. Oligospermia (a total sperm count of under 40 million per ejaculate) was induced by Ali A. Abbasi et al.[308a] in four out of five volunteers through dietary zinc restriction and then reversed after zinc was administered.

Furthermore, J. G. Bieri and E. L. Prival[309] found that a deficiency of either zinc or vitamin E in rats results in testes degeneration and an elevation of arachidonic acid in the testicular lipid. A study by Prithiva Chanmugam et al.[309a] has shown that a zinc-deficient diet causes, in rats, increased testicular levels, not only of arachidonic acid but also of prostaglandin 6-keto-PGF$_{1\alpha}$. Another rat study by the same group[309b] found that a zinc-deficient diet led to a decreased level of docosapentenoic acid in the testes and this deficiency did not appear to be correctable with dietary supplementation of docosapentenoic acid.

The essentiality of zinc for human male sexual function is shown by a double-blind trial of 20 male hemodialysis patients.[310] Ten received 50 mg. of elemental zinc as zinc acetate and ten received a placebo. At the end of six months there was a significant increase in plasma zinc, testosterone and sperm count of the zinc-treated group but not in those receiving the placebo. The zinc-treated group also had a significant decline in serum leuteinizing hormone and follicle-stimulating hormone. Patients receiving zinc had an improvement in potency and libido with an increased frequency of intercourse. This is not to say, however, that supplemental zinc will help improve the potency or libido of men not deficient in the mineral. (Often research such as this is used by the unscrupulous or the unaware to sell supplements to those who do not need them.)*

How about zinc and prostate health? F. K. Habib[311] reported that endocrine activity of the gland is dependent upon the zinc concentration in the tissue. Dr. Habib found, as had many earlier investigators such as G. Randolph Schrodt et al.[312] and Ferenc Györkey et al.,[313] that in benign hypertrophy there is a higher concentration of zinc, while in prostatic cancer there is a very low zinc concentration.

Habib[313a] found, in an *in vitro* study of the prostatic tissue of patients who had benign prostatic hypertrophy, that zinc concentrations lower than 10^{-8}M inhibited the activity of the enzyme 5 $\propto$-reductase which is needed to activate testosterone. Note, in Figure 15, that the percentage of unconverted testosterone favorably declines with an increase of zinc concentration from 10^{-9}M to about 10^{-5}M, but then shows a *reverse effect* and rises as the zinc becomes excessive. Habib speculated that the low zinc levels in neoplastic tissue and the subsequent fall in enzyme activity might account for the accumulation of testosterone in malignant tissue. Subsequently, Habib et al.[313b] raised the possibility that zinc manipulation of the gland might

---

* Zinc seems to affect cell membranes and in this connection inhibits histamine release from mast cells.[310a] (If the presumed orgasm promoting propensity of histamine were real as hypothesized by Carl C. Pfeiffer, Durk Pearson, Sandy Shaw and Saul Kent (references 42a-d of Chapter 5), then zinc would be an anti-libido mineral. On the contrary, many believe zinc to increase sexual powers (an idea which is probably valid only in the case of a zinc deficiency being overcome).

be used as an alternative to hormones in controlling both benign and malignant prostatic growth.

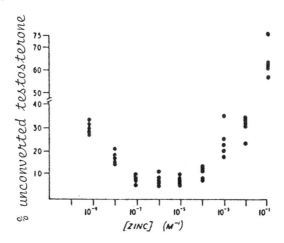

Figure 15. Results of an *in vitro* **study showing the effect of divalent zinc ions on the reduction of testosterone in the prostatic tissue of five patients with benign prostatic hypertrophy. Reproduced from F. K. Habib,** *Jrl. of Steroid Biochemistry* **(1978) 9: 403-407, with permission of the publisher, Pergamon Press, and of the author. Note the increased activation of testosterone (i.e., the percentage of unconverted testosterone declines) as the zinc concentration increases from 10^{-9} to 10^{-7} molar. Then, between 10^{-7}M and 10^{-5}M, a** *reverse effect* **sets in and the activation of testosterone is again decreased.**

Rodney V. Anderson[314] reports that very low concentrations of zinc are also associated with prostatitis. Dr. Anderson states that oral zinc fails to raise the zinc level in the prostatic gland or in the secretion. However, we noted a few pages back that the form of oral zinc has a great influence over which body tissues will take it up. I wonder if Dr. Anderson had used a different zinc supplement (he does not report what he used), or high-zinc foods such as herring or oysters, whether the results might have been different. Robert H. Rhamy[315] similarly states that, while zinc may enhance the binding of androgen to prostatic cells, the binding is not zinc-dependent. He believes there is no reason to use zinc therapy for either benign hypertrophy of the prostate or for prostatic cancer. (As suggested before, I think results may depend on the type of zinc used.)

Zinc is a component of acid phosphatase, an important component of prostatic fluid. The level of acid phosphatase in the human prostate is low in childhood but increases rapidly at puberty. The concentration of acid phosphatase correlates with androgenic activity,[315a] but its action is inhibited by calcium.[315b] Several studies show that its presence in the urine may be an indication of sexual arousal in men.* Furthermore, A. M. Barclay[317,318] found that men with a high sexual drive (as measured by the number of orgasms per month) secreted more acid phosphatase in the urine than men of lower sexual drive. Thus, we are provided with a possible rationale supporting zinc's reputation as a sex stimulant, although the presence of zinc at times of sexual arousal could, of course, be merely a concomitant rather than a causal phenomenon. In any event, do not assume that *more* is necessarily *better*. Sakari Kellokumpu and Hannu Rajaniemi[319] reported on an action of zinc that suggests caution in its overuse by men hoping to become more sexy. These scientists reported that, when zinc chloride was injected into the testicles of rats prior to injecting human chorionic gonadotropin, there was an increase in the uptake of the hormone by the testes, which is fine, but—and here is the big BUT—the primary testosterone response was reduced.

Although we have noted sufficient serum zinc seems to be an important factor in fertility, too much may exhibit a *reverse effect* and be detrimental. S. Aonuma et al.[320] found that mouse epididymal sperm (those not yet capacitated)** in the presence of zinc failed not only to penetrate the zona pellucida (the outside

---

* A. M. Barclay[316] concluded earlier that acid phosphatase in the urine is a specific indicator of sexual arousal rather than an indicator of general arousal (e.g., anger). Note that we are speaking of acid phosphatase in the *urine*. The test for *serum* acid phosphatase is used to detect metastatic cancer of the prostate.

** Sperm are not capable of fertilizing an ovum until they are capacitated, a process that ordinarily occurs only in the vagina of the female. Capacitation has been accomplished *in vitro*, however, in many species but is, as Reuben J. Mapletoft[320a] relates, "the most difficult aspect of *in vitro* fertilization."

envelope of the egg) and also failed to fuse with zone-free ova. There was, however, no effect observed on capacitated sperm. Furthermore, O. Johnson and R. Eliasson[321,322] have shown, with *in vitro* experiments using human sperm, that *removal* of zinc from sperm can be closely associated with capacitation and fertilization. Thus, men trying out for fatherhood should probably not overdo their zinc intake anymore than should those who would like to be hypersexy.

Furthermore, W. R. Sutton and Victor E. Nelson[323] reported that large amounts of dietary zinc markedly affected reproduction in rats. A diet of 1/2% zinc carbonate fed to female rats resulted in defective and dead offspring. After five months on the ration they ceased to become pregnant. (Interestingly, when salt was removed from their diet, reproduction became normal at the high 1/2% level of zinc.) Zinc at a level of 1/2% is, of course, a lot of zinc—equivalent to about 5 grams in a person eating 1 kg. (2.2 lbs.) of food daily. Small amounts of zinc are essential for health and for sex, but large amounts can be disastrous.

Leaving the subject of sex and reproduction, let us consider zinc in relation to heart health. Vernon E. Wendt et al.[324] reported on the effects of alcohol on the heart. In a study of 8 patients, 30 minutes after the ingestion of alcohol, 6 of these subjects showed a liberation of zinc by the myocardium (the middle muscular layer of the heart wall). With the loss of zinc there is an increased probability of a myocardial infarction. We also noted earlier that Ranjit Kumar Chandra[295a] reported excessive zinc detrimentally lowers HDL and raises LDL. Then too, zinc is present at higher levels in hypertensive persons according to G. Frithz and G. Ronquist.[325] Furthermore, Peter W. F. Fischer and Maurice W. Collins[326] observed that the serum zinc/copper ratio is positively correlated with diastolic blood pressure in women (but not in men). Similarly, this ratio in the hair was found, by Denis M. Medeiros et al.,[327] to be positively correlated with both systolic and diastolic pressures in members of a university community. On the contrary, William R. Harlan et al.[327a] recently reported that not only calcium but also zinc is inversely related to blood pressure in humans. Perhaps some of these studies are being influenced by the *reverse effect*. Could it be that some of the persons involved in these studies may have been exposed to cadmium and in these the zinc was working to lower pressure while tending to raise pressure in those without a cadmium burden? However, reports that zinc may help control the presumed blood pressure-raiser cadmium may be questionable. Joachim Manthey et al.[328] reported that cadmium "does not appear to be implicated as a major factor in the genesis of elevated blood pressure in humans." On the other hand, Stephen J. Kopp et al.[329] subsequently observed that a low intake of dietary cadmium showed dose-dependent functional and biochemical changes in the cardiovascular tissues of rats. Their data support the hypothesis that ingested or inhaled environmental cadmium could be a factor in human hypertension. Nevertheless, earlier, in regard to calcium and the hard- versus soft-water controversy, we noted that three studies[67a] show cadmium workers do not have elevated blood pressures.

Zinc is a component of alcohol dehydrogenase, an enzyme needed to metabolize alcohol. Alcohol dehydrogenase catalyzes the oxidation of ethanol, vitamin A alcohol and certain sterols using the niacin-based compound nicotinamide-adenine-dinucleotide (NAD) as a cofactor.[330] Those drinking excessive amounts of alcohol will lose zinc via the urine. This loss of zinc, through both alcohol metabolism and because of excessive excretion, may be a factor in the development of cirrhosis of the liver. A third factor working against the alcoholic's having sufficient zinc (or other minerals and vitamins) is that his dietary intake is likely to be low in nonalcoholic food. The alcoholic's zinc deficiency often results in a reduced libido, delayed ejaculation or complete failure to ejaculate, perhaps because the prostate cannot function without zinc. Eventually, the chronic alcoholic may become impotent.

When it comes to types of alcohol consumed, red wine may get a better rating in terms of its effect than do other forms of alcohol. Janet T. McDonald and Sheldon Margen[331] found that when either red zinfandel or dealcoholized zinfandel was consumed there was increased zinc absorption from dietary sources compared to absorption when either alcohol or water was taken. Presumably, a nonalcoholic constituent or constituents (congeners) of the red wine account for the favorable action. (Similar findings were reported earlier[332] for calcium, phosphorus and magnesium by the same scientists.*

A rather newly recognized difficulty, *hypogeusia,* may be helped with zinc. Hypogeusia is the name given to the condition whose symptom is inert taste buds. This condition is sometimes the result of a respiratory infection. In other cases the loss of taste comes on slowly and unaccountably and there is a tendency to prefer more spicy foods. Some of the victims become depressed and experience anxiety, vertigo and reduced libido. Sometimes malnutrition can set in because when food is tasteless there is little incentive to eat.

Robert I. Henkin of the National Heart and Lung Institute of Bethesda, Maryland, working with D. F. Bradley of Brooklyn Polytechnic Institute, has developed a possible cure for hypogeusia. Henkin finds that by giving zinc sulphate he can often awaken the sleeping taste buds. Henkin has reported that taste is a function not only of the tongue (as has long been thought to be the only site of the taste buds) but also of the palate, pharynx and larynx. (This, if true, would explain why those with dentures may have some trouble tasting food.) A related disorder, hyposmia (impaired smelling ability), has been found by Henkin to also be benefitted by zinc therapy. The principal salivary protein, called *gustin,* contains zinc, so it seems reasonable that zinc should have gustatory significance.

The studies of Henkin do not, however, seem to be applicable to older persons according to the work of J. L. Greger and A. H. Geissler.[334] In a double-blind study using 49 aged institutionalized persons, Greger and Geissler fed one group 15 mg. of supplemental zinc daily and the other group received no zinc supplementation. The zinc hair levels of the supplemented group rose significantly. The detection thresholds for sodium chloride and sucrose improved

---

* Alcohol-free wine and beer have been on sale for several years.[333] Since many studies suggest alcohol in moderation may be health-promoting, the main value of the new products may be in bringing excessive alcohol consumption down closer to optimal range.

slightly but not significantly among those receiving zinc supplementation. Greger and Geissler also reported that taste acuity was not correlated with diet, hair zinc level, smoking habits or use of dentures. In another study of patients on dialysis (average age 51 years), Sudesh K. Mahajan et al.[335] reported that upon daily supplementation with 50 mg. of zinc acetate their threshold of taste detection for salt and sweet and bitter, but not for sour, improved significantly in all patients. Zinc supplementation will not, however, help everyone with a taste problem. Robert I. Henkin et al.[336] found that, in a randomized, double-blind crossover study of 106 patients with taste and smell disfunction, supplementing with zinc sulphate achieved results no better than did administration of a placebo. Henkin[336a] has recently published a review of zinc in the taste function. Zinc may sometimes be useful, but many abnormalities of taste and smell functions do not seem amenable to zinc therapy. Even more recently, W. W. Dinsmore et al.[336b] have presented data suggesting that zinc metabolism is disturbed in anorexia nervosa. The absence of appetite may, perhaps, be related to reduced zinc absorption and consequent reduction in taste sensation. D. Bryce-Smith and R. I. D. Simpson[336c] have also reported some success in treating anorexia nervosa with supplements of zinc sulphate (50 mg., three times daily). They explain that starvation (as is the case with other stresses) increases urinary zinc excretion. The resulting zinc shortage impairs the zinc-dependent senses of taste and smell, thereby further decreasing the desire to eat.

Michele Garrett-Laster et al.[336d] studied taste and olfaction senses in 37 vitamin A-deficient patients with alcoholic cirrhosis. Eleven of these also had low serum zinc levels. When these patients were given supplemental vitamin A there was significant improvement in detection and recognition thresholds for bitter and salty taste and for pyridine olfaction regardless of zinc status. As we saw in Chapter 4, the retinal binding protein contains zinc so that it is reasonable to presume that a shortage of either zinc or of vitamin A might produce detrimental taste and olfactory effects.

There are many other possible uses for zinc. Large amounts of zinc and ascorbic acid can be used to chelate cadmium and lead out of the body, perhaps obviating the need for chelation therapy with EDTA or penicillamine (as will be discussed in Chapter 8). A deficiency of zinc may also be a cause of epilepsy according to Dr. Andre Barbeau.[340] A study by H. George Ketola[340a] with rainbow trout showed that a zinc deficiency caused cataracts. (Remember, however, that the physiology of a fish may only remotely resemble that of a human.) This work was followed by at least six other studies relating to cataractogenesis in trout and also in salmon that, in 1986, were analyzed in *Nutrition Reviews*.[340b] The problem seems to arise partially because of the calcium richness of fish meals and the fact that they contain plant-derived phytates. The calcium presumably enhances the formation of zinc phytates which are poorly absorbed, thus causing the zinc deficiency which, in turn, leads to the formation of cataracts. *Nutrition Reviews* "wonders whether zinc is needed for some special requirement of the fish lens, or if a suitably monitored and prolonged study of zinc deficiency in warm-blooded species would reveal opacities."

Then too, recent studies suggest the probable presence of a moderate zinc deficiency in adults having sickle-cell anemia. G. L. Brewer et al.[341] have reported that zinc supplementation decreases the number of irreversible sickle cells *in vivo*. *Nutrition Reviews*[342] tells about a typical case of a favorable response to zinc supplementation in a sickle-cell patient. Ananda S. Prasad and Zafrallah T. Cossack[342a] also experienced favorable results in treating patients with sickle-cell disease. M. Cassandra Matustik et al.[342b] reported that zinc excretion, ordinarily elevated in sickle-cell patients, was favorably decreased by increasing sodium intake.) Recent, preliminary observations by Pierre Reding et al.[342c] suggest, however, that the improvement of sickle-cell anemia by zinc supplementation is apt to be of short duration.

Possible Rhythms in Blood Zinc Levels

The blood concentration of zinc may be subject to a circadian rhythm. R. I. Henkin[343] observed that the level of serum zinc was higher than the mean between 2 A.M. and 6 A.M. The serum zinc level *rose* after breakfast (6 A.M. to 10 A.M.) and after dinner (6 P.M. to 10 P.M.). The research of R. D. Bhattacharya[344] supports

Henkin's study. However, it seems obvious to me after looking at both studies that dietary zinc shows up rather promptly in the blood—thus acting as a perturbation to any real cycle if such exists. (This conclusion of mine is at complete variance with that of Morton K. Schwartz[345] who says in regard to serum zinc that "values less than the fasting concentrations are observed 2 to 3 hours after the ingestion of food.") O. Guillard et al.[346] reported on variations in diurnal zinc concentration in fasting subjects. Their data show rises at 9 A.M. and 6 P.M. with a low at 3 P.M. Contrary to some of the conclusions they drew, I think their data is in fairly good agreement with Henkin. Nevertheless, if one ignores the Guillard study (which was based on just 14 subjects whose individual serum zinc values were often at wide variance with the group as a whole), one might be tempted to deny the existence of a circadian rhythm in serum zinc, choosing instead to ascribe the variations found by Henkin and by Bhattacharya to a rather prompt reaction to dietary zinc.

Whether or not a diurnal rhythm, independent of diet, exists in serum zinc, there is a rhythm—not daily, but monthly—relating to the concentration of zinc and copper in the blood of women. The concentration of zinc and copper in the blood varies with the time of the menstrual cycle according to M. G. Ioskovich.[347] In the first half of the cycle—the follicular phase—there is an increased concentration of copper and a decrease in the zinc. After ovulation—the luteal phase—the concentration of zinc tends to reach a maximum on the 22nd day of the cycle. Women on the Pill have, by the way, an increased requirement for zinc.

Zinc from Food or Supplements—Factors Affecting Absorption

What foods should one eat to assure an adequate zinc intake? Oysters contain generous amounts of zinc. Other sources for zinc are organ meats such as liver (especially pork liver) and pancreas, herring, other seafoods, spices, brewer's yeast, nuts, sunflower seeds, pumpkin seeds, wheat germ, wheat bran, oatmeal and other whole grains, milk, egg yolk, beets, beans, carrots, onions, peas, spinach, watercress, mushrooms, gelatin, maple syrup and cocoa. When vegetables are cooked zinc will be lost if the cooking water is discarded. Then too, the grains and other seeds contain fiber and phytic acid, which may join with some of the zinc and also with some of the manganese, copper, molybdenum, calcium, magnesium and iron to make these elements partially unavailable to the body.* For example, it has been reported that just 44% of zinc in soy protein is available.[348] (Sprouting, however, makes the zinc and other elements more available.) Therefore, even though these foods may contain fair amounts of zinc, in many cases half or less is usable. However, *The Miller Message*[348] says, "Addition of animal protein products to a diet prevents zinc deficiency symptoms, largely because of the presence of chelating agents that facilitate increased zinc absorption during digestion."** Dorothy Latta and Michael Liebman,[348a] in studying vegetarian and nonvegetarian males, found that crude fiber intake was negatively correlated with zinc levels in the red blood cells. (There was, however, no correlation between dietary iron or crude fiber intakes and any iron-status parameter.) A relatively high percentage of vegetarians (33%) had low plasma zinc levels (below 65 µg/dl) compared to 22% of nonvegetarians.

Zinc deficiency is obviously bad, but too much zinc may be bad also. Although phytic acid, as we said, inhibits absorption of various minerals, it inhibits absorption of zinc over that of copper. Leslie M. Klevay[350] reports that phytic acid will lower the ratio of zinc to copper absorbed from the intestinal tract, thus, according to Klevay, working to prevent hypercholesterolemia.

Absorption of zinc was reported to be inhibited by inorganic iron but not by heme iron.[351] The effect was not observed, however, when zinc, as oysters, was consumed. It is known that there are separate body pools for heme and nonheme iron and this study suggests the possibility there could be separate pools for organic and inorganic zinc. Furthermore, inorganic iron and inorganic zinc may share a common pool.

---

* Not all fiber inhibits the bioavailability of zinc. N. T. Davies[347a] reported that, in rats, cellulose, pectin and hemicellulose were without effect on the intestinal absorption of zinc.

** In an interesting display of "body wisdom," urinary zinc is much lower in those consuming low-protein diets, thus acting to conserve body stores of this mineral.[349]

Animal experiments have shown that calcium inhibits zinc absorption. Herta Spencer et al.[352] found, on the other hand, that when calcium intake in patients was increased six- to ten-fold there was no significant change in absorption of zinc, but the study did not consider the effects of the phytate/zinc ratio. Later, using animal experiments, Donald Oberleas and Barbara F. Harland[353] presented evidence to indicate that diets with a phytate/zinc molar ratio of 10 or less (i.e., with a ratio of phytate/zinc that is under 100:1) probably provide adequate dietary zinc, but those with a molar ratio consistently above 20 may jeopardize zinc status. Other experiments indicating the importance of the phytate/zinc ratio at varying levels of dietary calcium are cited by Frank W. Hogarth. [354] A recent study of 36 adult males by Herta Spencer et al.,[354a] again ignoring phytate, found that the simultaneous intake of high amounts of calcium (up to 2,000 mg./day) and of high amounts of phosphorus (up to 2,000 mg./day) had no effect on the zinc balance.

Most persons take their supplements with or following meals. It should be observed, however, that this will not in all cases assure maximum assimilation and utilization. Some nutrients, zinc being a prime example, will sometimes be utilized better if taken on an empty stomach. A. Pecoud et al.[355] noted that large doses of zinc sulphate were better tolerated when taken with meals rather than in the fasting state, but utilization of this mineral was negatively affected by the presence of many varieties of food. Foods rich in calcium and phosphorus (e.g., milk and cheese) or in fiber and phytate (e.g., whole grain foods) were very detrimental to zinc absorption. * Meat did not hurt zinc availability. Coffee cut zinc availability to about 50%. Other studies of foods markedly inhibiting zinc uptake were made by Noel W. Solomons.[360] Solomons concurs, in fact, with the

---

* To illustrate the complications of nutrition, another study showed that the addition of calcium in the form of milk products improved the absorption of zinc from a meal with wholemeal bread.[356] Gary W. Evans and Elaine C. Johnson[357] reported that human milk contains a zinc-binding ligand, picolinic acid. This may be yet another superior feature of human milk that helps assure breastfed infants of an adequate zinc supply even through human milk and cow's milk contain almost the same amounts of this mineral. (Picolinic acid is a product of tryptophan metabolism, but vitamin B 6 is required for the

assumption of the Expert Committee of the World Health Organization, Geneva, that the bioavailability of zinc in human diets ranges from 10% to 40%. It is interesting to note, however, that Bonnie M. Anderson et al.[361] reported the iron and zinc storage of Seventh Day Adventist vegetarian women seemed to be adequate in spite of their low intake of easily absorbable iron and zinc from flesh sources and in spite of their high consumption of foods containing fiber and phytate. Such studies are useful in that they clearly indicate one of the easily forgotten facts of nutrition, namely, that there are many factors that go into creating the big difference that generally exists between the amount of a nutrient that is consumed and the amount subsequently assimilated and utilized by the body. Furthermore, when one is attempting to decide if a given individual is getting the RDA of any particular mineral or vitamin many subtleties must be considered.

So, while vegetarians may thrive on far less than the RDA of zinc, let's give an example of a group that probably requires much more than the RDA. Persons with chronic diarrhea are reported by S. L. Wolman et al.[362] to need up to five times as much dietary zinc to maintain balance as those without diarrhea.

Some More Adverse Effects

Let's give just a brief word of warning before we leave the subject of zinc. I suggest, again, that you not be carried away with the idea, if you are a man, that you will become hypersexy if you take enormous amounts of zinc. Remember, in spite of all the popular literature heralding zinc as a sex-fostering mineral, we noted studies suggesting the opposite may sometimes be true. Zinc may help your sex life as we have discussed, but too much zinc can interfere with iron, copper and selenium metabolism, so take it easy! The toxicity of excessive amounts of zinc has been known at least since the time of Aristotle (384-322 B.C.).[362a]

---

reactions to occur. This is suggested as the reason B₆ and protein, to supply tryptophan, help zinc assimilation of foods and supplements not containing picolinic acid.) However, L. S. Hurley and B. Lönnerdal[358] argue rather convincingly that it is zinc citrate, not zinc picolinate, that accounts for the superiority of human milk as a source of highly available zinc. In addition, Eric W. Ainscough et al.[359] found that the iron-binding protein of human breast milk, lactoferrin, also transports zinc.

A high zinc supply increases urinary copper excretion and results in depleting the body of its store of this mineral.[363,364*] Rats fed a high-zinc diet (.75%—i.e., equivalent to 750 mg. in a person eating 1 kg. of food daily) developed defective red blood cells having only one-third the normal life expectancy.[365] It is known that copper as ceruloplasmin (ferroxidase) enters into formation of red blood cells, so perhaps the effect derives from the excess zinc depressing supplies of available copper. In a more recent experiment with healthy adult men, Peter W. F. Fischer et al.[365a] concluded that an oral supplement of 50 mg./day of zinc gluconate (given as 25 mg., twice a day) decreased copper status as measured by plasma ceruloplasmin and erythrocyte Cu Zn SOD. To the extent this copper reduction might interfere with the synthesis of hemoglobin, anemia and lack of sexual power might result. Hypersexiness is not achievable through a hyperintake of zinc! The *reverse effect*—hyposexiness could be the result. Furthermore, Kenneth H. Neldner [365b] notes that gastroenteritis, gastrointestinal bleeding, hypocupremia, microcytosis, relative neutropenia and hypoceruloplasminemia have been documented in patients receiving moderate-dose daily zinc supplements of 40 to 120 mg. Zinc tablets of 100 mg. are available, a fact which suggests that many could be overdosing. In addition, several epidemiological studies have shown that large amounts of zinc can abolish the cancer protection provided by selenium.[366]

Furthermore, E. L. Andronikashvili et al.[367] found that in the DNA and RNA purified from sarcomas, the zinc level remained constant after transplantation, while levels of iron, antimony, chromium, cobalt and selenium decreased. They concluded that zinc was required for growth of the tumor, while the other elements were not. Relatedly, Daniel T. Minkel et al.[367a] found that a zinc deficiency retarded growth of Ehrlich ascites tumors in mice. K. B. Olson et al.[368] observed increased liver zinc concentration in cancer patients and L. D. McBean

---

* Even a relatively small excess above the RDA may detrimentally affect copper retention. Melody D. Festa et al.[364a] found that, "an intake of zinc only 3.5 mg./day above the RDA for men reduced apparent retention of copper at an intake of 2.6 mg./day."

et al.[368a] also found increased liver and kidney zinc in patients with various cancers. I. L. Mulay et al.[368b] in one study, and A. E. Schwartz et al.[368c] in another, reported elevated zinc concentrations in cancerous lung and breast tissue. In yet another study, J. Borovansky et al.[369] reported a high zinc uptake by melanomas and the specific binding of zinc by melanosomes. I think we should, however, resist concluding that just because zinc—and also copper and manganese for that matter—may often be associated with cancerous tissue, it is likely to be a cause of cancer. Isn't it possible that the body may be mustering zinc, or copper or manganese, to fight the cancer? (In keeping with this line of reasoning, Gamal N. Gabrial et al.[370] found that zinc deficiency significantly enhanced tumor incidence in rats that were given a carcinogen.) Furthermore, a zinc deficiency is reported by L. Y. Y. Fong and P. M. Newberne[371] and also by Fong et al.[371a] to increase the incidence of nitrosamine-induced esophageal and forestomach tumors in rats. To the contrary, K. Wallenius et al.[371b] concluded from their studies with rats that a zinc-supplemented diet accelerated and a zinc-deficient diet retarded the development of chemically induced oral cancer. In light of this highly confusing group of contradictory experiments, it seems obvious that zinc and cancer are associated and that the golden mean should govern our intake of this mineral.

Some of the confusion regarding the interpretation of zinc studies may be due to failure to consider possible chronobiological effects. Moon K. Song et al.[371c] found that the time at which zinc supplementation began had a significant effect on the longevity of mice inoculated with tumor cells. When 4-week-old mice were inoculated with MOPC-104E tumor cells and immediately fed a zinc-deficient diet (.5 µg Zn/g) their longevity was significantly reduced compared to inoculated rats fed a control diet (37.5 µg Zn/g). However, when the zinc-deficient diet (.5 µg Zn/g) was begun on the 11th day after inoculation, longevity was significantly increased compared to controls. Astonishingly, excessive zinc intake (1 mg Zn/g) starting with the 11th day also significantly prolonged mean survival time. Thus, new confusion is introduced in the zinc-cancer connection, but the study also suggests that chronobiology will make great contributions to nutrition science.

Those interested in examining the large body of research suggesting zinc as a possible carcinogen, the role of zinc in increasing *or* decreasing tumor incidence and still other studies showing a negligible effect of zinc on tumor history are referred to the many references cited by Richard S. Beach et al.[372] and by Walter J. Pories et al.[373] Out of a correlation of such studies may come an elucidation of zinc's *reverse effect* that could be important in cancer prevention and therapy. Perhaps zinc could sometimes be operating like selenium which, in acting to inhibit tumorigenesis, is taken up readily by rapidly growing tumors. Morton K. Schwartz[345] suggests that, "the presence of selenium in the tumor cell may successfully compete with the carcinogen for binding places of the protein and thereby prevent carcinogenesis." It has also been suggested[373a] that there may be two different mechanisms of action by which zinc influences carcinogenesis at its different phases. Perhaps, in the early stages of carcinogenesis zinc may act through the immune system to overcome the cancer. However, if carcinogenesis should develop to the cell proliferation stage, then zinc may work to foster such proliferation and a zinc deficiency would, instead, be beneficial. Our ignorance is great. In light of these confusing facts it seems very important, however, to not overdose on any one or any two nutrients. In the absence of a known copper burden, wounds, relevant skin problems or other physiological conditions amenable to zinc therapy, the RDA of 15 mg. should probably not be exceeded.

In some individuals, elevated plasma zinc may be a heritable anomaly. J. Cecil Smith et al.[373b] found a case of hyperzincemia in five out of seven members of one family and in two out of three second generation individuals. They reported that zinc in the plasma seems to be bound to serum proteins, but the persons affected had no apparent clinical symptoms or abnormalities. However, I wonder about possible negative effects if a person who unknowingly had hyperzincemia were to take zinc supplements.

It is possible that zinc supplementation may sometimes be appropriate for older persons since they (or at least men) seem to have much less ability to absorb this mineral. Judith Turnlund and Sheldon Margen[374] observed that, although adult men, 65 to 74 years of age, seemed to absorb iron as well as younger men, zinc was much more poorly absorbed in the older subjects. The conclusion that more supplementation is required may or may not be warranted. It is always possible that "body wisdom" is shutting off the zinc supply for reasons not yet understood. Remember, zinc is associated with tumor formation, but animal experiments suggest that, depending on dosage and experimental design, it can either inhibit or enhance carcinogenesis. The *reverse effect* of zinc may quite possibly be due to zinc's influence on prostaglandin synthesis (as discussed in Chapter 3).[374a] Obviously, it is yet another case of both our ignorance as to what may constitute optimal nutrition and also our ignorance as to how *reverse effects* can be understood for the maximal benefit of any given individual.

Those fasting will lose large amounts of zinc in the urine. A 54-day study of urinary excretion of nitrogen, phosphorus, zinc and magnesium during starvation was reported by Herta Spencer et al.[375] During the first six days there were small increases in the urinary excretion of magnesium and calcium and a large increase in the excretion of zinc while excretion of nitrogen and phosphorus declined. After six days urinary zinc continued to increase while excretion of the other elements declined. Perhaps this loss of zinc is a reason for the diminished libido men generally experience during fasting, although I speculate libido loss may sometimes be due to an attendant drop in blood pressure.

If you plan to use zinc supplements, you may prefer to take them several hours apart from any iron* or selenium pills since these minerals compete with zinc for assimilation. Some scientists have reported zinc and copper to be antagonistic. However, a rat study by N. F. Adham and M. K. Sung[376] showed that copper had no effect on the zinc content of rat internal organs, whereas excess calcium decreased the organ's zinc content by 40%. Thus, one might presume that separating zinc and calcium supplementation by several

---

* Leslie S. Valberg et al.[375a] found, however, that while both inorganic iron and heme iron inhibited zinc absorption from zinc chloride, they did not inhibit zinc absorption from a test meal of turkey.

hours would be sensible.* On the other hand, based on rat experiments, the transport of zinc may be beneficially influenced by ascorbic acid.[379]**

Supplements of zinc and of folic acid may interfere with each other's assimilation. In Chapter 5 we noted that Wilson and, independently, Milne (references 147c,d of that chapter) reported folic acid can depress zinc assimilation. Recently, in 1986, Fayez K. Ghishan et al.[379b] not only confirmed the work of Wilson and of Milne, but also found that zinc depresses assimilation of folic acid. The inhibition was found to exist at the site of intestinal transport, a fact suggesting that if supplements of zinc and folic acid are being used they should be taken at least several hours apart.

In the event you are under a doctor's care and have been prescribed a tetracycline, be sure to tell him if you are supplementing with zinc. The effect of tetracyclines (except doxycycline and minocycline), under the influence of zinc, may be decreased if taken within two hours of each other.[379c] Plasma and erythrocyte zinc is decreased in women using oral contraceptives,[171b] possibly due to the concomitant increase in copper.

If you are a devotee of multivitamin supplements, you will be interested in an observation made by Noel W. Solomons and Robert A. Jacob.[380] The authors studied the 24 supplements listed in the 1977 *Physician's Desk Reference* and found only three had an iron/zinc ratio under 3:1. They concluded that the iron content of 21 of these 24 preparations might interfere with the availability of the

---

* Herta Spencer et al.[377] reported that they could not demonstrate a calcium-zinc antagonism in humans. Failing to demonstrate that such antagonism exists is, of course, different than demonstrating that the antagonism does not exist. In this regard, we noted earlier that zinc antagonizes the *in vitro* action of calcium in histamine secretion by human basophils. Furthermore, there is preliminary evidence that zinc inhibits functions of calmodulin.[378] (George J. Brewer[378a] has cited considerable evidence that zinc is an inhibitor of the calcium-activated calmodulin function.) Whether or not calcium and zinc compete for absorption, zinc inhibits (for better or for worse) many calcium-activated functions of the cell. If one greatly increases calcium intake, it would seem reasonable to also increase the consumption of zinc.

** Benjamin M. Sahagian et al.[379a] also reported that ascorbic acid enhanced zinc *transport* in rats. However, the *uptake* of zinc (and also of manganese) was depressed by L-ascorbate and dehydroascorbate.

zinc. Their work also indicates a fact we noted earlier, that heme iron is far less antagonistic than nonheme iron to the absorption of zinc.

Zinc as a Possible Anti-aging Element

Let's close this section on zinc with an optimistic note from Doron Garfinkel[380a] who, in 1986, published an article entitled "Is Aging Inevitable? The Intracellular Zinc Deficiency Hypothesis of Aging." Garfinkel maintains that a review of the relevant literature (his article has 85 references) suggests that an intracellular zinc deficiency may be the primary cause of the aging process. He points out that zinc-metaloenzymes play an important role in cellular metabolism, including DNA replication, repair and transcription. Garfinkel speculates that if we could find the right zinc compound (I think he should have said *compounds*), it might be possible to avoid development of intracellular zinc deficiency and thereby perhaps retard the aging process.

Garfinkel quotes A. S. Prasad[380b] as saying: "One should not expect that the zinc-dependent enzymes are affected to the same extent in all tissues of a zinc-deficient animal. Differences in the sensitivity of enzymes are evidently the result of differences in both zinc-ligand affinity of the various zinc-metaloenzymes and in their turnover rates in the cells of the affected tissues." Garfinkel goes on to say, "The response of a cell to zinc deficiency will depend upon the specific metabolic pathway regulated by its most vulnerable zinc-enzyme or zinc-enzymes. If zinc were involved with aging, the rate and manifestations of aging would be expressed differently by different tissues."

This brings to mind the work of Bergman and Soremark[269] discussed earlier in regard to the problems of hair analysis. Recall, they found that, in mice, the uptake by the pituitary gland of zinc administered as zinc benzoate was considerable, but that zinc given as zinc chloride did not accumulate in this gland. Does this suggest that unless mice (and perhaps humans) consume zinc in the form of the benzoate the pituitary might age more rapidly? Probably not, but I think it argues in favor of consuming zinc (and other nutrients) in a wide variety of forms from an array of zinc-concentrated foods and supplements. Regrettably, a wide array of zinc supplements, including zinc benzoate, is not readily available. Perhaps some supplier will take the hint and put a dozen forms of zinc in a single pill.

Sodium Chloride

People have been eating supplementary salt for at least five thousand years. It has always exerted great importance over human affairs, and wars have been fought to protect or obtain sources of supply. Men have been paid in salt for their labors and thus the word *salary* originated. History and tradition have joined to reinforce the practice of eating excessive amounts of salt—a habit highly detrimental to health.

Salt is essential for the body. However, cutting down one's salt intake may sometimes be a good move, but only if it can be done without reducing one's calcium consumption. Excessive salt can increase body weight not just through promoting water accumulation but (and this could be especially important to diabetics) through stimulating absorption of sugars.[380ba, 400a]

We previously stated, in connection with calcium, that Laragh and Pecker hold that only hypertensive persons with low levels of the kidney hormone renin (about 30% of those having high blood pressure) are likely to benefit from decreased levels of sodium intake.[57a,b] Most persons probably can use salt with impunity, but 20% or more* of Americans (the ones who develop high blood pressure) may be detrimentally affected by high levels of salt and, in some cases, the excessive salt could have caused or helped to cause the problem. Alta M. Engstrom and Rosemary C. Tobelmann[380c] reported that because of the increased awareness that sodium may be related to hypertension, many valuable foods are being eliminated from the diet. As a result, according to Tobelmann, a significant proportion of the population is consuming less than 66% of the RDA for calcium, iron,

---

* The percentage is a matter of how one defines "high blood pressure."

magnesium and vitamin B6. At any rate, unprocessed foods* naturally contain about the right amount of salt so the salt shaker, if it is to be used at all, should be used sparingly.

Excessive salt is implicated in many diseases. Several studies associate salted food with gastric cancer and some associate salt with other digestive tract cancers.[381] Ailsa Goulding and Dianne Campbell[382] suggest that, based on rat experiments, sodium chloride could even exacerbate bone loss, especially in postmenopausal women. In rats, increased salt causes decreased renal tubular reabsorption of calcium and thus lowered amounts of ionized calcium in plasma. This, in turn, stimulates parathyroid hormone secretion which results in bone resorption. It is this series of reactions that may make salt a threat in the development of osteoporosis in humans.

As we discussed in Chapter 3, inhibition of prostaglandin synthesis decreases renal excretion of sodium. We learned that linoleic and gamma-linolenic acids can encourage prostaglandin synthesis and the excretion of sodium and that this sometimes results in the lowering of blood pressure.

Sodium-potassium-dependent ATPase, which moves sodium and potassium in and out of the cells, must operate efficiently to normalize blood pressure. A number of investigators[383-385] have postulated the existence of circulating inhibitors of Na-K-ATPase. Vanadate, as discussed later in this chapter under vanadium, is an example of such an inhibitor. (Recently, Fuminori Masugi et al.[386] have developed a sensitive assay method to evaluate the inhibition provided by these factors.) A. M. Heagerty et al.[387] have pointed out, however, that there are many types of abnormalities in membrane handling of electrolytes, only one of which is defective sodium pump activity.

Studies made in various parts of the world have shown that the mean sodium intake is related to the prevalence of hypertension. However, studies within populations do not indicate a clear relationship between sodium consumption and individual blood pressure. Contrary to what you have heard, and strictly from the standpoint of hypertension, the majority of Americans probably do

---

* If they have been processed, excessive amounts of salt may have been added.

not have to worry about their salt intake. [388] Salt retention causes hypertension only when it also increases the volume of extracellular fluid. [388a] Interestingly, a study by David L. Longworth et al. [389] showed that in 28% of outpatients blood pressure rose at least 5 mm Hg when sodium was restricted.* Longworth et al. reported that, upon sodium restriction, patients whose blood pressure declined generally had low-renin hypertension. Those whose blood pressure rose upon restricting sodium generally had high-renin hypertension. A. Mark Richards et al. [412a] also found variable effects in hypertensive patients put on a sodium-restricted diet. Lower blood pressure readings were found in seven patients, higher levels in five, with a nonsignificant overall reduction of 4 mm. in mean pressure. However, this study was conducted over only a brief period of about four weeks and Alan J. Silman, [412b] criticizing the protocol, says the hypotensive effect of sodium restriction is generally effective only after a much longer period of time. Studies by C. A. Farleigh et al., [389d] by Jacqueline J. M. Castenmiller et al., [389e] and many other studies cited by David A. McCarron [404aa] have reported that sodium intake has no effect on normotensive humans.

Experiments with rats suggest that it is not sodium as such, but sodium chloride, that may be at fault in elevating blood pressure. In a study by Theodore W. Kurtz and R. Curtis Morris, Jr., [390] blood pressure of rats increased much more with a given dietary intake of sodium chloride than with equivalent intakes of sodium in the form of sodium bicarbonate, sodium ascorbate or a combination of these

---

* Earlier, David Robertson et al., [389a] studying normal subjects, found that sodium restriction increased supine plasma norepinephrine by 37% and ambulatory plasma norepinephrine by 22%. The most potent stimuli of norepinephrine were treadmill exercise, orthostasis (standing upright), caffeine, the cold pressor test (the left hand was placed in a pan containing equal parts of water and ice for 60 seconds), sodium restriction and handgrip exercise, in descending order. Another study of David Robertson et al. [389b] showed that in nine healthy, young, noncoffee drinkers maintained in sodium balance throughout the study period, caffeine (250 mg.) increased plasma renin activity by 57%, plasma norepinephrine by 75% and plasma epinephrine by 207%. Mean blood pressure rose 14/10 mm Hg one hour after caffeine ingestion. A follow-up study by David Robertson et al. [389c] reported that no long-term effects on blood pressure, heart rate, plasma renin activity, plasma catecholamines or urinary catecholamines could be demonstrated.

two chemicals. Studies by T. A. Kotchen et al.[390a] and by Shirley A. Whitescarver et al.[390b] similarly concluded that sodium chloride, not sodium as such, is the pressor chemical.[*] Kurtz and Morris[390e] subsequently reported that while sodium chloride induces persisting hypercalciuria as well as hypertension in rats, sodium carbonate does not. As the doctrine that the problem is not excessive sodium but rather excessive *sodium chloride* receives wider acceptability, it seems likely that low-sodium diets and tables showing the sodium content of foods will need revision. For example, breads and cakes have rather high amounts of sodium due to their baking powder or baking soda, but a relatively low content of sodium chloride.

Haralambos Gavras,[390f] in 1986, published his hypothesis regarding the mechanism by which salt raises blood pressure in affected persons. Gavras proposed the theory that "sodium exerts its hypertensive action by decreasing the state of affinity of the $\alpha2$-adrenergic receptors of the central nervous system for locally occurring agonist neurotransmitters, which results in disinhibition of sympathoinhibitory neurons and leads to the hyperadrenergic state characteristic of salt-induced hypertension." Interested readers who seek clarification of that "mouthful" are encouraged to request a photostatic copy of the Gavras article from their local library.

Belding H. Scribner[390g] points out the great need for a test to determine which of us are sensitive to increased salt intake.[**] In the absence of such a test he suggests that any person likely to develop hypertension should restrict salt intake. Among those he cites are:

---

[*] R. J. Shneidman and D. A. McCarron,[390c] interestingly, have found that sodium can act synergistically to *lower* blood pressure in hypertensive rats. In another study, S. A. Hahn et al.[390d] found that sodium restriction exacerbated blood pressure in rats and blunted the pressure-lowering effect of *calcium*. (Regrettably, neither report shows the type of sodium that was administered.) People do not necessarily react as do rats, but the studies of David L. Longworth[389] cited above show that even some hypertensives may be detrimentally affected by severe sodium restriction.

[**] John H. Laragh and Mark S. Pecker[57b] would argue, as we noted earlier, that such a test (for renin levels) already exists. Renin is a proteolytic enzyme in the kidney that acts on renin substrate to liberate angiotensin I, the precursor of the more active angiotensin II. The angiotensins are pressor-vasoconstrictors.

1. Any person with chronic renal disease;[*]
2. Any person with one or both hypertensive parents;
3. Certain racial groups, especially black males; and
4. Most persons older than 50 years. (Ability of kidneys to handle a sodium load decreases with age.)

So, while combating too extensive use of the salt shaker is not all there is to reducing hypertension, I think it is usually a good idea to make this a first step. Nutritional approaches to treating hypertension will be found under potassium, which immediately follows our discussion about sodium chloride.

The Chloride Content of Salt

Generally it is the sodium component of salt that is denounced, the chlorine content usually escaping condemnation. The chloride component of salt is useful in making the stomach's hydrochloric acid which is required for protein digestion. Chloride also helps the liver in its detoxifying action, although an excess will tend to destroy vitamin E. Chloride is a constituent of enzymes used for digesting fat and starch. Adequate chloride seems to be especially important in the case of potassium deficiency. Hans Kaunitz and Ruth Ellen Johnson[390i] reported that, in the absence of chloride, and regardless of whether sodium was present, potassium-deficient rats developed advanced testicular degeneration.

The way the body handles chloride may be related to the development of cystic fibrosis. Gina Kolata[391] relates that, based to a large degree on the research of Paul Quinton of the University of California at Riverside, it is speculated that cystic fibrosis may be caused by a genetic defect affecting the channels by which chloride enters and leaves the cells. The salty sweat that is characteristic of cystic fibrosis helps support the speculation. Kolata reported that Richard Boucher of the University of North Carolina at Chapel Hill has found the chloride in nasal epithelia of cystic fibrosis patients is

---

[*] On the other hand, renal tubular necrosis is more likely to occur with salt depletion[390h]—a possible *reverse effect*. Excessive salt restriction could be harmful to persons with a tendency toward this condition.

half that of controls. Thus, it seems likely that cystic fibrosis involves a deficiency of chloride within the cells.

Chloride sources other than salt are kelp, watercress, avocado, chard, tomatoes, cabbage, endive, cucumbers, asparagus, pineapples, cherries, oats, wheat germ, milk, butter, oysters, lamb, mutton, gizzard, okra, collards, spinach, marjoram, egg white and saltwater fish. Chlorine is also one of the constituents of vitamin B1.

Adverse Effects of Chlorine

We saw earlier that chlorine, rather than sodium, may be the detrimental constituent of salt.[*]   Chlorine has other bad aspects. Robert Harris, author of the Environmental Defense Fund study published by the Environmental Protection Agency, is very concerned about the carcinogenic properties of chlorine. He is quoted in *Science*[392] as saying that chlorination "could conceivably be an important cause of cancer, probably not as important as cigarettes but maybe not dramatically less." *Science* goes on to explain, "The reason is that chlorine has recently been found to react with the humic acids often present in water to produce a family of compounds known as trihalomethanes, one of which is chloroform, a confirmed cause of cancer in animals."[**] J. R. Meier et al.[393] have also studied chlorination of humic acids and cite many references for the common occurrence of mutagenic chemicals in finished drinking water. To further add to the problem of obtaining pure drinking water, potentially hazardous compounds, dihaloacetonitriles (DHANs), are formed when halogens, such as chlorine, react with amino acids and other organic materials in water during the process of disinfection.

---

[*] Shirley A. Whitescarver et al.[391a] found that, while blood pressure increased in rats fed 4% sodium chloride, it did not increase in those fed equivalent amounts of chloride as glycine chloride. They concluded that the development of hypertension is dependent not on sodium or chloride but on sodium chloride. However, John C. Passmore et al.[391b] (in a group that included Whitescarver) concluded that chloride independently contributed to sodium chloride-induced hypertension in rats. Whitescarver,[391c] in a subsequent study done in 1986 with salt-sensitive rats, again concluded that chloride loading (without sodium) does not alter blood pressure in either salt-sensitive or renin-dependent hypertension.

[**] A recent study by Charles E. Lawrence et al.[392a] of white schoolteachers in upstate New York found, on the contrary, that there was no evidence relating trihalomethanes in drinking water to colorectal cancer.

Dichloroacetonitrile, the most prominent member of the class, has been found to be mutagenic by the Ames test.[394]

Other studies show increased evidence for an association between chlorinated water and the incidence of rectal, colon and bladder cancer. The Council on Environmental Quality[394a] reported a 13% to 93% increase in tumor incidence when chlorinated water is regularly drunk. Thomas H. Maugh II[395] states that most epidemiologists that were interviewed agree that there is persuasive evidence to link chlorinated contaminants in drinking water with an increased cancer incidence, but what to do about it is not clear. (This preceded the study by Lawrence et al.[392a] referred to in the subnote. Nevertheless, Robert J. Morin and Peter Barna[392b] subsequently reviewed, in 1986, various studies pointing to the possibility that an increased incidence of various cancers may be associated with the drinking of heavily-chlorinated water.) Chlorination of water has virtually eliminated cholera epidemics, so hasty solutions may be regretted later. Ozonation is costly but a possible alternative. Granular-activated carbon filters will do the job, but how could one install such a filter on every drinking water tap? Meanwhile, federal regulations are now in effect to mandate that concentrations of trihalogenated methanes in public drinking water must remain below 100 parts per billion.

Another possible solution would be to treat drinking water with chlorine dioxide rather than with chlorine itself since chlorine dioxide does not interact with organic compounds to form trihalomethanes. However, chlorine dioxide, in reacting with water, forms chlorite. Certain persons, primarily blacks or whites of Mediterranean origin, may have a deficiency of the enzyme G6PD and because of this deficiency could be at particular risk in being exposed to chlorite. G. S. Moore et al.[396] reported that when such persons are exposed to chlorite they are three or four times more likely to develop hemolytic anemia.

Even fresh water, depending on its source, has been found to contain chemicals known to be or suspected to be mutagenic or carcinogenic. Chlorination further exacerbates the possible problem since other chemicals in water can be converted by chlorination to more reactive forms. Hypochlorite and chloramine, to name two of these, have both been shown to be mutagenic. Swimming pool water, with its organic contaminants such as sweat, epithelial cells, urine, menstrual blood, hair and cosmetics, when chlorinated has been found to be mutagenic. Reports of this finding and other references relating to the mutagenicity of chlorinated water are given by W. G. Honer et al.[397]

Chlorinated swimming pool water also presents a threat of corneal edema. A study by Jeffrey R. Haag and Richard G. Gieser[398] showed that 47 out of 50 subjects exposed to chlorinated swimming pool water had corneal epithelial erosions, although none experienced a measurable decrease in visual acuity.

The chlorinous smell emanating from swimming pools is caused not by chlorine gas but by nitrogen trichloride (an intense irritant) and to a lesser extent by monochloramine and chloroform.[398a] These compounds are produced when chlorine, in solution as hypochlorus acid, reacts with urea, creatine and other organic substances introduced into the pool by swimmers. These chlorinous gases can produce wheezing in sensitive persons and the problem is exacerbated by heat reclamation systems that recirculate pool air.[398a] The alternative is for pools to use ozone in addition to chlorine as a disinfectant, but modification of existing disinfecting systems is reported to be expensive.[398a]

Yet another danger of chlorine compounds exists in typewriter correction fluids (e.g., Liquid Paper®, Wite-Out®, Snopake®, etc.). A rather recent form of substance abuse is the inhalation of their fumes. The trichloroethylene and perchloroethylene in these products, when inhaled,[398b] can cause cardiovascular, respiratory, hepatic and renal damage, and mental phenomena such as delerium.[398c]

Problems of Too Little Sodium

Earlier we condemned an excess of sodium, at least an excess in the form of sodium chloride. A sodium deficiency, on the other hand, is also detrimental and can cause flatulence, muscle shrinkage and impaired metabolism. W. P. Kennedy, reporting on research with rats, indicated that a sodium deficiency caused a reduction in fertility. Sodium (as well as calcium) plays a role in cholinergic transmission, the depolarizing effect of acetylcholine being due mainly to the movement of sodium ions into the cells. [399] In addition, sodium is responsible, in part, for the intestinal transport of calcium.[400] Sodium is also an important factor aiding the intestinal transport of glucose and of some amino acids. [400a] Furthermore, sodium controls 90%-95% of the effective osmotic pressure of the extracellular fluid. Sodium is also required for renal absorption of glucose and phosphate.[401] In these and other ways a modest amount of sodium is vital to body chemistry. Food sources of sodium are dairy products (especially whey, butter and cheddar cheese), margarine, mayonnaise, olives, meat, fish, celery, beans, beets, beet greens, dandelion greens, carrots, cucumbers, okra and swiss chard.

Sodium enters our diet not only as salt but because of foods preserved in sodium nitrite* and in Chile saltpeter (sodium nitrate) instead of the more expensive true saltpeter (potassium nitrate). It also is present in monosodium glutamate, used with particular prominence in Chinese cooking. Still other sources of sodium are baking powder (in cakes, etc.), baking soda, soy isolates, hydrolyzed vegetable protein, sodium benzoate, sodium hydroxide, sodium propionate (in bread and crackers) and sodium alginate.

More Adverse Effects of Salt

Sodium and potassium tend to be balanced in the blood. Either in excess causes the other to be lost via the urine. When potassium is deficient in the diet, excessive sodium chloride tends to be retained. Excessive salt can, in some cases, not only lead to hypertension, but it can cause edema. Excessive salt may also sometimes be implicated in hair loss, hives, epilepsy, colds, sinus trouble, insomnia and nervous tension. Salt may sometimes also exacerbate many other conditions such as kidney disease, dropsy, liver disease, arthritic swelling, migraine headaches and tooth decay (by causing the body to lose calcium). Excessive amounts of sodium (whether from salt or

---

* Michael W. Pariza[401a] points out that use of nitrite at the legal limit in the curing of meats will not inhibit botulism unless sufficient salt is present. The current trend to curtail salt consumption, if it leads to a drastic lowering of salt levels in cured meats, might increase the danger of botulism.

other sources) can also result in a false-positive indication on the Diagnex blue test for impaired gastric function.

Drinking the proverbial eight glasses of water per day is usually healthful, but excessive drinking (polydypsia) could be a sign that one may be eating too much salt. [402] David F. Bohr[402] speculates that hypertension arises from a defect in calcium binding of the plasma membrane in cells of the pressure-regulating center in the hypothalamus. This causes altered sodium permeability. Bohr found that when blood pressure was reversed on a low-salt diet, polydypsia was also reversed.

It may be especially important not to oversalt the baby's food. Experiments with rats[403] showed that the animals were more prone to develop hypertension if they were fed high-salt diets at the time of weaning than if fed similar amounts of salt (proportioned to body weight) later in life. If such results have human application, it may be especially important to not salt an infant's food in accordance with the mother's possibly jaded taste sense. James Weiffenbach et al.[404] have reported that taste acuity for salt and bitter (but not for sweet and sour) declines with age. The sodium content of human breast milk decreases after parturition and reaches low levels after a few months.[404a] Nature is sending us a message we should heed.

It may be wise to taper off in your use of salt. However, if the "sodium and salt scare" leads one to cut back on a strong calcium source such as cheese, higher rather than lower blood pressures may result (and also, perhaps, osteoporosis).* Nevertheless, instead of the salt shaker, you might consider using powdered Norwegian kelp. (Being a sea plant, it does, of course, contain salt. Kelp has, however, much less sodium chloride and a far greater amount of valuable minerals than sea salt. Observe, nevertheless, warnings later in this chapter regarding excessive intake of iodine which is, of course, concentrated in kelp.) If you have been drinking artificially softened water, you may be drinking a weak saline solution. When cooking, experiment with the use of spices instead of salt. Let me

---

* Ask your librarian to obtain photostats of the recent debate between David A. McCarron[404aa] and Graham A. MacGregor[404ab] regarding the relative importance of sodium and of calcium in the pathogenesis of hypertension.

stress, however, that while some persons may be helped by salt restriction, others could be harmed. We must not ignore the fact that a modest amount of salt in the diet has a positive value.[404b]

Both sodium and chloride excretion generally reach a maximum somewhat before noon (but the cycle is reversed in night workers). Under the theory one should not thwart body rhythms, salting food at breakfast might be especially unhealthful since the body is trying to dispose of both sodium and chloride during the morning hours.

If you can't seem to leave the salt shaker alone (and you are sure it's not a problem of *hypogeusia* as discussed in connection with zinc), consider using potassium chloride instead or use a product such as Morton's Lite Salt®—a combination of sodium chloride and potassium chloride—but observe warnings given below in the potassium section. Avoid sea salt since it is apt to differ from the salt of ancient seas (that is mined by the big salt companies) only in its lack of additives, that possible "plus" being offset by its greater concentration of heavy metals—the latter factor being a result of today's pollution of our oceans. Better yet, use *rock salt* (also known as *earth salt*) which is mined from ancient seas but is without the additives found in the usual commercial variety. It is available at some specialty food shops.

In this section we have been considering sodium and chloride but mostly as sodium chloride. However, an interesting use of sodium bicarbonate has recently surfaced. Soda loading or buffer boosting is an ergogenic aid in athletic competition.[404c] The evidence indicates it can be used to enhance performance by reducing the lactic-acid buildup, and oral consumption of sodium bicarbonate is the favorite vehicle. D. P. M. MacLaren and G. D. Morgan[404d] have, in fact, reported a 12% longer time to exhaustion than with a placebo and this was determined to be a significant increase. Diarrhea, however, may be an undesirable result. Although soda loading has not yet been banned in athletic competition, it obviously contravenes the policy on doping.* When detection techniques are developed, soda loading most likely will be forbidden.

---

* Some of the legal and ethical problems of blood doping have been discussed by Harvey G. Klein[404e] and by Allan J. Ryan.[404f]

Potassium

It is speculated that the potassium content in the Precambrian oceans was much higher relative to the sodium content than it was even a relatively few years later. Since life arose at that time, this is suggested as a reason potassium is the major intracellular element. It is further speculated that when life emerged from the sea the sodium content of the oceans had already greatly increased relative to their potassium content and thus sodium became the major extracellular element.

That all seems very hypothetical. Perhaps it is more practical and potentially more valuable to study the relative dietary consumption of potassium and sodium for humans as contrasted with that of animals. S. Heyden and C. G. Hames[405] point out that, whereas the human dietary consumption of sodium is three to six times higher than our potassium intake, the reverse is true of the natural diet of lower animals. They state that carnivores consume four to five times as much potassium as sodium and herbivores consume 12 to 20 times as much. S. Boyd Eaton and Melvin Konner[26a] have estimated that the dietary ratio of potassium to sodium in paleolithic man was about 16 to 1. Generally, food processing greatly reduces potassium content and tremendously increases sodium content. Only recently have processors, because of consumer demand, generally reduced the amount of sodium they add to food.

Potassium and sodium interact within the body. Potassium is present primarily inside the cells with only a little existing in the fluids outside the cells. Sodium, on the other hand, is found largely outside the cells with only a small quantity in the cells' interior. Potassium holds water within the cells; sodium holds it between the cells. Good health is dependent on the free transport of sodium and potassium across the cell's membrane. One of the very negative aspects of lead is that, when present, it will interfere with this process. Harlan & Mann,[406] Sagnella & MacGregor[406a] have reported there is a factor in food which *in vitro* experiments show impairs the Na-K$^+$-ATPase-dependent ion pump. The factor is found in tea, cocoa, red wines and in some other dietary components. Various other studies have observed that sodium-potassium-ATPase activity may be lower in obese persons, but one study concluded the activity was higher in the obese. Ernest Beutler et al.[407] found that obesity was irrelevant to the operation of this enzyme but that its activity was a function of a person's ethnic origin. Non-Jewish white subjects, especially those with some Scandinavian ancestry, had the highest activity in this enzyme. Operation of the sodium-potassium pump is facilitated by adequate intake of potassium, magnesium and gamma-linolenic acid.[407a]

Potassium is also needed in the process whereby glucose is converted to glycogen for storage in the liver. When there is a deficiency of potassium to the extent that glucose metabolism is impaired, muscles cannot perform properly. A study by R. W. Hubbard et al.[408] showed that potassium-deficient rats run to exhaustion accomplished less than one-half the work done by controls. Persons doing hard physical work will, like the rats, require more potassium than those who are more sedentary.

Potassium-deficient diets of some elderly persons may contribute to the muscular weakness they sometimes display. The heart is, of course, a muscle and potassium serves a very important function in helping the heart maintain a regular beat. A deficiency of potassium in the coronary muscles may be a cause of heart disease and S. Bertil Olsson[409] has reported that decreased atrial muscle potassium in human patients greatly increases the occurrence of atrial fibrillation. Bowel action is also related to the strength of the intestinal muscles and so a potassium deficiency can be a cause of sluggish bowels and related pains due to excessive gas.

In connection with the nonvitamin B_{17}(laetrile) we noted a possible rationale for the Gerson high-potassium treatment of cancer. Mark F. McCarty[410] speculates that the Gerson diet of high potassium, low sodium should enhance the body's level of aldosterone. He suggests that some tumors may be sensitive to mineralocorticoids and this could help explain the success of the Gerson diet. Cope,[410a] citing work of Ling, holds that a high-potassium diet aids repair of toxin-caused tissue damage.

Potassium and the Problem of Hypertension

A moderate increase in potassium intake may be beneficial in reducing hypertension. In lowering blood pressure, potassium may be acting as a diuretic agent and thereby reduce extracellular volume which, in turn, could reduce blood pressure. On the other hand, potassium could alter renin-angiotensin activity and reduce angiotensin influence on vascular, adrenal or renal receptors. There are yet other possible explanations for this action of potassium and those interested are referred to a review by Janet Treasure and David Ploth[410b] of potassium's role in the treatment of hypertension.

Graham A. MacGregor et al.[411] reported that a group of 23 unselected patients with mild to moderate essential hypertension were entered into a double-blind randomized crossover study of one month's treatment with slow-release potassium pills without altering dietary sodium or potassium intake. After four weeks, mean supine blood pressure of the supplemented group had fallen 4% compared with the placebo group. However, not all patients had a fall in blood pressure with potassium supplementation. The investigators observed that the increase in potassium intake could have been achieved without pills by using a potassium-based salt substitute and by increased consumption of fruits and vegetables. The same scientists had earlier demonstrated a 6% average drop in blood pressure in a group undergoing moderate sodium restriction alone.

Osamu Iimura et al.[412] also reported that orally administered potassium greatly reduced the mean arterial pressure in a group of patients from an average of 114 to an average of 103. Mean Arterial Pressure (MAP) was calculated as the sum of diastolic pressure and one-third of pulse pressure (the difference between systolic and diastolic blood pressures) and was expressed as the average during the first five days. The reduction in MAP was also accompanied by a reduction in body weight and body fluid volume. The reduction in MAP of patients with low plasma renin activity was significantly greater than in persons with normal plasma renin activity.

On the other hand, A. Mark Richards et al.,[412a] whose work was reported on earlier in connection with sodium, found that, like sodium restriction, potassium supplementation had variable but nonsignificant effects on blood pressure. However, the Richards study was conducted over only a brief period of about four weeks and Alan J. Silman,[412b] in commenting on this research, states the hypotensive effect of potassium might, like sodium restriction, be effective only after a much longer time interval. Nevertheless, Stephen J. Smith et al.[412c] have maintained that potassium supplementation is not generally useful to those already restricting their sodium intake. After a two-month placebo-controlled trial of 20 patients with mild to moderate hypertension who had been moderately restricting their sodium intake, they concluded that potassium chloride supplementation did not significantly change supine or standing systolic and diastolic blood pressures.* However, patients deficient in potassium due to use of diuretics may be benefitted by potassium supplementation. A study by Norman M. Kaplan et al.[412d] with patients having diuretic-induced hypokalemia, found that supplementary potassium chloride may induce a significant fall in blood pressure. Interestingly, only a tiny amount of potassium chloride was given (six 10-nanomole tablets daily) for a six-week period. Regrettably, only 16 patients were involved, their diet was not controlled and individual results were not shown.

A study by Kay-Tee-Khaw et al.[412e] of 685 men and women aged 20 to 79 years found dietary intake of potassium estimated from 24-hour recall dietary history to be significantly and negatively correlated with age-adjusted systolic pressure in both men and women and age-adjusted diastolic pressure in men. In women, negative correlations of potassium intake with blood pressure increased after excluding those taking sex hormones.

Orna Ophir et al.[413] studied a group of 98 confirmed adult vegetarians and examined them against a control group for the prevalence of arterial hypertension. The average blood pressure was 126/77 for the vegetarians and 147/88 for the control group. The vegetarians showed significantly lower blood pressure in every decade of age. Only 2% of the vegetarians had hypertension (higher than

---

* Smith reminds us that chloride ions may increase hypertension. (We saw, in the previous section, that sodium chloride was a pressor but other forms of sodium were not.) Perhaps potassium in forms other than potassium chloride, for example fruits and vegetables, might be more useful since not only would the chloride ion be minimal, but the higher fiber content and lower saturated fat content would be additionally beneficial.

160/95) as compared with 26% of the nonvegetarians. A related study found that Buddist vegetarians had significantly lower systolic blood pressures than nonvegetarian matched subjects.[414] In this case, it seems to me, the tranquility of Buddhist life could be an additional factor working to achieve a favorable level of blood pressure. A study by Ray M. Acheson and D. R. R. Williams[415] showed in an epidemiological survey that population groups 45-64 years of age who consumed large amounts of fruits and vegetables had the lowest mortality due to cerebrovascular disease. Those eating large amounts of fruits and vegetables had a high potassium intake and this may be a reason for their generally low incidence of hypertension and their excellent heart health. Olov Lindahl et al.[415a] studied 29 patients who had had essential hypertension for an average of eight years, all receiving long-term medication for this condition. They went on a vegan diet for one year and in almost all cases medication was withdrawn or drastically reduced. There was a significant decrease in their systolic and diastolic blood pressure.

However, Ian L. Rouse et al.[416] would disagree that the increase in potassium/sodium ratio was responsible for the good effects. They reported, as had the other studies, that diastolic blood pressures fell significantly in a group who normally ate an omnivorous diet after they changed to a lacto-ova-vegetarian diet. Blood pressures rose again when they returned to an omnivorous diet. However, the scientists concluded that the effects were not mediated by changes in sodium or potassium intake. They maintained the view that the vegetarian diet, being lower in total fat but richer in linoleic acid, worked to lower blood pressure by increasing the synthesis of vasodilatory and natriuretic prostaglandins. (This would tie in with comments made in Chapter 3.) Nevertheless, Mark S. Paller and Stuart L. Linas[417] reported that potassium has a direct vasodilatory effect on arterial smoothe muscle cells rather than on either sodium balances or pressor hormone activity.

Then too, potassium supplementation may be beneficial in reducing the occurrence of strokes even when blood pressure remains unchanged. At any rate, L. Tobian et al.[417a] reported that adding potassium to the chow of stroke-prone, spontaneously hypertensive rats significantly reduced mortality even when there was no drop in blood pressure.

Potassium intake is no exception to the concept of the golden mean. Barbara Chipperfield and John R. Chipperfield[417b] have reported that a potassium/sodium ratio of 2.8 to 3.0 in the heart muscle seems to be optimum. Up to that ratio , additional potassium in the heart muscle increases survival from arteriosclerosis; thereafter there is a *reverse effect* and a further rise in this ratio increases mortality rates. The Chipperfields found a significant increase in myocardial potassium in people dying suddenly from ischemic heart disease.* Although soft drinking water is not generally rich in potassium, it is often also deficient in magnesium and the Chipperfields speculate that this magnesium deficiency may bring on cell-membrane changes to cause the cell to retain both magnesium and potassium.

In this regard, it seems apparent that studies regarding the effect of potassium on hypertension and on other cardiovascular effects should (but usually fail to) control for magnesium. Burton M. Altura and Bella T. Altura,[418] in a paper titled "New Perspectives on the Role of Magnesium in the Pathology of the Cardiovascular System" presented at the 12th French Colloquium on Magnesium (and published with 376 references in the journal *Magnesium*), make this statement: "The data suggest, *albeit* most indirectly, that Mg^+ can to a large extent regulate the cellular and subcellular distribution and the intracellular concentration of K^+."

(Continued on page 686)

---

* Many animal experiments have shown that a potassium deficiency can produce a *reverse effect* and lead to vasodilation and decreased blood pressure. Some of the many experiments that demonstrate this *reverse effect* are cited by Mark S. Paller and S. L. Linas.[417] More recently, Richard L. Tannen[418a] has similarly reported that potassium *depletion* can not only cause hypotension in normotensive animals but can sometimes show a *reverse effect* by lowering blood pressure in hypertensive animals and humans. However, please do not attempt to reduce your blood pressure by restricting your intake of magnesium or potassium. The physiological implications of the *reverse effect* must be understood before it can find therapeutic application.

Some Factors in Essential Hypertension

There are factors other than reduced sodium and increased potassium intake that relate to the genesis and treatment of high blood pressure. Increasing consumption of high-fiber foods[418b] such as fruits, vegetables and cereals (especially rice)[418c] while reducing the consumption of red meats may be useful. Some studies suggest that vitamin C may be associated with a lowering of blood pressure in hypertensives. Earlier, we noted a study of this effect by Eunsook T. Koh and another by Mitsuki Yoshioka et al. (references 111a and 111b of Chapter 6). David A. McCarron et al.,[418d] in an epidemiological study, found that reduced consumption of vitamin C (as well as of vitamin A, calcium and potassium) characterize the group of hypertensive persons in America. Insofar as McCarron's study relates to vitamin C, it seems quite possible that low intake of fruit (and only incidentally low intakes of vitamin C) might characterize hypertensives as a group. It could be low fiber or some other factor rather than low vitamin C that may at least partially account for this finding. Nevertheless, a study by Mitsuki Yoshioka et al.[418e] with rats discovered that when they were fed 200 ppm ascorbic acid in the diet, their mean blood pressure was 18-19 mm Hg lower than controls. Among rats fed 1,000 ppm in the diet the mean blood pressure was 30-40 mm Hg below controls. The researchers speculated that ascorbic acid acts on blood pressure through its effect on calcium metabolism and hormones related to calcium metabolism, such as parathyroid hormone and 1,25(OH)$_2$D.

Increased intake of onions and garlic, widely reported to have hypotensive action, and also ginger, according to K. C. Srivastava et al.,[419] may be effective. It may be useful to increase consumption of linoleic and gamma-linolenic acid (via evening primrose oil) to foster production of prostaglandin E$_1$ (as discussed in Chapter 3). Supplementary calcium and also zinc, through its possible stimulus of prostaglandin E₁-synthesis and its action as a vasodilator, may also be useful. It may also be appropriate to use supplementary magnesium to stimulate the potassium-sodium pump.* Recent animal experiments by A. Berthelot and J. Esposito[419b] have shown that with dietary magnesium depletion the heart rate accelerated and hypertension developed more rapidly. Magnesium loading, in contrast, increases sodium excretion in man and in the rat.[419c-419e] Denis M. Medeiros et al.[420] reported a positive association between the hair calcium/magnesium ratio and blood pressure. According to them, the higher the hair calcium relative to the magnesium content, the more likely is it that blood pressure will be elevated. (Let me remind you that high amounts of calcium in the hair do not necessarily reflect high concentrations in the body tissues.) Medeiros and Barbara J. Brown[420a] found that higher dietary copper intakes were associated with higher systolic and diastolic blood pressures, while higher dietary zinc intakes were associated with lower pressures. Supplementary tyrosine, GTF, vitamin B₆ and ubiquinone (coenzyme Q) have also been successfully used to lower excessive blood pressure.[421-421j]** Some of the remarkable *pressure-lowering* results with coenzyme Q₁₀ are thought to be brought about by normalization of peripheral resistance rather than by a cardiac-regulating mechanism.[421d] Aspartame, by the way, has been found to increase brain tyrosine levels in rats and the action is enhanced if the animals receive an insulin-releasing carbohydrate. As a result, their blood pressure was found to be significantly lowered.[422]

Furthermore, beware of those possible blood-pressure raisers:

---

* I. S. Cohen,[419a] on the contrary, suggests that intracellular sodium will not rise if the Na/K pump is inhibited. I am holding with majority opinion on this one, at least for now.

** Supplementary use of any amino acid, such as tyrosine, can increase uric acid formation (which, as we will see in Chapter 9, is not necessarily bad). Then too, more studies are needed before supplementary ubiquinone can be generally recommended since its reactions with vitamins, alcohol as well as with prescription and nonprescription drugs are, to a large degree, unknown.[421g,h] Warnings about excessive use of GTF and vitamin B₆ appear elsewhere in this book.

1. Coffee. A study from the University of Tromso in Norway conducted by Dag S. Thelle et al.[422a] implicates coffee as a long-term former of serum cholesterol. This study showed that men drinking nine or more cups of coffee daily had 14% more cholesterol in their blood than persons who averaged less than one cup. Their findings are contrary to those of Boston University's Framingham Heart Study. An editorial in *Lancet*[422b] speculated that the fact the majority of Tromso residents brew their coffee by boiling, an uncommon practice world-wide, may be a factor in producing the different result. However, a study in Jerusalem by J. D. Kark et al.[422c] confirmed the Tromso results and, in addition, found the association applied to women also. The increase of cholesterol due to coffee was primarily in the LDL fraction. Coffee drinking could therefore be a long-term factor in hypertension. However, Arthur L. Klatsky et al.[423] reported that persons drinking more than six cups of coffee daily tended to have lower blood pressures than those drinking less than six cups daily. Denis M. Medeiros[424] concluded that caffeine had no effect on blood pressure after adjusting for other factors.

Many studies, nevertheless, have found that coffee significantly increased blood pressure, although most have shown that the effect is temporary.* S. Freestone and L. E. Ramsay[425] found that coffee increased blood pressure for a period of at least 2 1/2 hours (the limit of their study). They also reported that coffee drinking combined with cigarette smoking resulted in a much greater pressor effect than coffee or smoking alone. H. P. T. Ammon et al.[426] found that eight cups of coffee per day increased catecholamine excretion and raised mean blood pressure about 5 mm Hg. After the fifth day no significant increase in catecholamine was observed. The investigators concluded that heavy coffee drinking by

---

* A transient increase is not necessarily innocuous. Furthermore, those who drink coffee throughout the day may have their blood pressure almost continuously elevated. How many strokes occur soon after coffee is consumed?

young persons does not appear to lead to hypertension. P. B. Dews[427] found that mean systolic blood pressure of adults given 250 mg. caffeine (equal to about three cups of coffee) rose from 106 mm Hg to 120 mg Hg and diastolic pressure rose from 75 to 85 mm Hg. The heart rate decreased and then increased (contrary to what would be expected under *Marey's Law*). When the subjects were given 250 mg. of caffeine three times a day (i.e., equal to about nine cups of coffee daily) for seven days, the effects ceased to occur. David Robertson et al.[389c,428] also found the blood pressure rises associated with coffee drinking were short-lived and did not exist beyond the third day. There is considerable epidemiological evidence that coffee does not increase the incidence of hypertension, myocardial infarction or sudden death.[428-432] In a massive study[429] involving 81,000 initial and 51,000 follow-up examinations of IBM Corporation employees, no specific correlation could be found between coffee drinking and blood pressure in those studied. (Interestingly, however, among the possible side effects of caffeine is hypotension,[432a] i.e., caffeine might be showing a *reverse effect* by *lowering* the blood pressures of some persons and this effect could be masking a possible direct correlation of caffeine consumption and blood pressure in most persons.)

A mice study by Prince McCann et al.[433] suggests, however, that coffee drinking may be less safe in women taking oral contraceptives. Mice fed ethinyl estradiol (1 mcg./kg. for 28 days) showed a progressive increase in blood pressure (30 mm Hg above controls). Then caffeine (15 mg./kg.) was added for 14 days in addition to the ethinyl estradiol regime. A rapid additional rise in blood pressure (60 mm Hg above controls) resulted. The amount of caffeine (15 mg./kg.) that was used is high but, nevertheless, the results suggest caution.

2. Sugar. Experiments with normotensive rats support the idea that chronic ingestion of *excessive* amounts of sucrose

inhibits pancreatic insulin and elevates systolic blood pressure by 10-15 mm Hg and also increases the pulse rate.[434] When rhesus monkeys were fed enormous amounts of sugar (76.5% of their calories) and spider monkeys were fed sugar to the extent of 38% of their calories, they showed significant increases in blood pressure.[434a] Harry G. Preuss and Richard D. Fournier[434b] have reviewed several experiments showing large amounts of sucrose raised blood pressure in animals (although one experiment concluded that honey did not). In yet another study, it was found by S. R. Srinivasan et al.[434c] that dietary sugar acted synergistically with salt to induce hypertension in spider monkeys. Curiously, however, Denis M. Medeiros and Robert F. Borgman[435] reported that young persons who disliked sweets and desserts had higher systolic and diastolic pressures than those who liked such items. (I suspect this is not because sugar is a "health item" but because it exemplifies the *pleasure concept*. Those who enjoy life tend to be healthier. At any rate, it would not be strange to find that sugar fed in huge amounts to rats and monkeys might display a *reverse effect* if fed to rats and monkeys in the normal amounts of the human diet.)

Serum cholesterol, often associated with blood pressure, may be beneficially *decreased* when consumption of sugar increases. P. J. Palumbo et al.,[435a] in dietary studies of 148 patients with coronary artery disease (CAD), found that diets containing 2 g. of simple carbohydrate (predominantly either sucrose or glucose) per kg. of body weight per day had no significant effect on fasting plasma glucose, serum triglycerides or serum free fatty acids. However, diets with 4 g. of simple carbohydrate (predominantly glucose) or 2 g. of fructose per kg. of body weight per day produced a significant rise in serum triglycerides with decreases in plasma glucose and fatty acids. They reported that, "Serum cholesterol diminished in all the diet groups, probably because of decreased fat and cholesterol intakes." The increase of serum triglycerides in the CAD patients was significantly greater than in normal control subjects fed the same diet, but no significant correlation could be found between changes in serum triglycerides and the extent of CAD as determined from coronary angiograms.

3. Alcohol. Arthur L. Klatsky et al.[423,423a] reported that alcohol had little effect on those consuming two or fewer drinks per day. In fact, women of all races who drank two or fewer drinks per day showed a lower blood pressure than nondrinkers. A recent study by Carlos A. Camargo et al.[435b] suggests that the association of moderate alcohol consumption and reduced risk of coronary heart disease may be mediated in part by increased levels of apolipoproteins A-I or A-II or both. These factors are found primarily in the HDL₃ fraction which, along with HDL₂, is considered to be heart protective. Camargo et al. warn, however, that "generalizations on the effects of alcohol must be avoided, since the nature of most associations with either health or lipoproteins is determined by the amount consumed." With an increased alcohol consumption to three or more drinks daily there seems to be a *reverse effect* and alcohol becomes a hypertensive factor.[423,436,436d]* It has been contended that some studies may have failed to consider that subjects generally take no alcohol before seeing their doctor. A higher blood pressure may result from this temporary withdrawal from alcohol. On withdrawal, urinary epinephrine increases while plasma norepinephrine, arginine, vasopressin and renin activity also increase, any of which could explain the temporary

---

* Richard P. Donahue et al.[436b] of the Honolulu Heart Program, in 1986, reported that there are risk factors for stroke occurrence in alcohol consumption that are independent of hypertensive status. Although they found no significant relationship between use of alcohol and thromboembolic stroke, the risk of hemorrhagic stroke more than doubled for light drinkers (1 to 14 ounces of alcohol per month) and nearly tripled for heavy drinkers (40 ounces or more per month). Elevated alcohol consumption is also associated with an increased risk of cancer. Joyce A. D'Antonio et al.,[436c] in 1986, speculated that the reason for this association may relate to lowered blood levels of cholesterol, vitamin A (carotene and retinol) and vitamin E in heavy consumers of alcohol.

increase in blood pressure.[437] Thus, alcohol could sometimes get unwarranted blame as a hypertensive agent. Nevertheless, J. F. Potter and D. G. Beevers[438] reached a contrary conclusion after studying 16 men with hypertension who drank up to 80 grams of alcohol daily. Antihypertensive treatment ceased two weeks before they were hospitalized for a seven-day study. Half of the men continued their usual alcohol consumption for four days after entering the hospital and their blood pressure remained high. During the next four days no alcohol was taken and both systolic and diastolic pressures dropped significantly. The other half of the group had no alcohol for three days after admission and their blood pressure declined slightly. Then they resumed alcohol consumption and both systolic and diastolic pressures rose significantly. The investigators concluded that hypertension is more likely due to alcohol than to the pressor response produced by alcoholic withdrawal. In keeping with this finding, Victoria Cairns et al.[439] reported that the odds for developing high blood pressure for men drinking 80 grams of alcohol per day (equivalent to about two quarts of beer) were 1.49 compared to nondrinking men. In women drinking one quart of beer daily there was an average increase in diastolic pressure of 2.4 mm Hg. I. B. Puddey et al.[439a] have reported a direct pressor effect of regular alcohol consumption not only among hypertensives but also in 46 normotensives who were moderate drinkers. They speculated that alcohol, therefore, "could be playing a major role in the genesis of the early stages of raised blood pressure." John R. Taylor et al.[439b] reported that alcohol was associated with hypertension in stroke patients and that they were more likely to be current drinkers than controls and were more likely to have been drinking heavily within 24 hours of admission to the hospital.

N. Conway[440] found that alcohol may acutely drop blood pressure. Other studies have, on the contrary, reported little acute effect or even increases in blood pressure. [423,423a,440a] Conway studied the effects of alcohol, 18, 32 and 44 minutes after ingestion—long enough to observe the blood pressure drops he reported, but not long enough to detect the later supranormal rise. Contrasted with these short-term effects, chronic alcohol ingestion detrimentally alters the fatty acid composition of heart, liver and brain (at least in animals).

Many investigators have observed that long-term alcohol consumption increases linoleate and decreases arachidonate. The effects seem to be mediated by alcohol's effect on the desaturases that are instrumental in converting the polyunsaturated fatty acids into prostaglandins. [441] M. S. Manku et al. [442] cite considerable evidence for alcohol enhancing the conversions of dihomo-gamma-linolenic acid (DGLA) to prostaglandins without much affecting the conversion to arachidonic acid. Since DGLA products inhibit platelet aggregation while many products of arachidonic acid enhance aggregation, this may be a "plus" for alcohol. However, after alcohol has mobilized body stores of DGLA there may be insufficient DGLA left for efficiently performing body processes, one characteristic of a "hangover." This action of alcohol provides yet another example of the virtue of the golden mean.

Prostaglandin E_1 from DGLA (and its immediate precursor gamma-linolenic acid, as found in evening primrose oil) is a dilator of coronary and other blood vessels. The Manku group [442] state, "If alcohol is in part exerting its effect by converting DGLA to PGE_1, the combination of alcohol and polyunsaturates would seem particularly desirable." They go on to note that PGE_1 may regulate thymus and T-lymphocyte function and cite references to support this possibility. They conclude, "The control of infections by alcohol consumption may prove to have a scientific basis!" Nevertheless, I am concerned about the results of many studies showing that those habitually drinking excessive amounts of alcohol tend to have supranormal blood pressures. A drink or two daily is probably healthful, but moderation is the "way to go."*

If you have a blood pressure problem, make certain, via hair analysis, that you do not have an excessive burden of lead or other heavy metals that might have pressor effects.[443a,b] There are many nondietary factors in hypertension, e.g., lack of exercise,[443c,d] obesity,[444-446d]** a negative mental attitude*** and an inability to adequately handle stress. (A study by M. Colgan[448] has shown that a patient could be taught biofeedback procedures so that he was able, at will, to significantly lower or raise his systolic blood pressure.)**** Similarly, W. Stewart Agras et al.[449] found that relaxation techniques lowered systolic blood pressure an average of 17 mm Hg. Neither biofeedback nor relaxation training was shown effective in lowering diastolic pressure.***** Later experiments by Betsy C. Little et al. [449c] concluded that, among hypertensive pregnant women, biofeedback and relaxation techniques lowered both systolic and

---

* Cynthia Baum-Baicker[443] has recently done an excellent review (with 106 references) of the health benefits of moderate alcohol consumption.

** A recent study by Christopher L. Melby[446d] concluded that the lower blood pressure in vegetarians they studied "appeared to be best explained by their lower body mass index."

*** A study by G. M. Saunders and Huldah Bancroft[447] shows that among the native population of the Virgin Islands, where the pace of life is very relaxed and racial tensions are low, there is a very high prevalence of hypertension. A good mental attitude helps but is not enough, in itself, to keep one healthy!

**** Many phenomena transiently raise blood pressure. Sue A. Thomas[448a] reported that even the excitement of children reading aloud in school significantly raises both their blood pressure and heart rate. Erika Friedman et al.[448b] found that even speaking rapidly may raise the blood pressure of normotensive individuals. Kenneth L. Malinow et al.[448c] observed the blood pressure of deaf persons while signing and reported, in 1986, that communication, independent of vocalization, has significant effects on the cardiovascular system.

***** A widespread but seemingly false idea exists that holds diastolic pressure to be the more important number. The Framingham study and actuarial statistics indicate that systolic pressure is the more significant.[449a] Nevertheless, a study by Yukiko Shimizu et al.[449b] concluded, "Cerebral hemorrhage was more strongly related to diastolic than to systolic blood pressure, while cerebral infarction appeared to be more strongly related to systolic than to diastolic blood pressure." C. M. Fisher[449ba]

The Reverse Effect

diastolic pressures. Those especially interested in biofeedback and relaxation techniques are likely to also find studies by Bernard L. Frankel et al.,[449d] by James P. Henry,[449e] by Iris B. Goldstein et al.,[449f] by Herbert Benson[449g] and by Chandra Patel[449h] to be valuable. A study by Dean Ornish et al.,[449i] although not employing strictly mental techniques, is also of interest. The Ornish group used a combination of dietary changes, meditation and guided imagery in a controlled experiment with cardiovascular patients, 23 of whom received the therapy and 23 of whom did not. The experimental group demonstrated a 44% mean increase in duration of exercise, a 55% mean increase in work performed, a 20.5% mean decrease in cholesterol and a 91.0% mean reduction in angina episodes. The control group remained essentially unchanged in the various parameters. A general review of nondrug treatment of hypertension by Norman M. Kaplan[449j] will be useful to laymen and to the physicians who guide them. A report by Michael J. Horan et al.[449k] on challenges in nutrition in regard to hypertension will also be useful.

Older persons should have their blood pressure measured at least three times since variability increases with age.[450]****** Blood pressure in older persons should be taken both sitting and standing since the incidence of orthostatic hypotension (postural hypotension), i.e., a drop in pressure when standing, increases with age.[450] One other astonishing development is that high blood pressure in the elderly (85 years and up) seems to improve chances for further longevity[451-453] (Figure 16). Interestingly, J.

---

goes so far as to recommend the "elimination of diastolic readings, at least for routine monitoring." Alan Gilston,[449bb] writing in 1986, notes that the capability of doing the diastolic measurement greatly adds to the cost of automatic blood pressure recorders. He says: "Although physiologically the diastolic pressure is important (e.g., in the context of coronary blood flow) the systolic or mean blood pressure, to which it is so closely linked, is always our practical guide. It is time we abandoned this academic and expensive measurement." Ramsay and Waller disagree.[449bc]

****** At any age, blood pressure may range widely throughout the day. Readings should therefore be taken at appropriate intervals to arrive at average values. Many articles dealing with the circadian rhythms in blood pressure were published in a recent issue of *Chronobiologia*.[451a]

R. A. Mitchell[453] says, "In the very elderly low pressure may be a monument to cardiovascular problems which have already happened." The crossover ages (when higher blood pressure starts to work in one's favor) could be as low as 70 for men and 80 for women.

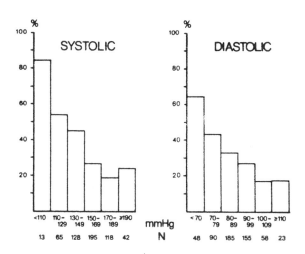

Figure 16. Two-year mortality according to systolic blood pressure in people aged 85 years or more. Reproduced from S. Rajala et al., *Lancet* (Aug. 27, 1983): 520-521, with permission of the publisher and of the author.

Sometimes, lowering of blood pressure in stroke victims might be even more fraught with danger. Patrick Lavin,[453a] treating two stroke patients that were well under the age of 85 (actually 59 and 70), reported in 1986 that, "Lowering systemic blood pressure in patients with acute cerebral infarction may produce clinical deterioration." Interestingly, in a study of 452 stroke survivors, the Hypertension-Stroke Cooperative Study Group[453b] concluded, "The hypothesis that antihypertensive therapy for hypertensive stroke survivors would alter the stroke recurrence rate was not statistically supported by the data." They also reported that, "No statistically significant reduction occurred

in the number of endpoints due to cardiovascular disease except
for congestive heart failure, in which the drug-treated group
exhibited a statistically significant reduction."

Problems of pseudohypertension in the elderly (where
diastolic pressure may be incorrectly measured as being elevated
by 30 mm Hg or more) have been discussed by J. D. Spence et
al.[453c] Their answer to the problem is to employ direct intra-
arterial blood pressure measurements rather than the standard,
but indirect, cuff and manometer technique. In the direct
measurement method a needle is inserted into an artery and
pressures recorded on an arterial/venous tranducer and digital
display system. The interested reader may check the reference
cited.

I have ignored discussing antihypertensive drugs. Many
drugs are subject to *reverse effects,* a fact which accounts for
some of the side effects which often include one or more
conditions the drugs are attempting to correct.
Hydrochlorothiazide is often prescribed to alleviate hypertension.
Among its side effects are purpura and "paradoxical pressor
response."[453d] Purpura indicates that capillaries have broken and
the leaking blood has discolored the skin. The likely cause is a
"paradoxical pressor response," i.e., an increase in blood
pressure, the condition we were trying to correct.

(Continued from page 674)

Circadian Rhythms in Body Potassium

The concentrations of various hormones, minerals and vitamins
in the body undergo circadian rhythms (rhythms that are
approximately one day in length) and the body's potassium
concentration is no exception. Healthy persons retiring at 11 P.M.
and rising at 7 A.M. generally have a peak potassium excretion late in
the morning, whereas the greatest concentration of this mineral in the
red blood cells tends to occur at about 7 P.M. This potassium cycle
affects the activity of the adrenal glands and the operation of the
nervous system.

One of the problems medical research will be asked to solve is the question of whether body rhythms of a particular nutrient, enzyme or hormone should be emphasized or whether, instead, a steady state should be preferred. Earlier, when discussing the diurnal rhythm in serum iron, I suggested that we should foster rather than thwart body cycles. In the case of potassium, also, I believe that potassium-rich foods (such as fruits—including orange juice) may be bad foods for breakfast since they would add to the body's potassium stores while the body is trying to excrete that mineral.[*] On the other hand, perhaps potassium-rich foods should be consumed at lunchtime when the body is starting to excrete less potassium and at a time, therefore, when the body apparently needs more of this mineral. Not much is known in regard to whether the dietary need of the body for potassium is greater at certain times. There is a possibility, however, that diets of the future will be planned according to the circadian rhythm in the usage of potassium and of other major nutrients. The study of circadian rhythms is certainly in its infancy and, as far as I know, I am the first to suggest that nutrition take cognizance of these rhythms in the preparation of diets. (On the contrary, there may be times when we desire to counteract body cycles. For example, men may wish to modify the body's circadian rhythm of testosterone—which usually peaks in the blood about 8 o'clock in the morning—because of our socially induced tendency to perform sex when men [and possibly women also] are least able, namely at night. A supplement such as folic acid that might foster the androgenic action of testosterone, as mentioned in Chapter 5, would then be taken in the afternoon or evening.)

Causes of Potassium Deficiency

Alcohol and coffee increase the amount of potassium excreted via the urine. Alcohol is especially bad in this connection since it depletes the body's magnesium supply, and in order for potassium to

---

[*] Chronobiologic concern over just urine and/or blood levels of various substances may be simplistic. Vasopressin concentrations in the cerebrospinal fluid of cats shows a large daily rhythm with high concentrations during daylight hours, but a similar fluctuation was not detected in the blood.[453e] Perhaps minerals and other nutrients may have meaningful circadian rhythms in cerebrospinal fluid or in various other body fluids of humans and these rhythms may interest nutritionists of the future.

be held in the cells magnesium must be present. A rat experiment by E. Cotlove et al. [453f] demonstrated that magnesium depletion results in a loss of skeletal muscle potassium. Drugs, including aspirin, may also increase the need for potassium.

A deficiency of potassium can also be produced by eating too many refined foods, too much salt and too few of the foods listed below. Such a deficiency may cause not only a slow and irregular heartbeat but can help produce high blood pressure, insomnia, nausea, vomiting, nervousness, irritability, muscle spasms, kidney stones, kidney malfunction and infantile gastroenteritis.*

The potassium content of the body tends to decrease with age and with lowered body weight. Therefore, as one ages one should possibly increase his or her intake of this mineral. (This reasoning could be simplistic; perhaps "body wisdom" is dictating a benefit to decreased availability!)

A shortage of potassium brought on by rapid growth during adolescence may be a contributing cause of acne since the shortage may have a negative impact on the adrenal glands. When it is realized that the more salt in the diet the more potassium is required, then the fact that teenagers tend to eat lots of salty french fries and potato chips makes a potassium shortage even more probable. The candy and ice cream they consume with its surfeit of sugar also exacerbates a potassium shortage since the metabolism of sugar uses up potassium.

Potassium in Foods; Dangers of Supplements

Bran and wheat germ are concentrated sources for potassium, as are kelp, dulse, molasses, brewer's yeast, peanuts, nuts, seeds, figs, prunes, dates, dried currants and raisins. Meats, fish (especially sardines and halibut) and eggs contain generous quantities also. Other good sources for potassium are fruits and vegetables of all kinds, some of the best being potatoes (especially eaten with their

---

* Until a few years ago many brands of canned baby foods contained excessive salt, designed to appeal to the mother's jaded taste buds. Such excess of salt sometimes induced potassium deficiency which, in turn, resulted in colic. Concerned, nutritionally minded persons eventually effected its elimination. Consumers have great power to effect change!

skins on), avocados, bananas, cantaloupes, figs, carrots, soybeans, yams, parsley, spinach, beet greens, dandelion greens, swiss chard, parsnips, celery, tomatoes, dried beans, lima beans and mushrooms. Carrot juice, orange juice, grapefruit juice and tomato juice also contain a great deal of potassium. Much potassium is lost, however, when vegetables are soaked or boiled and the potassium-laden water is discarded. Therefore, steam fresh vegetables in preference to boiling them.

Potassium chloride is available and may be of value as a salt substitute if one's hair analysis indicates a low potassium level. (I have not seen studies, however, that indicate how reliably the hair reflects body stores of this mineral. In fact, M. R. Laker[454] believes that hair levels of potassium and sodium—and perhaps even of calcium—do not reflect body stores.) Furthermore, if the chloride ion rather than the sodium ion is the culprit in sodium chloride, then supplementing with potassium chloride may be a questionable practice.

Pills are available as potassium gluconate, potassium orotate and as potassium complexed with protein. However, Chris Lecos[455] points out that concentrated potassium chloride can corrode the intestinal lining and so, if it is to be used, it must be diluted to prevent damage. Then too, potassium pills in both the discontinued enteric-coated variety that dissolves in the intestinal tract and the uncoated type that disintegrates in the stomach can produce ulcers and other serious side effects. (These side effects are discussed in several references cited by M. S. Harris.[456] The modern pills in a waxy matrix are, however, somewhat safer.)[456a,b] D. H. Lawson[457] cautions that potassium supplements may be especially dangerous if taken by those who already have hyperkalemia and should be used cautiously, if at all, by the elderly, those with uremia and those taking diuretics.* Potassium supplements should, I believe, be used only upon a doctor's advice for treating such conditions as acute

---

* Patients with renal failure must strictly limit their potassium intake in accordance with their physicians' instructions. William H. Bay and Judith A. Hartman[458] report unexplained hyperkalemia in several patients during dialysis. The problem arose because of a manufacturer's increase in the potassium content of his low-sodium soup. Such patients must read labels with great care.

diarrhea, congenital renal alkalosis with diarrhea, aldosteronism, hypokalemic type of periodic familial paralysis and diabetic coma or by patients taking digitalis. The problems associated with potassium pills may be reduced through the development of slow-release capsules. These capsules are discussed by Harris[456] and also by J. Arnold et al.[459] However, the safety of slow-release potassium pills, like other potassium pills, may also be questionable.[460,461] At any rate, simply eating additional amounts of fruits and vegetables will put far more potassium in your body than you could safely obtain from pills. If potassium supplements are used, however, it may be advisable to take them several hours before or after calcium supplements. J. Wrobel et al.[462] report that, while sodium facilitates calcium transport into the body, such movement is inhibited by potassium.

If potassium chloride is prescribed for you, both you and your doctor should be aware that its use can cause a false-negative indication on the test for glucose fasting level if perchance you are scheduled to be given this test. Large amounts of supplemental potassium can also give a false-positive indication on the Diagnex blue test for impaired gastric function. Excessive potassium chloride, by lowering the pH of the ileum, can also inhibit absorption of vitamin B_{12}.[463,464] As indicated above, if potassium supplements are taken, they should be used with respect. Charles V. Wetli and Joseph H. Davis[465] report on two cases where death resulted from overdosage of potassium chloride. Potassium chloride overdosage can be especially dangerous in persons with compromised renal or cardiac function. Furthermore, the *Drug Interaction Index* edited by Ben R. Gant and Thomas D. Gant[466] warns that enteric-coated potassium chloride may be especially dangerous if taken with antacids or milk and its products which, being alkaline, might cause premature dissolution in the stomach. Jerome P. Kassirer and John T. Harrington[466a] warn that "diabetics, the elderly and patients receiving any of several widely used drugs (beta-adrenergic blocking agents, certain non-steroidal antiinflammatory agents, and captopril) are also susceptible to hyperkalemia when given potassium loads."

Physicians who prescribe potassium supplements to patients taking diuretics are referred especially to an article by Gina Kolata.[467] It is entitled "Should Hypertensives Take Potassium?" and points up the dangers of what may be an all too common practice of potassium prescribing by doctors or of self-prescribing by laymen. Many other articles (e.g., "Our National Obsession with Potassium" by John T. Harrington et al.)[468] cite the dangers of potassium supplementation. Physicians who find it necessary to recommend supplementary potassium should consider prescribing it as a liquid.[469]

Drug Facts and Comparisons[496a] warns that potassium supplementation is subject to these contraindications: "Severe renal impairment with oliguria; anuria or azotemia; untreated Addison's disease; hyperkalemic familial periodic paralysis (adynamia episodica hereditaria); acute dehydration; heat cramps. Potassium intensifies the symptoms of myotonia congenita. Potassium should not be administered to patients receiving potassium sparing diuretics (spironolactone, triamterene or amiloride) or aldosterone-inhibiting agents." *Drug Facts and Comparisons* also warns that in persons "with impaired mechanisms for excreting potassium, the administration of potassium salts can produce death through hyperkalemia, cardiac depression or arrest." *Drug Facts and Comparisons*[469b] observes that "this occurs more commonly in patients given potassium by the IV route, but may also occur in patients given potassium orally. Potentially fatal hyperkalemia can develop rapidly and be asymptomatic." Let's resolve to get our potassium through eating more fruits and vegetables!

The literature also contains warnings about the possible dangers of salt substitutes.[470-473] Ali Haddad and Evan Strong[472] suggest the name "salt substitute" be changed to "medical salt" to inform persons they are taking a drug, not an inert substitute for salt. These "salt substitutes" generally contain the chloride ion and, as we have seen, chloride rather than sodium is the possibly negative element in sodium chloride, at least from the standpoint of hypertension. (Actually, sodium chloride, not sodium alone or chloride alone, is a probable cause of hypertension in sensitive persons.) Those desiring to study various problems relating to potassium metabolism in greater depth are referred to "Disorders of Potassium Homeostasis" by H. John Reineck.[474]

Iodine

Iodine, in the form of iodide, is essential for the manufacture of thyroxin by the thyroid gland. A deficiency of iodine (or of vitamin E, lack of which inhibits the thyroid's absorption of iodine) can lead to goiter. Goiter is the enlargement of a thyroid gland which is trying desperately to produce thyroxin from insufficient raw material. Eating sufficient amounts of good protein is also essential since the amino acid tyrosine, which protein contains, is needed (along with vitamins B6, C and choline) to make thyroxin. When thyroxin is in short supply it leads not only to goiter problems, but to such symptoms as fatigue, headache, cold hands and feet, thickening and drying of the skin, low blood pressure, excess blood cholesterol, nervousness, irritability, obesity, slow physical and mental reactions, irregular and/or excessive menstruation and diminished interest in sex.

The nonendocrine biologic effects of iodide are listed by Orville J. Stone[475] as follows:

1. Increases the movement of polymorphonuclear leukocytes into areas of inflammation, both systemic and local.
2. Improves phagocytosis of bacteria by polymorphonuclear leukocytes.
3. Improves the ability of polymorphonuclear leukocytes to kill bacteria.
4. Concentrates in granulomas.
5. Decreases the size of noninfectious granulomas.
6. Decreases the size of some infectious granulomas.
7. Cures sporotrichosis.
8. Increases glandular secretion.
9. Increases proteolytic effect of polymorphonuclear leukocytes.

10. Redistributes in tumor patients and concentrates around the tumor.
11. Redistributes after mast cell rupture or injection of histamine or serotonin.
12. Increases the tendency of mast cells to rupture.
13. In large quantities, it ruptures mast cells.

Another possible use for iodide is in dental prophylaxis. Ernest Newbrun et al.[476] report that flossing with iodide reduces the proportion of caries-causing *Streptococcus mutans* in plaque when these organisms are present in large numbers. There appeared to be no difference whether the iodide was dried on the floss or the floss was dipped into a solution of .2% iodine and 2% potassium iodide.

Iodine may be valuable for women—even more so if they are taking the Pill. Iodine (along with protein and various B vitamins but diminished fat consumption) seems to protect the breast from the possibly harmful effects of estrogen. Dr. Bernhard A. Eskin,[477] working both with rats that had been given estrogen and with women on the Pill, reported iodine to be effective in reducing the occurrence of breast cysts and cancer. Dr. Eskin related that in areas where iodine is lacking in the soil, not only is there a high incidence of goiter but also increased deaths due to breast cancer. Iodine was actually used during the 19th century for treating breast cancer.[478] However, Eskin[479] stated that large amounts of iodine do not seem to have a valid treatment basis in breast cancer therapy.

Iodine may affect hair coloring and texture. It has been suggested that Japanese, living in Japan, generally retain their dark hair into old age. It has been noted further that if Japanese men and women come to the United States their hair often begins to fall out and begins to turn gray just as does that of most other inhabitants. The important difference may be that their diet while they lived in Japan contained much larger quantities of iodine in the form of fish and seaweed. However, ascribing the retention of dark hair color by the Japanese into advanced age to their large intake of iodine is strictly hypothetical. Seaweed contains many other minerals (including copper), so one should really not jump at easy but perhaps erroneous conclusions. Anyway, Japanese who consume massive quantities of kelp are reported to suffer a high incidence of thyroid dysfunction—a high price for nongray hair if, in fact, kelp is related to hair color.

G. Norris Bollenback[479a] reported, in 1986, that a sugar-iodine salve (called "Sugardine") has been developed by Richard A. Knutson, a surgeon with the Delta Medical Center in Greenville, Mississippi. Sugar has great healing power, as discussed in a subnote of Chapter 10, but this salve may represent a good improvement since it is reported to stay on the wound better and thus increase the pace of healing. Microorganisms do not survive in concentrated solutions of sugars (or of salts) since osmosis cannot occur at a normal rate.

Problems with Excessive Iodine

It is possible that Occidentals also would benefit from a modestly increased intake of iodine. However, although small amounts of iodine, in the form of iodide, can be beneficial to the thyroid gland, large amounts can, as we have seen, inhibit its function. Furthermore, I would be wary about assuming that levels of a dietary component, namely iodine, which Orientals may have become accustomed to through hundreds of generations, necessarily provide a safe dietary model for Occidentals. At any rate, rats can certainly get too much iodine. J. Wolff, I. L. Chaikoff et al.[480,480a] found that the capacity of the thyroid of rats to synthesize organic iodine increased as iodide was supplied but then, upon being supplied further amounts of iodide, the ability of the thyroid to produce organic iodine rapidly declined. This phenomenon, which you will recognize as a *reverse effect,* has become known as the *Wolff-Chaikoff effect.*

As far as a goiter is concerned, it seems that both too low and too high an intake of iodine can lead to this condition. Although the prevalence of goiter has been markedly reduced since the introduction of iodized salt, it is still reported present in American children. Frederick L. Trowbridge et al.[481,482] are of the opinion that these goiters cannot be explained in terms of iodine deficiency. Jan Wolff[483] had, in fact, pointed out in a review many years earlier that chronic ingestion of iodine or iodide-generating organic compounds in amounts ten or more times the daily requirements for hormone biosynthesis leads to goiter in some persons. Trowbridge also states that in study areas of highest goiter incidence there was a higher iodine excretion among goitrous children and adults. Thus, we have an example of a *biphasic reverse effect:* the detrimental influence of an iodine deficiency on the thyroid is reversed (normalized) by modest quantities of the element while megadoses, in turn, reverse the gland's normal function and have a detrimental influence. In cases of hyperthyroidism it may be just as erroneous to conclude that iodine should be withheld. J. Wolff and I. L. Chaikoff[484] cautioned doctors of a generation ago that "failure to maintain high enough levels of plasma iodine may account for the exacerbation of patients suffering from hyperthyroidism." Nutrition is seldom as simple as we often suppose.

An interesting inverse correlation between the amount of iodine in hair and intelligence is suggested by a report by Adon A. Gordus et al.[264b] In studying students at the Naval Academy, this group found that cumulative grade averages were, in general, highest among the students with lowest amount of hair iodine. They suggested that the difference may be due to thyroidal uptake and utilization of iodine. Those with thyroids that efficiently used iodine performed better academically and less iodine was deposited in the hair.

Either a deficiency or an excess of iodine may even be a cancer factor.[373] A high incidence of thyroid cancer has been reported to exist in areas such as Switzerland and parts of Colombia where the populations are iodine deficient. On the other hand, high-incidence areas for thyroid cancer exist where the inhabitants get too much iodine, such as those living along the coast of Norway and the people of Iceland, Newfoundland, Hawaii and Japan.* It seems to

---

* The low incidence of breast cancer in Japan may be related to the habit of consuming seaweed. Jane Teas[485] reported that seaweed extract had an antitumor effect against sarcoma-180 in mice. I wonder if an excessive intake of seaweed would produce a *reverse effect* in mice and in women? Jane Teas [486] has also proposed, based on epidemiological and biological data, that Lamineria, a brown kelp seaweed, may be an important factor in contributing to the relatively low breast cancer incidence in Japan. Subsequentiy, Teas et al.[486a] reported that a diet including 5% of Lamineria was useful in reducing mammary

be an example of a *biphasic reverse effect*. The carcinogenicity of too little iodine is reversed at nominal intake, which is reversed again at excessive intake to once again be carcinogenic.

G. I. Vidor,[487] analyzing iodine consumption, concludes that for most persons an intake of 100-300 mcg./day is desirable, although 500-1,000 mcg./day would more adequately ensure against iodine deficiency.** He also concludes that a total intake of 2,000 mcg./day may, for many persons, be toxic with a resultant inhibition of thyroid activity. (For pregnant women to take an amount of iodine perhaps ten times the RDA might result in a rebound deficiency effect in their offspring if the baby's diet is at more normal levels. In fact, Marjorie Safran and Lewis E. Braverman cite J. Wolff[487b] as saying, "the oral administration of pharmacologic quantities of iodine to pregnant women is occasionally associated with sporadic iodine-induced hypothyroidism and goiter in the newborn.") In addition, Thomas H. Shepard[488] cites many references showing that excess iodine causes defective animal offspring. One other warning, if you are undergoing tests and are taking supplemental iodine, tell your doctor. Iodine can cause a false-positive benzidine test for renal damage or blood in the urine.

J. E. Fulton, Jr. and E. Black[489] warn that those with acne should be especially cautious about their iodine intake. Iodine, circulating in the bloodstream, is excreted through the oil glands of the skin. This can result in irritation of the pores, skin eruptions and inflammation. Excessive intake of iodine can even cause acne in those not having the condition. Iodine may be detrimental not only to patients with acne but to those with dermatitis herpetiformis and

---

adenocarcinomas in rats. They postulated that the active ingredient in the seaweed might be the sulphated polysaccharide, fucoidan. Furthermore, Masato Ohshima and Jerrold M. Ward[486b] found that male rats injected with the carcinogen N-nitrosomethylurea had a significantly increased incidence of thyroid follicular adenomas if fed an iodine-deficient diet. On the other hand, recent rat experiments by Bandaru S. Reddy et al.[486c] suggest that dietary seaweed increases the risk for colon tumors. It may be yet another example of the benefits derived from obeying the dictate of the golden mean.

** According to the Committee on Dietary Allowances,[487a] "An intake in adults between 50 and 1,000 mg of iodine can be considered safe."

pustular psoriasis. Orville J. Stone[475] gives some 20 additional side effects and contraindications of iodides. In addition, Marshall B. Block and Salvatore J. DeFranceso[492] reported on a case of hyperthyroidism they suspected was induced by the iodine in a multivitamin pill. Such anecdotal speculation appearing in a respected journal should not overly concern one any more than one should rush to act on anecdotes in a popular "health" magazine. However, it seems quite likely to me that if you are supplementing your diet with iodized salt and with kelp you may be getting too much rather than too little iodine.

Perhaps a special word of warning is in order in regard to vaginal douching with polyvinylpyrrolidone-iodine (PVP). PVP with iodine is frequently prescribed as a topical germicide. Marjorie Safran and Lewis E. Braverman[490] reported that use of such a douche causes iodine to be absorbed across the vaginal mucosa with a subsequent increase in serum iodine and serum thyrotropin. They found no evidence, however, of overt thyroid dysfunction in these women. I wonder, however, if it could be dangerous to use such a douche along with oral consumption of iodized salt, kelp and other sources of iodine.

Kelp and dulse are strong sources of iodine, as are seafoods, including green turtle, which is an especially potent source. Iodine is also found in fresh pineapple, barley, tomatoes, garlic, kidney beans, rhubarb and in many other fruits, cereals and vegetables. However, if fruits, cereals and vegetables are grown on iodine-deficient soil they will contain very little of the mineral. Soil is iodine-deficient around the Great Lakes and in the Pacific Northwest, two famous "goiter belts" so named because persons living there, prior to the availability of iodized salt, were apt to develop goiter due to iodine deficiencies in both the food and water. (Food now travels widely, however, and so those in the "goiter belts" might in some cases be eating some high-iodine foods while those in "protected regions" might be eating some foods grown in the "goiter belts.") Why should anyone doubt that the quality of the soil determines the quality of the fruits or vegetables grown on it? A word of warning: if one eats considerable amounts of brassicas (cabbage, kale, cauliflower, brussels sprouts, rutabaga, etc.), their thiocyanate may inhibit uptake of iodine by the thyroid, thus possibly leading to goiter.*

Should one add kelp to the diet? Perhaps it may be desirable, especially if one eats large quantities of vegetables of the *Brassica* genus and fails to eat generous amounts of seafood. However, analyses of kelp show it may sometimes contain lead and cadmium. When deciding if you should supplement your diet with kelp to achieve an iodine intake in G. I. Vidor's optimal range, [487] do not ignore the iodine content in other foods, including the iodized salt you may be using.

Let me warn again about the possibility of excessive iodine consumption. Recent research by N. Bagchi et al. [491a] suggests that "excessive consumption of iodine in the United States may be responsible for the increased incidence of autoimmune thyroiditis." Bagchi and his colleagues cite a study by C. P. Barsano [491b] showing that daily intake of iodine in the United States is two to five times the RDA.

The increased incidence of thyrotoxicosis in the endemic goiter regions of Tasmania when iodine was added to the bread showed that supplemental iodine may not always be safe. [492a] Nevertheless, Richard F. Gillum [493] suggests that persons on low-sodium diets may become iodine deficient. Radioactive isotopes of iodine from nuclear power plants and nuclear weapons tests could be taken up by the thyroid in persons having low amounts of iodine in the diet and thyroid cancer might result. Gillum observes that most persons receive their iodine from table salt (not from manufactured food in which iodine is generally absent). It's an interesting speculation to counter the many beneficial aspects of avoiding use of the salt shaker.

---

* I am, of course, not suggesting one avoid cruciferous vegetables. Lee W. Wattenberg [491] has shown that the indoles therein offer good protection against chemical carcinogens. It's another example of the merit of moderation. Related comments appear later in this chapter in regard to sulphur.

Fluoride

It is interesting to note that fluorine in the form of fluoride is a common element in the earth's crust, being even more common than chlorine. However, whereas chlorine (as sodium chloride) is very common in the oceans, fluoride is quite rare. As a nutritional element, its requirement in man seems to correspond to its ocean level rather than to its land concentration. Perhaps this is an atavistic carry-over, like the sodium chloride content of the blood, to our primordial origin in the water of the oceans. Let's look, in turn, at the "pluses" and "minuses" of fluoride.

Studies by Daniel S. Bernstein et al.[494] showed that the incidence of osteoporosis, especially among women, was substantially higher in areas where the drinking water contained low levels of fluoride. They concluded that fluoride consumption is important in the prevention of osteoporosis and that it may also play a role in preventing calcification of the aorta. Recently, Olli Simonen and Ossi Laitinen[494a] similarly found that bone fragility was significantly less in a town that had fluoridated its water supply since 1959 compared to a town showing a low fluoride level in its drinking water. On the other hand, Jennifer Madans et al.[494b] reported that they found no evidence of protection against osteoporosis when the drinking water contained .7 ppm of fluoride, the level recommended for prevention of dental caries. They did, however, find some indication of a protective effect at higher fluoride levels for groups with a high incidence of osteoporosis. They warned, nevertheless, that the safety of higher doses would have to be tested. They noted that, "If a much higher level of fluoride is necessary for the prevention of osteoporosis than for prevention of dental caries, it may be more feasible for fluoride to be administered on an individual basis to those at high risk."

Jenifer Jowsey et al.,[495] in commenting on these effects, observed that fluoride in both men and animals can stimulate bone formation. The bone, however, is poorly mineralized when fluoride is used alone and osteomalacia, as well as secondary hyper-parathyroidism, often occur. In studying variable levels of fluoride administration in patients with osteoporosis, the Jowsey group found that a daily regimen of 50 mg. of sodium fluoride and at least 900 mg. of calcium plus a weekly intake of 50,000 units of vitamin D was beneficial. They attributed the relative absence of osteomalacia in their patients to the protective effect of vitamin D. In confirmation of Jowsey's treatment, O. Grove and B. Halver[496] reported results of a prospective randomized clinical trial of 22 postmenopausal women with backache, loss of calcium from the spine and fractures. Treating them with sodium fluoride, calcium and vitamin D and using a control group treated only with placebo, they reported significant reduction of pain and infirmity. In recent years, two vitamin D compounds incorporating fluorine—24,24-F_2-25-OH-D_3 and 24,24-F_2-1,25$(OH)_2D_3$—have been synthesized.[497,497a] The latter compound is reported to be ten times more active than 1,25$(OH)_2D_3$ in intestinal organ cultures *in vitro*[497b] and in intestinal calcium transport, bone calcium mobilization and the mineralization of bone,[497c,d] as well as being active for longer periods.[497,497a] Thus, it may have a therapeutic advantage over 1,25$(OH)_2D_3$.[497,497a]

W. A. Rambeck,[497e] in 1986, published a report showing that a third fluorine-substituted compound of 1,25$(OH)_2D_3$, namely 24R-F-1,25$(OH)_2D_3$, had only about 25% to 50% of the potency of 1,25$(OH)_2D_3$ in rats, chickens and in Japanese quails. Due to its wider therapeutic dosage range, however, Rambeck and his co-workers speculated that it could be of clinical value.

A controlled study using estrogen plus fluoride and calcium as compared with the same treatment without estrogen showed that estrogen was also important in increasing the bone mass in postmenopausal osteoporosis.[498] B. Lawrence Riggs et al.[498a] similarly concluded that the combination of calcium, fluoride and estrogen was more effective than any other combination. A study by Joseph M. Lane et al.[498b] also, "demonstrated the significant ability of sodium fluoride, calcium and physiologic vitamin D to increase bone mass, decrease fractures and improve the well-being of osteoporotic patients." However, possible problems with supplementary estrogen are being widely discussed and fluoride, if it is to be used, must also be used with care. R. G. Van Kesteren et al.[499] stated that more than 100 fatal acute fluoride intoxications were reported between the years 1935 and 1981. One case they described in detail involved a woman who had accidentally taken 225 mg. of sodium fluoride during a six-week period instead of the 75 mg. prescribed for her osteoporosis. At any rate, since there are reports that fluoride treatment produces abnormal patterns of calcification and may even lead to osteomalacia (perhaps because of insufficient calcium supplementation), the sodium fluoride-calcium treatment of osteoporosis has not yet been approved by the FDA. So while experimental results and fluoride therapies in other nations look promising, FDA approval awaits the result of clinical trials supported by the National Institutes of Health. John A. Kanis and Pierre J. Meunier[499a] have recently reviewed the use of fluoride in treating osteoporosis.

Fluoride may also benefit the cardiovascular system. A study by D. S. Bernstein et al.,[500] another by H. Luoma et al.,[501] and a third by D. R. Taves[502] showed that the number of persons with cardiovascular disease was significantly lower in areas where the water contained high amounts of fluoride.

The most beneficial use of supplemental fluoride may be in reducing the incidence of tooth decay.* Large numbers of studies support this conclusion in spite of the fact that the antifluoridationists continue to muster arguments denying their validity. A study by A. J. Rugg-Gunn et al.[503] confirms the anticariogenic property of fluoride. Their seven-year study examined five-year-olds in four urban communities of England and found excellent inverse correlation between fluoride content of the water supplies and the incidence of caries.**

Hannu Hausen et al.[503b] have, however, reported some surprising findings regarding fluoridated water, toothbrushing and

---

* A *reverse effect* can be exhibited by administering fluoride at very high concentrations (far above those present in fluoridated water). When pregnant mice were given large amounts of fluoride, detrimental changes in the structure of the jaws and teeth occurred in the offspring.[502a]

** J. Afseth et al.[503a] found that copper sulfate and fluoride topically applied to rats' teeth resulted in significantly less caries than occurred in the teeth of rats when either fluoride alone or copper alone was applied.

sugar consumption. Among children exposed to fluoridated water, the daily brushers developed more caries than did occasional brushers. (The Hausen group speculated that dental plaque may beneficially serve as a means of introducing fluoride into enamel.) On the other hand, daily brushers among children whose teeth were exposed to topical fluoride developed fewer caries lesions than occasional brushers. Hausen and coworkers stated that "Toothbrushing produced a stronger effect, positive or negative, on caries occurrence in frequent sugar consumers than in occasional sugar consumers in both fluoride exposure groups." Frequent sugar consumption increased caries incidence in those exposed to fluoridated water (no surprise) but (perhaps surprisingly) decreased caries incidence in those given topical fluoride. Other references regarding possible dental benefits of sugar were cited earlier in this chapter.[75a-e]

When, earlier in this chapter, you read about the dangers of chlorine in our water, did you get the idea that antifluoridationists may be concentrating on the wrong chemical? Well, maybe not.

Negative Aspects of Fluoride—and Some "Positives"

Though the benefits of fluoridated water are obvious, its dangers may be more subtle. It should be observed, however, that although the antifluoridationists are correct in pointing out fluoride's detrimental effect on many of the body's enzyme systems, they are not correct in singling out sodium fluoride as the "unnatural form" and calcium fluoride as the "natural form." Henry A. Schroeder[504] in *The Trace Elements and Man* relates that almost all the fluoride in the sea is in the form of sodium fluoride, while calcium fluoride is virtually insoluble.* Life has thrived for billions of years on the 1.846 billion tons of sodium fluoride present in the ocean. This is not to say, however, that life will thrive on artificially fluoridated water.

Fluoride, as we have reported, is especially important in strengthening tooth enamel, but too much can cause mottling

---

* Actually, Schroeder is not quite correct. The ocean's fluoride exists, not as sodium fluoride but as sodium ions and fluoride ions.

(fluorosis) of the teeth. By combining with magnesium to form magnesium fluoride, which is not absorbed by the body, this excess fluoride may lead to a deficiency of magnesium and all that portends in regard to heart disease and other problems. Fluoride will combine with numerous other chemicals and may cause other difficulties. An excess of fluorides may contribute to the incidence of goiter. Dr. Thaddeus Mann[505] cites studies showing that sodium fluoride interferes with the utilization of fructose (fructolysis) by sperm. A study by I. Rapaport[506] in the 1950s linked the incidence of Down's syndrome with the fluoride content of drinking water. Subsequent studies, however, pointed out defects in the protocol of Rapaport's work. Properly designed studies have shown no connection between fluoride and Down's syndrome.[507]

Fluoride inhibits a number of metabolic enzymes,[507a] although not necessarily at the concentrations present in fluoridated water. To cite just one example, fluoride inhibits cholinesterases *in vitro* but only at much higher levels than exist in fluoridated water. [507b] On the other hand, Frederick J. Bloomfield and Marjorie M. Young [507e] showed that fluoride increases tissue levels of cyclic adenosine monophosphate (cAMP). Cyclic AMP acts as an enzyme activator and thus helps to control intracellular concentration of ATP. Many hormones affect cells by first causing cAMP to be formed in those cells. Thus, it is an important intracellular hormone mediator.[507d] Excess amounts of cAMP may, however, be detrimental to neutrophil function. Several studies show that neutrophil adhesiveness, phagocytosis, degranulation and chemotaxis are all inhibited by above-normal levels of cAMP.[507e]

Statistics compiled by John Yiamouyiannis and Dean Burk, as cited by Yiamouyiannis,[508] suggested that, among U.S. cities having a population of 1,000,000 or more, the incidence of cancer was greater in those cities where the water was fluoridated. The statistical validity of the Yiamouyiannis and Burk study has, however, been widely criticized.[509] Studies by the National Cancer Institute, the U.S. Center for Disease Control, the National Heart, Lung and Blood Institute and Canada's Health and Welfare Ministry each found an absence of evidence showing a link between fluoride and cancer. Interestingly, however, a study by C. M. Goodall[509a] in New Zealand showed that fluoridated areas had better records than unfluoridated areas in regard to cancer deaths of persons aged 45 and over. In unfluoridated areas there was an increase in cancer deaths from 1961 to 1976 of 29% for males and 2% for females. In fluoridated areas there was just a 10% increase for males and a *decline* of 5% for females.

An epidemiological appraisal is given by John S. Neuberger[510] and concludes that "current evidence does not support the hypothesis that fluoride is associated with cancer, much less causes it." Nevertheless, Irwin H. Herskowitz and Isabel L. Norton[511] reported that sodium fluoride increased the incidence of melanotic tumors in *Drosophila melanogaster*. Furthermore, the potential of leukocytes to develop cancer when exposed to excessive fluoride will be discussed later.[522b] In another series of experiments, Alfred Taylor and Nell Carmichael Taylor[512] reported that when sodium fluoride is introduced at very low levels (.00001-.0005 mg.) growth of mouse mammary tumors in eggs accelerated. However, when sodium fluoride is added to tumor suspensions at relatively high levels (.4-.8 mg. per mouse or .1-.8 mg. per egg) before implantation in mice or in eggs there is a *reverse effect* and the tumor growth is inhibited.

Fluoride interacts with the metabolism of calcium, magnesium, iron, zinc, copper and manganese.[513] Then too, John J. Miller[514] pointed out the negative effects of fluoride on the enzyme systems of the body. Dr. Miller cited research showing that blood hemoglobin may be decreased by the presence of fluoride, and also that fluoride may interfere with pituitary function and thus with the operation of the thyroid gland. His other citings of detrimental effects of fluoride are numerous and I cannot begin to cover them here. On the other hand, D. B. Ferguson[514a] has reported that the reduction in enzyme activity may be only temporary. Many studies[515,516] have found, other than beneficial effects on the teeth, no significant differences (either beneficial or detrimental) in the health of persons in towns drinking fluoridated water and those in towns where the water was not fluoridated. However, just because populations in general may be unaffected by supplemental fluoride, I think it premature to conclude that given individuals might not be affected for better or for worse.

For example, in areas of India where the fluoride level of the drinking water is very high (16 parts/million) bladder stone disease is very common. A. Anasuya[517] has shown that rats fed excessive fluoride (23 parts per 1,000 in their food) develop urinary bladder stones. Humans are not generally exposed to such excesses but, judging from the experience in India, some individuals might develop bladder stones from high dietary fluoride intake. Where the drinking water contains excessive amounts of fluoride and fluorosis is common, magnesium and calcium may be useful in inhibiting absorption of fluoride[518] (but see page 710, reference 527a).

As pointed out earlier, fluoride has both negative and positive aspects. H. H. Messer et al.[521] reported that female mice fed a low-fluoride diet over two generations showed a progressive decline in litter production. Addition of fluoride to their diet, however, restored their reproductive capacity. H. H. Messer et al.[522] observed that pregnant mice with a too-low fluoride intake developed anemia. They also found that fluoride was required by the mice to maintain normal hematocrit levels during the stress of pregnancy (Figure 17). Furthermore, mouse pups born to mothers having low dietary fluoride had depressed hematocrit levels during the first 20 days of their lives (Figure 18). Fluoride intake obviously should be subject to the golden mean—*moderation in all things.* Whereas small amounts of fluoride are probably biologically essential, large amounts are health threatening. Individuals, not governments, should decide the optimal amounts for themselves. Remember, those who desire fluoride to protect their teeth can use fluoride toothpaste or mouthwash.

In Chapter 9 we will discuss the oxygen free-radical superoxide in more detail. It may be interesting to note at this time, however, that fluoride affects the generation of superoxide by polymorphonuclear leukocytes (an important component of their microbicidal function). W. L. Gabler and P. A. Leong[522a] have found that generation of superoxide by polymorphonuclear leukocytes (PMNs) is inhibited

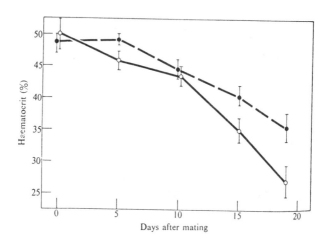

Figure 17. Hematocrit values of tail blood of pregnant mice given low (○) and high (•) dietary fluoride intakes. When fluoride is at too low a level, pregnant mice develop a lower hematocrit and anemia. It has been suggested that fluoride may play a role in hemopoiesis that is manifested only under the stress of pregnancy. Reproduced from H. H. Messer et al., *Nature New Biology* (Dec. 13, 1972) 240: 218-219, with permission of the publisher, Macmillan Journals Limited, and of the authors.

at low, .01-10 milli mole (mM) concentrations of fluoride (Figure 19). At 10 mM there is a very large, 50%, inhibition. Then, increased fluoride shows a *reverse effect* and at 20 mM the superoxide generation is roughly the same as it is with no fluoride present. In a *biphasic reverse effect,* another inhibition sets in and, at 35 mM concentration of fluoride, the 50% inhibition level is once again reached. Subsequent studies relating to fluoride's effect on the superoxide generation of human neutrophils during phagocytosis have been conducted by Denis English et al.[519] and Jan G. R. Elferink.[520] The importance of dose-response relationships is obvious. We obviously cannot say that fluoride either activates or

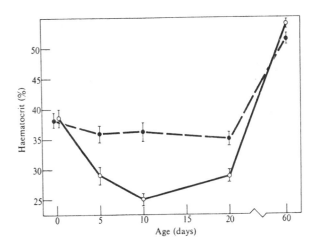

Figure 18. Hematocrit values from birth to 60 days of tail blood of mouse pups born to mothers with low (○) or high (•) dietary fluoride intakes. The maternal fluoride level did not influence the hematocrit of the pups at birth or at 60 days of age. However, while the pups were fed the mothers' fluoride-deficient milk, their hematocrit declined and they were anemic. After weaning at ten days, their condition improved, presumably after being fed a diet containing normal amounts of fluoride. Reproduced from H. H. Messer et al., *Nature New Biology* (Dec. 13, 1972) 240: 218-219, with permission of the publisher, Macmillan Journals Limited, and of the authors.

inhibits superoxide generation. *It does both*. Nutritional concepts of the future must be stated in terms of dose-response relationships.

The importance of delineating dose-response relationships between fluoride and leukocytes is suggested by experiments with mice done by S. R. Greenberg.[522b] He reported that young leukocytes chronically exposed to elevated fluoride levels have the potential for an irreversible shift toward the formation of a neoplasm. Takeki Tsutsui et al.[522c] found that sodium fluoride is genotoxic and capable of inducing neoplastic transformation in Syrian hamster embryo cells in culture. They noted, however, that the carcinogenic risk of fluoride to humans "may be reduced by factors regulating *in vivo* dose levels." In related studies, Tsutsui et al.[522d,e] reported on

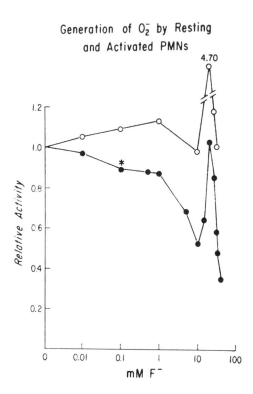

Figure 19. The effect of F⁻ on generation of 0⁻₂ by resting (○) and activated (•) PMNs. Each point represents the average of at least six runs. A *biphasic reverse effect* is in evidence, the turning points being at fluoride concentrations of about 10 mM and 20 mM. Reproduced from W. L. Gabler and P. A. Leong, *Jrl. of Dental Research*, (1979) **58:** 1933-1939, with permission of the publisher.

work suggesting that "sodium fluoride causes DNA damage in human diploid fibroblasts in culture."

Regardless of the positives and negatives of fluoride when consumed orally, it may not be safe when introduced via the lungs. (We should remain alert to the fact that, although substances may be safe if taken by mouth, they could be very dangerous when taken via other routes.) Philip R. N. Sutton,[522f] in 1986, speculated that the fluoride in cigarette smoke may be a factor in the incidence of lung cancer. He cited T. Okamura and T. Matsuhisa[522g] as finding that cigarettes contain between 35 and 640 ppm of fluoride and that the average American cigarette has 224 µg., i.e., about 5 mg. in 22 cigarettes.

Food Content of Fluoride

Food sources of fluoride are bonemeal, steel-cut oats, bran, beets, yams, sunflower seeds, whey, milk, cheese, garlic, green vegetables, kelp and small fish eaten with the bones (which are a rich source of fluoride). The fluoride content of gelatin may be in the toxic range.[523] Sodium silicofluoride spray (an insecticide) remains in the peel of oranges,[524] and many marmalades contain orange peel. (Peel unadulterated by fluoride may, however, be of value. R. Dalbak et al.[525] showed that citrus-peel oil has valuable antibacterial properties. Furthermore, T. H. Maltzman et al.[525a] reported, in 1986, that orange peel is effective in suppressing the development of mammary tumors in DMBA-treated rats.) A cup of tea may contain .1 to .2 mg. of fluoride, thus perhaps giving to habitual tea drinkers what may be an enzyme-inhibiting amount of fluoride. In Germany, fluoride is added to packaged salt[526] and in some Cantons of Switzerland it is added to bread.[526a] Additions to salt or to bread, rather than to the water supply, obviously make it far easier for individuals to exercise freedom of choice regarding fluoride consumption.

Vegetables grown in gardens using fluoridated water do not seem to have significantly more fluoride in them than those grown with nonfluoridated water. K. Toth and Edit Sugar[527] reported that, in studies made over a period of 30 years, only minor differences in fluoride content could be detected in vegetables, cereals or dishes of cooked meat, whether the water used in producing the food was fluoride-rich or fluoride-poor. However, Toth and Sugar found that the water in which the vegetables were cooked made a great difference. Vegetables cooked in fluoridated water averaged .40 mg. per kg., whereas those cooked in nonfluoridated water averaged only .20 mg. per kg. Those desiring to reduce fluoride consumption may desire to avoid not only fluoridated water but to minimize their consumption of foods cooked in such water.

Calcium, phosphorus and magnesium, while decreasing the intestinal absorption of fluoride in animals, reportedly have no such effect in man.[527a] Aluminum-containing antacids, however, greatly decrease the intestinal absorption of fluoride[527a] and might thus interfere with any therapy for osteoporosis employing fluoride.

Copper

Copper is hypothesized to have been introduced into living systems relatively late in evolutionary development. The first life forms to use copper are believed to have evolved during the middle of the Proterozoic era.[527b]

About 90% of plasma copper is in the form of an alpha-globulin, ceruloplasmin, with the remaining 10% being loosely bound to albumin or amino acids. Ceruloplasmin is required to release iron from ferritin, for the incorporating of iron into transferrin and for releasing the heme molecule to form hemoglobin. Thus, a deficiency of this mineral can cause anemia. The role of ceruloplasmin in connection with iron metabolism, providing protection both against pro-oxidant effects of iron and against iron overload, was discussed earlier in this chapter. Copper is also required in the body's production of neutrophils and in cases of copper deficiency may be associated with neutropenia—i.e., with a reduced number of neutrophils.[528]

Several studies report that ceruloplasmin is a powerful inhibitor of lipid peroxidation and a scavenger of superoxide.[529] B. Halliwell and J. M. C. Gutteridge,[530,531] however, deny that ceruloplasmin scavenges superoxide but believe the antioxidant action relates to its ability to inhibit metal-ion-catalyzed peroxidation even when superoxide is not involved in this process. In any event, Osamu Itoh et al.[529,532] reported that ceruloplasmin inhibits the growth of sarcoma-180 in mice and, although not directly cytotoxic, can enhance cytotoxic reactions against tumor cells.

Copper is also essential to the formation of one of the superoxide dismutases we will discuss more thoroughly in a later chapter. This copper-zinc compound was formerly called *erythrocuprein*, *hepatocuprein* and *cerebrocuprein*. A number of studies show that the level of superoxide dismutase (SOD) in the erythrocytes is dependent on copper but not on the zinc status. [533,534] A confusing situation is, however, pointed out by K. A. Andrewartha and I. W. Caple. [535] Although 60% of normal human erythrocyte copper is in the form of SOD, there apparently is no relation between SOD activity and erythrocyte copper concentration in either normal persons or in rheumatoid patients (who generally have low erythrocyte copper levels).[*] In a study using rats, Dawn L. Ellerson and Doris M. Hilker[535b] found that thiamin increased plasma ceruloplasmin and erythrocyte SOD when copper was deficient but had no effect when ceruloplasmin was normal or high. (Liver copper was decreased by high thiamin in rats having low or high copper but increased in those with normal copper.)

An interesting example of compensation which occurs when the copper supply of rats is depleted was reported by Wolfram Bohnenkamp and Ulrich Weser.[533] Copper depletion resulted in a drop in Cu Zn superoxide dismutase, which is not surprising, but note this example of "body wisdom": The levels of catalase (an iron-based enzyme), after dropping for two weeks, began to rise, exceeded the control value after six weeks, and by the eighth week were 30% above the control value. (Catalase, by neutralizing hydrogen peroxide and the hydroxyl ion, performs functions related to those of superoxide dismutase.)

In various animal experiments a copper deficiency has caused not only anemia but lameness, skin sores, defects of the aorta, brittle, easily fractured bones, myocardial fibrosis and general weakness. Copper deficiency can suppress the immune response and may be accompanied by bacterial infections.[536] Copper is also a factor in protein metabolism and in healing.

---

[*] A recent study by Sofia G. Ljutakova et al.[535a] may have a bearing on these facts. SOD activity may be enzymatic or nonenzymatic. Nonenzymatic copper *in vivo* may have a pro-oxidant effect rather than an antioxidant effect.

Copper is needed for the manufacture of ribonucleic acid (RNA) that is present in the nucleus of cells. It plays a part in the synthesis of phospholipids. On the other hand, lipid peroxidation has been reported by Dr. L. B. Lee[537] to proceed more rapidly in the presence of copper. Thus, copper in excess, unless controlled by antioxidants such as superoxide dismutase, ascorbic acid, vitamin E, selenium or BHT, may be an aging factor. However, more recent research has shown—as we will cover in Chapter 9—that many copper chelates exhibit superoxide dismutase activity and thus inhibit lipid peroxidation. Numerous copper chelates are reported as potentially useful anti-inflammatory, antiarthritic, antiulcer agents.[538,538a] We must, however, resist the temptation to conclude that inflammation does not serve useful functions. (Nature's processes are seldom without "wisdom.") John R. J. Sorenson[538b] has pointed out that an inflammatory response causes an increase in the body's production of Cu Zn superoxide dismutase. A historical review of the treatment of rheumatoid and other degenerative diseases, including the use of Permalon (a sodium salicylate and copper chloride mixture with various copper chelates), has been provided by John R. J. Sorenson and Werner Hangarter.[538c] In addition, Sorenson [538d] has made an in-depth report of copper complexes as antiarthritic drugs. He concludes, "The possibility that rheumatoid diseases are associated with deficits in Cu-dependent processes also suggests that the etiology and/or chronicity of these diseases may result from a quasi Cu deficiency or the lack of low molecular weight complex forms of Cu."

There are many copper-based enzymes in addition to superoxide dismutase. Copper is required to activate the enzyme that works to remove excess histamine which might otherwise lead to allergic reactions. A copper-containing enzyme is thought to be involved in the process that produces collagen (the fibrous protein which is the chief constituent of the fibrils of connective tissue) and elastin (a protein similar to collagen that is the main constituent of elastic fibers). Copper is also a component of *dopamine-beta-oxidase* that converts dopamine to norepinephrine.

Studies by K. G. D. Allen and L. M. Klevay[539, 539a] have reported that copper deficiency in rats produced high cholesterol levels. Brad W. C. Lau and Leslie M. Klevay,[540] as well as W. Harvey and Kenneth G. D. Allen,[541] reported that the effect is caused by a decrease in activity of the enzyme *cholesterol acyltransferase* when copper is deficient. These findings were questioned, however, by the work of Peter W. F. Fischer and Maurice W. Collins.[542] They found a negative correlation between HDL cholesterol and serum copper, just the opposite of the Allen-Klevay findings. Klevay[543] answered the seeming contradiction by stating that plasma copper can, at times, be maintained at the expense of liver copper. Thus, normal values of copper and zinc in the plasma do not constitute a basis for optimism unless the levels are confirmed by hair analysis.

Ny Wu et al. [543a] later reported that copper deficiency in rats led to increased cholesterol levels and a lower HDL as a percentage of total cholesterol (thus supporting Allen and Klevay rather than Fischer and Collins).* At the same time, Wu et al.[543a] and Denis M. Medeiros et al.[543c] of the same laboratory found that rats with low and marginal copper had lower blood pressures than those with adequate copper. Medeiros et al.[543c] also found increased copper concentration in the heart tissue of coronary victims. Denham Harman,[543d] years earlier, reported the same fact and attributed the phenomenon to increased lipid peroxidation of serum and aorta deposit lipids brought on by the higher copper concentrations. Harman[543e] further speculated that "peroxidation of fatty streak lipids may enhance the rate of conversion of fatty streaks to fibrous plaques." We have seen earlier in this chapter, however, that ceruloplasmin can act as an inhibitor of lipid peroxidation, can act as a scavenger of superoxide and can protect against pro-oxidant effects of iron.[528,529] Obviously, much work needs to be done regarding the role of copper in meeting nutritional needs of animals and of man.

---

* On the contrary, data from recent work by S. C. Croswell and K. Y. Lei[543b] suggested that in rats "the hypercholesterolemia observed in copper deficiency was associated with marked increases in cholesterol and apolipoprotein contents of apo E-rich HDL." (See Chapter 3 regarding the apolipoproteins.)

Hair analysis may be of particular value in trying to decide if one's body stores of copper are optimal. Hair analysis, although not always a reliable index to the minerals in various body tissues, is reported to be a good indicator of the liver's copper content. [544] Hair copper levels do not, however, reflect liver copper content in patients with primary liver cirrhosis.[545] Then too, T. Stephen Davies[546] points out that cold waving increases copper levels (and reduces zinc levels) in the hair. Thus, this suggests another possibility for a misleading hair analysis in addition to those we noted earlier. Furthermore, in cutting hair for analysis of mineral content it is well known that the cutting should be taken close to the scalp (usually from the nape of the neck). K. Michael Hambridge[547] has shown that this cutting technique is essential in analyzing for copper. Hambridge reported that copper levels in hair increase as one gets further from the scalp, thus suggesting that, since the part of the hair exposed longest to the external environment contains the most copper, it is likely that exogenous copper contributes to the hair content of this element.[*]

Copper's ability to help alleviate arthritic pain through being absorbed by the body from bracelets and necklaces may not be the superstition it is often thought to be. The widespread idea that wearing a copper bracelet can beneficially affect an arthritis sufferer is, however, given little credence by scientists. Nevertheless, an investigation by W. R. Walker and Daphne M. Keets[548] indicated that this long-standing folk remedy may have merit. The investigators concluded that some of the copper may have entered the body since the weights of the bracelets were reduced, but also they concluded that the psychological element could not be ruled out. Rationale for the beneficial action, if it is beneficial, might relate to the formation of anti-inflammatory copper compounds of benefit to the synovial membrane.

Copper and Gray Hair

The human body on a normal diet contains about 100 to 150 mg. of copper. The highest concentration of this mineral occurs in the

---

[*] Masae Yukawa[547a] reported that the concentrations of iodine, magnesium and calcium also increased, while those of chlorine and of bromine decreased from the scalp end to the tip.

hair, skin, liver, muscle and lung. The high concentration in the hair, especially if pigmented, suggests that copper may be important if one is to avoid graying of the hair.

Graying of the hair may or may not be of concern. But one should be concerned with the deficiencies of which it is a symptom. Pigment is formed by the copper-containing enzyme *tyrosinase* acting on the amino acid *tyrosine*. T. B. Fitzpatrick et al.[549] reported that graying is the result of a gradual loss of tyrosinase activity and this judgment was echoed by Jess H. Mottaz and Alvin S. Zelickson.[550] It seems reasonable that a copper deficiency could be a cause of diminished tyrosinase activity. Experiments with sheep, reported by Henry A. Schroeder,[551] have shown that when copper intake is low and molybdenum consumption is high, the hair of black sheep will turn white. This phenomenon has not, however, been demonstrated in man.

Nevertheless, a study by Henry A. Schroeder and Alexis P. Nason[552] showed that men with gray or white hair had somewhat less copper, and women with gray or white hair had far less copper, than their counterparts with naturally-colored hair.* Hirosi Yosikawa[552a] had earlier reported that white hairs from gray-haired men 50 to 65 years of age had far less copper than the black hairs of the same individuals. H. Kikkawa et al.[553] similarly found that the copper content of pigmented hair (of animals and of men) was higher than that of unpigmented hair. These results in regard to copper and hair color have not, however, been confirmed by all investigators. Ewin A. Eads and Charles E. Lambdin[276] reported that copper was inversely related to hair color, but H. Gross and M. M. Green,[554] in contrast, found no relation between copper and hair pigmentation. So contradictions remain to be resolved.

Graying of hair, for any given age, is correlated with increased pulse rate according to A. Damon and J. Roen[555] and lower pulse

---

* The same study showed that women, but not men, with gray or white hair had significantly *less* lead and cadmium in their hair than did their counterparts with naturally-colored hair. Since lead and cadmium are generally considered to be poisons and gray hair a sign of either aging or diminished health, might this argue that the *low* levels of lead and cadmium in the hair sometimes indicate *higher* levels in the rest of the body?

rates are thought to be an indication of better health. G. Lasker and B. Koplan,[556] in a study of 480 Mexican adults, found that the 91 who died of natural causes had grayer hair than those of equivalent age and sex. Graying of hair, since it suggests nutritional deficiencies, in some cases including copper, may be related to senescence. Speaking of nutritional deficiencies, there may be an even more important factor in loss of hair pigment than the effects of copper and other mineral shortages on enzyme systems. That factor could be melanocyte damage caused by free radicals from internal or external sources. Frequent washing will reduce the concentration of peroxides present in scalp lipids and detrimental free-radical effects. Antioxidants may also be useful in preventing graying, as well as hair loss, and F. A. J. Thiele[556a] speculates that suitable preparations will be developed by the cosmetic industry. Perhaps internal antioxidants in the form of vitamin E or of the various antioxidants discussed in Chapter 9 might also be useful.

Adverse Effects of Excess Copper

Excesses of copper may be just as dangerous as deficiencies. Carl C. Pfeiffer[557] has postulated that a principal cause of one type of schizophrenia, namely *histapenia*, is an excess of copper; and women with this problem who use the Pill, thus sending their blood copper even higher, may take an additional risk of psychoses. (M. H. Briggs et al.[558] reported that the copper content of hair of women taking oral contraceptives was strikingly higher than that of other women.)[*] Then too, according to Dr. Thaddeus Mann,[559] copper inhibits the metabolism of sperm. Furthermore, the copper in the intrauterine device (I.U.D.) affected both motility and cervical mucus penetration by human sperm, at least *in vitro*.[560][**] Copper has also been used, in rat experiments, to inhibit male fertility. S. S. Riar et al.[561] reported

---

[*] About 1% of persons in one study (done in England) had green plasma because of the elevated content of the blue plasma-protein ceruloplasmin. Most of this 1% group were women taking oral contraceptives.[558a] Sheila C. Vir et al.,[558b] contrary to Briggs, reported that there was no correlation between oral contraceptive use and hair copper. However, they found use of the Pill was associated with a marked increase in serum copper levels.

[**] Many I.U.D. failures—where conception resulted—may have been caused by the ingestion of aspirin or other drugs and the resulting modulation of prostaglandin synthesis.[560a]

that copper deposited by the process of iontophoresis into the vas deferens was subsequently slowly released and acted as a spermicide. They anticipate the procedure could be used to inhibit human male fertility.

Copper and Cancer

Serum copper levels are generally high in melanoma patients according to G. L. Fisher et al.[562] and the pigment melanin is formed through the action of the copper-containing enzyme tyrosinase. Serum copper is also generally above normal in cases of breast cancer, leukemia and Hodgkin's lymphoma.[563] Ehad J. Margalioth et al.[563a] recently reported that serum copper levels are also high in cases of ovarian carcinoma. Interestingly, they found that the serum copper levels declined as the disease activity was reduced through chemotherapy. The copper does not, however, seem to be a causal factor in these diseases but simply reflects the extent of tumor activity. Copper is beneficial, in fact, in several tumor-fighting applications. As we noted earlier, in Chapter 6, copper, along with vitamin C, has been found toxic to mouse and to human melanoma cells. We saw also that the use of a combination of copper and vitamin C resulted in greatly enhanced survival in mice having melanoma. Furthermore, Morton K. Schwartz[345] tells of the role of copper in increasing the cytotoxicity of an anticancer drug. However, Morton K. Schwartz[345] and G. N. Schrauzer et al.[564] report independently that epidemiological studies indicate there is a direct proportionality between dietary copper and several types of cancer. Since large amounts of copper (like zinc and cadmium) induce symptoms of selenium deficiency in animals, perhaps the absence of the cancer-protecting properties of selenium causes the problem. Regarding copper and cancer, it seems, once again, to be an example of the virtue of moderation.

The complexities of the serum copper: zinc ratio in terms of the stage of cancer development are indicated by a study by G. L. Fisher et al.[564a] Levels of serum copper were high in both primary and metastatic osteosarcoma patients. The ratio between serum copper and zinc was found to be higher in metastatic osteosarcoma patients than in those with primary osteosarcoma. (Fisher and his colleagues

suggested that the serum copper: zinc ratio may be usable as an index
to discriminate the primary from the metastatic stage of the disease.
What is significant about the stage in cancer development at which
the copper: zinc ratio shows a *reverse effect* ? Could metastasis be
prevented in a patient with primary osteosarcoma through thwarting
the reversal in the serum copper: zinc ratio by putting him on a low-
copper diet and by administering large amounts of zinc?) Serum
copper increases markedly not only in cases of osteosarcoma and of
melanoma but also increases during infections, in rheumatoid arthritis
(as we have already noted), in pregnancy and following virtually any
form of tissue injury.[565] It may be that ceruloplasmin functions as a
circulating anti-inflammatory protein. Perhaps it is an example of
"body wisdom" with increased copper, through antioxidant action,
attempting to combat disease.

Possible Effect in G6PD Deficiency

Earlier, we reported that either vitamin C or chlorite (formed
when drinking water is treated with chlorine dioxide) can present an
increased risk of hemolytic anemia in those with a deficiency of the
enzyme G6PD in their red blood cells. About 13% of American black
males are reported to have such a deficiency and Caucasians whose
ancestors originated in the Mediterranean area may also be affected.
Edward J. Calabrese et al.[566] have reported that copper can also cause
increases in the levels of methemoglobin (the oxidized form of
hemoglobin which is not able to combine reversibly with oxygen)
and decreases in the activity of the enzyme acetylcholinesterase in the
red cells of G6PD-deficient individuals. G. S. Moore and E. J.
Calabrese[567] speculate that the copper could potentiate the effect of
chlorite in persons having a G6PD deficiency.

Other Interesting Effects

The copper concentration in the blood's serum undergoes an
interesting circadian rhythm. R. I. Henkin[343] reported that the level of
serum copper is higher than the mean from 10 A.M. to 2 P.M.,
significantly below the mean from 2 P.M. to 6 P.M. and equal to the
mean from 6 P.M. to 10 P.M. The line of reasoning I presented in
relation to iron and to potassium might also suggest to future

dieticians the time of day it might be best to provide the body with high-copper foods or supplements.

Earlier, we reviewed Robert I. Henkin's research regarding the effects of zinc on the sense of taste. Henkin[343] has also studied the effect of copper on taste. Of his patients being treated with D-penicillamine (which chelates copper out of the body), 32% developed hypogeusia. Henkin observed that taste sensitivity returned to normal in every patient treated with copper after serum copper and ceruloplasmin concentrations normalized.

If a hair analysis shows copper to be present to excess in your body, taking supplemental zinc and manganese may promote increased excretion of copper via the urine. Furthermore, when the water supply is acid and the pipes that carry it are of copper, there may be toxic amounts of copper present in that water. It should not be drunk. Use bottled spring water instead.

Copper and ascorbic acid show various interactions with each other. Copper increases the inhibitory actions of vitamin C on the enzyme catalase, as pointed out in Chapter 6. We noted, on the other hand, that copper may promote the antihistaminic action of vitamin C. H. Scheinberg and I. Sternlieb[568] have shown that ascorbic acid also favorably affects the incorporation of copper into ceruloplasmin. Nevertheless, excessive consumption of ascorbic acid is antagonistic to copper status.[568a] (If both are used as supplements, it may be wise to take them at widely separated intervals.) Antacids have also been reported to cause a severe copper deficiency.[568b]

Copper in Food and in Supplements

Food sources for copper are nuts, thyme, black pepper and other spices, calves' liver (a far better source for copper than beef liver), kidney, brain, fish, oysters, shrimp, corn oil, margarine, chocolate, molasses, egg yolk, dried beans, peas, prunes, pomegranates, berries, dried fruit (especially apricots and figs), rice bran, wheat bran, whole grains, cauliflower, mushrooms and green leafy vegetables if grown on copper-rich soil. The absorption and retention of copper by humans fed a high-protein diet is reported by J. L. Greger and S. M. Snedeker[569] to be much greater than it is in subjects fed a low-protein diet.

Tablets of copper glutamate or of the amino-acid chelate are available, but they should probably be avoided unless a hair analysis clearly indicated you are deficient in this mineral. If you require copper supplementation, take it not only several hours away from vitamin C (as already suggested) but also away from any zinc or manganese supplements you may be using or absorption will be reduced. If you take supplemental copper and are undergoing tests, tell your doctor about the copper (and about the other minerals and vitamins) you are taking. Copper can cause false-positive indications in the benzidine and guaiac tests for occult blood.

Manganese

Manganese enters into many body reactions, including some involving vitamins B_1 and E. It activates a large number of metal-enzyme complexes involving transferase, hydrolase, lyase, isomerase and ligase reactions.[570] Manganese activates the cardiac enzyme adenyl cyclase according to G. I. Drummond et al.[571] (as does magnesium, cobalt and fluoride). However, at higher concentrations, Drummond et al. found that manganese exhibits a *reverse effect* on this enzyme and is inhibitory.

Manganese is especially highly concentrated in the bones, liver, pancreas, kidney and pituitary gland. It is also present in tears—about 30 times the serum concentration of the subjects that were tested.[572]

An important form of superoxide dismutase contains manganese and we must take in sufficient amounts of this mineral for the body to form this vital enzyme. David I. Paynter[572a] reported that, in rat experiments, the greatest reduction of MnSOD, following a decrease in dietary manganese, occurred in the heart. The increase in manganese and in MnSOD concentrations in heart tissue as dietary manganese was increased are shown in Figure 20. In this study CuZnSOD remained essentially unchanged. Interestingly, L. Hurley[573] reported that in chicks fed a manganese-deficient diet the activity of CuZnSOD increased as that of MnSOD declined. Daret Kasemset and Larry W. Oberley[573a] found, by means of *in vitro* experiments, that intraperitoneal injection of glucose depressed MnSOD and CuZnSOD in mouse heart. The MnSOD and CuZnSOD were maximally depressed at a glucose concentration of 4.5 mg./kg. (In a similar *in vitro* experiment glucose also depressed SOD activity in mouse brain. Curiously, the glucose suppression effect on MnSOD activity in the heart was partially alleviated by x-irradiation.)

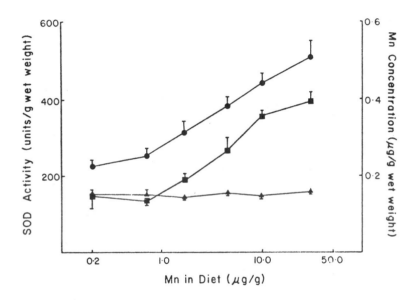

Figure 20. Effect of dietary manganese concentration on MnSOD activity (circle), CuSOD activity (triangle) and manganese concentration (square) in heart tissue of rats fed the diets for ten weeks. Values for diets supplemented with 4.5 and 29.5 mg. Mn/kg. are the means (±SEM) of four rats. For all others, values are means (±SEM) of six rats. Reproduced from David I. Paynter, *Jrl. of Nutrition* (1980) 110: 437-447, with the permission of the copyright owner, the American Institute of Nutrition, and the author.

Both MnSOD and CuZnSOD exist as isoenzymes.[574] Isoenzymes (isozymes) are electrophoretically distinct forms of an enzyme representing different polymeric states but having the same function. We will consider SOD further in Chapter 9.

A Mineral of Many Uses

Manganese is probably a factor in the metabolism of carbohydrates. G. L. Everson and R. E. Shrader[575] found that manganese-deficient guinea pigs showed a diabetic-like response to glucose loading that reversed when manganese was given. Perhaps a deficiency of manganese may contribute to the onset of diabetes in humans. K. Hermansen and J. Iversen,[575a] in related work, reported that dog experiments showed the manganese ion inhibited the release of both insulin and glucagon during the first three to four minutes of infusion. This depressing action was followed by an *increase* in the release of these hormones. Janet E. Merritt and Barry L. Brown[575b] have referenced studies showing other "paradoxical stimulatory effects" (which are *reverse effects*) of manganese on adrenaline and amylase secretion. They also have reported their own research on such "paradoxical effects" of manganese on the body's production of prolactin.

Manganese is required for the body to join the sugars xylose and galactose in producing various glycoproteins (such as heparin) that are vital to body chemistry. Manganese is concentrated in melanocytes that are responsible for pigmentation of the skin and hair.[570] Manganese is also reported to be valuable in assuring normal function of ligament tissues. D. Meissner[570a] reported, in 1986, that manganese may be useful also in treating arteriosclerosis.

Manganese is used by the thyroid gland in the production of thyroxin. Along with calcium, manganese is important in the efficient functioning of the mammary glands during lactation. Manganese, through its enzyme *arginase,* is also involved in the metabolism of the amino acid arginine to ornithine and urea.

Manganese, or a lack thereof, is a factor in a potpourri of other functions and diseases. A deficiency of manganese in a pregnant rat can lead to congenital deformities in her offspring.[575c] Experiments with mice have shown that the presence of ample manganese can, as I. J. T. Davies[576] says, "alter the expression of harmful genes." Manganese is required in the building of strong bones and it also promotes health of the nerves. Below-normal levels of manganese have been found in the hair of patients having schizophrenia.[577] Peter E. Sylvester[577a] and, later, P. J. Barlow and P. E. Sylvester[577b] reported that hair levels of manganese (and also of calcium and copper) were low in children with Down's syndrome.

Manganese is also a factor in the immune response. Mark F. McCarty[577c] observes that the ability of manganese to increase levels of coenzymes Q and to potentiate antibody production in rodents to antigen challenge is analogous to the action of selenium. However, a number of animal experiments indicate that either a deficiency or an excess of dietary manganese can decrease antibody production.[577d] Thus, a deficiency of manganese that might cause a depressed immune response may show a *reverse effect* as manganese approaches optimal levels. Then, as manganese continues to increase, to excessive amounts, another *reverse effect* may set in and the immune system may once again be depressed.

Manganese and Cancer

E. J. Underwood[121] cites a number of studies showing that patients who died of lung cancer had much less manganese in the cancerous tissue than in other tissues of either the involved lung or the uninvolved lung. Is it possible that lung cancer developed because of the shortage of MnSOD in the lungs? On the other hand, I. L. Mulay et al.[578] showed that malignant breast tissue had higher concentrations of manganese than did homologous normal tissue. In 1971, MnSOD had not yet been discovered. I wonder if Mulay's manganese was really in the SOD form and whether "body wisdom" was sending it there to fight the cancer. But, if so, why doesn't "body wisdom" send MnSOD to cancerous lungs? Recently, Larry W. Oberley and Terry D. Oberley[578a] have presented a hypotheses relating MnSOD to chemical carcinogenesis and gene amplification. There are obviously many mysteries yet to be solved.

Preliminary work by T. F. Parkinson et al.[579] has indicated higher concentrations of manganese and copper in melanoma biopsies (although markedly lower zinc concentrations in basal cell carcinoma biopsies). As we noted earlier, in connection with Fisher's confirmation of the high concentration of copper in melanomas, the presence of copper or of manganese (or the absence of zinc) does not appear to be a causal factor in the generation of the cancers. In fact, an epidemiological study by G. N. Schrauzer et al.[564] showed that dietary intake of manganese was inversely correlated with cancer mortality, especially with death due to cancer of the pancreas, an organ which normally contains a large amount of this mineral.

Nevertheless, manganese in high concentrations is a mutagen and a carcinogen.[580] That fact is, however, no reason to fear this absolutely essential mineral; on the contrary, the theory of the *reverse effect* suggests that in modest amount manganese could be cancer protective. This is probably the case, protection being provided by manganese-based superoxide dismutase and also by various manganous complexes if the *in vitro* experiments of Frederick S. Archibald and Irvin Fridovich[581] are applicable *in vivo*.

Other Effects of Manganese

Various investigators, as cited by E. J. Underwood,[121] have reported that the manganese content of the black hair of cattle was much higher than the white hair of the same animal. In Hereford cattle the red hair consistently contained significantly more manganese than did the white hair of the same animal. Similarly, Vlado Valkovic[582] reported that analysis of black and gray hair of men showed the gray hair contained much lower levels of manganese. Having an adequate level of manganese may be one of the factors if one is to avoid or reduce graying of the hair.

According to the popular (but misleading) book, *Biological Transmutations,* by Louis C. Kervran[583] some manganese is transmuted into iron by the body. I question this; hair analysis shows, on the contrary, that excessive manganese can suppress iron (and other minerals) in the body. If you use manganese supplements, have periodic hair analyses to determine the effect on your body's other vital minerals. However, throughout this book I have cited problems in connection with hair analysis. Some hairsprays contain manganese which will not come out in the washing process done by hair analysts.[577]

Excessive manganese may not only depress the level of other minerals but it may be detrimental to the teeth. J. L. Hardwick and C.

J. Martin[584] have shown that manganese, in a concentration similar to that present in dental plaque, increased the amount of lactic acid produced by each of seven strains of *Streptococcus mutans,* thought to be a major factor in causing caries. Subsequently, M. E. Martin et al.[584a] reported that manganese is required for *Streptococcus mutans* to move from anerobic niches to regions of elevated oxygen in the mouth. Thus, increased manganese in the mouth should lead to greater proliferation of this organism and thus increase dental caries. David Beighton[585] reported that manganese stimulated utilization of glucose by *Streptococcus mutans* and by several other oral *Streptococci* species. He also found that fluoride inhibited utilization of glucose by these bacteria, thus providing a rationale (other than that of tooth hardening) for the beneficial dental effect of fluoride.

Manganese seems to have some importance in the reproductive function. A deficiency in male rats and rabbits is reported to cause decreased libido, decreased semen and degeneration of the seminal tubules. George C. Cotzias[586] found that there is a high correlation between manganese and dopamine in the brains of rats. Sexual stimulation in men has been reported when levodopa (prescribed for parkinsonism) was converted in the brain to dopamine (which, in turn, forms norepinephrine). Thus, perhaps this is the reason for the reports that manganese can act as a sexual stimulant.

On the other hand, studies with mice and rats cited by Leon Earl Gray, Jr. and John W. Laskey[587] have shown that huge amounts of manganese can cause retardation in sexual development. Gray and Laskey also cite a report by J. Rodier who studied Moroccan miners who developed manganese poisoning. He reported that 81% of these patients had reduced levels of urinary 17-ketosteroids made by the Leydig cells of the testes. Thus, we have another example of the *reverse effect.* Modest amounts of manganese are beneficial for sex; large amounts are detrimental.

Manganese inhibits absorption of many other metals, including iron. Thus, an excess of manganese could be a cause of anemia. Low iron or calcium intakes or increased alcohol consumption promote manganese absorption (at least in rats).[587a] Food sources for manganese are tea and spices (especially cloves, cardamom, ginger and bay leaves), wheat germ, rice bran, wheat bran, whole grains, nuts (especially walnuts), seeds, beans, spinach, parsley and kelp. Manganese is also available as tablets in gluconate and amino-acid chelated forms.

Chromium and the Glucose Tolerance Factor (GTF)*

Chromium in the form of the glucose tolerance factor is involved in the body's use of insulin, and its lack may be a contributing cause of diabetes, hypertension and atherosclerosis. The biologically active form of chromium is GTF but this, according to D. Shapcott et al.,[588] is a minor component of the circulating chromium. W. Mertz and E. E. Roginski have defined biologically active chromium as compounds that potentiate the insulin-dependent conversion of glucose to carbon dioxide *in vitro*. However, studies should be made in the attempt to expand that definition to include other biological functions.

GTF is a compound probably consisting of a chromium molecule plus two niacin molecules plus glutamic acid, glycine and cysteine. Methods of extracting GTF from brewer's yeast (which contains very little GTF activity) are discussed in a patent of Andrew Szalay.[588a] GTF can be made by the body but not always in sufficient amounts to meet body needs. Cihad T. Gürson[589] suggests that older persons may have particular difficulty in converting inorganic chromium to GTF.

---

* Steven J. Haylock et al.,[587b] in 1983, held that if chromium is an essential part of the GTF structure, it constitutes a minor component with the bulk of the material being nicotinic acid or other extraneous substances. Then, later in that year, they assumed a much more radical stance. Haylock et al.[587c] in this later study insisted that the glucose tolerance factor could no longer be regarded as a chromium complex. The long association of chromium and GTF activity has persisted, they stated, because of inadequate separation procedures. They said GTF is also not tyramine (which constituted about 90% of their GTF) but an unidentified substance which represented probably less than 10% of the material they had isolated. If this work is replicated it will obsolete much of what I say here, and what others say, about chromium and GTF. (You may desire to check Haylock periodically in *Citation Abstracts*.)

Chromium in the form of GTF, since it reduces plasma glucose, has been used in the treatment of diabetes.* Chromium, as the glucose tolerance factor, greatly increases the hormonal effect of insulin, about three-fold according to Mark F. McCarty.[591] GTF has also been reported to be beneficial in the treatment of hypoglycemia. However, Mark F. McCarty[591] points out a possible risk in the use of GTF. McCarty states that if GTF has value in treating reactive hypoglycemia, this benefit must be weighed against the risk of possibly worsening the condition by the reduction in plasma glucose. Recently, Alice E. Hunt et al.[591a] reported that chromium, given as brewer's yeast, greatly increased the hair chromium concentrations in diabetes patients (as well as in nondiabetics), but no significant effects were noted in fasting blood glucose, fasting serum insulin, hemoglobin A_1, total serum cholesterol, HDL-cholesterol or serum triglyceride concentrations.

GTF may be useful in many other therapies. Mark F. McCarty[591] develops a line of reasoning that would suggest GTF could have a very broad spectrum immunostimulant action. It may be an aid in treating arthritis and periodontitis. In animal experiments, a deficiency of chromium caused cataracts. In experiments performed by Henry A. Schroeder[591b] rats fed extra chromium had lower cholesterol and lived longer. Chromium is found in nucleic acids and it is probable that the body's use of some amino acids is facilitated by its presence.

Well over a decade ago it was predicted by H. A. Schroeder et al.[592] that a shortage of chromium might eventually be determined to be a cause of atherosclerosis. Then R. J. Doisy et al.[593] reported a decrease in cholesterol levels of persons on brewer's yeast supplementation and suggested that the effect was due to the chromium content. A study by Howard A. I. Newman et al.[594] found that a group with coronary artery disease had significantly lower serum chromium levels than persons with normal arteries. They concluded, in fact, that chromium levels were the best predicator for coronary artery disease. Then too, Michel Cote and Denis

---

* Synthetic chromium compounds have been prepared which reduced plasma glucose by 9% to 20% compared with a reduction of 36% when GTF was used.[590]

Shapcott[594a] reported that men with arteriosclerotic disease had significantly lower chromium in their hair compared to men with normal coronary arteries. In addition, Abraham S. Abraham et al.[595] discovered that when rabbits were fed a 1% cholesterol diet there were much lower serum cholesterol levels in those that were also injected with potassium chromate than in those not treated with chromium. Not only does chromium seem to be a well-established hypocholesterolemic factor, but Rebecca Riales and Margaret J. Albrink,[596] in a study of healthy adult men, presented data to support the hypothesis that chromium supplementation raises high-density lipoprotein. This data also suggests that chromium supplementation improves insulin sensitivity in those with insulin resistance but normal glucose tolerance. J. C. Elwood et al.[596a] confirmed that high-chromium brewer's yeast significantly decreased serum cholesterol while significantly increasing HDL levels in groups of hyperlipidemic and of normolipidemic adults. Following supplementation, the triglyceride levels in blood were not changed in either group.

Esther G. Offenbacker and F. Xavïer Pi-Sunyer[597] reported that when chromium-rich brewer's yeast was fed to elderly persons, including some with noninsulin-dependent diabetes, they showed an improved glucose tolerance and every member of the group achieved a reduction in serum cholesterol.* A control group fed chromium-poor torula yeast did not show improved glucose tolerance, but some showed an improvement in serum cholesterol, thus suggesting the presence of a hypocholesterolemic factor other than chromium in torula yeast. (For noninsulin-dependent diabetics, the only proven treatment is weight loss[597a] although rat studies [*Science* (Aug. 21, 1987) 237: 885-887] suggest fish oil may be useful. Contrarily, *Medical World News* [June 8, 1987] 28:104 reports fish oil may harm diabetics.)

---

* A study by R. F. Borgman et al.[598] showed hair content of chromium was positively correlated with the incidence of hypertension (although not with heart mortality). Confusing, since chromium, to the extent it is hypocholesterolemic, should work to reduce hypertension. The study also showed positive correlations between the incidence of hypertension and the hair levels of lead, selenium and copper but no correlation for cadmium. Perhaps no conclusion should be drawn except to note that the study helps demonstrate that hair stores of an element may not always be well correlated with body stores of that element but, instead, may sometimes be better correlated with body excretion. These facts illustrate the primitive state of hair analysis. Hair analyses can be interesting, but interpretations should not be taken too seriously.

GTF may be of some value in dieting. Insulin has been shown to stimulate the hypothalamic satiety center and Mark F. McCarty[591] has suggested that this implies supplemental GTF might have a useful hunger-suppressant action during calorie-deficit dieting. He observed that this suggestion assumes, however, that any accompanying reduction in plasma glucose levels (perhaps through stimulating hunger) will not negate the value of the presumed effect. In working to prevent a high/low effect in blood sugar and in helping to assure a more steady flow of glucose to the brain and to the rest of the body, GTF may not only be a satiety factor that could help control appetite, but at the same time it could contribute to a sense of well-being.

It is widely reported that body stores of chromium tend to decline as we get older and our refined foods (from which chromium has been lost) are held to be responsible. Furthermore, according to Richard A. Anderson,[599] some highly processed foods, including sucrose, stimulate urinary excretion of chromium and thus further deplete body stores. At any rate, persons living in countries not yet widely exposed to refined foods—e.g., the Far East, the Middle East and Africa—are reported to have much higher chromium levels in their bodies than do Americans. On the other hand, the story that aging depletes body chromium content would seem to be questionable in light of the research of A. S. Abraham et al.[600] Abraham's group found that the mean serum chromium level of men under 60 years of age was lower than that of those over 60, although women showed no change in level with increasing age. It should be noted that this research reported on *total* serum chromium, not on GTF, so Gürson's suggestion, noted earlier, that older persons may have difficulty converting inorganic chromium to GTF may still be valid. Perhaps the refined-food story may also have validity if GTF rather than total chromium is being considered.

The greatest concentration of chromium occurs in the ovaries. When men are given radioactive chromium by injection there is a rapid absorption by the testes, suggesting that the element is used in forming spermatozoa. Chromium is, therefore, probably related to fertility and/or sexuality. Women on the Pill require greater amounts of chromium and should, perhaps, increase their intake by consuming more foods that contain it or by using supplementary tablets.

The hair content of chromium in parous women (those who have given birth to children), and presumably the chromium content of the rest of their bodies as well, has been reported to be lower than that of nulliparous women (those who have not given birth). However, D. Shapcott et al.[601] measured hair chromium levels of 432 women at delivery and observed that, although levels in general were lower than in nonpregnant women, there was no correlation between hair chromium level and age or number of pregnancies. * If lack of chromium were a contributing cause of diabetes it might help explain why multiparous women—those who have given birth to many children—are more apt to contract diabetes than are nulliparous women. However, individuals with diabetes absorb more chromium than nondiabetic persons, and insulin-requiring diabetics excrete more chromium than normal persons.[599] The problem seems to be one of nonutilization of chromium by persons with diabetes rather than a lack of the element. Anderson[599] states that mildly diabetic persons often respond to chromium supplementation but severely diabetic persons do not.

Levels of hair chromium are reported to be normal in persons with maturity-onset diabetes but below normal in those with the juvenile-onset type.[577] This helps support the conclusion that these types of diabetes have different causes.

Richard A. Anderson et al.[601a,b] reported that chromium, probably since it is involved in glucose metabolism, and also zinc are lost in increased amounts in the urine during strenuous exercise. Janet S. Borel et al.[601c] discovered that within 24 hours of trauma, patients showed an elevated urinary chromium concentration of several-fold. Perhaps supplementation might be useful in such cases of extreme body stress.

Chromium is found in brewer's yeast (by far the best source of biologically available chromium), spices (especially thyme and to a

---

* Hair chromium values, however, may be of only limited value in assessing body content of the element, particularly for individuals in a state of protein and energy malnutrition.[602]

lesser degree pepper and some others),* organ meats (especially liver), cheese, wheat germ, whole grains, mushrooms, parsnips, corn oil (far more than in corn itself), lecithin, butter, nuts, maple syrup, sugar beet, molasses, grape juice and tomatoes if cooked in stainless steel kettles. Beer, depending on the brand, may be a poor but at other times may be an excellent source of chromium, apparently because of the stainless steel brewing vessels that are sometimes used. Wine is generally a good source of chromium and this may be one of the factors in the decreased heart risk enjoyed by wine (and by beer) drinkers.[603] Cigarette smoke also contains chromium, but it is the hexavalent, toxic form of the metal rather than the trivalent variety found in foods. It is the trivalent form that is so important to our well-being. If a chromium supplement is used, it should be taken several hours away from any zinc supplement since these metals will compete with each other for assimilation.

However, as important as chromium is, it is unlikely that supplementation via pills is required by most persons, especially if they will include modest amounts of chromium-rich foods (such as brewer's yeast) in their diets. Richard A. Anderson[599] relates that, contrary to many reports and contrary to the GTF-pill pushers, the chromium requirements of normal persons can be met through the chromium complexes found widely in foods. Thus, the form of dietary chromium does not appear to be as vital as was postulated earlier by Walter Mertz. However, inorganic chromium compounds must be converted by the body to a biologically active form in order for chromium to perform its functions.

Possible Dangers of Excessive Chromium

It is possible that chromium supplements could sometimes pose a threat to health. Mutagenic and carcinogenic activity of chromium has been found primarily in the hexavalent compounds. A. Leonard and R. R. Lauwerys[604] point out, however, that trivalent chromium appears to be inactive in the assay systems used to detect

---

* Spices such as thyme and pepper are more concentrated sources of chromium than is brewer's yeast, but one cannot easily consume such spices in generous amounts.

mutagenicity (and, therefore, possible carcinogenicity). Note these disturbing words of Leonard and Lauwerys:

> It can be considered as evident, however, that the ultimate mutagen, which binds to the genetic material, is the trivalent form produced intracellularly from hexavalent chromium, the apparent lack of activity of the trivalent form being due to its poor cellular uptake.

To add to our concern, G. N. Schrauzer et al.[564] provide epidemiological data from 28 countries suggesting a direct association between dietary chromium and several types of cancer. They say, "Although it would be premature to conclude that dietary chromium stimulates human cancer development, experimental studies should be performed to test the possibility." Meanwhile, how safe is it to overload the body with chromium in the form of GTF pills as some "health enthusiasts" are now doing? It seems especially weird if Steven J. Haylock et al. [587c] are eventually proved correct in their thesis that chromium is not contained in GTF!

Sulphur

Sulphur has been called the "beauty mineral" because it helps keep hair glossy and smooth and aids one in maintaining a smooth and youthful complexion. It also fosters healthy fingernails.

Sulphur enters our bodies when we eat proteins containing the amino acids methionine, cystine, cysteine and taurine. These sulphydryl amino acids are important antioxidants, all being essential except possibly taurine. Taurine is widely reported to be nonessential (which, of course, does not mean it is unneeded by the body but merely that the body can make it from other essential amino acids). Apparently taurine *is* nonessential for lower animals. On the other hand, Gerald E. Gaull and David K. Rassin[605] found that taurine is essential in man. The human infant, especially, needs a dietary supply of taurine to synthesize the bile salt *taurocholate*. Gaull and Rassin reported that taurine appears to be an important component of the developing brain and that it must be supplied to humans in their diet.

Sulphur is present in the body in some mucopolysaccharides (including heparin and dermatan sulphate) and in glycolipids and in the form of sulphate esters in various metabolites. It is a component of coenzyme A which we discussed in connection with pantothenic acid and the Krebs cycle in Chapter 5. Sulphur accumulates as chondroitin sulphate in benign prostatic hyperplasia,[606] but the significance of this fact is yet to be explained. We must resist the temptation to conclude, however, that a substance associated with a disease implies causality. "Body wisdom" could just as conceivably be using the substance to mollify the condition. At any rate, accumulation of chondroitin sulphate might be beneficial in combating atherosclerosis. K. Nakazawa and K. Murata[606a] have reported orally administered chondroitin polysulphate has demonstrated its antilipemic and antithrombogenic properties in elderly patients with atherosclerosis.

Sulphur is also a constituent of insulin and of a number of other body chemicals. The oral hypoglycemic drug tolbutamide is a sulfonylurea compound. Sulphur is present in homocysteine and in cystathionine, both of which were discussed earlier in connection with vitamin B6 and its role in obviating a possible cause of atherosclerosis. DMSO, which contains sulphur, destroys free radicals (hydroxyl radicals). In doing its work it is, however, changed into a sulfoxide free radical so vitamins E or C or another free radical scavenger should be taken when DMSO is used. Topical applications of DMSO have been reported to sometimes lead to relief from arthritic pain.

Sulphur is also a component of glutathione, the tripeptide which is so important in regulating oxygen supply to the cells and helps protect the body from damage by free radicals.[607] In Chapter 3 we observed that glutathione is involved in prostaglandin and leukotriene synthesis. Then too, glutathione may be very important for eye health. Kartar Singh et al.[608] have reported that reduced glutathione in normal lenses was present in a much greater concentration than in cataractous lenses. Reduced glutathione also plays an important role in our avoiding liver toxicity. L. F. Prescott[609] relates that the hepatotoxity of many compounds including cocaine, and possibly even ethyl alcohol, can be diminished or prevented by reduced glutathione precursors and related sulphydryl compounds. Furthermore, Noriko Tateishi et al.[610] have proposed that the liver stores glutathione as a reservoir of the amino acid cysteine. Yet another "plus" for reduced glutathione is the part it has been shown to play in causing regression of aflatoxin B-induced tumors in rats.[611]

About one-third of the amino acids of metallothionein, protein compounds which seem to protect the body from toxic minerals,[611a] contain the sulphur-based amino acid cysteine.[611b]* The metallothioneins are proteins of small size, in the range of polypeptides, with a molecular weight of about 6,600 daltons.[611d] Adjusting for the metal content of five to seven gram atoms per mole of protein, the metal-free polypeptide (called thionein) has a molecular weight of about 6,000 daltons.[611d] With an excess of sulphur a *reverse effect* sets in and metallothionein levels are decreased.[611b] Paul J. Thornalley and Milan Vasak[611e] have reported that metallothionein appears to be an extraordinarily efficient hydroxyl-radical scavenger. Interestingly, ethyl alcohol induces biosynthesis of metallothionein (at least it does so in the liver of the mouse).[611h] Zinc, cadmium or copper administration also increases the concentration of metallothionein[611f,g]

Sulphur, in the form of sulfatide, may be a lipid requirement for the sodium pump of the red blood cell.[612] However, sulfatide in excess can lead to sulfatidosis (as occurs in leukodystrophy). Sulphur compounds, alone and used with vitamin C, show great potential for combating acetaldehyde poisoning occasioned by alcoholism and smoking. In this regard, interesting and potentially very valuable research was published by Herbert Sprince et al.[613] Used individually, thiamin (vitamin B₁), l-cysteic acid, sodium metabisulfite and N-acetyl-l-cysteine were especially effective, while ascorbic acid was reasonably good in protecting against acetaldehyde poisoning in rats. Used in combination, l-ascorbic acid, l-cysteine and thiamin chloride were

---

* Metallothionein also stores and carries nontoxic metals. Kirk B. Nielson et al.[611c] showed that at least 18 different metals are associated with these proteins.

completely effective and another combination, l-ascorbic acid, N-acetyl-l-cysteine and thiamin chloride was almost as good. The scientists caution, however, that further animal research should be performed before considering long-term, high-dosage use for humans.

An ascorbic acid metabolite, *ascorbate 3 sulfate,* is present in the urine. Vitamin C may, in some cases, remove valuable amounts of sulphur from the body. This suggests the possibility that those taking large amounts of vitamin C might consider eating increased amounts of sulphur-containing foods.

Sulphur is present in many of the cruciferous plants (those of the mustard family and having leaves or petals in the form of a cross), including cabbages, brussels sprouts, cauliflower, broccoli, turnips, kale, radishes and mustard. The sulphur is present in the form of glucosinolates, and about 65 of these compounds have been isolated, the more common among which are sinigrin, sinalbin and progoitrin. Upon hydrolysis of the glucosinolates, thiocyanate is formed and, as we noted in relation to iodine, it can act as a goiterogenic agent. However, there is a positive side to eating cruciferous vegetables. Saxon Graham et al.[614] have reported that the risk of colon and rectum cancer increases with decreases in the frequency with which vegetables (especially cabbage, brussels sprouts and broccoli) are eaten.* Graham[614a] subsequently confirmed the value of consuming cruciferous vegetables in reducing cancer incidence of the colon, rectum and bladder.** On the contrary, Gail E. McKeown-Eyssen and Elizabeth Bright-See,[614ab] in an international epidemiological survey, found no evidence linking colon cancer mortality and the availability of cruciferous vegetables. Disulphides derived from cysteine sulfoxides are found in some members of the *Liliaceae* family, especially

---

* These same scientists found that increased consumption of peanut butter increases the risk of rectum cancer. However, they reported that consumption of meat, which is often thought to increase the risk of cancer, was not associated with the incidence of either colon or rectal carcinogenesis.

** Kazuyoshi Morita et al.[614aa] had earlier screened factors from crucifers and from other vegetables and fruits for natural desmutagens. Juices from cabbage, broccoli, green pepper, eggplant, apple, burdock, shallot, ginger, pineapple and mint leaf were found to have strong capacities of inactivating mutagenicity of tryptophan pyrolysis products.

those of the *Allium* genus. Allylthiosulfinate (allicin) is present in garlic and is garlic's antibacterial principle.[614ac-ad] Various other sulphates are found in onions and chives. Only if consumed in large amounts is it possible that those foods might contribute to the incidence of goiter.

The yolk of eggs is an excellent food source for sulphur. Good sources, in addition to the crucifers already mentioned, include meat, fish, oysters, poultry, clams, cheese, wheat germ, bran, peanuts, brazil nuts, chestnuts, red currants, cranberries, pineapples, celery, swiss chard, string beans, watercress, endive and sorrel. Sulphur is one of the constituents, not only of vitamin B 1 as we have already pointed out, but also of biotin. Sulphur is also a component of "vitamin U,"* the antiulcer vitamin found in cabbage leaves and in other green vegetables.[614b] The S-methylmethionine sulfonium chloride form of vitamin U given orally was found to significantly ameliorate plasma cholesterol and phospholipid levels in rats and was an effective treatment for nephrotic syndrome.[614c]

Sulphur in the form of sulphur dioxide, sulphurous acid and salts of sulphite and bisulphite shows antioxidant and antimicrobial properties and so these chemicals are often used as preservatives in certain foods and beverages. Sulphite and bisulphite are widely used in winemaking as selective inhibitors of yeasts and bacteria and they are often present in finished wine. They are also used in dehydrated fruits, vegetables and soups; fruit juices; cider; vinegar; sausages; pickles; mushrooms; potato chips and beer. Prior to July, 1986 bisulphiting agents were used by restaurants to extend the life of lettuce and other salad vegetables as well as salad dips.[614d]** Bisulphite is used as an antioxidant in pharmaceuticals, including preparations of epinephrine, apomorphine and sodium salicylate.[614da] Stanley I. Wolf and Richard A. Nicklas[614db] give an extensive list of medications containing sulphites. Furthermore, they state that sulphites may be

---

* "Vitamin U" is listed in *The Merck Index*[614b] but is not considered to be a vitamin by the Committee on Dietary Allowances.[614ba]

** In July, 1986 the FDA extended suphite labeling requirements on packaged foods and banned use of sulphites as a preservative for fruits and vegetables in restaurant and supermarket salad bars. This ban did not affect use of sulphite on fresh potatoes or in wine and beer. The FDA actions are described in the *Federal Register* of July 9, 1986.

present even in the vitamin B complex. (If you are sensitive to sulphite and are taking the vitamin B complex, ask your supplier to check the disclosure manual to see if the product is sulphite-free.)

Possible Danger of Excessive Sulphur

Ingested sulphite (sulfite) is cleared in the body by the enzyme sulphite oxidase. To the extent sulphite is not cleared by the body, it could pose problems by inhibiting the sulphatases. For some persons (those short of the molybdenum-based enzyme sulphite oxidase) the presence of bisulphiting agents added to food has resulted in allergic reactions.[614e-h] William A. Pryor[614i] speculates that sulphite may increase the rate of conversion of arachidonic acid to eicosatraene hydroperoxides (HPETES)—which we met in Chapter 3. If so, this would explain the sensitivity of asthmatics to sulphite. On the other hand, Rhoda Papaioannou and Carl C. Pfeiffer[614j] speculate that molybdenum deficiency may be a cause.

Although in low concentrations, sulphite and bisulphite act as antioxidants, in larger concentrations they can show *reverse effects* and act as pro-oxidants. Bunji Inouye et al.[614k] reported that lipid peroxidation was induced by sulphite, depending on concentration, in rat lung extracts, liver microsomes and mitochondria. Peroxidation was accelerated by iron or vanadium. Hemolysis of human erythrocytes was induced *in vitro* during incubation in the presence of sulphite and the action was exacerbated when vanadium was also present.

Hikoya Hayatsu and Akiko Miura[614l] reported that sodium bisulphite has mutagenic activity. A. F. Gunnison[615] speculates that sulphite might even be a cocarcinogen. However, although bisulphite enhances ultraviolet-induced mutagenesis in *E. coli* and in Chinese hamster cells and *in vitro* transformation of Syrian hamster cells, many *in vivo* animal tests of sulphite and bisulphate indicate noncarcinogenicity and low toxicity.[615a] In fact, small amounts (300 ppm or less) of sulphite or bisulphite inactivated the mutagenicity of coffee (possibly by interacting with its diacetyl).[615a] Thus, it seems likely that sulphite and bisulphite might, under proper experimental conditions, exhibit *reverse effects* by both enhancing and inhibiting mutagenesis in the same entity. If true, the sulphites and bisulphites might be candidates for possible anticancer action.

Cobalt

Cobalt is an important constituent of vitamin B_{12} and gives that vitamin its pink color. In addition to its function in the formation of vitamin B_{12}, cobalt is a component of the biotin-dependent enzyme transcarboxylase, each molecule of which usually consists of two atoms of cobalt and four of zinc. (Although the sum of the cobalt and zinc content is constant, the ratio between the two metals can vary.)[616] Experiments have shown that cobalt can replace zinc, not only in transcarboxylase but also in a number of other zinc enzymes. Cobalt also activates a number of enzymes and in pharmacologic doses stimulates production of red blood cells.[617] Cobaltous chloride has been used in treating certain anemias, but such treatment may have side effects, including thyroid enlargement[617a] and a depressing effect on cytochrome P-450 concentration in the liver.[617b]

Cobaltous chloride has been reported by Tadashi Inoue et al.[617c] and by Hajime Mochizuki and Tsuneo Kada[617d] to act as an antimutagen. The Inoue group speculated that cobaltous chloride may correct the error-proneness of DNA replicating enzyme(s) by improving its (their) fidelity in DNA synthesis. When, in animal experiments, either cobaltous chloride or sodium cobaltinitrite is administered in conjunction with the topical application of the carcinogen methycholanthrene, the tumorigenic response is significantly decreased. Gerald P. O'Hara et al.[618] found, however, that these cobalt compounds had no effect on the growth of established epithelial tumors.

Cobalt was formerly added to beer as a foam stabilizer and was present to the extent of about 1.2 ppm. Some individuals who drank large quantities of beer developed congestive heart failure due to cardiopathy induced by the cobalt. They also experienced polycythemia (an increase in the number of red blood cells, i.e., the opposite of anemia), thyroid hyperplasia (increased thyroid tissue) and neurological problems. Thankfully, cobalt is no longer used in the manufacture of beer.

There are other negative aspects of cobalt. As we noted earlier in this chapter,[10] calcium is an essential factor in secreting insulin. Claes B. Wollheim and Danilo Janjic,[618a] in a rat experiment, found that cobalt ions abolish glucose-induced calcium-ion uptake and insulin release. A study by Colette N. Thaw et al.,[618b] using cell cultures, suggested that cobalt ions also inhibit prolactin secretion. Then too, cobalt-chromium alloy constructions used in dentistry might sometimes pose a threat. Torsten Stenberg and Bo Bergman[618c] showed that cobalt was released from subcutaneous implants of such alloys. They suggest the possibility that the corrosive milieu of the oral cavity might also cause the release of cobalt. Brushing can increase the release of cobalt. But, perhaps more significant, Joaquin Fontes de Melo et al. [618d] showed that dental enamel, impacting on a cobalt-chromium prosthesis, can cause a cobalt release of 13 to 14 times higher than caused by brushing.

Seafood is by far the strongest source for this mineral. Other, but less concentrated, sources were shown in Chapter 5 in connection with vitamin B_{12}. Most diets furnish enough cobalt so that bacteria in the colon can synthesize vitamin B_{12} but, as related in Chapter 5, whether or not that vitamin is made available to the body from this source is problematical.

Molybdenum

Molybdenum is a constituent of several enzymes: aldehyde oxidase, sulfite oxidase, xanthine oxidase and xanthine dehydrogenase. Xanthine oxidase may be involved in the release of iron from ferritin and is definitely a factor in the oxidation of purines to uric acid.

An *in vitro* rat liver membrane experiment by Jon M. Richards and Norbert I. Swislocki[618e] has shown that molybdate, like fluoride, stimulates the activity of the enzyme adenylate cyclase by inhibiting a phosphatase and the stimulatory effects are additive to the effect produced by glucagon. As indicated in Figure 21, the stimulation (as

measured by the concentration of cyclic AMP) increases up to a
molybdate concentration of about 20 mM, at which point a *reverse
effect* sets in and, as the molybdate concentration continues to
increase, the stimulation declines.

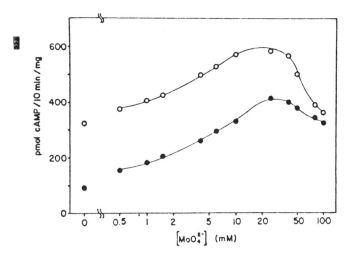

Figure 21. Effects of molybdate, with (○) glucagon, and
without (•) glucagon, on adenylate cyclase activity. Reprinted
from Jon M. Richards and Norbert I. Swislocki, *Biochimica
et Biophysica Acta* (1981) 678: 180-186, with permission of
the publisher, Elsevier Biomedical Press B. V. Amsterdam, and
of the authors. Observe the *reverse effect* that set in at a
molybdate concentration of about 20 mM.

Experiments with rats[619] have shown that excess molybdenum in
the diet resulted in above-normal xanthine oxidase activity and thus
increased uric acid production. A study showed that areas in
Armenia, U.S.S.R., having a high incidence of gout* also had high
concentrations of molybdenum in their soil and plants.[619]

On the other hand, a study made in China by X. M. Luo et al.[619a]
(and discussed on the Public Broadcasting System program

---

* One of the ways physicians have of suppressing *hyperuricemia*, excessive uric acid,
which is present in gout, is by inhibiting the molybdenum-based enzyme xanthine
oxidase through use of the drug *allopurinol*.

"NOVA") showed that there is a correlation between a soil *deficiency* of molybdenum and the development of cancer of the esophagus. Luo et al. found that low soil levels of molybdenum led to lower levels of vitamin C in the crops grown on that soil. This, in turn, led to lessened protection against the nitrates and nitrites present in the food being converted into nitrosamines, which then produced cancer. Furthermore, molybdenum is a cofactor of the enzyme nitrate reductase which affects the nitrate and nitrite contents of plants. Luo et al. demonstrated negative correlations between mortality rates for esophageal cancer and the molybdenum, zinc, magnesium, silicon, nickel, iron, phosphorus, potassium and sodium in cereals and drinking water. Lower levels of molybdenum were found in the serum, hair and urine of inhabitants of the high-risk area compared with those from the low-risk areas. Luo et al. also found that molybdenum supplementation reduced the incidence of N-nitrososarcosine ethyl ester-induced forestomach cancer in mice and esophageal and forestomach cancer in rats. J. W. Burrell et al.[620] reported that a molybdenum soil deficiency, which showed up as a deficiency in garden plants, was associated with the incidence of esophageal cancer in the Bantu of Transkei, South Africa.

Molybdenum is thought to be a growth-control factor. It has been observed that peoples such as the Mexicans and Chinese, subsisting primarily on beans and other legumes high in molybdenum, tend to be short. Carl C. Pfeiffer[620a] has suggested that molybdenum may be the key to Bergman's Law in anthropology. (Peoples in mountainous regions and in cold climates tend to grow taller, while those on the flood plains and living in warmer climates tend to be shorter.) Those on the flood plains, says Pfeiffer, often eat bean curd and rice (which are high in molybdenum), while those living at the higher altitudes generally eat eggs, meat, nuts and dairy products (which are low in molybdenum). Molybdenum interacts with copper (a growth stimulant) and with sulphur amino acids to reduce growth.

Molybdenum has been reported to contribute to the prevention of tooth decay, but this now seems to be in doubt. A high ratio of molybdenum to copper in the soil has been hypothesized as being associated with an increased risk of multiple sclerosis[621] We have seen, then, that both a deficiency or an excess of molybdenum in the soil (and, of course, in the vegetables grown in such soil) can be detrimental to human physiology.

Molybdenum may be related to sexuality. *In vitro* experiments have shown that molybdate markedly enhances the number of androgen-binding sites in the excised prostate glands of rats[622] and in excised human hyperplastic prostate glands.[623] Restrain yourself, however, if you are a man, from concluding that molybdenum will make you hypersexy. Too much might work to make you impotent. J. W. Thomas and Samuel Moss[624] reported that sodium molybdate fed to two Holstein male calves caused them to exhibit lack of sexual interest. This may be another example of the *reverse effect.* Perhaps small amounts of molybdenum might foster sex (although this has not been shown), while large amounts, at least in the case of cattle, seem to diminish sexuality. Experiments with the uterine material of calves have demonstrated that molybdate also interacts with estrogen receptors, sometimes exhibiting *reverse effects.* [625]

Earlier we reported a copper-molybdenum interaction. Experiments with chicks also show that molybdenum reduces plasma levels of silicon, and silicon reduces molybdenum tissue retention[626]

Molybdenum is concentrated primarily in the liver, kidney and in the adrenal glands. Liver, kidney, scallops, wheat germ, whole cereals (especially buckwheat), dark green vegetables, peas, lima beans and other legumes are good sources of this element. Tablets of molybdenum bound to yeast are available at health food stores. Mol-Iron, a source of molybdenum and iron for adding to milk or water, is available at pharmacies. I am, of course, in no sense recommending these nonfood sources of molybdenum.

Silicon

Silicon occupies an interesting place in the periodic table of the elements. It lies between aluminum and phosphorus in the third period and under carbon in group IV. Like carbon, it forms chains, branched chains, rings, polymers and macromolecules.[627] Next to oxygen, it is the most common element of the earth's crust.

Silicon probably enters into bone building, growth of skin, nails, hair and the creation of strong tooth enamel. Edith M. Carlisle [628] suggests that silicon is associated with calcium in an early stage of calcification. Brittleness of bones in older persons may be due not only to a calcium deficiency but also to a lack of silicon. A deficiency is reported to also cause weak, thin and brittle fingernails, flabbiness of the skin, falling hair and sties on the eyelids. Klaus Schwarz [629] noted considerable differences in skull size and bone structure in rat littermates raised with and without dietary silicon. Edith M. Carlisle and William F. Alpenfels[630] reported that experiments with chicken embryos demonstrated the requirement for silicon in formation of articular cartilage. They concluded that silicon is required for collagen biosynthesis in the formation of normal cartilage. Furthermore, Carlisle and Alpenfels[630a] have suggested that silicon may be involved in mitochondrial synthesis of proline precursors. Their suggestion is supported by the finding of silicon in the mitochondria of the osteoblast.

Schwarz also reported that silicon shows catalytic effects on peptides. According to Schwarz, silicic acid in bound form is also present in acid mucopolysaccharides and polyuronides and it serves as a cross-linking agent in forming connective tissue. Thus, silicon may contribute to both the architecture and resilience of such tissue. Klaus Schwarz[631] also determined that a high level of bound silicon is found in the hyaluronic acid from umbilical cord (but not in the hyaluronic acid from vitreous humor).

Silicon may play a preventive role in atherosclerosis. [632,633] J. Loeper et al.[634] found that the silicon content of the normal human aorta decreases with age. The Loeper group[635] also reported that the concentration of silicon in the aortic wall decreases prior to the appearance of lipid deposits. Silicon increases the impermeability of the endothelium, which results in lesser penetration of lipids. J. Loeper et al.[636] also observed that silicon administered intravenously or by mouth to rabbits inhibits atheromas normally induced by an atheromatous diet. On the contrary, a study by Klaus Schwarz et al.[637] reported an inverse relation between silicon in drinking water and atherosclerosis in Finland. Furthermore, C. H. Becker and A. G. S. Janossy[637a] discovered that the peripheral blood vessels of the colon, heart and nephron of acute hypertensive rats contained two to three times more silicon compared to control animals.

Abnormal silicon metabolism may be a factor in hypertension. C. H. Becker[638] found that old rats with chronic hypertension had relatively low amounts of silicon in their blood vessel walls and also a shortage of collagen fibers which appeared to need silicon-based hyaluronic acid for their formation.

Good food sources are pectin, milk (especially goat's milk), honey (especially dark honey), rice hulls, oat hulls, wheat bran, soybean meal, whole grains (especially oats and buckwheat), liver, alfalfa, mushrooms, apples, strawberries, grapes, pumpkins, watermelon, cabbage, green leafy vegetables, carrots, tomatoes, beets, onions, parsnips, lentils, asparagus, wild rice, cucumbers, savoy cabbage, marjoram, horseradish, the skin of potatoes and the herbs oat-straw and horsetail. Horsetail, also known as *shavegrass,* is an especially strong source for silicon, in the form of alginic acid, but horsetail cannot be recommended since it contains the enzyme thiaminase which destroys vitamin B1.

Some Possible Negatives

Tablets containing silicon are available at health food stores. A liquid sold under the trade name Calphonite®, contains calcium, phosphorus and manganese, along with bentonite. Bentonite is a volcanic rock containing montmorillonite, a complicated chemical composed of silicon and many other elements. Possibly the silicon plays a part in promoting calcium absorption by the body. However, aluminum is also present in montmorillonite and aluminum may be dangerous if the body absorbs it. (Aluminum may be implicated in Alzheimer's disease—early senility—and silicon may be implicated also.[639] J. H. Austin[640] reported that some, but not all, Alzheimer patients had up to ten times as much silicon in the corpora amylacea of their nervous systems compared to controls.) Therefore, one wonders if bentonite should be taken to put calcium and silicon into the body, a purpose for which Calphonite® is recommended.

Calphonite® is, by the way, produced under a patent[641] which states that bentonite is present to occasion shattering of the calcium diphosphate crystals, presumably to aid assimilation. (Actually, the patent's main claims refer to its use as a metal polish, not as a nutritional supplement.)*

An example of silica toxicity is shown in research done by S. Nadler and S. Goldfischer.[642] Using macrophages of mice, it was shown that lysosomal contents were released into the cytoplasm following ingestion of silica by the mice. D. A. Levison et al.[643] have reported the presence of silica stones in the urinary bladder following ingestion of magnesium trisilicate, an antacid to treat indigestion. Then too, studies of Klaus Schwarz[644] indicate that silicon may interfere with fluoride utilization. Silicon, in the form of sodium metasilicate, has been shown to inhibit the effect of fluoride on growth. If silicon supplements are to be taken, it should be with the knowledge that the numerator of the risk/benefit ratio is not zero. Silicon levels in the blood are normally low, very similar to silicon's concentration in ocean water. In light of our small requirements for this element and, in view of the fact that silicon is a common constituent of cereals, there would seem to be no good reason to take it as a supplement. Silicon appears to be biologically essential, at least in animals, but perhaps its relative resistance to assimilation is what helps make it a "safe" element. In fact, recent studies by A. W. Varnes and W. H. Strain[645] indicated that silicon accumulates, with aging, in the paratracheal lymph nodes. These scientists concluded that a silicon accumulation, not a deficiency, is associated with aging.

Furthermore, Allen J. Natow[645a] warned, during 1986, that talc, a magnesium silicate used to dust diapered babies and by many women to dust their own perineal areas, may be associated with an

---

* Bentonite is sometimes used as an intestinal cleanser. In this connection it is interesting to note J. Walter Wilson[641a] reported that mice fed a diet consisting of 50% bentonite (a huge amount) had their growth almost completely suppressed and they developed liver tumors. Wilson concluded that the hepatomas were a result, in part, of a choline deficiency brought on by the ingestion of the bentonite. Studies by D. H. Laughland and W. E. J. Phillips[641b] showed that in rats fed very modest amounts of bentonite (.5% to 2.5% of the diet) absorption and storage of vitamin A in the liver were inhibited.

increased risk of ovarian cancer. Studies have shown that particles of powder introduced into the vagina can be found in the fallopian tubes within 30 minutes and may subsequently enter the ovaries to act as a carcinogen. Talc used as a cosmetic, however, seems to be safe except for occasional reports of chronic overdose of talcum powder leading to pulmonary fibrosis.

Selenium

At one time we heard and read that selenium was strictly a poison. Then later we were told that selenium in small amounts is essential but that there was no real evidence to show that humans are ever deficient in this mineral. Then, late in the 1970s, reports came from China regarding Keshan disease, a fatal cardiomyopathy in children.[646] It is speculated that the absence of selenium from the heart's myocardium is what leads to free-radical damage of the cellular membranes.[646a] A study by P. V. Luoma et al.[646b] related low levels of the selenium-based enzyme glutathione peroxidase to coronary risk. Keshan disease, first identified in Keshan county, affects large numbers of children (and some adults) in a wide area of China where the soil is very deficient in selenium. The children there eat a vegetarian diet with cereals—rice, wheat and soya beans—containing very low amounts of selenium (because the soil in which they are grown is low in selenium). Hair analysis indicated that human hair from 27 places affected by Keshan disease averaged just .12 ppm. Hair from persons living in nearby areas not having Keshan disease averaged .20 ppm, while hair from areas of China far away from the affected area averaged .25-.60 ppm. In recent years, selenium in the form of sodium selenite has been administered to children of the affected area. When selenium is taken regularly the disease is now almost nonexistent.[646c] Recent reviews have been provided by Guanggi Yang et al.[646d] and by Xu Guang-lu et al.[646e]

Selenium may have a role in the biosynthesis of ubiquinone (coenzyme Q) but this has not yet been demonstrated. (You will recall that the ubiquinones function as electron carriers in the mitochondrial electron transport system.) Ubiquinone in the normal heart is at a higher level than in most other tissues and, as suggested by the facts regarding Keshan disease, selenium may be important for all of us to preserve heart health.[647] Furthermore, in a matched-pair longitudinal study conducted in Finland, Jukka T. Salonen et al.[648] found that serum selenium deficiency was associated with risk of death from coronary heart disease. As pointed out in Chapter 3, a deficiency of selenium has been reported to suppress formation of prostacyclin. If true, this may be relevant to the Salonen finding and to the etiology of Keshan disease. In possibly-related work, but with male rats, W. L. Stone et al.[648a] discovered, in 1986, that selenium deficiency significantly elevated the low-density lipoprotein cholesterol.

A selenium deficiency may be a cause of other heart-related problems. Selenium is present in the myosin of muscle and is especially concentrated in heart muscle. As shown by Raymond F. Burk et al.,[649] selenium is needed for heme metabolism in the liver. It was at one time thought that selenium might help reduce high blood pressure, but this now seems doubtful. (Selenium combats cadmium and cadmium may be an elevator of blood pressure.)

Selenium deficiency in cattle has been associated with Heinz (pronounced *hints*) bodies and anemia.[650] Heinz bodies, named after the German physician, are defects in red blood cells resulting from oxidative injury and precipitation of hemoglobin. Cells with this flaw are associated with hemolytic anemia. Up to now there have not, however, been reports of Heinz body formation in human selenium deficiency.

Selenium plays a vital role in activating the enzyme glutathione peroxidase* which acts as an antioxidant, destroying peroxides before they can injure the membrane of the cells. Vitamin E acts primarily by reducing production of peroxides, while glutathione peroxidase neutralizes those that are formed.** Thus, selenium, in

---

* There are several glutathione peroxidases. The selenium-dependent enzyme destroys both hydrogen peroxide and organic hydroperoxides.[651] Non-selenium glutathione peroxide does not metabolize hydrogen peroxide.[649]

** Nai-Yen Jack Yang and Indrajit Dayalji Desai[652] have reported that both a vitamin E deficiency and a vitamin E excess depress glutathione peroxidase activity in the liver,

protecting the cells, is an antiaging factor that may help us to significantly increase our life span. Glutathione peroxidase has been found to be at depressed levels in the blood of otherwise healthy persons who have various skin disorders. L. Juhlin et al.[653] reported that this enzyme was at low levels in patients with psoriasis, eczema, atopic dermatitis, vasculitis, mycosis fungoides and dermatitis herpetiformis. Many other diseases are associated with a deficiency of this enzyme. Based on *in vitro* rat experiments, even the incidence of candidiasis may be increased by a shortage of glutathione peroxidase.[654] Glutathione itself, the sulfhydral tripeptide so important in tissue oxidations, is influenced by selenium concentrations. In an interesting example of the *reverse effect* using *in vitro* cultures of human breast cancer cells, sodium selenite at 10^{-8} M stimulated glutathione levels, but at higher concentrations glutathione was depressed in a dose-dependent manner.[654a] Glutathione's cancer-fighting power may be helped by modest amounts of selenium while being reduced at higher levels of the mineral.

We have just described some problems associated with a shortage of glutathione peroxidase. In Down's syndrome patients there is, on the other hand, an increased activity of this enzyme in their erythrocytes and fibroblasts. (As we will see in Chapter 9, superoxide dismutase activity is also increased in Down's syndrome patients.) Furthermore, a positive correlation exists between erythrocyte glutathione peroxidase and the I.Q. of these individuals.[655]

In some ways selenium acts very much like vitamins C and E. Raymond J. Shamberger and his colleagues have demonstrated that it is possible to protect animals from cancer caused by irritating chemicals by giving them vitamins C and E along with selenium. In one series of Shamberger experiments,[656] selenium (along with BHT and vitamins C and E) was shown to be effective in blocking the muta-genicity of malonaldehyde that is present in large

---

plasma, uterus and erythrocytes of female rats. This *reverse effect* gives us another good reason to keep our vitamin E intake at nominal levels.)

amounts in beef. G. N. Schrauzer[657] has reported that subtoxic amounts of selenium added to drinking water lowered the incidence of spontaneous mammary tumors in mice.

It has been shown that, in tissue cultures, selenium and other antioxidants such as vitamins C and E (along with the synthetic BHT that is often used as a preservative) reduce the incidence of chromosome breakage, a factor in causing birth defects and cancer. Whenever the selenium content of the soil is high, people are far less apt to get cancer of those organs that come into contact with dietary selenium—the pharynx, esophagus, stomach, intestines, rectum, kidney and bladder. [657a,b] the incidence of breast cancer is also much lower in regions having large amounts of selenium in the soil. The human cancer death rate was reported by Raymond J. Shamberger and Charles E. Willis[657b] to be inversely related to the amount of selenium in the blood (Figure 22). A worldwide epidemiological study by G. N. Schrauzer et al.[657c,d] inversely correlated mortalities from cancers at all sites with apparent dietary selenium intake. Larry C. Clark has recently reviewed many of the studies showing that decreased selenium status is associated with an increased risk of cancer.[657e]*

Selenium has at least three modes of action in cancer control. First, the selenium-based enzyme glutathione peroxidase, which catalyzes the destruction of peroxides in the cell and thus helps to reduce damage from free radicals, may be a contributing mechanism.[657f] Second, selenium alters the metabolism of neoplastic cells and inhibits growth of transplanted tumors.[657f] And third, studies by Julian E. Spallholz et al.,[657g,h] by Werner A. Baumgartner[657i] and by others have shown that selenium is involved in immune mechanisms. Results indicate that one to three ppm selenium (as sodium selenite) may potentiate the synthesis of circulating antibodies.

Experiments with mice indicate that selenium inhibits the genesis of mammary tumors. Gerhard N. Schrauzer and Debra Ishmael[658]

---

* We cannot be certain, however, that low selenium status is a cause of cancer. It could be an effect of cancer or it is possible that another factor could be the cause of both low selenium status and of cancer.

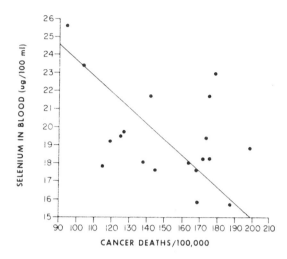

Figure 22. The 1962-66 average human cancer death rate and the blood selenium content in 19 cities of the United States. Reprinted from Richard J. Shamberger and Charles E. Willis, *Critical Reviews in Clinical Laboratory Sciences* (1971) 2: 211-221, with permission of the copyright owner, CRC Press, Inc., Boca Raton, Florida.

found that the incidence of spontaneous mammary tumors in female virgin mice fed two ppm selenite in their drinking water was lowered to 10% relative to an incidence of 82% in controls. Based on this and other studies, G. N. Schrauzer et al. [659,659a] reported that selenium in the form of selenite, in subtoxic and toxic ranges, significantly inhibited tumorigenesis in animals. They noted that the effect of selenium was, however, counteracted by zinc (which gives us a good reason to not excessively supplement the diet with zinc).

Many studies by R. J. Shamberger[659b,c] have also shown that selenium significantly reduces tumor production in mice and rats. In another experiment, Carmia Borek[660] studied the effects of selenium on chemical- and irradiation-induced transformations in mice cells. Such cells, when preincubated with selenium and then treated with either benzo(a)pyrene, pyrolysate or radiation, showed a marked inhibition of cell transformation compared with cells not preincubated with selenium. Daniel Medina et al.[661] found that mice fed 2.0 ppm dietary selenium developed only 16% DMBA-induced mammary tumors contrasted with 56% in those fed just .2 ppm dietary selenium. They concluded that the chemopreventive property of selenium could not be attributed to maintaining high levels of glutathione peroxidase. Henry J. Thompson et al.[661a] found that sodium selenite was more effective and less toxic than selenomethionine in inhibiting mammary carcinogenesis in rats. Maryce M. Jacobs[661b] studied the effect of selenium on colon carcinogenesis induced by 1,2-dimethylhydrazine (DMH). Thirty-one weeks after the first of ten weekly injections of DMH, or at death if it occurred earlier, both control rats and those given 4 ppm of selenium in the form of sodium selenite (Na_2SeO_3) were analyzed for colon tumors. Whereas the DMH-only controls had a tumor incidence of 29%, those given the selenium showed a tumor incidence of just 3%. (Selenium's anticancer power may be nulli-fied by excess vitamin C.)[661ca]

Work with cell cultures also bears out selenium's anticancer effects. Malay Chatterjee and Mihir R. Banerjee,[661d] working with organ culture of the whole mammary glands of mice, found that selenium in inhibiting carcinogenesis seems to act "principally at the promotion stage of transformation of the mammary cells *in vitro.*" They noted, however, that a modifying influence of selenium at the initiation stage also remains a possibility. Daniel Medina and Carol J. Oborn,[661e] using a cell culture of preneoplastic mouse mammary epithelial cells, reported that a low concentration of $5 \times 10^{-8}M$ selenium (as sodium selenite) stimulated cell growth, whereas a higher concentration of $5 \times 10^{-6}M$ showed a *reverse effect* and delayed cell growth, while $5 \times 10^{-5}M$ was cytotoxic. They concluded that "one of the mechanisms of selenium-mediated inhibition of carcinogenesis may be due to an inhibition of cell proliferation of responsive cells." (But note that at $5 \times 10^{-8}M$ selenium stimulated growth of preneoplastic cells. We will examine other possible negatives of selenium in regard to cancer shortly.)

Selenium may be useful not only in reducing cancer incidence but also in obviating or treating other conditions relating to an immune deficiency. R. Boyne and J. R. Arthur[661g] reported, in 1986, that a selenium deficiency exacerbated *Candida* infections in mice after they had been injected with *Candida albicans* as compared with infections in injected mice given a selenium supplemented diet. Boyne and Arthur also demonstrated, by *in vitro* tests, that a selenium deficiency impaired the ability of mouse neutrophils to kill *Candida albicans*. (Regrettably, mice fed a normal diet, neither deficient in selenium nor selenium supplemented, were not studied. Thus, this research does not suggest more than the possibility that selenium supplementation might benefit mice and humans with *Candida*.)

Although epidemiological studies show that persons living in areas where the soil is high in selenium are less prone to cancer, different studies indicate that such persons may have other problems. Those living in areas where the soil is high in selenium sometimes show a loss of hair, brittleness of nails, nail sloughing, a garlic-like breath due to excretion of dimethyl sulphide, dermatitis, gastrointestinal disturbances, jaundice, arthritis and tooth decay. Arthur W. Kilness[661f] has even reported a possible association between a high-selenium environment and the onset of amyotrophic lateral sclerosis. However, let's not dwell on negatives until later but, instead, let's cite more of selenium's benefits or possible benefits.

It has been speculated, particularly by Joel Wallach, that if sufficient selenium were present in a pregnant woman's diet, cystic fibrosis could be eliminated as a birth defect. However, Ricardo O. Castillo et al.[662] reported no significant difference in serum selenium levels between children with CF and other children. L. O. Plantin et al.[662a] also observed that selenium values for cystic fibrosis patients did not differ from controls. Furthermore, studies of normal subjects in New Zealand, where the crops are low in selenium, show that their blood levels are far below those of typical CF patients in the U.S., yet the New Zealanders give no evidence of morbidity relating to this condition.* The lay press (the "health" magazines) have made

---

* It is tissue levels, however, rather than blood levels of various nutrients that may be important for health. Thus, while CF patients may have blood selenium levels below

much of the Wallach hypothesis, but more evidence will have to be presented before a selenium deficiency can be considered to be an important cause of cystic fibrosis.

Most CF patients have problems in absorbing fat and therefore many have low levels of vitamin E. Persons with low vitamin E levels are more subject to selenium toxicity, so the advice that CF children take large supplemental amounts of selenium could be dangerous, especially if their vitamin E intake is not increased accordingly.

Selenium has been shown to protect against the toxic effect of mercury. H. E. Ganther et al.,[663a-d] at the University of Wisconsin, fed 10 ppm of methyl mercury to a group of rats and fed the same amount of methyl mercury plus .5 ppm of selenium to another group. All the rats fed the mercury without the selenium died, but those fed the same diet with selenium were all alive at the end of six weeks. Incidentally, tuna fish contains from 1.71 to 3.40 ppm of selenium, sufficient to protect against the mercury it also contains.[663a] (Interestingly, tuna with low mercury content was found to contain lower amounts of selenium, about 1.91 ppm, while high mercury tuna averaged 2.91 ppm selenium.)[663a] Selenium is also reported to be useful in detoxifying silver, cadmium, arsenic and sometimes lead.

Selenite does not, however, always protect against mercury poisoning. Toshima Nobunaga et al.[663e] found that a total of 55.4% of mice fetuses showed malformations after their mothers had been fed high levels of mercury during gestation. Surprisingly, at these high levels of methylmercury a dosage of selenite (11.4 nmol./ml.), which was significantly (but not completely) protective at lower levels of mercury, showed a *reverse effect* and *increased* the percentage of fetuses showing malformations to 60.7% (Table 1). It's yet another example of the importance of stating nutritional principles in terms of dose-response relationships. The fact is that the toxicity of methylmercury may be decreased (usually) or increased (sometimes) by selenite, depending on dosages.

---

those of typical New Zealanders, that may not be true of comparative tissue levels. Joan M. Braganza[663] has discussed this subject in a recent issue of *Lancet*.

TABLE 1. TERATOGENIC EFFECTS OF METHYLMERCURY AND SELENITE ON DAY 18 OF GESTATION

	Number of fetuses	Cleft palate	Hare lip	Micrognathia	Number of Fetus with malformation
Control	92	0	0	0	0
Methylmercury (15.9 nmol/g)	114	19	1	1	21
		16.7%	1%	1%	18.4%
Methylmercury (31.9 nmol/g)	74	41	0	3	41
		55.4%		4.0%	55.4%[a]
Selenite (11.4 nmol/ml)	112	0	0	0	0
Selenite (22.8 nmol/ml)	88	2	0	1	2
		2.38		1%	2.3%
Methylmercury (15.9 nmol/g) and selenite (11.4 nmol/ml)	117	8 6.8%	0	0	8 6.8%
Methylmercury (31.9 nmol/g and selenite (11.4 nmol/ml)	56	34 60.7%	0	2 3.6%	34 60.7%
Methylmercury (31.9 nmol/g) and selenite (22.8 nmol/ml)	76	65 85.5%	0	1 1.3%	65 85.5%

Modified from Toshima Nobunaga et al., *Toxicology and Applied Pharmacology* (1979) 47: 79-88, with permission of the publisher, Academic Press, and of the authors.

Dietary selenium also seems to offer some protection against paraquat poisoning, acting apparently through the enzyme glutathione peroxidase.[663f] Paraquat is a widely used, broad-spectrum herbicide which may cause pulmonary lesions in animals and humans. Some marijuana plants have been sprayed with paraquat and represent a threat to pot smokers.

Animal experiments have shown that either selenium or vitamin E must be present to prevent muscular dystrophy but, as noted earlier, this is not the same disease that occurs in humans. It has also been suggested that selenium may be useful in preventing cataracts. Richard A. Lawrence et al.[664] found that selenium deficiency in rats decreased glutathione peroxidase activity in the lens of the eye. This enzyme protects against the detrimental effects of oxygen by repairing damage that free radicals do to membrane liquids, so adequate intake of selenium may be important to protect against cataracts.[*]

---

[*] I. Ostadalova et al.[665,666] showed that sodium selenite injected into young male rats produced cataracts. Older rats who survived such injections were not affected with

Selenium is a factor in the growth of cells. Daniel Medina et al.[661] cites W. M. Lewko and W. P. McConnell[664a] as having found that at low concentrations of selenite (10^{-9} to 10^{-7}M) synthesis of type IV collagen was stimulated. However, at higher concentrations (10^{-5} to 10^{-3}M) there was a *reverse effect* (my language) and the synthesis of collagen was decreased.

Selenium may be useful in treating some types of arthritis. It has been suggested that a combination of selenium and vitamin E may be especially beneficial for achieving relief of knee pain. Seletoc®, which is composed of 1,000 mcg. of selenium with 68 I.U. of vitamin E, is sometimes given orally or intravenously to dogs with hip dysplasia and lameness.

Dandruff is probably related to a selenium (or zinc) deficiency, and shampoo consisting of a 1% solution of selenium sulphide is often recommended for dandruff control. However, R. W. Grover[669] observed that prolonged use of selenium sulphide shampoo caused baldness. Then too, G. Nanjappa Chetty et al.[670] have reported that hair shaft abnormalities resembling *Trichorrhexis nodosa* were found in two patients using selenium shampoo.

Selenium has a sexual significance for men, and, to a lesser degree, probably also for women. Raymond F. Burk and Daniel G. Brown[671] showed that, in rats, the selenium supply of males is concentrated in the testicles and in the epididymis. (No such uptake was found in the females' ovaries or uteruses. However, many animal experiments, reported by Eric J. Underwood,[672] indicate that selenium is important in both male and female fertility.) The investigators speculate that the reason male rats get liver necrosis (a disease that may be caused by an insufficiency of selenium and vitamin E) might be because their reproductive organs require so

---

cataracts. Thomas R. Shearer[667] found that not only did injected sodium selenite cause cataracts in 100% of young rats, but that oral administration also caused cataracts. These studies, however, do not contradict the idea that selenium may help prevent cataracts. As we have seen, many substances act, in large doses, just the opposite to the way they act in small dosages, i.e., they exhibit a *reverse effect*. Nevertheless, there is a disturbing finding by Kailash C. Bhuyan et al.[668] that the selenium level is significantly increased in human senile cataract. If this finding is replicated by other scientists, it must be reconciled with the Lawrence study. Perhaps selenium was present in the Bhuyan experiment in a form that blocked the action of glutathione peroxidase.

much selenium that there is not enough left for normal liver functioning.* Several studies with male rats and mice, as reported by Edward J. Calabrese,[621] have shown that selenium protects the testes from cadmium-induced damage. (Amazingly, however, the selenium *increased* the amount of cadmium in the testes, implying the formation of a selenium-cadmium complex.) In men also, selenium concentrates in the sexual organs, and it seems probable that their sexual health is related to the presence of this mineral.

Selenium is important in maintaining sperm motility and is thus a factor in fertility. It is now known that during spermatogenesis selenium is incorporated in the mid-piece of the sperm in the form of *selenoflagel* (selenoflagellin), a protein having a molecular weight of about 16,000 daltons. Selenium is lost in the semen, so sexually active men may wish to make sure that their supply is continually replaced. However, men should not be overly concerned about the possibility of developing a testicular selenium deficiency. Dietrich Behne et al.[673] found that, in experiments with rats, the supply of sufficient selenium to the testes has priority over the supply to other tissues. In a study with boars, E. C. Segerson et al.[673a] reported that those fed a selenium-deficient diet showed no apparent impairment of sperm morphology or viability.

Excellent food sources for selenium are lobster, cod, tuna, herring, menhaden, anchovetta and other seafoods, although the mercury in them may tie up some of the selenium and make it unavailable. Other good selenium sources are brewer's yeast, beef liver, beef kidney and other meats, eggs, nuts, spices, sesame seeds, wheat germ, kelp, whole grains, mushrooms, garlic and onions. Additional sources are bran, broccoli, onions, cabbage, asparagus and tomatoes. The selenium content of these foods will, of course, vary with the selenium concentration in the soil on which they are grown. Then too, K. Alterman[674] has reported that much of the selenium in vegetables is lost in the cooking water if it is discarded.

---

* The fact that selenium goes preferentially to the reproductive organs is one of many examples of the policy of nature to choose survival of the species over survival of the individual.

Could Selenium Sometimes Cause Cancer?

The many health advantages of adequate dietary selenium are obvious and we have seen how it helps protect against cancer, but selenium consumption can be overdone. Selenium in the diets of female rats at 10 ppm has resulted in liver tumors. [675] (Males need more selenium to stay healthy and they are also less prone to selenium toxicity.) The propensity of selenium to cause tumor formation in rats was confirmed by L. A. Cherkes et al. [676] The Cherkes group fed 40 rats sodium selenate at a level of 10 mg./kg. of food, with the result that ten developed tumors. Then, Henry A. Schroeder and Marian Mitchener[677] fed rats selenate and selenite in their drinking water at levels of 2 and 3 ppm. A large number of animals (313) were used plus 105 controls. The scientists found selenite to be extremely toxic, suppressing growth and causing early death. Selenate was not toxic in terms of growth or longevity, but in older rats it was reported as being both tumorigenic and carcinogenic. The same researchers, [678] performing similar experiments with mice, found selenite and selenate at levels of 3 ppm to be nontoxic and there was no significant increase in incidence of tumors. Subsequent animal studies by H. L. Kling and C. M. Hendrick and by J. R. Harr et al., as cited in the *Federal Register*,[679] showed an absence of carcinogenic activity.

The FDA, in the *Federal Register*,[680] seems to conclude, based on a consideration of the above and other experiments, that selenium is not tumorigenic. They dismiss the studies that show selenium may be of possible danger because those experiments contained extraneous variables. Although the FDA is not generally known as being overly sympathetic to dietary supplementation, I wonder if they were not a bit hasty in implying that selenium presents a negligible threat of tumorigenicity. (It should be observed, however, that the FDA was commenting on the safety of selenium as an animal, not as a human, supplement.)

Selenium, as we have noted, can help protect one against cancer. However, in accordance with the theory of the *reverse effect,* selenium, if it aids in preventing cancer, might, at a different concentration, be expected to help *induce* cancer. Although we saw earlier[661a] that selenium can exert antimutagenic effects against mutagens such as malonaldehyde, it can also increase DNA fragmentation and chromosome aberrations in human cell cultures. K. Nakamuro et al.[681] reported that chromosome breaking was significantly higher for the 4-valent selenium compounds (selenites) and less so for the 6-valent ones (selenates). On the other hand, G. Löfroth and B. Ames[681a] (as cited by C. Peter Flessel)[681b] reported mutagenic activity in selenate but not in selenite. Later, Makoto Noda et al.[682] and others showed both selenite and selenate to be mutagenic on the Ames test.* Still later, Gordon R. Russell et al.[683] discovered that the organic form selenomethionine also has a reactive DNA effect. James H. Ray et al.[683a] found a three-fold increase in sister-chromatid exchange in human whole blood cultures at high concentrations (7.90 x 10^{-6}M and 1.19 x 10^{-5}M) of sodium selenite. L. W. Lo et al. [683b] observed that sodium selenite induced DNA fragmentation, DNA-repair synthesis, chromosome aberrations and mitotic inhibition in cultured human fibroblasts.** Selenate was less active but was able to significantly induce DNA-repair synthesis. Lo et al. pointed out that many studies show a correlation between the carcinogenic property of a compound and its capacity to give a positive response with the DNA-repair assay. They say that this test "would thus support the claim that selenium is a carcinogen." At an excessive level, the selenite ion no longer acts as an antioxidant but shows a *reverse effect* by becoming a pro-oxidant.[683d] (At high levels selenium no longer acts as a synergist with vitamin E but becomes antagonistic to it.)[683c] S. Knuuttila[683e] expresses concern that high dietary selenium may potentiate "carcinogen-induced cancer in tissues with low oxygen tension such as the bone marrow." These facts seem to suggest that the FDA may have been premature in concluding that selenium is not tumorigenic. Selenium may have not only a protective power against cancer

---

* Earlier in this section we noted Medina and Oborn[661e] found that low concentrations of selenite stimulated growth of preoplastic mouse mammary epithelial cells while high concentrations showed a *reverse effect* and were cytotoxic.

** Robert F. Whiting et al.[683c] reported that glutathione (which some take as a supplement for its antioxidant action) strongly enhanced unscheduled DNA synthesis in cultured human fibroblasts by inorganic selenium compounds. It also enhanced the DNA-damaging effect of selenocystine.

but also, at a different concentration, could possibly have a carcinogenic potential.

What Might Be the Optimal Selenium Intake?

Selenium is probably detrimental at far lower intakes than used in the Nelson, the Cherkes and the Schroeder experiments. Whereas J. R. Spallholz et al.[684,685] showed that the immune response in mice improved when the dietary intake of selenium in the form of selenite was increased up to 1.25 ppm, they found that the immune response slowly declined (a *reverse effect*) as the selenium intake was raised to higher levels. However, it was still above normal at a selenium level of 10 ppm (a level shown as being dangerous to rats by Nelson, by Cherkes and by Schroeder). Many other experiments indicate that selenium is more toxic to rats than it is to mice.

Another rat experiment, this one by Pamela Toy et al.[686] is also interesting. Toy et al. found that rats fed sodium selenite in their drinking water showed increased glutathione peroxidase activity in the liver at levels up to 1 ppm and then that activity decreased (a *reverse effect*) at higher levels.

To cite just one more relevant experiment, performed by J. A. Milner et al,[687] mice drinking water with 1 ppm of selenium had a 6% increase in longevity. Supplementing with 3 ppm increased longevity by 30%, but further raising the selenium intake to 5 ppm and 10 ppm showed a *reverse effect* by increasing their longevity to just 19% and 10% respectively. For mice, then, it would appear that in terms of longevity 3 ppm may be optimal.

In attempting to decide what selenium intake might be optimal for humans we must keep in mind that people do not necessarily react as do animals. Most of the above experiments were performed using inorganic selenium, whereas if you take selenium supplements you may be using organic selenium. Many studies[688] indicate little difference between organic and inorganic selenium as far as growth in animals or incorporation into the enzyme glutathione peroxidase are concerned. However, M.L. Scott[689] has shown that the selenium in alfalfa has greater bioavailability (in chickens) than selenite or selenium in brewer's yeast. On the other hand, selenium in tuna is less available (at least to the rat) than selenium from selenite, wheat or yeast as measured by glutathione peroxidase response in platelets, plasma or liver and selenium concentration in liver and plasma.[587a]

Furthermore, the optimal supplemental selenium intake will depend on other elements in our diet. For example, if we are taking large amounts of zinc or copper (which inhibit selenium absorption), then our optimal supplemental selenium intake will be higher than if we consume only small amounts of these nutrients. Then too, selenium toxicity is exacerbated in cases of vitamin E deficiency, and so the optimal level of selenium in one consuming adequate "E" is possibly (but not necessarily) higher than it would be for a person who is vitamin E deficient. (At any rate, this was demonstrated by G. F. Combs, Jr. and G. M. Pesti[690] to be true in chicks.) Research by L. A. Witting and M. K. Horwitt[691] has shown that the toxicity of a large intake of selenium is reduced by methionine. Thus, it would seem likely that the optimal selenium intake of those consuming foods containing large amounts of methionine (a constituent of many proteins such as casein and egg albumen) might be higher than normal. On the other hand, if we eat large amounts of seafood, brewer's yeast or cereals grown on seleniferous soil, the amount of selenium we should get from supplements will obviously be reduced. Even the amount of flaxseed meal (if any) in the diet can probably be a factor in what happens to the selenium in the diet. Ivan S. Palmer et al.[692] showed that the cyanogenic glycosides (linustatin and neolinustatin) in flax protect against excessive selenium consumption and so presumably these glycosides would, if present in the diet, increase the amount of supplemental selenium intake that might be desirable. (Laetrile is a cyanogenic glycoside but does not seem to have an appreciable effect on selenium levels.)

Selenium supplementation may be especially valuable to those consuming excessive amounts of alcohol. Brad M. Dworkin and William S. Rosenthal[692a] reported extremely low selenium levels in the whole blood, plasma and red blood cells of alcoholics with somewhat more favorable, but still depressed, levels in detoxified alcoholics. H. Korpela et al.[692b] found that alcoholics with normal liver histology had significantly lower serum selenium levels than healthy controls. They suggested that selenium deficiency could play a role in the pathogenesis of alcoholic liver disease. Considering the various animal experiments and the variables cited, I conservatively estimate the optimal intake of organic selenium in humans may be about .5 ppm. If a person eats 1 kilogram (2.2 lbs.) of food daily, which is 1,000,000 mg. or 1,000,000,000 mcg., then .5 ppm of selenium would amount to 500 mcg. Food sources probably account for about 100 to 180 mcg. of selenium intake daily, so supplementation at the level of about 300 to 400 mcg. might theoretically be beneficial. However, there is a danger in this reasoning. Animals are not persons and, even if the "ideal" dietary amount of selenium for a rat might be equivalent to 500 mcg. in a human, that does not prove 500 mcg. would be beneficial to a human. If selenium in excess poses a possible threat of cancer, then we have a good reason to restrict our intake to the amount found in a well-balanced diet.

The toxic levels and the nutritional levels of selenium are closer together than corresponding levels for most other substances, so considerable thought should attend any decision to use selenium supplements. The Food and Nutrition Board[693] recommends 50 to 200 mcg. as a safe and adequate range for daily ingestion of selenium, but this includes the amount we get from food and many of us are already getting this much without supplementing.* Because of selenium's relatively narrow range between its nutrient and toxic levels and because the law of biological individuality (and individual toxicity) has not been repealed, you may prefer to avoid supplementation. Since no one knows what is the best selenium intake on average, yet alone for you in particular, erring on the side of caution may be wise.

If one is planning to take selenium supplements it may be wise to get the mineral in a variety of forms (as occurs when one eats selenium-rich foods). There are physiological "pluses" and "minuses" associated with each of selenium's various compounds. Selenite is often recommended in preference to selenium yeast for those with a *Candida* problem. For other problems, selenate may

---

* On the other hand, H. Lithell et al[693a] reported that vegans (strict vegetarians) in their study did not even get 20-30 mcg. daily.

sometimes be more effective. Orville A. Levander et al.[694] found that men fed either selenium-rich wheat or selenium-rich yeast showed higher platelet glutathione peroxide activity than men fed sodium selenate. At times, selenomethionine may be better. Christine D. Thomson et al.[695] observed that men and women whose diets were supplemented with selenomethionine showed higher selenium concentrations in the whole blood, erythrocytes and plasma than did those supplemented with selenite.* Perhaps more seriously, enzyme activity of one of the four subjects given 500 mcg. selenite daily was unchanged despite a great increase in plasma selenium. A study by Gerhard N. Schrauzer and James E. McGinness[696] found that, while ingestion of selenium yeast efficiently put selenium into the blood, so-called selenium ascorbate was worthless.** The investigators pointed out that ascorbic acid reduces sodium selenite rapidly to elemental selenium which, they say, cannot be absorbed. Recently, however, Kern L. Nuttall[696a] has speculated that glutathione reductase may be able to mediate the reduction of colloidal selenium to hydrogen selenide which is biologically active. Furthermore, Marja Mutanen and Hannu M. Mykkänen,[696b] studying female university students, found that ascorbic acid increases the bioavailability of selenium in foods (but did not seem to affect the availability of supplemental sodium selenate).

In spite of what you have just read downgrading selenate and selenite relative to other forms of selenium, I would not completely rule out use of selenate and selenite if one's decision is to use supplemental selenium. We have already seen some examples of how the forms of selenium vary in their ability to perform specific functions, but let's cite a few more. Selenomethionine is reported to be four times as effective as selenite in preventing pancreatic fibrosis. On the other hand, J. A. Milner et al.[687] reported that selenite, but not selenomethionine, caused cancer regression in many types of

---

* Don R. Swanson[695a] has pointed out that selenomethionine, while beneficial in being more easily absorbed, could be potentially hazardous since experiments by O. A. Levander et al.[695b] and by C. D. Thomson et al.[695c] suggest that this form of selenium may build up indefinitely in the body.

** In Chapter 6 I speculated on the possible nonexistence of some of the ascorbates advertised to be in some commercial products.

transplanted tumors in mice. Then too, selenium in tuna has only one-third the value of selenite in preventing exudative diathesis in chickens.[689] Thus, we are likely to learn from future research that selenium in different forms may have different clinical applications and may also offer variable protection against diseases. Diets of the future are likely to include selenium from diverse sources. Not only sodium selenite, but also sodium selenate and selenium dioxide (all inorganic forms) have been found effective in preventing tumor development.[687] It is interesting that the organic form, selenomethionine, seems to be lacking in this power (a good reason perhaps for not limiting our selenium intake to organic forms). However, selenomethionine in high-selenium bread was more effective than selenite in raising human blood selenium levels, but both forms raised equally the whole blood glutathione peroxidase levels.[696c] Xianmao Luo et al.,[696d] in working to reduce the incidence of Keshan disease, also found that supplementary selenomethionine increased selenium and glutathione peroxidase levels of the plasma and of the red blood cells more rapidly than occurred with a sodium selenite supplement.

Do not let the experiments at high levels of selenium unduly frighten you. Selenium protects against cancers and is vital in many other ways. It is true that selenium is named after the moon goddess *Selene* and, like the moon, it has both a light and a dark side. However, Klaus Schwarz[697] said, "...selenium deficiency appears to be a much more serious problem in the United States than selenium toxicity." With our greatly increased consumption of seafood, I wonder if anyone of the status of Schwarz would make a similar statement today.

If you are going to use selenium supplements, take them several hours away from any zinc or copper supplements you may be using since they can inhibit selenium's assimilation. Walter Mertz[698] said that "vitamin C...*in vitro* renders selenium totally unavailable." G. F. Combs, Jr. and G. M. Pesti[690] found, to the contrary, that in chicks oral doses of ascorbic acid promoted the enteric absorption of selenium. As we noted earlier, Mutanen and Mykkänen[696b] concluded that ascorbic acid increases the bioavailability of selenium in food but not of supplemental sodium selenate. We have here an example of why scientific conclusions sometimes look contradictory: the scientists are referring to different substances (in this case, selenium in food and selenium as selenate).

Germanium

The research of Kazuhiko Asai[699] suggests that sesquioxide compounds of germanium may have valuable health applications. The age-old curative properties of ginseng and garlic—and of many Chinese herbs such as *shelf fungus* that are relatively unknown in the West—may be due, at least in part, to their great concentration of germanium.

In the production of energy the body produces carbon dioxide, which is given off by the lungs, and hydrogen, which normally combines with body supplies of oxygen to form water. Asai maintains that when germanium sesquioxide compounds are consumed their oxygen will combine with available hydrogen and thus conserve the body stores of oxygen that would ordinarily be used up in combining with that hydrogen. Thus, more oxygen is made available to cells throughout the body.

It seems apparent that many body ailments hinge on a lack of oxygen at the cellular level that could possibly be corrected with germanium supplementation. The Nobel laureate Otto Warburg postulated that cancer is often caused or exacerbated by this lack of oxygen. Asai's work would seem to support the Warburg theory. Asai reported that in 20 cases of lung cancer all 20 were completely cured through the use of compounds of germanium sesquioxide and the ability of those compounds to oxygenate the cancerous tissues. Different forms of cancer and a long list of other diseases, including epilepsy, cirrhosis of the liver, arthritis and hypertension have reportedly been cured or alleviated with germanium therapy. Asai has, in fact, postulated that *all* diseases are due to a deficiency of oxygen.* Insofar as that hypothesis is valid, it would seem that

---

* On the contrary, many diseases are caused by a superfluity of oxygen in the form of free radicals.

germanium sesquioxide compounds might be valuable nutrients. However, other scientists have been unable to replicate Asai's work.

Masayoshi Kanisawa and Henry A. Schroeder[700] found that mice receiving germanium in the form of sodium germanate in their diet (and also those receiving sodium arsenate) had a decreased incidence of tumors (but without significant difference in malignant tumors). A similar experiment by the same scientists,[701] but with rats, showed significantly fewer tumors at many sites in those fed germanium. However, longevity was adversely affected by the germanium (while being benefitted by arsenic). The careful reader of the original papers will note some discrepancies in the research of Kanisawa and Schroeder. (The number of mice and rats in various subdivisions of these studies do not add up to the number in the total groups.) Nevertheless, the work of Kanisawa and Schroeder may throw doubt on the findings of Asai (other than his work in treating cancer). Furthermore, H. A. Schroeder et al.[701a] found in another study that rats fed germanium showed many adverse changes, including proteinuria and fatty livers and decreased life span in both sexes.

Then too, F. Caujolle et al.[702] reported that dimethyl germanium oxide is teratogenic in chick embryos. It should be observed, however, that sodium germanate and dimethyl germanium oxide would not be expected to necessarily act as the sesquioxide compounds of germanium do and, furthermore, a *reverse effect* may be applicable and thus Asai's work could be valid. However, Nobuko Kumano et al.[703] observed that carboxyethylgermanium sesquioxide (G E -132) had only a time-delaying action against tumors in mice. (The G E -132 was, by the way, supplied by the Asai Germanium Institute, Tokyo, whose director is Dr. K. Asai.) At the end of 100 days the mice injected with G E -132 had a tumor incidence of just 50% compared with a 90% incidence in the controls. However, at the end of 150 days the G E -132 group caught up and all groups had virtually a 100% tumor incidence. I think there is some cancer-fighting virtue in the use of germanium, but Asai's enthusiasm should properly be tempered with some skepticism.

Spirogermanium also exhibits antitumor activity. Many reports, such as one by Bridget T. Hill et al.,[704] suggest that spirogermanium may have possibilities in cancer fighting. However, it is toxic to cultured rat neurons, which means that human use might prove to be dangerous. Furthermore, Daniel R. Budman et al.[705] reported the results of a clinical trial of spirogermanium in breast adenocarcinoma. Toxic effects were noted in 50% of the patients and no major favorable responses were seen. More recently, Alison M. Badger et al.[705a] reviewed various studies showing spirogermanium to be cytotoxic for tumor lines both *in vitro* and *in vivo*. They also reported on their own work with rats showing that spirogermanium can suppress adjuvant-induced arthritis and can induce suppressor cells which inhibit the proliferative response of normal spleen cells to concanavalin A. Thus, spirogermanium could have a future not only in cancer therapy but also in treating autoimmune arthritic disease.

Other research suggests a youth-fostering role for germanium. Norito Kuga et al.[706] noted that mice fed 300 mg./kg. of organic germanium since five weeks of age did not develop amyloidosis. The mechanism for the action has not been elucidated, but if germanium can inhibit formation of amyloid it could be of considerable interest to gerontologists. The dosage of 300 mg./kg. is huge, however, and large dosages of anything suggest the possibility of side effects. When the experiment was repeated at a level of just 30 mg./kg. daily over a 22-month period, half the mice developed amyloidosis. Thus, germanium's possible application in human longevity programs would still seem to be in question.

The most concentrated, readily available food sources for germanium are garlic and ginseng. A somewhat less powerful but strong source is the popular herb comfrey, but it cannot be recommended because of its content of poisonous pyrrolizidine alkaloids.* Tablets of germanium bound to yeast are available at

---

* Comfrey (*Symphytum officinale*) was reported by Iwao Hirono et al.[706a] to be carcinogenic in rats when the roots were fed at levels of 1% of the diet or more or when the leaves were fed at 16% of the diet or more. (Only one tumor developed in a group of 28 rats fed leaves at a level of 8% of the diet, i.e., cancer occurred in this group at approximately the same level as in the controls—5 tumors in 129 rats.) Hepatocellular adenomas were commonly found in rats fed comfrey root or leaves at the 16% or higher

health food stores, but let me stress again that my notice of availability is not a recommendation to act.

Other Trace Elements

Other elements possibly play a role in the chemistry of the body. Indicated among these are aluminum, arsenic, barium, boron, bromine, cesium, lithium, nickel, silver, rubidium, tin, titanium, tungsten and vanadium. These trace elements, and the others we have discussed in this chapter, are all available in kelp and dulse.

Nickel

Nickel seems to be a factor in the production of adrenaline by the adrenal glands and also in the production of hormones by the thyroid gland. It could be involved in membrane metabolism. Nickel may, to a modest extent, take the place of cobalt in aiding the bone marrow's production of red blood cells. It is present in a serum protein called *nickeloplasmin.* Hyprogeusia (taste impairment) can sometimes be corrected, according to R. I. Henkin and D. F. Bradley,[707] not only by zinc and copper but also by nickel. M. Anke et al.[708] reported that nickel-deficient goats show increased iron excretion, which suggests that iron absorption is decreased when nickel is deficient. Nickel not only affects iron absorption and metabolism but one's iron status affects nickel metabolism.[709] Forrest H. Nielsen[709a] has provided findings of other studies, and related references, demonstrating nickel's probable essentiality for humans.

Grains and vegetables are sources of dietary nickel, but fiber or phytate (especially in the grains) may bind it and thus decrease its availability for intestinal absorption. Very little nickel is present in

---

level and hemangioendothelial sarcomas of the liver occurred less frequently. Pyrrolizidine alkaloids were presumed to be the responsible agents. Consuming comfrey leaves in modest amounts would seem to be safe. The *theory of the reverse effect* suggests that small amounts of comfrey leaves might be a protective factor against cancer. However, I cannot encourage anyone to consume a carcinogen until dose-response studies demonstrate whether or not a protective *reverse effect* exists. At any rate, if there is a component in comfrey that combats cancer, I suspect that it is not germanium but one or more of the pyrrolizidine alkaloids working through the *reverse effect*.

foods of animal origin. Absorption of nickel was suppressed by the presence of cow's milk, coffee, tea, orange juice and ascorbic acid, but not by a cola beverage.[710] Nickel absorption was hurt by a typical breakfast of eggs, bacon, toast, margarine and coffee but, surprisingly, phytate did not seem to show an effect.[710]

Nickel is toxic in anything beyond very minute quantities. (Even in very low concentration it causes coronary vasoconstriction and a significant increase in diastolic pressure.[711] Nickel, in excess, may detrimentally affect the liver, kidneys and brain and bring on symptoms such as headaches, vertigo and mental depression, tremors, kidney problems, constipation and loss of appetite. Nickel may enter our bodies via margarine (which could contain a residue of the catalyst used in the hydrogenation process), drinking water, cigarette or coal fumes, insecticides and dental alloys. Use in dentistry is, in fact, far more common than it was years ago in spite of the fact that nickel allergy is quite common. In Sweden, use of nickel in dental casting alloys has been condemned by The Swedish National Board of Health and Welfare.[712] It is suspected that alloys used for dental crowns may pose a long-term threat of nickel poisoning. A study by David W. Eggleston[712a] suggests that dental nickel alloys can adversely affect the quantity of T-lymphocytes. According to anecdotal reports, even piercing of the ears may cause a nickel sensitivity. Once sensitized, such women, it is said, may react not only to earrings containing free nickel (and thus must wear hypoallergenic earrings) but they may be sensitive to nickel-chrome door handles, "carbonless" business forms or even five-cent coins.

Tin

Tin, when missing from the diet of laboratory animals, causes growth retardation and so may be of use in human nutrition. Larger amounts can, however, negatively affect zinc utilization.[713] It may, therefore, be to our benefit that less tin is entering our bodies since the tin coating of cans has to a large degree been replaced with lacquer. J. M. Barnes and H. B. Stoner[714] make a strong case for tin's toxicity. Subsequently, Attallah Kappas and Makin D. Maines[715] reported that tin enhances heme breakdown in the kidney, thus impairing heme-dependent cellular functions such as P-450 mediated drug biotransformation. Nevertheless, the reported fact, as pointed out by Morton K. Schwartz,[716] that tin levels in some cancer tissues are lower than in homologous normal tissues may have a significance that is not yet understood. Furthermore, tin could find a therapeutic use in preventing neonatal jaundice. A rat study by George S. Drummond and Attallah Kappas[716a] suggests that tin-protoporphyrin may be useful in treating excessive bilirubin levels in the newborn. The brain barrier is permeable to many substances, including the potentially toxic bilirubin, immediately after birth, and this tin compound might prevent in humans, as it does in rats, the jaundice that may otherwise occur. A book edited by Nate F. Cardarelli,[716b] and dealing with tin as a vital nutrient, was published in 1986.

Silver

Some have speculated that silver may have nutritional value, but the possibility seems remote. On the other hand, silver has been shown by several different studies to be toxic to various types of animals through its interference with the selenium enzyme glutathione peroxidase. Then too, dietary silver, according to A. T. Diplock et al.[717] produces a copper deficiency in chicks and might have a similar action in humans. By the way, baby's silver cup is probably safe when used for drinking milk. But could it become dangerous if used for an acid beverage such as orange juice?

Cesium and Rubidium

Cesium and rubidium may be factors in the control of cancer. A. Keith Brewer[718] reports that the Hopi Indians of Arizona and the Indians of certain areas of Central America and Peru—groups which are said to have a low incidence of cancer—eat diets high in rubidium. Brewer also stated that the Hunzas of Pakistan, where cancer is also said to be relatively rare, have a diet high in cesium. According to Brewer, these minerals, when present in the cancer cell, raise its pH. As I have pointed out in connection with the nonvitamin B 17, cells malfunction and die when their pH deviates greatly from the normal value of 7.35.

Brewer[718] reported on experiments involving rubidium carbonate and mice. Tumors after the mice were fed rubidium carbonate for 13 days along with standard mouse chow were only one-eleventh the size of tumors in a control group. Both cesium and rubidium, bound to yeast, are available from health food suppliers, but availability does not mean use of such supplements should be encouraged. Animals tolerate feeding of rubidium or cesium very well for about two weeks but then toxicity symptoms, chiefly of neuromuscular irritability and growth cessation, appear.[719] This toxicity would appear to limit preventive or therapeutic use of rubidium or of cesium. An excellent review entitled "Rubidium: Overview and Clinical Perspectives" was authored by Ronald R. Fieve and Kay R. Jamieson.[720] They relate that patients on rubidium therapy experience a slowing of the pulse and an increase in blood pressure. They envision, however, an increased role for rubidium in medicine.

Aluminum

Aluminum is a very plentiful and reactive element, so it is surprising that a useful physiological function is yet to be discovered. (The possibility that such a discovery may be made is the reason aluminum is treated here rather than in Chapter 8.)* Aluminum is absorbed by the duodenum, probably in two ways. Andrew J. Adler and Geoffrey M. Berlyne[720b] have reported that its absorption seems to occur by a nonsaturable mechanism and also by a vitamin D-dependent saturable mechanism, for which it may compete with calcium.

Although a minute amount of aluminum may eventually be shown useful to body chemistry, it should be avoided. Aluminum has been implicated as a possible causal factor in amyotrophic lateral sclerosis, parkinsonism and Alzheimer's disease.[721] Research has

---

* Mice experiments by Nobutoshi Kobayashi et al.[720a] indicated that the presence of aluminum (as $AlCl_3$), either via inhalation or subcutaneous injection, reduced the incidence of lung adenomas induced by 4-nitroquinoline 1-oxide. Furthermore, J. J. Nagyvary et al.[720aa] found that alginate and pectin became hypocholesterolemic in rats only if the aluminum ion Al^{3+} was added to the diet. They also reported that carrageenan and pectic acid, although hypocholesterolemic without Al^{3+}, had their activity enhanced by the addition of this ion. Nagyvary and his coworkers concluded that "the possibility still exists that Al^{3+} might be a useful adjuvant in the human diet."

shown that aluminum binds to DNA.[722] Another study presented spectrometric evidence that aluminum accumulates in neurofibrillary tangles.[723] This laboratory work provides a rationale for the widely held opinion that aluminum is involved in Alzheimer's disease. However, John R. McDermott et al.[724] reported that brain aluminum concentration appears to increase with age regardless of whether or not a person has *Alzheimer's dementia*. The McDermott group found no statistically significant differences in brain aluminum concentration between ten patients with Alzheimer's disease and nine nonneurological controls. (Papers published during 1986 by J. M. Candy et al.[724a] and by Peter O. Yates and David M. A. Mann,[724b] however, continue to implicate aluminum in the form of aluminosilicates in the etiology of Alzheimer's disease.)* The concept that Alzheimer's disease could be caused by prions—very tiny, rod-shaped, fiber-like, protease-resistant proteins or something else that destroys cholinergic neurons—may be a more meaningful approach to developing a therapy for this disease.[724e,f] A review of various aspects of the disease was published in 1986 by Robert Katzman.[724g]

Aluminum binds with inorganic phosphorus in the intestines, which results in an increase in fecal phosphate and a decrease in phosphate available to the body. Aluminum can interfere with iron metabolism.[724h] However, there may be a *reverse effect*. J. M. C. Gutteridge et al[725] found that *in vitro* aluminum ions accelerated iron-stimulated lipid peroxidation. This phenomenon could partially account for the toxicity of aluminum in nervous tissue.

Intestinal absorption of aluminum can produce toxicity in children having excessive amounts of nitrogenous compounds in the blood, a condition called azotemia.[725a,b] Symptoms of aluminum poisoning include gastrointestinal irritation, muscle twitching and loss of appetite. Aluminum in the dialysate water of kidney patients may be especially threatening.[725c] Aluminum poisoning from

---

* R. D. West[724c] has suggested that a calcium deficiency might lead to the presence of the aluminum silicate in the plaques of Alzheimer's disease. Ian J. Deary and A. G. Hendrickson,[724d] in 1986, further developed this thesis and suggested that calcium supplementation might provide some protection not only in Alzheimer's disease but also in benign senescence.

intravenous therapy may also be a possibility and Aileen B. Sedman et al.[725d] found that premature infants receiving such therapy may be especially vulnerable. Herta Spencer and Lois Kramer[725e] point out that aluminum, especially from antacids, may interfere with intestinal absorption of fluoride and calcium and thus could contribute to bone loss and osteoporosis. In light of the ability of aluminum to complex with calcium and fluoride in the intestinal tract, it can have detrimental effects whether or not it is absorbed.

Cooking in aluminum kettles is probably safe, but its safety has been questioned.[726] The *FDA Consumer*[726a] warns against retaining salty or highly acidic foods such as tomato sauce and sauerkraut, as well as beverages, including citrus juices and carbonated drinks, in such cookware for several days. Similarly, acidic or salty foods should not be stored in aluminum foil. Aluminum may be found in baking powder, cake mixes, frozen doughs, pancake mixes, self-rising flour, pickled vegetables, antacids, buffered aspirin and in toothpaste.[726b] It may also be present in some table salt and in some grated Parmesan cheeses (and in some other grated cheeses) to enhance pourability. Deodorants are still other sources of possible aluminum poisoning. Aluminum, in the form of its sulphite, may even be added to your city water supply.

Vanadium

Vanadium is an element that may deserve more attention. Vanadates resemble inorganic phosphates and this is probably the reason they affect many enzymes, including human alkaline phosphatase.[709]

Several experiments with rats and chickens, as referenced by Forrest H. Nielsen,[727] showed that too little vanadium intake adversely affected the animals. A deficiency of vanadium in these animals reportedly led to an impairment of growth, of reproduction and of bone and lipid metabolism. Vanadium's biochemical function is thought to be that of an oxidation-reduction catalyst. However, some of the animal experiments are confusing and even contradictory.

In vitro experiments by Graham Carpenter[728] showed that vanadate added to human fibroblasts stimulated thymidine incorporation into DNA and produced an increase in cell numbers. Carpenter reports that the stimulation of DNA synthesis by vanadate is less than that provided by the epidermal growth factor, but vanadate appears to act synergistically with that factor. However, at concentrations of 20 ppm—at least in chick experiments—vanadate depressed growth (a *reverse effect*), but this depression of growth was overcome by feeding chromium at the same time.[729]

Vanadium compounds have been used therapeutically in treating anemia, tuberculosis, syphilis and various chronic diseases. Vanadate is reported to have a digitalis-like action on the heart.[730] An insulin-like action of vanadate has also been observed by several groups of investigators, including Torben Clausen et al.[731] Shinri Tamura et al.,[731a] in studying adipocytes from rat epididymal tissue, concluded that "vanadate enhances the phosphorylation of the insulin receptor by stimulating the kinase reaction in a similar but not identical manner to insulin." Subsequently, Clayton E. Heyliger et al.[731b] found that vanadate controlled the high blood glucose in diabetic rats and prevented the decline in cardiac performance associated with diabetes. Moreover, Anthony White[732] has reported that vanadium, in affecting cell membrane processes, increased the levels of cyclic AMP and NADH.

Strong dietary sources of vanadium, as reported by A. R. Byrne and L. Kosta,[733] are the liver and kidneys of beef, pork and chicken, oysters, gelatin, parsley, radishes, mushrooms, rice, wheat and buckwheat. Beverages—tea, cocoa, wine and beer—are very strong sources. Their study showed large concentrations in bones of various animals (including man) and also in human teeth and hair. Large concentrations in the feces, which they also reported, would seem to suggest low absorbability. Duane R. Myron et al.[734] found that chicken light meat has about twice as much vanadium as the dark meat. They reported that egg yolk, cod fish, scallops, peanut butter, white bread (more so than whole wheat), beans and gluten, dill seed and black pepper are strong sources. Myron et al. state that most processed foods are relatively high in vanadium and so the average intake of this metal may be increasing as more and more such foods are consumed.

Vanadium is also available bound to yeast as a "health-food" supplement, but there may be a problem in its use. Many studies cited by J. S. Larsen and O. Thomsen[735] give good evidence for vanadate being a powerful vasoconstrictor that acts directly on the blood vessel wall. Although Larsen and Thomsen question whether this phenomenon has physiologic importance, I think it might argue against vanadium supplementation. Vanadium, as vanadate, is a potent inhibitor of Na^+, K^+-ATPase and thus may affect the Na^+-K^+ pump responsible for moving sodium and potassium in and out of cells.[736,736a]* Because of this inhibition of Na^+, K^+-ATPase, and because plasma levels of vanadate are raised during mania, D. A. T. Dick et al.[737] and G. J. Naylor et al.[738] have postulated that vanadium may have a detrimental effect in affective disorders. I will have more to say about the negative aspects of vanadium in connection with manic-depressive patients when we consider lithium in the pages immediately following.

Although it has been suggested that vanadium may lower blood pressure, the Robert P. Steffen group[736a] found that uninephrectomized rats (i.e., those with one kidney removed) that were fed sodium orthovanadate in their drinking water showed a gradual increase in systolic blood pressure. Rats fed a level of dietary vanadate of 200 ppm had a higher systolic blood pressure than those fed at 100 ppm (Figures 23 and 24).

Although vanadium is considered to be essential for growth,[739] Steffen found that an excess shows a *reverse effect* by inhibiting growth. There may be yet other problems with vanadium. *Lancet,*[740] while pointing out that vanadium in the form of vanadate might not affect the sodium-potassium pump *in vivo* because glutathione may reduce the vanadate to vanadyl, warns that vanadate can inhibit

---

* Small amounts of vanadium in foods might beneficially act to control ATPase, while supplementary amounts might act to shut down the enzyme action. Furthermore, I. S. Cohen[736b] suggests the possibility that inhibiting the Na or K exchange pump might lead to a *reduction* of intracellular sodium (rather than a *rise* of sodium as is generally held). Since sodium is now believed to often be relatively irrelevant in affecting blood pressure, the Cohen hypothesis may be more tenable than it might have been if presented earlier.

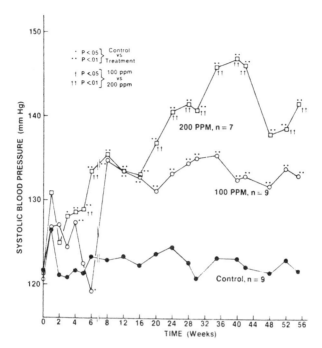

Figure 23. Effect of two levels of dietary vanadate treatment on systolic blood pressure of uninephrectomized Sprague-Dawley rats drinking tap water. After six weeks, each symbol represents the mean of four weekly measurements. Reproduced from Robert P. Steffen et al., *Hypertension* (1981) 3: 1173-1178, with permission of the publisher, the American Heart Association.

various enzymes. Among those inhibited are acid phosphatase, alkaline phosphatase, myosin ATPase, calcium ATPase, adenylate kinase and phosphofructokinase, but adenyl cyclase, on the other hand, is stimulated. Furthermore, H. U. Meisch and H. J. Bielig [739] state that vanadium inhibits cholesterol synthesis, increases cysteine metabolism (thereby reducing the level of coenzyme A needed to run the Krebs cycle) and inhibits monamine oxidase.

Then too, blood levels of vanadium are reported to be elevated in cancer patients,[730] but whether this helps bring on the disease or is an example of "body wisdom" in fighting the disease is not known.

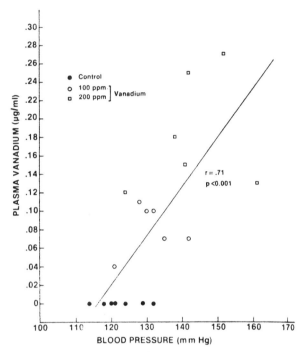

Figure 24. Relation between the last recorded systolic blood pressure and vanadium concentration in plasma obtained upon sacrificing the animal. Each symbol represents one uninephrectomized Sprague-Dawley rat drinking tap water and receiving no vanadate or one of two levels of vanadate in the diet. Reproduced from Robert P. Steffen et al., *Hypertension* (1981) 3: I173-I178, with permission of the publisher, the American Heart Association.

Danuta Witkowska and Jacek Brzezinski [740a] have reported that vanadium affected the normal equilibrium of brain monoamines: noradrenaline decreased while dopamine and 5-hydroxytryptamine increased. They consider these to be early signs of toxic action on the function of the central nervous system. In treating manic-depressive illness, a restricted vanadium intake and lowering of plasma vanadate levels seems especially desirable. [740b] Anthony White [732] suggests use of ascorbic acid, glutathione and a number of specific vanadium chelators to reduce intracellular levels of vanadate. I think supplementation of vanadium, unless it is prescribed by a physician aware of the problems, is inadvisable and, pending arrival of more information, must be considered to be potentially dangerous.

A summary of the Symposium presented by the American Society for Pharmacology and Experimental Therapeutics regarding the role of vanadium in biology was published in 1986 by *Federation Proceedings*.[741]

Lithium

Lithium salts have been used in medicine since the last half of the 19th century. Then, in 1949, John F. J. Cade[741a] reported on studies that resulted in his suggesting a role for lithium in managing and preventing psychogenic excitement. His and subsequent studies have shown that lithium can play an important role in the restoration of mental health. The findings that lithium and other drugs could empty our mental hospitals is rated by *Science 84* [741aa] as one of the 20 great discoveries of the 20th century.

Earl B. Dawson et al.[741b,742] of the University of Texas Medical Branch in Galveston studied the rate of admissions to mental hospitals in Dallas, a city which has very little lithium in its drinking water, and in El Paso where there is a generous amount of lithium (130 micrograms per liter) in the drinking water. On a per capita basis in the two cities, Dallas had three times as many admissions for psychosis, six times as many for neurosis and three times as many for personality problems. Dawson and his co-workers have studied 24 Texas communities and found a similar correlation between the presence of lithium in the water and a decreased rate of mental disease. However, Alex D. Pokorny et al.[742a] have pointed out that the high-lithium counties of Texas are mainly from the Rio Grande River Valley, a sparsely populated area far away from the nine state hospitals. Pokorny shows that the likeliness of entering a mental hospital is inversely related to the distance one must come. Pokorny holds that Dawson was really measuring not lithium, but distance to a hospital.

It is now known that lithium can have a remarkably beneficial effect on manic and depressive patients, but seems to be without similar value for other mental patients. Furthermore, a more recent study of drinking water (in North Carolina) showed no correlation between lithium content of the water and the occurrence of manic and depressive illness. Why not? Because the concentrations of lithium that are likely to occur in drinking water are far below levels now considered to be effective.[742aa]

The mental disorder of displaying excessive aggression is amenable to treatment with lithium. Michael H. Sheard[742b] was first to report successful use of lithium to control the behavior of violent prisoners. M. H. Sheard and G. K. Aghajanian[742c] had found earlier that lithium enhances the metabolism of serotonin, a chemical that reduces aggression. Suzanne Knapp and Arnold J. Mandell[743] also reported that lithium stimulates the uptake of tryptophan in the brain and its conversion to serotonin. (A similar role that calcium plays in converting tryptophan to serotonin is well known.) They also suggest that after about ten days the therapeutic efficacy of lithium chloride in treating mania is partially due to a decrease in brain tryptophan hydrolase.

The use of lithium compounds in treating bipolar affective psychosis involves an incompletely understood mechanism. It is believed, however, that the interference of lithium with processes involving cyclic adenosine monophosphate (cAMP) is a factor. In depressive illness the red blood cells show decreased Na^+, K^+-ATPase activity with a resulting rise in intracellular sodium.[742d] G. J. Naylor et al.[742e] reported lithium increases the activity of erythrocyte Na^+, K^+-ATPase without increasing the number of Na^+, K^+-ATPase molecules and they speculate this could be due to lithium's reducing the inhibitory effect of vanadate. Then too, the lymphocytes of manic-depressives have a greatly reduced ability to produce new action sites for Na^+, K^+-ATPase pump activity.[742f] The fact (as cited earlier) that magnesium encourages the operation of this pump[419b-e] and that vanadium decreases the pump's action[736,736a] makes one wonder if therapy for manic-depressives should not employ supplemental magnesium while restricting the consumption not only of salt but of high-vanadium foods. D. A. T. Dick et al.[737] have, in fact, found that there was a significant negative correlation between the body's vanadium concentration and the ratio of Na^+, K^+-ATPase to Mg ATPase in 72 manic-depressives but not in 23 controls. Large dosages of ascorbic acid can reduce vanadate to the vanadyl ion, which has much less ability than vanadate to inhibit the potassium-sodium pump. Naylor and Smith[738] discovered that the severity of illness among 11 manic and 12 depressed patients was alleviated by orally administering 3 grams of vitamin C daily. In a separate experiment they found that a low-vanadium diet was also effective therapy.

Returning to the consideration of lithium once again, Ewen Mac Donald[742g] has reported that lithium showed no protective effect against vanadate inhibition of Na^+, K^+-ATPase. If this is true, it would seem that it may be especially important to treat manic-depressives not only with lithium but with vitamin C and to restrict dietary vanadium.* J. Ananth and R. Yassa[744] speculated that the importance of magnesium in treating mental illness may relate to an interaction with lithium. The fact that both magnesium and lithium stimulate Na^+, K^+-ATPase pump activity may be the connection about which they were speculating. A recent study by Jan A. Fawcett[745] at Rush-Presbyterian-St. Luke's Hospital, Chicago, reports good results using lithium in treating alcoholics.

Lithium carbonate is sometimes used in treating cluster headache, perhaps the beneficial effect being due to an influence on brain neurotransmitters. E. Ferrari et al.[745a] reported that when 900 mg. of lithium carbonate was administered in the evening a significantly higher level of serum lithium resulted as compared to a similar dosage given earlier in the day. However, Ferrari and his associates did not observe any differences in the therapeutic effectiveness of lithium due to the timing of the treatment.

J. Boyle et al.[745b] recently reported success in treating seborrheic dermatitis topically with lithium succinate. They also observed that

---

* The potassium-sodium pump inhibitor found in certain foods (e.g., tea, cocoa and red wines)[406,406a] should also probably be avoided.

while *topical* treatment was useful for seborrheic dermatitis, *systemic* lithium exacerbated psoriasis.

Lithium has also been used in treating genital herpes. *In vitro,* lithium salts inhibit replication of herpes simplex and other DNA viruses.[746] G. R. B. Skinner[747] reported that local application of lithium succinate as an ointment provided good symptomatic relief and lowered viral excretion in genital herpes.

Adverse Effects of Lithium

The toxic symptoms of lithium include blurred vision, dry mouth, constipation, loss of memory, amnesia and disorientation, confusion, ataxia, delirium and hallucinations.[747a] Some studies have indicated that orally administering lithium can result in an undesirable slowing of thyroid activity.[748] The problem may be exacerbated if potassium iodide has also been prescribed.[748a] Dysregulation of body temperature often occurs when lithium salts are used, most persons having a consistently elevated temperature.[748b] We noted earlier in this chapter that lithium may thwart the role of zinc in catalyzing prostaglandin production. Then too, experiments with mice have shown that lithium reduces the number of acetylcholine receptors at neuromuscular junctions.[749]

Lithium may also have detrimental sexual effects, especially in regard to penile erections.[750] On the other hand, T. K. Banerji et al.[751] reported that plasma testosterone in mice showed a significant increase after seven days of lithium administration. However, there was no significant difference in testosterone levels between treated mice and controls after 21 days. The levels of leutenizing hormone were unchanged at 7 days and after 21 days. The mouse experiment gives no support, therefore, for the reported negative sexual findings in humans. Subsequently, however, Dwane H. Dean and Raymond H. Hiramoto,[751a] in another experiment with mice, supported clinical observations that lithium at therapeutic dosage may impair male sexual function. In this regard, M. Kolomaznik et al.[752] found that in some patients treated with lithium sexuality was disturbed while in others it was not. Different studies have shown that at concentrations 100-fold greater than those used in therapy lithium impairs the quality of sperm. However, J. Raboch et al.[753] observed that at therapeutic levels lithium does not affect sperm.

Another hazard of treatment with lithium carbonate may be a detrimental effect on the teeth. Aaron Gillis[754] reported increased incidence of dental caries in a number of patients under long-term treatment with lithium carbonate. Furthermore, Joseph Michaeli et al.[754a] have warned against the possibility that lithium salts may induce hypertension.

Sometimes, negative skin effects may result from internal use of lithium. Frederick J. Bloomfield and Marjorie M. Young[507e] have shown that lithium can induce granulation of neutrophils *in vitro* and they speculate that if this happens *in vivo* the release of inflammatory factors might account for the cutaneous side effects found during lithium therapy.

There are yet other negative features to lithium treatment. J. Perez-Cruet and J. T. Dancey[755] stated that chronic treatment with lithium chloride produced significant involution of the thymus gland and a persistent lymphopenia (reduction in the amount of lymph). The levels of corticosterone also increased without changes in adrenal weights. J. R. King et al.[755a] reported that thirst was prevalent in 67% of 87 patients being administered lithium.

Negative cardiac reports exist but are rare. There is also some evidence that lithium increases the incidence of congenital heart defects if given to pregnant women, especially in the first trimester. These and other facts relating to the role of lithium in medicine can be found in an article by Norman E. Rosenthal and Frederick K. Goodman.[756] In addition, an article entitled "Hazards and Adverse Effects of Lithium" by R. Bruce Lydiard and Alan J. Gelenberg[757] is especially detailed in elaborating on the negative effects.

The Lithium Information Center is available to clinicians and researchers for information on any aspect of lithium and its use in medicine.[757a] Clinicians are likely to find *Lithium Encyclopedia for Clinical Practice*[757b] to be a valuable reference. Individual sections are devoted to lithium physiology, therapeutic use, adverse effects and drug interactions. The book is based on three interacting computer programs: the Lithium Library, Lithium Index and Lithium Consultation.

Lithium, bound to yeast, is available in health food stores, but I should have said enough to keep you away from it unless it is prescribed by a physician. If lithium has been prescribed, a low-salt diet may increase its effect.[757c]

Bromine

How about the mineral bromine? A significant correlation has been found between bromine deficiency and the quality of sleep. P. L. Oe et al.[758] reported that when bromine was added to the dialysate of dialysis patients their sleep quality greatly improved. Most of us have no problems with a dietary bromine deficiency. On the other hand, since bromine is often added to gasoline, our environment could present us with a possible excess.

Boron

Much of the work with boron chemistry has been done by William Nunn Lipscomb, Jr., for which he was awarded the Nobel Prize for Chemistry in 1976, and by Herbert Brown, who shared the Nobel Prize for Chemistry with George Wittig in 1979. Boron may possibly be required in human nutrition, although this has not yet fully been demonstrated. However, Rex E. Newnham[759] cites evidence for its essentiality and usefulness in treating osteo- and rheumatoid arthritis. He states that boron and magnesium are synergistic. Sales of tablets containing magnesium carbonate and sodium borate seem to be substantial in his home country of Australia. U. Weser[760] has shown that giving borate to boron-deficient rats stimulated RNA synthesis by liver cells. Boron is found in green leafy vegetables, bee pollen and some honeys. Colostrum contains twice as much boron as later milk.[759]

Tungsten

Tungsten at present seems to have no status as a human nutrient. However, it may have some uses. At any rate, Alvin L. Moxon and Kenneth P. DuBois[761] showed that tungsten prevented selenium poisoning in rats.

Arsenic

Even arsenic, a powerful poison in modest quantities, may have value in the miniscule amounts contained in mineral waters. In 1786, Fowler introduced the use of potassium arsenite for treating various ailments and by 1912 it was considered the best agent in the Pharmacopoeia.[762]*

Arsenic's mode of action in the body is to take part in some of the reactions involving phosphate. Arsenic probably catalyzes the biosynthesis of glutathione, the remarkable anticancer metabolite we met earlier in connection with sulphur.[764] Arsenite, in nontoxic amounts, also influences the release of glutathione in the bile according to *in vitro* experiments on the livers of rats performed by Irene Anundi et al.[765] It is speculated that glutathione affects the bioavailability of ingested compounds and studies to test this hypothesis are now under way.

DuBois et al.[766] found that both sodium arsenite and sodium arsenate were able to reduce the toxicity in animals of several selenium compounds, including seleniferous wheat. O. H. Muth et al.[767] reported similar results of arsenic reducing selenium toxicity in lambs. These arsenic compounds are, however, too toxic for general usage on farms and ranches plagued with soil poisoned with excessive selenium.

G. N. Schrauzer et al.[768] reported that, although there was found to be a weak association between dietary arsenic and cancer of the buccal cavity and pharynx, there was an inverse relationship between dietary arsenic and lung cancer. Arsenic may, in fact, cause remission of human leukemias,[768a] although large doses can exhibit a *reverse effect* and *cause* leukemia in mice.[768b] Perhaps related to this latter finding is another murine study by G. N. Schrauzer et al.[769] which showed that arsenic abolished the anticarcinogenic effect of selenium. In this experiment arsenite caused a significant increase of the rate of tumor growth and increased the incidence of multiple tumors, although an earlier experiment[658] showed that arsenite

---

* H. F. Smyth, Jr., M.D.,[763] relates that his father, a physician, treated him many years ago with Fowler's Solution and thereby corrected his low hemoglobin.

The Reverse Effect

reduced tumor incidence by 27% while enhancing the rate of tumor growth. Thus, the status of arsenic as a poison and as a quasi nutrient is still confused. Nevertheless, it seems probable that the relatively recent reversal of attitude toward selenium (from poison to nutrient) may even now be helping to effect a change in attitude toward arsenic.

Arsenic, in small quantities of course, is an important ingredient of chicken feed and increases the egg production of hens. Arsenic deficiency in goats in the second or third generation led to sudden heart failure with a mortality of 71%.[770] On the other hand, Gillian R. Paton and A. C. Allison[771] have reported that arsenic induces chromosome damage in human cells. The golden mean, moderation in all things, will probably be found applicable to the two-faced nutritive-poisonous aspects of arsenic.

In spite of possible benefits, it will take considerable educating to overcome arsenic's strong reputation as a poison. An indication of the present low status of arsenic as a nutrient is shown by the advertising of one of the suppliers of *Spirulina algae* which says it is a good source of selenium but fails to mention arsenic. *Spirulina* may contain far more arsenic than selenium. [772] (Really, its content of arsenic and other minerals varies according to the mineral values of the water in which it is grown.) * However, in light of the quasi-good words I have said about arsenic, perhaps someday its presence will be a selling point of *Spirulina* marketers. Fish and other seafood are reasonably good sources of arsenic. [773] I presume that kelp might also be a strong source.

Nevertheless, arsenic is not an unmixed blessing. Henry A. Schroeder[774] reported that hundreds of people in Taiwan were poisoned by drinking naturally occurring arsenic in the water from deep wells. Many of them developed cancers of the skin. Organic arsenic is rapidly excreted via the kidneys, so excessive accumulation does not occur and it has low toxicity. Inorganic arsenic, on the other hand, does accumulate in the body and can be very poisonous indeed.

---

* In India *Spirulina platensis* is grown on raw sewage. [772a] It is used as chicken feed and is effective in making the yolks more yellow (which is considered desirable).

It is probable that the biologically essential trace elements are far more important than is generally realized. Agriculture books often contain illustrations of sad-looking plants along with a commentary as to what mineral deficiency or deficiencies were causal factors. If a lack of minerals can occasion such havoc in the health of a plant, isn't it reasonable to assume that mineral deficiencies could cause us to lose our health, youthfulness and vitality?

A Theory of How Side Effects Might Be Eliminated

Earlier, on page 164, we speculated as to how undesirable *reverse effects* might be obviated. Suppose we now hypothesize that side effects of nutrients and drugs are phenomena originating in organs where one or more *reverse effects* are occurring. Suppose further (as we speculated on page 164) that each molecule of a given nutrient or drug, instead of being administered in its raw state, could be administered coupled to a carrier that would be uncoupled by means of local enzymatic action only upon reaching the organ responsible for the diseased condition. In accordance with this scenario, we would eliminate the possibility of the substance being delivered anywhere except in the target organ. The nutrient or drug would not uncouple in any of the various organs in which *reverse effects,* leading to side effects, might occur if the corresponding raw substance were being used.

If side effects could be eliminated by this method of drug-nutrient delivery, any given nutrient or drug could be administered in much greater potency whenever such increased potency was considered to be desirable. Potency might be usefully increased as long as the concentration of the nutrient or drug after uncoupling in the target organ did not itself lead to an undesirable *reverse effect.*

"I rather think it proves that the discovery of new ideas follows other laws than laws of logical order; that knowledge of half the truth can be a sufficient directive for the creative mind on its path to the full truth, and that contradictory theories can be helpful only because there exists, though unknown at that time, a better theory which comprehends all observational data and is free from contradictions. While humans search, truth slumbers; it will be awakened by those who do not stop their search even when their path is obstructed by the brushwood of contradictions."
— Hans Reichenbach, *The Rise of Scientific Philosophy* (Berkely: University of California Press, 1964)

"Facts are probabilities which we trust until new data arrive."
— Walter A. Heiby, *Live Your Life* (New York: Harper and Row, 1966)

CHAPTER 8

Your Body Can't Sing if You Poison It

The previous chapter concerned itself primarily with the minerals vital to body chemistry. Now let us give some brief information about toxic,* possibly dangerous metals.

---

* The great metal chemist Klaus Schwarz has written: "The term 'toxic metal' is justified only from the pragmatic, practical point of view. Many, if not all metals, are toxic. In acute oral toxicity tests Cu, for instance, is just as toxic as Cd; Fe, Mo and Sb are more toxic than Pb; and the toxicity of Hg is surpassed by that of V in form of vanadate, and also by Se, both of which are proven to be essential."

The metals that are probably the greatest troublemakers are lead, mercury, strontium and cadmium. We have already considered these briefly, so you are probably already concerned that you minimize their entrance into your body. Other metals such as aluminum, arsenic and nickel have a quasi-nutrient, quasi-poison status and I commented on them in the preceding chapter. Many studies have shown that young mice and rats and also children have a greater capacity to absorb heavy metals than do adults of their species. It may, therefore, be especially important to have children's hair analyzed periodically to discover any latent problems.

Lead

It is possible that of the several poisonous metals the greatest body havoc is occasioned by lead. However, the poisonous nature of lead has not always been realized. Even in fairly recent times lead, in combination with opium, was actually prescribed by physicians to combat diarrhea.[1a] In the early part of the 20th century lead continued to be recommended for external use. In a popular "home-medical" book[2] it was suggested that "in painful bruises one of the best applications is lead and opium lotion." Interestingly, although lead is now almost universally condemned as a poison, Klaus Schwarz[3] said that lead "has many properties for an essential trace element. It is obvious from past experience that toxicity is no argument against potential essentiality." It seems appropriate to give the following additional quotation from the same article: "It can be calculated that one would have to go down by four to five orders of magnitude, into the area of parts per trillion, before coming to the threshold where only one atom of a specific element would be present for one specific gene in the chromosomes of a cell. I could conceive this as the extreme lower limit of biological trace element function." Klaus Schwarz was one of our greatest biochemists; in thinking "big" it is apparent that he was capable of thinking quite "small." He was also stretching to its philosophical limit the Arndt-Schultz Law which we met in Chapter 1.

As Schwarz suggested, in minute quantities lead may be of physiological value. A number of lead compounds inhibit lipoxygenase activity.[4] You will recall, as we related in Chapter 3, the lipoxygenase enzyme converts arachidonic acid into hydroperoxy derivatives and then into leukotrienes. There are both beneficial and detrimental aspects to the leukotrienes but, in many cases, inhibiting their production might be beneficial. Even if lead compounds might be useful in such applications, other side effects could limit their use. If we desire to inhibit lipoxygenase activity, other chemicals, including propyl gallate, flavonoids and vitamin E might be safer. Nevertheless, this effect on lipoxygenase could be a "plus" for lead, a metal which is so often thought to be strictly a poison.

Then too, Von Anna M. Reichlmayr-Lais and M. Kirchgessner[5] reported on lead deficiency(!) in rats. (Interesting idea, "lead deficiency," but it correlates with my concept of the *reverse effect*.) These scientists reported that lead-deficient rats showed increased alkaline phosphatase activity in serum and liver but decreased alkaline phosphatase activity in the femur. The activity of the transferases GOT and GPT in the liver was lower in lead-depleted rats compared with controls. Obviously, lead deficiency makes a difference. Do we know enough to call all these differences "bad"?

In addition, M. Kirchgessner and Anna M. Reichlmayr-Lais[6] reported that iron absorbability of lead-depleted rats was impaired. They concluded that there is a function for lead in iron absorption. Furthermore, these same scientists[7] reported on experiments showing that absence of lead induced growth depressions and other physiological abnormalities. Addition of lead abolished or prevented these abnormalities. In yet another study[7a] they found that lead-depleted rats showed reduced values of hematocrit by 11%, of hemoglobin by 15% and of mean corpuscular volume by 9%. Therefore, they concluded that lead is an essential element. However, in anything but the most minute quantities I think it reasonable to assume that lead is a poison.

H. W. Mielke et al.,[7b] in studying soil samples in metropolitan Baltimore, concluded, in 1983, that soil lead levels were unacceptable. Subsequently, Mielke et al.[7c] found that the soil of metropolitan Minneapolis—one of the top cities in terms of environmental quality—was also contaminated with lead. They discovered a 10-fold increase in soil lead near the city limits compared to the rural area and another 10-fold increase in the soil of downtown Minneapolis (for a 100-fold increase over that in the rural area). It is frightening to realize that some of the inhabitants are growing their vegetables in this soil.

A danger of lead poisoning exists in the solder used to join water pipes. Futhermore, even though the pipes in your house may be of galvanized steel, copper or polyvinyl chloride, the pipe leading from the water main to your house could be of lead. If your water is hard, calcium will be deposited on such pipes and thus provide a protective coating. If the water is soft, however, there may be more danger. Today, there is probably a reduced lead threat from paints and insecticides, but any decrease is more than made up by increased danger from cigarette smoking. (However, children continue to get lead poisoning by eating paint chips from peeling walls. Adults, scraping the paint off such walls may also breathe in some lead in the form of paint particles.) Lead glazes on dishes may also be a source of poisoning and such dishes should be discarded. (Lead-glazed pitchers filled with acid fruit juices may be especially threatening.) Obviously, working with lead (e.g., the pouring, by children, of lead to make toy soldiers or the forming, by an artist, of lead separators in what is to be a stained-glass window) may be especially hazardous. Cosmetics may also contain lead. The most threatening recent source of lead in our environment is probably automotive exhaust, but this has decreased with the use of nonleaded gasoline.

The life-styles of some ethnic groups may be a factor in saturnism (lead toxicity, derived from the archaic word for lead, saturn). A remedy called "Azarcon," a bright orange powder used by some Hispanic parents to treat indigestion in their children, was found to contain 86% to 93.5% lead tetroxide.[7d] Similarly, Hmong (Southeast Asian) refugees have been known to use as a remedy a reddish-orange powder called "pay-loo-ah" containing varying amounts of lead.[7d]

Food from soldered tin cans can be very polluted with lead and should be avoided. It may be especially dangerous to store opened cans of fruit juice in the refrigerator. A study by C. A. Bache and D. J. Lisk[7e] showed that orange juice stored in an opened, soldered, tinned can for 168 hours had a six-fold increase in lead content. Other types of packaged foods may also contain illegal amounts of lead. John J. Miller[8] reported on amounts of lead found in various foods: instant tea, 2.1 ppm, instant rice 1.4 ppm, baby foods 1.1 ppm, some fruit juices 1.5 ppm, canned and powdered milk from 1 to 1.4 ppm, bone meal up to 8.8 ppm, dolomite up to 28 ppm, desiccated liver 13.7 ppm and kelp 12.1 ppm. Not only canned and powdered milk, but also fresh milk, may present a lead problem. Lead retention in rats is increased about four times by a diet high in milk because milk increases lead absorption by the intestines.[9] Other foods from lead-soldered cans are likely to be contaminated with significant amounts of lead.[9a] Commercial drying and pulverizing, not only of milk but also of other foods, can greatly increase lead contamination.[9a]

The body's absorption of lead (and of other metals, both good and bad) may be increased during a period of fasting. Many health enthusiasts extol fasting in glowing terms. However, an increase in heavy metal absorption due to short fasts has been reported by many investigators. J. Quarterman and Elaine Morrison[10] cite much of the research in this area, as well as report on their own findings. Quarterman and Morrison found that when rats were given various heavy metals (via a tube directly into the stomach) after a fast of 16 to 24 hours, absorption of those metals was greatly increased. The finding held true for all metals that were examined—not only for such valuable minerals as copper, zinc, calcium and iron, but for the toxic metals, lead and mercury. The effects of a longer fast of 40 hours were variable—the metal retention sometimes being more and sometimes being less than during the shorter fasts. Since poisonous metals are always present in the environment—including our gastrointestinal tracts—this may provide a reason, among others, to question the wisdom of fasting.

Harold G. Petering[11] makes the point that lead toxicity can be expressed in two ways. Lead can act directly and detrimentally in biochemical and cellular processes or indirectly by interfering with the availability and function of nutrients such as copper and zinc. Lead is very upsetting to the body's enzyme systems. By stimulating the production of detrimental hyaluronidase, quantities of valuable hyaluronic acid are reduced, with possible negative effects on the synovial membranes and resulting in arthritis.[11a]* Adenosine triphosphate (ATP), which provides energy for body functions, was reported by E. J. Underwood[14] to be sensitive to lead. Gary W. Goldstein and Diane Ar[14a] propose that some of the toxic effects of lead may be explained by its interaction with calmodulin.

Some symptoms of lead poisoning are: mental retardation in children, hyperactivity,** loss of appetite, headaches, constipation, fatigue and sexual problems. Troels Lyngbye et al.[14c] cite several studies that implicate lead as a cause of sudden infant death. A number of these symptoms may be due to lead's interference with the enzyme involved in the synthesis of heme. Several investigators[15] have reported that lead causes carcinogenic effects in kidneys of rats. D. G. Beevers et al.[16] found that subclinical lead exposure from drinking water may be a factor in the development of hypertension. More recently, S. J. Pocock et al.[16a] concluded from their study that there was some suggestion of increased hypertension due to lead but

---

* I should not imply that hyaluronidase is without a valuable function. (Nature does not have the body produce substances that are strictly detrimental to her purposes.) D. McLean et al.[12] reported that, following coronary occlusions in rats, hyaluronidase produced significant reductions in infarct size. The finding may or may not be applicable to humans. (Obviously, we should not conclude that lead is indicated for treating coronary occlusions.) Hyaluronidase is also believed to be released by the acrosome of the sperm cell to facilitate its entrance into an egg[13]

** Bryan K. Yamamoto and Charles L. Kutscher[14b] reported that dietary lead produced hyperactivity in rats under certain conditions. The animals were fed a 1% lead acetate diet from the age of 100 days until the end of the experiment. After 82 days of lead feeding, behavioral tests were started. Lead produced no activity change when rats were not challenged. However, when challenged with either food deprivation (Figure 1) or with an injection of phenylethylamine (Figure 2) hyperactivity (as measured by wheel turning) greatly increased over that of controls that were fed a lead-free diet. This suggests that with conditions of fasting or undernutrition, lead poisoning in humans might be similarly exacerbated. It is also conceivable that lead might act synergistically not only with phenylethylamine (PEA) but with other drugs or perhaps even with nutrients.

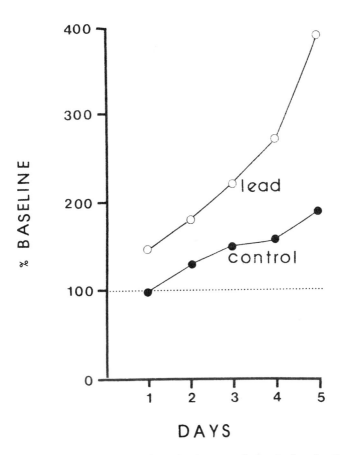

Figure 1. Daily wheel turning during total food deprivation as a percentage of daily predeprivation baseline. Reproduced from Bryan K. Yamamoto and Charles L. Kutscher, *Pharmacology, Biochemistry & Behavior* (1981) 15: 505-512, by permission of the publisher, Ankno International Inc., and of the authors.

it did not reach statistical significance. Nevertheless, William R. Harlan et al.[16b] found a direct relationship between blood lead levels and systolic and diastolic blood pressures in men and women and for white and black persons from 12 to 74 years of age. Blood lead

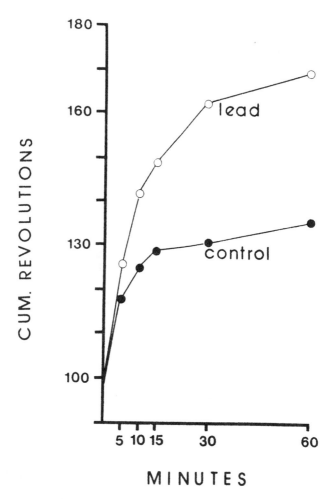

Figure 2. Wheel turning following PEA injection for rats on lead or control diet. Reproduced from Bryan K. Yamamoto and Charles L. Kutscher, *Pharmacology, Biochemistry & Behavior* (1981) 15: 505-512, by permission of the publisher, Ankno International Inc., and of the authors.

levels were significantly higher in younger men and women (aged 21 to 55 years) with high blood pressure but not in older men or women. Other studies in regard to lead and blood pressure have been reviewed by A. G. Shaper and S. J. Pocock.[16c]

In anything except miniscule amounts, lead is certainly a poison. The natural amino acid cysteine is an efficient chelating agent for removal of lead from the body.* Eating kidney and navy beans may also be helpful in ridding the body of lead through the action of their sulphur-amino acids (cysteine, cystine and methionine). Supplementation with calcium and zinc[17a,b] may also help reduce absorption of lead. Dietary use of pectin or sodium alginate** will allow these chemicals to combine with lead in the gut and prevent its entrance into the rest of the body.

Narayani P. Singh[18] reported that magnesium fed to rats helps mobilize lead from bone. Similarly, A. R. Krall et al.[19] found that magnesium infusions caused a more rapid excretion of lead from tissue as well as from bone. (However, they also observed that more rapid assimilation of lead from the diet occurred at the same time.)

Animal studies by Edward J. Calabrese[20] indicate that optimal (but *not* excessive) values of copper and iron may also be important in reducing lead toxicity. (Note the word *optimal*. Excessive amounts of copper concomitant with low amounts of iron can dramatically *increase* lead toxicity.) James C. Barton et al.[20a] have postulated that the two metals compete for similar binding sites on intestinal mucosal proteins that are involved in absorption of the metals. They subsequently reported discovering a protein weighing about 370,000 daltons that binds lead and iron. On the other hand, Peter R. Flanagan et al.[21] maintained that human lead retention was unrelated to either iron absorption or body stores. They reported, however, that lead retention was slightly increased by ingestion of fat. They also found that fasting in humans (as had been found earlier with rats) increased lead retention.

---

* This fact may account for cysteine's reported success in treating some cases of arthritis where lead has encouraged formation of hyaluronidase and subsequent interference with the synovial fluid in the joints. Cysteine, being a source of sulphur, may also be helpful in forming synovial fluid.

** Sodium alginate (algin) tremendously impairs calcium absorption in rats.[17] If it does so in humans, its use should probably not be encouraged.

Research by Gerald R. Bratton et al.[22a] suggests that thiamin may be useful in preventing accumulation of lead in the body. They administered vitamin B₁ in animals by injection[22] or orally[22a] and found it prevented tissue buildup of lead. On the contrary, Bratton, as part of the group of Lyle B. Sasser et al.,[22b] found that the tissue of rats injected with thiamin showed a two-fold increase in lead at 24 hours after dosing but returned to normal 24 hours later. R. T. Louis Ferdinand et al.[22c] similarly reported that thiamin caused an increase of the lead in the blood and bone of rodents after lead injection, but the effect disappeared two days later. Sasser et al.[22b] speculate that a lead-thiamin complex may have formed, preventing prolonged binding of lead by body tissues. Other members of the vitamin B complex (niacin, B₁₂ and folic acid) have also been suggested for treatment of lead poisoning. S. J. S. Flora et al.[22d] found administering the B complex to rats beneficially reduced lead-induced inhibition of various enzymes. Animals are not people, but thiamin and other members of the vitamin B complex may have value in conjunction with chelation therapy.

The belief that vitamin C may diminish lead toxicity is widespread and some research supports the idea. However, at least four studies prior to 1978 cast doubt on it. Then, in 1978, Marcel E. Conrad and James C. Barton[23] observed that ascorbic acid actually *enhanced* absorption of lead. Keeping the issue confused, S. Niazi and J. Lim[24] and also Flora and Tandon[24a] reported on experiments with rats showing that ascorbic acid does aid in the urinary clearance of lead. In science the last word on a given subject is never said. However, seldom does the answer to what should be a simple question remain in such a confused state over a period of many years.

A. E. Sobel and M. Burger,[25] in rat experiments, showed that vitamin D given with lead enhances lead absorption, causing a rise in blood lead. However, after lead administration stops, vitamin D, by causing a rise in serum phosphate, depresses the blood level of lead.[26] Vitamin D (in the form of 1,25 dihydroxycholecalciferol) increases intestinal absorption of lead (and also, of course, of calcium and phosphorus). However, high blood lead concentrations reduce the circulating levels of 1,25 dihydroxycholecalciferol, perhaps because lead concentrates in the kidney where this vitamin D metabolite is formed.[27] The body's shutting down production of 1, 25 (OH)$_2$D and thus lead absorption when excessive lead is already circulating is an interesting example of "body wisdom."

Selenium, according to F. L. Cerklewski and R. M. Forbes,[28] at low levels (i.e., .015, .05 and .50 ppm) is mildly protective for rats, but they found that rats given 1.0 ppm showed enhanced lead retention. Orville A. Levander et al.[28a] also found that selenium was slightly effective against lead poisoning in rats, but only if the selenium level was so high as to be toxic itself. They found, however, that vitamin E was far more valuable in protecting against lead. Flora et al.[29] confirmed that selenium can partially prevent or reduce the toxicity of lead during simultaneous administration. However, they speculated that a more toxic effect of lead might appear after cessation of selenium administration when the lead-selenide compound that was formed begins to dissociate and release its lead. (They speculated this also happens in the use of selenium to detoxify cadmium through the formation of, and subsequent dissociation of cadmium selenide.)

Removal of lead from the body is important, of course, but the detoxification process should not be viewed simplistically. When calcium, magnesium, zinc and other supplements are used to remove lead from the bone (where it resides probably rather innocuously) the procedure could result in dangerous levels of lead reaching the kidney and nervous tissue. This process should, therefore, not be hurried by taking unusually massive amounts of the detoxicants. More research is needed to develop a reliable protocol for lead removal by such means. In developing such a protocol it should be kept in mind that estrogen (for example in the form of the birth control pill) enhances the body's uptake of calcium and this could, in turn, result in accelerated, perhaps dangerously accelerated, removal of lead from bone. (For that matter, research should be done to determine if the Pill, while beneficially increasing absorption of calcium, may detrimentally increase absorption of undesirable metals.)

Mercury

Another poison, mercury, probably enters the body primarily from food and air. However, Hal H. Huggins, D.D.S., disagrees and believes that the amalgam in dental fillings is a major contributor to mercury poisoning. In fact, Huggins reports that cases of physical problems such as arthritis have been corrected by replacing dental amalgams with gold. Others[29a,b] have also reported on allergies resulting from amalgam fillings. Daniel H. Rosen,[29c] who maintains that the evidence supports Huggins' position, reminds us that if one decides to have his amalgam fillings removed, the removal process itself exposes one to increased mercury exposure that may increase toxicity symptoms for several days.

Henry A. Schroeder[29d] states, on the contrary, that dental fillings pose only a minor threat of mercury poisoning. Furthermore, a review of the problem by N. W. Rupp and G. C. Paffenbarger[29e] concluded that amalgams do not present a significant hazard to the patient. They admit, however, that "mercury in dental amalgam has contributed to allergic responses in the form of dermatitis in susceptible individuals." (If you are one of these mercury-sensitive persons, the possible fact that amalgams do not present a significant hazard may seem quite irrelevant.) The American Dental Association held (at least they held in 1971) that amalgam fillings posed a possible threat to the dentist but not to the patient.[29e]

The March 1986 issue of *Consumer Reports*[29f] discussed the antiamalgamists and the *Amalgameter*. This is an invention of Huggins that he maintains indicates the danger posed by any given filling. *Consumer Reports* takes a negative view of the supposed dangers of dental amalgam poisoning except for those allergic to mercury. Nevertheless, a more recent study by David W. Eggleston[29g] indicates that dental amalgam may adversely affect the quantity of T-lymphocytes. Furthermore, in 1986, Magnus Nylander,[29h] after doing necropsy studies, reported that dentists (and to a lesser degree patients with many amalgam fillings) had high levels of mercury in their pituitary glands.

The burning of coal, and mercury's use in paper, ointments, fumigants and fungicides are some of the ways this poison enters the environment. Mercury compounds in interior paints and the subsequent vaporization of the mercury in closed rooms is another source of contamination. Mercury's use as a coating for seeds to prevent growth of mold is another threat to our well-being. Anyone planning to sprout seeds should obtain them from a health food store rather than from other sources where the assumption is being made that they will be planted. Mercury's increasing industrial use has produced more contamination of air and water, leading, in turn, to greater amounts in fish. Fish have the ability to concentrate metals, beneficially in the case of zinc, but detrimentally in the case of mercury. It is reported, however, that sufficient selenium is generally present to protect icthyophagists. Nevertheless, Don R. Swanson,[29i] writing in 1986, points out that lakes in areas exposed to acid rain may be contaminated with methyl mercury sediment. He suggests that it would seem prudent to avoid eating fish from such lakes.

Mercury concentrates primarily in the brain, liver and in the kidneys and can be a threat to various body functions. Some symptoms are: emotional disorders, convulsions, tremors, swollen gums and loss of sense of pain and of appetite. Fatigue may also be present since mercury interferes with glucose entering the cell.

Mary M. Gilbert et al.[30] have discovered, in experiments with hamsters, that vitamin E has protective potential against chromosome damage caused by mercury. Some studies have suggested that selenium may also provide useful protection against mercury. J. Alexander et al.[31] reported that selenite offered good protection against mercury poisoning in rats even if the selenite was given three days after the mercury. K. Sumino et al.[31a] found that selenite injected into female rats resulted in free methylmercury being lowered in the kidney, but there were no changes in other organs. Mercury-selenium interaction in rats was found, by Jadwiga Chmielnicka et al.[32] to result in increased accumulation of both elements in membranes of liver mitochondria. Jens C. Hansen and Preben Kristensen[33] reported that, under the influence of selenium, mercury was eliminated much more slowly from the body and accumulated in certain organs, e.g., the spleen. They say: "This means the beneficial effect of selenium in the case of chronic exposure is questionable as it may increase mercury accumulation." If you have a possible mercury problem (as shown by hair analysis), it seems best to not unduly increase your selenium intake.

Sometimes vitamin C is also recommended to remove mercury from the body. However, studies by S. Blackstone et al.[34] and by D. R. Murray and R. E. Hughes[35] indicate that vitamin C *increases* tissue levels of orally administered mercury. Furthermore, Yohko Fujimoto et al.[35a] have found that methylmercuric chloride (MMC) stimulates lipid peroxidation in rabbit renal cortical mitochondria and that the peroxidation by MMC is increased markedly by ascorbic acid.

Strontium and Strontium-90

Strontium, immediately below calcium in the periodic table, sometimes acts like that metal. Eugene F. Ferraro et al.[35b] reported that either in high concentrations can stimulate bone formation. Several epidemiological studies (cited by M. E. J. Curzon and P. C. Spector)[35c] show that strontium tends to reduce dental caries, although animal studies have been equivocal. Curzon and Spector[34b] have reported that treatment of the teeth with a solution of strontium chloride and EDTA was associated with a subsequent reduction in enamel solubility. They also reported an association between strontium in drinking water and low caries prevalence in man. Curzon and Spector[35d] found that strontium may be associated with the inhibition of dental caries over and above the effect achieved through fluoridation. Their data (although sparse since it was developed from only seven towns, all in Wisconsin) suggests that caries prevalence may decrease with increasing strontium concentration in drinking water up to a level of 5-6 mg./liter. Then a *reverse effect* seems to set in and at higher strontium concentrations the effect is reduced or eliminated.

Valuable though strontium may be, the radioactive isotope strontium-90 is a body poison which has become a source of concern since the advent of the atomic bomb. Some plants will concentrate strontium and, if these plants are subsequently eaten by cattle, contaminated milk will result. Strontium-90 accumulates in various organs, but especially in the lungs and the kidneys. Still greater concentrations are found in bone, as might have been expected, since strontium has some of the properties of calcium. Calcium, pectin, kelp and various forms of alginates may help protect the body from strontium-90.

Cadmium

The last of the poisonous metals we will consider here is cadmium. Metallothionein, a protein containing variable percentages of cadmium and zinc (as much as 5.9% cadmium and 2.2% zinc), has been found in human kidneys and liver.* The large amount of cadmium in this compound argues in favor of a functional role for this metal. However, in anything beyond minor amounts it seems mandatory to consider it a poison. K. Schwarz and J. Spallholz[37] have, in fact, reported that cadmium enhanced the growth rate of rats. They infer that, at levels far below toxic amounts, cadmium may be essential. Perhaps apropos of cadmium's possible status as a quasi nutrient is a report of Ronald H. Jones et al.[38] This group found that when rats were injected intravenously with human gamma globulin, an injection of cadmium (.6 mg./kg.) initiated 14 and 7 days prior to the antigen injection enhanced and suppressed antibody synthesis, respectively.

Cadmium is directly associated with many types of cancer but, in an epidemiological study of men and women in 27 countries, dietary cadmium was found to be inversely related to the presence of liver cancer.[39] The theory of the *reverse effect* suggests that we be on the lookout for possible beneficial effects of cadmium at low levels that might act to cure the conditions brought on at the higher levels. Likewise, with lead, mercury and other "poisons."

---

* Metallothionein can exist as a copper-binding as well as a cadmium- and zinc-binding protein. It has been isolated from various tissues.[36]

Cadmium accumulates to some degree in the liver, arteries and lungs, but primarily in the kidneys and in the testes. A high concentration of cadmium relative to zinc may be implicated as a possible cause of hypertension according to Henry A. Schroeder.[40] Dr. Schroeder has also pointed out that in the kidneys of Americans there is an average of about 16 mg. of zinc to 11 mg. of cadmium, a ratio of 1.5. In the kidneys of primitive Africans the ratio is a much more healthful 6. The ratio in beef kidney is about 40 and pork kidney 72. Whereas in laboratory rats that were fed a low-cadmium diet the ratio was 464-500, in other rats fed cadmium to the point they developed hypertension the ratio was about 1 to 1.7. Note how close this ratio in *sick* rats (1 to 1.7) approximates that of the *average* American (1.5). Introducing zinc into the diet is perhaps an easier way to increase this ratio than trying to reduce cadmium intake (although this should be worked at also, especially through consumption of foods containing only low amounts of cadmium or those having a high zinc/cadmium ratio. It should be noted, however, that D. G. Beevers et al.[41] believe that reports of a cadmium-blood pressure link may be confounded by a failure to allow for cigarette smoking habits of the subjects who were studied. Then too, as we noted in connection with zinc, Joachim Manthey et al. have reported that cadmium does not seem to be a major factor in elevating human blood pressure. On the other hand, Stephen J. Kopp and Thomas Glonek[42] presented new evidence that cadmium may contribute to human hypertension. Aijiroh Tokushige et al.[42a] have recently shown that cadmium exerts a substantial inhibitory effect *in vitro* on the Na, K-ATPase of disrupted vascular smooth-muscle cells (but has no demonstrable effect on the Na-K pump in intact vascular smooth-muscle cells). Furthermore, H. A. Schroeder[42b] reported that 117 normotensive Americans who died in accidents had far less cadmium in their kidneys than 17 hypertensive Americans who died similar deaths. On the other hand, the fact that several studies cited by Luciano C. Neri and Helen L. Johansen[42c] reported cadmium workers do not suffer excess hypertension argues, I think, that cadmium presence in the kidney of hypertensives is a concomitant, but not causal, phenomenon. It seems to me that cadmium is probably either a real but perhaps minor factor in hypertension or, depending on its level, may be subject to a *reverse effect* that leads to the seemingly contradictory conclusions.

The seminiferous tubules of the testes of animals seem to be especially sensitive to cadmium poisoning, a condition which can result in sterility. Cadmium seems to inhibit the testicular blood supply. No sterility resulted when adult female animals were exposed to high levels of cadmium. Underwood,[42d] however, reported that when young female rats were maintained in a permanent state of estrus and exposed to high levels of cadmium, massive hemorrhagic necrosis occurred in nonovulating ovaries.

Cadmium, like zinc, has the ability to stimulate growth of human prostatic epithelium at low concentrations. Mukta M. Webber,[42e] during 1986, published a study relating to isolated prostatic cells that had been removed from human tissue at the time of surgery for prostatic hyperplasia. These cells were grown in a serum-free medium. Webber found that zinc chloride stimulated cell proliferation up to a maximum of 10^{-8}M. Then, at 10^{-7}M a *reverse effect* set in and zinc chloride became inhibitory and then toxic at concentrations between 10^{-5} and 10^{-4}M. Cadmium chloride stimulated cell proliferation between 10^{-9} and 10^{-7}M concentration. Then, at 10^{-6}M a *reverse effect* became effective and proliferation was inhibited with toxicity occurring at a concentration of 10^{-5} to 10^{-4}M. An increased incidence of prostatic cancer has been noted in men exposed to cadmium. This involvement in carcinogenesis may be related to cadmium's ability to replace zinc in the prostate.

Cadmium, which interferes with some enzyme systems requiring zinc, often occurs in the same foods that are rich in zinc. Henry A. Schroeder[43] shows an interesting table giving the zinc/cadmium ratio of various foods. A high ratio is, of course, desirable, as we have already indicated. Nuts, oysters, legumes, root vegetables and cereals have an especially high ratio. (However, if the oysters are from polluted waters they could contain considerable amounts of cadmium, which would make the ratio much lower.) Dairy products (perhaps because milk is stored in galvanized cans), margarine and other fats and oils all have a low ratio. Leafy vegetables and some fruits (with their exposure to contaminants in insecticides and in just ordinary air) also generally have a low ratio. However, orange juice (perhaps because the skin provides protection against contamination) has a very favorable ratio of 73. Whole rye and oatmeal have a very high, but white bread has an extremely low, ratio. Dr. Schroeder does not report on the zinc/cadmium ratio of raw honey. However, refined honey has a very undesirable ratio of just a little over 1. Lump sugar rates even poorer at a little under 1, whereas blackstrap molasses has a more favorable ratio of 10. Coffees of various types are shown in Dr. Schroeder's tables as having variable but generally undesirable ratios. Teas rate better in this regard (but of course could be bad for other reasons). Dry cocoa has a high ratio of 79, but if this were mixed with low-ratio milk, the resulting drink would probably rate about like coffee. Whiskey, gin and brandy have undesirable ratios of about 1, while wine at 17 and beer at 33 are more favorable (ignoring, of course, all factors other than the zinc/cadmium ratio). Grape juice, with a ratio of 44 (compared to wine's 17) gives my teetotaling readers some ammunition to use against those of us who like wine.

Dr. Schroeder warns, by the way, that food stored in galvanized containers may absorb cadmium. Acid drinks left in galvanized pails or ice trays may lead to acute cadmium poisoning. Galvanized and (astonishingly) even copper water pipes, according to Dr. Schroeder, may also provide a source of contamination and he expresses the opinion that cadmium is likely to be more readily absorbed from water and other fluids than from foods. Many types of canned foods, particles from auto tires and polluted air (especially in large industrialized cities) are other sources of cadmium. The lungs of smokers contain deposits of cadmium and this cadmium is thought to be one of the causes of emphysema. Whether we smoke or not, zinc will help protect us against cadmium poisoning, including protection not only of the lungs, but of the seminiferous tubules of the testes. Using vitamin B_1 to form a thiamin-cadmium-iron complex may be a possible means of treating cadmium poisoning. [43a] Vitamin C was reported by Benjamin M. Sahagian et al. [44] to depress the uptake of cadmium, whereas its transport was enhanced. Selenium is highly effective in combating cadmium toxicity. Iron, copper and protein may also be useful in protecting the body from this poison. On the other hand, vitamin D exacerbates a cadmium problem.[20]

In spite of all the negative things that are known about cadmium, could it have any redeeming value? At the present time this may seem to be a ridiculous suggestion. However, in the previous chapter it was pointed out that selenium increases the concentration of cadmium in the testes of male rats and mice, thus implying the formation of a possibly beneficial selenium-cadmium complex. Furthermore, a study by Masayoshi Kanisawa and Henry A. Schroeder[45] found that some male (but not female) rats fed cadmium lived longer than the controls. (Cadmium *increased* the life span of the longest-lived rats but *decreased* the life span of most of the animals.) Perhaps cadmium in minor amounts will eventually earn some status as a nutrient, but as of now we are quite right to try to minimize its presence in the body.

Chelation Therapy

If cadmium, lead or other heavy metals are a problem, your doctor, if he knows of chelation therapy (also called chemo-endarterectomy), may suggest using it. A metal chelator such as EDTA, DTPA or penicillamine is administered in a solution via slow intravenous infusion. A series of perhaps 20 such infusions may be given at the rate of 2 per week over a period of 10 weeks. The procedure is designed to chelate the unwanted metals for subsequent removal via the urine. This technique is reported to work wonders in effecting the removal of heavy metals from the body. Chelation therapy has also been used for reducing heart valve calcification and for many other applications.

Those interested in chelation therapy will want to read "Chelation as a Mechanism of Pharmacological Action" by Maynard B. Chenoweth,[46] "Synthetic Chelating Agents in Clinical Medicine" by Theodore N. Pullman et al.,[47] "The Medical Applications of Chelating Agents" by Murray Weiner[48] and "Chelation: Stability and Selectivity" by Arthur E. Martell.[49] "The Pharmacology of Some

Useful Chelating Agents" by Harry Forman[50] will also be useful. Forman reports on the toxic complications of the various EDTA-type chelating agents and how the occurrence of such toxicities can be minimized. A book, *The Scientific Basis of EDTA Chelation Therapy* by Bruce W. Halstead,[50a] is useful as an introduction to the subject.

R. P. Agarwal and D. D. Perrin[51] discuss a computer-based approach to chelation therapy. They point out limitations of the most widely used chelating agent, EDTA, and warn that prolonged treatment, even at low levels of this agent, leads to zinc deficiency. Agarwal and Perrin comment on the advantages of the thiosemicarbazones as chelating agents. Gerald R. Peterson[52] has also reported on the negative effects of chelation therapy using EDTA. Testing various chelating agents in mice, Louis R. Cantilena, Jr. and Curtis D. Klaassen[52a] reported on how they affected the excretion of some of the valuable minerals—zinc, copper, magnesium, manganese, iron and calcium. The undesirable excretion of essential minerals along with the toxic ones should be, of course, a major concern when using chelation therapy.

Physicians using chelation therapy will be interested in an article entitled "A Hypothesis for the Selection of Chelate Antidotes For Toxic Metals" by Mark M. Jones and Mark A. Basinger.[53] The authors divide therapeutic chelating agents into six categories and discuss the structural features of these agents and their relative effectiveness depending upon the objectives. In addition, the use of meso-dimercaptosuccinic acid (DMSA), of the sodium salt of 2, 3-dimercapto-1-propanesulfonic acid (DMPS), of 2, 3-dimercaptosuccinic acid or of dimercaptopropane sulfonate has been the subject of various studies and reviews.[53a-d] Obviously, the tendency of some physicians to always employ EDTA regardless of the problem must be viewed as being rather simplistic. Such physicians will benefit from studying the works cited here. A related article, "Computer Simulation of Chelation Therapy" by Peter M. May and David R. Williams,[54] will also be of value.

A new technique, *mixed ligand chelate therapy,* has been developed by Drs. Jack Schubert and S. Krogh Derr of Hope

College, Holland, Michigan.[55] This method, which employs salicylic acid in addition to EDTA or DPTA, has thus far been used only on animals. It seems to be far superior to former chemo-endarterectomy methods. Regrettably, a lengthy interval is sometimes involved before the results of animal research are applied in human therapies. (Technical note: A *ligand* is defined as any ion or molecule that by donating one or more pairs of electrons to a central metal ion is coordinated with it to form a complex ion or molecule. The Nobel laureate Henry Taube of Stanford (California) University showed that a ligand temporarily forms a bridge between ions. Its bond to the original metal ions later breaks away to cause a movement of the electrons. In *mixed ligand chelate therapy* ligands are formed between the unwanted metals and salicylic acid, as well as between the metals and EDTA, or DPTA; hence the term "mixed ligand.")

W. H. Betts et al.[55a] have studied the *in vitro* effects of three chelating agents (EDTA, penicillamine and bishomopenicillamine) on hyaluronic acid (HA). As the concentration of the chelator increased, the viscosity of 1 mg./ml. hyaluronic acid solutions in an enzyme system at first decreased and then, at a chelator concentration of about 1.0 mM, showed a *reverse effect* and increased (Figure 3). Additional studies will be needed to gauge the effects of this phenomenon *in vivo* and its possible implications in chelation therapy.

The general opinion of chelation therapy in the medical community is that it has an undesirable risk/benefit ratio. However, there are many physicians throughout the world who, to the contrary, believe that this therapy has considerable merit. T. J. Baily Gibson,[56] writing about chelation therapy, says: "It has been shown to relieve angina and to improve ECG tracings. It has been shown to improve claudication and to benefit small vessel disease in the diabetic. Recently it has been shown to produce significant improvement in the left ventricular ejection fraction. One of its mechanisms of action may be related to its ability to increase mitochondrial ATP production. It lowers intracellular calcium and thus another of its mechanisms of action may be, like the calcium antagonists, on the slow channel. It has also been shown to mobilize

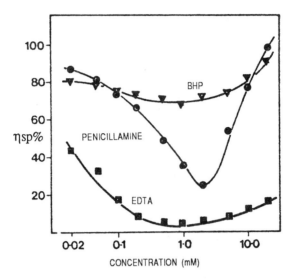

Figure 3. Effect of increasing concentrations of penicillamine
(●), bishomopenicillamine (▼) and EDTA (■) on viscosity of 1
mg./ml. HA solutions in the enzymatic system (η sp %).
Reproduced from W. H. Betts et al., *Agents and
Actions* (1984) 14, no. 2: 283-290, by permission of the
publisher, Birkhäuser, Verlag Basel.

atherosclerotic plaque in vitro." Dr. Gibson cites references to support
each of his statements.

Chelation therapy is probably valuable, but only if two caveats are
observed: (1) Since the therapy removes the good as well as the bad
minerals, a supplement program must be employed; and (2) the old
dietary mistakes must be corrected or the arteries will once again
become choked and a new series of chelation treatments may be
needed.

"Method of Investigation: As soon as we have thought something, try to see in what way the contrary is true."
— Simone Weil, *Gravity and Grace* (New York: G. P. Putnam's Sons, 1952)

"Were science the mere description of what is immediately observable, poetry, rather than physics, would be the better science of the brook."
— F. S. C. Northrup, "The Function and Future of Poetry," *Furioso* (1941) Vol. 1, no. 4

"The great difference, intellectually speaking, between one man and another is simply the number of things they can see in a given cubic yard of world."
— Gilbert Murray, *Tradition and Progress*, (London: George Allen & Unwin Ltd., 1922)

CHAPTER 9

The Antioxidants—Keys to Superlongevity?

I would much prefer to eat a food that has a preservative in it than to eat a food that is rancid. Interestingly, it seems that not everyone agrees. W. L. Porter[1] says that, "Most consumers, judged by taste panel results, prefer the fresh to the rancid odor and taste, although some have so adapted to poorly stored products that they prefer slight rancidity like that of the carrots in dried soup mixes." If that seems strange, imagine how a traveler from outer space might react to the fact that some of us prefer the product of "rotten" grapes to the fresh grapes themselves.

Preservatives are not necessarily bad. Many preservatives are completely natural products. The antioxidant properties of numerous herbs and spices have been reported. Some examples are extracts from cocoa shells, coffee (caffeic acid and quinic acid), oats, barley, malt and rice bran. Yellow, brown and green pigments from teas functioned in margarine, vegetable oil and bakery products at .1% to .2% basis fat as well as BHT did at the .02% level.[1a] V. Bracco et al.[1b] have reported that extracts of rosemary and sage are particularly strong antioxidants. In their study, these extracts showed antioxidant activity comparable to that of the much-maligned BHA and BHT. The antioxidants carnosol, rosmanol and rosmaridiphenol that are found in rosemary leaves act as antioxidants in lard with an effectiveness comparable with BHT.[1c] Recently, R. E. Kramer[1d] identified gallic acid and eugenol as major antioxidants in clove. The comparative antioxidant activity of nine different herbs and of eight different naturally occurring antioxidants is given by Winifred M. Cort.[2] Extracts of dried cranberry leaves containing a tannincatechin complex have been reported to be effective in preventing oxidation of butter, milk, margarine and hydrogenated fats.[2a] Antioxidants sometimes act, not merely additively, but synergistically. S. J. Bishov and A. S. Henick[2b] reported, for example, that when aqueous extract or oregano was coupled with BHA, 30% of the antioxidant effect was due to synergism.

Natural antioxidants can, in fact, be prepared from herbs and patent #3,732,111 by D. L. Berner and G. A. Jacobson covers the process of such an extraction from rosemary. The process, however, makes use of such carcinogens as benzene and ethylene dichloride. If remnants of these chemicals are left in the "natural" product, I'd prefer to take my chances with BHA or BHT. Among the other antioxidants (which we will not treat here) are osage orange, vegetable oils, algae, fermented soybean products such as tempeh, amino acids, cinnamic acids (in soybeans and elsewhere), peptides, polyphenols, sodium benzoate, coenzyme Q_{10} (one of the class of chemicals called *ubiquinones*) and menadione (vitamin K_3). As we shall soon see, preservatives may in some cases preserve not only our food but preserve us as well.

Many of the flavonoids, which we met in Chapter 6, are good antioxidants. Albert Szent-Györgyi and his associates,[2c] in 1936, claimed that some of the flavonoids acted as a vitamin which they called "vitamin P." This "vitamin" does not seem to meet the current definition of a vitamin (although, as pointed out in Chapters 6 and 4, respectively, vitamins C and D perhaps do not either). Nevertheless, while the bioflavonoids may not be indispensable for maintaining life, they have health-promoting qualities. Of the over 800 flavonoids thus far discovered, the flavonol and catechin subgroups provide the best protection for vitamin C, the anthocyanidins being less efficient in this regard, while the flavanones and flavones have very little power to protect ascorbic acid. Flavonoids also provide strength for the capillaries in addition to acting as antioxidants.

The strongest of the flavonoid antioxidants are quercitin, myricetin, quercetagetin and gossypetin.[2d] The flavanones (e.g.,hesperidin) are inactive.[2d] Among foods, red and yellow (but not white) onions[2e] and also garlic are especially rich in flavonoid antioxidants. The improved keeping quality of foods containing onions, garlic and various herbs and spices is due to their antioxidant content. Soybeans, potatoes and sweet potatoes are among the other foods that contain antioxidants.[2f] Some of the naturally occurring flavonoids—centaureidin, eupatin, eupatorein, tetramethyl-scutellarein (from thyme), quercetagitrin and patulitrin—are active cytotoxic agents *in vivo* and *in vitro* against various human carcinoma cells.[2d] R. E. Henze and F. W. Quackenbush[2g] reported the presence of antioxidant(s) in tomato lipids, although they did not characterize it (them) beyond a determination that two fractions exist (the primary antioxidant and a synergistic substance). They found the tomato antioxidant(s), in terms of keeping time in lard, to be superior to NDGA, gossypol and ∝-tocopherol. I speculate that the substance(s) may belong to the flavonoid family.

The antioxidants not only postpone aging through acting to reduce cross-linking, as covered in Chapter 2, but also through reducing the formation of peroxides from lipid (fatty) substances due to some of the body's own enzymes or to the action of free radicals. A free radical, as we know from earlier chapters, consists of a nonionic atom or group of atoms having one or more unpaired electrons. They are, therefore, highly reactive intermediaries in chemical reactions. They fly about and cause destruction of cells or, short of complete destruction of the cell, the free radicals may damage its DNA or RNA so that defective proteins are produced. Normally, the presumed biofeedback mechanism of the cell's membrane (one of perhaps some 100,000 biofeedback mechanisms in the body) senses the presence of nearby cells, thus causing the cell to refrain from dividing and proliferating into nonavailable space. If free radicals damage a cell's membrane, the membrane's delicate mechanism will no longer "tell" the cell about the presence of other nearby cells and the cell may rapidly divide and proliferate—a phenomenon we call *cancer.* Understanding this postulated biofeedback mechanism might be a key to cancer control.*

Free radicals can develop during the cell's mitochondrial respiration and self-oxidation of biological chemicals. Free radicals are formed, and have just a transient presence, when oxygen and various minerals in the cell are exposed to x-rays, cosmic rays, radioactivity, microwaves or ultraviolet light. They can be formed also when nitric and nitrous oxides, excessive polyunsaturated fatty acids, alcohol, rancid foods, ozone, tobacco smoke,** automobile exhaust and other pollutants react with cellular material. Experimental evidence of the *in vitro* free-radical scavenging efficiency of 21 antioxidants and their mixtures is given by Richard D. Lippman.[24]

Free radicals interact with fatty acids to produce lipid radicals, which can then form peroxy radicals by adding oxygen molecules. One such free radical of oxygen is called *superoxide.* Superoxide is generated during autoxidation of many substances relevant to body chemistry such as epinephrine, tetrahydropterins, leukoflavins, thiols, reduced ferredoxines and hemoglobin. It is generated by some oxidative enzymes, and by mitochondria, chloroplasts and by phagocytes.[25] One superoxide ion is even generated for each oxidized molecule of vitamin C.[26] Among other pro-oxidants that give rise to various free radicals are peroxides and heavy metals such as iron and

---

* Carcinogen-induced chromosomal breakage is decreased by antioxidants. Raymond J. Shamberger et al.[23] reported that chromosomal breaks in leukocytes induced by dimethylbenzanthracene were greatly reduced by the presence of antioxidants. The reductions were as follows: ascorbic acid, 31.7%; BHT, 63.8%; sodium selenite, 42.0%; and dl-alpha tocopherol, 63.2%

** According to William A. Pryor[23a] there are 10^{16} free radicals/puff in cigarette smoke.

copper. According to K. H. Eberhardt,[2h] as cited by F. A. J. Thiele,[160c] even sodium chloride can act as a pro-oxidant.

Furthermore, J. U. Skaare and T. Henriksen[26a] have reported that a free radical exists in ethoxyquin and we have seen that other antioxidants such as vitamins C and E also form free radicals. Perhaps free radicals are present in all antioxidants and may be essential to their function.

Antiaging Experiments

Nonnatural preservatives are not necessarily bad, nor are natural preservatives necessarily good. (Goodness and badness in biological chemicals, as suggested by the theory of the *reverse effect,* must necessarily be related to dosage.) Anyway, experiments suggest that the antioxidants BHA (butylated hydroxyanisole) and BHT (butylated hydroxytoluene) help prevent cross-linking of molecules within our cells, including DNA and RNA elements, and preventing this cross-linkage may be a factor in promoting longevity. Cross-linking of the body's collagen, causing it to become firmer and less pliable, is a normal process during infancy and youth. Although at maturity the body produces enzymes to slow this process, generally the firming of the collagen continues to occur. As the collagen stiffens, the capillaries may be constricted, oxygen, water and other nutrients have difficulty getting to the cells, the skin becomes leathery and we are aging *fast.*[*] The beneficial antiaging action of the antioxidants may also involve improved immune function. (Immune responses generally decline with age.) Antioxidants are thought to affect immunity through modulation of the arachidonic acid cascade.[3b]

---

[*] Leonard Hayflick[3] cites a listing of J. Bjorksten[3a] of naturally occurring known cross-linking agents found in living tissue: "aldehydes, sulfur cross-linkages, alkylating and acylating agents, quinones, free radicals, antibodies, polybasic acids and their esters, citric acid, polyvalent metals and cross-linkages formed as integral parts of reacting molecules such as conversion of specific lysine residues to aldehydes which react to cross-link collagen." The Hayflick article[3] provides a good review of current theories concerning the aging process.

The experiments of Denham Harman, M.D., Ph.D., Professor of Medicine and of Biochemistry of the University of Nebraska,[4] have shown that the mean longevity of mice receiving .50% by weight of BHT in the diet increased 30% to 40%. In another experiment Harman[5] found a 45% increase in longevity in mice receiving .50% by weight of BHT in their diet and a 29.2% increase in mean life span through the use of 1.0% by weight of another antioxidant, 2-MEA (2-mercapto-ethylamine hydrochloride).* In a different experiment, Dr. Harman[7] reported an amazing 72% increase in mean life span in mice by adding to their diet .25% of another antioxidant, ethoxyquin (1,2 dihydro-6 ethoxy-2, 2,4 trimethylquinoline). This superiority of ethoxyquin (Santoquin®) is shown in Figure 1.[7a]

Robert R. Kohn[8] reported on experiments with BHT and 2-MEA that resulted in findings similar to those of Harman. The antioxidants increased the mean survival times of animals, but the maximum life spans were not increased beyond optimal control values. Kohn concluded that the antioxidants he studied did not inhibit the processes which determine maximum life span, but do inhibit some harmful environmental or nutritional factors that cause longevity to be suboptimal.**

A more recent study by Neal K. Clapp et al.[9] substantiates the earlier work of Harman and Kohn in regard to mean life span extension in mice through the use of BHT. Dr. Clapp's group fed young adult mice for the rest of their lives a 75% BHT supplement in their standard laboratory chow. They found, as had Harman and Kohn, that maximum life spans of about 1,100 days were not extended, but the BHT treatment increased the mean survival time a maximum of 206 days in males and 174 days in females. Brief (three-week treatments) with BHT during early adult life also extended the mean life span. Dr. Clapp points out that, although the

---

* The related compound, 2-mercaptoethanol, enhances the immune responses of lymphocytes both *in vivo* and *in vitro*.[6]

** The protocol of this experiment, with 20 animals housed per cage, may be open to criticism. I should not, however, single out Kohn's work for such a comment—it is a common flaw of numerous experiments.

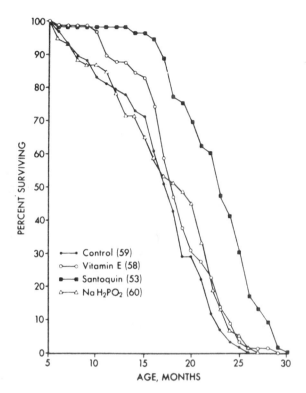

Figure 1. NZB male mice: effect of dietary antioxidants on the percent surviving as a function of age. Reproduced from Denham Harman, *Age* (1980) 3: 64-73, by permission of the author.

reason for the life-lengthening effect of BHT is not obvious, it is known that BHT beneficially modifies diethylnitrosamine-induced squamous forestomach cancers (but not lung tumors) in laboratory animals. It is also known that BHT modifies certain induced colon tumors in mice. An alternative explanation, as Dr. Clapp explains, is that BHT may either protect against loss of some not yet identified dietary factor or that it improves the metabolic-utilization process.

Antioxidants may not only act as life extenders but, as has been mentioned, they have been shown to sometimes inhibit tumor development. The effect of .3% BHT on inhibition of DMBA-induced mammary tumors in both polyunsaturated and saturated fat diets was studied by M. Margaret King and Paul B. McCay.[9a]* Their interesting results (Figure 2) clearly show that tumor growth, whether or not inhibited by BHT, proceeds at a faster rate on a diet containing large amounts of polyunsaturated fat (20% stripped corn oil) than one containing large amounts of saturated fat (18% coconut oil and 2% linoleic and methyl esters).** Note that polyunsaturated fat is a greater threat than is saturated fat for the development of mammary tumors (at least in rats). Like so many other studies, this research was done using uncooked fats. What if cooked fats were used? Would animals fed cooked fats (which contain many mutagens and carcinogens) show increased tumor formation at earlier elapsed times? I speculated in Chapter 3 that if, instead, tumor formation rates turned out to be lower when animals were fed cooked fats it would be a highly interesting example of the *reverse effect* and would send cancer research in a new direction. At least some of the carcinogens in cooked fats should, it seems to me, display a *reverse effect*.

Earlier, McCay et al.[9b] reported that BHA and alpha tocopherol, which inhibited DMBA-induced tumor growth in rats fed commercial rations, were not effective when given in purified diets. McCay et al.[9b] suggested that the purified diets may have contained some factor or factors which rendered the antioxidants ineffective. Later, King and McCay[9a] speculated that, whether or not the suppression of tumor activity is due to the antioxidant property of antioxidants, the suppression may be applicable only to certain carcinogens, the properties of which require the formation of reactive radicals. Furthermore, in some cases antioxidants can *increase* the probability that cancer may occur and thus exemplify the theory of the *reverse effect*. Hanspeter Witschi et al.[9c] reported that injections of 400 mg. BHT/kg. dissolved in corn oil *increased* the incidence of

---

* Both the group on the high polyunsaturated-fat diet and that on the high saturated-fat diet were fed 46% sucrose. Interestingly, other groups fed a low-fat diet with and without BHT—and in which fewer tumors developed—were fed huge amounts of sucrose to the extent of 64% of their diet!

** As in so many other studies, the rats were housed in groups of 10 or 15 per cage, which might conceivably have affected results.

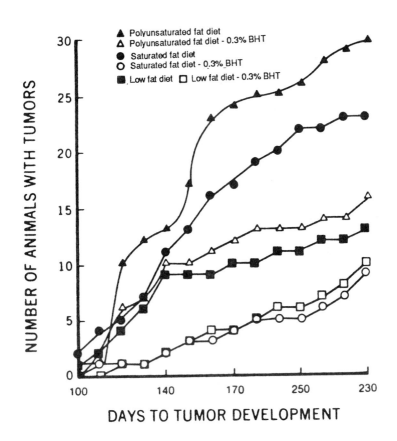

Figure 2. Comparison of the relative rates of mammary tumor development in the three dietary groups with and without BHT supplementation. DMBA-induced mammary tumor incidence in female Sprague-Dawley rats on various diets as a function of time (age of rats). Treated rats received 10 mg. DMBA in 1 ml. stripped corn oil at 50 days of age. Tumors include palpable ones as well as those not palpated which were discovered at necropsy. Only neoplasms which had been verified to be adenocarcinomas are included in this chart. (N = 30 for all groups). Abscissa, age of rats (days). Reproduced from M. Margaret King and Paul B. McCay, *Cancer Research* (1983) 43 Supp: 2485s-2490s, by permission of the copyright owner, Cancer Research, Inc., and of the authors.

lung cancer in mice. They stressed that their results do not nullify conclusions that dietary BHT is not harmful and may be beneficial by preventing some forms of carcinogenesis.

Dr. Denham Harman[10] has compared the life span of controls with male mice started on antioxidants at the age of six weeks. He fed the mice either alpha tocopherol acetate (vitamin E), ethoxyquin (Santoquin®) or sodium hypophosphate. After 25 months just 1.7% of the controls survived compared with 3.4%, 3.2% and 5.0%, respectively, among those fed the antioxidants. The mice were housed 10 to a cage (instead of individually as is proper) and so the dominant mice probably got the most food and some of the others may have starved.

Other experiments have shown that the offspring of rats fed antioxidants, starting one month before they were mated and continuing during pregnancy and until their offspring were weaned, had extended average life spans. Harman reported[11] that adding either .5% or 1.0% 2-MEA, 1.0% sodium hypophosphite or .1% BHT to the diets of mice during pregnancy and until their offspring had been weaned increased the average life span of the male offspring by 18.2%, 26.9%, 19.2% and 13.5%, respectively, compared with controls. The data for the female offspring was parallel to that of the males. These experiments show the importance of diet during pregnancy for producing long-lived offspring.

At least some of the increased longevity of animals that has been achieved through use of antioxidants is likely due to the effect of free-radical reaction inhibitors on the immune response. Denham Harman et al.[12] found that vitamin E had a greater effect than ethoxyquin (Santoquin®) on humoral responses (i.e., those relating to circulating antibodies, the globulin molecules that attack invaders). However, ethoxyquin was determined to be superior to vitamin E in fostering cell-mediated immunity (which relates to lymphocytes sensitized to destroy invaders).

Most of the life extension in animal experiments has involved an increase in mean life span, but the maximum life span of an experimental group is generally not improved. However, A. Comfort et al.[13] found that ethoxyquin increased not only the mean life span of mice but extended their maximum life span from 711 days to 887 days in males and from 722 days to 907 days in females.

We should mention another antioxidant, 2-dimethylamino-ethanol, known as DMAE and as deanol. DMAE not only acts as an antioxidant but, through stabilizing the membrane of the cells' lysosomes, it can prevent the often poisonous contents of the lysosomes from leaking—a major cause of aging, especially in later life. Administering DMAE to mice in their drinking water, R. Hochschild[14] reported median survival time increases of 30.8% and 49.5% over controls. Even more exciting, he found that maximum survival time of mice given DMAE was increased by 36.3% over controls. Using the related p-chlorophenoxy-acetate ester of DMAE (also called centrophenoxine and meclofenoxate), Hochschild[4a] reported median, mean and maximum survival time increases of 29.5%, 27.3% and 39.7%, respectively. The great increase in maximum life span (not just median life span) makes the Hochschild studies especially interesting.

Earlier, Carl Pfeiffer,[15] had reported that DMAE was a possible precursor of brain acetylcholine. If true, it could be expected to enhance cholinergic neurotransmission. Then C. C. Pfeiffer and H. B. Murphree[16] and Murphree et al.[16a] published studies on human research with DMAE. In a double-blind study, a group of students was given DMAE over a three-month period and then compared with a similar group given placebos. The DMAE group showed increased muscle tone, increased ability to concentrate and better sleep habits with generally less sleep being required. They also experienced a mild euphoria and a tendency to develop a more outgoing personality. No changes were noted in heart rate, blood pressure, muscle strength, hand steadiness, vital capacity or body weight. The DMAE stimulation reportedly lasted 24 to 48 hours after discontinuing the dosage and was not accompanied by any depression. Overdosage produced such adverse effects as insomnia, muscle tenseness and muscle twitches. Other studies have shown that DMAE also acts, as does niacin and as negative ion generators are reported to do, to prevent blood sludging (the tendency of erythrocytes to clump together and thus inhibit the transmittal of oxygen). Still other studies by K. Nandy and G. H. Bourne[17] and by K. Nandy[18] have shown that the DMAE ester removes the age-pigment lipofuscin from cells.*

DMAE is made naturally by the body and a good food source is reported to be fish. Powdered DMAE in the form of the bitartrate is available without prescription from several sources. (In powdered form it may, however, be difficult to measure and to limit the dosage to the 10-20 mg. amount that has been reported useful.) DMAE, even though it is a natural substance produced by the body and available in food, may have a pharmaceutical effect when taken as a supplement. DMAE can have toxic effects which may include headache, muscle tension, insomnia, pruritus and postural hypertension, and the substance should never be given to patients with grand mal epilepsy.[21] Other side effects of DMAE (listed as deanol), as well as abstracts of various relevant studies, can be found in *Martindale—The Extra Pharmacopoeia.*[21a] Obviously, if DMAE is to be used it should be used thoughtfully. "Thoughtfully" means asking how the health of a person taking it should be assessed. "Thoughtful" also means asking if this substance should be taken by "normals."

Another antioxidant, dihydroergotoxine (which is known as DHET and is the active compound in Hydergine®) has also been shown by K. Nandy and F. H. Schneider[22] to reduce formation of lipofuscin. The scientists speculate that, since lipofuscin seems to be a product of wear-and-tear within the cells, DHET probably works by reducing this intercellular action associated with aging.

The Superoxide Dismutases

We saw earlier, in Chapter 7, that superoxide dismutase (SOD) exists in copper-zinc and in manganese forms. The enzyme, Cu Zn

---

* Lipofuscin is variously called wear-and-tear pigment, chromolipid, hemofuscin, ceroid, lipochrome, cytolipochrome and cytolipofuscin. The words are not all synonymous, however. Lipofuscin contains more zinc than does ceroid, but ceroid contains more calcium, iron and copper![19,20]

superoxide dismutase (SOD), formerly called *erythrocuprein* or *hemocuprein* and known to geneticists as *tetrazolium oxidase*,[27] is found in the body's cells and is also available in food and as pills for sale by health food suppliers. Superoxide dismutase is a very unusual enzyme whose substrate is an unstable free radical which generally has an extremely short lifetime. Technical details regarding SOD's structure and mechanism of action are discussed by Giuseppe Rotilio et al.,[28] by Roger H. Pain,[29] by John A. Tainer et al.[29a] and by William C. Stallings et al.[29b] SOD functions by destroying excessive amounts of superoxide. Regrettably, although SOD is widely available in foods, in pills and as sublingual drops, it is probably worthless when taken by mouth. In fact, Irwin Fridovich,[29c] who is the codiscoverer of SOD, says, "oral SOD cannot be at all efficacious. This is the modern equivalent of snake oil." A study with mice has demonstrated that dietary supplementation of Cu Zn SOD showed no effect on Cu Zn SOD or Mn SOD activity in the intestine, liver, kidney or blood.[29d] A subsequent murine study by S. N. Giri and H. P. Misra[30] confirmed that dietary SOD does not affect tissue levels.

Some research indicates that small amounts of peptides may enter the bloodstream without being digested.[30a-s] However, this process is currently limited to molecules far smaller than SOD and, furthermore, may be accompanied by allergic symptoms. (An azopolymer film for protecting peptides, such as insulin and vasopressin, from digestion in the stomach and small intestine for release in the colon is, however, under development.)[30t] Like other enzymes, SOD in foods or pills is broken down to amino acids and then assimilated along with amino acids that are derived from other proteins in foods. SOD is a very common protein in the body so, even if SOD from a pill could survive the stomach acid and the duodenal alkalinity and pass the brush border of the intestines into the bloodstream and then into the cells (which it can't), the amount would be just a drop in the ocean since it is made inside the cells. It seems possible, however, that SOD might be useful in the excipient of vitamin pills or as an additive to various foods as a preservative.

Although the zinc-copper type of SOD contains both zinc and copper, a zinc deficiency[31] has little or no effect on the activity of

SOD in the red blood cells.* If we optimize our copper intake we should be able to produce adequate amounts of SOD. Effective, injectable forms of superoxide dismutase—known by the nonproprietary name of orgotein, assigned by the United States Adopted Names Council—are available to veterinarians as Palosein® and to physicians as Ontosein®**

Two major types of SOD have thus far been discovered: the blue-green Cu Zn SOD found in bovine and in human red blood cells and a red-colored Mn SOD found in the cell's mitochondria. Mn SOD had originally been thought to be concentrated only in the mitochondria. However, it has been shown that Mn SOD is also found in the cell's nucleus in the human liver and that up to 50% of this SOD lies outside the mitochondria.[33] Another Mn SOD has been found in the matrix of bacteria and a fourth type of SOD, containing iron, has also been found in bacteria. It exists in *Escherichia coli* that are present in the intestinal tract.[34] Since *E. coli* can cause such conditions as peritonitis and infections of the urinary tract, this use for iron, while beneficially protecting the bacteria, is probably detrimental to the bacteria's host, man.***

---

* The zinc site in the SOD molecule can be vacant or can be occupied with cobalt or mercury and the SOD activity will remain. However, no replacement for the copper has ever been discovered that would preserve the SOD activity.[31a,b] (On the other hand, Koiche Ishigame and Yoshikazu Nishi[31c] have cited the work of R. Boyne and J. R. Arthur[31d] showing a surprising relationship between copper, SOD activity and the killing power of granulocytes that is unlike the finding in the case of erythrocytes. Although granulocytes from steers fed copper-deficient diets had less killing ability than those of steers fed a copper-supplemented diet, the SOD activity of the copper-deficient group was the same as the SOD activity of the copper-supplemented group. Thus, poisoning of granulocytes by superoxide may not be the cause of decreased killing ability.)

** The half-life of SOD in the blood is only about six minutes, while its pharmacological effect lasts three to six hours.[31e] This suggests that SOD operates through an indirect effect. (SOD is rated in terms of McCord/Fridovich units, a measure of enzyme activity first defined by Joe M. McCord and Irwin Fridovich.[32] One such unit is approximately equal to .3 micrograms of pure Cu Zn SOD.)

*** Interestingly, while *E. coli* under anerobic conditions contain just the iron variety of SOD, when exposed to oxygen a Mn SOD and a new, previously undescribed, SOD (that appeared to contain iron) as well as catalase and peroxidase were reportedly induced.[35] Such a "chemistry laboratory" within a bacterium and the "knowledge" of how to use it makes it easy for me to invoke in myself a mystical mood—the mood that says, "God is a better chemist." Actually, other examples of SOD biosynthesis in response

The Cu Zn and Mn forms of SOD have several iso-enzymes.[37,38,39] Wheat germ, for example, contains a mangano-superoxide dismutase and two CuZn SOD isoenzymes. These latter enzymes have approximately the same molecular weight (about 31,000 daltons) but have different amino acid compositions. The leaf and stalk of the wheat plant were found to contain just one of these enzymes and it is not known what additional function the second enzyme might serve in the seed.[40] Stefan L. Marklund[40a,b] has recently found a new isoenzyme called EC-SOD. The EC-SOD molecule contains four copper atoms and possibly four zinc atoms and it has a molecular weight of about 135,000 daltons.[40a,b] EC-SOD is the major superoxide dismutase in the extracellular fluids of mammals and may also be found in tissues.[40a,b] As already noted, there also exist cobalt and mercury derivatives of bovine superoxide dismutase.[41,41a] The SOD family of enzymes continues to grow.

The total Cu Zn superoxide dismutase content of the body is estimated at 3,900 mg. (with Mn superoxide dismutase total contents about half that much). Although there is in the body about one-half as much Mn SOD as there is Cu Zn SOD, the dismutase activity of the Mn variety is far less than that of the Cu Zn SOD. Mn SOD, at least in rats, accounts for just 8% of the total dismutase activity while Cu Zn SOD accounts for 92%.[42] Human liver contains more of each than do other tissues, and SOD activity of the lymph is more than twice that of serum.[43]

There are also artificial superoxide dismutases such as copper salicylate complexes. One of these, copper aspirinate, may have a beneficial effect on arthritic joints that is not merely that of an anodyne. In addition, R. Fantozzi et al.[43a] have reported that a new nonsteroidal anti-inflammatory drug, imidazole 2-hydroxybenzoate, after forming complexes with copper, displays significant superoxide dismutase activity. Furthermore, many copper chelates with various amino acids show superoxide dismutase activity. Ceruloplasmin itself has been found to act as a superoxide free-radical scavenger.[44] Ceruloplasmin and other copper compounds may be especially important

---

to increased oxygen or superoxide occur in yeast, potato slices, endothelial cells, rat lung, etc.[36]

when their levels are elevated as in acute infections or late in pregnancy. The marked increase in the levels of ceruloplasmin and of other antioxidants in those with rheumatoid arthritis was studied by U. Ambanelli et al. [45] Furthermore, Shiro Yamashoji and Goro Kajimoto[46] reported that ceruloplasmin has an antioxidant effect independent of the superoxide-scavenging activity. The fact that serum and synovial fluid levels of copper compounds tend to be abnormally high in patients with rheumatoid arthritis* may be yet another example of "body wisdom." We must always resist the temptation to conclude that a phenomenon coexistent with a disease is causal.

Even copper alone may act as a superoxide dismutase. (In fact, Irwin Fridovich believes the reason that many copper chelates are active in this way is that the chelating agents are sufficiently weak to allow some free copper to be present in solution.) Copper (valence 2) effectively catalyzes the dismutation of superoxide in an acid pH but loses its activity as the pH is raised to neutral or to the alkaline range.[47] However, free copper is virtually nonexistent in biological systems because of the ubiquitous chelating agents.[48] Furthermore, although various copper compounds and also the iron compounds transferrin and ferritin have superoxide dismutase activities, such activity is at a very low level—respectively, 40,000, 350,000 and 330,000 times lower than that of the human blue-green enzyme, Cu Zn superoxide dismutase.[49] Nevertheless, Ira M. Goldstein[44] points out that Cu Zn SOD is almost exclusively an intracellular enzyme and so ceruloplasmin may be an important circulating scavenger of superoxide. (The extracellular fluids contain insignificant amounts of SOD or catalase. Thus, even if copper compounds show relatively little superoxide-scavenging ability, their action may be important at locations such as the joints. By combating superoxide—which, if allowed to exist

---

* Simultaneously, the copper content of the liver declines.[40a] Since the liver absorbs ingested copper quite rapidly and is the body's only copper-storage organ, its low level of copper in rheumatoid arthritis suggests that excretion may be excessive.[46a] On the other hand, the production of superoxide (which in excess is combated by SOD and other copper compounds) tends to be low in rheumatoid arthritis patients (and extremely low in those with Felty's syndrome—rheumatoid arthritis, splenomegaly, lymphadenopathy, granulocytopenia and anemia).[46b,c] Perhaps the level of copper compounds is high simply because they have not been "used up" neutralizing superoxide.

could react with hydrogen peroxide to form the inflammatory hydroxyl radicals—copper compounds may help protect the joints from arthritis.)[*] Manganese ions are also reported to have SOD activity and to be a very effective inhibitor of lipid peroxidation.[50] Thus, the number of entities showing SOD activity may be quite large.

Superoxide dismutase is especially effective in scavenging superoxide molecules (each of which has an unpaired electron) in a simultaneous oxidation-reduction process called *dismutation*.[**] (Two molecules of superoxide combine with two atoms of hydrogen to yield hydrogen peroxide and oxygen. Superoxide dismutase will catalyze the reaction and the enzymes catalase, glutathione peroxidase and myeloperoxidase will convert the hydrogen peroxide to oxygen and water.[51] It should be noted that superoxide, by reacting with the hydrogen peroxide has the ability to form the hydroxyl radical (OH) and this, rather than the superoxide itself, may be the more toxic agent.[***] (Charles W. Garner[51a] reported that peroxidase, in the form of horseradish peroxidase, potentiates the oxidative capacity of hydrogen peroxide and superoxide. Garner noted that oxidation of fatty acids by peroxidase took place at very low concentrations of hydrogen peroxide. Since peroxidase either neutralizes superoxide and hydrogen peroxide or potentiates their action, it seems to me that a *reverse effect* is involved.)

Hydrogen peroxide can also produce hydroxyl radicals through interacting with ferrous iron. Hydroxyl radicals may subsequently react with many physiological entities, including nucleic acids, proteins and lipids. Singlet oxygen, which can also be destructive, may be produced through the nonenzymatic dismutation of two superoxide radicals or through the interaction of superoxide and hydrogen peroxide.[53a] Superoxide dismutase, thus, through catalyzing the

---

[*] Not everyone agrees that SOD is an effective anti-inflammatory agent.[49a]

[**] The odd electron of a free radical is generally represented in the chemical formula as a dot. For example, superoxide is shown as $O_2^{\cdot -}$

[***] Ascorbic acid also reacts with hydrogen peroxide and helps protect against toxicity due to this and other hydroperoxides.[52] Ascorbic acid was shown by C. Winterbourne to accelerate the iron-catalyzed formation of hydroxyl radicals from hydrogen peroxide.[53]

dismutation reaction, can help destroy excess superoxide radicals which, as we have seen, generate the potentially more destructive hydroxyl radical and may also produce the possibly dangerous singlet oxygen. Thus, superoxide dismutase serves a vital body function and may be of importance in slowing the aging process. However, as we will see shortly, SOD in excess could exhibit a *reverse effect* and might be detrimental to body systems.

Richard G. Cutler[53b] has published an interesting graph (Figure 3) relating the tissue SOD activity ÷ the specific metabolic rate (SMR) to the species' maximum life span potential (MLSP). The MLSP of various species increases as the SOD activity per specific metabolic rate in the liver increases. A similar relationship exists for the antioxidant uric acid (urate), as will be shown later in this chapter, and also (but less strongly) for vitamin E and the other antioxidants DHEA, choline, glucose and cholesterol. The relationship, however, does not hold for ascorbic acid. (Thus, Cutler speculates, ascorbic acid may *not* have played an important role in determining the long, maximum life span potential of humans.) Curiously, a negative relationship exists between species' longevity and such tissue antioxidants as catalase, glutathione and glutathione peroxidase.[53b*] I speculate that perhaps this argues, under the doctrine that "ontogeny recapitulates phylogeny" (the history of the individual repeats the history of the species), against excessive selenium being a prolongevity mineral. Even though use of supplemental selenium is touted by many of the life-extension theorists, I think this finding of Cutler, specifically in regard to glutathione peroxidase, suggests that a high concentration of selenium does not promote longevity. (Why? Because selenium does much of its work through its enzyme glutathione peroxidase which we have just noted is negatively correlated with longevity.) In regard to SOD, Jerome L. Sullivan[53c] has argued against the proposal by

---

* We noted earlier, in Chapter 2, that large amounts of serum vitamin E will tend to depress the levels of other antioxidants. Perhaps large amounts of catalase, glutathione and glutathione peroxidase might similarly reduce the levels of more useful antioxidants. Cutler[53b] has stated, however, that "we have found two-fold differences between human individuals for urate, alpha-tocopherol and carotene, and yet there is no evidence of associated differences in their aging rates."

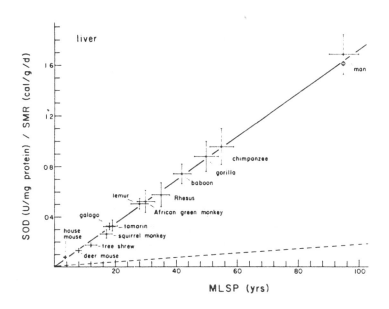

Figure 3. Correlation of superoxide dismutase (SOD) activity per specific metabolic rate (SMR) against MLSP in liver of primate and rodent species. Correlation coefficient, r = 0.998. Reproduced from Richard G. Cutler in *Free Radicals in Molecular Biology, Aging and Disease,* ed. D. Armstrong et al. (New York: Raven Press, 1984) pp 235-266, at 245, with permission of the publisher and of the author.

Julie M. Tolmasoff, Tetsuya Ono and Richard G. Cutler[53d] that the ratio of SOD to the specific metabolic rate as a function of maximum life span potential provides evidence that longevity may be partially controlled by SOD activity. Sullivan's article, Cutler's reply [53e] and a subsequent paper by Ono and Shigefumi Okada[54] make interesting reading.

Superoxide and Other Antimicrobial Systems

Before going any further, I think we should say a good word about superoxide and the other oxygen entities—which I have cast in the role of archdevils. Nature is not in the habit of creating worthless entities. Free radicals, such as superoxide, are important intermediaries in some biological reactions as we have already noted. As I reported in Chapter 6, the superoxide free radical is also produced when ascorbic acid undergoes oxidation. Sperm have been found, in experiments with rabbits, to produce superoxide and the sperms contain superoxide dismutase for protection against lipid peroxidation that would otherwise be caused by the superoxide.[54a] Phagocytic cells (neutrophils, monocytes, eosinophils, macrophages and large granular lymphocytes called killer cells*) give off superoxide in what is called the "respiratory burst."[55a,b] Current opinion is that superoxide itself is not directly responsible for microbicidal action and tissue damage. Instead, this antimicrobial activity and damage to tissues are probably caused by superoxide derivatives: hydrogen peroxide, hydroxyl radical and possibly singlet oxygen.[55b,c,d] Then too, polymorphonuclear neutrophils and macrophages not only give off superoxide, hydrogen peroxide and hydroxyl free radicals, but also generate hypohalous acids and N-chloroamines as one of their mechanisms by which they destroy bacteria.[56,56a**] These leukocytes consume oxygen which is transformed by membranous NADPH oxidase to superoxide.[59,60,61]

The burst of oxidative metabolism which accompanies phagocytosis by polymorphonuclear leukocytes is believed to be initiated at the cell surface. [62] This oxidative burst is accompanied by the generation of thromboxanes and prostaglandins from membrane fatty acids.[63,63a] (The generation of prostaglandin E as a function of

---

* Natural killer cells not only provide protection against viruses, but they may be involved in fetal growth. A retrospective survey by Kunihiro Okamura et al.[54b] found a negative correlation between natural killer cell activity during pregnancy and the birth weight of the baby. (There were no differences in natural killer cell activity between toxemic and nontoxemic women.) Natural killer cells may also be a factor in the regulation of hemopoiesis (formation of blood)[54b] and surveillance against neoplasia.[54b-d,55]

** Superoxide can also be produced by white blood cells when stimulated by immunoglobulins and by either mast cells or basophils when stimulated immunologically or nonimmunologically.[57,58] Superoxide by itself is only weakly bactericidal, but in combination with hydrogen peroxide produces the hydroxyl free radical which is highly toxic to many types of microorganisms. In rheumatoid arthritis patients (especially those with Felty's syndrome) there is an increased prevalence of infections. One of many causes may be the significantly lower rate of superoxide production in such persons.[55c,58a]

time is shown in Figure 4.)[63a] When engulfment is completed the respiratory burst ceases.[63f] The respiratory burst occurs in leukocytes not only during phagocytosis but also under various chemical influences.[63b]* Thus, it is conceivable that one could overload the body with SOD to the point of interfering with ascorbic acid oxidation, sperm production, thromboxane and prostaglandin generation, as well as with phagocytic action, and the latter has, in fact, been shown to occur. Research by Henry Rosen and Seymour J. Klebanoff[65] found that the bactericidal activity of the acetaldehyde-xanthine oxidase system was inhibited not only by SOD but by catalase, mannitol, uric acid and other chemicals. Bactericidal activity can also be inhibited if superoxide activity is diminished through disease. Studies were made of superoxide production from two patients with chronic granulomatous disease (a disease related to mature, granular leukocytes called *granulocytes*). In patients with this disease, superoxide production was found to be greatly reduced.[66]

The body has many antimicrobial systems, some oxygen-dependent and some oxygen-independent.[67] A major oxygen-dependent system is mediated by one of the peroxidases, *myeloperoxidase* (MPO), which catalyzes oxidation of a number of substances to hydrogen peroxide. (Myeloperoxidase is the peroxidase of neutrophils and the green color of pus is due to its presence.) The MPO system usually uses iodide from the thyroid hormones, thyroxine or triodothyronine, as a cofactor.** Sometimes other halides (bromide or chloride) act as cofactors instead of iodide and so this microbicide system is sometimes called the

---

* *In vitro* studies show that the addition of collagen, thrombin or arachidonic acid to human platelets also is accompanied by an oxidative burst associated with the generation of oxygenated products of arachidonic acid. Neil M. Bressler et al.[64] have reported that experiments using SOD and catalase indicate that endogenously produced superoxide radicals had no effect on collagen-induced oxygen burst or aggregation. They concluded that, since the oxidative burst in leukocytes is associated with the generation of superoxide radicals and hydrogen peroxide, it follows that leukocyte and platelet oxygen bursts are associated with different cellular functions.

** E. Siegel and B. A. Sachs[68] have reported that the uptake of iodide by human leukocytes is 1,200 times greater than the uptake by erythrocytes. They also reported that the leukocyte uptake of iodide by hypothyroid subjects is less than that of euthyroid (normal) subjects which, in turn, is less than that of hyperthyroids.

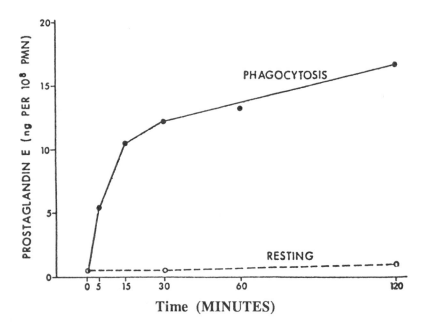

Figure 4. Prostaglandin release with respect to time. Polymorphonuclear leukocytes (PMN) were incubated at 37° C without (resting) or with (phagocytosis) zymosan. Each point represents the mean prostaglandin release of three different observations. Reproduced from Robert B. Zurier and Donna M. Sayadoff, *Inflammation* (1975) 1, no. 1: 93-101, with permission of the publisher, Plenum Publishing Corp., and of the authors.

myeloperoxidase-hydrogen peroxide-halide system. Stephen J. Weiss et al.[69] suggest that myeloperoxidase may have a role to play in the production of hydroxyl free radicals by granulocytes. However, whether or not this is true, once hydrogen peroxide exists, the hydroxyl radical can be produced through interaction with superoxide, via the Haber-Weiss reaction, or through interaction with ferrous iron as proposed by Kuo-Lan Fong et al.[70]* (The process by which ferrous

---

* The ability of phagocytes to generate the hydroxyl ions needs further study. However, they combat invaders by releasing other oxygen-derived metabolites (perhydroxyl radicals and

iron can reduce peroxide to hydroxyl radical is known as Fenton's reaction.)[71a] Leukocytes can use the MPO system not only to destroy bacteria, fungi and viruses, but also to destroy tumor cells. The role of hypochlorous acid in monocyte- and granulocyte-mediated tumor cell destruction has been discussed by Stephen J. Weiss and Adam Slivka.[72]

Other oxygen-dependent antimicrobial systems, unrelated to MPO, still rely on the production of hydrogen peroxide, superoxide anion, the hydroxyl radical and/or singlet oxygen to do the microbial killing. Still other of the body's systems for killing invaders that are not concerned with oxygen or any of its products involve lactic acid, lysozyme, lactoferrin and granular cationic proteins. The operations of these various systems is poorly understood, but an excellent review is presented by S. J. Klebanoff.[73] Generally, the body works on the principle of overkill and various systems will be operating to control microbial growth. When the various systems shut down or operate inefficiently, severe infection results.

Thus, we have seen that the superoxide free radical and other oxygen entities can have both a good and a bad aspect. I presume, however, that our bodies are usually benefited through an increase in SOD production by optimizing the body's copper-zinc ratio and its stores of manganese. Why? Because when polymorphonuclear neutrophils and macrophages come into proximity of body tissue that is low in SOD, problems may develop. The synovial membrane in the region of the joints is an example of such tissue. Without adequate protection supplied by antioxidants, as Joe M. McCord[74] first reported and as Robert A. Greenwald and Wai M. Moy[75] further developed, arthritis may occur. The disease process develops as the hyaluronic acid of the synovial fluid is destroyed through the action of the superoxide, hydrogen peroxide, hydroxyl radicals or singlet oxygen produced as a result of the phagocytic action of the various types of white blood cells. It is interesting to note that polymorphonuclear neutrophils contain some SOD and lymphocytes contain far more to protect the cells themselves from the superoxide being

---

hydrogen peroxide) and   the products of their intermediate reactions—HOCl, HOI and HOBr.[71]

produced.[76] M. I. Salin and J. M. McCord[77] have, in fact, reported that granulocytes commit suicide following phagocytosis as a result of the cytotoxic action of their own superoxide. By the way, *in vitro* experiments show that each human neutrophil, exposed to a stimulus, can generate enough superoxide to lyse (disintegrate) ten human erythrocytes if not protected by SOD.[78] Thus, the SOD in erythrocytes serves a vital function indeed.

The Hydroxyl Free Radical

It now appears, however, that superoxide is probably less of a threat to body health than had been earlier believed. It has been known for many years that two free radicals of superoxide combine with two ions of hydrogen to form normal oxygen and hydrogen peroxide. This is known, as we have noted, as the *dismutation reaction* and superoxide dismutase acts as its catalyst. As we also noted earlier, the hydrogen peroxide (unless denatured promptly with catalases or peroxidases) can then react with another superoxide free radical, in a process called the Haber-Weiss reaction,* to produce the highly active hydroxyl free radical. It is this hydroxyl ion, rather than the superoxide, that seems to cause at least some of the beneficial and also some of the damaging phenomena of which superoxide has been credited and accused. Hydroxyl radicals have never been observed directly in living organisms but their presence is inferred by some oxidative reactions and by the blocking action of hydroxyl radical scavengers.[80] Sodium benzoate and mannitol will scavenge the hydroxyl free radical but not superoxide.[81] If either sufficient superoxide dismutase is present to quench the superoxide or enough catalase is there to convert hydrogen peroxide to water, the possibly

---

* The Haber-Weiss reaction is widely accepted as being the source of the hydroxyl radical. However, Gidon Czapski and Yael A. Ilan[79] argue that this reaction proceeds very slowly. They believe that most of the hydroxyl ions are formed through the reduction by superoxide of ferric iron bound to biological compounds. In accordance with their theory, the reduced (ferrous) iron then reacts with hydrogen peroxide to yield hydroxyl free radicals.

dangerous hydroxyl radical will be safely controlled even if its specific scavengers are absent.

An enzymic flux of hydrogen peroxide and superoxide has caused breaks in DNA, probably because of the hydroxyl ion that was produced.[82,82a] Thus, the hydroxyl ion may be a root cause of evolution. (When such changes occur today, we call them genetic defects.) Such changes may also be related to cancer. A study by B. D. Goldstein et al.[81a] has explored the possible role of reactive oxygen species in tumor promotion.

Among the other damaging effects of the hydroxyl ion, as we have already seen, is its ability to degrade hyaluronic acid which, unless controlled, can result in arthritis. (The degradation appears to be mediated by iron chelates and possibly by copper chelates as well. This degradation action gives us a reason, among others presented in Chapter 7, for not going "overboard" in supplementing the diet with these minerals.) Chromosome breakage is observed in various autoimmune diseases and is reported to be a constant finding in many collagen diseases such as lupus erythematosus. Chromosome breaks are also formed in about two-thirds of rheumatoid arthritis patients.[83]

Chromosome aberrations increase with the severity of disease and with age. However, SOD added to cultures of human lymphocytes reduced the frequency of these chromosome breaks.[83] Drs. I. Emerit and J. P. Camus, in France, have used SOD in treating various diseases associated with chromosome breaks. Intramuscular injection of SOD has reportedly resulted in striking improvement in cases of lupus erythematosus, dermatomyositis, Crohn's disease and systemic sclerosis.[84] One of the little-noticed benefits of ethyl alcohol, of the often-maligned preservative benzoate, and also of DMSO* is that of hydroxyl scavenging[85] and thus these chemicals might, it seems to me, be an aid in treating diseases associated with chromosome breaks.

---

* The scavenging of the hydroxyl radical would account for the reputation of DMSO in protecting the synovial membranes and thus alleviating arthritis and also for its reputation in the treatment of a long list of other diseases. Unless prescribed by a physician, however, DMSO is likely to contain contaminants that could threaten the body.

However, just as superoxide has not only dangerous but also has valuable properties, so too hydroxyl free radicals, hydrogen peroxide and also singlet oxygen may be of value to the body. Studies by Bernard M. Babior[86] and others have suggested that hydrogen peroxide, the hydroxyl free radical and singlet molecular oxygen (generated by the removal of the unpaired electron from superoxide)—these various entities that are produced from the degradation of superoxide—may be more powerful bactericidal agents than superoxide itself. Many of these oxygen byproducts may arise from reactions involving xanthine oxidase and we have already mentioned one such reaction.* Xanthine oxidase, to the extent it produces superoxide and hence the hydroxyl free radical and hydrogen peroxide, can kill the bacteria *Staphylococcus epidermis.* ** Either SOD or catalase stops the bactericidal action which suggests that the hydroxyl free radical is the bactericidal agent. Xanthine oxidase may also be a factor in killing the bacteria *Escherichia coli* which, although a normal inhabitant of the intestines, can cause peritonitis and infections of the urinary tract. In this case, however,

---

* Coffee, tea and cocoa contain methyl xanthines and xanthine oxidase is an enzyme used to metabolize those methyl xanthines. Is it not possible that large amounts of methyl xanthines (in the form of coffee, etc.) might stimulate extra production of xanthine oxidase? If so, would coffee, tea and cocoa drinkers need more SOD to neutralize the resulting superoxide? (However, as we will see later, coffee and tea contain antioxidants that might be able to neutralize any excessive superoxide.) Nevertheless, this may all be irrelevant if H. A. Simmonds et al.[86a] are correct. They maintain that, although mouse macrophages contain abundant xanthine oxidase activity, human peritoneal macrophages do not. The Simmonds' group relate that "xanthine oxidase activity is confined almost exclusively to the liver and intestinal mucosa in man." They go on to say, "It would seem unlikely that xanthine oxidase is of any significance *in vivo* to the generation of toxic superoxide radicals in man."

** Harold P. Jones et al.[86b] have presented evidence, however, that "xanthine oxidase is not a major superoxide-generating system in activated neutrophils." The production of superoxide by phagocytosing neutrophils seems primarily to be due to the activity of the plasma enzyme NADPH oxidase (nicotinamide adenine dinucleotide phosphate oxidase). By the way, P. Daniel Lew and Thomas P. Stossel[86c] found that calcium in micromolar concentrations (i.e., at concentrations likely to exist in macrophage cytoplasm) inhibited the NADPH-dependent superoxide generating activity of phagocytic vesicles. B. Halliwell and J. M. C. Gutteridge[86d] cite relevant studies by M. G. Battelli et al. [86e] and by E. Della Corte and F. Stirpe.[86f] Halliwell and Gutteridge say: "Although the enzyme xanthine oxidase is frequently used as a source of O_2^- in experiments *in vitro*, almost all the xanthine-oxidizing activity present in normal tissues is (due to) a dehydrogenase enzyme that transfers electrons not to O_2, but to NAD^+, as it oxidizes xanthine or hypoxanthine into uric acid." The parenthetical words "due to" are mine.

catalase (but not SOD) stops the bactericidal action, which suggests that hydrogen peroxide is the bactericidal agent.[87]

A related study by Manikkam Suthanthiran et al.[87a] showed that hydroxyl radical scavengers—DMSO, thiourea, dimethylurea, tetramethylurea, benzoic acid, ethanol, methanol and ethylene glycol—inhibited the activity of natural killer (NK) cells. (The NK cells were in preparations containing .1% monocytes or polymorphonuclear leukocytes.) Catalase and SOD either alone or in combination did not inhibit NK cell activity. Thus, it seems probable that the hydroxyl radical (possibly generated via the lipoxygenase pathway, as noted in Chapter 3) is vital for the cytotoxicity of natural killer cells. Obviously, the hydroxyl free radical has many valuable uses in body chemistry. It follows that hydroxyl radical scavengers, including DMSO, ethyl alcohol, benzoic acid and benzoate, may sometimes detrimentally affect the action of natural killer cells and other lymphocytes in warding off body invaders.

Therapeutic Possibilities of SOD

As we have already seen, SOD serves many useful functions in the body. According to Drs. C. Cohen and R. E. Heikkila of the Mt. Sinai School of Medicine in New York City, SOD protects the brain's neurotransmitter norepinephrine from destruction by superoxide. (A shortage of norepinephrine may lead to mental depression and lack of sex drive.) Injected SOD (orgotein) is reported to be useful for supporting heart tissue after a heart attack.[87b] Injected SOD has been used to successfully treat patients having radiation cystitis as a consequence of radiation therapy for carcinoma of the cervix.[88] SOD injected into the eyes of dogs is reported to have dissolved cataracts,[89] so it seems reasonable that an increase in SOD production, if we can make it happen, might offer prevention for humans. However, Jay Brainard et al.[90] reported, on the contrary, no clearing of cataractous lenses in dogs using injected SOD. Not alcohol as such, but superoxide (which oxidizes that byproduct of alcohol metabolism, acetaldehyde, to acetate) may be a cause of cirrhosis of the liver and perhaps SOD may offer protection.[91] SOD has been injected subcutaneously (the FDA guidelines prohibit intravenous infusions of protein) in premature infants with respiratory distress syndrome, meconium aspiration or similar diseases in an attempt to avoid bronchopulmonary dysplasia and a blind, controlled investigation is now underway.[92] SOD has also been reported as effective in treating fibrotic lesions such as are present in Peyronie's disease.[71a] The work of Karen S. Guice et al.,[92a] published in 1986, suggests that SOD may be useful in treating pancreatitis. Another 1986 study, this one by Karin Przyklenk and Robert A. Kloner[92b] and with dogs, indicates that SOD (plus catalase) may find human application in improving contractile function in cases of "stunned myocardium."

Cancer cells have been reported to produce superoxide in abundance, and so it seems possible that treatment of cancer should involve an attempt to achieve increased production of SOD, catalase and peroxidases. On the other hand, the seeming abundance of superoxide produced by cancer cells may simply be due to the lesser amounts of Mn SOD they contain. (Tumor cells generally have lowered Cu Zn SOD activity and always have lower Mn SOD activity.)[93] A cancer therapy might, therefore, involve purposeful increase of superoxide within the body. Normal cells, with their greater content of superoxide dismutase, could withstand the onslaught; cancer cells, less well protected, would be killed. Conversely, introducing SOD activity into cancer cells might be expected to enable them to assume at least some characteristics of normal cells, such as growth control. The key might be in already-synthesized copper dismutases of low enough molecular size to enter the tumor cell.[93] Obviously, some of these approaches to cancer control seem contradictory but suggest exciting research to come. To cite just one example of such research, Thomas W. Kensler et al.[94] reported that a low molecular copper compound with SOD-activity inhibited actions of a tumor promoter in mouse epidermis. Such inhibition implicates oxygen radicals in the tumor promotion process.* The role of superoxide and of SOD and other

---

* Bruce N. Ames,[94a] in a definitive article entitled "Dietary Carcinogens and Anticarcinogens," says: "A common property of promoters may be their ability to produce oxygen radicals. Some examples are fat and hytrogen peroxide (which may be

antioxidants in the promotion and inhibition of cancer is discussed by Larry W. Oberley.[95] Subsequently, Oberley et al.[95a] found that a low-weight compound, copper diisopropylsalicylate, has SOD-like activity and shows antitumor effects. They reported that glutathione partially reduced its antitumor potency. This led them to hypothesize that the antitumor effect may be due to production of hydrogen peroxide. Other interesting possibilities for free radicals in combating cancer have been suggested by T. L. Dormandy.[96]

SOD may also be valuable, as we have already noted, in preventing and reversing rheumatoid arthritis, osteoarthritis and many other degenerative diseases. Synovial fluid in the joints of arthritis-free persons contains superoxide dismutase, but the enzyme is apt to be in short supply where the joint is affected by arthritis. Drs. Joe M. McCord and Kenneth Wong[97] of the University of Alabama have reported that superoxide dismutase, as well as the enzyme catalase and the sugar alcohol mannitol, prevents the degradation of synovial fluid. Klaus M. Goebel et al.[98,98a] have observed that injected (note, *injected, not oral*) superoxide dismutase (orgotein) is effective in treating rheumatoid arthritis** and they cite references for its effectiveness

---

among the most important promoters), TCDD, lead and cadmium, phorbol esters, wounding of tissues, asbestos, peroxides, catechol, mezerein and teleocidin B, phenobarbital, and radiation. Inflammatory reactions involve the production of oxygen radicals by phagocytes, and this could be the basis of promotion for asbestos or wounding." Ames continues by referring to "complete" carcinogens—those that are both initiating mutagens (DNA-damaging agents) and promoters of carcinogenesis after the DNA damage has occurred: "Many 'complete' carcinogens cause the production of oxygen radicals; examples are nitroso compounds, hydrazines, quinones, polycyclic hydrocarbons (through quinones), cadmium and lead salts, nitro compounds, and radiation. A good part of the toxic effects of ionizing radiation damage to DNA and cells is thought to be due to generation of oxygen radicals, although only a tiny part of the oxygen radical load in humans is likely to be from this source." Fat is often considered to be a cancer promoter, as indicated here by Ames. It is relevant to note, however, that C. M. Hasler and M. R. Bennink[94b] published, in 1986, an interesting finding as a result of experiments with MBBA-initiated mammary carcinogenesis in rats. They discovered that "the fat (energy) control of the diet during initiation was more critical than during promotion."

** Serum of patients with rheumatoid arthritis, lupus erythematosus, scleroderma or other collagen diseases contains an agent which produces chromosomal breakage in lymphocyte cultures of healthy persons. The aberration rate is reduced to normal by adding SOD to the culture medium. The breakage factor may act on chromosomes by producing toxic oxygen species. Breakage factors also exist in plasma of irradiated persons and of infectious hepatitis patients.[99] The *reverse effect* of radiation causing and curing cancer (and thereby acting as a cause of future cancer) thus has a rationale.

in osteoarthritis. By the way, orgotein's anti-inflammatory effects may be due not only to its ability to neutralize superoxide, and hence the hydroxyl ion, but to its power to inhibit prostaglandin formation.[100]*

SOD may even be related to fertility. Mammalian spermatozoa are very sensitive to oxygen-caused damage and in fertilization the sperm's membrane integrity is essential.[100c] Protection of sperm against the action of free radicals is provided by various antioxidants such as vitamin E and SOD. Sezione di Palma[100c] studied the antioxidant activity of the semen of three bulls. The data, although sparse, seemed to indicate a decrease in antioxidant activity with age. Di Palma suggested that the measure of antioxidant activity could be a basis for semen evaluation prior to artificial insemination.

Superoxide dismutase activity was found to decrease with the age of any particular erythrocyte[101] but—and this is especially interesting—the SOD activity of erythrocytes was independent of the age of human donors from 1 to 98 years of age.[102]** If this should be proved true of other SOD production sites (various other cells including those in the liver) it would argue that it might not be of use to increase one's SOD production as one ages. Rather than SOD activity in the liver declining with age, however, Kozo Utsumi, et al.[104]

---

* On the other hand, B. Halliwell and J. M. C. Gutteridge[100a] observe that, "Few of these experiments are accompanied by controls with the apoenzyme, however, and without such controls it cannot be ruled out that the result is a 'nonspecific protein effect' rather than the consequence of scavenging O_2^-. SOD has a well-established anti-inflammatory effect in several animal model systems yet there is increasing doubt as to whether this is mediated purely by scavenging of O_2^-. If it is then all types of SOD should be effective, but Baret, Jadot and Michelson[100b] found that rat copper-zinc SOD, or manganese SOD, did not suppress carrageenan-induced paw inflammation in the rat, whereas human and bovine copper-zinc SOD did so."

** More recently, A. Vanella et al.[103] have reported that Cu Zn SOD decreases in the cerebral center of a rat as he ages. However, the activity of Mn SOD *increases* with age. Perhaps this finding is true for humans and would be an interesting example of compensation. If the brain is a "pacemaker" of aging processes, this could be a noteworthy discovery. The body's production of Cu Zn SOD is controlled by chromosome 21 and that of Mn SOD by chromosome 6. However, activity of Mn SOD at least sometimes seems to be regulated by Cu Zn SOD or superoxide as shown by the fact that Down's syndrome patients, who produce 50% more Cu Zn SOD, have only one-third as much Mn SOD.[93]

reported that SOD activity is low in the liver of fetal rats, even lower in newborn rats and then increases to reach maximum in 60 days. David I. Paynter and Ivan W. Caple[104a] subsequently found that Cu Zn SOD and Mn SOD activities increased in the liver, lung, heart, kidney and skeletal tissue as lambs grew into adult sheep.

More SOD (which destroys excess superoxide) would be needed as animals and humans age if it could be demonstrated that the production of superoxide increases with age. Studies with rats by Hans Nohl and Dietmar Hegner[105] indicated that aging did increase detectable superoxide. If these findings apply to men and women, then it may be useful to attempt to encourage production in our bodies of additional SOD as we age by attempting to optimize, via hair monitoring, our intake of copper and of manganese.* The catalytic activity of copper-zinc SOD, but not of manganese SOD, is inhibited by cyanide.[106] SOD, although inactive when taken orally, is often recommended by the laetrile enthusiasts and laetrile, of course, contains cyanide. Thus, laetrile, while inactive against cancer, may destroy endogenous SOD, which, if left undestroyed, could be an aid in combating cancer. Then too, an *in vitro* study by Kenneth D. Munkres[105a] showed that bovine SOD was activated from 6-to 45-fold by the guanyl nucleotides, 3' 5'-cyclic GMP or 5'-GMP. Munkres speculates that the guanyl nucleotides might activate SOD *in vivo* and perhaps be therapeutic.

Danger of Excessive SOD

Although SOD has many benefits, in keeping with the dictum of the golden mean, it can be overdone. Therefore, physicians employing orgotein should monitor their patients for the possible occurrence of *reverse effects*. Abnormally high amounts of SOD can interfere with metabolic oxidation processes (logical since some require

---

* It appears, according to a study by H. Moustafa Hassan and Irwin Fridovich,[104b] that SOD synthesis is controlled directly or indirectly by the intracellular level of superoxide. (Glucose, except where the pH is low enough to cause a shift to nonfermentative metabolism, depresses the synthesis of SOD.)[104b]

superoxide to proceed). The gene for making Cu Zn SOD is located on the human chromosome 21, as we have noted, and therefore Down's syndrome persons—those having trisomy 21 (i.e., three chromosomes instead of two at position number 21)—have 50% more Cu Zn SOD.[107,108] This excessive SOD leads to accelerated production of hydrogen peroxide and hence to hydroxyl and singlet oxygen radicals. The brain has low levels of enzymes, such as glutathione peroxide, for removing hydrogen peroxide and thus brain damage is likely to occur.[109]* Patients with psychiatric diseases—schizophrenia, paranoid psychosis and other psychoses—also tend to have increased levels of SOD. The attempt to find opposing chemotherapeutic agents is underway.[84]

Another possibly negative effect of too much SOD is that, at least *in vitro,* it can inhibit vitamin K-dependent carboxylation reactions.[111] Vitamin K reacts with oxygen to produce superoxide and the fact that SOD inhibits the carboxylation mechanism implies that superoxide is

---

* The selenium-based enzyme, glutathione peroxidase, is also increased in trisomy 21, although it is produced, not on chromosome 21 but on chromosome 3. It is speculated that this is a regulatory effect, i.e., what I have called "body wisdom," in reaction to the increased production of hydrogen peroxide by the excessive SOD. Pierre M. Sinet[109a] has reported that erythrocyte glutathione peroxidase is positively correlated with I.Q. in Down's syndrome patients. Sinet et al.[109b] have also found that Down's syndrome subjects have low plasma selenium. (This might have been suspected since it goes into the formation of glutathione peroxidase.) Regrettably, however, the increased production of glutathione peroxidase in the brain is not generally sufficient for complete protection. Would vitamins E and C, BHT and other antioxidants, such as small-molecule copper synthetics, be therapeutically useful? If trisomy 21 were discovered in a fetus via chorionic villi sampling or via amniocentesis and abortion were declined, could vitamins E and C and some of the other antioxidants of small molecular size administered to the mother be able to pass the placental barrier and then the fetal brain barrier so as to avoid fetal brain damage? A few of the persons having the Down's syndrome stigmata do not, however, produce SOD in amounts significantly above normal individuals[10] and this minority, therefore, might not be benefitted by my suggested therapy. The great majority of Down's syndrome patients do, however, produce excessive amounts of SOD and, as a consequence, the ability of their polymorphonuclear neutrophils to generate superoxide is not sufficient.[110a]   This probably accounts, at least in part, for the increased susceptibility of Down's syndrome patients to infections with certain microorganisms, including *Candida.*[110] Adults with Down's syndrome develop neurological characteristics identical to those of Alzheimer patients.[110b-e] Thus, any resolution of the problems relating to the elimination of or successful treatment of Down's syndrome might also have application to patients with Alzheimer's dementia.

needed for these reactions. Thus, we see another instance in which superoxide is useful and too much SOD may be harmful.

Antioxidants Control Lipid Peroxidation

We noted earlier that copper and its compounds exhibit antioxidant activity. However, copper also acts as an efficient catalyst for the combining of oxygen with organic compounds in free-radical reactions. Therefore, although copper is required to make the zinc-copper type of superoxide dismutase and serves other valuable functions in the body, it is important that its level not be elevated above body requirements. Dr. Harman has found that easily oxidized amino acids such as histidine and lysine (at levels of 1% in the diet) also increase free-radical reactions and may thereby reduce life expectancy. On the other hand, superoxide dismutase, BHA, BHT, 2-MEA and ethoxyquin, as well as DMAE, vitamins E and A, the ascorbates and ascorbic acid (as well as its fat-soluble form, ascorbyl palmitate), selenium (through the action of the enzyme glutathione peroxidase of which it is a constituent), manganese and zinc (each of which also work through their respective enzymes), and the sulphur-based amino acids, methionine, cystine and cysteine—all act to keep those free radicals under control so that either they inhibit peroxides from forming or else they battle those peroxides if they are formed.

Excessive peroxides detrimentally affect the function of the mitochondrial membrane of the cells and may even cause cell death. Although death and birth of cells is going on continually, this excessive death of cells can be thought of as being a vital factor in aging. The Krebs cycle and the electron-transport chain, that are vital to the manufacture of ATP, occur in the mitochondria, and lipid peroxides can deactivate some of the components involved. Thus, excessive lipid peroxidation is a serious threat to healthful longevity and antioxidants are essential to keep it under control.

As we have seen, a number of interesting animal experiments using various antioxidants have shown that they have great (continued on page 843)

Possible Dangers of Hydrogen Peroxide Ingestion

A dangerous recommendation to ingest hydrogen peroxide to aid in the treatment of cancer and other diseases is being circulated. Hydrogen peroxide certainly has uses in the body as a potent antimicrobial agent in conjunction with the myeloperoxidase system. But can it be effective against cancer if introduced orally? R. A. Holman[139] reported that hydrogen peroxide given orally to rats caused the disappearance of implanted adenocarcinoma. He also reported that oral dosages led to an improvement in human cancers. Kanematsu Sugiura[140] reported many failures to regress tumors in mice using both oral and injected hydrogen peroxide, but a higher injected dose had a moderate inhibitory effect on sarcoma 180 ascites tumor. That's not much, however, on which to base a human therapy.

Hydrogen peroxide is a natural product made by the body through the dismutation of superoxide with superoxide dismutase acting as a catalyst, but that does not make hydrogen peroxide safe. (T. M. Nicotera et al.[140a] note that several reports concluded that hydrogen peroxide may inactivate SOD.) It seems probable that if hydrogen peroxide were ingested it would most likely dissociate into water and oxygen before it could be effective. To the extent that it did not dissociate it could be dangerous. Putting hydrogen peroxide in your body could lead to depletion of body stores of the valuable enzymes catalase and peroxidase required to convert it to innocuous oxygen and water. We have already seen that hydrogen peroxide is a probable cause of brain damage in Down's syndrome patients. Hydrogen peroxide damages uptake mechanisms for the biogenic amines and is believed to destroy nerve terminals.[141] Raymond J. Shamberger et al.[142] observed that "marked damage of DNA has been induced with H_2O_2 (hydrogen peroxide)." The research of Durga and Kailash

Bhuyan of the Department of Ophthalmology of the Mount Sinai School of Medicine of the City University of New York has shown that hydrogen peroxide may produce cataracts when the eye's stores of catalase, peroxidase and superoxide dismutase are depleted. K. C. Bhuyan et al[143] reported that hydrogen peroxide is doubled in cataractous lenses. John V. Fecondo and Robert C. Augusteyn[143a] also implicated hydrogen peroxide (and the superoxide radical) in formation of cataracts. Hydrogen peroxide is injurious to cells throughout the body probably because, on decomposition, it yields the extremely reactive hydroxyl radical which, as we have seen, can cause chromosome breaks that are associated with many diseases. Do *not* put hydrogen peroxide into your body!

(Continued from page 841)

possibilities for the successful treatment of atherosclerosis, cardiovascular disease, hypertension and cancer. In fact, the presence of the antioxidants as preservatives in foods may be an important cause for the decrease in the death rate due to stomach cancer. In 1930 when antioxidants such as BHT were first introduced as food preservatives, the death rate due to stomach cancer was 30 per 100,000; today it is just 10 deaths per 100,000. Death rates due to stomach cancer in other countries, where antioxidants are less widely used, have not declined to such a great degree. It seems likely that the increased consumption of fresh fruits and vegetables in the U.S. and the introduction of breakfast cereals rich in vitamin E may help account for the decreased incidence of stomach cancer. Nevertheless, it is interesting to speculate on the possibility of much more dramatic decreases in the incidence of cancer and of other degenerative diseases if larger amounts of the antioxidants were regularly ingested. Many of the antioxidants we have mentioned are, by the way, made available to life-extension experimenters through various suppliers. However, availability of products obviously does not in itself suggest that they are safe to use. *Caveat emptor!*

Are the Synthetic Antioxidants Safe?

What about the safety of BHT and the other synthetic antioxidants? H. Babich[112] has reviewed the positive and negative aspects of BHT. He points out that there have been very few human studies regarding the effects of BHT ingestion. He cites, however, the various animal studies that indicate BHT may show both detrimental and beneficial effects. He notes that BHT reduces the toxicity and carcinogenicity of some chemical and physical agents but, on the other hand, potentiates the toxicity and carcinogenicity of others. Babich also observes that, while BHT may increase the life span of some animals, it can have detrimental effects on the lungs, kidneys, myocardial cells, liver metabolism of lipids and on clotting factors. It is also a potential behavioral and developmental teratogen. If you are tempted to supplement with BHT, remember its many possible dangers.

Countless animal experiments indicate BHT is an anticarcinogen.* Many experiments, of Dr. Harman and others, indicate that it extends the mean life span in animals. But how about its safety?

BHT may be an important key to increasing human longevity, but it is vital to establish its levels of safety and of danger. It is true that BHT, and also BHA, have been found toxic as noted above. But remember, selenium can also be very toxic and yet is very valuable to the body in modest quantities. I think that eventually a similar judgment could also be widely accepted for various antioxidants such

---

* The words *carcinogen* or *carcinogenic* are often used where the terms *carcinosarcomagen* or *carcinosarcomagenic* might be more appropriate. *Carcinosarcomagenic* refers to the generation of any type of cancerous tumor. "Carcinogenic" ought to refer only to the generation of *carcinomas* (cancers of the epithelial cells lying within the connective tissue), with the word *sarcomagenic* being used in reference to production of *sarcomas* (cancers of the connective tissue). The word *carcinosarcomagenic,* though cumbersome, would often be a more accurate substitution for the word *carcinogenic* or even of the word *oncogenic* (which refers to the generation of either cancerous or benign tumors). Even so, we would be ignoring cancer of blood tissues, leukemia, but a neologism such as *carcinosarcomaleukemigenic* would be cumbersome indeed.

as BHA and BHT.[*] Perhaps this quotation of Dr. A. L. Branen, Department of Food Science and Technology, Washington State University, in regard to BHA and BHT will be convincing. Dr. Branen reviewed various experiments relating to pathological effects of BHA and BHT and the following is the entire abstract of his article entitled "Toxicology and Biochemistry of BHA and BHT":

Butylated hydroxyanisole and butylated hydroxytoluene are used extensively as food antioxidants. It is estimated that man consumes ca. 0.1 mg/kg body wt. daily of these antioxidants. At levels 500 times this level (50 mg/kg/day), both butylated hydroxyanisole and butylated hydroxytoluene appear to be free of any obviously injurious effects. However, at larger doses (500 mg/kg/day), both butylated hydroxyanisole and butylated hydroxytoluene result in certain pathological, enzyme, and lipid alterations in both rodents and monkeys, and butylated hydroxytoluene, in some cases, has been reported to have certain teratogenic and carcinogenic effects upon rodents. These alterations appear to differ markedly between rodents and monkeys, apparently as a result of differences which exist in the metabolism and excretion of butylated hydroxyanisole and butylated hydroxytoluene by these two species. However, in both animal species, the alterations appear to be physiological responses which are reversible upon removal of butylated hydroxyanisole and butylated hydroxytoluene from the diet. Long term chronic ingestion of butylated hydroxyanisole and butylated hydroxytoluene may be beneficial in sparing

---

[*] It seems possible, also, that BHT may become a standard treatment, or even a preventative agent, for herpes infections. Wallace Snipes et al.[113] show that herpes viruses (as well as other viruses of high lipid content) have been inactivated *in vitro* at levels that could easily be achieved through oral ingestion of BHT (Figure 5). They caution, however, that animal studies are needed before we might consider this use of BHT in human therapy or prevention. The effectiveness of a 5% and of a 15% solution of BHT applied topically to herpes cutaneous infections in mice is reported by Alec D. Keith et al.[114] The value of BHT in combating other lipid-containing viruses was reported by P. Wanda et al.[115] They found that calcium ions potentiated the effect of BHT.

vitamin E and in modifying the acute toxicity of a number of mutagenic and carcinogenic chemicals.[117]

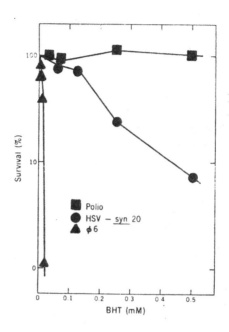

Figure 5. Inactivation of viruses by different concentrations of BHT. Virus stocks were diluted to approximately (2 to 4) X 10[7] plaque-forming units per milliliter in appropriate buffered solutions. A 0.1-ml. portion of a BHT solution in 95% ethanol was added to 5 ml. of buffer, and this was added, after mixing, to a 5 ml. sample of the virus. After 30 minutes, the samples were diluted and assayed for plaque-forming units on appropriate host cells. The abscissa indicates the BHT concentration present during the 30-minute exposure. Reproduced from Wallace Snipes et al., *Science* (1975) 188: 64-65, by permission of the copyright owner, The American Association for the Advancement of Science, and the authors.

In the *Code of Federal Regulations* (often referred to as the *CFR*),[118] BHT is listed as an acceptable food preservative at the level of .02%. This contrasts with a value of only half that (.01%) shown as the acceptable level some years ago (1963) in the *Kirk-Othmer*

Encyclopedia of Chemical Technology. [119] Perhaps the trend to increasing the acceptable level of BHT will continue. If a person eats three pounds (1,360 grams) of food daily, then .02% of that amount would be equal to 2.72 grams of 2,720 mg., considerably more BHT than is at present being ingested by people in general. This line of reasoning can, of course, be very misleading. The government's .02% figure takes into account the fact that most persons will be consuming large amounts of food (meat, fish, eggs, fruits, vegetables, etc.) that contain no BHT and so they can easily tolerate .02% in those relatively few foods that contain it.

What might be the effective amount of BHT in human terms to achieve a significant increase in life span and yet be safe? (Many studies have reported toxicity and so we know that the possible occurrence of *reverse effects* must be considered.) Experiments with animals have shown, as reported above, that a daily intake of 500 mg. of BHT/kg. of body weight is injurious and a daily intake of 50 mg./kg. produces no obviously injurious effects. For a 70 kg. (approximately 150 lb.) person (assuming man reacts to BHT as do animals) a highly injurious level of BHT would be 500 X 70 or 35,000 mg. per day. However, just because a BHT daily intake of 50 mg./kg. may be safe for animals, it is not necessarily safe at that level for humans. The safe human level could be considerably lower (or, of course, it could be higher).

Now, let us examine Dr. Harman's animal research and speculate what it may mean in human terms. Dr. Harman found, as I have reported, that mice receiving .50% by weight of BHT in their diet had significantly extended mean life spans. In human terms, assuming a person eats 1,500 grams (about three pounds) of food daily, .50% would be equal to 7.5 grams or 7,500 mg. Consuming 3,500 mg. of BHT daily might appear to be reasonably safe (if humans react to BHT as do animals, *but this is obviously an unwarranted assumption*). Anyway, the human theoretical life-extending level of BHT, as shown by Dr. Harman's experiments with mice, would be about double this or 7,500 mg. So even though 3,500 mg. of BHT daily could be dangerous for humans, it might not be enough to significantly extend the mean life span. What we need is animal research showing how various antioxidant synergists used with lowered levels of BHT might affect human life span. *In vitro* experiments reported by W. M. Cort[120] have shown, in fact, that ascorbyl palmitate and BHT used together can greatly reduce the formation of peroxides compared to either alone. Cort reported that ascorbyl palmitate also worked synergistically with the antioxidants BHT, thiodipropionic acid (TDPA) and norihydroguaiaretic acid (NDGA) to provide protection against formation of peroxides. It seems likely to me that if Dr. Harman's experiments were repeated with lower levels of BHT but using ascorbyl palmitate at the same time, significant life-extension might be achieved at these lower, perhaps completely safe, levels of BHT.* However, the potential of BHT as an *in vivo* antioxidant is limited by its poor absorption. Less than one part per million was deposited in the liver of rats fed .5% in their diet.[119a] (Caution: No one should experiment with BHT until all appropriate animal testing has been completed and its safety and effectiveness proven. To use it prematurely may present a risk for liver, kidney and thyroid functions.)

Not only may BHT be life-lengthening, but studies show, as we have noted, that it inhibits chemically-induced carcinogenesis in animals.[119a,b,120a,b] On the other hand, H. Witschi and S. Lock [120c] have shown that, in urethane-induced adenoma in mouse lung, BHT can increase the number of tumor-bearing animals and also the number of tumors formed per lung. Then, Witschi et al.[120d,e] demonstrated that BHT may enhance development of lung tumors induced by carcinogens other than urethane and that the effect occurs whether BHT is injected, gavaged or ingested in the diet. These studies and their possible relevance to humans have been reviewed by C. Roston.[120f] Subsequently, R. Djurhuus and J. R. Lillehaug [120g] showed that BHT has tumor-promoting activity in an *in vitro* two-stage carcinogenesis assay. To those of us on the lookout for *reverse effects* it should come as no surprise. Until dose-response *reverse*

---

* Perhaps better results might be achieved at *lower* levels of BHT, with or without ascorbyl palmitate. The work of J. Cillard et al. (reference 227 of Chapter 2) indicated that high levels of BHT can show what I call a *reverse effect* and can act as a pro-oxidant rather than as a desirable antioxidant.

effects can be delineated, BHT should not be used in supplement form.

A review of recent work relating to BHT has been made by Alvin M. Malkinson.[120h] He noted that the Delaney amendment did not apply to BHT since it was considered to be noncarcinogenic. (The Delaney amendment relates to cancer initiators and ignores cancer promoters.)* Malkinson suggested that new laws will be required to afford protection against tumor promoters. But will such proposed laws work against substances that could possibly provide cancer *protection* at certain dosages?

Life-extension experimenters who desire to achieve results with their own bodies need not feel it is essential to consume BHT. Why? Because *in vitro* experiments reported by W. M. Cort[120] using ascorbyl palmitate have shown that it very effectively reduces lipid peroxidation—it is far superior, in fact, to BHT. Animal experiments using not only ascorbyl palmitate but also vitamin E, vitamin A and selenium, along with sulphur-amino acids, might yield very exciting results. Lecithin, which acts as an antioxidant synergist, and the other antioxidants tabulated later in this chapter might also help increase mean life span. Disappointingly, one such experiment with mice fed a mixture of antioxidants and nutrients (vitamins E and C, BHT, methionine and sodium selenite) resulted in a significant reduction of fluorescent products in the testes and the heart but the mortality rate was unaffected.[121] Many more experiments, with varying ratios of antioxidants, should be performed.

The use of BHT, ethoxyquin and the other synthetics brings on the burden of their detoxification. The trade-off between the resulting body stress and the benefit of antioxidant protection is a problem that needs resolving. It seems possible, however, that the highly effective trio of ascorbyl palmitate, vitamin E and BHT (plus additional

---

* When BHT is administered either prior to or at the time of carcinogen exposure, it inhibits carcinogenesis. Unknown to Malkinson when he wrote the above, Preben Olsen et al.[120i] found that BHT can also show a *reverse effect* (my language) and act as a carcinogen. Thus, BHT can act not only as a cancer promoter but, depending on dosage, can act either to initiate or to inhibit carcinogenesis. (Theoretically, the use of BHT as a food additive should now be discontinued in accordance with the Delaney amendment. The Delaney amendment, however, has seldom been invoked.)

synergistic effects of the other antioxidants listed below) might yield results that could be superior to those achieved in Dr. Harman's animal research. These superior results, which I visualize as a good possibility, might be achievable, in my view, using enough BHT to provide an optimal synergistic action among the other antioxidants but at a level far less than that employed by Dr. Harman. An objective of those of us interested in life extension should be to include large amounts of antioxidants in the diet and in such proportional relationships so as to approach achievement of optimal synergistic effects. If this can be done, cross-linking of DNA and RNA as well as lipid peroxidation, leading to cell destruction, should be greatly reduced. The result could be an increase in human mean life span, and possibly even in maximum life span. On the other hand, amateur life-extension experimenters, using excessive amounts of antioxidants before *reverse effects* are delineated and dose-response relationships are subject to more accurate estimates, run the risk of detrimentally affecting their health and life span.

Commonly Consumed Antioxidants

Listed below are the antioxidants many persons consume, and in a few cases I comment on some that are produced endogenously. Used in excess, they may, however, be detrimental to health and longevity.*

Ascorbic Acid:

Ascorbic acid is an effective antioxidant, but ascorbate-iron chelates at low concentrations (100 ppm) act as pro-oxidants. Ascorbic acid and copper can also produce a pro-oxidant effect. Higher concentrations of vitamin C (2,000 ppm) appear to prevent this negative effect.[122] However, at extremely high concentrations, attended by only marginally adequate vitamin E,

---

* C. D. H. Evans and J. Hubert Lacey,[121a] in 1986, published a quite complete list of the toxic effects of excessive vitamins. The other antioxidants, in excess, also pose dangers, and in many cases these dangers are discussed throughout this book. (Refer to the index.)

a pro-oxidant effect may occur and lipid peroxidation increase. (Linda H. Chen, reference 161 in Chapter 6.) Whether vitamin C acts as a pro-oxidant or as an antioxidant depends, not only on the presence or absence of metals, but also on the concentrations of oxygen, polyunsaturated lipids, hydroperoxides and other pro-oxidants and antioxidants.[123] Review Chapter 6.

Ascorbyl Palmitate:

This form of ascorbic acid is somewhat soluble in fat and much more readily soluble in alcohol, but is only slightly soluble in water. The synergistic effect of ascorbyl palmitate on the antioxidant activity of various food ingredients is reported by W. M. Cort[2] and by H. Kläui and G. Pongracz.[123a]

Vitamin A:

V. N. R. Kartha and S. Krishnamurthy[124] report that the antioxidant function of vitamin A becomes apparent only when large amounts are used. However, Kartha and Krishnamurthy seem to contradict this statement in at least two later reports, one of which states: "In the present study, it is shown that both retinol and retinyl acetate are in fact more potent inhibitors than alpha-tocopherol in preventing the lipid peroxidation of rat brain homogenates."[125] Nevertheless, even more recent work still seems to show vitamin A to be only a weak antioxidant. P. Sanjeev Kumar et al.[126] found that a single dose of 400,000 I.U. of retinyl palmitate, fed before challenging rats with carbon tetrachloride, acted as an antioxidant. That dosage, however, would be equivalent to many millions of I.U. in a person—obviously a very dangerous level. Jules Duchesne holds that whether or not vitamin A has significant antioxidant effects, vitamin A could, contrary to virtually "everyone," accelerate aging. (See Chapter 4 and reference 54 of that chapter.)

While retinol and retinoic acid show antioxidant action, they can also display a *reverse effect* in activating superoxide production by the polymorphonuclear leukocytes. H. Hemilä and M. Wikström[126a] have reported that this activation occurs at extremely low (micromolar) concentrations of the vitamin A compounds.

Beta Carotene:

Beta carotene, a vitamin A precursor, first acts as an antioxidant and then as a pro-oxidant.[127] Beta carotene, canthoxanthin and other carotenoid pigments scavenge singlet oxygen and other free radicals.[128-131] H. W. Renner[131a] reported that beta carotene (but not retinol) showed dose-dependent anticlastogenic effects (i.e., it inhibited chromosome breakage) *in vivo* on chemically induced aberrations in bone marrow cells of hamsters. Review Chapter 4.

Vitamin E:

Many of the cytotoxic drugs used in cancer therapy contain the quinone group (which we first met in Chapter 2 in connection with vitamin E). Quinone-containing antitumor agents such as adriamycin, daunorubicin and streptonigrin may act by generating free radicals.[131b,c] Asher Begleiter[131c] states in regard to the quinone antitumor compounds bis (dimethylamino) benzoquinone and benzoquinone dimustard that "the cytotoxicity was inhibited significantly by catalase, an enzyme that removes hydrogen peroxide from the cell, but was not affected by superoxide dismutase, which removes superoxide radicals. This result provided evidence that the cytotoxic activity of these compounds, at least in part, involves active oxygen species such as hydrogen peroxide. The lack of inhibition observed with superoxide dismutase suggests that the mechanism of action of these agents may not involve superoxide radical." Interestingly, as pointed out in Chapter 2, while vitamin E can act as an anticancer agent, it can, on the other hand, increase the toxicity (on bone marrow) of adriamycin (reference 215 of Chapter 2). *

---

* Other animal experiments,[131d-f] however, have shown that vitamin E can reduce the harmful effect that adriamycin may have on the heart. To the contrary, J. G. S. Breed et

We also noted in Chapter 2 that vitamin E, in acting as a scavenger of superoxide, is converted to a quinone (reference 151 of Chapter 2). We saw in Chapter 4 that vitamin K (whose various forms are quinones or quinone derivatives) can act as an anticancer agent. Quinones, whether in the form of drugs or of vitamins, seem to be cancer inhibitors perhaps because they produce oxygen species such as hydrogen peroxide. Thus, the cancer-fighting power of vitamin E seems to relate, not to its superoxide-scavenging ability, but to the formation of a quinone that can, in turn, generate other oxygen species such as hydrogen peroxide.

Herman Baker et al.[131j] showed, in 1986, that twice-a-day supplements of 400 I.U. dl-$\propto$ tocopheryl acetate (all-rac-$\propto$ tocopheryl acetate) or d-$\propto$ tocopheryl acetate (RRR-$\propto$ tocopheryl acetate) depressed plasma gamma tocopherol to one-third its initial values. If gamma tocopherol has physiological uses distinct from alpha tocopherol, it might be advisable to take supplements in the form of mixed tocopherols.

Vitamin B Complex:

Vitamins B2 and B12 are antioxidants.[132] PABA acts as a scavenger of hydroxyl free radicals.[133,134] Folic acid also scavenges hydroxyl free radicals.[135] Choline, generally found in B complex pills, may also act as an antioxidant. Lipoperoxidation products (such as ceroid) have been found in livers of long-term choline-deficient rats. BHA and BHT have protected choline-deficient rats

---

al.[131g] reported that, in rabbits, vitamin E failed to protect against adriamycin-induced cardiotoxicity. Sheri Zidenberg-Cherr and Carl L. Keen[31h] showed, in a 1986 study, that the antioxidant status of an animal may influence adriamycin toxicity. They found that not only vitamin E sufficiency but also a manganese-sufficient diet (probably through promoting synthesis of manganese SOD) was heart protective in animals treated with adriamycin. If free-radical production (and the resulting lipid peroxidation) is the mechanism whereby adriamycin may injure heart, bone marrow and cancer cells, then could antioxidants—while offering protection against adriamycin-induced body damage—reduce the cancer-fighting power of the drug? If we used antioxidants to protect the heart and bone marrow of a cancer patient from adriamycin toxicity might we be hastening the patient's death from cancer? Perhaps not; vitamin E enhances the chemotherapeutic effect of adriamycin on human carcinoma cells *in vitro*. [131i]

against vascular damage, thus suggesting that the synthetic antioxidants took over a function normally performed by choline![136]

Selenium:

This mineral promotes the formation of glutathione peroxidase which destroys lipid peroxides and repairs the damage free radicals do to membrane lipids. Glutathione peroxidase destroys hydrogen peroxide. (Hydrogen peroxide, in the presence of unsaturated fats along with a deficiency of vitamin E, produces malonaldehyde, which can react with DNA to produce mutations or cancer.)[137]

Ubiquinone (Coenzyme Q):

Scavenges singlet oxygen.[137a]

Zinc:

Milos Chvapil et al.[137b] reported that zinc acts as an antioxidant and controls lipid peroxidation in such tissues as the liver and the red blood cells.

Copper-Zinc Superoxide Dismutase (SOD):

Worthless when taken by mouth. We probably cannot salvage any of the enzyme from tablets or from foods. Superoxide dismutase is, however, made by the human liver as well as by cells throughout the body, but adequate amounts of copper must be present. In copper-deficient lambs, SOD was linearly related to serum copper concentration. When the animals were fed 10-14 mg./kg. of copper the SOD level optimized and did not significantly increase as more copper was given.[138] Man eats about 1 kg. of food a day, but the official RDA for copper is not 10-14 mg. but 2-3 mg. (Men are not sheep, so one must not quickly conclude that the intake of copper should be increased many-fold.)

Manganese-based Superoxide Dismutase:

Supplemental manganese may aid the body in making this type of SOD.

Catalase:

Worthless when taken orally. The catalase molecule is very large (240,000 daltons) and so would have no chance of entering the body from an oral source even if it were not digested as, of course, all enzymes and other proteins are. However, catalase production in the body is probably encouraged by the presence of adequate iron. Catalase converts sometimes harmful hydrogen peroxide as well as the sometimes dangerous hydroxyl radical to innocuous oxygen and water. It is a red, crystalline, iron-based enzyme consisting of a protein complex combined with hematin—a compound derived from oxidized heme (which we met in Chapter 7 in connection with iron).

Fluoride:

As we saw in Chapter 7, fluoride can act as an antioxidant to inhibit superoxide production of polymorphonuclear leukocytes or can show a *reverse effect* by promoting such action (references 519, 520 and 522a of Chapter 7).

Cysteine Hydrochloride:

Cysteine is one of the sulphur-amino acids available as a supplement. Dr. Harman reported that the mean life span of male mice was increased by 15% when large amounts (1%) of cysteine were added to their diet. Simion Oeriu and Elena Vochitu[144] found that subcutaneous injection of cysteine increased the survival of male mice and female guinea pigs but not of female rats. Cysteine has, however, been found to be mutagenic in the Ames test.[144a] Glutathione, a tripeptide of cysteine, glutamic acid and glycine (that is important in the activation of some enzymes and in oxidation-reduction processes) is also mutagenic in the Ames test even at concentrations found in mammalian tissues.[144a]

Lecithin:

H. Bollmann patented lecithin as an antioxidant in Germany in 1923[145] and in the U.S. in 1926.[146] Actually, lecithin seems to be an antioxidant synergist (with ethoxyquin for example) rather than a primary antioxidant.[147] Luther L. Yaeger and Johann Bjorksten have shown that lecithin, in the presence of vitamin E, acts as an antioxidant. However, in another study, lecithin plus ascorbic acid was no more effective than ascorbic acid alone.[148] L. R. Dugan reports that cephalin (predominantly *phosphatidylethanolamine* and a constituent of lecithin) is more effective than lecithin.[149]

Coffee, Caffeine and Caffeic Acid:

Caffeine is present in coffee and tea. Caffeic acid is found in coffee, oats, green pepper seeds and in other plants. A study by W. L. Porter[150] showed caffeic acid to be only a little less effective than BHA (and more effective than BHT and vitamin E) as an antioxidant. Possibly on the negative side, however, caffeic acid reportedly causes chromosome breaks using *in vitro* tests with Chinese hamster ovary cells but not if a mixture of copper and manganese ions is present.[151] Methylglyoxal, also present in coffee, is mutagenic on the Ames salmonella test. However, U. Friederich et al.[151a] found that the mutagenic activity of methylglyoxal was abolished by the enzymes glyoxalase I and II and reduced glutathione, all of which are present in mammalian cells. These enzymes reduced the mutagenicity of coffee, however, by only 80%. (Interestingly, Friederich and his co-workers discovered that, using the Ames test, the number of TA100 revertants rose as the concentration of coffee increased up to 30 mg. per plate but then a *reverse effect* set in and at a 50 mg. concentration the number of revertants were back to the level present when coffee was absent. (The number of TA102 revertants increased with coffee concentration and showed no *reverse effect* within the range of concentrations that were studied.)

B. A. Kihlman[151b] points out that caffeine itself was shown to be mutagenic over one-third of a century ago by E. M. Witkin and, independently, by N. Fries and B. Kihlman. A. Ronen and M. Marcus[151c] note that caffeine has been found by D. Weinstein et al.[151d] to be clastogenic in human tissue cultures at a concentration of 250 µg./ml. Its concentration, however, never becomes this high *in vivo* by drinking coffee. (Such concentration can, nevertheless, be achieved *in vitro* in treating sperm with caffeine for artificial insemination.)[151c] The theory of the *reverse effect* suggests that, just as the mutagenicity of caffeine conceivably might be a causal factor in cancer,* so that very mutagenicity is what may give caffeine its antineoplastic properties. In Chapter 4 (references 36a and b, as well as Figure 3) we saw how caffeine can increase the antitumerigenic effect of vitamin A and of the drug BCNU. (Perhaps vitamin A or BCNU enhances caffeine's mutagenic properties.) The mutagen caffeic acid also shows a *reverse effect* by suppressing stomach cancer in mice.[151ka]

In a possibly related study, Taisel Normura et al.[151l] found that caffeine, among other tumor inhibitors, when given to pregnant mice, significantly suppressed chemically-induced fetal malformations. Our state of knowledge obviously does not allow us to suggest that pregnant women drink coffee, but is this an eventual possibility? There are many other uses or possible uses for caffeine such as control of breathing in infant apnea (including those having "near-miss Sudden Infant Death

---

* Caffeine administration in animals is reported by some investigators[151e-h] to be carcinogenic and by others [151b-j] to be antineoplastic. Denda et al.[151h] reported a dose-dependent biphasic effect of caffeine on chemically-induced (4-HAQO) pancreatic tumorigenesis in partially pancreatectomized rats. Injecting the maximum tolerated dose of caffeine (120 mg./kg. body wt.) every 12 hours decreased the number of nodules, whereas treatment with one-fourth as much caffeine every 12 hours showed a *reverse effect* (my language) with an increased number of nodules. A study was published in 1986 by Abraham Nomura et al.[151k] that involved coffee consumption of 7,355 men clinically examined from 1965 to 1968. It showed that coffee intake did not increase the risk of any of the cancers that were studied. (However, they reported a beneficial, but weak, negative association between coffee drinking and rectal cancer.)

Syndrome"),[151m] use in treating bronchial asthma[151n-p] and opening airways for asthmatics.[151q] We have previously noted other benefits of caffeine. In a footnote of Chapter 7 (reference 10b of that chapter) we saw how caffeine may increase physical performance. J. L. Ivy et al.[151r] and D. L. Costill et al.[151s] similarly found caffeine useful in combating fatigue through its enhancement of the rate of lipid metabolism and through its positive influence on nerve transmission.

Tea, Theophylline and Phenolics (Including Tannins):

K. C. D. Hickman has said: "It was Professor Mattill and his various pupils who showed us that an unprotected oil that might go rancid in an hour (in the Swift Tester) could be, for instance, protected for eight (8) hours with ∝-tocopherol, for fifty (50) hours with ∝-tocopherol plus phospholipid, for two hundred (200) hours with ∝-tocopherol, phospholipid and ascorbic acid and for three hundred (300) hours with all the above plus tannins. Thus, was offered an insight into how nature stabilizes vegetable fats for relative vast periods with meager supplies of antioxidants."[152] The antioxidants epigallocatechin gallate and gallic acid (as well as caffeine as noted earlier) have also been found in tea leaf.[152a] Chocolate lovers will be glad to learn that the tannins in cocoa, possibly acting through an antioxidant effect, seem to inhibit plaque formation, while cocoa fat may protect the teeth through formation of an antibacterial coating.[152b,c] (Any beneficial dental effect is probably more than offset, however, by negatives associated with the sugar likely to be present in cocoa products.) Excessive consumption of tannins, on the other hand, is associated epidemiologically with both esophageal and stomach cancer.[152d] The *reverse effect* suggests, to me, a possible beneficial action at lower dosages. In fact, K. Rothwell[151j] has pointed out that P. K. Reddi and S. M. Constantinides[152e] showed tumor production can be partially suppressed *in vivo* by theophylline. Then too, Hans F. Stich et al.[152f] reported that *in vitro* studies showed that "a Japanese, a Chinese and a Ceylonese tea prevented the formation of mutagenic nitrosated fish products at doses that are usually consumed by man." Various phenolics, catechin, chlorogenic acid, gallic acid, pyrogallol and tannic acid—which are found in teas—suppressed the formation of mutagenic nitrosation products. (Interestingly, saliva also exerted an inhibitory effect.)

Govind J. Kapadia et al.[152g] have discussed the tannins to be found in herbal teas such as those made from bayberry, calamus, coltsfoot, comfrey, golden ragwort and sassafras and the danger of esophageal cancer when they are consumed to excess. (On the other hand, the *theory of the reverse effect* suggests to me that the antioxidant property of the tannins in these teas might work for cancer protection. Use of herbal teas dates back to primitive cultures. The doctrine of "survival value" suggests they may be efficacious.)

Quercetin, Quercitrin, Quercetin 3-Triglucoside, Quercetin 3-Monoglucoside, Quercetin 3-Diglucoside, Myricetin and Myricetin 3-Monoglucoside:

Modest amounts of these bioflavonoid antioxidants may be obtained by eating green onion tops, green pepper pods and seeds and potato peels. Potato peels contain the poison *solanine* and so should be eaten only in moderation.[153] Quercitrin is also present in citrus fruits. Myristicin also occurs not only in the vegetables cited above but in celery and in oils of nutmeg and mace.[154]

The mutagenicity of the flavonoids was discussed in Chapter 6 (references 59a-f of that chapter). Quercitrin's mutagenicity, according to M. Nagao et al.[154a] and Ikuko Ueno et al.,[154b] is enhanced by Cu Zn SOD. (In addition, James F. Hatcher and George T. Bryan[154c] found that the mutagenicity of the related flavonoid quercetin may sometimes be enhanced by both SOD and by ascorbate.)* On the other hand, Mendel Friedman and G.

---

* Could it also be that quercetin and the other bioflavonoids might enhance the mutagenicity of ascorbate? To the extent that ascorbate might be therapeutic in cancer

860   The Reverse Effect

A. Smith[154d] reported that ferrous and copper sulphates inactivate quercetin's mutagenicity. (A review of various studies suggesting genetic and carcinogenic effects or lack of effects of various flavonoids has been provided by James T. MacGregor.)[154e] The *reverse effect* suggests that flavonoids, at some dosage, might offer cancer protection or therapeutic possibilities, and we noted in Chapter 6 that this is the case (references 60a-c of that chapter).

Alcohol:

There are many benefits to modest alcohol consumption, one of which is to scavenge hydroxyl free radicals which can attack DNA.** (Alcohol will not, however, attack either superoxide or hydrogen peroxide. Superoxide and hydrogen peroxide react to produce the hydroxyl ion.)[155] On the other hand, R. Fink et al.[155a] suggested that chronic alcoholism may induce a detoxifying mechanism that is associated with a great increase in free radical activity. (This seems to involve another *reverse effect.* Modest amounts of alcohol reduce free radicals; large amounts increase them.) Shinji Kubota et al.[155b] have shown that, perhaps as a response to the increase in free radicals, Mn SOD is elevated in persons with alcoholic liver injuries. C. L. Keen et al.[155c] reported that long-term ethanol consumption in humans resulted in increased erythrocyte Cu Zn SOD activity.

Uric Acid:

Bruce N. Ames et al.[156] hypothesize that uric acid, an end product of purine metabolism, provides an antioxidant defense

---

therapy because of its chromosome-damaging property, could the bioflavonoids provide a beneficial synergism?

** Protecting the DNA is a beneficial function of the ethanol that is produced by the body. On the other hand, although we properly view DNA modification as generally destructive, it is this plus one or two billion years that turned the amoeba into man. A genetic defect may sometimes be a matter of perception. Imagine, some ten million years ago, a father or mother primate, having observed a "genetic defect" in his/her offspring, might have thought: "Something's wrong with our kid. He's using only two of his legs for walking."

against oxidant- and radical-caused aging and cancer. They suggest that, during the evolution of the primates when the ability to make ascorbate was lost, urate replaced some of the antioxidant functions of ascorbate. Today, the plasma urate level is considerably higher than the ascorbate level. Several other lines of evidence support the hypothesis that uric acid may be an important antioxidant in humans.[157] However, in hyperuricemia uric acid is in excess, gout may occur and degeneration of bone (osteolysis) is often present.[158] Monosodium urate crystals *in vitro* stimulate production of arachidonic acid metabolites by human neutrophils and platelets.[158] Nobuchika Ogino et al.[158a] have found that uric acid stimulates the conversion of prostaglandin G_1 to prostaglandin H_1 and C. Deby et al.[157a] speculate that uric acid may be acting as a hydroxyl radical scavenger in enhancing this reaction. Deby et al.[157a] explain gout osteolysis in terms of the increased prostaglandin synthesis.

Richard G. Cutler[53b] reported that the levels of plasma urate divided by specific metabolic rate (SMR) for various species are related to species maximum life span potential (MLSP) and the relationship is shown in Figure 6. As we saw earlier with SOD (Figure 3), we now see that as the urate levels of various species rise, so does their maximum life span potential. Cutler points out that uric acid is structurally similar to caffeine and other neural stimulants. He also observes that men who have suffered from gout (i.e., men who have a high level of uric acid) are often very successful. Brain urate levels in terms of the specific metabolic rate rises in the primates from lower levels in the squirrel monkey to higher levels in the chimpanzee and orangutan to the highest levels in man. Cutler has reported that the increase in uric acid levels with increased species maximum life span potential is related to a loss in uricase enzyme activity. However, we must not assume, in reference to uric acid, that ontogeny (the history of the individual) will necessarily recapitulate phylogeny (the history of the species).

T. Glazer et al.[158b] found that the addition of urea to monocytes of healthy subjects caused a marked reduction in their production

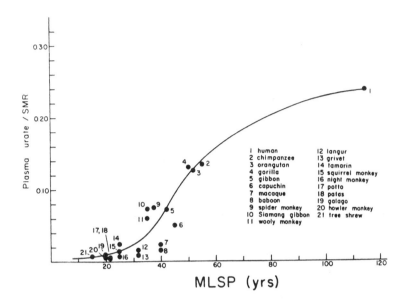

Figure 6. Plasma urate levels and urate level per SMR in primates as a function of MLSP. Values taken from the literature. Correlation coefficient, r = 0.82. Reproduced from Richard G. Cutler in *Free Radicals in Molecular Biology, Aging and Disease,* ed. Donald Armstrong et al. (New York: Raven Press, 1984) pp. 235-266, at 250, with permission of the publisher and of the author.

of superoxide—so important for phagocytic activity. Recently, J. H. Peters et al.[158c] reported uric acid shows mutagenic activity. Furthermore, mice studies by Mark A. Reynolds et al.[158d] failed to indicate a positive correlation between serum uric acid and life span. B. Pence and F. Buddingh,[158e] using rat dietary studies, reported, in 1986, no significant correlations between either serum uric acid or lipid peroxide levels and tumor incidence, multiplicity or total size.

It is interesting to note that "urine therapy," which involves the drinking of urine,[159,160] is believed, by a tiny minority, to be beneficial. This is probably faddist and extremist but, nevertheless, it seems possible that the "pluses" of modestly increased uric acid as cited above [156,157] might sometimes outweigh the "minuses."[158-158d] Whether or not "urine therapy" has any relation to serum uric acid, a quick way to increase serum uric acid might be to simply eat more sugar. J. T. Solyst et al.[160a] found that serum uric acid was increased when humans consumed a diet containing 30% of the calories as sucrose compared to controls getting 30% of their calories from starch. Could this be a possible "plus" for sugar?

Other Antioxidants, Their Synergists and Controllers of Free Radicals:

Rutin and other bioflavonoids (in addition to those mentioned above), various herbs and grains and the sulphur-amino acids, methionine and cystine (in foods such as eggs). Some foods, especially cereals, contain vitamin E. In addition, many other foods contain various antioxidants so this list is, obviously, far from complete. Even glucose and cholesterol may act as antioxidants.[53b] Cutler[53b] speculates that catecholamines, found in high concentrations in the brain, may be potentially important antioxidants, "deficiencies of which may lead to free radical damage associated with Parkinson's and Alzheimer's disease." Chlorophyllin, the sodium and copper salt of chlorophyll, is an antioxidant. Tong-man Ong et al.[160b] reported, in 1986, on their own and on other studies showing that chlorophyllin has antimutagenic properties. Finally, gossypol (the cotton product being tested as a male contraceptive) is an antioxidant.[160c] However, Yu Chen et al.[160d] reported, in 1986, that gossypol increases the frequency of DNA-strand breaks in human leukocytes *in vitro*. Since free radicals are likely involved as a pro-oxidant, we have a *reverse effect.*

I believe that the preceding pages dealing with antioxidants and the possibility of an increased human life span (shocking as some of this material will seem to many traditionally oriented health enthusiasts who believe "unnatural chemicals" must always be bad for the body) may be among the most thought provoking in this book. To give balance to my enthusiasm, however, there could be a negative side to excessive consumption of antioxidants. Food antioxidants, even in low concentrations, inhibit both PGE1 and PGE2 prostaglandins *in vitro*.[161] Such action is, however, probably subject to dose-response subtleties including *reverse effects*. At any rate, animal experiments suggest the excellent possibilities for a greatly increased human mean life span and maybe even an increase in maximum life span. Harman[161a] calls for future studies to include "a search for free radical reaction inhibitors that have only a slight depressing effect on ATP production at levels which significantly inhibit adverse free radical reactions elsewhere in the body."

New derivatives of BHT, of the tocopherols and of other antioxidants may provide an even better opportunity to give us an increase in maximum life span, not just in mean life span.[162] None of the known antioxidants can penetrate the inner membrane of the mitochondria, the source of over 95% of the free radicals generated by living systems. Richard D. Lippman[162] speculates that these new derivatives might be able to penetrate this inner membrane. Then too, he suggests that carnitine, the normal *in vivo* carrier of fatty acids into the inner membrane of the mitochondria, might be employed to put the new derivatives where we want them. Imagine the exciting possibilities that lie ahead!

That Jekyll-and-Hyde Element—Oxygen

Let us conclude this chapter by dealing in greater depth with some of the good and bad effects of oxygen. The benefits of oxygen are obvious and a series of 10 or 15 hyperbaric oxygen treatments may perform wonders for many conditions, including burns, gangrene, senility, strokes, osteomyelitis and multiple sclerosis, but the health-destroying properties of oxygen are more subtle. Vergil H. Ferm[163] has reported on the teratogenic effects of hyperbaric oxygen on hamsters and mice (although rats seem to be unaffected). Let's look at some of oxygen's other negative properties.

The possibility that oxygen might be dangerous to human beings should not strike one as being unusually strange. (Even in hyperbaric oxygen therapy there exists the danger of excessive lipid peroxidation.) Animals breathing an atmosphere of pure oxygen at normal pressure develop tracheitis within a few hours. Within a few days they experience lung damage and—amazingly—die of anoxia, i.e., a lack of oxygen. (The body shuts off the supply of poisonous oxygen.) We all know that oxygen attacks many materials. Plastics decay, rubber cracks, paper crumbles, metals rust, animal tissue degrades and foods become rancid. But the activity of oxygen, drastic as it is, is minor compared with the action of the superoxide radical with which we have been dealing in this chapter.[*] Ideally, oxygen should be employed by the cells of the body in enzymatic reactions under tight metabolic control. But often superoxide forms and the body must be protected by SOD and other antioxidants, as we have been discussing, or aging will be accelerated and disease will occur. Alan B. Weitberg et al.[165] presented evidence that oxygen metabolites have a primary role in the generation of sister chromatid exchanges (that we discussed in Chapter 6). Atmospheric oxygen, an important environmental mutagen, is even being suggested as a major carcinogen.[166]

Prior to the arrival on earth of the plants, and the byproduct of their photosynthesis, oxygen, it is probable that this element was rare in our planet's atmosphere. Before that event, life on earth existed under essentially anaerobic conditions for several hundred million years. These primitive organisms lived on organic material created in the early atmosphere by the interaction of ultraviolet light, methane, ammonia, water vapor and hydrogen. They were not, however, nearly so numerous as the creatures that exist everywhere in the oceans today.

By the way, descendants of these organisms still exist, but only in anaerobic niches, and are called *obligate anaerobes*. There are a large number of families of anerobic bacteria, including some that reside in the intestinal tract. *Bergey's Manual of Determinating*

---

[*] As I did earlier in this chapter, I think I should once more give balance by coming to the defense of superoxide. E. W. Kellogg III et al.[164] theorize that negative air ions have the formula $(O_2^-)(H_2O)n$ and are thus a beneficial species of superoxide. (I. Rosenthal,[164a] on the other hand, holds that the effects of negative ion generators can be explained in terms of reactions of the carbonate radical anion.)

Bacteriology[167] should satisfy—if not amaze—my more curious readers. An all-too-common example of such an anerobic microbe is *streptococcus mutans,* one of the types of bacteria that form plaque on our teeth. It was suggested, way back in 1924 by J. K. Clarke, [168] that this bacterium is related to dental caries. Brushing and flossing introduce oxygen into their colonies, thus inhibiting propagation. I predict that bathrooms of the future will have oxygen applicators for use following flossing in order to provide improved protection against cavities.*

Let's return to the early story of the earth. After several hundreds of millions of years, during which time there were only anaerobic life forms, organisms evolved and developed—about two billion years ago—the ability to use the energy of ordinary visible light to make food out of water and carbon dioxide. These cyanophytes of the family *myxophyceae*—which reproduce by fission and in this way are related to bacteria—still exist today. Photosynthesis, with oxygen as a byproduct, set the stage for the development of life forms—the animals—that were to employ oxygen in their metabolism. The process probably began in shallow pools and then spread throughout the oceans, with the resulting oxygen beginning to accumulate in the oceans and in the atmosphere. Subsequently, some of the oxygen was converted to ozone in the atmosphere and it screened off ultraviolet light, thus making it impossible for evolution to ever again begin on earth in the same way.

When the green plants appeared on earth the various life forms that had evolved prior to that event must have faced tremendous challenges in adapting their biological systems to utilize oxygen in energy-producing metabolic pathways. Life forms were forced to simultaneously employ defenses from the free radicals that were readily generated from that oxygen. As Denham Harman[169] says:

---

* Future vacination against caries may make the idea obsolete before it is adopted. Relatedly, several reports cited in 1986 by Jose O. Alvarez and Juan M. Navia[168a] showed that a higher incidence of caries in the deciduous teeth seems to be followed by less caries in the permanent teeth. Interestingly, one more carious tooth surface at the age of 8 results, on average, in about five fewer carious surfaces at age 16. It is believed that children with a higher incidence of caries in their "baby teeth" acquire a stronger immunity to the causative agent(s). Discovery of the mechanism for this effect might contribute to the development of an effective vaccine against dental caries.

"...life originated as a result of free radical reactions, selected free radical reactions to play major metabolic roles, and utilized them to provide for mutation and death, thereby assuring evolution." The antioxidants, and primarily superoxide dismutase,[*] were and are now used to provide life forms, including man, with defenses against the free radicals and this two-faced angel-devil called oxygen. (Parenthetically, it should be noted that astronomers and biologists who believe that life forms "out there" will be found only where oxygen exists are myopic—being deprived of the farsighted backward vision to appreciate the conditions under which life arose on our own planet.)

Just as oxygen was incorporated into life systems when the green plants arrived on earth, so various other elements and compounds have been included in the metabolic pathways of animals evolving toward man as the eons passed. Someday it seems likely that an increasing number of antioxidants such as BHT, 2 MEA, DMAE and ethoxyquin will be used beneficially by the body to continue the battle against various free radicals, including forms of that Jekyll-and-Hyde element known as oxygen. BHT and the other synthetic antioxidants may be thought of as future nutrients that have been absent until recently from the diet of living creatures. Such antioxidants should be incorporated efficiently into the body's metabolic pathways a lot faster than the billions of years it has taken oxygen to achieve its present quasi-poison, quasi-nutrient status. Great benefits may accrue through the use of these new antioxidants in the body's metabolic machinery.

---

[*] Early life forms were protected by the manganese and iron forms of SOD but, as related in Chapter 7, copper (and therefore Cu Zn SOD) had probably not yet been incorporated into living systems.

Bilirubin as an Antioxidant

Bilirubin, the principal pigment of bile and endproduct of heme metabolism, is generally considered to be a potentially cytotoxic substance that should be excreted. "Bilirubin lights" have attracted attention for treating the jaundiced neonate because their use results in the formation of bilirubin isomers that can be excreted more readily. (A photoisomer of bilirubin was also detected in the plasma of healthy adults after they had been exposed to sunlight.)[170] By this procedure, the risk of encephalopathy caused by high concentrations of the pigment, especially in the brain, can be reduced. Excessive bilirubin concentrations can be responsible, not only in children but also in adults, for the symptoms of kernicterus.

Over 30 years ago it was suggested that bilirubin (and also biliverdin) may serve vital functions by protecting vitamin A and linoleic acid from oxidation in the intestinal tract.[171, 172] Roland Stocker et al.[173] (a group that included Bruce N. Ames) published, in 1987, results of a study showing that at low but physiological oxygen concentrations bilirubin is a powerful antioxidant. At a 2% oxygen concentration in liposomes, bilirubin suppresses oxidation better than vitamin E which is generally considered to be the best *in-vivo* antioxidant. Bilirubin, previously thought to be merely a waste product, may in reality be one of nature's most vital, life-fostering antioxidants. If it can be shown that the encephalopathy occasioned by bilirubin at high concentrations is caused by a pro-oxidant effect and if bilirubin at low concentrations demonstrates an antioxidant effect we will have yet another example of the *reverse effect*.

"What do you want out of life, Wally?" I want to experience everything worth experiencing that I have not yet tried and repeat many of the experiences I have already had. For the rest of my life I want to *live* my life! My objective is to grow in sensitivity to all phases of life and living. I want to do what I can to change, for the better, myself and the world.
— Walter A. Heiby

CHAPTER 10

A Long Life of Lifelong Happiness!

What promises does the future hold for the human race? The future is always an intriguing topic. As Charles Kettering said: "I am vitally interested in the future. After all, I'll be spending the rest of my life there."

Through eating better, through learning to meet stress better and through exercising more, or (sometimes) perhaps through exercising *less,* we can increase our chances for a long life. Does the idea that exercising *less* might increase longevity strike you as being strange? See the adjoining boxed-in copy entitled "Does Lethargy Promote Longevity? Does Excessive Exercise Diminish Health?"

Long-lived ancestors would tend to increase the probability that we may also experience longevity. (Natural selection, however, does not favor genes that promote longevity. It is interesting to speculate on possible increases in average human longevity if sexual desire, sexual desirability and reproductive capacity peaked, rather than diminished, at advanced ages.) We can't choose our ancestors, but there are many other ways we can help assure that we will live long, vigorous lives.

(continued on page 876)

Does Lethargy Promote Longevity? Does Excessive Exercise Diminish Health?

Exercise and activity usually get very good notice; inactivity and lethargy generally do not. It has been speculated that exercise can reduce excessive blood pressure, can diminish the probability of a first or recurrent heart attack, can reduce the probable occurrence of other atherosclerotic diseases and that it might even increase longevity.[1,2] Psychological benefits such as a reduction in depression, a better control of stress and anxiety and better appetite control have been described.[1-4] As far as weight control is concerned, any benefit may depend on whether exercising is done before or after meals. K. Willcutts et al.[4a] reported, in 1986, that fat utilization was greater in physically fit young women (men were not studied) during exercise in the fasted state than during exercise begun 60 and 90 minutes after a meal. If you are trying to lose weight, exercise when you're hungry! Furthermore, G. Kaminori et al.[4b] reported, also in 1986, that caffeine ingestion by obese young men (women were not studied) can assist the mobilization and metabolism of free fatty acids for energy during the latter stages of prolonged submaximal exercise.

Harvey B. Simon[5] reported that exercise beneficially produced an increase in circulating pyrogen in humans which appears to be identical with interleukin-1, a product of mononuclear cells that enhances lymphocyte function. Several studies[6-9] with rats and mice have concluded that exercise slows tumor growth. The many other benefits of exercise are well known.* Nevertheless, there are negatives associated with too much of anything, including exercise.

---

* Some of the well-known "benefits" of exercise may, however, be nonexistent. Even the value of sit-ups in reducing abdominal fat has been questioned. F. I. Katch

Steven Seely[10] maintains that the most lethargic species live longer. The orangutan,** the most lethargic of the primates with a life span of 50 years, has a longevity second only to man among the related animals. Man's long life, according to Seely, is positively correlated with his inactivity. Seely speculates, however, that "the true danger of sedentary life is not in inactivity, but in the failure to reduce food intake with the reduction of needs." *** Furthermore, R. S. Sohal[11] has reported that house flies allowed to live in large jars where they can fly have shortened maximum life spans compared to flies kept in small vials where they cannot fly. Flies not allowed to fly can have maximum life span extensions as great as 260%. In more recent work with adult male houseflies, Sohal et al.[12] reported that, while superoxide dismutase and catalase were not appreciably affected by physical activity, the concentrations of inorganic peroxides and of glutathione were increased. (Sohal et al. found that solitary confinement of the male flies was essential. Otherwise, the persistent homosexual copulatory attempts they made on each other enhanced their physical activity.)

Experiments showing life extensions among restricted mice and rats are described and referenced by Ben E. Sheffy and Alma J. Williams.[13] Mice experiments by Elizabeth Steinhagen-Thiessen et al.[14] have shown that exercise diminishes activity of the amino acid creatine and of the enzymes kinase, aldolase, superoxide dismutase and catalase in older animals (while increasing the activities of creatine and of those enzymes in younger animals). Steinhagen-

et al.[9a], as reported in *Sports Medicine*, found that "a programme of sit-up exercise does not selectively decrease fat cell diameter or the amount of subcutaneous fat in the abdominal area." Furthermore, B. Gutin et al.[9b] hypothesize that hyper-estrogenemia may be the major predisposing factor for coronary heart disease (CHD) in men and that a high estradiol: testosterone ratio may cause the expression of risk factors. They found that the estradiol: testosterone ratio was significantly lower in the trained group but they speculate that "exercise training may decrease risk factors for coronary heart disease without decreasing the risk of coronary heart disease."

** The word orangutan is derived from the French *orang*, man or person, and *hutan*, forest, i.e., man or person of the forest.[10a]

*** It seems improper to ignore the environment in which the animals live. If man lived naked in the rain and snow, would he be the longest lived of the primates?

Thiessen et al. conclude that their results support the idea "that there is 'threshold of age' beyond which exercise becomes detrimental to the aging organism."

In men and women, testosterone and prolactin are reduced by long-distance running according to Garry D. Wheeler,[15] although Sidney Alexander,[1] on the contrary, holds that aerobic exercise increases testosterone in women.[*] Amenorrhea is a frequent symptom of female runners and William B. Fears et al.[15a] report that it is sometimes associated with *anorexia nervosa.* T. W. Boyden et al.[16] speculate that menstrual dysfunction occurs in endurance-trained women due to a synergy between individual susceptibility, changes in body weight and a malfunction in gonadotrophin responsiveness. Hale has tabulated the values of five reproductive hormones as originally published by E. Dale and D. H. Gerlach.[17a] Dale and Gerlach found that 51% of multiparous runners and 21% of nulliparous runners had developed an irregularity of their cycle. (David C. Cumming and Robert W. Rebar[17] maintain, however, that "exercise-associated defects in reproduction are not serious and can be reversed by changes in life-style"—i.e., by reducing the amount of exercise.)

J. G. Stewart et al.[17c] have reported that long-distance running can cause loss of blood in the gastrointestinal tract. They found that fecal hemoglobin levels increased significantly from .99 mg./g. before to 3.95 mg./g. after the race. Male and female runners had significantly lower mean hemoglobin, serum ferritin concentrations and hematocrit than controls. The Stewart group concluded that the gastrointestinal blood loss could contribute to the iron deficiency and/or anemia found in some athletes. Whether it is an iron deficiency or some other factor or factors that could be

---

[*] David C. Cumming and Robert W. Rebar[17] have published graphs showing that both women who are untrained and amenorrheic runners show a testosterone increase for the first 30 minutes following exercise and then a decrease. The graph of testosterone in normal cycling (i.e., nonamenorrheic) runners shows a decrease following exercise, then an increase, followed by another decrease. In a related study of amateur wrestlers, Richard H. Strauss et al.[17b] reported that, "Low serum testosterone levels were significantly correlated with low body fat, large loss of body fat and large weight loss." They concluded that "dietary restriction practiced by some wrestlers may affect serum testosterone levels adversely."

causal, athletic training may diminish immunological status. Ernest Jokl[17d] cites studies suggesting that training may render athletes more susceptible to infections.

The anemia of athletes, even if it may decrease their immune function, could have a health-serving purpose and therefore we must not too quickly conclude that they should take iron supplements. B. Halliwell and J. M. C. Gutteridge[17e] have speculated that the excretion of copper and iron in sweat (and the resulting anemia) may be a protective mechanism. It may be a mechanism that decreases the rate of metal-dependent lipid peroxidation or of hydroxyl free radical formation during periods of high production of oxygen free radicals. Should iron supplementation sometimes be avoided even in cases of apparent deficiency? Nutrition may be a very subtle subject indeed!

Lead pollution is a little-appreciated hazard to which marathon runners are exposed. S. R. Grobler et al.[17f] examined the whole-blood lead levels of athletes who participated in the 1984 Two Oceans Marathon held in Cape Town, South Africa. In a control group the mean lead level was $9.7\,\mu g/dl$. In the experimental group the level was $46\,\mu g/dl$ before the race and $53\,\mu g/dl$ after the race. Interestingly, Joseph D. Wassersug,[18] while holding that running does not prolong life or improve health, speculates that arm exercise might be health promoting. He cites the great longevity of orchestra conductors, virtuoso violinists and concert pianists to support his thesis. (Musicians are, however, prone to develop their own varieties of physical problems.) [18a,b]

As the pulse and blood pressure drop in the three minutes following running and other strenuous exercise, adrenaline and norepinephrine (which stimulate the heartbeat) rise to as much as ten times the resting norm.[19] This can sometimes lead to a fatal irregularity of the heartbeat.[19] C. F. Chester and C. P. Conlon[19a] have reported case studies of serious cerebrovascular complications from strenuous exercise. R. Tyler Frizzell and Gilbert H. Lang[19b] published, in 1986, a study involving two cases where ultramarathon runners even developed hyponatremic encephalopathy. (They cited a study by T. D. Noakes et al.[19c] of four runners in which "water intoxication" due to an abnormally low level of blood sodium (hyponatremia) was corrected in three of them after they were advised to drink less.) Raul Artal et al.[19d] have found that even fetal bradycardia (slowed heartbeat) may occur during maternal exercise and the condition is believed to be mediated by catecholamines. However, it appears to be transitory and is perhaps harmless.

We noted earlier in this chapter that Simon[5] had reported exercise, possibly through increasing interleukin-1, may enhance lymphocyte function. Many share Simon's belief that exercise may sometimes strengthen the immune system, but Simon[5] himself asks, "can exercise adversely affect infection in man?" He notes that B. G. Gatmaitan et al.[19e] had found forced swimming increased the severity of myocarditis in mice with experimental Coxsackie virus B3 infections and Simon[5] cautions that, while there are no similar findings in man, "these observations should have a sobering effect on athletes who have systemic viral illnesses." Daniel R. Neuspiel,[19b] writing in 1986, expresses particular concern about exercise-caused sudden deaths from myocarditis in children and adolescents. How does strenuous exercise cause such dire events? Heyward L. Nash[19g] quotes Peter G. Hanson, professor of medicine in the division of cardiology at the University of Wisconsin-Madison, as saying, "Exhaustive exercise may be a stressor that depresses the mucociliary blanket and allows germs into the body." Too little, like too much, protective mucus can be detrimental to the body.

A number of studies have shown that exercise can induce asthma attacks in sensitive persons.[20-23] E. R. McFadden, Jr. and R. H. Ingram, Jr.[24,25] state that heat loss, through an unknown mechanism, can initiate airway obstructions in persons with asthma. Allen P. Kaplan[26] has reported on exercise-induced hives. Other studies, including one by Ellen M. Buchbinder[27] show that, as a result of excessive exercise, food-dependent anaphylaxis is sometimes induced. The anaphylaxis is the result of an IgE antibody-mediated reaction caused by the ingestion of the antigenic substance by a previously sensitized person.[28] James M. Kidd III et al.[28] cite fish, shrimp, nuts and celery as being among those foods precipitating exercise-induced anaphylaxis. (A. Bundgaard[28a] maintains, however, that exercise is not hazardous to asthmatics. He states that while almost all asthmatics have exercise-induced asthma, physical training may be beneficial.)

Thomas R. Friberg and Robert N. Weinreb[29] have warned of the dangers to the eye in gravity inversion exercise through the use of devices that suspend a person by the feet or ankles in a head-down position. They found that intraocular pressure more than doubled on such inversion. Friberg and Weinreb also reported that "pressures in the central retinal artery underwent similar increases." They warned: "Patients with retinal vascular abnormalities, macular degeneration, ocular hypertension, glaucoma, and similar disorders refrain from inversion altogether. Whether normal individuals will suffer irreversible damage from inversion is uncertain, but it seems prudent to recommend that prolonged periods of inverted posturing be avoided." Injuries such as sprained ankles, pulled muscles and "tennis elbow" resulting from other types of activity are too common to require comment.

L. A. Kuehn[30] and S. Corrsin[31] have developed a theory of life span based on the hypothesis of a fixed total number of heartbeats and upon a reduction of the resting heart rate due to exercise.* They conclude that their theory suggests a life span increase for moderate amounts of exercise and a decrease for very large amounts. Victoria Persky et al.,[32] by the way, maintain that increased heart rate is an independent risk factor for cancer mortality in man.

Chapter 9 dealt with the dangers of excessive amounts of free radicals and their control by means of antioxidants. Excessive exercise may pose an increased health threat from free radical formation and earlier in this section we noted that the excretion of

---

* A sign of "overtraining" in athletes is for the "basal morning heart rate" to show a *reverse effect* by increasing to a higher base level.[31a]

copper and iron in sweat (and the resulting anemia) might help protect against free-radical damage. Kelvin J. A. Davies et al.[33] reported a two-to-three-fold increase in free radical concentration of muscle and liver in animals following exercise to exhaustion. Exhaustive exercise also produced decreased mitochondrial respiratory control, loss of sarcoplasmic reticulum and endoplasmic reticulum integrity and an increase in lipid peroxidation products. Endurance in animals deficient in vitamin E was 40% less than in controls. A. T. Quintanilha[34] also found that rats had an increased requirement for vitamin E during endurance exercise training. Mitsuru Higuchi et al.[34a] reported that mitochondrial superoxide dismutase (SOD) increased only 14% to 37% in muscles adapted to endurance exercise, whereas the constituents of the mitochondrial respiratory chain increased two-fold. In other words, the ratio of SOD to respiratory chain constituents is reduced in mitochondria of muscle that has adapted to endurance exercise. Higuchi and his associates concluded their report with these words: "Thus, expressed in terms of the muscles' capacity for aerobic metabolism, mitochondrial SOD activity is actually decreased, making it unlikely that an increased capacity for enzymatic scavenging of superoxide radicals represents a major protective adaptation against free radical damage and accelerated aging in endurance-trained muscle." Lester Packer,[35] in connection with free radicals formed by exercise, has written most provocatively in pointing out possible dangers of excessive exercise. Packer asks, "Does physical exercise cause spreading of oxy-radical damage, increase the incidence of cancer, decrease the incidence of heart disease, and decrease life span?"

(Continued from page 869)

Healthfully meeting the stresses of life with calmness; minimizing the poisons taken in with our air, water and food; avoiding a noisy environment as much as possible; getting adequate exercise; observing proper weight control; avoiding youth destroyers such as nicotine and adequately feeding our cells with amino acids, vitamins, minerals and antioxidants—these are some of the ways to keep the cells of our bodies alive and fully operational. However, even the "good" nutrients must not be overconsumed to the point *reverse effects* may occur.

Immortality—Is It Necessarily Impossible?

Perhaps some of us will live long enough to reach the day when immortality—living forever, barring serious accidents—can become a reality. Dr. Leonard Hayflick of Stanford University has been widely cited for his research showing that human cells can live for a period of 50 replications—which would require about 150 years. However, human longevity may not necessarily be bound to any such upper limit. If we are able to find the genetic determiner we might be able to manipulate it so as to extend the number of replications. While we await this great leap forward in influencing longevity, there are other possibilities. Lester Packer and Kathy Fuehr[36] found that when human diploid cells divide in a medium where oxygen is present in reduced amounts their life span is extended. Grace C. Yuan and R. Shihman Chang[37] have reported that the life span of human amnion cells *in vitro* can be extended by hydrocortisone, corticosterone, dexamethasone, fluocinolene, trimcinolone, prednisolone and aqueous extract of *Panax ginseng*.

It continues to be reported by the vitamin E sellers that, in September of 1974, Lester Packer and James R. Smith[38] announced that they were able to get human lung tissue cells to divide, not just 50 times, *but 120 times* by adding vitamin E to their environment. Furthermore, the study stated that the cells were still continuing to divide at the time these scientists made their report. The facts are that no one, not even Packer and Smith, have been able to replicate their results in subsequent experiments.[39-41] Regrettably, we are forced to ignore this intriguing report.

However, Robert R. Krohn[42] points out that cells of mice tongue epithelium have shown an average of 565 doublings over the life span with no significant difference between young and old animals.

Dr. Krohn notes that G. M. Martin et al.[43] found, similarly, that there was no significant difference in doubling capacity of cells from human donors 20 to 90 years of age. Furthermore, I. L. Cameron[44] reported that in tissues exhibiting lessened cell proliferation with age there was no dying out or loss of cells. In addition, James G. Rheinwald and Howard Green[45] found that when epidermal growth factor (a polypeptide with molecular weight of 6,045 and a known amino acid sequence) was added to epidermal cells of human neonates their lifetime increased from 50 to 150 generations. It seems apparent that the Hayflick limit is subject to many exceptions and, shortly, we will cite some more of them.

How did Hayflick arrive at his findings? Drs. R. Holliday, L. I. Huschtscha, G. M. Tarrant and T. B. L. Kirkwood,[46,47] in connection with their *Commitment Theory of Cellular Aging,* suggested that the finite life span of Hayflick's cells may have been due to the decline and loss of a subpopulation of immortal cells. Thus, under proper conditions cell immortality may be achievable and the Hayflick hypothesis of limited cell replication may need modification. An important distinction should be made, however, between the property of cell cultures to divide indefinitely and the as-yet-unachievable individual immortality of a multicellular organism. Dr. Leonard Hayflick[48] has stated: "If all the multitude of animal cell types were continually renewed, without loss of function or capacity for self-renewal, one would expect that the organs composed of such cells would function normally indefinitely and that their host would live on forever. Unhappily, however, renewal cell populations do not occur in most tissues, and when they do a proliferative finitude is often manifest."

C. A. Reznikoff et al.,[49] in studying culture conditions of immortalized lines of mouse fibroblast cells, discovered that such cultures could be made to attain "immortalization" after about ten doublings (which ordinarily corresponds with their normal life span). Subsequently, A. Macieira-Coelho et al.[50] found that low-dose irradiation accelerated the acquisition of unlimited growth potential in mouse fibroblast cells. (This, you will appreciate, is an example of the *reverse effect,* since with increasing amounts of radiation not only will growth stop but death will occur.) More recently, Laura Curatolo et al.[51] have reported on varying culturing procedures that can lead, or fail to lead, to immortalization.

The results of a study by Jennifer D. Hall et al.[52] suggest that the DNA repair mechanisms of human skin fibroblast cells (which act on a variety of lesions, including cross-links) do not decline with age. If true, this is fully as exciting as Krohn's research showing no significant difference in doubling capacity of human cells regardless of the age of the donor and the "immortalization" of cell cultures.

Dean P. Loven et al.[53] discovered that Mn SOD was completely absent in immortal lines of both normal and malignant human fibroblast cells that they examined. They also found that the immortal normal cell lines had Cu Zn SOD activity which was modulated by thyroid hormone. The immortal malignant lines, on the other hand, had Cu Zn SOD activity which was unaffected, or less strongly affected, by the presence of thyroid hormone. It seems especially interesting that the loss of the ability to induce Mn SOD is related to the acquisition of immortality. It is also interesting that the loss of ability to induce Cu Zn SOD activity is associated with the loss of growth control and the attainment of malignancy. These discoveries may represent important steps in our search for immortality and cancer control.

The fact that cancer cells will live and continue to divide forever if they are fed and they have enough room, suggests that gerontologists through studying them may learn to give normal cells a greater life span. Through the process of fusing normal and cancerous cells, a single cell is produced that has the combined DNA of both parent cells. One such study was published by Gretchen H. Stein and Rosalind M. Yanishevsky.[54] They reported that when human diploid cells were fused with malignant T98G human glioblastoma cells or to RK13 rabbit kidney cells, the human diploid cells were transformed to immortality. This came about through loss of a normal regulatory factor, yet the diploid cells retained some characteristics of normal cells.

In regard to physical immortality, it takes little imagination to presume that cloning of humans will become possible. (For many years it has been done with lower animals.)* Then it will be feasible to have, in cryo-storage, clones of oneself as a spare-parts bank. Organ after organ could be replaced to keep the body operating at youthful efficiency. Or perhaps the brain could be transplanted into a clone for a completely new body. For even wilder dreaming, listen to the imaginings of Albert Rosenfeld.[55]

In *The Second Genesis—The Coming Control of Life,* Albert Rosenfeld speculates on the possibility of re-creating a person not merely from his original chemicals, but from *raw information.* If such information were stored, any number of copies could be made. Under this concept there would be no need to keep cells alive for cloning purposes. One could simply store oneself on tape and in the event of an accident (including old age, which might by then be considered to be an accident) he or she could duplicate himself or herself as a healthy adult by playback of the tape. This would become merely an operational procedure of what Richard Landers of Thompson Ramo Wooldridge, Inc. has called *dybology* (from the Hebrew word *dybbuk* meaning "unassigned soul")—a field that is a hybrid between biology and engineering. Let's keep our bodies youthful with antioxidants and with the other techniques discussed in this book while we wait for gerontologists or bioengineers to give us immortality!

If we can come close enough to discovering the meaning of "optimal" in relation to our own personal nutrition and other life-style factors so that we can succeed in living to the age of 120, it seems likely that gerontology may have given us, by that time, techniques to live to 200, perhaps through shutting off of a possible "death hormone."** This death hormone is hypothesized to be triggered by

---

* Five of the many relevant articles of the past five years are those by Karl Illmensee and Peter C. Hoppe,[53a] by Jean L. Marx,[53b] by George E. Seidel, Jr.,[53c] by Anne McLaren [53d] and by James McGrath and David Solter.[53e] Each of these followed in *Citation Abstracts* will keep you informed of future developments.

** W. D. Denckla has shown that the pituitary gland produces a substance that he calls the "decreasing oxygen consumption hormone (DECO)." DECO causes a fall in the basal metabolic rate as we age and is often referred to as the "death hormone." On the contrary, A. Yabrov[55a] speculates that it could be a "longevity hormone." He points out that the higher the oxygen intake for a given body weight, the shorter the life span. Furthermore, Yabrov notes that

the essential neurotransmitter serotonin that is present in too-great-a-quantity. Perhaps we will discover a means of controlling autoimmune responses—where leukocyte antibodies are misdirected to act against our own white blood cells. At the same time, perhaps chemical stabilizers can prevent the lysosomes of cells from spilling their garbage and upsetting cell activities.*** Perhaps more efficient anti-cross-linking agents will keep our collagen youthful and also help avoid cross-linking of our DNA and of our RNA so they can continue giving faithful instructions for protein synthesis. Perhaps we will discover ways to remove the excessive histone accumulation that clings to DNA as we age and causes errors in transmitting genetic information to the RNA that in turn affects our ability to accurately produce new proteins.**** Perhaps hormonal agents can help keep our glands performing youthfully.

Your Relationship With Your Doctor

No matter how healthy you are because of good heredity, good nutrition and good ability to meet stress healthfully, there will be times when you need medical assistance. There are many fine, competent doctors, of course. They are correcting the defects in their education by intensively studying nutrition and other modalities of holistic health. However, if you are a layman with an excessive degree of trust in all doctors, you might find *Confessions of a Medical Heretic* by Robert S. Mendelsohn, M.D., *The Medicine*

---

mice exposed to cold temperatures throughout their lives had a 40% decrease in oxygen consumption and a marked increase in longevity. Should we inhibit or foster the production of DECO?

*** It may be hard to realize, but most of our knowledge of the cells is based on rather recent research that dates to the 1940s. During this period, Albert Claude discovered mitochondria, George Palade, ribosomes, and Christian de Duve, lysosomes. These researchers shared the 1974 Nobel Prize for Medicine or Physiology.

**** Histones are nucleoproteins that serve a useful function in that they mask the genetic information that is not needed in any given process. Later, when information is needed that is blocked by histones, those histones are removed by other nucleoproteins called *nonhistones*. Defective cell replication may occur if the nonhistones do not effectively remove histones from an area of the DNA that is needed for accurate transmitting of information.

Men by Leonard Tushnet, M.D., *The Unkindest Cut* by Marcia Millman, *How to Avoid Unnecessary Surgery* by Lawrence P. Williams, M.D., *Medical Nemesis* by Ivan Illich, *The Solid Gold Stethoscope* by Edgar Berman, M.D., and *The Doctors* by Martin L. Gross to be eye-openers. If you are a woman you'll probably find *Male Practice—How Doctors Manipulate Women* by Robert S. Mendelsohn, M.D., and *The Hidden Malpractice—How American Medicine Mistreats Women* by Gena Corea to be especially disturbing. Most of these books are, however, simply examples of social criticism and not based on definitive studies showing how orthodox therapies could be inferior. Thus, these books may ask interesting questions about patient-doctor relationships but provide little guidance as to where confused patients might turn.

If your faith in doctors is what I would characterize as being excessive, you might check the words *iatrogenic* and *nosocomial* in an unabridged dictionary. (The change in attitude toward doctors and hospitals is illustrated by the fact that these words are defined in Webster's Third New International Dictionary but not in the earlier Second Edition.) * My objective is not to make you *iatropistic* (having little faith in doctors), a word that has not yet found its way into most dictionaries, but simply to make you *realistic*.

I hope your doctor is not the "typical doctor" who is unaware of nutritional principles. If you have a highly miseducated doctor, you may desire to search for a physician who is enthusiastic about the ability of good nutrition and other holistic health modalities to help cure and to help prevent disease. If you do not have or are unable to find such a doctor, the burden of remaining healthy will be completely yours. Doctors regrettably are, in general, only experts in disease; few are experts in the maintenance of health.

In fact, most doctors' idea of *practicing preventive medicine* (as contrasted with their active specialty of *treating disease*) is to insist

---

* Ivan Illich has coined the interesting expression *social iatrogenesis*. He defines this as the disabling impact of modern medicine and technology which develops in people a feeling of inability to attend to their own well-being. The antithesis, self-responsibility in matters of health, is essential for optimizing health.

that you have a yearly checkup. Just what is the value of the yearly physical? To detect a disease without symptoms is very difficult. Most periodic checkups are virtually without value and may, in fact, be harmful. The constant worry about *disease* (as contrasted with a continual concern about *health*) can bring on the diseased condition one is trying to prevent.

Then too, a study was made over the period of 1964 to 1973 on members of the Kaiser Health Plan in California.[56] Two comparable groups, each of which consisted of about 5,000 randomly selected people, were analyzed for the value of frequent physical examinations. One group was encouraged to have frequent checkups; the other was not, but all of the members were free to use the service as they desired. Members of the group urged to come in frequently came in for examinations far more often than those in the group not encouraged to do so. However, physicians who evaluated the health status of the two groups over the period of seven years could find no significant differences between them in the incidence of disease, disability or death.

Periodic checkups, however, may be of value in some cases. If one's physician is well versed in preventive techniques, his interpretation of blood, urine and hair analyses made at regular intervals might be very valuable. So, I would not want to make a blanket condemnation of all regular checkups. They certainly have value in the examples cited and probably in other cases also. But I believe their importance, *if one has no symptoms,* has been blown out of proportion. Physicians themselves virtually never go in for annual checkups.[56a] However, when you have actual symptoms of disease, get to your physician in a hurry!

If your doctor prescribes drugs, ask him if there is a nondrug approach that might correct your condition. If he insists on use of one or more drugs, get him to show you his copy of the *Physicians' Desk Reference* (often simply called the *PDR*) and read to you the side effects of the drug or drugs he has prescribed. Perhaps the *PDR* will frighten him into prescribing a nondrug approach! I do not mean to imply, however, that I am strictly antidrug and provitamins. Drugs are often lifesaving, while vitamin and mineral supplements, as we have seen throughout this book, can sometimes have pharmacological effects and may be even health threatening.

Each of us must be the principal guardian of our own health and that of our family. Each of us can show our doctor nutritional references, preferably from scientific sources that he may be more inclined to give serious consideration. If he cannot be convinced, you may have to proceed on your own, for your health and that of your family is more important than your doctor's injured feelings.

Anyway, it will be a maturing experience to lose the infantile notion that a doctor will watch over your well-being. Read more books about health and study contrary opinions. Make your own decisions or decide consciously to keep a decision in abeyance pending the arrival of more information. Be a questioner; think for yourself!

Ultimately, you may find it more health serving to switch to a tomorrow-type doctor than to fight with your yesterday-type doctor. A nutrition-conscious, holistically-minded physician—one in tune with both the realities of science today and with the possibilities of tomorrow—can be very important to you in meeting your objective of living a long, youthful life. Such a physician will undoubtedly exemplify the original definition of the word *physician*—it derives from the Greek word *physis* which means "nature." He is apt to be the sort of doctor that Dr. Erasmus Darwin, grandfather of the great naturalist Charles Darwin, envisioned when he said, "The science of medicine will someday resolve itself into a science of prevention rather than a matter of cure."

Searching for a holistically-oriented doctor can present some difficulties. Doctors are often relatively untrained in nutrition or in other alternative health modalities and, as we have said, are not used to thinking in terms of health. They are generally disease-oriented and their minds are often closed regarding matters relating to maintaining and improving health. Ranjit Kumar Chandra[56b] writing in 1986, said: "It is ironic that traditional and ancient systems of medicine, such as the *Ayurveda,* regard nutrition as fundamental to good medical practice. The modern medicine system should take lesson from that, and look to the East for fresh guidance and new light." Those interested in studying the availability of nutritional classes in the training of future physicians are referred to the book *Nutrition Education in US Medical Schools*.[56c] Findings published by Roland L. Weinsier et al.[56d] in 1986 showed the significant range in nutritional knowledge among medical students as measured by an examination given to seniors in ten medical schools. Eighty-five percent of these students were reported to be dissatisfied with the quantity and 60% with the quality of their medical-nutrition education. Another 1986 study, this one by Aileen Brett et al.,[57] also reported current medical school teaching of nutrition to be inadequate.

I must, however, be wary of giving the impression that I think vast numbers of doctors are completely oblivious to nutrition. (It would certainly be even more dangerous to be treated by a physician oblivious to the occasional need for lifesaving drugs.) At any rate, just because many doctors have little knowledge of nutrition, that does not mean the knowledge is unavailable. Doctors will often engage the services of a nutritionist, although some may stubbornly insist that nutrition is nonsense.* Even at that, doctors are often more knowledgeable than food faddists seem to think they are. Nutritional principles are incorporated in many of the courses leading to the M.D. degree. Massive numbers of nutritional articles appear in the journals read by physicians.** What is sometimes meant by statements decrying the nutritional knowledge of doctors is that they are unaware of the "fact" that vitamins are panaceas.

---

* Dietitians are trained to analyze information about food but, regrettably, they often have only limited expertise in applying the nutritional implications of drug usage. I hope your physician is acquainted with books such as *Drug-Induced Nutritional Deficiencies* by Daphne A. Roe[57a] and *Nutrition and Drugs*, edited by Myron Winick,[57b] as well as with the journal *Drug-Nutrient Interactions,* so he can help tailor your diet, as well as your vitamin and mineral supplementation, in light of the nutritional effects of the drugs he may have prescribed. As Daphne A. Roe[57c] has pointed out, the advice physicians often give their patients to take medications with food may increase the risk of drug-nutrient reactions and the adverse outcomes of such reactions.

** In the past 15 years over 100,000 articles relating to nutrition have appeared in the journals covered by *Index Medicus, Excerpta Medica* and *Nutrition Abstracts.*

Health Freedom and Balanced Information

Let us digress to the important subject of health freedom. We have heard much about the four freedoms—*freedom of speech, freedom of the press, freedom from want* and *freedom from fear*. As important as these freedoms are, there is another great freedom—*freedom of choice*. However, freedom of choice is a dangerous doctrine unless full information is available and one has the ability to make a valid choice. Should a child have the "freedom of choice" to play with matches? Should an adult have the "freedom of choice" to select an unorthodox treatment while being as innocent as the child as to the possible harm that might be done? Does one have enough information to have "freedom of choice" if he is unaware of laetrile's mutagenicity or of DMSO's teratogenicity? (Thomas H. Shepard in his *Catalog of Teratogenic Agents*[58] cites many references that might disturb a DMSO enthusiast. Such a person should realize that DMSO suppresses the immune system. This, however, may be detrimental or it may be beneficial.)* There can be no basis for "freedom of choice" unless the brain is first freed of informational polarization.

Orthodox therapies are continually scrutinized in scientific journals and the articles contain judgments as to both the negatives and the positives of those treatments. Unorthodox practitioners, on the other hand, often traffic in generalities and let glowing testimonials substitute for reality. They often fail to point out the negatives associated with their therapies. Instead, they frequently invoke the idea that they are being harassed by the authorities and by traditional medical doctors. Especially, beware of those promoting the "conspiracy theory" that the National Cancer Institute and the American Cancer Society, with the collusion of the AMA, are attempting to suppress information about cures so their jobs in cancer research will not be terminated. Consider the possibility that the promulgators of the conspiracy

---

* Alan Pestronk and Daniel B. Drachman[59] reported that DMSO decreases antibody titres. They noted that this suggests it "might be effective in the treatment of diseases such as myasthenia gravis where antibodies have an important pathogenic role."

theory may themselves be conspiring to maintain their flow of profits from questionable remedies.

Risk/benefit ratios of standard therapies are a continual concern of medical practitioners and are subject to frequent review in the scientific journals. Unorthodox practitioners, on the other hand, often pretend that risks associated with their therapies are minimal and that the benefits may approach the miraculous. One must be informed of the risk/benefit ratios of various therapies for treatment of disease, as well as various approaches to health maintenance before one has, in fact, a basis for "freedom of choice." And when we speak of a risk/benefit ratio we should be referring to personal, public or environmental health rather than to the healthfulness of industrial or practitioner profits. Choice is only an illusion in the absence of full information.

Information is never really "full" and never will be.* What we should seek is *balanced information.* We must be careful that our information represents a reasonable assortment of both pro and con positions. We must be wary of being victims of *managed information.* It is just such managed information that is continually purveyed by so many unorthodox practitioners. If you, right now, are one of those persons who thinks of the FDA as being at all times a stupid meddler, are you unknowingly under the influence of one or more persons with a financial "axe to grind"? (To cite just one example, the FDA's work in opposing the nonvitamin B 15 benefitted the cause of better health, but was opposed by many members of the public who were under the influence of those having commercial interests in such products.) It is not easy to know how many of our views—whether orthodox or unorthodox—are influenced by those who have money to lose or to gain.

How many of your views and my views are influenced by a pseudo-science that has been presented cleverly to look like science? What is pseudo-science? According to Oliver Wendell Holmes,[60] "A Pseudo-science consists of a nomenclature, with a self-adjusting

---

* "Proof of safety" is a concept that exemplifies the fact that we can never have "full information." Only risks can be demonstrated; "safety" can never be "proved" except in terms of an absence of known risks.

arrangement by which all evidence, or such as favors its doctrines, is admitted, and all negative evidence, or such as tells against it, is excluded. It is invariably connected with some lucrative practical application."

Paul Kurtz[60a] has written:

...one should make a distinction between the open mind and the open sink. The former uses certain critical standards of inquiry and employs rigorous methodological criteria that enable one to separate the genuine from the patently specious, and yet to give a fair hearing to the serious heretic within the domain of science. Isaac Asimov has made a useful distinction between *endoheresies,* which are deviations made *within* science, and *exoheresies,* which are deviations made *outside* of science by those who do not use objective methods of inquiry and whose theories cannot be submitted to test, replication, validation, or corroboration. Even here one must be extremely cautious, for an exoheretic may be founding a new science. A protoscience may thus be emerging that deserves careful appraisal by the scientific and intellectual community. Or the exoheretic may simply be a crank—even though he or she may have a wide public following and be encouraged by the powerful effects of extensive media coverage. Simple neutrality in the face of this may be a form of self-deception.

As an aid in distinguishing between science and pseudoscience it may be useful to read the entire article "Debunking, Neutrality and Skepticism in Science" by Paul Kurtz[60a] from which the above quote was taken. In addition, the following articles may also serve as useful guides: "What is Pseudoscience?" by Mario Bunge, [60b] "A Measure for Crackpots" by Fred J. Gruenberger[60c] and "Demarcation of the Absurd" by Petr Skrabanek.[60d]

When reading about or listening to a presentation of an unorthodox therapy, we must be willing to be open-minded in regard to "facts" the promulgator would have us believe to be obvious. You may believe you "know" that $3 + 4 = 7$. But, in vector mathematics $3 + 4$ may assume values between -1 and 7. Furthermore, $3 + 4$ is not necessarily equal to $2 + 5$ (since $2 + 5$ can assume values between -3 and 7). *When faced with the obvious, look for a hidden truth.*

Computer devotees have a saying, "Garbage in, garbage out." This philosophy applies not only to computer technology but to the workings of the brain. If you expose yourself to views—whether it be in the popular "health literature" or at a health convention—and those views are polarized to exclude arguments opposed to the views being expounded, then you can expect nothing but polarized views to come out of your brain. Beware of putting garbage in; you will most surely get only garbage out. If, on the other hand, you get a good balance of information from all sides of an issue (including a literature search of the scientific journals) then, in coming to a decision, you will surely have "freedom of choice." However, in forming a decision, keep open to the possibility that new facts, not yet available to you, may rightfully cause you to change your mind. Furthermore, realize that the purveyor of an unorthodox "cure" will often support his claims with "science" and experiments generally having defective protocols and therefore unpublishable in respected scientific journals. Question the validity of the laboratory protocol or the line of reasoning that leads any investigator to new "facts." Those who do not understand the "miracles" of science often find it easy to believe in the "reality" of science fiction. On the other hand, do not reject out of hand creative ideas that may go counter to the current scientific consensus. Imagination is an important ingredient in science's fact-finding process. As Albert Einstein is credited with saying, "Imagination is more important than knowledge."

Be a Label Reader

In your search for increased health be an inveterate label reader. Know what is in the foods you eat. Ingredients of packaged foods are listed in order of their concentration; the one present in the greatest quantity is listed first, the one present in the second largest concentration, second, etc. If sugar is high on the list, you may prefer to avoid that product! However, often sugar equivalents may be listed separately under various names such as raw sugar, brown sugar, dextrose, glucose, levulose, fructose, corn syrup and corn sweetener so as to keep sugar out of the number one position on the list of ingredients. (If the FDA were to require that the concentration of each ingredient be shown, it would be easy to total the amounts of the sugar equivalents.) Perhaps someone will discover that the term "crystalized beet juice" might be still another way to fool the consumer.* On the other hand, a "left-handed" sugar (LHS) that contains the same atoms as ordinary sugar but arranged in a mirror image of the common substance has been developed by Biospherics, a research firm of Bethesda, Maryland. [67] Small amounts of LHS occur in some plants such as seaweed, berries and bananas. LHS tastes like common sugar, but the body cannot absorb it and neither can the bacteria that cause tooth decay. A synthetic sucrose polyester (SPE) has also been developed. It feels like vegetable oil or margarine but is not digestible by the enzymes in the small intestine.

---

* In light of my willingness throughout this book to say bad words about nutritional friends, let me say a good word about sugar—often castigated as a nutritional enemy. The fact that it may be bad for the teeth does not mean sugar is devoid of quasi-redeeming qualities. Sugar may help protect one against cirrhosis of the liver and even help protect against cancer of the liver and of the stomach. Gerhard N. Schrauzer[61] correlated age-corrected mortalities from cancer at 17 sites with consumption of 12 major food items in different countries. Although consumption of sugar correlates with mortality from many sites of cancer (which is no surprise), there is a strong *inverse* correlation between sugar consumption and mortality due to cancers of the liver and of the stomach and also due to liver cirrhosis! We should stress, however, that a correlation does not prove a causal relationship. To repeat, although cancer mortality seems to be increased by increased sugar consumption, sugar may help protect one from stomach and liver cancers and from liver cirrhosis. Is it possible that sugar could be a bad food for most of us, yet be protective for an alcoholic? But if sugar is really a bad food, how do you explain the fact that many experiments show animals, infants and even fetuses have a preference for sucrose and for sweet foods in general?[62] Sugar and honey have been used as antimicrobial agents in wound healing for hundreds of years and are still used today.[63-66a] (Mark K. Addison and Juan N. Walterspiel[66b] point out, however, that sugar is not always sterile.) Honey treatment has even been used for wound healing after a radical operation for carcinoma of the vulva.[66c] A recent study by Jean Louis Trouillet et al.[66d] found that patients with acute mediastinitis (inflammation of the space in the middle of the chest between the two pleurae) after cardiac surgery were discharged from the hospital on average in 54 days if their wound had been treated with granulated sugar as compared with a stay of 85 days when the wound was not treated with sugar. The Trouillet article cites many other studies showing benefits of sugar in the healing of wounds. Various benefits of sugar can be found elsewhere in this book. Consult the index.

The bacteria of the colon, which ordinarily convert bile acids and cholesterol into possibly carcinogenic substances, cannot make this undesirable conversion when SPE is consumed instead of ordinary fats. SPE, with zero calories, is now on the market. Anal leakage (possibly correctable with palmitic acid) and reduced vitamin A liver storage, however, may be undesirable side effects of SPE.[67a-c]

Let's also consider labeling of vitamins and of other health-food products. Although we often hear about the superiority of natural vitamins, there could be circumstances under which synthetic vitamins might be better. Why? We noted in Chapter 6 that vitamin C is often made from corn, and those allergic to this grain may have difficulty with such a vitamin. Then too, vitamin tablets may contain lactose as a filler and many persons are sensitive to this sugar. Other "health" products may pose similar problems. If you have any known allergies, study the manufacturer's disclosure manuals to determine if the products you are considering are apt to pose any problems. You may decide that a synthetic product is better for you than a natural one.

Ascorbic acid may be assimilated more efficiently if bioflavonoids are not present (and they will be present if a natural source is being used). O. Pelletier and M. O. Keith[67d] reported that synthetic ascorbic acid without rutin caused a significantly greater increase in the blood of total ascorbic acid plus dehydroascorbic acid than the ingestion of ascorbic acid with rutin or with orange juice.

The theory that "natural" is superior to "synthetic" is ridiculous. As Edward J. Cafruny says,[68] "It seems that when plants rearrange the elements of our planet, the resultant drugs are considered natural and therefore good—apt to prolong life; when humans rearrange the same elements, the resultant drugs are synthetic and therefore suspect—apt to shorten life." Cafruny might have added after his words "natural and good" a few examples of those great natural herb products such as coffee, tobacco, heroin, opium, marijuana and cocaine. Nature, it seems, is as clever as man in creating toxic drugs. Nature is, of course, neutral to our aims and desires. Her laws, however, work inexorably and it behooves us to cooperate with such laws to further our own ends.[69]

Forget About Your Chronological Age!

If we can approach optimum values in the various nutrients with which we supplement our diet we should achieve robust health and improve our chances for increased longevity. However, it is not simply a long life that should be our objective. Far better to live youthfully all the days of one's life—whether or not one's life span approaches or even, perhaps, greatly exceeds the 100-year mark.

Let me give you a final exhortation to stop thinking about your chronological age. Chronological age is simply the number of times the earth has gone around the sun since once's birth. Why should this mere movement of the earth around the sun assume such an overwhelming importance to us? Think instead about your biological age and your psychological age—how young you feel; how, day by day, your health is improving.* That great, ageless black ball player, Satchel Paige, who had a fantastic career in the minor leagues prior to the major league's liberation of the blacks, is known for his philosophic sayings. Paige asked: "How old would you be if you didn't know how old you was?" T. L. Dormandy[78] has said: "'Old' and 'young' have non-chronological connotations which are understood by every child but not by scientists."

When you hear the master of ceremonies at the circus addressing "children of all ages," is the expression strange and meaningless? If you can't see the advantage of your being childlike, you are aging fast! Your psychological age and then, in turn, your biological age

---

* The assessment of biological age using a profile of physical parameters is discussed by Gary A. Borkan and Arthur H. Norris.[70] A specific program for measuring the human aging rate, citing many relevant parameters, has been proposed by Alex Comfort.[71] Relatedly, Richard L. Sprott and Edward L. Schneider[71a] have provided a list of 29 human biomarkers of aging. In another study, Charles L. Rose and Michel L. Cohen[72] cite many factors influencing longevity. That longevity correlates with a low incidence record of illnesses, absence of smoking and of worry offers no surprise. Perhaps astonishing, however, is the fact that an appearance of being of a younger age was found to be more important for longevity than any of the other factors studied. Gary L. Grove[73] cites G. A. Borkan and A. Norris[74] as having found that "certain individuals who appeared old for their age were in fact biologically older in a series of physical tests and expected to die sooner than their chronological peers." Grove and his co-workers[73,75-77] have been especially active in studies involving the skin as an indicator of biological age.

tend to become what you think they are! I hope that the creativity of the pro-and-con approach to health exemplified in this book has helped you. I hope this creative exercise has helped you to learn how to *grow older* without *growing old.*[*]

Recently someone asked me: "Wally, how old are you?" I replied, "Nineteen years and some months!" And, unless you are 18 or younger, that's your age too. Say your age out loud right now! *Nineteen and some months.*

We all know young people of 80 or 90 and old fogies of 40. Our democracy, remember, is based on respect for the individual. One should be judged on oneself and not on one's chronological age, and that includes judging of yourself by yourself. If you are 60 years old and want to do something you think more appropriate for a 20-year-old, do it! If you're young at heart, show it!

May you remain youthful no matter what your years and may you be a prime example of my basic tenet that biological age can be quite unrelated to chronological age. Best wishes to you for a long, vibrantly healthy, happy, fulfilling life.

Your attitude toward life and health will be caught by others who will, in turn, pass on your influence. Good health is contagious!

---

[*] I do not mean to comply with the "youth-is-all attitude" so prevalent in our society. Many things increase in value with age: wine, cheese, stamps, coins, art and furniture to name just a few. Why not aging persons? Why is there such little recognition of the wisdom that often comes with years of living? When will Western civilization venerate the aged—as the Chinese have done since the earliest times?

"It is important that students bring a certain ragamuffin, barefoot irreverence to their studies. They are not here to worship what is known, but to question it."

— Jacob Bronowski

"And no concept is final: concepts are made and remade. Gravitation does not become a lie when Einstein substitutes something else for it; it becomes part of the wider concept of relativity."

— Jacob Bronowski

"No science can ever give an exact picture of the universe—of any of its parts or of any of its processes. Science continually strives, however, for more exact statements of the operations of nature. Science is a key for unlocking nature's secrets, but the door has an infinite number of locks. Perfection in the understanding of the laws of nature is an impossible goal. Science is the name we call the struggle to achieve that goal."

— Walter A. Heiby

"When you see yourself as part of the solution rather than as being part of the problem, you make a decision to *affect* life rather than merely *reflecting* it. Happiness is a byproduct of devoting one's life to something or someone other than oneself."

— Walter A. Heiby

REFERENCES

Lengthy reference lists will almost certainly contain many errors in spite of heroic efforts to keep such errors at a minimum. Gerald de Lacey et al., writing in the *British Medical Jrl.* (Sept. 28, 1985, vol. 291: 884-886), have analyzed the accuracy of references in six major medical journals published during January, 1984. They reported that "errors in citation of references occurred in 24% of the articles, of which 8% were major errors—that is, they prevented immediate identification of the source of the reference." Great care has been taken in the present volume to minimize errors and I hope there are none of the "8% variety."

If you find an incorrect reference in this book, assume that most of the reference is correct. Perhaps the year cited is wrong but the volume number is right or vice versa. Perhaps the beginning page number of a range is in error but the final page number may be correct. The spelling of the first scientist's name could be inaccurate but the second name (if any) may be right. Often the journal being cited will have an index at the end of the year and that may be helpful. Then too, *Citation Abstracts* or *Index Medicus* might be useful if the spelling of the author's name (or the name of at least one of the authors) is correct. (Remember, however, that the publishing of these volumes lags behind that of the article by about six months and may lag even longer.) As an alternative, the computer—operated by a librarian—may be a more rapid means of resolving the error.

Introduction—153 References

1. Peter Mc Cullagh, *Medical Jrl. of Australia.* (1985) 142: 328–329.
1a. Adolph Grünbaum, *Psychological Medicine* (1986) 16: 19–38.
1b. Michael L. Burr, *Human Nutrition: Applied Nutrition* (1984) 38A: 329–334.
2. Philip W. Lavori et al., *New England Jrl. of Medicine* (1983) 309, no. 21: 1291–1299 at 1291–1292.
3. Thomas A. Louis, *Annual Review of Public Health* (1983) 4: 25–46.
4. John C. Bailar III et al., *New England Jrl. of Medicine* (1984) 311, no. 3: 156–162.
5. Lincoln E. Moses, *New England Jrl. of Medicine* (1985) 312, no. 14: 890–897.
6. S. A. Barnett and J. Burn, *Nature* (1967) 213: 150–152. Cited by S. Michael Plaut, *Pediatric Clinics of North America* (1975) 22, no. 3: 619–631, at 626.
7. Robert Ader, *Psychosomatic Medicine* (1980) 42, no. 3: 307–321, at 312.
7a. *Neural Modulation of Immunity,* ed. Roger Guillemin, Melvin Cohn and Theodore Melnechuk (New York: Raven Press, 1985).
7b. *Psychoneuroimmunology,* ed. Robert Ader (New York: Academic Press, 1981).
7c. *Mind and Immunity: Behavioral Immunology,* ed. S. E. Locke and M. Hornig-Rohan (New York: Praeger, 1983).
7d. *Mind and Immunity: Behavioral Immunology (1976–1982) An Annotated Bibliography* by Steven Locke and Mady Hornig-Rohan (New York: Institute for the Advancement of Health, 1983).
7e. *Stress, Immunity and Aging,* ed. Edwin Cooper (New York: Marcel Dekker, Inc., 1984).
7f. *Psychoneuroimmunology,* ed. Steven E. Locke et al. (Hawthorne, N.Y.: Aldine Pub., 1984).
7g. J. Edwin Blalock, *Jrl. of Immunology* (1984) 132, no. 3: 1067–1070.
7h. Jean L. Marx, *Science* (1985) 227: 1190-1192.
8. Marvin Stein et al., *Science* (1976) 119: 435–440.
9. Nicholas Pavlidis and Michael Chirigos, *Psychosomatic Medicine* (1980) 42, no. 1: 47-54.
10. Jay R. Kaplan et al., *Science* (1983) 220: 733–735.
11. R. H. Gisler et al., *Cellular Immunology* (1971) 2: 634–645.
12. Stanford B. Friedman et al., *Psychosomatic Medicine* (1965) 27: 361–368. Cited by Robert Ader, *Psychosomatic Medicine* (1980) 42, no. 3: 307–321, at 314.
12a. Steven Greer, *British Jrl. of Psychiatry* (1983) 143: 535–543.
13. Benjamin H. Newberry et al., *Psychosomatic Medicine* (1972) 34, no. 4: 295-303.
13a. Lawrence S. Sklar and Hymie Anisman, *Science* (1979) 205: 513–515.
13b. Madelon A. Visintainer et al., *Science* (1982) 216: 437–439.
14. Benjamin H. Newberry et al., *Psychosomatic Medicine* (1976) 38, no. 3: 155–162.
15. Andrew A. Monjan and Michael I. Collector, *Science* (1977) 196: 307–308.
16. Malcolm P. Rogers et al., *Jrl. of Rheumatology* (1983) 10, no. 4: 651–654.
17. Marcus M. Jensen and A. F. Rasmussen, *Jrl. of Immunology* (1963) 90: 17-20.
17a. I. S. Chohan et al., *Thrombosis and Haemostasis* (1984) 51, no. 1: 22–23.
18. Ernest A. Peterson, *Jrl. of Animal Science* (1980) 30: 422–439.
18a. P. Rachootin and J. Olsen, *Jrl. of Occupational Medicine* (1983) 25: 394–402. Cited by Donna Day Baird, *JAMA* (1985) 253: 18: 2643–2644.
19. Vernon Riley et al. in *Psychoneuroimmunology,* ed. Robert Ader (New York: Academic Press, 1981) pp. 45-46.
19a. Marcus M. Jensen and A. F. Rasmussen, *Jrl. of Immunology* (1963) 90: 21–23.
19b. A. R. Turnbull et al., *British Jrl. of Surgery* (1975) 62: 657.
19c. George F. Solomon et al., *Proc. of the Society for Experimental Biology and Medicine* (1967) 126: 74-79.
20. J. F. Spalding et al., *Laboratory Animal Care* (1969) 19, no. 2: 209–213.

21. John Nash Ott in *Environmental Variables in Animal Experimentation,* ed. Hulda Magalhaes (Lewisburg: Bucknell University Press, 1974) pp. 39–57.

22. James T. Marsh et al., *Science* (1963) 140: 1414–1415.

23. Susan R. Burchfield et al., *Physiology & Behavior* (1978) 21: 537–540.

24. Benjamin H. Newberry and Lee Sengbusch, *Cancer Detection and Prevention* (1979) 2, no. 2: 225–233.

25. Malcolm P. Rogers, *Arthritis & Rheumatism* (1980) 23, no. 12: 1337–1342.

26. H. M. Weiss et al., *Jrl. of Comparative and Physiological Psychology* (1976) 90: 257–259. Cited by Lawrence S. Sklar and Hymie Anisman, *Psychological Bulletin* (1981) 89, no. 3: 369–406, at 358.

27. F. H. Bronson and B. E. Eleftheriou, *Jrl. of Gerontology* (1965) 20: 239. Cited by James P. Henry et al., *Psychosomatic Medicine* (1971) 33, no. 3: 227–237.

28. B. L. Welch and A. S. Welch, *Proceedings of the National Academy of Sciences* (1969) 64: 100. Cited by James P. Henry et al., *Psychosomatic Medicine* (1971) 33, no. 3: 227–237.

29. George F. Solomon et al., *Psychotherapy and Psychosomatics* (1974) 23: 209–217.

30. Vernon Riley, *Science* (1975) 189: 465–467.

31. P. Ebbesen and R. Rask-Nielsen, *Jrl. of the National Cancer Institute* (1967) 39: 917–932.

32. David A. D'Atri et al., *Psychosomatic Medicine* (1981) 43, no. 2: 95-105.

33. Stanford B. Friedman and Lowell A. Glasgow, in *Health and the Social Environment,* ed. Paul M. Insel and Rudolf H. Moos (Lexington, Mass: D. C. Heath and Co., 1974) pp. 169–191, at 175. Originally appeared in *Pediatric Clinics of North America* (May, 1966) 13, no. 2: 315–335.

34. Ethel Tobach and Hubert Bloch, *American Jrl. of Physiology* (1956) 187: 399–402.

35. Howard B. Andervont, *Jrl. of the National Cancer Institute* (1944) 4: 579–581.

36. O. Muhlbock, *Acta Int. Union Against Cancer* (1951) 7: 351. Cited by Richard C. LaBarba, *Psychosomatic Medicine* (1970) 32, no. 3: 259–276.

37. J. L. Barnett et al., *General and Comparative Endocrinology* (1981) 44: 219–225.

38. Vernon Riley, *Science* (1984) 212: 1100–1109.

38a. Joseph T. King et al., *Proc. of the Society for Experimental Biology and Medicine* (1955) 88: 661–663.

39. Doreen Berman and Barbara E. Rodin, *Pain* (1982) 13: 307–311.

40. G. S. Wiberg and H. C. Grice, *Science* (1963) 142: 507.

41. James P. Henry et al., *Psychosomatic Medicine* (1975) 37, no. 3: 277-283.

42. James Rollin Slonaker, *American Jrl. of Physiology* (1935) 112: 176–181.

43. E. P. Durrant, *American Jrl. of Physiology* (1935) 113: 37.

44. David R. Lamb et al., *Laboratory Animal Care* (1966) 16, no. 3: 296–299.

45. H. M. Bruce, *British Medical Bulletin* (1970) 26: 10–13.

46. S. Michael Plaut et al., *Psychosomatic Medicine* (1969) 31: 536–552.

47. V. Riley and D. Spackman, *Proc. Amer. Assn. Cancer Res.* (1979) 18: 173. Cited by M. Chevedoff et al., *Food and Cosmetic Toxicology* (1980) 18: 517–522, at 521.

48. June Marchant, *British Jrl. of Cancer* (1967) 21: 576–585, at 584.

49. Patricia F. Hadaway et al., *Psychopharmacology* (1979) 66: 87–91.

50. George F. Solomon et al., *Nature* (1968) 220: 821–822.

51. G. Newton et al., *Jrl. of Nervous and Mental Disease* (1962) 134: 522. Cited by ref. 50.

52. S. Levine and C. Cohen, *Proceedings of the Society for Experimental Biology and Medicine* (1959) 102: 53. Cited by ref. 50.

53. Stanford B. Friedman et al., *Psychosomatic Medicine* (1967) 29, no. 4: 323–328.

54. Robert M. Nerem and Murina J. Levesque, *Science* (June 27, 1980) 208: 1475–1476.

54a. Robert Ader and Stanford B. Friedman, *Jrl. of Comparative and Physiological Psychology* (1965) 59, no. 3: 361–364.

55. Robert Ader, *Psychosomatic Medicine* (1970) 32, no. 6: 569–580.

56. Stephen H. Vessey, *Proc. of the Society for Experimental Biology and Medicine* (1964) 115: 252–255.

57. David E. Davis and John J. Christian, *Proc. of the Society for Experimental Biology and Medicine* (1957) 94: 728–731.

58. Paul Brain, *Life Sciences* (1975) 16: 187–220.

59. P. D. McMaster and R. E. Franzl, *Metabolism* (1961) 10: 990. Cited by Stanford B. Friedman and Lowell A. Glasgow in *Health and the Social Environment,* op. cit. (ref. 33) p. 175.

60. E. D. Kilbourne et al., *Nature* (1961) 190: 650. Cited by Stanford B. Friedman and Lowell A. Glasgow in *Health and the Social Environment,* op. cit. (ref. 33) p. 175.

61. I. E. Bush, *Pharmacological Reviews* (1962) 14: 317. Cited by Stanford B. Friedman and Lowell A. Glasgow in *Health and the Social Environment,* op. cit. (ref. 33) p. 176.

61a. W. Cassell et al., *Proc. of the Society for Experimental Biology and Medicine* (1967) 125 supp.: 676–679.

61b. B. Jencks, unpub. doctoral dissertation, University of Utah (1962). Cited in ref. 61a.

62. F. H. Bronson and B. E. Eleftheriou, *General and Comparative Endocrinology* (1964) 4: 9 as cited by John W. Mason, *Psychosomatic Medicine* (1968) 30, no. 5. (Part III): 576–607, at 579.

63. J. W. Mason, J. V. Brady and M. Sidman, *Endocrinology* (1957) 60: 741, cited by John W. Mason, *Psychosomatic Medicine* (1968) 30, no. 5: (Part III) 576–607 at 579.

64. Robert Ader and Nicholas Cohen, *Psychosomatic Medicine* (1975) 37, no. 4: 333–340.

64a. Robert Ader et al., *Trends in Pharmacological Sciences* (1983) 4, no. 2: 78–80.

65. Michael Russell et al., *Science* (1984) 225: 733–734.

66. S. Michael Plaut, *Pediatric Clinics of North America* (1975) 22, no. 3: 619–631, at 628.

66a. Carl Peraino et al., *Cancer Research* (1971) 31: 1506–1512.

67. Robert Ader in *Environmental Variables in Animal Experimentation,* ed. Hulda Magalhaes (Lewisburg: Bucknell University Press, 1974) pp. 109–135, at 123.

68. Robert Ader, *Psychosomatic Medicine* (1967) 29, no. 4: 345–353.

69. R. Ader and S. B. Friedman, *Neuroendocrinology* (1968) 3: 378–386.

70. Alexander H. Freidman and Charles A. Walker, *Jrl. of Physiology* (1968) 197: 77–85.

71. M. P. Rogers et al., *Psychosomatic Medicine* (1979) 41, no. 2: 147–164 at 151.

72. Stanford B. Friedman et al., *Annals of the New York Academy of Sciences* (1969) 164: 381–393.

73. D. H. Sprunt and C. C. Flanigan, *Jrl. of Experimental Medicine* (1956) 104: 687–706. Cited by Stanford B. Friedman et al., ibid.

74. Robert Ader in *Environmental Variables in Animal Experimentation,* ed. Hulda Magalhaes (Lewisburg: Bucknell University Press, 1974) pp. 109–135, at 119–120.

74a. E. A. Emken, *Annual Review of Nutrition* (1984) 4: 339–376, at 365–367.

75. Morton Rothstein, *Biochemical Approaches to Aging* (New York: Academic Press, 1982) p. 258.

75a. S. Mitchell Harman et al., *Endocrinology* (1978) 102, no. 2: 540–544.

76. G. Miescher and C. Böhm, *Schweiz med. Wschr.* (1947) 77: 821–826. Cited by Annie M. Brown in *Animals for Research,* ed. W. Lane-Petter (New York: Academic Press, 1963) pp. 271 and 283.

76a. *Merck Index,* 10th ed. (Rahway, N.J.: Merck & Co., 1983) p. 3147.

77. John B. Jemmott, III et al., *Lancet* (June 25, 1983): 1400–1402.

78. Ziad Kronfol et al., *Life Sciences* (1983) 33: 241–247.

79. Stanley M. Bierman, *Western Jrl. of Medicine* (1983) 139, no. 4: 547–552.

80. Sharon Warren et al., *Jrl. of Chronic Diseases* (1982) 35: 821–831.

81. Stanislav V. Kasl et al., *Psychosomatic Medicine* (1979) 41, no. 6: 445–466.

82. Richard B. Shekelle et al., *Psychosomatic Medicine* (1981) 43, no. 2: 117–125.

83. Cary L. Cooper, *Jrl. of Human Stress* (1984) 10, no. 1: 4–11.

84. Steven Greer, *British Jrl. of Psychiatry* (1983) 143: 535–543.

85. Lawrence E. Hinkel, Jr. et al., *Psychosomatic Medicine* (1958) 20, no. 4: 278–295, at 295.
86. Richard H. Barnes et al., *Federation Proceedings* (1963) 22: 125–128.
87. Roman Kulwich et al., *Jrl. of Nutrition* (1953) 39: 639–645.
88. Richard H. Barnes et al., *Jrl. of Nutrition* (1957) 63: 489–498.
89. Richard H. Barnes and Grace Fiala, *Jrl. of Nutrition* (1958) 65: 103–114.
90. Richard H. Barnes et al., *Jrl. of Nutrition* (1959) 67: 599–610.
91. M. J. Sharkey, *Mammalia* (1971) 35: 162–168.
92. B. K. Armstrong and A. Softly, *British Jrl. of Nutrition* (1966) 20: 595–598.
92a. S. E. Olpin and C. J. Bates, *British Jrl. of Nutrition* (1982) 47: 577–588.
92b. R. J. Neale, *Laboratory Animals* (1984) 18: 119–124.
93. Frederick Hoelzel and Esther DaCosta, *Amer. Jrl. of Digestive Diseases* (1941) 8, no. 7: 266–270.
93a. Vernon Riley et al., *Cancer Detection and Prevention* (1979) 2, no. 2: 235–255.
93b. John K. Inglehart, *New England Jrl. of Medicine* (1985) 313, no. 6: 395–400.
93c. Thomas D. Overcast and Bruce D. Sales, *JAMA* (Oct. 11, 1985) 254, no. 14: 1944–1949.
94. Douglas K. Obeck, *Laboratory Animal Science* (1978) 28, no. 6: 698–704.
94a. Maxine Briggs in *Recent Vitamin Research,* ed. Michael H. Briggs (Boca Raton, Florida: CRC Press, 1984) p. 46.
95. M. W. Fox in *Environmental Variables in Animal Experimentation,* ed. Hulda Magalhaes (Lewisburg: Bucknell University Press, 1974) pp. 96–108, at 108.
95a. S. B. Friedman and R. Ader, *Neuroendocrinology* (1967) 2: 209–212.
95b. A. Wise and D. J. Gilburt, *Food and Cosmetic Toxicology* (1980) 18: 643–648.
95c. B. H. Ershoff, *American Jrl. of Clinical Nutrition* (1974) 27: 1395. Cited in ref. 95b.
95d. B. H. Ershoff, *Jrl. of Nutrition* (1977) 107: 822. Cited in ref. 95b.
95e. D. Kritchevsky, *Federation Proceedings* (1977) 36: 1692. Cited in ref. 95b.
95f. David M. Klurfeld et al., *Federation Proceedings* (March 5, 1986) 45, no. 4: 1076.
95g. Victor Herbert, *Science* (April 4, 1986) 232: 11.
95h. L. R. Jacobs, *Cancer Research* (1983) 43: 4057. Cited in ref. 95g.
95i. Hugh J. Freeman et al., *Cancer Research* (1980) 40: 2661–2665.
95j. Hugh J. Freeman in *Carcinogens and Mutagens in the Environment,* vol. 2, ed. Hans F. Stich (Boca Raton, Fla.: CRC Press, 1983) pp. 129–137, at 130.
95k. K. Wakabayashi et al., *Cancer Letters* (1978) 4: 171. Cited in ref. 95j.
95l. K. Watanabe et al., *Cancer Research* (1978) 38: 4427. Cited in ref. 95j.
96. R. A. Hinde, *Animal Behavior: A Synthesis of Ethology and Comparative Psychology,* 2nd ed. (New York: McGraw Hill, 1970.) Cited by S. Michael Plaut, *Pediatric Clinics of North America,* (1975) 22, no. 3: 619–631, at 620.
96a. Noel W. Solomons and Fernando E. Viteri in *Ascorbic Acid: Chemistry, Metabolism and Uses,* (Washington, D.C.: American Chemical Society, 1982) pp. 560–561.
97. S. A. Barnett, *Newsweek* (Dec. 3, 1973): 6–8. Cited by S. Michael Plaut, *Pediatric Clinics of North America* (1975) 22, no. 3: 619–631, at 621.
98. Panel on Non-human Primate Nutrition of the National Research Council of the National Academy of Sciences, *Nutrient Requirements of Nonhuman Primates* (Washington, D.C.: National Academy of Sciences, 1978).
99. Lowell A. Glasgow et al., *American Jrl. of Medicine* (July 20, 1982) 73, supp. 1A: 132–137.
99a. Mathew M. Ames et al., *Research Communications in Chemical Pathology and Pharmacology* (Oct., 1978) 22, no. 1: 175–185.
99b. John C. Bailar III, *New England Jrl. of Medicine* (Oct. 24, 1985) 313, no. 17: 1080–1081.
100. H. Babich, *Environmental Research* (1982) 29: 1–29, at 9.
100a. Elliot S. Vesell et al., *Federation Proceedings* (1976) 35: 1125–1132.
101. C. M. Brubaker et al., *Life Sciences* (1982) 30, no. 23: 1965–1971.

102. John B. Barnett, *International Archives of Allergy and Applied Immunology* (1981) 66: 229–232.
103. Carl J. Bodenstein, *Pediatrics* (1984) 73, no. 5: 733–736.
104. T. C. Chamberlin, *Jrl. of Geology* (1897) 5: 837–848. Cited by S. Michael Plaut, *Pediatric Clinics of North America* (1975) 22, no. 3: 619–631, at 628.

Chapter 1—220 References

1. Robert P. Heaney, *Jrl. of Laboratory and Clinical Medicine* (1982) 100: 309.
2. F. C. Redlich, *Jrl. of Medicine and Philosophy* (1976) 1, no. 1: 269–280.
3. Michael H. Kottow, *Medical Hypotheses* (1980) 6: 209–213.
4. George E. Vaillant, *New England Jrl. of Medicine* (1979) 301: 1249–1254.
5. S. Greer et al., *Lancet* (Oct. 13, 1979): 785–787.
5a. Keith W. Pettingale, Steven Greer et al., *Lancet* (March 30, 1985): 750.
6. J. Paget, *Surgical Pathology*, 2nd ed. (London: Longmans Green, 1870). Cited by S. Greer, *Psychological Medicine* (1979) 9: 81–89 at 82.
7. Lawrence LeShan, *Jrl. of the National Cancer Institute* (1959) 22, no. 1: 1–18.
8. Lawrence LeShan, *Annals of the New York Academy of Sciences* (1966) 125: 780–793.
9. Constance Holden, *Science* (1978) 200: 1363–1369.
10. Phillip Shaver et al., *American Jrl. of Psychiatry* (1980) 137, no. 12: 1563–1658.
11. Erik Agduhr, *Acta Medica Scandinavica* (1939) 99, no. 5: 387–424.
12. D. Drori and Y. Folman, *Experimental Gerontology* (1969) 4: 263.
13. D. Drori and Y. Folman, *Experimental Gerontology* (1976) 11: 25–32.
14. H. F. Smyth, Jr., *Food Cosmetic Toxicology* (1967) 5: 51–58.
15. Loren J. Chapman et al., *Jrl. of Abnormal Psychology* (1976) 85, no. 4: 374–382.
16. Martin Harrow et al., *American Jrl. of Psychiatry* (1977) 134, no. 7: 794–797.
17. Soon D. Koh et al., *Schizophrenia Bulletin* (1981) 7, no. 2: 292–307.
18. Mark Cook and Fredie Simukonda, *British Jrl. of Psychiatry* (1981) 139: 523–525.
19. Robert F. Simons, *Psychophysiology* (1982) 19, no. 4: 433–441.
20. Jan Fawcett et al., *Archives of General Psychiatry* (1983) 40: 79–84.
21. Robert H. D. Dworkin and Kathleen Saczynski, *Jrl. of Personality Assessment* (1984) 48, no. 6: 620–626.
22. Paul E. Meehl, *Bulletin of the Meninger Clinic* (1975) 39, no. 4: 295–307, at 299–300 and 305.
23. William S. Edell and Loren J. Chapman, *Jrl. of Consulting and Clinical Psychology* (1979) 47, no. 2: 379–384.
24. W. E. Penk et al., *Jrl. of Consulting and Clinical Psychology* (1979) 47, no. 6: 1046–1052.
25. Charles G. Watson, *Jrl. of Abnormal Psychology* (1972) 80, no. 1: 43–48.
25a. Charles G. Watson et al., *Psychological Reports* (1970) 26: 371–376.
26. E. Cuyler Hammond, *Jrl. of the National Cancer Institute* (May, 1964) 32: 1161–1188. Cited in *Wine of Life* by Harold J. Morowitz (New York: St. Martins Press, 1979).
27. Stephen L. Taylor, *New York Times* (Feb. 10, 1982).
28. Robert M. Nerem et al., *Science* (June 27, 1980) 208: 1475–1476.
28a. B. S. Gow, M. E. McCaskill and M. J. Legg, *Atherosclerosis* (1982) 44: 121–122.
28b. M. J. Legg, B. S. Gow and M. R. Roach, *Proc. Aust. Physiol. Pharmacol. Soc.* (1981) 12: 130 P. Cited in ref. 28a.
28c. S. Michael Plaut et al., *Psychosomatic Medicine* (1974) 36, no. 4: 311–320.
28d. S. Michael Plaut, *Developmental Psychology* (1970) 3, no. 3: 157–167.
29. W. B. Gross and Paul B. Siegel, *American Jrl. of Veterinary Research* (1982) 43, no. 11: 2010–2012.
30. W. B. Gross and P. B. Siegel, *American Jrl. of Veterinary Research* (1982) 43, no. 1: 137–139.
31. Jay R. Kaplan et al., *Arteriosclerosis* (1982) 2: 359–368.
32. John N. Edwards and David L. Klemmack, *Jrl. of Gerontology* (1973) 28, no. 4: 497–502.
33. Judith G. Rabkin and Elmer L. Struening, *Science* (1976) 194: 1013–1020.

34. Michael G. Marmot and S. Leonard Syme, *American Jrl. of Epidemiology* (1976) 104, no. 3: 225–247.
35. John G. Bruhn et al.,*Southern Medical Jrl.* (1982) 75, no. 5: 575–580, at 580.
36. Dianne Timbers Fairbank and Richard L. Hough,*Jrl. of Human Stress* (1979) 5: 41-47.
37. Jerry Suls et al., *Jrl. of Psychosomatic Research* (1979) 23: 315–319.
38. Irwin G. Sarason et al., *Psychosomatic Medicine* (1985) 47, no. 2: 156–163.
39. Rafaella M. A. Osti et al., *Psychotherapy and Psychosomatics* (1980) 33: 193–197.
39a. Carol W. Buck and Allan P. Donner, *Jrl. of Chronic Diseases* (1984) 37, no. 4: 247–253.
39b. T. Theorell, *Psychotherapy and Psychosomatics* (1980) 34: 135–148.
39c. D. G. Byrne, *British Jrl. of Medical Psychology* (1981) 54: 371–377.
39d. L. N. Gupta and R. K. Verma, *Indian Jrl. of Medical Research* (1983) 77: 697–701.
39e. Ralph Carasso, *International Jrl. of Neuroscience* (1981) 14: 223–225.
40. Thomas H. Holmes and Richard H. Rahe, *Jrl. of Psychosomatic Research* (1967) 11: 213–218.
41. Janice K. Kiecolt-Glaser et al., *Psychosomatic Medicine* (1984) 46, no. 1: 7–14.
42. Steven E. Locke et al., *Psychosomatic Medicine* (1984) 46, no. 5: 441–453.
42a. R. W. Bartrop et al., *Lancet* (April 16, 1977): 834–836.
42b. S. J. Schleifer et al., *JAMA* (1983) 250: 374–377.
42ba. Harold Levitan, *Psychosomatics* (Dec., 1985) 26, no. 12: 939–94.
42c. William A. Greene, *Jrl. of the American Medical Women's Assn.* (1965) 20, no. 2: 133–141, at 137.
42d. Knud J. Helsing et al., *American Jrl. of Public Health* (1981) 71, no. 8: 802–809.
43. W. P. Cleveland and D. T. Gianturco, *Jrl. of Gerontology* (1976) 31: 99–102. Cited in *Bereavement-Reactions, Consequences and Care,* ed. Marian Osterweis, Fredric Solomon and Morris Green (Washington, D.C.: National Academy Press, 1984).
43a. Guilia I. Perini et al., *Psychotherapy and Psychosomatics* (1984) 41: 48–52.
43b. Nancy A. Williams and Jerry L. Deffenbacher, *Jrl. of Human Stress* (1983) 9: 26–31.
43c. Barry Glassner and C. V. Halipur, *American Jrl. of Psychiatry* (1983) 140, no. 2: 215–217.
43d. G. H. B. Baker, *Psychotherapy and Psychosomatics* (1982) 38: 173–177.
43e. Richard Totman et al.,*Jrl. of Psychosomatic Research* (1980) 24: 155–163.
43f. Steven Lehrer, *Psychosomatic Medicine* (1980) 42, no. 5: 499–502.
43g. Francis Creed, *Lancet* (June 27, 1981): 1381–1385.
44. Kenneth B. Matheny and Penny Cupp, *Journal of Human Stress* (June, 1983): 14–23.
45. Paul J. Rosch, *JAMA* (1979) 242, no. 5: 427–428.
46. Hans Selye, *Stress and Distress* (New York: J. B. Lippincott, 1974).
46a. Rickey S. Miller and Herbert M. Lefcourt, *American Jrl. of Community Psychology* (1983) 11, no. 2: 127–139.
46b. W. D. Gentry et al., *Psychosomatic Medicine* (1982) 44: 195–202.
46c. Steven Greer and Maggie Watson, *Social Science and Medicine* (1985) 20, no. 8: 773–777.
46d. K. W. Pettingale et al., *Jrl. Psychsoc. Oncol.* In press. Cited in ref. 46c.
46e. L. Temoshok and B. H. Fox in *Impact of Psychoendocrine Systems in Cancer and Immunity,* ed. B. H. Fox and B. H. Newberry (New York: C. J. Hogrefe, 1984). Cited in ref. 46c.
46f. M. Watson et al., *Advances in the Biosciences, vol. 49—Psychological Aspects of Cancer,* ed. M. Watson and T. Morris (Oxford: Pergamon Press, 1984). Cited in ref. 46c.
46g. L. V. Holdeman et al., *Applied and Environmental Microbiology* (1976) 31, no. 3: 359–375.
46h. Marcia Angell, *New England Jrl. of Medicine* (1985) 312, no. 24: 1570–1572.
46i. Robert B. Case et al., *New England Jrl. of Medicine* (1985) 312, no. 12: 737–741.
47. Barrie R. Cassileth et al., *New England Jrl. of Medicine* (1985) 312, no. 24: 1551–1555.

47a. Austen Clark, in *Examining Holistic Medicine,* ed. Douglas Stalker and Clark Glymour (Buffalo, N.Y.: Prometheus Books, 1985) pp. 67–106.

47b. Edward R. Friedlander, in *Examining Holistic Medicine,* ibid., pp. 273–285.

48. Reubin Andres, *International Jrl. of Obesity* (1980) 4: 381–386.

49. A. R. Dyer et al., *Jrl. of Chronic Diseases* (1975) 28: 109–123. Cited by Ancel Keys in *Nutrition in the 1980's,* ed. Nancy Selvey and Philip L. White (New York: Alan R. Liss, 1981) pp. 31–46, at 39.

50. R. J. Garrison et al., *JAMA* (1983) 249: 2199–2203. Cited by Artemis P. Simopoulos, *Nutrition Reviews* (1985) 43, no. 2: 33–40.

50a. JoAnn E. Manson et al., *JAMA* (Jan. 16, 1987) 257, no. 3: 353-358.

50b. Ulf Smith, *Medical World News* (Feb. 11, 1985) 26, no. 3: 74.

51. Bernard Fisher et al., *New England Jrl. of Medicine* (1985) 312, no. 11: 665–673.

52. M. Alice Ottoboni, *The Dose Makes the Poison* (Berkeley, CA: Vincente Books, 1984) pp. 91–92.

53. Ibid., p. 94

54. *Federal Register* (Oct. 5, 1983) 48, no. 194: 45508.

55. W. W. Duke, *JAMA* (Nov. 6, 1915) 65, no. 19: 1600–1610.

56. Lawrence P. Garrod, *British Medical Jrl.* (Feb. 3, 1951): 205–210.

57. G. E. Foley and W. D. Winter, *Jrl. of Infectious Diseases* (1949) 85: 268. Cited by ref. 56.

58. T. D. Luckey, *Federation Proceedings* (Feb., 1978) 37, no. 2: 107–109.

58a. Committee to Study the Human Health Effects of Subtherapeutic Antiobiotic Use in Animal Feeds, National Research Council, *The Effects on Human Health of Subtherapeutic Use of Antimicrobials in Animal Feeds* (Washington, D.C.: National Academy of Sciences, 1980) p. XIII.

58b. Ibid., p. 7

58c. Ibid., pp. 22–23.

58d. Scott D. Holmberg et al., *New England Jrl. of Medicine* (1984) 311, no. 10: 617–622.

58e. N. V. Medunitsyn, *Zh. Mikrobiol. Epidemiol. Immunobiol.* (1960) 31: 742–743.

59. Frank R. George et al., *Pharmacology, Biochemistry and Behavior* (1983) 19: 131–136.

60. Robert E. Hodges et al., *American Jrl. of Clinical Nutrition* (Aug., 1962) 11, no. 2: 85–93.

61. M. L. Smith and W. A. Loqman, *Archives of Andrology* (1982) 9: 105–113.

62. M. C. Chang, *Jrl. of Andrology* (1984) 5: 45-50.

63. C. Selli et al., *European Urology* (1983) 9: 109–112.

64. Robert T. Rubin et al., *Jrl. of Clinical Endocrinology and Metabolism* (1978) 47, no. 2: 447–452.

65. S. P. Ghosh et al., *Jrl. of Reproduction and Fertility* (1983) 67: 235–238.

66. P. Marrama et al., *Maturitas* (1982) 4: 131–138.

67. Herbert Y. Meltzer, *Jrl. of Pharmacology and Experimental Therapeutics* (1983) 224, no. 1: 21–27.

68. John T. Clark et al., *Science* (Aug. 24, 1984) 225–847–849.

69. Mark F. Schwartz et al., *Biological Psychiatry* (1982) 17, no. 8: 861–876.

70. A. Rocco et al., *Archives of Andrology* (1983) 10: 179–183.

71. L. C. Garcia Diez and J. M. Gonzalez Buitrago, *Archives of Andrology* (1982) 9: 311–317.

72. D. Ayalon et al., *Int. Jrl. of Gynaecology and Obstetrics* (1982) 20: 481–485.

72a. John Bancroft in *Biological Determinants of Sexual Behavior,* ed. J. B. Hutchison (New York: John Wiley & Sons, 1978) pp. 493–519, at 511.

72b. L. Lidberg, *Pharmakopopsychiat.* (1972) 5: 187. Cited in ref. 72a.

72c. L. Lidberg, *Hormones* (1972) 5: 273. Cited in ref. 72a.

72d. L. Lidberg and V. Sternthal, in prep. Cited in ref. 72a (p. 511).

73. Anon, *Science Digest* (July, 1982) 9: 94.

74. J. C. Theiss, *International Colloquium on Cancer,* Houston: M. D. Anderson Hospital and Tumor Institutes, 1981. Cited by*Lancet* (Dec. 11, 1982): 1317–1318.
75. Michael L. Kleinberg and Michael J. Quinn, *Amer. Jrl. Hosp. Pharm.* (1981) 38: 1301–1303.
76. Hanna Norppa et al., *Scand. Jrl. Work Envir. Health* (1980) 6: 299–301.
77. R. P. Bos, *Int. Arch. Occup. Environ. Health* (1982) 50: 359–369.
77a. Marja Sorsa et al., *Mutation Research* (1985) 154: 135–149.
78. S. Venitt et al.,*Lancet* (Jan. 14, 1984): 74–76.
79. *Lancet* (Dec. 11, 1982): 1317–1318.
80. J. F. Gibson et al., *Lancet* (Jan. 14, 1984): 100–101.
81. *Lancet* (Jan. 28, 1984): 203.
82. Luci A. Power and Michael H. Stolar,*Lancet* (March 10, 1984): 569–570.
82a. Sherry G. Selevan et al., *New England Jrl. of Medicine* (Nov. 7, 1985) 313, no. 19: 1173–1178.
82b. Eula Bingham, *New England Jrl. of Medicine* (Nov. 7, 1985) 313, no. 19: 1220–1221.
82c. Robert Hoover and Joseph F. Fraumeni, Jr., *Cancer* (1981) 47, no. 5: 1071–1080.
83. M. A. Firer et al., *British Medical Jrl.* (1981) 283: 693–696.
84. E. R. Stiehm et al., *Annals of Internal Medicine* (1982) 98: 80–93, cited by Richard D. de Shazo and John E. Salvaggio, *JAMA* (Oct. 26, 1984) 252, no. 16: 2198–2201.
84a. Gene P. Siegal et al., *Proceedings of the National Academy of Sciences* (1982) 79: 4064–4068.
85. Frederick Hoelzel and Esther DaCosta, *Amer. Jrl. of Digestive Diseases and Nutrition* (1937) 4: 325–331.
85a. James C. White, *New England Jrl. of Medicine* (1985) 312, no. 4: 246–247.
86. T. D. Luckey, *Health Physics* (1982) 43, no. 6: 771–789.
87. *Encyclopaedia Britannica,* 15th ed., vol. 15, "Radiation, Effects of" (Chicago: Encyclopaedia Britannica, 1979) pp. 378–392 at 386.
88. G. W. Beebe et al., cited by Alice M. Stewart, *Jrl. of Epidemiology and Community Health* (1982) 36: 80–86.
89. L. P. Breslavets et al., *Biophysics* (1960) 5, 86–87.
90. L. D. Carlson et al., *Radiation Research* (1957) 7: 190.
90a. Carolyn Ferree, *JAMA* (Dec. 6, 1985) 254, no. 21: 3036
91. Roy E. Albert et al.,*Radiation Research* (1961) 15: 410–430.
92. Wheeler P. Davey, *Jrl. of Experimental Zoology* (1919) 28, no. 2: 447–458.
93. T. D. Luckey, *Hormesis with Ionizing Radiation* (Boca Raton, Florida: CRC Press, 1980).
94. R. L. Sullivan and D. S. Grosch,*Nucleonics* (1953) 11: 21, cited by Luckey (ref. 93).
95. E. Lorenz et al., in *Biological Effects of External X and Gamma Radiation,* Part 1, ed. R. E. Zirkle (New York: McGraw Hill, 1954) p. 24, cited by Luckey (ref. 93).
96. J. J. Morris et al., *Effects of low level X radiation upon growth of mice,* unpublished report (1963), cited by Luckey (ref. 93).
97. L. P. Breslavets and A. S. Afanasyeva, *Vestn. Rentgenol. Radiol.* (1935) 14: 302 and *Cytologia* (1935) 8: 110, cited by Luckey, (ref. 93).
98. R. K. Schulz in *Survival of Food Crops and Livestock in the Event of Nuclear War,* ed. D. W. Benson and A. H. Sparrow (Oak Ridge, Tenn.: U.S. Atomic Energy Commission, 1971) p. 370, cited by Luckey (ref. 93).
99. I. Fendrik, *Stim. Newsletter* (1970) 1: 8, cited by Luckey (ref. 93).
100. A. S. Pressman, *Electromagnetic Fields and Life* (New York: Plenum Press, 1970) pp. 156–157.
101. C. M. Southam and J. Ehrlich,*Pythopathology* (1943) 33: 517–529.
102. T. D. Luckey in *Heavy Metal Toxicity, Safety and Hormology* by T. D. Luckey, B. Venugopal and D. Hutcheson (New York: Academic Press, 1975) p. 103.
103. House of Representatives no. 2284, 85th Congress, Second Session (1958).
103a. *Chicago Tribune* (June 28, 1985).

103b. Marjorie Sun, *Science* (1984) 223: 667–668.

103c. Marjorie Sun, *Science* (1985) 229: 739–741.

103d. David A. Kessler, *Science* (1984) 223: 1034–1040.

103e. W. Gary Flamm in *Carcinogens and Mutagens in the Environment*, vol. 1, ed. Hans F. Stich (Boca Raton, Florida: CRC Press, 1982) pp. 275–281.

104. Minna Alice Ottoboni, *The Dose Makes The Poison* (Berkeley, CA: Vincente Books, 1984) p. 99.

105. National Center for Toxicological Research, *Jrl. of Environmental Pathology and Toxicology* (1980) 3, no. 3. Cited in ref. 104.

106. Society of Toxicology Committee, *Fundamental and Applied Toxicology* (1981) 1, no. 1: 27–128. Cited in ref. 104.

107. *Physicians' Desk Reference*, 39th ed. (Oradell, N.J.: Medical Economics Co., 1985).

107a. David F. Horrobin, *Medical Hypotheses* (1981) 7: 115–125.

107b. *Physicians' Desk Reference*, 39th ed. (Oradell, N.J.: Medical Economics Co., 1985) pp. 1723–1724.

107c. Ibid., pp. 538 and 540.

107d. Ibid., p. 1051.

107e. Ibid., p. 532.

107f. Ibid., p. 1940.

107fa. *AMA Drug Evaluations*, 5th ed. (Chicago: American Medical Assn., 1983).

107fb. *Drug Facts and Comparisons* (St. Louis, Mo.: Facts and Comparisons, Inc., 1985).

107g. Joseph Meites et al., *Proceedings of the Society for Experimental Biology and Medicine* (1971) 137: 1225–1227.

107h. C. Huggins, *Cancer Research* (1965) 25: 1163. Cited in ref. 107g.

107i. R. I. Dorfman, *Methods in Hormone Research* (1965) 4: 165. Cited in ref. 107g.

107j. J. Hayward, *Recent Results in Cancer Research* (Berlin: Springer-Verlag, 1970) p. 69.

108. Mary E. Caldwell and Willis R. Brewer, *Cancer Research* (Dec., 1983) 43: 5775–5777.

108a. D. R. Stoltz et al., *Environmental Mutagenesis* (1984) 6: 343–354.

108b. S. Morris Kupchan and E. Bauerschmidt, *Photochemistry* (1971) 10: 664–666.

108c. Thomas S. Kuhn, *The Structure of Scientific Revolutions* (Chicago: University of Chicago Press, 1962) p. X.

108d. Ibid., p. 6.

108e. Ibid, p. 24.

108f. John Pfeiffer, *The Changing Universe* (New York: Random House, 1956) p. 142.

109. A. J. Clark, *The Mode of Action of Drugs on Cells* (London: Edward Arnold, 1933) cited by D. F. Horrobin, *Prostaglandins* (1977) 14, no. 4: 667–677.

110. E. J. Ariens et al., *Pharmacological Reviews* (1957) 9: 218–236.

111. J. M. Von Rossum in *Molecular Pharmacology*, vol. 2, ed. E. J. Ariens (New York: Academic Press, 1964) pp. 199–255. Do not confuse this book with the journal of the same name.

112. W. D. M. Paton, *Proc. of the Royal Society* (1961) 154B: 21–69.

112a. Richard N. Zare, *Science* (Oct. 19, 1984) 226: 298–303.

113. Seymour L. Romney et al., *Gynecologic Oncology* (1985) 20: 109–114.

114. Erhard Haus et al., *Science* (July 7, 1972) 177: 80–82.

115. F. Hallberg et al., *Experientia* (1973) 29, no. 8: 909–934.

116. L. E. Scheving et al., in *Chronobiology*, ed. Lawrence E. Scheving, Franz Halberg and John E. Pauly (Tokyo: Igaku Shoin Ltd., 1974) pp. 213–217.

117. Karel M. H. Philippens, in *Chronobiology*, ibid., pp. 23–28.

118. G. Brubacher et al., *Bibliotheca Nutri, Dieta* (1981) 30: 90–99.

119. R. L. Gross and P. M. Newberne, *Physiological Reviews* (Jan., 1980) 60: 188–302, at 260.

119a. C. M. Leevy et al., *American Jrl. of Clinical Nutrition* (1965) 17: 259. Cited by ref. 119.

120. D. J. Smithard and M. J. S. Langman, *British Jrl. of Clinical Pharmacology* (1978) 5: 181–185.

120a. K. Bartlett, *Advances in Clinical Chemistry* (1983) 23: 141–198.

121. S. Harvey Mudd, *Jrl. of Clinical Pathology* 27 (Supplement *Royal College of Pathology,* 1974) 8: 38–47.

122. Charles Scriver, *Pediatrics* (1970) 36, no. 4: 493–496.

123. S. Harvey Mudd, *Advances in Nutritional Research,* vol. 4, ed. Harold H. Draper (New York: Plenum Pub., 1982) pp. 1-34.

124. E. Cheraskin and W. M. Ringsdorf, Jr., *New Hope for Incurable Diseases* (Jericho, N.Y.: Exposition, 1971).

124a. Noel S. Weiss, *New England Jrl. of Medicine* (Sept. 5, 1985) 313, no. 10: 632–633.

124b. Samuel M. Lesko et al., *New England Jrl. of Medicine* (1985) 313, no. 10: 593–596.

124c. Jon J. Michnovicz et al., *New England Jrl. of Medicine* (Nov. 20, 1986) 315, no. 21: 1305-1309.

124d. Cope, G. F., et al., *British Medical Jrl.* (Aug. 23, 1986) 291: 481.

124e. Roger Lewin, *Science* (Dec. 5, 1986) 234: 1200-1201.

125. Committee on Dietary Allowances of the Food and Nutrition Board, *Recommended Dietary Allowances,* 9th ed. (Washington, D.C.: National Academy of Sciences, 1980).

126. Eliot Marshall, *Science* (Oct. 25, 1985) 230: 420–421.

127. Henry Kamin, *Science* (Dec. 20, 1985) 230: 1324, 1326.

128. Robert E. Olson, *Science* (Dec. 20, 1985) 230: 1326.

129. Frank Press, *Science* (Dec. 20, 1985) 230: 1326, 1410.

130. Edward L. Schneider et al., *New England Jrl. of Medicine* (Jan. 16, 1986) 314, no. 3: 157–160.

131. Victor Herbert, *Federation Proceedings* (March 1, 1986) 45, no. 3: 477 (abstract no. 1885).

132. *Nutrition Today* (Nov./Dec., 1985): 4-23.

133. Food and Nutrition Board, *Jrl. of Nutrition* (1986) 116: 482–488.

134. Henry Kamin, *American Jrl. of Clinical Nutrition* (1985) 41: 165–170.

135. E. J. van der Beek, *Sports Medicine* (1985) 2: 175–197, at 179.

Chapter 2—402 References

1. Mary Louise Quaife and Mei Yu Dju, *Jrl. Biological Chemistry* (1948) 180: 263, cited by J. Bjorksten, *Rejuvenation* (1975) 3: 38–51.

1a. Willy A. Behrens et al., *Amer. Jrl. of Clinical Nutrition* (1982) 35: 691–696.

1b. Willy A. Behrens and Rene Madere, *Nutrition Research* (1985) 5: 167–174.

1c. Ella Haddad et al., *Amer. Jrl. of Clinical Nutrition* (1985) 41: 599–604.

2. J. F. Pennock et al., *Biochem. Biophys. Res. Comm.* (1964) 17: 542–548.

3. S. Kasparek in *Vitamin E,* ed. Lawrence J. Machlin (New York: Dekker, 1980) p. 14.

3a. Herman Baker, *American Jrl. of Clinical Nutrition* (Sept., 1985) 42: 568.

3b. Paris Constantinides and Martha Harkey, *Virchows Archiv. A. Pathological Anatomy and Histology* (1985) 405: 285-297.

4. Erling F. Week, et al., *Jrl. of Nutrition* (1952) 46: 353–359.

5. E. E. Edwin et al., *Biochemical Jrl.* (1961) 79: 91–105.

6. Archives of *Biochemistry and Biophysics* (1974) 165: 6–8.

7. *European Jrl. Biochemistry* (1974) 46: 217–219.

8. *European Jrl. Biochemistry* (1982) 123: 473–475.

9. *U.S. Pharmacopeia* (1980) XX.

9a. Stanley R. Ames, *Jrl. of Nutrition* (1979) 109: 2198–2204.

9b. H. Baker et al., *Federation Proceedings* (1985) 44, no. 4: 935 (abstract no. 3063).

10. Rao V. Panganamala, *Prostaglandins* (1977) 14, no. 2: 261–271.

11. C. W. Birky and J. A. Power, *Amer. Jrl. of Clinical Nutrition* (1980) 33: 1856–1860.

12. M. K. Horwitt, *Amer. Jrl. of Clinical Nutrition* (1980) 33: 1856–1860.

13. Philip L. Harris et al., *Jrl. of Biological Chemistry* (1944) 156: 491–498.

14. T. Leth and H. Sondergaard, *Internat. Jrl. Vit. Nutri. Res.* (1983) 53: 297–311.

15. Philip L. Harris and Marion I. Ludwig, *Jrl. of Biological Chemistry* (1949) 180: 611–614.

16. Torben Leth and Helge Sondergaard, *Jrl. of Nutrition,* (1977) 107: 2236–2243.

17. H. Weiser and M. Vecchi, *Internat. Jrl. Vit. Nutri. Res.* (1981) 51: 100–113.

18. J. Bunyan et al., *Jrl. of Nutrition* (1976) 106: 124–127.

19. Bernard Century and M. K. Horwitt, *Federation Proceedings* (1965) 24: 906–911.

20. Leo Friedman et al., *Jrl. of Nutrition* (1958) 65: 143–160.

21. M. K. Horwitt, *Amer. Jrl. of Clinical Nutrition* (1980) 33: 1856–1860.

22. H. Weiser et al., *Science* (1963) 140: 80.

22a. Cora J. Dillard et al., *Jrl. of Nutrition* (1983) 113: 2266–2273.

23. Abbas E. Kitabchi and Jay Wimalasena, *Biochimica et Biophysica Acta* (1982) 684: 200–206.

23a. C. J. Dillard et al., *Jrl. of Nutrition* (1983) 113, no. 11: 2266–2273. Cited in *Nutrition Abstracts* (1984) series A, 54, no. 5: 372.

24. Max K. Horwitt, *Vitamin E,* ed. Lawrence J. Machlin (New York: Dekker, 1980) p. 630.

25. H. Dam and E. Sondergaard, *Z. Ernahrungswiss* (1964) 5: 73–79.

26. W. L. Marusich et al., *Poultry Science* (1967) 46: 541–548.

27. Stanley R. Ames, *Lipids* (1971) 6: 251–290.

28. E. L. Hove and Philip L. Harris, *Jrl. of Nutrition* (1947) 33: 95–106.

29. M. L. Scott and I. D. Desai, *Jrl. of Nutrition* (1964) 83: 39–43.

30. L. D. Matterson and W. J. Pudelkiewicz, *Jrl. of Nutrition* (1974) 104: 79–83.

31. L. J. Machlin et al., *Jrl. of Nutrition* (1982) 112: 1437–1440.

32. W. J. Pudelkiewicz et al., *Jrl. of Nutrition* (1960) 71: 115–121.

33. Hugo E. Gallo-Torres in *Vitamin E,* ed. Lawrence J. Machlin (New York: Dekker, 1980) p. 209.

34. G. W. Burton and K. U. Ingold, *Jrl. of the Amer. Chemists Soc.* (1981) 107: 6472–6477.

34a. L. H. Chen and R. R. Thacker, *Nutrition Research* (1985) 5, no. 4: 431–434. Abstracted in *Nutrition Abstracts and Reviews,* Series A (1985) 55, no. 9: 6: 636 (abstract no. 5576).

35. C. K. Chow and H. H. Draper, *Internat. Jrl. Vit. Nutri. Res.* (1974) 44: 396–403.

35a. W. Heimann and H. von Pezold, *Fette-Seifen Anstrichmittel* (1957) 59: 330. Cited in ref. 35.

35b. P. Lambelet and J. Löliger, *Chemistry and Physics of Lipids* (1984) 35: 185–198.

36. John G. Bieri and R. Poukka Evarts, *Amer. Jrl. of Clinical Nutrition* (1974) 27: 980–986.

36a. J. G. Bieri and R. P. Evarts, *Amer. Jrl. of Clinical Nutrition* (1975) 28: 717–720.

36b. M. K. Horwitt, *Amer. Jrl. of Clinical Nutrition* (1976) 29: 569–578.

36c. I. R. Peake et al., *Biochimica et Biophysica Acts* (1972) 260: 679–688.

36d. Coy D. Fetch and J. Friedrich Diehl, *Proc. of the Soc. for Experimental Biology and Medicine* (1965) 119: 553–557.

37. V. N. R. Kartha and S. Krishnamurthy, *Internat. Jrl. Vit. Nutri. Res.* (1978) 48: 38–43.

38. Kenji Fukuzawa et al., *Archives of Biochemistry and Biophysics* (1981) 206, no. 1: 173–180.

39. C. D. Fitch et al., *Archives of Biochemistry and Biophysics* (1965) 112: 448–493.

40. Stanley R. Ames, *Lipids* (1971) 6: 281–290.

41. E. L. Hove and Zelda Hove, *Jrl. of the Biological Society* (1944) 156: 623–632.

41a. Max K. Horwitt et al., *Amer. Jrl. of Clinical Nutrition* (1984) 40: 240–245.

42. Franklin Bicknell and Frederick Prescott, *The Vitamins in Medicine,* 3rd ed. (Milwaukee, Wisc.: Lee Foundation For Nutritional Research, 1962).

43. H. Kläui and G. Pongracz, *Vitamin C,* ed. J. N. Counsell and D. H. Hornig (New York: Elsevier—Published in England by Applied Science, 1981) p. 163.

43a. A. Seher and St. A. Ivanov, *Fette Seifen Anstrichmittel* (1973) 75: 606–608.

44. T. W. Anderson, *Canadian Medical Jrl.* (1974) 110: 401–406.

45. Manfred Steiner and John Anastasi, *Jrl. of Clinical Investigation* (1976) 57: 732–737.

45a. P. C. Huijgens et al., *Acta Hematologica* (1981) 65: 217–218.

45b. M. Steiner, *Thrombosis and Haemostasis* (1983) 49: 73–77.

45c. Jun Watanabe et al., *Tokoku Jrl. of Exp. Med.* (1984) 143: 161–169.

46. M. Steiner, *Biochimica et Biophysica Acta* (1981) 640: 100–105.

47. A. Chadwick Cox et al., *Blood* (1980) 55: 907–914.

48. D. W. Wooley, *Jrl. Biological Chemistry* (1945) 159: 59.

49. J. D. Kanofsky and Paul B. Kanofsky, *New England Jrl. of Medicine* (1981) 305: 173–174.

50. E. Agradi et al., *Prostaglandins* (1981) 22, no. 2: 255–266.

51. R. E. Olson, *Circulation* (1973) 48: 179–184.

52. Joseph Gomes et al., *Amer. Heart Jrl.* (1976) 91: 425–429.

53. Hyman J. Roberts, *JAMA* (1981) 246, no. 2: 129–130.

53a. P. Bostwick and M. M. Mathias, *Federation Proceedings* (1985) 44, no. 4: 929 (abstract no. 3033).

54. William J. Hermann, Jr. et al., *Amer. Jrl. of Clinical Pathology,* (Nov., 1979) 72: 849-852.

55. William J. Hermann, Jr., *Annals of the N.Y. Academy of Sciences* (1982) 393: 467-472.

56. Peter L. Schwartz and Ian M. Rutherford, *Amer. Jrl. of Clinical Pathology* (1981) 76: 843-844.

57. L. J. Hatam and H.J. Kayden, *Amer. Jrl. of Clinical Pathology* (1981) 76: 122-124.

58. Donald R. Howard et al., *Ibid:* 86-89.

59. Meir J. Stampfer et al., *Amer. Jrl. of Clinical Pathology* (1981) 76:86-89.

60. W. Marx, *Archives of Pathology* (1949) 47: 440.

61. O.A. Levander et al., *Jrl. of Nutrition* (1973) 103: 536.

61a. N.R. DiLuzio and F. Costales, *Experimental and Molecular Pathology* (1965) 4:141-154.

910 **The Reverse Effect**

61b. Joyce E. Redetzki et al., *Jrl. of Toxicology—Clinical Toxicology* (1984) 20, no. 4: 319-331.
62. H. Paul Ehrlich et al., *Annals of Surgery* (1972) 175:235-240.
63. James O. Woolliscroft, *DM—Disease-A-Month* (1983) 25:1-56.
64. Peter L. Scardino and Perry B. Hudson, *Annals of the N.Y. Academy of Sciences* (1949) 52, art. 3: 425-427.
65. Peter L. Scardino and William Wallace Scott, Ibid: 390-396.
65a. R. J. Morgan and J.P. Pryor, *British Jrl. of Urology* (1978) 50: 111-113.
65b. J. P. Pryor and J.M. Fitzpatrick, *Jrl. of Urology* (1979) 122: 622-623.
66. H.J. Roberts, *Angiology* (Mar., 1979) 30: 169-177.
67. Archie A. Abrams, *New England Jrl. of Medicine* (1965) 272: 1080-1081.
68. David Solomon et al., *Annals of the N.Y. Academy of Sciences* (1972) 203: 103-110.
69. G. S. Sundaram et al., *Jrl. of the Amer. Oil Chemists' Society* (1981) 58: 765A.
69a. W.J. Serfontein et al., *Amer. Jrl. of Clinical Pathology* (1983) 5: 604-606. *Cited in Nutrition Abstracts and Reviews, Series A* (May, 1984) 54, no. 5: 372 (Abst. No. 2347).
69b. Timo Kuusi et al, *Lancet* (Nov. 17, 1984): 1163.
69c. Maret G. Traber and Herbert J. Kayden, *American Jrl. of Clinical Nutrition* (Oct. 1984) 40: 747-751.
70. G.S. Sundaram et al, *Cancer Research* (1981) 41: 3811-3813.
70a. K. Larry smith et al., *Jrl. of Dairy Science* (1984) 67: 1293-1300.
70b. P.P. Nair and H.J. Kayden, editors, *International Conference on Vitamin E and its Role in Cellular Metabolism* (New York: New York Academy of Sciences, 1972). Cited by M. Briggs in ref. 165.
70c. J.P. Minton et al., *Surgery* (1979) 86, no. 1: 105-109.
70d. J.P. Minton et al, *American Jrl. of Obstetrics and Gynecology* (1979) 135, no. 1: 157-159.
71. Philip G. Brooks et al., *Jrl. of Reproductive Medicine* (1981) 26: 279-282.
72. Siegfried Heyden. *Surgery* (1980) 88: 741-742.
73. V.L. Ernester et al., *Amer. Jrl. of Epidemiology* (1981) 114: 421.
74. James Marshall et al., *Public Health Briefs* (1982) 72, no. 6: 610-612.
74a. Collen A. Boyle et al., *Jrl. of the National Cancer Institute* (1984) 72, no. 5: 1015-1019.
74aa. Flora Lubin et al., *JAMA* (1985) 253: 2388-2392.
74ab. J.P. Minton, *JAMA* (Nov. 1, 1985) 254, no. 17: 2408.
74ac. Flora Lubin et al., *JAMA* (Nov. 1, 1985) 254, no. 17: 2408-2409.
74ad. Michael F. Jacobson and Bonnie F. Liebman, *JAMA* (March 21, 1986) 255, no. 11: 1438-1439.
74ae. Jason Pozner, *JAMA* (Feb. 14, 1986) 255, no. 6: 748.
74b. R. London, G.S. Sundaram et al., *Jrl. of the Amer. College of Nutrition* (1984) 3, no. 3: 264 (Abstract 95).
74ba. Virginia L. Ernester et al., *Surgery* (1985) 97, no. 4: 490-494.
74c. Robert V.P. Hutter, *New England Jrl. of Medicine* (1985) 312, no. 3: 179-181.
74d. S.M. Love et al., *New England Jrl. of Medicine* (1982) 307: 1010-1014. Cited in ref. 74c.
74e. Helmuth Vorherr, *New England Jrl. of Medicine* (1985) 312, no. 19: 1258.
75. Seth L. Haber and Robert W. Wissler, *Proc. of the Soc. for Experimental Biology and Medicine* (1962) 111: 774-775.
76. S.A. Burobina and E.A. Nefakh, *Transactions of the Moscow Soc. of Naturalists* (1970) 32: 56-61.
77. Gerald Shklar, *Jrl. of the National Cancer Institute* (1982) 68, no. 5: 791-793.
78. Woranut Weerapradist and Gerald Shklar, *Oral Surgery* (1982) 54: 304-12.
79. Martin G. Cook and Peter McNamera, *Cancer Research* (1980) 40: 1329-1331.
80. Clement Ip, *Carinogenesis* (1982) 3: 1453-1456.
80a. Paula M. Horvath and Clement Ip, *Cancer Research* (Nov., 1983) 43: 5335-5341.

80b. W.J. Mergens et al., from *N-Nitroso Compounds: Analysis, Formation and Occurrence,* ed. E.A. Walker, M. Castegnaro, L. Griciute and M. Borzsonyi (Lyon, France: IARC Scientific Publication no. 31, 1980) pp. 250-267.

81. William J. Mergens, *Annals of the N.Y. Academy of Sciences* (1982) 393: 61-69.

81a. C.K. Chow et al., *Toxicology Letters* (1984) 23: 109-117.

82. Michael P. Kurek and Laurence M. Corwin, *Nutrition and Cancer* (1982) 4: 128-139.

82a. Toshima Yasunaga et al., *Nippon Geka Hokan, Archiv für Japanishe Chirurgie* (1984) 53, no. 2: 312-323.

83. Kedar N. Prasad et al., *Proc. of the Soc. for Experimental Biology and Medicine* (1980) 164: 158-163.

83a. Ifor D. Capel et al., *Cancer Research* (1983) 3:59-62.

83b. Takashi Kokunai et al., *Neurologia medico-chirurgica* (1983) 23, no. 6: 421-427.

83c. Richard F. Wagner et al., *International Jrl. of Dermatology* (1984) 23, no. 7: 453-457.

83d. K.N. Prasad and J. Edwards-Prasad, *Cancer Research* (1982) 42: 550. Cited in ref. 83c.

84. A. Lopez and B.Y. LeGardeur, *Clinical Research* (1982) 30, no. 2: 623A.

84a. N.J. Wald et al., *British Jrl. of Cancer* (1984) 49: 321-324.

85. A. Kagerud and H.I. Peterson, *Acta Radiologica Oncology* (1981) 20: 97-100.

86. C. Beckman et al., *Mutation Research* (1982) 105: 73-77

87. I.R. Telford, *Annals of the N.Y. Academy of Sciences* (1949) 52: 130.

88. M.H. Briggs, *Lancet* (Feb. 9, 1974): 220.

88a. Onatolu Odukoya et al., *Nutrition and Cancer* (1986) 8, no. 2: 101-106.

89. Rollin H. Heinzerling et al., *Infection and Immunity* (1974) 10:1292-1295.

90. K. Folkers, *Int. Jrl. for Vitamin and Nutrition Research* (1969) 39: 334.

91. Emile Bliznakov et al., *Experientia* (1970) 26: 953-954.

92. Andria C. Casey and E. Bliznakov, *Chem. Biol. Interactions* (1972) 5: 1-12.

93. Emil G. Bliznakov, *Mechanisms of Ageing and Development* (1978) 7: 189-197.

93a. Emil G. Bliznakov in *Biomedical and Clinical Aspects of Coenzyme Q,* vol. 3, ed. K. Folkers and Y. Yamamura (Amsterdam: Elseveier/North Holland Biomedical Press, 1981) pp. 311-323.

93b. Emil G. Bliznakov et al., *Jrl. of Medicine* (1978) 9, no. 4: 337-346.

94. Mark F. McCarty, *Medical Hypotheses* (1981) 7: 515-518.

94a. D. Jones et al., *Internat. Jrl. Vit. Nutr. Res.* (1971) 41: 215-220.

94b. Th. M. Farley et al., *Internat. Z. Vit. Forshung,* now called *Internat. Jrl. Vit. Nutr. Res.,* (1968) 38: 355-361.

94c. Yuichi Yamamura in *Biomedical and Clinical Aspects of Coenzyme Q,* vol. 1, ed. K. Folkers and Y. Yamamura (Amsterdam: Elsevier Scientific Publ. Co., 1977) pp. 281-298.

94d. Ryo Nakamura et al., *Proc. National Academy of Sciences* (1974) 71: 1456-1460.

94e. Edward G. Wilkinson and Ralph M. Arnold, *Research Communications in Chemical Pathology and Pharmacology* (Sept., 1975) 12, no. 1: 111-124.

94f. Edward G. Wilkinson and Ralph M. Arnold, in *Biomedical and Clinical Aspects of Coezyme Q,* vol. 1, op. cit. (ref. 94c) pp. 251-266.

94g. Inge L. Hansen et al., *Research Communications in Chemical Pathology and Pharmacology* (1976) 14, no. 4: 729-738.

94h. Edward G. Wilkinson et al., *Research Communications in Chemical Pathology and Pharmacology.* (1976) 14, no. 4: 715-719.

94i. Karl Folkers and Tatsuo Watanabe, *Jrl. of Medicine* (1977) 8, no. 5: 333-348.

94j. Yoshiro Nakamura et al., *Cardiovascular Research* (1982) 16: 132-137.

94k. Masahara Takenaka et al., *Transplantation* (1981) 32, no. 2: 137-141.

94l. Karl Folkers et al., *Research Communications in Chemical Pathology and Pharmacology* (1978) 19, no. 3: 485-490.

94m. Karl Folkers, *International Jrl. for Vitamin and Nutrition Research* (1969) 39: 334-352.

94n. T. Farley, J. Scholler and K. Folkers, *Biochem. Biophys. Res. Commun.* (1966) 24: 299. Cited by ref. 94m.

912 The Reverse Effect

94o. J. Scholler, T. Farley and K. Folkers, *International Jrl. for Vitamin and Nutrition Research*, (1968) 38: 369. Cited by ref. 94m.

95. Toshima Yasunaga et al., *Jrl. of Nutrition* (1982) 112: 1075-1084.

96. Cheryl F. Nockels, *Federation Proceedings* (1979) 36: 2134-2138.

97. T.S. Lim et al., *Immunology* (1981) 44: 289-295.

98. Laurence M. Corwin and Richard K. Gordon, *Annals of the N.Y. Academy of Sciences* (1982) 393: 437-451.

98a. Naoki Inagaki et al., *Jrl. of Pharmacobiodynamics* (1984) 7, no. 1: 70-74.

99. William R. Beisel, *Amer. Jrl. of Clinical Nutrition* (Feb., 1982) 35: 417-468 at 431-433.

100. J. Siva Prasad, *Amer. Jrl. of Clinical Nutrition* (1980) 33: 606-608.

101. Alan C. Tsai et al., *Amer. Jrl. of Clinical Nutrition* (1978) 31: 831-837.

101a. Adrianne Bendich et al., *Jrl. of Nutrition* (1986) 116: 675-681.

102. J.S. Goodwin and P.G. Garry, *Clin. Exp. Immunol.* (1983) 51: 647-653.

103. J. Green, *Annals of the N.Y. Academy of Sciences* (1972) 203: 29-44, at 41.

104. M. Passeri and D. Provedini, *Acta Vitaminol Enzymol* (1982) 5: 53-63.

104a. R.L. Holman, *Proc. Soc. for Experimental Biology and Medicine* (1947) 66: 307-309.

105. Toshikazu Yoshikawa et al., *Biochemical Medicine* (1983) 29:227-234.

105a. J.Watanabe et al., *Thrombosis and Haemostasis* (1984) 51, no. 3: 313-316.

106. Samuel Ayres, Jr. and Richard Mihan, *Cutis* (1979) 23: 49-54.

107. Arthur Voglesang, *Angiology* (April 1970) 21:·275-279.

108. A.E. Harding et al., *Annals of Neurology* (1982) 12: 419-429.

109. D.P.R. Muller et al., *Lancet* (Jan. 29, 1983): 225-228.

110. Knut Haeger, *Amer. Jrl. of Clinical Nutrition* (1974) 27: 1179-1181.

111. Phillip M. Farrell, *Vitamin E,* ed. Laurence J. Machlin (New York: Dekker, 1980) pp. 588-592.

112. Conor T. Keane and Rosemary Hone, *Lancet* (March 16, 1974): 458.

113. Robert Semple, *Lancet* (April 20, 1974): 735.

114. James O. Woolliscroft, *DM—Disease-A-Month* (1983) 29: 1-56.

115. Samuel Ayres, Jr. and Richard Mihan, *Southern Medical Jrl.* (1974) 67: 1308-1312.

115a. Robert S. London et al., *Jrl. of the Amer. College of Nutrition* (1983) 2: 115-122, 287.

115b. Keiji Ono, *Nephron* (1985) 40: 440-445.

116. Laurence Corash et al., *New England Jrl. of Medicine* (Aug. 21, 1980) 303: 416-420.

117. Laurence Corash et al., *Annals of the N.Y. Academy of Sciences* (1982) 393: 348-360.

118. Gerhard J. Johnson et al., *New England Jrl. of Medicine* (1983) 308: 1014-1017.

119. Johannah G. Newman et al., *Clinical Biochemistry* (1979) 12, no. 5: 149-151.

120. John W. Eaton et al., *Nature* (1976) 264: 758-760.

120a. *Nutrition Reviews* (1984) 42, no. 5: 195-196.

121. C.L. Natta et al., *Amer. Jrl. of Clinical Nutrition* (1980) 33: 968-971.

122. Danny Chiu et al., *Annals of the N.Y. Academy of Sciences* (1982) 393: 323-335.

123. William M. Ross et al., *Canadian Jrl. of Ophthalmology* (1982) 17, no. 2: 61-66.

124. John R. Trevithick, William R. Ross et al., *Investigative Ophthalmology and Visual Science* (March 1981) 20, no. 3 supp: 219.

124a. Kailash C. Bhuyan et al., *Annals of the N.Y. Academy of Sciences* (1982) 393: 169-171.

125. P.P. Guptz et al., *Indian Jrl. of Experimental Biology* (1984) 22: 620-622.

125a. S.D. Varma et al., *Photochemistry and Photobiology* (1982) 36: 623-626.

125b. S.D. Varma et al., *Invest. Ophthalmol. Vis. Sci.* (1980) 19: 13 as cited in S.D. Varma et al., Ibid: 626.

125c. S.D. Varma et al., *Ophthalmic Res.* (1982) 14: 167-175.

125d. R.H.T. Edwards et al., *Medical Biology* (1984) 62: 143-147.

125e. G. Fitzgerald and B. McArdle, *Brain* (1941) 64: 19-42. Cited in ref. 125d.

125f. J.N. Walton and F.J. Nattrass, *Brain* (1954) 77: 169-231. Cited in ref. 125d.

125g. L.Z. Stern et al., *Archives of Neurology* (1982) 39: 342-346. Cited in ref. 125d.

126. Arthur C. Guyton, *Textbook of Medical Physiology,* 5th ed. (Philadelphia: W.B. Saunders Co., (1976) p. 984.

127. Franklin Bicknell and Frederick Prescott,*The Vitamins in Medicine,* 3rd ed. (Milwaukee, Wisc.: Lee Foundation for Nutritional Research (1962) p. 636.

127a. M.C. Farber et al., *Physiol. Chem.* (1953) 295: 318, cited in ref. 127b.

127b. E. Sondergaard and H. Dam, *Zeitschrift für Ernährungswissenschaft* (1970) 10, no. 1: 71-78.

128. K.L. Blaxter et al., *British Jrl. of Nutrition* (1953) 7:337.

129. H.H. Draper and A. S. Csallany, *Proc. of the Society for Experimental Biology and Medicine* (1958) 99: 739-742.

130. Benjamin N. Berg, *Jrl. of Gerontology* (1959) 14: 174-180.

131. K.L. Blaxter et al., *British Jrl. of Nutrition* (1953) 7: 287.

132. J.W. Safford et al., *Amr. Jrl. of Veterinary Research* (1956) 17: 503.

132a. M.J. Jackson et al., *Jrl of Inherited Metabolic Disease* (1985) 8, Supp. no. 1: 84-87.

133. O.A. Levander et al.,*Jrl. of Nutrition* (April 1973) 103: 536-547.

134. W.J. Rhead et al., cited by Douglas V. Frost and Paul M. Lish, *Annual Reviews of Pharmacology* (1975) 15: 259-284.

134a. Gerhard N. Schrauzer et al., *Annals of Clinical and Laboratory Science* (1975) 5, no. 1: 31-37.

134b. Sidney L. Saltzstein, *Lancet* (May 10, 1975): 1095.

135. Ashley Montagu, *Touching—the Human Significance of the Skin* (New York: Harper and Row, 1978).

136. William J. Goldwag, *Bestways* (Dec. 1977).

136a. I. Gontzea et al., *Arch. Franc. Ped.* (1970) 27: 733-741.

136b. Malcolm L. Chiswick et al., *British Medical Jrl.* (July 9, 1983) 287: 81-84.

136c. Q.S. Zhu et al.,*Biochimica et Biophysica Acta* (1982) 680: 69-79.

136d. Francisco J. Aranda and Juan C. Gomez-Femandez, *Archives of Biochemistry and Biophysics* (1982) 218, no. 2: 525-530.

137. E.L. Hove et al., *Archives of Biochemistry* (1945) 8: 395-404.

138. Edward J. Calabrese, *Nutrition and Environmental Health,* vol. 1 (New York: Wiley Interscience, 1980).

139. M.G. Mustapha,*Nutrition Reports International* (1975) 11:473.

140. Jack D. Hackney et al., *Jrl. of Toxicology and Environmental Health* (1981) 7: 383-390.

140a. John K. Timtim et al., *Hawaii Medical Jrl.* (1983) 42, no. 7: 160-164.

140b. L.N. North and J. Judson McNamara,*Aviation, Space and Environmental Medicine* (1984) 55, no. 7: 617-619.

141. *Advertising Age* (Oct. 15, 1973).

142. R. Hayakawa et al., *Acta Vitaminologica et Enzymologica* (1981) 3n.s. 31-38.

143. Stanley Starasoler and Garry S. Haber,*N.Y. State Dental Jrl.* (1978) 44: 382-383.

144. Jungman Ego Kim and Gerald Shklar, *Jrl. of Periodontology* (1983) 54: 305-308.

144a. Robert L. Ruberg, *Surgical Clinics of North America* (1984) 64, no. 4: 705-714 at 709.

144b. William A. Pryor in *Free Radicals in Biology,* ed. Donald Armstrong et al. (New York: Raven Press, 1984) pp. 13-41, at 15-16.

145. G.W. Burton, et al., *Lancet* (Aug. 7, 1982): 327.

145a. Albert A. Barber and Frederick Bemheim, *Advances in Gerontological Research* (1967) 2: 355-403 at 379.

145b. E.G. Hill, *Jrl. of the Amer. Oil Chemists' Society* (1963) 40: 360-364. Cited in ref. 145a.

145c. J.G. Bieri and A.A. Anderson, *Archives of Biochemistry and Biophysics* (1960) 90: 105-110. Cited in ref. 145a.

146. Richard D. Lippman,*Jrl. of Gerontology* (1981) 36: 550-557.

146a. Toshihiko Ozawa et al., *Biochimica et Biophysica Acta* (1978) 531:72-78.

146b. E.N. Frankel, *Jrl. of the American Oil Chemists' Society* (1984) 61, no. 12: 1908-1917, at 1910.

146c. A.L. Tappel, *Annals of the New York Academy of Sciences* (1980) 355: 18-31.

146d. B. Halliwell and J.M.C. Gutteridge,*Molecular Aspects of Medicine* (1985) 8: 89-193, at 119.

147. Denham Harman in *Free Radicals in Molecular Biology,* ed. Donald Armstrong et al. (New York: Raven Press, 1984) pp. 1-12 at 7.

147a. Joe M. McCord, *New England Jrl. of Medicine* (1985) 312, no. 3: 159-163.

147b. Shunichi Fujimoto et al., *Surgical Neurology* (1984) 22: 449-454.

148. F. Z. Meerson et al., *Basic Research Cardiology* (1982) 77: 465-485.

149. C. W. Karpen et al., *Prostaglandins* (Oct., 1981) 22: 651-661.

149a. T.L. Dormandy, *Lancet* (Oct. 29, 1983): 1010-1014.

149b. Toshihiko Ozawa and Akira Hanaki, *Biochemistry International* (1983) 6, no. 5: 685-692.

149c. T.L. Dormandy, *Annals of the Royal College of Surgeons of England* (1980) 62: 188-194.

149d. G.W. Burton et al., *Biochemical Society Transactions* (1983) 11: 261-262.

149da. Rao V. Panganamala and David Cornwell, *Annals of the New York Academy of Sciences* (1982) 393: 376-389.

149e. Richard G. Cutler in *Free Radicals in Molecular Biology,* ed. Donald Armstrong et al. (New York: Raven Press, 1984) pp. 235-266, at 255, at 259-260, and at 261-262.

149f. J. Hallfrisch et al., *Federation Proceedings* (March 5, 1986) 45, no. 4: 828 (abstract no. 3922).

150. M.A. Warso and W.E.M. Lands,*British Medical Bulletin* (1983) 39: 272-280.

150a. Beverly D. Lyn-Cook and Rosalyn M. Patterson, *Nutrition Research* (1984) 4: 989-993.

151. Paul B. McCay and M. Margaret King,*Vitamin E,* ed. Laurence J. Machlin (New York, Dekker, 1980) p. 295.

152. Morimitsu Nishikimi et al., *Biochimica et Biophysica Acta* (1980) 627: 101-108.

152a. Toshihiko Ozawa and Akira Hanaki, *Chemical & Pharmaceutical Bulletin* (1983) 31, no. 8: 2535-2539.

153. Irwin Fridovich, *Acta Physiologica Scandinavica* (1980) supp. 492: 142.

154. Johann Bjorksten, *Rejuvenation* (1979) 7, no. 2: 33-36.

155. Robert L. Baehner et al., *Blood* (Aug. 1977) 50: 327-335.

155a. G. Balla et al., *Acta Paediatrica Academiae Scientiarum Hungaricae* (1982) 23, no. 3: 319-325.

155b. Hans Nohl and Dietmar Hegner,*European Jrl. of Biochemistry* (1978) 82: 563-567.

156. R.O. Recknagel and A.K. Ghoshal, *Laboratory Investigation* (1966) 15: 132-146. Cited in ref. 155b.

156a. M. Wartanowicz et al., *Annals of Nutrition and Metabolism* (1984) 28: 186-191.

156b. Etsuo Niki et al.,*Jrl. of Biological Chemistry* (1984) 259, no. 7: 4177-4182.

157. A.D. Blackett and D.A. Hall, *Age and Ageing* (1981) 10: 191-195.

158. L. Green, *Annals of the New York Academy of Sciences* (1972) 203: 29-44.

159. William A. Pryor, *Annals of the New York Academy of Sciences* (1982) 393: 1-22.

160. Lloyd A. Witting, *Amer. Jrl. of Clinical Nutrition* (1974) 27: 952-959.

160a. B. Halliwell and John M.C. Gutteridge,*Lancet* (June 23, 1984): 1396-1397.

160b. Luis Garcia-Bunuel,*Lancet* (Sept. 8, 1984): 577.

160c. Iswar S. Singh and Jagat J. Ghosh, *Lancet* (Sept. 8, 1984): 577.

160d. B. Halliwell and J.M.C. Gutteridge,*Lancet* (Nov. 10, 1984): 1095.

161. Laurence M. Corwin and Janet Shloss, *Jrl. of Nutrition* (1980) 110: 2497-2505.

162. A.M. Butler et al.,*Prostaglandins and Medicine* (1979) 2: 203-216.

162a. Robert O. Likoff et al., *Amer. Jrl. of Clinical Nutrition* (1981) 34: 245-251.

163. A.N. Siakotos and N. Koppang,*Mechanisms of Ageing and Devel.* (1973) 2: 177.

163a. A. Saari Csallany et al., *Jrl. of Nutrition* (1977) 107: 1792-1799.

164. Patricia Kruk and Hildegard E. Enesco, *Experientia* (1981) 37: 1300-1301.

164a. A. Salminen et al., *Experientia* (1984) 40: 822-823.

164b. B. Zaspel Menken et al., *Jrl. of Nutrition* (1986) 116: 350-355.

165. Michael Briggs, *Mecical Jrl. of Australia* (1974) 1: 434-437.

165a. Daniel W. Nebert, *British Medical Jrl.* (Aug. 22, 1981) 283: 537-542, at 538.

166. D. Lees et al., *Jrl. of Reproduction and Fertility* (1982) 66: 543-545.

166a. J.P. Mather et al., *Acta Endocrinologica* (1983) 102: 470-475.

167. Wilbur H. Miller and Alice M. Dessert, *Annals of the New York Academy of Sciences* (1949) 52, art 3: 167-179.

168. Roman J. Kutsky, *Handbook of Vitamins, Minerals and Hormones* (New York: Van Nostrand Reinhold, 1981) p. 30.

168a. Edmond J. Farris, *Annals of the New York Academy of Sciences* (1949) 53, art. 3: 409-410.

169. N.Y. J. Yang and I.D. Desai, *Experientia* (1977) 33: 1460-1461.

170. C. Raychaudhwi and I.D. Desai, *Science* (1971): 1028.

171. W. Gullickson, *Annals of the New York Academy of Sciences* (1949) 52, art. 3: 256-259.

172. F.C. van der Kaay et al., *Annals of the New York Academy of Sciences* (1949) 52 art 3: 276-283.

173. Edward Herold et al., *Archives of Sexual Behavior* (1979) 8: 397-403.

174. Evan Shute, *The Heart and Vitamin E* (London, Canada: Shute Foundation for Medical Research, 1963).

175. I.M. Sharman, *British Jrl. of Nutrition* (1971) 26: 265-276.

176. Ivan M. Sharman and Michael G. Down, *Jrl. of Sports Medicine* (1976) 16: 215-223.

177. Thomas Kirk Cureton, *The Physiological Effects of Wheat Germ Oil On Humans in Exercise* (Springfield, Ill: Charles C. Thomas, 1972).

178. Ezra Levin in *The Physiological Effects of Wheat Germ Oil on Humans in Exercise* by Thomas Kirk Cureton, ibid.

178a. Melvin H. Williams, *Nutritional Aspects of Human Physical and Athletic Performance* (Springfield, Ill.: Charles C. Thomas, 1976) pp. 218-225.

179. *IARC Monographs on the Evaluation of the Carcinogenesis Risk of Chemicals to Humans,* vol. 20 (Lyon, France: International Agency for Research on Cancer, World Health Organization, 1979) pp. 429-448.

179a. Bruce Ames, *Science* (1979) 204, no. 11: 587-593.

179b. U.S. patent numbers 2,374,219, and 2,503,313 and 3,509,933.

180. L.G. Rowntree, *Amer. Jrl. of Cancer* (1937) 31, no. 3: 359-372.

180a. L.G. Rowntree and W.M. Ziegler, *Proceedings of the Society for Experimental Biology and Medicine* (1943) 54: 121-123.

180b. Christopher Carruthers, *Proceedings of the Society for Experimental Biology and Medicine* (1939) 40: 107-108.

180c. Paul N. Harris, *Cancer Research* (1947) 7: 26-34.

181. Werner G. Jaffee, *Experimental Medicine and Surgery* (1946) 4: 278-282.

182. Patent number 3,031,376 issued to Ezra Levin.

182a. Roy J. Shephard, *Jrl. of Sports Medicine* (1983) 23: 461-470.

182b. Y. Kobayaski, as cited by E.R. Buskirk, *Ann. Rev. Nutr.* (1981) 1: 319-350.

183. A.T. Quintanilha, *Biochemical Society Transactions* (1984) 12: 403-404.

183a. Wilfrid E. Shute, *Annals of the New York Academy of Sciences* (1949) 52: 354-357.

183b. R.D. Wigley and M. Vlieg, *AJEBAK* (1978) 56, part 5: 631-637. Note: *AJEBAK* is also known as the *Australian Jrl. of Experimental Biology and Medical Science.*

183c. Wilfrid E. Shute et al., *Medical Record* (1947) 203: 230-234.

184. Jane Kinderlehrer, *Prevention* (Aug. 1975).

185. Francis A. Hellebrandt et al., *Amer. Jrl. of Digestive Disease and Nutrition* (1936) 7: 477, cited in *A Devotion to Nutrition* by Frederick Hoelzel (New York: Vantage Press, 1954) p. 85.

186. M.S. Losowsky et al., *Annals of the New York Academy of Sciences* (1972) 203: 212-222.
187. M. Akerib and W. Sterner, *Int. Jrl. Vit. Nutr. Res.* (1971) 41: 42.
188. N.E. Alderson et al., *Jrl. of Nutrition* (1971) 101: 655.
189. Hugo E. Gallo-Torres in *Vitamin E,* ed. Lawrence J. Machlin, op. cit. (ref. 24) p. 181.
189a. L. Jansson et al., *Acta Paediatrica Scandinavica* (1984) 73: 329-332.
189b. N.E. Bateman and D.A. Uccellini, *Jrl. Pharm. Pharmacol.* (1984) 36: 461-464.
189c. Ursula Kocher-Becker and Walter Kocher, *Zeitscrift für Naturforshung* (1981) sec. C, 36: 904-906.
189d. John B. Barnett, *Int. Archs. Allergy appl. Immun.* (1981) 66: 229-232.
189e. C.M. Brubaker et al., *Life Sciences* (1982) 30, no. 23: 1965-1971.
189ea. Emanuela Masini et al., *Agents and Actions* (1985) 16, no. 6: 470-477.
189f. Carl J. Bodenstein, *Pediatrics* (1984) 73, no. 5: 733.
189g. John Butler et al., *American Jrl. of Hospital Pharmarcy* (1984) 41: 1514, 1516.
189h. *Physicians' Desk Reference* (Oradell, N.J.; Medical Economics Co., Inc., 1983) p. 2414.
189i. R.E. Brown et al., *JAMA* (May 9, 1986) 255, no. 18: 2445.
190. Fritz Weber, *Prog. Clin. Biol. Res.* (1981) 77: 119-135.
191. Franklin Bicknell and Frederick Prescott, *The Vitamins in Medicine,* op. cit., pp. 644-645.
192. Evan Shute, *The Summary,* (Dec., 1973).
193. R.E. Kirk and. D.F. Othmer, *Encyclopedia of Chemical Technology,* supp. 1 (New York: Interscience Publishers, Inc., 1957) pp. 77-78.
194. Victor Herbert, *Nutrition Reviews* (June 1977) 35: 158.
195. Harold M. Cohen, *New England Jrl. of Medicine* (1973) 289: 980.
196. Michael Briggs, *New England Jrl. of Medicine* (1974) 290: 579-580.
197. Samuel Ayers, Jr. and Richard Mihan, *New England Jrl. of Medicine* (1974) 290: 580.
197a. K. Narayanareddy and P. Bala Krishna Murthy, *Nutrition Reports International* (1982) 26, no. 5: 901-906.
198. O.K. Melhorn and S. Cross, *Jrl. of Pediatrics* (1971) 79: 581-588.
199. Neil N. Finer et al., *Lancet* (May 15, 1982): 1087-1090.
200. Robert E. Kalina, *New England Jrl. of Medicine* (April 8, 1982) 306: 867.
200a. Solomon Sobel et al., *Jrl. of Medicine* (April 8, 1982) 306: 867.
200b. Neil N. Finer et al., *Ophthalmology* (May, 1983) 90, no. 5: 428-435.
200c. Arnall Patz, *Ophthalmology* (May, 1983) 90, no. 5: 425-427.
200d. Neil N. Finer et al., *Pediatrics* (1984) 73, no. 3: 387-392.
200e. David B. Schaffer et al., *Ophthalmology* (1985) 92, no. 8: 1005-1011.
201. Hyman J. Roberts, *JAMA* (July 10, 1981) 246, no. 2: 129-130.
202. Philip M. Farrell and John G. Bieri, *Amer. Jrl. of Clinical Nutrition* (1975) 28: 1381-1386.
203. Jeffrey Bland et al., *Physiological Chemistry and Physics* (1975) 7, no. 1: 69-75.
203a. Joseph L. Napoli et al., *Archives of Biochemistry and Biophysics* (1984) 230, no. 1: 194-202.
203b. J.C. Somogyi, "Anti-Vitamins, Report of the Committee on Food Production, Food and Nutrition Board, National Research Council," in *Toxicants Occurring Naturally in Foods* (Washington, D.C.: National Academy of Sciences, 1973) pp. 254-275.
204. W.J. Pudelkiewicz et al., *Jrl. of Nutrition* (1964) 84: 113-117.
205. L. Arnich and V.A. Arthur, *Annals of the New York Academy of Sciences* (1980) 355: 109-118.
206. J.E. Packer et al., *Nature* (1979) 278: 737-738.
206a. Linda H. Chen, *Nutrition Reports, Int'l* (1976) 14, no. 1: 89-96
207. E. Ginter et al., *Internatl. Jrl. Vit. Nutr. Res.* (1982) 52: 55-59.
208. Linda H. Chen, *Amer. Jrl. of Clinical Nutrition* (1981) 34: 1036-1041.
208a. Hon-Wing Leung et al., *Biochimica et Biophysica Acta* (1981) 664: 266-272.

208b. Paul B. McCay, *Annual Review of Nutrition* (1985) 5: 323-340.

209. Arthur Vogelsang, *Angiology* (April, 1970) 21: 275-279.

210. *Nutrition Reviews* (1982) 40: 180-182.

211. James J. Corrigan, *Annals of the New York Academy of Sciences* (1982) 393: 361-368.

212. Roman J. Kutsky, *Handbook of Vitamins, Minerals and Hormones*, op. cit., p. 24.

213. C.G. MacKenzie, *Science*, (Aug. 29, 1941) 94: 216-217.

214. W.M. Cort et al., *Jrl. of Food Science* (1978) 43: 797-798.

215. D.S. Alberts et al., *Biomedicine* (1978) 29: 189-191.

216. H.A. Nadiger, *Nutrition and Metabolism* (1980) 24: 352-356.

217. H.A. Nadiger et al., *Clinica Chimica Acta* (1981) 116: 9-16.

217a. H.A. Nadiger et al., *International Jrl. for Vitamin and Nutrition Research* (1984) 54: 307-311.

218. W.V. Applegate, *Internat. Jrl. for Vitamin and Nutrition Research* (1979) 43-50.

219. Jack Bauernfeind in *Vitamin E*, ed. Lawrence J. Machlin, op. cit. (ref. 24) p. 119.

220. Irvin E. Liener, ed., *Toxic Constituents of Plant Foodstuffs*, 2nd ed. (New York: Academic Press, 1980) p. 444.

221. J.G. Bieri, *Annals of the New York Academy of Sciences* (1972) 203: 181-191.

222. M.S. Losowsky et al., *Annals of the New York Academy of Sciences* (1972) 203: 212-222.

222a. Joanna Lehmann, *American Jrl. of Clinical Nutrition* (1981) 34: 2104-2110.

222b. Herman Baker et al., *Nutrition Reports International* (1980) 21, no. 4: 531-536.

222c. Hugo E. Gallo-Torres, *Lipids* (1969) 5, no. 4: 379-384.

222d. M.T. MacMahon and G. Neale, *Clinical Science* (1970) 38: 197-210. Cited in ref. 222b.

222e. J.G. Bieri and P.M. Farrell, *Vitamins and Hormones* (1976) 34: 31. Cited in ref. 222b.

222f. Garry J. Handelman et al., *Jrl. of Nutrition* (1985) 115: 807-813.

222g. Telegdy Kovats and E. Berndorfer-Krazner, *Nahrung* (1968) 12, no. 4: 407-414.

223. G. Pongracz, *International Jrl. for Vitamin and Nutrition Research* (1973) 43: 517-525.

224. K. Taufel et al., *Nahrung* (1958) 2: 853, cited in ref. 223.

225. Jenifer A. Lindsey et al., *Lipids* (1985) 20, no. 3: 151-157.

226. J. Cillard et al., *Jrl. of the American Oil Chemists' Society* (1980) 57, no. 8: 252-255.

227. J. Cillard et al., *Jrl. of the American Oil Chemists' Society* (1980) 57, no. 8: 255-261.

228. J.P. Koskas, J. Cillard and P. Cillard, *Jrl. of the American Oil Chemists' Society* (1984) 61, no. 9: 1466-1469.

229. David R. Blake et al., *Annals of the Rheumatic Diseases* (1983) 42: 89-93, at 92.

230. L.H. Chen and. R.R. Thacker, *International Jrl. of Vitamin and Nutrition Research* (1986) 56: 253-258.

Chapter 3—620 References

1. Martin Press et al., *Lancet* (April 6, 1974): 597-599.
2. *The Pharmacological Effect of Lipids* (Alternate title: *Symposium on the Pharmacological Effect of Lipids*), ed. Jon J. Kabara (Champaign, Ill.: Amer. Oil Chemists' Soc., 1978).
3. Ralph T. Homan, *Amer. Jrl. of Clinical Nutrition* (1982) 35: 617-623.
3a. E.G. Hammond and W.R. Fehr, *Jrl. of the Amer. Oil Chemists' Soc.* (Nov., 1984) 61, no. 11: 1713-1716.
4. W.M.F. Leat et al., *Quarterly Jrl. of Experimental Pathology* (1983) 68: 221-231.
5. Brack A. Bivins et al., *Jrl. of Parenteral and Enteral Nutrition* (1983) 7, no. 5: 473-478.
6. T. Tinoco, *Progress in Lipid Research* (1982) 21: 1-45.
6a. R.B. Wolf et al., *Jrl. of the American Oil Chemists' Soc.* (Nov., 1983) 60, no. 11: 1858-1860.
6b. N. Chetty and B.A. Bradlow, *Thrombosis Research* (1983) 30: 619-624.
6c. Helmut Traitler et al., *Lipids* (1984) 19, no. 12: 923-928.
7. J. Dyerberg et al., *Lancet* (Jan. 26, 1980): 199.
7a. Mary Ann Van Duyn et al., *American Jrl. of Clinical Nutrition* (1984) 40: 277-284.
7b. O. Adam et al., *Fette Seifen Anstrichmittel* (1984) 86, no. 5: 180-183. Cited in *Nutrition Abstracts and Reviews,* Series A (Oct., 1984) 54, no. 10: 885 (abstract no. 6240).
8. *Nutrition Reviews* (May 1982) 40: 144-147.
9. A.D. Challen et al., *Human Nutrition: Clinical Nutrition* (1983) 373C: 197-208.
10. S. Gudbjarnason and J. Hallgrimsson, *Acta Med. Scand.* (1975) suppl. 587: 17-26.
11. D.A. Peterson et al., *Medical Hypotheses* (1981) 7: 1390-1395.
12. H.B. Demopoulos et al., *Acta Physiologica Scandinavica* (1980) supp. 492: 91-119.
12a. Aaron J. Marcus, *New England Jrl. of Medicine* (1983) 309, no. 24: 1515-1517.
13. Rao V. Panganamala et al., *Prostaglandins* (1976) 11: 599-607.
13a. William E. Rosenblum and Farouk El-Sabban, *Stroke* (1982) 13, no. 1: 35-39.
13b. J.M.F. Thomas et al., *Thrombosis Research* (1984) 34: 117-123.
14. A.L. Willis, *Nutrition Reviews* (1981) 39: 289-301.
14a. P. Kutsky et al., *Prostaglandins* (1983) 26, no. 1: 13-21.
14b. Charles N. Serhan et al., *Biochemical and Biophysical Research Communications* (1984) 118: no. 3: 943-949.
14c. Charles N. Serhan et al., *Proc. of the National Academy of Sciences* (1984) 81: 5335-5339.
14d. S.M.F. Lai and P.W. Manley, *Natural Products Reports* (1984) 1: 409-441 at 409.
14e. H.Kikuchi et al., *Tetrahedron Letters* (1982) 23: 5171. Cited in ref. 14d.
14f. M. Kobayashi et al., *Tetrahedron Letters* (1982) 23: 5331. Cited in ref. 14d.
15. Claudio Galli in *Advances in Nutritional Research,* vol. 3, ed. Harold H. Draper (New York: Plenum Press, 1980) p. 95-126 at 96.
15a. Kerin O'Dea and Andrew J. Sinclair, *American Jrl. of Clinical Nutrition* (1982) 36: 868-872.
15b. R.G. Ackman in *Nutritional Evaluation of Long Chain Fatty Acids in Fish Oil,* ed. S.M. Barlow and M.E. Stansby (London: Academic Press, 1982) pp. 25-28. Cited by R.A. Gibson et al., *Comp. Biochem. Physiol.* (1984) 78C, no. 2: 325-328.
16. Gene Bylinsky, *Fortune* (June, 1972).
16a. S. Moncada and J.R. Vane, *Pharmacological Reviews* (1979) 30: 293-331.
16b. Dwight R. Robinson, *DM—Disease-a-Month* (1983) 30, no. 3: 2-47.
16c. Norman A. Nelson et al., "Prostaglandins and the Arachidonic Acid Cascade," a special report of the Upjohn Co., reprinted from *Chemical and Engineering News* (Aug. 16, 1982) 60: 30.
16d. Niels H. Lauersen et al., *Obstetrics and Gynecology* (1976) 47, no. 4: 473-478.

17. Niels H. Lauersen and Kathleen H. Wilson, *Obstetrics and Gynecology* (1974) 44, no. 6: 793-801.

17a. Kaare M. Gautvik and Mojmir Kriz, *Endrocrinology* (1976) 98: 352-358.

17b. Rashida A. Karmali, *CA-A Cancer Jrl. for Clinicians* (Nov.-Dec., 1983) 33: 322-332.

17ba. R.R. Brenner, *Molecular and Cellular Biochemistry* (1974) 3, no. 1: 41-52.

17bb. B.J.F. Hudson, *Jrl. of the Amer. Oil Chemists' Soc.* (1984) 61, no. 3: 540-543.

17c. R.A. Gibson and G.M. Kneebone, *Amer. Jrl. of Clinical Nutrition* (1981) 34: 252.

17d. B.J.F. Hudson and I.G. Karis, *Jrl. Sci. Food Agric.* (1974) 25: 759, cited in ref. 17f.

17da. B.W. Nichols and B.J.B. Wood, *Lipids* (1968) 3, no. 1: 46-50.

17e. M.B. Bohannon and R. Kleiman, *Lipids* (1976) 11, no. 2: 157-159.

17f. B.J.F. Hudson, *Jrl. Amer. Oil Chemists' Society* (1984) 61, no. 3: 540-543.

17g. Sara M. Actis Dato et al., *Lipids* (1973) 8, no. 1: 1-6.

18. D.F. Horrobin et al., *Medical Hypotheses* (1979) 5: 969-985.

18a. Raul O. Peluffo et al., *Lipids* (1984) 19, no. 2: 154-157.

18b. Simon N. Meydani and Jacqueline DuPont, *Jrl. of Nutrition* (1982) 112: 1098-1104.

18c. S.C. Cunnane, *Progress in Lipid Research* (1981) 20: 601-603.

18d. Alan C. Fogerty et al., *Nutrition Reports International* (Nov., 1985) 32, no. 5: 1009-1019.

19. D.F. Horrobin, *Progress in Lipid Research* (1981) 20: 539-541.

19a. D.R. Robinson et al., *Annals of the N.Y. Academy of Sciences* (1979) 332: 279-294.

19b. Donald J. Wolff, *Jrl. of the Medical Society of New Jersey* (1984) 51, no. 6: 503-505.

20. Rao V. Panganamala and David G. Cornwell, *Annals of the N.Y. Academy of Sciences* (1982) 393: 376-391.

20a. A.J. Vergroesen, *Progress in Lipid Research* (1981) 20: 469-470.

20b. J. Booyens, *Medical Hypotheses* (1983) 12: 195-201.

20c. David F. Horrobin, *Medical Hypotheses* (1980) 6: 785-800.

21. L. Mathers Dunbar and J. Martyn Bailey, *Jrl. of Biological Chemistry* (1975) 250: 1152-1153.

22. J. Dwight Stinnett, *Nutrition and the Immune Response* (Boca Raton, Fla.: CRC Press, 1983) p. 20.

23. F.A. Kuehl et al., *Nature* (1977) 265: 170-173.

24. Daljeet Singh et al., *Amer. Jrl. of Hematology* (1981) 11: 233-240.

24a. Manikkam Suthanthiran et al., *Nature* (1984) 307: 276-278.

24b. M. Tien et al., *Federation Proceedings* (1981) 40: 179-182.

24c. A. Rahimtula and P.J. O'Brien, *Biochemical and Biophysical Research Communications* (1976) 70: 893.

24d. Richard S. Bodaness and Phillip C. Chan, *Biochemical Pharmacology* (1980) 29: 1337-1340.

24e. J. Baumann and G. Wurm, *Prostaglandins, Leukotrienes and Medicine* (1984) 14: 139-152.

25. Gerald Weissman et al., *Advances in Inflammation Research* (1979) 1: 95-112.

25a. K.C. Srivastava and K.K. Awasthi, *Prostaglandins, Leukotrienes and Medicine* (1982) 9: 669-684.

25b. Steven J. Taussig, *Medical Hypotheses* (1980) 6: 99-104.

25c. A.N. Makheja, *Lancet* (April 7, 1979): 781.

25ca. Sidney Belman, *Carcinogenesis* (1983) 4, no. 8: 1063-1065.

25d. D.P. Mikhailidis et al., *New England Jrl. of Medicine* (Aug. 23, 1984) 311, no. 8: 537-538.

25da. R. Landolfi and M. Steiner, *Blood* (1984) 64: 679.

25db. D.P. Mikhailidis et al., *Blood* (1985) 65, no. 3: 777.

25dc. M. Steiner and R. Landolfi, *Blood* (1985) 65, no. 3, 777.

25e. G.G. Fenn and J.M. Littleton, *Thrombosis and Haemostasis* (1984) 51, no. 1: 50-53. Cited in *Nutrition Abstracts and Reviews*, Series A (1984) 54, no. 11: 972 (item 6877).

25f. A.S. St. Leger et al., *Lancet* (May 12, 1979): 1017-1020.
25g. Charles H. Hennekens et al.,*JAMA* (1979) 242, no. 18: 1973-1974.
25h. T.W. Meade et al., *British Medical Jrl.* (1985) 290: 428-432.
25i. Matti Hillbom et al., *Stroke* (1985) 16, no. 1: 19-23.
25j. Akio Yoshimoto et al., *Jrl. of Biochemistry* (1970) 68: 487-499.
26. C. Galli and A. Socini, *Acta Vitaminol. Enzymol* (1982) 4: 245-252.
26a. W.C. Hope et al., *Prostaglandins* (1975) 10, no. 4: 557-571.
26b. Muslim Ali et al., *Prostaglandins and Medicine* (1980) 4: 79-85.
26c. J.R. Beetens and A. G. Herman,*Arch. Int. Pharmacodyn* (1982) 259: 300-302.
26d. K.C. Srivastava, *Prostaglandins, Leukotrienes and Medicine* (1985) 18: 227-233.
27. Peter Polgar and Linda Taylor, *Prostaglandins* (1980) 19, no. 5: 693-700.
27a. T. Masukawa et al., *Experientia* (1983) 39: 405-406.
27b. N.W. Schoene et al., *Federation Proceedings* (March 1, 1984) 43, no. 3: 477.
27c. Elisabeth Schafer and Lotte Amrich,*Jrl. of Nutrition* (1984) 114: 1130-1136.
27d. Mohsen Meydani et al., *Prostaglandins, Leukotrienes and Medicine* (1985) 18: 337-346.
27da. Pauline M. Herold and John E. Kinsella, *American Jrl. of Clinical Nutrition* (1986) 43: 566-598, at 570.
27e. E. Mahmud et al., *Prostaglandins, Leukotrienes and Medicine* (1984) 16: 131-146.
27f. Philip K. Moore and Richard J. Griffiths, *Prostaglandins* (Oct., 1983) 26, no. 4: 509-517.
28. J.M. Iacono et al., *Progress in Lipid Research* (1981) 20: 349-364.
28a. Alvin C. Chan et al., *Jrl. of Nutrition* (1980) 110: 66-73.
29. Frederick A. Kuehl, Jr. and Robert W. Egan,*Science* (1980) 210: 978-984.
29a. Garret A. Fitzgerald et al.,*New England Jrl. of Medicine* (1984)
29b. D.P. Mikhailidis et al.,*British Medical Journal* (Nov. 19, 1983) 287: 1495-1498.
29c. Peter Hoffmann and Werner Förster,*Advances in Lipid Research* 18: 203-227.
29d. Graham W. Taylor and Howard R. Morris, *British Medical Bulletin* (1983) 39, no. 3: 219-222.
29e. Gerald Weissmann, *Cellular Immunology* (1983) 82: 117-126.
29ea. William F. Stenson and Charles W. Parker, *Clinical Reviews of Allergy* (1983) 1: 369-384.
29f. Stewart A. Metz, *Medical Hypotheses* (1983) 12: 341-357.
29g. Mark McCarty *Medical Hypotheses* (1984) 13: 45-50.
29h. L.B. Klickstein et al., *Jrl. of Clinical Investigation* (1980) 66: 1166-1170, cited by Edward J. Goetzl, *Medical Clinics of North America* (1981) 65, no. 4: 809-828.
29i. Ephraim T. Gwebu et al., *Research Communications in Clinical Pathology and Pharmacology* (1980) 28, no. 2: 361-376.
30. Edward J. Goetzl, *Nature* (1980) 288: 183-185.
30a. Andreas Jorg et al.,*Jrl. Experimental Medicine* (1982) 155: 390-402.
30b. T. Jones et al.,*Prostaglandins* (Nov., 1983) 26, no. 5: 833-843.
30c. K. Bernstroem and S. Hammarström, *Biochem. Biophy, Res. Commun.* (1982) 109: 800-804. Cited by L.G. Letts et al.,*Prostaglandins* (Nov., 1984) 28, no. 5: 602-604.
31. Michael A. Crawford, *British Medical Bulletin* (1983) 39: 210-213.
32. Bengt Samuelsson, in *Advances in Prostaglandin, Thromboxane and Leukotriene Research*, vol. 9, ed. Bengt Samuelsson and Rudolfo Paoletti (New York; Raven Press, 1982) p. 1-17.
33. G.C. Folco et al., *Advances in Prostaglandin, Thromboxane and Leukotriene Research*, vol. 9, op. cit., pp. 153.
33a. B. Samuelsson and S. Hammarström, *Vitamins and Hormones* (1982) 39: 1-30.
33b. A.J. Marcus et al., *Annals of the N.Y. Academy of Sciences* (1982) 401: 195-202.
33c. Carol A. Rouzer et al.,*Proc. National Academy of Sciences* (1982) 79: 1621-1625.
34. John G. Gleason et al., *Advances in Prostaglandin, Thromboxane and Leukotriene Research* vol. 9, op. cit., pp. 243-250.
34a. A.L. Willis, *Lancet* (Sept. 22, 1984): 697.

34b. J.M. Bailey et al., in *Leukotrienes and Other Lipoxygenase Products*, ed. B. Samuelsson and R. Paoletti (New York: Raven Press, 1982), cited in ref. 34a.

34c. A.W. Ford-Hutchinson, *Jrl. of Allergy and Clinical Immunology* (1984) 74, no. 3, part 2: 437-440.

35. S.A. Rae et al., *Lancet* (Nov. 20, 1982): 1122-1124.

36. Robert M. Goldman et al., *Hospital Practice* (Sept., 1983) 18, no. 9: 186-192.

37. Susan D. Brain et al., *Lancet* (Oct. 2, 1982): 762-763.

37a. T. Ruzicka et al., *Lancet* (Jan. 28, 1984): 223.

37b. Tak H. Lee et al., *New England Jrl. of Medicine* (1985) 312: 1217-1224.

37c. Joel M. Kremer et al., *Lancet* (Jan. 26, 1985): 184-187.

37d. Hideki Sumimoto et al., *Biochimica et Biophysica Acta* (1984) 803: 271-277.

37e. Jeffrey K. Beckman et al., *Lipids* (1985) 20, no. 5: 318-321.

37f. W. Martin et al., *Agents and Actions* (1985) 16, no. 1/2: 48-49.

38. David R. Webb et al., *Biochemical and Biophysical Research Comm.* (1982) 104: 1617-1622.

39. Priscilla J. Piper, *British Medical Jrl.* (1983) 39: 255-259.

39a. Sven Hammarström, *Jrl. of Biological Chemistry* (1981) 256, no. 5: 2275-2279.

39b. Takao Shimizu et al., *Proc. National Academy of Sciences* (1984) 81: 689-693.

40. Richard L. Maas et al., *Advances in Prostaglandin, Thromboxane and Leukotriene Research*, vol. 9, op. cit., (ref. 32) pp. 29-44.

41. O. Rädmark et al., ibid, pp. 61-70.

41a. Jan Ake LIndgren et al., ibid, pp. 53-60.

41aa. R. Reich et al., *Prostaglandins* (1983) 26, no. 6: 1011-1020.

41b. M. Chopra et al., *Prostaglandins* (Nov., 1984) 28, no. 5: 667.

41ba. C.R. Pace-Asciak and J.M. Martin, *Prostaglandins, Leukotrienes and Medicine* (1984) 16: 173-180.

41bb. C.R. Pace-Asciak et al., *Jrl. of Biological Chemistry* (1983) 258: 6835. Cited in ref. 41ba.

42. Eva B. Cramer et al., *Proc. Natl. Academy of Sciences* (1983) 80: 4109-4113.

43. Michael A. Bray, *British Medical Bulletin* (1983) 39: 249-254.

43a. Edward J. Goetzl et al., *Jrl. of Clinical Immunology* (1984) 4, no. 2: 79-84.

43b. Takashi Terano et al., *Prostaglandins* (Nov., 1984) 28, no. 5: 668.

44. B.J.R. Whittle and S. Moncada, *British Medical Bulletin* (1983) 39: 232-238.

44a. Frank H. Valone, *Cancer Research* (1983) 43: 5695-5698.

45. Hans-Erik Claesson, *FEBS Letters* (1982) 139: 305-308.

46. Arthur C. Guyton, *Textbook of Medical Physiology*, 5th ed., (Philadelphia: W.B. Saunders Co., 1976) pp. 990-991.

47. R.L. Singhal et al., in *Normal and Abnormal Growth of the Prostate*, ed. Martin Goland (Springfield, Il.: Charles C. Thomas, 1975) pp. 445-493.

48. Helen G. Morris, *Biochemical and Biophysical Research Communications* (1981) 103: 774-779.

48a. *Nutrition Reviews* (1982) 40, no. 11: 338-340.

48b. *Nutrition Reviews* (1981) 39, no. 8: 317-320.

48c. T.P. Clay and P. Miller, *Practitioner* (May, 1984) 228: 510-513.

48d. Lawrence Levine and Nancy Worth, *Jrl. of Allergy and Clinical Immunology* (1984) 74, no. 3, part 2: 430-436.

49. Karen G. Rothberg and Margaret Hitchcock, *Prostaglandins, Leukotrienes and Medicine* (1983) 12: 137-147.

49a. D.M. Pugh et al., *British Jrl. of Pharmacology* (1975) 53: 469p.

50. E. Agradi et al., *Prostaglandins* (1981) 22: 255-266.

51. Alvin R. Sams et al., *Advances in Prostaglandin, Thromboxane and Leukotriene Research*, vol. 9, op. cit., pp. 19-28.

51a. Kenneth R. McLeish et al., *Jrl. of Immunopharmacology* (1982) 4, no. 1 and 2: 53-64.

51aa. Katsuhiko Mirazawa et al., *Japanese Jrl. of Pharmacology* (1985) 38: 199-205.

51b. P. Ramwell et al., in *Advances in Prostaglandin, Thromboxane and Leukotriene Research*, vol. 12, ed. B. Samuelsson, R. Paoletti and P. Ramwell (New York: Raven Press, 1983) pp. 229-234.

51ba. J. Van Wauwe and J. Goossens, *Prostaglandins* (1983) 26: 725-730. Cited by Istvan Lepran and Allan M. Lefer, *Circulatory Shock* (1985) 15: 79-88.

51c. Yuhei Hamasaki and Hsin-Hsiung Tai, *Biochimica et Biophysica Acta* (1985) 34: 37-41.

51ca. Tanihiro Yoshimoto et al., *Biochemical and Biophysical Research Communications* (1983) 116, no. 2: 612-618.

51d. Per Hedqvist et al., *Prostaglandins* (Nov., 1984) 25, no. 5: 605-608.

52. Daniel H. Hwang and Judith Donovan, *Jrl. of Nutrition* (1982) 112: 1233-1237.

52a. R. Mower and M. Steiner, *Prostaglandins, Leukotrienes and Medicine* (1983) 10: 389-403.

52b. *Nutrition Reviews* (May 1982) 40, no. 5: 157-159.

52c. N.K. Boughton-Smith et al., *Gut* (1983) 24: 1176-1182.

52d. Stewart Metz et al., *Jrl. of Clinical Investigation* (1983) 71: 1191-1205.

52da. Stewart A. Metz, *Prostaglandins and Medicine* (1981) 7: 581-589.

52db. Sumer Pek et al., *Diabetes* (1978) 27: 801-809.

52dc. L. Best and W. J. Malaisse, *Diabetologia* (1983) 25: 299-305.

52e. D.H. Nugteren et al., *Recueil Des Travaux Chimiques Des Pays-Bas* (1966) 85: 405-419.

52f. J.Y. Westcott and Robert C. Murphy, *Prostaglandins* (1983) 26, no. 2: 223-239.

52g. P.K. Varma and T.V.N. Persaud, *Prostaglandins, Leukotrienes and Medicine* (1982) 8: 641-645.

53. D. Wilson et al., *Clinical Research* (1973)21: 829.

54. J. Lieb, *Prostaglandins and Medicine* (1980) 4: 275-279.

55. C. Zioudrou et al., *Jrl. Biological Chemistry* (1979) 254: 2446-2449.

56. K.S. Stone et al., *Lipids* (1979) 14: 174-180.

57. P.B.A. Kernoff et al., *British Medical Jrl.* (Dec. 3, 1977): 1441-1444.

57a. M.B. Feinstein et al., *Prostaglandins* (1977) 14: 1075-1094.

57b. J.E. Shaw and P.W. Ramwell, *Worcester Foundation for Exp. Biol.* (1967): 55-64. Ctied by ref. 58.

57c. A.K. Banerjee et al., *Nature New Biology* (1972) 238: 177-179. Cited by ref. 58.

57d. R. Befrits and C. Johansson, *Prostaglandins* (1985) 29, no. 1: 143-152.

57e. Jan Nilsson and Anders G. Olsson, *Atherosclerosis* (1984) 53: 77-82.

57f. M.A. Bach and J.F. Bach in *Prostaglandin Synthetase Inhibitors*, ed. H.J. Robinson and J.R. Vane (New York: Raven Press, 1974) pp. 241- 248. Cited by Horrobin et al. (ref. 18).

57g. R.B. Zurier et al., *Federation Proceedings* (1975) 34: 1029. Cited by Horrobin et al. (ref. 18).

58. I.L. Bonta and N.J. Parnham, *British Jrl. of Pharmacology* (1978) 62: 417-8P. Cited by Horrobin et al. (ref. 18).

58a. M.S. Manku et al., *Prostaglandins* (1977) 13, no. 4: 701-710.

58b. M.S. Manku et al., *Biochemical and Biophysical Research Comm.* (1978) 83, no. 1: 295-299.

58c. M.S. Manku et al., *Endocrinology* (1979) 104, no. 3: 774-779.

59. F. ten Hoor, *Nutrition and Metabolism* (1980) 24, supp. 1: 162-180.

60. P.Hoffman et al., *Prostaglandins, Leukotrienes and Medicine* (1983) 11: 43-44.

60a. Cedrick H. Hassall and Stephen J. Kirtland, *Lipids* (1984) 19, no. 9: 699-703.

61. Peter Oster et al., *Research in Experimental Medicine, Berlin* (1979) 175: 287-291.

62. H.U. Comberg et al., *Prostaglandins* (1978) 15: 193.

63. P. Oster et al., *Progress in Food Nutr. Sci.* (1980) 4: 39-40.

64. Murray C. MacDonald et al., *Canadian Jrl. of Physiology and Pharmacology* (1981) 59: 872-875.

64a. A.J. Vergroesen et al., *Acta Biologica et Medica Germanica* (1978) 37: 879-883.

64b. Olaf Adam and Gunther Wolfram, *American Jrl. of Clinical Nutrition* (1984) 40: 763-770.

65. P. Singer et al., *Acta Biologica et Medica Germanica* (1982) 41: 215-225.

66. G. J. Mogenson and B.M. Box, *Ann. Nutr. Metab.* (1982) 26: 232-239.

67. Rainer Düsing et al., *Amer. Jrl. of Physiology* (1983) 224: H228-H233.

68. Tetsuji Okuro et al., *Hypertension* (1982) 4: 809-816.

69. Christopher L. Melby, *Medical Hypotheses* (1983) 10: 445-449.

70. Louis Tobran et al., *Hypertension* (1982) 4, supp. II: II 149-II 153.

71. Carin Larsson and Erik Änggard, *Jrl. Pharm. Pharmac.* (1973) 25: 653-654.

72. Gregory J. Dusting et al., *European Jrl. of Pharmacology* (1978) 49: 65-72.

73. P. Hoffmann et al., *Arch. int. Pharmacodyn. Ther.* (1982) 259: 40-58.

73a. N.W. Schoene et al., as cited by P.C. Weber et al., *Klinishe Wochenschrift* (1982) 60: 479-488.

74. James M. Iacono, *Hypertension* (1982) 4, supp. III: III 34-III 42.

75. Pekka Puska et al., *Lancet* (Jan., 1983): 1-5.

76. D.A. Wood et al., *British Medical Jrl.* (Dec. 11, 1982) 285: 1738.

77. Ancel Keys, *British Medical Jrl.* (Oct. 30, 1982) 285: 1275.

77a. Gerald Hornstra, *Progress in Lipid Research* (1981) 20: 407-413.

77aa. David F. Horrobin in *Clinical Uses of Essential Fatty Acids,* ed. David F. Horrobin (Montreal: Eden Press, 1982) pp. 89-96, at 91.

77ab. P. Hoffman et al., *Acta Biol. Med. Germ.* (1978) 37: 863, cited by David F. Horrobin, ibid pp. 3-36, at 25.

77b. A.E. Harper, *Amer. Jrl. of Clinical Nutrition* (1983) 39: 669-681.

78. G.A. Collins et al., *Prostaglandins* (1979) 18, no. 4: 591-603.

78a. H.-J. Mest and W. Förster, *Arch. Int. Pharmacodyn* (1975) 217: 152-161.

78b. A. Swift et al., *Prostaglandins* (1975) 15, no. 4: 651-657.

78c. M. Karmazyn and N.S. Dhalla, *Experientia* (1980) 36: 996-998.

79. H.-J. Mest and W. Förster, *Prostaglandins and Medicine* (1981) 7: 411-419.

79a. David G. Menter et al., *Cancer Research* (1984) 44: 450-456.

79b. P.H. Rolland et al., *Jrl. National Cancer Institute* (1980) 64: 1061-1070, cited by Menter et al., ref. 79a.

79c. A. Bennett et al., *British Jrl. Pharmacology* (1979) 66: 415P, cited by Menter et al., ref. 79a.

79ca. S. Nigam et al., *Prostaglandins* (1985) 29, no. 4: 513-528.

79cb. P.K. Heinonen and T. Metsä Ketelä, *Gynecologic and Obstetric Investigation* (1984) 18: 225-229.

79d. M. Rita Young and Sarah Knies, *Jrl. of the National Cancer Institute* (1984) 72, no. 4: 919-922.

79e. James S. Goodwin, *Medical Clinics of North America* (1981) 65, no. 4: 829-844.

79f. R.A. Karmali et al., *Pharmacological Research Communications* (1979) 11, no. 1: 69-75.

79g. Eric J. Werner et al., *Cancer Research* (1985) 45: 561-563.

80. D.F. Horrobin, *Medical Hypotheses* (1979) 5: 849-858.

81. D. Bhana et al., *Cancer* (1971) 2: 233-237.

82. P.M. Grimley et al., *Jrl. of the National Cancer Institute* (1969) 42: 663-680.

83. M.G. Santoro, *Nature* (1976) 263: 777-779.

84. D.F. Horrobin, *Medical Hypotheses* (1980) 6: 469-486.

85. Eduardo N. Siguel, *Nutrition and Cancer* (1983) 4: 285-291.

86. D.F. Horrobin, *Medical Hypotheses* (1979) 5: 599-620.

87. Nola Dippenaar, *South African Medical Jrl.* (1982) 62: 505-509.

88. W.P. Leary et al., ibid.: 681-685.

89. Nola Dippenaar et al., ibid.: 683-685.

90. C.F. van der Merwe, *South African Medical Jrl.* (1983) 63: 304.

90a. C.F. van der Merwe, *South African Medical Jrl.* (1984) 65, no. 4: 113-114.

924 The Reverse Effect

90b. *Chemical Abstracts* (1984) 100: 144997 m.

90c. K.M. Robinson and J.H. Botha, *Prostaglandins, Leukotrienes and Medicine* (1985) 20: 209-221.

90d. J. Booyens et al., *Prostaglandins, Leukotrienes and Medicine* (1984) 15: 15-33.

91. Kenneth V. Honn, *Science* (1981) 212: 1270-1272.

92. Thomas Simmet and Bernard M. Jaffe, *Prostaglandins* (1983) 25: 47-53.

93. Cezar M. Popescu, *Prostaglandins and Medicine* (1981) 7: 321-325.

94. R.L. Aspinal and P.S. Cammarata, *Nature* (1969) 224: 1320-1321.

95. R.B. Zurier and F. Quagliata, *Nature* (1971) 234: 304-305.

96. R.B. Zurier and Maurice Ballas, *Arthritis and Rheumatism* (1973) 16: 251-258.

96a. Arthur C. Guyton, *Textbook of Medical Physiology*, 6th ed., (Philadelphia: W.B. Saunders Co., 1981) p. 76.

97. Louis M. Pelus and Helen R. Strausser, *Life Sciences* (1977) 20: 903-914.

98. Troels Mork Hansen et al., *Scan. Jrl. Rheumatology* (1983) 12: 85-88.

98a. J.P. Kelly and C.W. Parker, *Jrl. of Immunology* (1979) 122: 1556-1562. Cited by J. Mertin, *Progress in Lipid Research* (1981) 20: 851-856.

98b. B.D. Bower and E. A. Newsholme, *Lancet* (March 18, 1978): 583-585.

98c. M.I. Gurr, *Progress in Lipid Research* (1981) 20: 851-856.

99. A. J. Houtsmuller et al., *Progress in Lipid Research* (1981) 20: 377-386.

100. A.J. Houtsmuller et al., *Prog. Food Nutrition Science* (1980) 4: 41-46.

100a. M. Yusoff Dawood, *Comprehensive Therapy* (1982) 8, no. 6: 9-16.

100aa. M.A. Lumsden et al., *British Jrl. of Obstet. Gynaecol.* (1983) 90: 1135. Cited by R.W. Kelly et al., *Prostaglandins, Leukotrienes and Medicine* (1984) 16: 69-78.

100ab. H.P. Zahradnick and M. Breckwoldt, *Archives of Gynecology* (1984) 236: 99-108.

100b. James R. Dingfelder, *Amer. Jrl. Obstet. Gynecol.* (1981) 14, no. 8: 874-879.

100c. M.Y. Dawood, *Drugs* (1981) 22: 42-56.

100ca. Penny Wise Budoff, *Jrl. of Reproductive Medicine* (1983) 28, no. 7: 469-478.

100d. R. Carraher et al., *Prostaglandins* (1983) 26, no. 1: 23-32.

100da. M. G. Brush in *Clinical Uses of Essential Fatty Acids,* ed. David F. Horrobin (Montreal: Eden Press, 1982) pp. 155-161.

100db. U.S. Patent no. 4,415,554 (Nov. 15, 1983) and 4,302,477. Great Britain patent application 78/2,642 (Jan. 23, 1978). Cited in *Chemical Abstracts* (1984) 100: 10911w.

100dc. David F. Horrobin, *Jrl. of Reproductive Medicine* (1983) 28, no. 7: 465-468.

100dd. Jukka Puolakka et al., *Jrl. of Reproductive Medicine* (1985) 30, no. 3: 149-153.

100e. Guy E. Abraham and Michael M. Lubran, *Amer. Jrl. of Clinical Nutrition* (1981) 34: 2364-2366.

100f. Joshua Backon, *Amer. Jrl. of Clinical Nutrition* (1982) 36: 386.

100g. Burton V. Caldwell and Harold R. Behrman, *Medical Clinics of North America* (1981) 65, no. 4: 927-936.

100h. N.L. Pashby et al., *British Jrl. of Surgery* (1981) 68: 801.

100i. Alan C. Fogerty et al., *Amer. Jrl. of Clinical Nutrition* (1984) 39: 201-208.

101. H.C. Meng, *Amer. Jrl. of Clinical Nutrition* (1983) 37: 157-159.

102. R.T. Holman et al., *Amer. Jrl. of Clinical Nutrition* (1983) 37: 159-160.

103. Julian Lieb, *Prostaglandins, Leukotrienes and Medicine* (1983) 10: 361-367.

104. David F. Horrobin and Mehar S. Manku, *British Medical Jrl.* (June 7, 1980): 1363-1366.

104a. D.F. Horrobin et al., *Psychological Medicine* (1978) 8: 43-48.

104aa. D.F. Horrobin, *Lancet* (Mar. 10, 1979): 529-531.

104b. Parviz Malek-Ahmadi and Margaret A. Weddle, *General Pharmacology* (1982) 13: 467-469.

105. O. Sahap Atik, *Prostaglandins, Leukotrienes and Medicine* (1983) 11: 105-107.

106. D.F. Horrobin, *Medical Hypotheses* (1980) 6: 225-232.

107. D.F. Horrobin, *Medical Hypotheses* (1979) 5: 365-378.

107a. K.S. Vaddadi, *Prostaglandins and Medicine* (1979) 2: 77-80.

107b. K.S. Vaddadi, and D.F. Horrobin, *IRCS Medical Science* (1979) 7:52.

107c. Donald N. Paty, *Archives of Neurology* (Oct. 21, 1983) 40: 693-694.

107d. S.C. Cunnane et al., *British Jrl. of Nutrition* (1985) 53: 441-448.

108. S. Wright and J.L. Burton, *Lancet* (Nov. 20, 1982): 1120-1122.

108a. M.S. Manku et al., *British Jrl. of Dermatology* (1984) 110: 643-648.

108b. D.V. Johnston and L.A. Marshall, *Progress in Food and Nutrition Science* (1984) 8: 3-25.

109. H.H. Evans et al., *Jrl. of Biological Chemistry* (1934) 106: 445-449.

110. R.O. Pellufo et al., *Amer. Jrl. of Physiology* (1970) 218: 669-673.

111. R.W. Kelly et al., *Nsture* (1976) 260: 544-545.

111a. R.J. Aitken and R.W. Kelly, *Jrl. of Reproduction and Fertility* (1985) 73: 139-146.

111b. W. McLean Grogan, *Lipids* (1984) 19, no. 5: 341-346.

112. Sixta Arjala et al., *Jrl. of Lipid Research* (1973) 14: 296-305.

113. C. Pudelkewicz et al., *Jrl. of Nutrition* (1968) 64: 138-146.

114. L.J. Machlin, *Jrl. of the Amer. Oil Chemists' Society* (1963) 40: 368-371.

114a. Hans Kaunitz in *Symposium on the Pharmacological Effect of Lipids,* ed. Jon J. Kabara (Champaign, Il.: American Oil Chemists' Society, 1978) pp. 203-210.

114b. H. Kaunitz and R.E. Johnson, Proc. 9th International Congress on Nutrition, Mexico, 1972, 1: 362 (1975). Cited in ref. 114a.

114c. R.G. Ackman and S. N. Hooper, *Jrl. of the American Oil Chemists' Society* (1974) 51: 42-49.

114d. A. Kiritsakis, *Jrl. of the American Oil Chemists' Society* (1985) 62, no. 5: 892-896.

114e. Wilbur A. Parker and Daniel Melnick, *Jrl. of the American Oil Chemists' Society* (1966) 43: 635-638.

115. Antti Ahlstromm and Ritva Jarvinen, *Chemical Abstracts* (Sept. 17, 1973) 79: item 64971 f.

115a. Granville A. Nolen et al., *Jrl. of Nutrition* (1967) 93: 337-348.

115aa. Jen-Kun Lin et al., *Nutrition and Cancer* (1984) 6, no. 3: 148-159.

115b. L.F. Bjeldanes et al., *Food, Chem. Toxicol.* (1982) 20: 357-363.

115ba. Neil E. Spingam and John H. Weisburger, *Cancer Letters* (1979) 7: 259-264.

115bb. C.A. Krone and W.T. Iwaoka, *Mutation Research* (1984) 141: 131-134.

115bc. *Longevity Letter* (Dec., 1985) 3, no. 12:2.

115c. S. L. Taylor et al., *Jrl. of the American Oil Chemists' Society* (1983) 60, no. 3: 576-580.

115d. S.L. Taylor et al., *Food, Chem. Toxicol.* (1982) 20: 209, cited in ref. 115c.

115e. Michael W. Pariza et al., *Cancer Research* (1983) 43 supp: 2444s-2446s.

116. S.S. Chang, *Jrl. of the Amer. Oil Chemists' Society* (1978) 55: 718-727.

117. F.A. Kummerow, *Science News* (April 20, 1974) 105: 253.

117a. F.A. Kummerow, *American Jrl. of Clinical Nutrition* (1981) 34: 601-602.

117b. T. Mizuguchi, F.A. Kummerow et al., *Fed. Amer. Soc. Exp. Biol.* (1974) 235 (abst. 183). Cited in ref. 117a.

117c. J.L. Beare-Rogers et al., *Amer. Jrl. of Clinical Nutrition* (1979) 32: 1805-1809.

117d. S.P. Kochhar and T. Matsui, *Food Chemistry* (1984) 13 no. 2: 85-101.

117e. H.T. Slover et al., *Jrl. of the American Oil Chemists' Society* (1985) 62, no. 4: 775-766.

117f. M. G. Enig et al., *Jrl. of the American Oil Chemists' Society* (1983) 60, no. 10: 1788-1795.

118. J.B. Ohlrogge et al., *Jrl. of Lipid Research* (1981) 22: 955-960.

119. Matthias Sommerfeld, *Prog. in Lipid Research* (1983) 22: 221-223.

119a. Walter H. Meyer, *Amer. Jrl. of Clinical Nutrition* (1981) 34: 603-605.

119b. Steven M. Royce, F.A. Kummerow et al., *Amer. Jrl. of Clinical Nutrition* (1984) 39: 215-222.

119c. L.H. Thomas et al., *J. Epidemiol. Commun. Health* (1983) 57: 22-24. Cited by E. A. Emken, *Ann. Rev. Nutri.* (1984) 4: 339-376.

119d. J.E. Kinsella et al., *Amer. Jrl. of Clinical Nutrition* (1981) 34: 2307-2318.

119e. Remi de Schrijver and Orville S. Privett, *Lipids* (1982) 17, no. 1: 27-34.

119f. Miriam D. Rosenthal and Mark A. Doloresco, *Lipids* (1984) 19, no. 11: 869-874.

119g. M.M. Mahfouz et al., *Acta Biologica et Medica Germanica* (1982) 41: 355-363.

120. David Kritchevsky, *Federation Proceedings* (1982) 41: 2813-2817.

121. Herbert Ruttenberg et al., *Jrl. of Nutrition* (1983) 113: 835-844.

121a. John C. Kabara, *Jrl. of the Amer. Oil Chemists' Society* (1984) 61, no. 2: 397-403.

121b. Remi de Schrijver and Orville S. Privett, *Jrl. of Nutrition* (1984) 114: 1183-1191.

122. Mary G. Enig et al., *Federation Proceedings* (1978) 37: 2215-2220.

122a. Mary G. Enig et al., *Federation Proceedings* (1979) 38: 2437-2439.

122b. K.K. Carroll, *Jrl. of the American Oil Chemists Soc.* (Dec., 1984) 61, no. 12: 1888-1891.

122c. Patricia L. Kraft, *Regulatory Toxicology and Pharmacology* (1983) 3: 239-251.

123. J. Edward Hunter, *Jrl. of the National Cancer Institute* (1982) 69: 319-321.

124. R.B. Alfin-Slater et al., *Jrl. of Nutrition* (1957) 63: 241-261.

125. R.B. Alfin-Slater and L. Aftergood in *Geometrical and Positional Fatty Acid Isomers*, ed. E. A. Emken and H.J. Dutton (Champaign, Il.: Amer. Oil Chemists' Society, 1979) pp. 151-175.

126. T.H. Applewhite, *Jrl. of the Amer. Oil Chemists' Society* (1981) 58: 260-269.

126a. Kikuko Nishiyama et al., *Lipids* (1985) 20, no. 5: 325-327.

126b. Atif Awad, *Jrl. of the National Cancer Institute* (1981) 67, no. 1: 189-192.

126c. Sandra L. Selenskas et al., *Cancer Research* (1984) 44: 1321-1326.

126d. Kent L. Erickson, *Food & Nutrition News* (1984) 56, no. 2: 9-12.

127. T.H. Applewhite, *Lipids* (1981) 16, no. 9: 703-704.

127a. D. Chobanov and R. Chobanova, *Jrl. of the American Oil Chemists' Society* (1977) 54: 47-50.

127b. B. Sreenivasan, *Jrl. of the American Oil Chemists' Society* (1978) 55: 796-805.

127c. D.G. Chobanov and M.R. Topalova, *Jrl. of the American Oil Chemists' Society* (1979) 56: 581-584.

127d. Y.C. Lo and A.P. Handel, *Jrl. of the American Oil Chemists' Society* (1983) 60, no. 4: 815-818.

128. H. Kaunitz and R.E. Johnson, as reported by David Kritchevsky, *Federation Proceedings* (May, 1979) 38: 2001-2006.

129. Elspeth B. Smith, *Lancet* (March 8, 1980): 534.

129a. Patrick Tso et al., *Lipids* (1984) 19, no. 1: 11-16.

129b. R.F. Heller et al., *Atherosclerosis* (1983) 48: 185-192.

129c. P.N. Durrington, *Clinical Science* (1979) 56: 501, cited in ref. 129b.

129d. A. H. Conney et al., *Clinical Pharmacology and Therapeutics* (1976) 20: 633. Cited in ref. 129b.

129e. David A. Snowdon et al., *Preventive Medicine* (1984) 13: 490-500.

130. Robert Baker et al., *Cancer Letters* (1982) 16: 81-89.

130a. S. Krishnamurthy et al., *Acta Vitaminologica et Enzymologica* (1983) 5, no. 3: 165-170.

130b. J. Szepsenwol, *Proceedings of the Society for Biology and Medicine* (1963) 112: 1073-1076.

130c. J. Szepsenwol, *Proceedings of the Society for Biology and Medicine* (1964) 116: 1136-1139.

130d. J. Szepsenwol, *Proceedings of the Society for Biology and Medicine* (1966) 121: 168-171.

131. Scott M. Grundy, *Annual Review of Nutrition* (1983) 3: 71-96.

131a. R. Ross and J.A. Glomset, *Science* (1973) 180: 1332-1339. Cited by Keith E. Suckling and Eduard F. Stange, *Jrl. of Lipid Research* (1985) 26: 647-671, at 661.

131b. P. Helgerud et al., *European Jrl. of Clinical Investigation* (1982) 12: 493-500. Cited by Keith E. Suckling and Eduard F. Stange, *Jrl. of Lipid Research* (1985) 26: 647-671, at 658.

131c. Francis Heller et al., *American Jrl. of Clinical Nutrition* (1985) 41: 748-752.

132. Roslyn B. Alfin-Slater and Lilla Aftergood in *Modern Nutrition in Health and Disease,* ed. Robert S. Goodhart and Maurice E. Shils, Philadelphia: Lea & Febiger, 1973) pp. 132-134.

133. T. Takatori et al., *Lipids* (1976) 11, no. 4: 272-280.

134. Carolyn E. Moore et al., *Jrl. of Nutrition* (1980) 110: 2284-2290.

135. Michihiro Sugano et al., *Jrl. of Lipid Research* (1984) 25: 474-485.

136. Ancel Keys, *Amer. Jrl. of Clinical Nutrition* (1984) 40: 351-359.

137. Hirotsuga Ueshima et al., *Preventive Medicine* (1979) 8: 104-111.

138. Harold D. Chope and Lester Breslow, *American Jrl. of Public Health* (Jan. 1956) 46: 61-67.

139. M.F. Oliver, *Lancet* (Sept. 18, 1982): 655.

140. W.B. Kannel and T. Gordon, *Lancet* (Aug. 11, 1982): 374-375.

141. Albert B. Lowenfels, *Nutrition and Cancer* (1983) 4, no. 4: 280-284.

142. Zivi N. Berneman, *JAMA* (July 22/29, 1983) 250, no. 4: 483.

143. Geoffrey Rose et al., *Lancet* (Feb. 9, 1974): 181-183.

143a. Paul J. Nestel, *American Jrl. of Clinical Nutrition* (1986) 43: 752-757.

144. Donald J. McNamara (and a reply by Ancel Keys), *American Jrl. of Clinical Nutrition* (1985) 41: 657-659.

144a. Suk Y. Oh and Lorraine T. Miller, *American Jrl. of Clinical Nutrition* (1985) 42: 421-431.

145. Paul J. Nestel et al., *New England Jrl. of Medicine* (1973) 288, no. 8: 379-382.

146. David H. Blankenhorn, *New England Jrl. of Medicine* (1985) 312, no. 13: 851-853.

146a. Judith Krzynowek, *Food Technology* (1985) 39, no. 2: 61-68.

147. Nobuko Iritani et al., *Jrl. of Nutritional Science and Vitaminology* (1979) 25: 205-211.

147a. Santhirasegaram Balasubramaniam et al., *Jrl. of Lipid Research* (1985) 26: 685-689.

147b. M. Sugano et al., *American Jrl. of Clinical Nutrition* (1980) 33: 787-793.

147c. J.J. Nagyvary et al., *Nutrition Reports International* (1979) 20, no. 5: 677-684.

148. Daan Kromhout et al., *New England Jrl. of Medicine* (1985) 312, no. 19, 1205-1209.

149. Theodore P. Labuza in *CRC Critical Reviews in Food Science and Technology* (1971) 2: 355-405, at 389.

149a. Stein E. Vollset et al., *New England Jrl. of Medicine* (Sept. 26, 1985) 313, no. 13: 820-821.

149b. J. David Curb et al., *New England Jrl. of Medicine* (Sept. 26, 1985) 313, no. 13: 821.

149c. Richard B. Shekelle et al., *New England Jrl. of Medicine* (Sept. 26, 1985) 313, no. 13: 820.

149ca. William S. Harris et al., *Metabolism* (1984) 33, no. 11: 1016-1019.

149cb. D. Roger Illingworth et al., *Arteriosclerosis* (1984) 4: 270-275.

149cc. L.A. Simons et al., *Atherosclerosis* (1985) 54: 75-88.

149cd. Beverley E. Phillipson et al., *New England Jrl. of Medicine* (1985) 312, no. 19: 1210-1216.

149ce. G. Schonfeld et al., *Diabetes* (1974) 23: 827. Cited in ref. 149cf.

149cf. Ikuo Nishigaki et al., *Biochemical Medicine* (1981) 25: 373-378.

149cg. Ad Hoc Committee to Design a Dietary Treatment of Hyperlipoproteinemia (Antonio M. Gotto, Jr., et al.), *Circulation* (1984) 69: 1067A-1090A.

149ch. E. Schimke et al., *Biomedica and Biochimica Acta* (1984) 43, no. 8, 9: S351-S353.

149d. Simin N. Meydani et al., *New England Jrl. of Medicine* (Sept. 26, 1985) 313, no. 13: 822.

149e. C.G. Mackenzie et al., *Jrl. of Nutrition* (1941) 21: 225-234. Cited in ref. 149d.

150. *Nutrition Reviews* (1985) 43, no. 2: 43-44.

151. D. Kromhout, *American Jrl. of Clinical Nutrition* (1983) 38: 591-598. Cited in ref. 150.

151a. D.P. Baar, E.M. Russ and H.A. Eder, *American Jrl. of Medicine* (1951) 11: 480-491. Cited by Hans Dieplinger et al., *Jrl. of Lipid Research* (1985) 26: 273-282.

152. GIna Kolata, *Science* (Sept. 16, 1983) 221: 1164-1166.

153. Richard J. Havel, *Jrl. of Lipid Research* (1984) 25: 1570-1576.

154. Yitzchak Oschry et al., *Jrl. of Lipid Research* (1985) 26: 158-167.

154a. Michael S. Brown and Joseph L. Goldstein, *Jrl. of Clinical Investigation* (1983) 72: 743-747.

154b. Joseph L. Goldstein et al., *New England Jrl. of Medicine* (1983) 309, no. 5: 288-296.

154c. Jean L. Marx, *Science* (Nov. 8, 1985) 230: 649-651.

155. Michael S. Brown and Joseph L. Goldstein, *Scientific American* (Nov., 1984) 251, no. 5: 58-66.

155a. Joseph L. Goldstein and Michael S. Brown, *Jrl. of Lipid Research* (1984) 25: 1450-1461.

155b. Olafur G. Björnsson et al., *Archives of Biochemistry and Biophysics* (1985) 238, no. 1: 135-145.

155c. Akiro Endo, *Advances in Experimental Medicine and Biology* (1985) 183: 295-310.

155d. Akiro Endo et al., *Jrl. of Antibiotics* (1976) 29: 1346-1348. Cited in ref. 155c.

156. Lipid Research Clinics Program, *JAMA* (1984) 251, no. 3: 351-364.

157. Lipid Research Clinics Program, *JAMA* (1984) 251, no. 3: 365-374.

158. Robert I. Levy et al., *Circulation* (1984) 69, no. 2: 325-337.

159. W. Virgil Brown, *Amer. Jrl. of Cardiology* (1984) 54: 27C-29C.

160. Günter Schlierf et al., *American Jrl. of Cardiology* (1983) 52: 17B-19B.

160a. R.F. Heller, *Lancet* (Dec. 5, 1981): 1258-1260.

161. Fiona C. Ballantyne et al., *Metabolism* (1982) 31, no. 5: 423-437.

161a. Mark A. Kantor et al., *Medicine and Science in Sports and Medicine* (1985) 17, no. 4: 462-465.

162. Richard E. Gregg, *Jrl. of Lipid Research* (1984) 25: 1167-1176.

163. Shlomo Eisenberg, *Jrl. of Lipid Research* (1984) 25: 1017-1058 at 1020.

163a. William Stoffel, *Jrl. of Lipid Research* (1984) 25: 1586-1592, at 1586.

163b. Pascal Puchois et al., *Clinica Chimica Acta* (1984) 185: 185-189.

164. Guisepe Cazzolato et al., *Arteriosclerosis* (1985) 5: 88-92.

165. R. J. Deckelbaum et al., *Jrl. of Lipid Research* (1982) 23: 1274-1282. Cited by Shlomo Eisenberg, *Jrl. of Lipid Research* (1984) 25: 1017-1058 at 1020.

166. J.W. Gofman et al., *Circulation* (1966) 34: 679-697. Cited in ref. 161.

167. James J. Maciejko et al., *New England Jrl. of Medicine* (1983) 309, no. 7: 385-389.

168. Peter O. Kwiterovich and Allan D. Sniderman, *Preventive Medicine* (1983) 12: 815-834.

168a. M.F. Reardon et al., *Circulation* (May, 1985) 71: 881. Cited by Margene A. Wagstaff, *Jrl. of the American Dietetic Assn.* (Sept., 1985) 85, no. 9: 1238.

169. J. Scott et al., *Lancet* (1985): 771-773.

170. G. Fager et al., *Arteriosclerosis* (1981) 1: 273-279. Cited in ref. 169.

171. E. Pilger et al., *Arteriosclerosis* (1983) 3: 57-63. Cited in ref. 169.

172. C.H. Chen and J.J. Albers, *Arteriosclerosis* (1983) 3: 489a. Cited in ref. 169.

172a. Armin Steinmetz and Gerd Utermann, *Jrl. of Biological Chemistry* (1985) 260, no. 4: 2258-2264.

173. C.E. Jahn et al., *FEBS Letters* (1981) 131: 366-368. Cited in ref. 169.

174. A.N. Orekhov et al., *Lancet* (Nov. 17, 1984): 1149-1150.

175. R. Saynor et al., *Atherosclerosis* (1984) 50: 3-10.

176. Beverley E. Phillipson et al., *New England Jrl. of Medicine* (1985) 312, no. 19: 1210-1216.

177. William S. Harris et al., *Metabolism* (1983) 32, no. 2: 179-184.

178. T.A.B. Sanders and Michele C. Hochland, *British Jrl. of Nutrition* (1983) 50: 521-529.

179. Richard S. Cooper,. et al., *Atherosclerosis* (1982) 44: 293-305.

180. Fred H. Mattson, AOCS Mongraph 10, *American Oil Chemists' Society* 1983. Cited by Don R. Swanson, *Amer. Longevity Assn. Longevity Letter* (1985) 3, no. 1: 12.
181. P. Couzigou et al., *Ann. Nutr. Metabl.* (1984) 28: 377-384.
182. Joanne E. Cluette et al., *Proc. of the Society for Experimental Biology and Medicine* (1984) 176: 508-511.
182a. J.K. Allen and M.A. Adena, *Annals of Clinical Biochemistry* (1985) 22: 62-66.
183. William J. Haskell, *Preventive Medicine* (1984) 131: 23-26.
184. Naruhiko Nagao et al., *Jrl. of Sports Medicine* (1984) 24: 219-224.
184a. E. Ernst et al., *British Medical Jrl.* (1985) 291: 139.
185. Paul J. Nestel in *Drugs Affecting Lipid Metabolism*, ed. Remo Fumagalli, David Kritchevsky and Rodolfo Paoletti (Amsterdam: Elsevier/North Holland Biomedical Press, 1980) p. 161.
186. John R. L. Masarei et al., *Amer. Jrl. of Clinical Nutrition,* (1984) 40: 468-479.
187. Frank M. Sacks et al., *New England Jrl. of Medicine* (1975) 292, no. 22: 1148-1151.
187a. Frank M. Sacks et al., *JAMA* (Sept. 13, 1985) 254, no. 10: 1337-1341.
188. Paul T. Williams, *JAMA* (1985) 253, no. 10: 1407-1411.
189. D.S. Thelle et al., *New England Jrl. of Medicine* (1983) 308: 1454-1457.
190. Olav Helge Forde et al., *British Medical Jrl.* (1985) 290: 893-895.
191. Ancel Keys, cited by John Henahan, *JAMA* (1981) 246: no. 20: 2311-2315.
192. Russell L. Holman, *Federation Proceedings* (1946) 5: 223-224.
192a. Robert S. Gordon, *JAMA* (1980) 244, no. 1: 25.
193. Victor Herbert, *Amer. Jrl. of Clinical Nutrition* (Apr., 1981) 34: 592-593.
194. International Collaborative Group, *JAMA* (1982) 248, no. 21: 2853-2859.
195. Manning Feinleib, *Cancer Research* (1983) 43 supp.: 2503s-2507s.
196. David P. Horrobin, *Medical Hypotheses* (1980) 6: 469-486.
197. Leland L. Smith, in *Autoxidation in Food and Biological Systems,* ed. Michael G. Simic and Marcus Karel (New York: Raven Press, 1980) supp. 119-132.
197a. Lee Shin Tsai and Carol A. Hudson, *Jrl. of Food Science* (1985) 50: 229-231, 237.
198. C.B. Taylor et al., *Amer. Jrl. of Clinical Nutrition* (1979) 32: 40-57.
199. R.W. Turner, *Lancet* (Apr. 9, 1983): 827.
200. J.A.L. Gorringe, *Lancet,* (May 21, 1983): 1165.
201. M.J. Hill, *Cancer Research* (1975) 35: 3398-3402.
202. M.J. Hill, *Lancet,* (Mar. 8, 1975): 535-539.
203. Lucien R. Jacobs and Joanne R. Lupton, *Jrl. of the National Cancer Institute* (1973) 51: 1765-1779.
204. W. Haenszel et al., *Jrl. of the National Cancer Institute* (1973) 51: 1765-1779.
204a. Barbara Olds Schneeman, *American Jrl. of Clinical Nutrition* (Nov., 1985) 42: 966-972.
205. Gail E. McKeown-Eyssen and Elizabeth Bright-See, *Nutrition and Cancer* (1984) 6, no. 3: 160-170.
206. W. Forth et al., cited by M.A. Eastwood, *Medical Hypotheses* (1975) 1: 46-53.
207. Denham Harman, *Jrl. of Gerontology* (1971) 26, no. 4: 451-457.
207a. C.B. Wood, *British Medical Journal* (1985) 291: 163-165.
207b. R.J. Booyens and L. Maguire, *Medical Hypotheses* (1985) 17: 351-362.
207c. Samuel H. Preston, Nathan Keyfitz and Robert Schoen, *Causes of Death* (New York: Seminar Press, 1972) pp. 332, 334, 412, 414, 768, 770.
208. Denham Harman, *Clinical Research* (1969) 17: 125.
209. Charles F. Aylsworth et al., *Jrl. of the National Cancer Institute* (1984) 72, no. 3: 637-645.
210. Eva Kwong et al., *Jrl. of Nutrition* (1984) 114: 2324-2330.
211. Miroslav Ledvina and Milena Hodanova, *Experimental Gerontology* (1980) 15: 61-71.
212. Thomas H. Jukes, *Nature* (Feb. 9, 1978) 271: 499.
213. E.B. Lillehoj et al., *Science* (1976) 193: 495-496.
214. Denham Harman et al., *Jrl. of the Amer. Geriatrics Society* (1976) 27, no. 7: 301-306.

215. Alan F. Hofmann et al., *New England Jrl. of Medicine* (1973) 288: 46-47.
216. R.A.L. Sturdevant et al., *New England Jrl. of Medicine* (1973) 288: 24-27.
217. George W. Melchior et al., *Federation Proceedings* (1974) 33: 626.
218. Leslie J. Schoenfield et al., *Annals of Internal Medicine* (1981) 95, no. 3: 257-282.
218a. William Lijinsky, *Cancer Research* (1983) 43 supp.: 2441s-2443s.
219. Gina Kolata, *Science* (Jan. 23, 1987) 235: 436.
219a. William Fears et al., *Jrl. of Adolescent Health Care* (1983) 4: 22-24.
219b. R.A. Frisch in *Anorexia Nervosa*, ed. R.A. Vigersky (New York: Raven Press, 1977) pp. 149-161. Cited in ref. 219a.
220. D. Hollander et al., *Jrl. of Lipid Research* (1984) 25, no. 2: 129-134. Cited in *Nutrition Abstracts and Reviews,* Series A (1984) 54, no. 9: 786 (item 5524).
221. Garry J. Hopkins and Clive E. West, *Life Sciences* (1976) 19: 1103-1116.
222. P.C. Chan et al., *Proc. Soc. for Experimental Biology and Medicine* (1975) 149: 133-135, cited by ref. 221.
223. D.F. Horrobin, *Medical Hypotheses* (1979) 5: 599-620, at 611.
224. P.C. Chan and Leonard A. Cohen, *Jrl. of the National Cancer Institute* (1974) 52, no. 1:25-30.
225. H.L. Newmark et al., *Jrl. of the National Cancer Institute* (1984) 72, no. 6: 1323-1325.
226. P. Stevens et al., *Progress in Lipid Research* (1981) 20: 751.
227. S. Boyd Eaton and Melvin Konner, *New England Jrl. of Medicine* (Jan. 31, 1985) 312, no. 5: 283-289.
228. H.O. Ledger, *Symp Zool. Soc., London* (1968) 21: 289-310. Cited in ref. 227.
229. M.A. Crawford, *Lancet* (1968) 1: 1328-1333. Cited in ref. 227.
230. C.K.W. Wo and H.H. Draper, *Amer. Jrl. of Clinical Nutrition* (1975) 28: 208-213. Cited in ref. 227.
231. M.A. Crawford et al., *Biochemical Jrl.* (1969) 115: 25-27. Cited in ref. 227.
232. J. Dyerberg et al., *Lancet* (1978) 2: 117-119. Cited in ref. 227.
233. R.M. Feeley et al., *Jrl. Amer. Diet Assn.* (1972) 61: 134-149. Cited in ref. 227.
234. U.S. Select Committee on Nutrition and Human Needs, United States Senate. *Dietary Goals for the United States* (Washington D.C.: Government Printing Office, 1977). Cited in ref. 227.
235. Nutrition Committee of the American Heart Assn., *Circulation* (1982) 65, no. 4: 839A-854A.
235a. Constance Kies, cited in *Medical World News,* (June 25, 1984) 25: 41.
236. A.S. Milton, *Trends in Pharmaceutical Sciences* (Dec., 1982): 490-492.
237. G.J. Roth and P.W. Majerus, *Jrl. of Clinical Investigation* (1975) 56: 624-632.
238. Gerald J. Roth et al., *Proc. of the National Academy of Sciences* (1975) 72, no. 8: 3073-3076.
239. Gerald J. Roth and Chester J. Siok, *Jrl. of Biological Chemistry* (1978) 253, no. 11: 3782-3784.
240. *International Symposium on Fever,* ed. James M. Lipton (New York: Raven Press, 1980).
241. Mathew J. Kluger, *Fever—Its Biology, Evolution and Function* (Princeton, N.J.: Princton Univ. Press, 1979).
241a. I. Gery et al., *Jrl. of Immunology* (1971) 107: 1778-1785. Cited in ref. 241d.
241b. S.K. Durum and R.K. Gershon, *Proceedings of the National Academy of Sciences* (1972) 79: 4747-4750. Cited in ref. 241d.
241c. J.J. Oppenheim and I. Gery, *Immunology Today* (1982) 3: 113-119. Cited in ref. 241d.
241d. Gordon W. Duff and Scott K. Durum, *Yale Jrl. of Biology and Medicine* (1982) 55: 437-442.
241e. K.A. Smith et al., *Jrl. of Experimental Medicine* (1980) 151: 1551-1556. Cited in ref. 241d.
242. Harvey B. Simon, *JAMA* (Nov. 16, 1984) 252, no. 19: 2735-2738.
242a. Vincenzo Rossi et al., *Science* (1985) 229: 174-176.

243. J.R. Vane, *Nature New Biology* (June 23, 1971) 231: 232-235.
244. J.B. Smith and A.L. Willis, ibid: 235-237.
245. S.H. Ferreira, S. Moncada and J.R.Vane, ibid: 237-239.
246. S. Moncada and J.R. Vane, *British Medical Bulletin* (1978) 34: 129-135.
247. R. Neal Pinckard,*Monographs in Pathology* (1982) 112: 38-53, at 45.
247a. William F. Stenson and Charles W. Parker, *Clinical Reviews of Allergy* (1983) 1: 369-384 at 375.
247b. M.I. Siegel et al., *Proc. of the National Academy of Sciences* (1979) 76: 3774-3778. Cited in ref. 247a.
247c. M.I. Siegel et al., *Proc. of the National Academy of Sciences* (1980) 77: 308-312. Cited in ref. 247a.
247d. M.I. Siegel et al., *Biochemical and Biophysical Research Communications* (1980) 92: 688-695. Cited in ref. 247a.
248. Gerald Weissmann, *Cellular Immunology* (1983) 82: 117-126.
249. *Nutrition Reviews* (1983) 41, no. 3: 90-91.
249a. M. Fletcher-Cieutat et al.,*Prostaglandins, Leukotrienes and Medicine* (1985) 18: 255-259.
250. A.A. van Kolfschoten et al., *Naunyn-Schmiedeberg's Archives of Pharmacology* (1984) 325: 283-285.
251. J.G. Collier and R.J. Flower, *Lancet* (Oct. 16, 1971): 852-853.
252. A.K. Didolkar et al., *International Jrl. of Andrology* (1980) 3: 585-593.
253. H.U. Comberg et al., *Prostaglandins* (1978) 15: 193-197.
254. E.C. Huskisson, *Seminars in Arthritis and Rheumatism* (1977) 7, no. 1: 1-20.
255. A. Szczeklik, *Bulletin Europeen di Physio Pathologie Respiratoire* (1983) 19: 531-538.
255a. Amy L. Daniels and Gladys J. Everson,*Proc. of the Society for Experimental Biology and Medicine* (1936) 35: 20-24.
255b. H.S. Loh and C.W.M. Wilson, *International Jrl. for Vitamin and Nutrition Research* (1975) 41: 258.
256. G.B. West, *Jrl. Pharm. Pharmacol.* (1964) 16: 788-793.
257. S. Sayama et al., *Proc. of the National Academy of Sciences* (1981) 78: 7327. Cited by R. Yoshida and O. Hayaishi,*Methods in Enzymology* (1984) 105: 61-70.
258. A. Kimchi et al.,*Proc. of the National Academy of Sciences* (1979) 76: 3208. Cited by R. Yoshida and O. Hayaishi,*Methods in Enzymology* (1984) 105: 61-70.
259. John Baum, *Amer. Jrl. of Medicine* (June 14, 1983): 10-15.
260. Alan K. Done, ibid: 27-35.
261. Ryunosuke Kumashiro et al.,*American Surgeon* (1983) 49, no. 8: 423-427.
262. A. Robert, *Gastroenterology* (1974) 66: 765.
263. Edward Cotlier et al.,*Amer. Jrl. of Medicine* (June 14, 1983): 33-90.
264. James J. Kolenick et al., *Lancet* (Sept. 30, 1972): 714.
265. Gabriel Gasic et al., *Proc. Amer. Assn. for Cancer Research* (March, 1973) 14: 87.
266. Gabriel J. Gasic et al., *Proc. of the National Academy of Sciences* (1968) 61: 46-52.
267. G.A. Jamieson, editor, *Interaction of Platelets and Tumor Cells* (New York: Alan R. Liss, 1982), especially G. J. Gasic and T. B. Gasic, pp. 429-444.
268. Gabriel J. Gasic et al., *Cancer Research* (1978) 38: 2950-2955.
269. Ferdinando Laghi et al.,*Tumori* (1983) 69: 349-353.
270. Hamid Al-Mondhiry et al., *Thrombosis and Haemostasis* (1983) 50, no. 3: 726-730.
271. P.M. Evans and F. P. Cowie, *Cell Biology International Reports* (1983) 7, no. 9: 771-778.
272. Edward Pearlstein et al., *Jrl. of Laboratory and Clinical Medicine* (1979) 93, no. 2: 332-344.
273. Kailash C. Agarwal and Robert E. Parks, Jr.,*International Jrl. of Cancer* (1983) 32: 801-804.
273a. Hans-Inge Peterson, *Invasion Metabolism* (1983) 3: 151-159.

274. G.A. FitzGerald and Sol Sherry in *Prostaglandins and the Cardiovascular System,* ed. John A. Oates, vol. 10 of *Advances in Prostaglandin, Thomboxane and Leukotriene Research Series* (New York: Raven Press, 1982) pp. 107-171.

275. John C. Hoak, *Thrombosis Research* (1983) supp. 4: 47-51.

276. R.B. Philp and M.L. Paul, *Prostaglandins, Leukotrienes and Medicine* (1983) 11: 131-142.

277. G.A. FitzGerald et al., in *Advances in Prostaglandin, Thromboxane and Leukotriene Research* , vol. 11, ed. B. Samuelsson, R. Paoletti and P. Ramwell (New York: Raven Press, 1983) pp. 265-266.

278. C. Patrono et al., ibid., pp. 493-498.

279. P. Patrignani, ibid., pp. 259-264.

280. S.P. Hanley et al., *British Medical Jrl.* (1982) 285: 1299-1302.

281. F. Eric Preston et al., *New England Jrl. of Medicine* (1981) 304, no. 2: 76-79.

282. Edwin W. Salzman, *New England Jrl. of Medicine* (1982) 307, no. 2: 113-115.

283. Aaron J. Marcus, *New England Jrl. of Medicine* (1983) 309, no. 24: 1515-1517.

284. H. Daniel Lewis, Jr., *New England Jrl. of Medicine* (1983) 309, no. 7: 396-403.

285. G. D'Andrea et al., *Thromb. Haemostas.* (1983) 49, no. 2: 153.

286. Margareta Thorngren et al., *Haemostasis* (1983) 13: 244-247.

287. Margareta Thorngren and Anders Gustafson, *Amer. Jrl. of Medicine* (1983): 66-71.

288. Garret A. FitzGerald et al., *Jrl. of Clinical Investigation* (1983) 71: 676-688.

289. Carlo Patrono, *New England Jrl. of Medicine* (1984) 310, no. 20: 1326.

290. Paulette Mebta, *New England Jrl. of Medicine* (1984) 310, no. 20: 1326-1327.

291. Mark Fisher, *New England Jrl. of Medicine* (1984) 310, no. 20: 1327.

292. Aaron J. Marcus, *New England Jrl. of Medicine* (1984) 310, no. 20: 1327.

293. P.C. Elwood, *Drugs* (1984) 28: 1-5.

294. R.L. Lorenz et al., *Lancet* (June 9, 1984) 1261-1264.

295. R. Simrock et al., *Thrombosis and Haemostasis* (1984) 51, no. 2: 269-271.

296. S.P. Hanley et al., *Lancet* (1981) 1: 969-71. Cited in ref. 298.

297. J. Kaliman et al., *Wien Klin. Wochenschr.* (1983) 95: 615-617. Cited in ref. 298.

298. P. Patrignani et al., *Jrl. of Clin. Investigation* (1982) 69: 1366-1372.

299. H. Sinzinger et al., *New England Jrl. of Medicine* (Oct. 18, 1984) 311, no. 16: 1052.

300. *Physicians' Desk Reference* (1984) 38th ed. (Oradell, N.J.: Medical Economics Co., 1984) n. 989.

301. *AMA Drug Evaluations* (1983) 5th ed.: 91.

302. Don R. Swanson, *Longevity Letter* (1984) 2, nos. 1 and 2.

303. J.R. A. Mitchell, *British Medical Bulletin* (1983) 39: 289-295.

303a. The American-Canadian Co-Operative Study Group, *Stroke* (1985) 16, no. 3: 406-415.

303b. H.C.S. Wallenburg et al., *Lancet* (Jan. 4, 1986): 1-3.

304. Elizabetta Dejana et al., *Thrombosis Research* (1983) supp. 4: 153-159.

305. J.L. Humes et al., *Proc. National Academy of Sciences* (1981) 78: 2053-2056.

306. E Dejana et al., *Jrl. Clinical Investigation* (1981) 68: 1108-1112. Cited in ref. 181.

307. Domenico Rotilio et al., *European Jrl. of Pharmacology* (1984) 97: 197-208.

308. Marja-Liisa Dahl et al., *Prostaglandins, Leukotrienes and Medicine* (1983) 12:21-28.

309. E. Walter et al., *Klinische Wochenschrift* (1981) 59: 297-299.

310. Steven A. Rosenberg et al., *New England Jrl. of Medicine* (Dec. 5, 1985) 313, no. 23: 1485-1492.

311. Beverly Merz, *JAMA* (Sept. 12, 1986) 256, no. 10: 1241, 1244.

312. Michael T. Lotze et al., *JAMA* (Dec. 12, 1986) 256, no. 22: 3117-3124.

313. Charles G. Moertel, *JAMA* (Dec. 12, 1986) 256, no. 22: 3141.

Chapter 4—376 References

1. Gary L. Peck, *Gynecologic Oncology* (1981) 12: S331-S340.
1a. S. Smith and D. Goodman, *Federation Proceedings* (1979) 38: 2504-2509. Cited by B. Mazieres in *Clinical Rheumatology* (1982) 1, no. 4: 239-242.
2. David E. Ong and Frank Chytil, *Jrl. of Biological Chemistry* (1975) 250: 6113-6117.
3. David E. Ong and Frank Chytil, *Proc. of the Natural Academy of Sciences* (1976) 73: 3976-3978.
4. J. Ganguly et al., *Vitamins and Hormones* (1980) 38: 1-54.
4a. David E. Ong, *Nutrition Reviews* (Aug., 1985) 43, no. 8: 225-232.
5. Dewitt S. Goodman, *Federation Proceedings* (1979) 38, no. 11: 2501-2503.
6. W.J. Pudelkiewicz et al., *Jrl. of Nutrition* (1964) 84: 113-117.
7. John G. Bieri et al., *Jrl. of Nutrition* (1981) 111: 458-467.
8. John G. Bieri and Teresa J. Tolliver, *Jrl. of Nutriton* (1982) 112: 401-403.
9. J.A.D. Anderson and I.H. Stokoe, *British Medical Jrl.* (Aug. 3, 1963): 294-296.
10. Samuel Ayers, Jr. and Richard Mihan, *International Jrl. of Dermatology* (1981) 20: 616.
10a. Albert M. Kligman et al., *International Jrl. of Dermatology* (1981) 20, no. 4: 278-285.
10b. Howard L. Sofen, *Lancet* (Jan. 7, 1984): 40.
10c. Waun Ki Hong et al., *New England Jrl. of Medicine* (Dec. 11, 1986) 315, no. 24: 1501-1505.
11. Gerald Shklar, *New England Jrl. of Medicine* (Dec. 11, 1986) 315, no. 24: 1544-1546.
11a. Paul J. Banke, *JAMA* (1984) 251, no. 24: 3267-3269.
11b. Reba Michels Hill, *Lancet* (June 30, 1984): 1465.
11c. Christopher S. Conner, *Drug Intelligence and Clinical Pharmacy* (April, 1984) 18: 308-309.
12. D. Tsambaos and C.E. Orfanos, *Pharm. Ther.* (1981) 14: 355-374.
13. *Amer. Family Physician* (1983) 28, no. 4: 359.
14. *Physicians' Desk Reference,* 37th ed. (Oradell, N.J.: Medical Economics Co., 1983) pp. 1643-1644.
14a. Peter E. Pochi, *New England Jrl. of Medicine* (1983) 308, no. 17, 1024-1025.
14b. *Medical Letters* (1983) 25, issue 649: 105-106.
14c. A. Ward et al., *Drugs* (1984) 28: 6-37.
14d. Edward J. Lammer et al., *New England Jrl. of Medicine* (Oct. 3, 1985) 313, no. 14: 837-841.
14da. Emmilla Hodak et al., *British Medical Jrl.* (Aug. 16, 1986) 293: 425-426.
14e. W. Grote et al., *Lancet* (June 1, 1985): 1276.
14f. C. Vahlquist et al., *British Jrl. of Dermatology* (1985) 112: 69-76.
14g. Susan Bershad et al., *New England Jrl. of Medicine* (Oct. 10, 1985) 313, no. 16: 981-985.
14h. Peter E. Pochi et al., ibid: 1013-1014.
14i. John J. DiGiovanna et al., *New England Jrl. of Medicine* (Nov. 6, 1986) 315, no. 19: 1177-1182.
15. Alfred Sommer et al., *Lancet* (Sept. 10, 1983): 585-588.
15a. V. Reddy et al., *Acta Paediatr. Scand.* (1979) 68: 65-69.
15b. K. Vijayaraghavan et al., *Lancet* (July 21, 1984): 149-151.
16. Salin Bishara, *British Jrl. of Ophthalmology* (1982) 66: 767-770.
16a. M.D. Kendall, *Experientia* (1984) 40: 1181-1185.
16b. Eli Seifter et al., *Federation Proceedings* (1973) 32: 947 Abs.
16c. Allan L. Goldstein, *Antibiotics and Chemotherapy* (1978) 24: 47-59.
16d. Allan L. Goldstein, *Jrl. of the Reticuloendothelial Society* (1978) 23: 253-266.
16e. Ronald Ross Watson: "Regulation of Immunological Resistance to Cancer by Beta Carotene and Reinoids" in *Nutrition, Disease Resistance and Immune Function* (New

York: M. Dekker, Inc., 1984). Cited by Ronald Ross Watson, *Arizona Medicine* (Oct. 1984) 41, no. 10: 671-673.

17. M.D. Appleton et al., *Amer. Jrl. Mental Defic.* (1964) 69: 324-327.
18. M. Jurin and I.F. Tannock, *Immunology* (1972) 23: 282-287.
19. Benjamin E. Cohen and L. Kelman Cohen, *Jrl. of Immunology* (1973) 111: 1376-1380.
20. Benjamin E. Cohen and Ronald J. Elin, *Jrl. of Infectious Diseases* (1974) 129: 597-600.
21. Umberto Saffiotti et al., *Cancer* (1967) 20: 857-864.
22. Umberto Saffiotti, *Amer. Jrl. of Clinical Nutrition* (1969) 22: 1088.
23. Elizabeth W. Chu and Richard Malmgren, *Cancer Research* (1965) 25: 884-895.
23a. A. Lopez, *Clinical Research* (1982) 30, no. 2: 623A.
24. S. Atukorala et al., *British Jrl. of Cancer* (1979) 40: 927-931.
24a. Miroslav Malkovsky, *Proc. of the National Academy of Sciences* (1983) 80: 6322-6326.
25. Seymour L. Romney et al., *Amer. Jrl. of Obstetrics and Gynecology* (1981) 141: 890-894.
25a. Arnold Bernstein and Beth Harris, *Amer. Jrl. Obstet. and Gynecology* (1984) 148, no. 3: 309-312.
25b. Clement Ip and Margot M. Ip, *Carcinogenesis* (1981) 2, no. 9: 915-918.
26. R.C. Moon and C.J. Grubbs, *Nature* (1977) 267: 620.
27. Clifford W. Welsh et al., *Jrl. of the National Cancer Institute* (1981) 67: 935-938.
28. Richard C. Moon et al., *Cancer Research* (1979) 30: 1339-1346.
29. Andre Lacroix and Marc E. Lippman, *Jrl. of Clinical Investigation* (1980) 65: 586-591.
30. Hisako Ueda et al., *Cancer* (1980) 46: 2203-2209.
31. Reuben Lotan, *Cancer Research* (1979) 39: 1014-1019.
32. Frank L. Meyskens, Jr. and Sydney E. Salmon, *Cancer Research* (1979) 39: 4055-4057.
33. Frank L. Meyskens, Jr. and Bryan B. Fuller, *Cancer Research* (1980) 40: 2194-2196.
34. J. Gouveia et al., *Lancet* (1982) 1: 710-712.
35. Beverly A. Pawson et al., *Jrl. of Medicinal Chemistry* (1982) 25: 1269-1277.
35a. W. Bollag, *Lancet* (April 16, 1983): 860-863.
36. Saxon Graham, *Jrl. of the National Cancer Institute* (Dec., 1984) 73, no. 6: 1423-1428.
36a. Shigetoshi Hosaka et al., *Gann* (1984) 75: 1058-1061.
37. Lee W. Wattenberg, *Cancer Research* (1983) 43 supp.: 2448s-2453s.
37a. Reuben Lotan, *Biochimica et Biophysica Acta* (1980) 605: 33-91.
37b. Reuben Lotan, *Jrl. of Cell Biology* (Nov. 1978) 79: 29a (Abstract CD 144).
38. Samuel Baron et al., *Jrl. of National Cancer Institute* (July, 1981) 67: 95-97.
38a. Anton M. Jetten and M.E. Jetten, *Nature* (March 8, 1979) 278: 180-182.
38b. Anton M. Jetten et al., *Experimental Cell Research* (1979) 124: 381-391.
38c. Sidney Strickland and Vijak Mahdavi, *Cell* (1978) 15: 393-403.
38d. Lawrence Levine and Kazuo Ohuchi, *Nature* (Nov. 16, 1978) 276: 274-275.
38e. E.L. Wilson and E. Reich, *Cell* (1978) 15: 385-392.
38f. Anton M. Jetten, *Nature* (April 17, 1980) 284: 626-629.
39. I.S. Levij et al., *Cancer* (1968) 22: 300-306.
40. I.S. Levij et al., *Jrl. of Investigative Dermatology* (1969) 53: no. 8: 228-231.
41. David M. Smith et al., *Cancer Research* (1975) 35: 11-16.
41a. T. Narisawa et al., *Cancer Research* (1976) 36: 1379-1383. Cited in ref. 41b.
41b. David E. Ong and Frank Chytil, *Vitamins and Hormones* (1983) 40: 105-143.
42. Edward W. Schroder and Paul H. Black *Jrl. of the National Cancer Institute* (1980) 65, no. 4: 671-674.
43. David Gaudin et al., *Biochemical and Biophysical Research Communications* (1971) 45, no. 3: 630-636.
44. H.J. Juhl et al., *Mutation Research* (1978) 58: 317-320.
45. S. Qin et al, *Environmental Mutagenesis* (1985) 7: 137-146.
45a. Jeremy D. Kark et al., *Jrl. of the National Cancer Institute* (1981) 66, no. 1: 7-16.
45aa. Izchak Peleg et al., *Jrl. of the National Cancer Institute* (Dec., 1984) 73, no. 6: 1455-1458.

45b. H.B. Stähelin, *Lancet* (Feb. 13, 1982): 394-395.

45c. Walter C. Willett, *New England Jrl. of Medicine* (1984) 310: 633-638.

46. Thomas Kummet et al., *Nutrition and Cancer* (1983) 5, no. 2: 96-106.

46a. T. Moore, *Vitamine A* (Amsterdam: Elsevier, 1957). Cited by Richard G. Cutler in *Intervention in the Ageing Process, Part B*, ed. William Regelson and F. Marott Sinex (New York: Alan R. Liss, 1983) p. 112.

47. Richard B. Shekelle et al., *Lancet* (Nov. 28, 1981): 1185-1189.

48. Leonard E. Gerber and John W. Erdman, Jr., *Jrl. of Nutrition* (1982) 112: 1555-1564.

49. Micheline M. Mathews-Roth, *Oncology* (1982) 39: 33-37.

49a. R.W. Shearer in *Modulation and Medication of Cancer by Vitamins*, ed. F.L. Meyskens and K.N. Prasad (Basel, Switzerland: Karger, 1983) pp. 89-94.

49b. Curtis Mettlin et al., *Jrl. of the National Cancer Institute* (June, 1979) 62: 1435-1438.

50. E. Bjelke, *Int. Jrl. of Cancer* (1975) 15: 561-565.

51. Gunnar Kvale et al., *Int. Jrl. of Cancer* (1983) 31: 397-405.

52. Takeshi Hirayama, *National Cancer Institute Monographs* (1979) 53: 149-155.

52a. Martin Y. Heshmat et al., *Prostate* (1985) 6: 7-17.

52b. Abraham M.Y. Nomura et al., *Cancer Research* (1985) 45: 2369-2372.

52c. Carlo La Vecchia et al., *International Jrl. of Cancer* (1984) 34: 319-322.

52d. Richard G. Cutler in *Free Radicals in Molecular Biology, Ageing and Disease*, ed., D. Armstrong et al., (New York: Raven Press, 1984) p. 252.

53. R. Peto et al., *Nature* (1981) 290: 201-208.

53a. Christopher S. Foote et al., *Jrl. of the American Chemical Society* (Aug. 26, 1970) 92, no. 17: 5216-5219.

53b. G. W. Burton and K.U. Ingold, *Science* (1984) 224: 569-573.

53c. John Rhodes, *Jrl. of the National Cancer Institute* (1983) 70, no. 5: 833-837.

53d. Guiseppe Rettura et al., *Federation Proceedings* (1983) 42: 786.

53e. L. Santamaria et al., *Experientia* (1983) 39: 1043-1045.

54. Jules Duchesne, *Medical Hypotheses* (1981) 7: 429-432.

54a. Walter C. Willett et al., *New England Jrl. of Medicine* (Feb. 16, 1984) 310, no. 7: 430-434.

54b. Gina Kolata, *Science* (1984) 223: 1161.

54c. Don R. Swanson, *Longevity Letter* (Sept., 1985) 3, no. 9: 9-10.

54d. Charles H. Hennekens, *Jrl. of the National Cancer Institute* (Dec., 1984) 73, no. 6: 1473-1476. Cited in ref. 54c.

54e. Charles H. Hennekens et al., *Preventive Medicine* (1985) 14: 165-168.

55. T. Benedek, *Acta Rheumatol. Scand.* (1958) 4: 178, cited by Roger J. Williams in *Nutrition Against Disease* (New York: Pitman Publ. Corp. 1971) p. 127.

56. Constance E. Brinckerhoff, *Science* (1983) 221: 756-758.

56a. Edward D. Harris, Jr., *Annals of Internal Medicine* (1984) 100, no. 1: 146-147.

57. Isobel Jennings, *Vitamins in Endocrine Metabolism* (Springfield, Il.: Thomas, 1970).

57a. Stanley M. Levenson et al., in *Relevance of Nutrition to Sepsis—Report of the Third Ross Conference of Medical Research* (Columbus, Ohio: Ross Laboratories, 1982) pp. 112-113.

58. H. Paul Ehrlich and Thomas K. Hunt, *Annals of Surgery* (1968) 167: 324-328.

59. Thomas K. Hunt et al., *Annals of Surgery* (1969) 170: 633-641.

60. Henry C. Sherman et al., *Proc. Nat. Acad. of Sciences* (1945) 31, no. 4: 107-109.

61. Roger J. Williams, *Nutrition Against Disease* (New York: Pitman Publ. Corp., 1971) p. 57.

61a. Emmanual Unni et al., *Indian Jrl. of Experimental Biology* (1983) 21: 180-192.

62. David H. Van Thiel et al., *Science* (Dec. 6, 1974) 18: 941-942.

63. Noel W. Solomons, *Prog. Clin. Biol. Res.* (1981) 67: 97-127.

63a. Charles S. Lieber in *Nutrition and Drugs*, ed. Myron Winick (New York: John Wiley & Sons, 1983) pp. 58-59.

63b. M.A. Leo, M. Sato and C.S. Lieber, *Clin. Res.* (1981) 29: 266. Cited in ref. 63a.

64. H.F.S. Huang and W.C. Hembree, *Biology of Reproduction* (1979) 21: 891-904.
65. M.R.S. Rao et al., *Biochemical and Biophysical Research Communications* (1980) 94, No. 1: 1-8.
66. Rina Singer et al., *Archives of Andrology* (1982) 8: 61-64.
67. B. Ahluwalia et al., *Federation Proceedings* (1973) 32: 947 Abs.
68. Johnathan Cohen and S. Burt Walbach, *A.M.A. Archives of Pathology* (1953) 56, no. 4: 333-340.
69. J. Cecil Smith, Jr. et al., *Science* (Sept. 7, 1983) 181: 954-955.
70. J. Cecil Smith, Jr., et al., *Jrl. of Laboratory Medicine* (1974) 84: 692-697.
70a. F.S. Messiha, *Neurobehavioral Toxicology and Teratology* (1983) 5: 233-236.
71. J. Glover, *World Rev. Nutr. Diet* (1978) 31:21.
72. Maija H. Zile and Malford E. Cullum, *Proc. of the Soc. for Experimental Biology and Medicine* 1983) 172: 139-152.
73. David E. Hatoff et al., *Gastroenterology* (1982) 82: 124-128.
74. Richard N. Podell, *Postgraduate Medicine* (Sept., 1983) 74, no. 3: 297-301.
74a. Edward Shmunes, *Archives of Dermatology* (1979) 115: 882-883. Cited by *Nutrition and the M.D.* (Oct. 1979): 4.
75. J.W. Millen and D.H.M. Woolam, *Nature* (Oct. 4, 1958) 182: 940.
75a. Myron J. Adams, Jr., *New England Jrl. of Medicine* (Sept. 27, 1984) 311, no. 13: 860.
76. *CRC Handbook Series in Nutrition and Food,* section E, vol. 1, ed. Miloslav Rechcigl (Cleveland, Ohio: CRC Press, 1978) p. 74.
77. Maria Anna Leo et al., *Gastroenterology* (1982) 82: 194-205.
77a. *Nutrition Reviews* (1983) 41, no. 7: 224-226.
78. Gary L. Peck, *Arch. Dermatol.* (March, 1980) 116: 283-284.
78a. G. Rettura et al., *Jrl. of the American College of Nutrition* (1984) 3, no. 3: 291-292 (abstract no. 162).
79. Eric W. Martin, *Hazards of Medication* (Philadelphia: J.B. Lippincott Co., 1971).
79a. Frances Talaska Fischbach, *A Manual of Laboratory Diagnostic Tests,* 2nd ed. (Philadelphia: J.B. Lippincott Co., 1984).
80. Philip. d. Hansten, *Drug Interactions* (Philadelphia: Lea & Febiger, 1979) p. 506.
81. L. Ovesen, *Drugs* (1979) 18: 278-298.
81a. Richard Harkness, *Drug Interactions Handbook* (Englewood Cliffs, N.J.: Prentice Hall, 1984) p. 20.
81aa. Ekkehard Kemmann et al., *JAMA* (1983) 249, no. 7: 926-929.
81ab. D.V. Vakil et al., *Nutrition Research* (1985) 5: 911-917.
81ac. Peter Reich et al., *New England Jrl. of Medicine* (1960) 262, no. 6: 263-269.
81b. S.R. Ames, *Amer. Jrl. of Clinical Nutrition* (1969) 22: 934-935.
81c. Walter C. Willett et al., *Amer. Jrl. of Clinical Nutrition* (Oct., 1983) 38: 559-566.
81d. M. Frigg and J. Broz, *International Jrl. for Vitamin and Nutrition Research* (1984) 54: 125-134.
81e. Samuel Ayers, Jr., *Dermatology* (Nov., 1983) 22, no. 9: 548-549.
81f. Samuel Ayers, Jr. et al., *Cutis* (1979) 23: 600-603, 689-690.
82. J.M. Lewis et al., *Jrl. of Pediatrics* (1947) 31: 496-508.
83. Warren J. Warwick et al., *Clinical Pediatrics* (1976) 15: 807-810.
84. Daniel Hollander, *Jrl. of Laboratory and Clinical Medicine* (April 1981) 97, no. 4: 449-462.
84a. Daniel Hollander et al., *Age* (1986) 9, no. 2: 57-60.
85. William A. Farris, *JAMA* (Mar. 5, 1982) 5: 1317-1318.
86. Victor Herbert, *Amer. Jrl. of Clinical Nutrition* (1982) 36: 185-186.
86a. *Nutrition Reviews* (1982) 40, no. 9: 272-274.
86b. Jo Freudenheim et al., *Federation Proceedings* (March 5, 1984) 43, no. 4: 990, (abstract 4122).
86c. Johnnie L. Underwood and Hector F. De Luca, *Amer. Jrl. of Physiology* (1984) 246: E493-E498.

87. R. H. Wasserman et al., *Science* (1976) 194: 853-855.

87a. R.H. Wasserman et al., *Jrl. of Nutrition* (1976) 106: 457-465.

87aa. Ricardo L. Boland, *Nutrition Reviews* (Jan., 1986) 44, no. 1: 1-8.

87b. W. Farnsworth Loomis, *Science* (Aug. 4, 1967) 157: 501-506.

87c. Michael F. Holick et al., *Biochemistry* (1979) 18: 1003-1008.

87d. *Nutrition Reviews* (1979) 37, no. 6: 203-205.

87e. M.F. Holick et al., *Science* (1980) 210: 203-205.

87f. M.F. Holick et al., *Science* (1981) 211: 590-593.

88. *Nutrition Reviews* (1984) 42, no. 10: 341-343.

88a. M.S. Cohen and T. K Gray, *Proc. of the National Academy of Sciences* (1984) 81: 931-934.

88b. M.S. Cohen and T.K. Gray, *Annals of Internal Medicine* (1984) 100, no. 4: 611-612.

88ba. Homer S. Black and Wan-bang Lo, *Nature* (1971) 234: 306-308.

88bb. Homer S. Black and David R. Douglas, *Cancer Research* (1973) 33: 2094-2096.

88bc. Homer S. Black and Jarvis T. Chan, *Jrl. of Investigative Dermatology* (1975) 65: 412-414.

88c. Egil Haug et al., *Molecular and Cellular Endocrinology* (1982) 28: 65-79.

89. Gershon W. Hepner et al., *Digestive Diseases* (1976) 21: 527-532.

89a. Michael R. Wills and John Savory, *Annals of Clinical and Laboratory Science* (1984) 14, no. 3: 189-197.

89b. David R. Fraser in *Vitamins in Medicine,* vol. 1, ed. Brian M. Barker and David A. Bender (London: William Heinemann Medical Books Ltd., 1980) p. 81.

90. Norman H. Bell et al., *Jrl. of Clinical Investigation* (Oct., 1984) 74, no. 4: 1540-1541.

90a. Russell T. Turner et al., *Biochemistry* (1983) 22: 1073-1076.

90b. N.A. Breslau et al., *Annals of Internal Medicine* (1984) 100: 1-7.

90c. Stavos C. Manolagas and Leonard J. Deftos, *Annals of Internal Medicine* (1984) 100: 144-146.

90ca. M. Davies et al., *Lancet* (May 25, 1985): 1186-1188.

90d. Rebecca S. Mason et al., *Annals of Internal Medicine* (1984) 100: 59-61.

90e. Joseph Zimmerman et al., *Annals of Internal Medicine* (1983) 98, no. 3: 338.

90f. R.C. Brown et al., *Lancet* (July 7, 1984): 37.

90g. G.L. Barbour et al., *New England Jrl. of Medicine* (1981) 305: 440-443. Cited by ref. 90h.

90h. Jacob Lehmann, Jr. and Richard W. Gray, *New England Jrl. of Medicine* (Oct. 25, 1984) 311, no. 17: 1115-1117.

90i. T.L. Frankel et al., *Jrl. of Clinical Endocrinology and Metabolism* (1983) 57: 627-631.

91. D.E.M. Lawson and M. Davie, *Vitamins and Hormones* (1979) 37: 1-67.

91a. K.S. Tsai et al., *Clinical Research* (1984) 32: 411A.

91b. B. Riis et al., *Acta Vitaminol. Enzymol.* (1984) 6, no. 2: 77-82.

92. R. Bouillon and H. Van Baelen, *Calcified Tissue International* (1981) 33: 451-453.

93. John G. Haddad, Jr. in *Advances in Nutritional Research* (1982) 4: 35-38.

94. V.M. Duncombe and J. Reeve, *Clinics in Gastroenterology* (1981) 10: 653-670.

94a. John Cunningham and Louis V. Avioli, *Advances in Experimental Medicine and Biology* (1982) 151: 333-339.

94b. Anthony W. Norman et al., *Endocrine Reviews* (1982) 3, no. 4: 331-366.

94ba. D.F. Guillard-Cumming et al., *Clinical Endocrinology* (1985) 22: 559-566.

94c. Stephen J. Marx et al., *Vitamins and Hormones* (1983) 40: 235-308 at 253.

94d. A.W. Norman et al., *Science* (1980) 209: 823, cited by ref. 94b.

95. Hector F. DeLuca and Heinrich K. Schnoes, *Ann. Rev. Biochem.* (1983) 52: 411-439.

96. Russell W. Chesney, *Clinical Orthopaedics and Related Research* (1981) 161: 285-314.

96a. L. Tjellesen et al., *Calcified Tissue International* (1984) 36, supp. 2: S45 (item 157).

97. S.W. Stanbury, *Proc. Nutrition Society* (1981) 40: 179-186.

97a. A.M. Parfitt et al., *Jrl. of Clinical Investigation* (1984) 73: 576-586.

97b. W.G. Goodman et al., *Calcified Tissue International* (1984) 36: 206-213.

97c. Y. Meller et al., *Clinical Orthopaedics and Related Research* (1984) 183: 238-245.
97d. Louis V. Avioli and John G. Haddad,*New England Jrl. of Medicine* (1984) 311, no. 1: 47-49.
97e. Anthony B. Hodsman et al.,*American Jrl. of Medicine* (1983) 74: 407-414.
97f. H.L. Henry and A.W. Norman, *Science* (1978) 201: 835-837. Cited by Stephen J. Marx et al., *Vitamins and Hormones* (1983) 40: 235-308.
97g. David R. Fraser, in *Vitamins in Medicine,* vol. 1, 4th ed., ed. by Brian Barker and David A. Bender, (London: William Heinemann Medical Books, 1980) pp. 52-54. This is a more recent edition of the famous book of the same title by Franklin Bicknell and F. Prescott.
97h. Bernard P. Halloran and Hector F. DeLuca, *Archives of Biochemistry and Biophysics* (1981) 208, no. 2: 477-486.
98. A. Michael Parfitt et al., *Amer. Jrl. of Clinical Nutrition* (1982) 36: 1014-1031.
99. William F. C. Rigby et al., *Jrl. of Clinical Investigation* (Oct., 1984) 74, no. 4: 1451-1455.
99a. Jacques M. Lemire et al., *Jrl. of Clinical Investigation* (Aug., 1984) 74, no. 2: 657-661.
100. A.M. Reed et al., cited in *The Vitamins in Medicine* by Franklin Bicknell and Frederick Prescott (Milwaukee, Wisc.: Lee Foundation for Nutritional Research, 1962) p. 533.
101. Adelle Davis, *Let's Get Well* (New York: Harcourt, Brace World, 1965) pp. 305-306.
102. J.C. Gallagher et al.,*Clinical Research* (1979) 27: 366A.
102a. R.R. Ghose and D. Wynford-Thomas, *Postgraduate Medical Journal* (1980) 56: 785-786.
102b. David M. Slovik et al.,*New England Jrl. of Medicine* (1981) 305, no. 7: 372-374.
103. J.C. Gallagher et al., *Proc. of the National Academy of Sciences* (1982) 79: 3325-3329.
103a. Cedric Garland et al.,*Lancet* (Feb. 9, 1985): 307-309.
103b. Chisato Miyaura et al.,*Biochemical and Biophysical Research Communications* (1981) 102, no. 3: 937-943.
103c. Yoskio Honma et al., *Proceedings of the National Academy of Sciences* (1983) 80: 201-204.
103d. M.R. Haussler et al., *Calcified Tissue International* (1983) 35: 694.
103e. R.J. Majeska and G.A. Rodan, *Jrl. Biological Chemistry* (1982) 257: 3362-3365, cited by Stephen J. Marx et al., *Vitamins and Hormones* (1983) 40: 253-308.
103f. Robert U. Simpson et al., *Federation Proceedings* (March 1, 1984) 43, no. 3: 468 (abstract no. 1177).
103g. H.C. Freake et al., *Cancer Research* (1984) 44: 3627-3631.
103h. K. Colston et al.,*Endocrinology* (1981) 108: 1083. Cited in ref. 103i.
103i. Richard F. Wagner et al., *International Jrl. of Dermatology* (1984) 23, no. 7: 453-457 at 454.
103j. R.J. Frampton et al., *Cancer Research* (1983) 43: 4443. Cited in ref. 103i.
103k. J.A. Eisman et al., in *Modulation and Mediation of Cancer by Vitamins,* ed. F.C. Meyskens and K.N. Prasad (Basel, Switzerland: Karger, 1983) pp. 282-286.
104. Mark R. Haussler, *JAMA* (Feb. 12, 1982) 247: 841-844.
105. H.F. DeLuca, *Clinical Biochemistry* (1981) 14, no. 5: 213-222.
106. J.A. Kanis, *Jrl. of Bone and Joint Surgery* (1982) 64B: 542-560.
107. H.F. DeLuca, *Nutrition Reviews* (1980) 38: 169-182.
107a. Yoko Tanaka et al., *Proc. National Academy of Sciences* (1980) 77, no. 11: 6411-6414.
107b. Norio Ohnuma and Anthony W. Norman,*Archives of Biochemistry and Biophysics* (1982) 213, no. 1: 139-147.
107c. Helen L. Henry and Anthony W. Norman, *Annual Review of Nutrition* (1984) 4: 493-520 at 499.
108. Hector F. DeLuca, *Harvey Lectures* (1980) 75: 333-379.
108a. Hector F. DeLuca,·U.S. Patent no. 4, 217,288 (Aug. 12, 1980).
109. M.F. Holick and J. MacLaughlin, *Age* (1981) 4: 140.

110. M. F. Baker et al., *Age and Ageing* (1980) 9: 249-252.
110a. J.R. Bullamore et al., *Lancet* (Sept. 12, 1970) 2: 535-537.
110b. D.V. Havlir et al., *Calcified Tissue International* (1983) 35: 695.
110c. J.C. Gallagher et al., *Clinical Research* (1978) 25: 415A, cited by J.C. Gallagher et al., *Jrl. of Clinical Investigation* (1979) 69, 729-736.
110d. M. Davie and D.E.M. Lawson, *Clinical Science* (1980) 58: 235-242.
111. D.E.M. Lawson et al., *British Medical Jrl.* (Aug. 4, 1979): 303-305.
112. R.M. Neer et al., *Nature* (1971) 279: 255-257.
113. M.S. Devgun et al., *Age and Ageing* (1980) 9: 117-120.
114. John L. Omdahl et al., *Amer. Jrl. of Clinical Nutrition* (1982) 36: 1225-1233.
115. *American Jrl. of Clinical Nutrition* (1983) 38: 335-339.
115a. Daniel Hollander and Hella Tarnawski, *Jrl. Lab. Clin. Med.* (1984) 103: 462-469.
115b. Claus Christiansen and Paul Rodbro, *Calcified Tissue International* (1984) 36: 19-24.
115c. J. Lemann et al., *Calcified Tissue International* (1984) 36: 139-144.
115d. B.E. Christopher Nordin et al., *American Jrl. of Clinical Nutrition* (Sept. 1985) 42: 470-474.
116. David R. Fraser, *Lancet* (April 30, 1983): 969-972.
117. Rajiv Kumar et al., *Digestive Disease and Sciences* (1981): 242-246.
117a. Howard M. Saal et al., *Clinical Pediatrics* (1985) 24: 452. Cited by Alexander Grant, *Healthwise* (Oct., 1985) 8, no. 10: 1.
118. Elmer M. Nelson, *JAMA* (1959) 171, no. 8: 1103.
119. Tetsuya Takahashi and R. Yamamoto, *Yakugaku Zasshi* (1969) 89: 903-913.
119a. Joseph A. Johnston, *Amer. Jrl. of Diseases of Children* (1944) 67: 265-274.
120. A. Michael Parfitt et al., *Amer. Jrl. of Clinical Nutrition* (1982) 36: 1014-1031.
121. *Recommended Dietary Allowances* , 9th ed. (Washington, D.C.: National Academy of Sciences, 1980).
122. K.R. Johnson et al., *Age and Ageing* (1980) 9: 121-127 as cited in ref. 120 above.
123. Fred A. Kummerow, *Amer. Jrl. of Clinical Nutrition* (1979) 32: 58-83.
123a. Ross P. Holmes and Fred A. Kummerow, *Jrl. of the Amer. College of Nutrition* (1983) 2: 173-199.
123b. R. Bouillon, *Jrl. of Steroid Biochemistry* (1983) 19, no. 1: 921-927.
123c. Iris Robertson et al., *British Jrl. of Nutrition* (1981) 45: 17-22.
123d. Paul J. Drinka and Wolfram E. Nolten, *Jrl. of the American Geriatrics Society* (1984) 32, no. 5: 400-407.
124. Peng Shi-Kaung et al., *Pario Arterielle* (1978) 4, no. 4: 229-243.
125. E.G. Knox, *Lancet* (June 30, 1973): 1465-1467.
125a. Robert F. Light et al., *Jrl. of Biological Chemistry* (1931) 92: 47-51.
126. Sharon Monahan Miller, *Amer. Jrl. of Medical Technology* (1983) 49: 27-37.
127. J.A. Karis, *Jrl.. of Bone and Joint Surgery* (1982) 6B: 542-560.
128. G. Finn Jensen et al., *Clinical Endocrinology* (1982) 16: 515-524.
128a. R. Neer et al., *Jrl. of the Amer. College of Nutrition* (1982) 1: 105.
128b. K.S. Tsai et al., *Jrl. of Clinical Investigation* (June 1984) 73, no. 6: 1668-1672.
128c. J. Reeve et al., *Acta Endocrinologica* (1982) 101: 636-640.
129. Zalman S. Agus et al., *Amer. Jrl. of Medicine* (1982) 72: 473-487.
130. Edward J. Calabrese, *Nutrition and Environmental Health,* vol. 1 (New York: Wiley Interscience, 1980).
131. Solomon Garb, *Laboratory Tests in Common Use* (New York: Springer, 1976).
131a. Carla Bazzani et al., *Life Sciences* (1984) 34: 461-466.
132. Roman J. Kutsky, *Handbook of Vitamins, Minerals and Hormones* (New York: Van Nostrand Reinhold, 1981) p. 213.
132a. Daphne A. Roe, *Nutrition Reviews* (April, 1984) 42, no. 4: 141-154.
132b. Marielle Gascon-Barre et al., *Jrl. of the Amer. College of Nutrition* (1984) 3: 45-50.
133. H.O. Bang et al., *Amer. Jrl. of Clinical Nutrition* (1980) 33: 2657-2662.
133a. C.R.M. Hay et al., *Lancet* (June 5, 1982): 1269-1272.

133b. *Nutrition Reviews* (May, 1982) 40: 151-159.
133c. J. Dyerberg et al., *Prostaglandins* (1981) 22, no. 6: 857-862.
133d. S. Fischer and P.C. Weber, *Nature* (1984) 307: 165-168.
133e. K.L. Black et al., *Prostaglandins* (1984) 28, no. 4: 545-556.
133f. N.A. Begent et al., *Jrl. of Physiology* (1984) 349: 69P. Cited in *Nutrition Abstracts and Reviews* Series A (October, 1984) 54, no. 10: 886 (abstract no. 6244).
133g. P. Needleman et al., *Science* (1976): 163-165. Cited in ref. 133m.
133h. P. Needleman et al., *Proceedings of the National Academy of Sciences* (1979) 76: 944-948. Cited in ref. 133m.
133i. R.J. Gryglewski et al., *Prostaglandins* (1979) 18: 453-478. Cited in ref. 133m.
133j. J. Dyerberg et al., *Lancet* (1978) 2: 117-119. Cited in ref. 133m.
133k. E.G. Nidy et al., *Tetrahedron Letters* (1978) 27: 2375-2378. Cited in ref. 133m.
133m. Sven Fischer and Peter C. Weber, *Nature* (1984) 307: 165-168.
133n. Terano Takashi et al., *Prostaglandins* (Nov. 1984) 28, no. 5: 668.
134. William S. Harris and William E. Connor, *Transactions Assn. of Amer. Physicians* (1980) 43: 148-155.
134a. Denham Harman, *Jrl. of the Amer. College of Nutrition* (1982) 1: 27-34.
134b. William S. Harris et al., *Metabolism* (1983) 32, no. 2: 179-184.
134c. T.A.B. Sanders et al., *Clinical Science* (1981) 61: 317-324.
134d. R. Saynor et al., *Atherosclerosis* (1984) 50: 3-10. Cited in ref. 134e.
134e. R. Saynor, *Lancet* (Sept. 22, 1984): 696-697.
134f. Bonnie H. Weiner, *New England Jrl. of Medicine* (Oct. 2, 1986) 315, no. 14: 841-846.
135. D.B. Jones and T.M.E. Davies, *Lancet* (July 24, 1982): 221.
135a. C.R.M. Hay, A.P. Durber and R. Saynor, *Lancet* (1982) 1: 1269-1277. Cited in ref. 135ab.
135ab. R. Saynor and D. Verel, *Lancet* (June 11, 1983): 1335.
135ac. G. Hornstra et al., *Lancet* (Nov. 17, 1979): 1080.
135b. H.M. Sinclair, *Progress in Lipid Research* (1981) 20: 897-899.
136. *Nutrition Reviews* (1984) 42, no. 5: 189-191.
136a. Jorn Dyerberg and Kaj Anker Jorgensen, *Progress in Lipid Research* (1982) 21: 255-269.
136b. Rudi Scherhag et al., *Prostaglandins* (1982) 23, no. 3: 369-383.
136c. Reinhard Lorenz et al., *Circulation* (1983) 67, no. 3: 504-510.
136d. J.Z. Mortensen et al., *Thrombosis and Haemostasis* (1983) 50, no. 2: 543-546.
136da. Heinz Juan and Wolfgang Sametz, *Prostaglandins, Leukotrienes and Medicine* (1985) 19: 79-86.
136e. Paul J. Nestel et al., *Jrl. of Clinical Investigation* (1984) 74, no. 1: 82-89.
136f. B.E. Woodcock et al., *British Medical Jrl.* (Feb.25, 1985) 288: 592-594.
136g. P. Singer et al., *Experientia* (1985) 41: 462-464.
136h. Peter Singer et al., *Atherosclerosis* (1985) 56: 111-118.
136i. Dwight R. Robinson et al., *Prostaglandins* (1985) 30, no. 1: 51-75.
137. Erik Agduhr and Nils Stenström, *The Appearance of the Electrocardiogram in Heart Lesions Produced by Cod-Liver Oil.* (Uppsala, Sweden: Almquist and Wiksells Boktryckeri, 1930).
138. K.L. Blaxter et al., *British Jrl. of Nutrition* (1953) 7: 287-298.
138a. C.G. MacKenzie et al., *Science* (Aug. 29, 1941) 94: 216-217.
138b. Simin N. Meydani et al., *New England Jrl. of Medicine* (Sept. 26, 1985) 313, no. 13: 822.
139. Yoshiki Kobatake et al., *Jrl. of Nutritional Science and Vitaminology* (1984) 30: 357-372.
139a. Denham Harman, *Age* (Oct., 1984) 7: 111-131.
139b. F. Sundholm and A. Visapaa, *Lipids* (1978) 13, no. 11: 755-757.
140. F. Peckel Möller, *Cod Liver Oil Chemistry* (London: Peter Möller Co., 1895).
141. G.R. Mizuno et al., *Jrl. of Agricultural and Food Chemistry* (May-June, 1966).

141a. Rashida A. Karmali et al., *Jrl. of the National Cancer Institute* (1984) 73, no. 2: 453-461.

141b. Vicki E. Kelley et al., *Jrl. of Immunology* (1985) 134, no. 3: 1914-1919.

141c. Richard N. Podell, *Postgraduate Medicine* (1985) 77, no. 7: 65-72.

141ca. R.A. Gibson, *Proc. of the Nutrition Society of Australia* (1985) 10: 181. Cited in *Nutrition Abstracts and Reviews, Series A* (1986) 56, no. 10: 732.

141d. N. Chetty and B.A. Bradlow, *Thrombosis Research* (1983) 30, 619-624.

141da. Tibor Zemplengi in *Frontiers in Longevity Research,* ed. Robert J. Morin (Springfield, Il., Charles Thomas, 1985) p. 40.

141e. James J. Corrigan, in *Advances in Pediatrics* , vol. 28, ed. Lewis A. Barness (Chicago: Year Book Medical Publishers, 1981) pp. 57-74.

141f. Robert E. Olson in *Modern Nutrition in Health and Disease,* 5th ed., ed. Robert S. Goodhart and Maurice E. Shils (Philadelphia: Lea & Febiger, 1973) p. 17.

142. Geoffrey J. Blackwell et al., *Thrombosis Research* (1985) 37: 103-114.

142a. V. Egilsson, *Lancet* (July 30, 1977): 245-255.

142b. P. Hilgard, *Lancet* (Aug. 20, 1977): 403.

142c. P. Hilgard, *British Jrl. of Cancer* (1977) 35: 891-892.

142d. Kedar N. Prasad et al., *Life Sciences* (1981) 29: 1387-1392.

143. R.T. Chlebowski et al., in *Modulation and Medication of Cancer by Vitamins,* ed. F.L. Meyskens and K.N. Prasad (Basel, Switzerland: Karger, 1983) pp. 276-281.

143a. Rowan T. Chlebowski et al., *Cancer Treatment Reviews* (1985) 12: 49-63.

144. A.C. Casey and E.G. Bliznakov, *Chem. Biol. Interactions* (1972) 5: 1-12.

145. John I. Gallin et al., *Jrl. of Immunology* (1982) 128: 1399-1408.

146. R.L. Merkel, *Amer. Jrl. of Obstetrics and Gynecology* (1952) 64: 416. Cited in ref. 148.

147. Jonathan V. Wright, *Amer. Jrl. of Obstetrics and Gynecology* (1984) 149, no. 1: 107.

147a. M. René Malinow et al., *Science* (April 23, 1982) 216: 415-417.

147b. Marie M. Cassidy et al., *Amer. Jrl. of Clinical Nutrition* (1981) 34: 218-228.

148. James O. Woolliscroft, *DM—Disease-A-Month* (1983) 29, no. 5: 46.

148a. Robert E. Olson, *Annual Review of Nutrition* (1984) 4: 281-337 at 320-321.

149. *Health and Longevity Report* (April 15, 1984) 2, no. 8: 3.

150. J.W. Cook et al., *British Medical Bulletin* (1958) 14, no. 2: 132-135.

151. Hans Olaf Bang and Jorn Dyerberg in *Advances in Nutritional Research,* vol. 3 (New York: Plenum Press, 1980) pp. 1-22 at 17-18.

152. M.C. Ehrström, *Acta Medica Scandinavica* (1951) 140: 416. Cited by Claudio Galli in *Advances in Nutrition Research,* vol. 3 (New York: Plenum Press, 1980) pp. 95-126, at 106.

153. N. Kromann and A. Green, *Acta Med. Scand.* (1980) 208: 401-406. Cited by Howard R. Knapp and Garret A. FitzGerald, *New England Jrl. of Medicine* (Oct. 2, 1986) 315, no. 14: 892-893.

154. George L. Royer et al., *American Jrl. of Medicine* (July 13, 1984): 25-34.

Chapter 5—502 References

1. H.E. Sauberlich, *Annals of the N.Y. Academy of Sciences* (1980) 355: 80-97.
2. H. Baker and O. Frank, *Jrl. of Applied Nutrition* (Spring, 1981).
3. Herman Baker et al. *Cancer* (1981) 47: 2883-2886.
4. Eric W. Martin, *Hazards of Medication* (Philadelphia: J.B. Lippincott Co., 1981) p. 255.
4a. Harold H. Sandstead in *Modern Nutrition in Health and Disease*, 5th ed., ed. Robert S. Goodhart and Maurice E. Shils (Philadelphia: Lea and Febiger, 1973) pp. 593-596.
4b. C.R. Scriver, *Jrl. of Inherited Metabolic Disease* (1985) 8, supp. 1: 2-7.
5. R. Prasad et al., *Ann. Nutr. Metab.* (1982) 26: 324-330.
5a. P. Szüts et al., *Lancet* (May 12, 1984): 1072-1073.
5b. M. Duran and S.K. Wadman, *Jrl. of Inherited Metabolic Disease* (1985) 8, supp. 1: 70-75.
6. Ruth Flinn Harrell, *Effect of Added Thiamin On Learning* (New York: AMS Press, Inc., 1973). Reprint of 1943 edition.
6a. Ruth Flinn Harrell et al., *Metabolism—Clinical & Experimental* (1956) 5: 552-562.
6b. Ruth F. Harrell et al., *Proc. National Academy of Sciences* (1981) 78, no. 1: 574-578.
6c. George Ellman et al., *Amer. Jrl. of Mental Deficiency* (1984) 88, no. 6: 668-691.
6d. Caislin Weathers, *Amer. Jrl. of Mental Deficiency* (1983) 88, no. 2: 214-217.
6e. Forrest C. Bennett et al., *Pediatrics* (1983) 72, no. 5: 707-713.
7. Jay Chanowitz et al., *American Jrl. of Mental Deficiency* (1985) 90, no.2: 217-219.
7a. *Nutrition Reviews* (Oct., 1982) 40, no. 10: 316-318.
7b. Edward R. Asregadoo, *Annals of Ophthalmology* (1979) 11: 1095-1100.
7c. Donald J. Connor, *Biological Psychiatry* (1981) 16, no. 9: 869-872.
7d. O. Michelsen et al., in *Modern Nutrition in Health and Disease*, ed. Robert S. Goodhart and Maurice E. Shils (Philadelphia: Lea & Febiger, 1973) pp. 413-433 at 422.
7e. Gary D. Tollefson, *Jrl. of Clinical Psychiatry* 1983) 44: 280-288.
7f. A. Theron et al., *Clinical and Experimental Immunology* (1981) 44: 295-303.
8. Walter G. Strauss et al., *Amer. Jrl. of Tropical Medicine and Hygiene* (1968) 17, no. 3: 161-164.
8a. Derrick Lonsdale and Raymond J. Shamberger, *Amer. Jrl. of Clinical Nutrition* (1980) 33: 205-211.
9. Irvin E. Liener in *Toxic Constituents of Plant Foodstuffs*, ed. Irvin E. Liener (New York: Academic Press, 1980) p. 445.
9a. Pintip Ruenwongsa and Supakorn Pattanavibag,*Life Sciences* 34: 365-370.
9b. F. Tencconi et al., *Bollettino Chimico Farmaceutico* (1983) 122, no. 1: 27-44
9c. K.C. Hayes and D. Mark Hegsted in *Toxicants Occurring Naturally in Foods*, 2nd ed., Frank M. Strong, Chairman Subcommittee on Naturally Occurring Toxicants in Foods (Washington, D.C.: National Academy of Sciences, 1973) p. 247.
9d. R.C. Rose, *Jrl. of Inherited Metabolic Disease* (1985) 8, supp. 1: 13-16.
10. M.W.J. Older and J.W.T. Dickerson,*Age and Ageing* (1982) 11: 101-107.
11. Y. Itokawa in *CRC Handbook Series in Nutrition and Food, Section E, Vol. 1*, ed. Miloslav Rechcigl (Cleveland, Ohio: CRC Press, 1978) p. 3.
12. Donald J. Connor, cited by James O. Woolliscroft, *DM—Disease-a-Month* (1983) 29, no. 5: 23.
13. Joseph R. DiPalma and David M. Ritchie, *Annual Review of Pharmacol. Toxicol.* (1977) 17: 133-148.
14. Yoshinori Itokawa et al.,*Metabolism* (1972) 21, no. 5: 375-379.
15. Roman J. Kutsky, *Handbook of Vitamins, Minerals and Hormones* (New York: Van Nostrand Reinhold, 1981) p. 44.
15a. Leo H. Criep, *Allergy and Clinical Immunology* (New York: Grune & Stratton, 1976) p. 516.

15b. R.E. Davis et al., *New England Jrl. of Medicine* (1980) 303: 462. Cited by Richard E. Davis and Graham C. Icke in *Advances in Clinical Chemistry* (1984) 23: 93-140.

16. M. Soukop and K.C. Calman, *British Jrl. of Cancer* (1978) 38: 180.

16a. M.K. Horwitt in *Modern Nutrition in Health and Disease,* 5th ed., ed. Robert S. Goodhart and Maurice S. Shils (Philadelphia: Lea & Febiger, 1973) pp. 191-197.

17. S.K. Srivastava and E. Beutler,*Experientia* (1970) 26: 250.

18. Harold W. Skalka and Joseph T. Prchal, *Amer. Jrl. of Clinical Nutrition* (1981) 34: 861-863.

19. Shambhu D. Varma et al., *Proc. National Academy of Sciences* (1979) 76: 3504-3506.

20. M. Atkinson, cited in *The Vitamins in Medicine,* 3rd ed. by Franklin Bicknell and Frederick Prescott (Milwaukee, Wisc.: Lee Foundation for Nutritional Research, 1962).

21. G.V. Reddy et al., *Jrl. of the National Cancer Institute* (1973) 50: 815-817.

22. F.J. Lemonier et al., *Jrl. of the National Cancer Institute* (1975) 1085-1089.

23. Richard S. Rivlin, *New England Jrl. of Medicine* (1970) 283: 463-472.

24. M. Lane and F.E. Smith, *Proc. Amer. Assn. Cancer Research* (1971) 12: 85A.

25. Richard S. Rivlin, *Cancer Research* (1973) 33: 1977-1986.

25a. N. Pelliccione et al., *Clinical Research* (1983) 31: 621A, cited by Richard S. Rivlin et al., *American Jrl. of Medicine* (1983) 75: 843-854.

25b. Amy Z. Belko et al., *Amer. Jrl. of Clinical Nutrition* (1983) 37: 509-517.

26. Ernest Beutler, *Science* (Aug. 9, 1969) 165: 613-615.

27. Solomon Garb, *Laboratory Tests in Common Use* (New York: Springer, 1976).

27a. Frances Talaska Fishbach,*A Manual of Laboratory Diagnositc Tests* (Philadelphia: J.B. Lippincott Co., 1984).

27b. *Merck* Index, 10th ed., (Rahway, N.J.: Merck, 1983): 1184.

27c. N.E. Bateman and D.A. Uccellini, *Jrl. Pharm. Pharmacol.* (1984) 36: 461-464.

27d. M.K. Horwitt in *Modern Nutrition on Health and Disease,* op. cit. (ref. 16b) pp. 198-202.

27e. William M. Petrie and Thomas A. Ban,*Drugs* (1985) 30: 58-65.

28. Anders G. Olsson et al., *Lancet* (Sept. 3, 1983): 565-566.

29. N. Svedmyr et al., *Acta Pharmacol et Toxicol.* (1977) 41: 397-400.

30. Jonathan K. Wilkin et al.,*Clin. Pharmacol. Ther.* (1982) 31: 478-482.

30a. Richard A. Kunin,*Jrl. of Orthomolecular Psychiatry* (1976) 5, no. 2: 89-100.

30b. Brita Eklund et al., *Prostaglandins* (1979) 17: 821-830.

31. Gunnar Aberg and Nils Svedmyr,*Arneimittel Forschung* (1971) 21: 795-796.

32. T.A. Ban, *Canadian Psychiatric Assn. Jrl.* (1971) 16: 413-431.

33. George Serban, *Nutrition and Mental Functions* (New York: Plenum Press, 1975) pp. 245-270.

34. A. Moncrieff, *Lancet* (1942) 1: 633.

35. The Coronary Drug Project Research Group,*JAMA* (Jan. 27, 1975) 231, no. 4: 360-381.

35a. M.F. Oliver et al.,*British Heart Jrl.* (1978) 40: 1069-1118.

36. John P. Kane, et al., *New England Jrl. of Medicine* (1981) 304: 251-258.

37. J. Ferreira-Marques, cited in *The Vitamins in Medicine,* 3 ed., op. cit. (ref. 20), pp. 375-376.

38. William Kaufman, *Connecticut State Medical Jrl.* (1953) 17: 584-587.

38a. Walter B. Shelley and E. Dorinda Shelley,*Lancet* (Sept. 8, 1984): 576.

39. Robert A. Wilson, *Sex and Drugs* (Chicago: Playboy Press, 1973).

39a. W. Hotz, *Advances in Lipid Research* (1983) 20: 195-207.

40. Gay Gaer Luce, *Biological Rhythms in Psychiatry and Medicine* (Mineola, N.Y.: Dover Press, 1971).

41. Norman A. Christensen et al.,*JAMA* (1961) 177: 546-550.

42. David Hawkins in *Orthomolecular Psychiatry,* ed. David Hawkins and Linus Pauling (San Francisco: Freeman, 1973).

42a. Carl C. Pfeiffer, *Mental and Elemental Nutrients* (New Canaan, Conn.: Keats Publ., 1975) pp. 469-472.

944 The Reverse Effect

42b. Durk Pearson and Sandy Shaw, *Life Extension* (New York: Warner Books, 1982) pp. 204, 754.

42c. Durk Pearson and Sandy Shaw, *The Life Extension Companion* (New York: Warner Books, 1984) pp. 143-144.

42d. Saul Kent, *Your Personal Life-Extension Program* (New York: William Morrow and Co., 1985) pp. 190-191.

43. Hirotaka Araki et al., *The Prostate* (1983) 4: 253-264.

44. Loren R. Mosher, *Amer. Jrl. of Psychiatry* (1970) 126: 1290-1296.

45. Victor Herbert, *Jrl. of the Amer. Pharmaceutical Assn.*(Dec., 1977).

45a. James C. Woodard, *Jrl. of Nutrition* (1970) 100: 1215-1226.

45b. Leslie Alhadeff et al., *Nutrition Reviews* (1984) 42, no. 2: 33-40.

46. Morris Smithberg, *Univ. of Minnesota Medical Bulletin* (Nov., 1961) 33: 62-72.

47. R. Schoental, *Cancer* (1977) 40, no. 7: 1833-1840.

48. D.M. Shapiro et al., *Cancer Research* (1957) 17: 600-604.

48a. A.S. Truswell, *Proc. Nutr. Soc.* (1976) 35: 1-14.

48b. David A. Bender, in *Vitamins in Medicine*, vol. 1, 4th ed., ed. by Brian M. Barker and David A. Bender, (London: William Heinemann Medical Books, 1980) p. 35.

48c. K. Dakshinamurti, in *Determinants of the Availability of Nutrients to the Brain*, vol. 1 of *Nutrition and the Brain*, ed. Richard J. Wurtman and Judith L. Wurtman (New York: Raven Press, 1977) pp. 251-318, at 284.

48d. B. Shane and E.E. Snell, *Biochem, Biophys. Research Commun.* (1975) 66: 1294-1300. Cited by George P. Tryfiates et al., *Anticancer Research* (1981) 1: 263-268.

48e. A.D.G. Gunn, *Internationale Zeitschrift für Vitamin und Ernahrungs Forshung Beiheft* (1985) 27: 213-224.

48f. Carolyn D. Ritchie and Ratree Singkamani *Human Nutrition: Clinical Nutrition* (1986) 40C: 75-80.

49. Karen Schuster et al., *Human Nutrition: Clinical Nutrition* (1985) 39C: 75-79.

49a. David A. Bender and Lena Totoe, *Jrl. of Neurology* (1984) 43, no. 3: 733-736.

49b. Steven L. Ink and LaVell M. Henderson, *Annual Review of Nutrition* (1984) 4: 455-470 at 465.

49c. Yoon S. Shin et al., *Lancet* (Oct. 13, 1984): 871-872.

50. J. McKierhan et al., *Clinical Pediatrics* (1981) 20: 208-211.

51. Guy E. Abraham et al., *Jrl. of Clinical and Laboratory Science* (1981) 11: 333-336.

52. James O. Woolliscroft, *DM—Disease-a-Month* (1983) 29, no. 5: 28.

52a. A. Bankier et al., *Archives of Disease in Childhood* (1983) 58: 415-418.

52b. M. Ebadi et al., *Neuropharmacology* (1983) 22, no. 7: 865-873.

52c. Joseph R. DiPalma and David M. Ritchie, *Ann. Rev. Of Pharmacol. Toxicol.* (1977) 17: 133-148.

52ca. J.S. Kroll, *Developmental Medicine and Child Neurology* (1985) 27: 377-379.

52d. Herbert Schaumberg et al., *New England Journal of Medicine* (1983) 309: 445-448.

52e. *Nutrition Reviews* (Feb., 1984) 44-46, 49-51.

53. *Nutrition Reviews* (1976) 34: 188-189.

53a. S.C. Cunnane et al., *Jrl. of Nutrition* (1984) 114: 1754-1761.

54. Craig G. Burkhart, *Archives of Dermatology* (Aug., 1982) 118: 535.

55. M.A. Packham and S. C-T. Lam, *Lancet* (Oct. 10, 1981): 809-810.

56. U.N. Das, *Lancet* (Sept. 19, 1981): 638.

56a. *Lancet* (June 13, 1981): 1299-1300.

56b. Miriam Zahavi et al., *Life Sciences* (1984) 35: 1497-1503.

56c. K.S. McCully, *Amer. Jrl. of Pathology* (1969) 56: 11-122.

56d. Kilmer S. McCully and Robert B. Wilson, *Atherosclerosis* (1975) 22: 215-227.

56e. P.H. Proctor and J.E. McGinness, *Age* (1984) 7, no. 4. Cited by Denham Harman, *Age* (1984) 7: 111-131.

56f. Phyllis A. Cohen et al., *Jrl. of Nutrition* (Jan., 1973) 103, no. 1: 143-152.

57. Edward J. Calabrese, *Medical Hypotheses* (1984) 15: 361-367.

57a. David E. L. Wilcken et al., *New England Jrl. of Medicine* (1983) 309, no. 8: 448-453.
57b. L.A. Smolin et al., *Jrl. of Pediatrics* (1981) 99: no. 3: 467-472.
57c. Philip L. Hooper et al., *Internat. Jrl. for Vitamin and Nutrition Research* (1983) 53: 412-419.
57d. J.V. Murphy et al., *Jrl. of Inherited Metabolic Disease* (1985) 8, supp. 2: 109-110.
57e. I. Yoshida et al., *Jrl. of Inherited Metabolic Disease* (1985) 8: 91.
57f. Lars E. Brattström et al., *Metabolism* (Nov., 1985) 34, no. 11: 1073-1077.
58. G. LeLord et al., *Acta Vitaminol Enzymol.* (1982) 4, no. 1-2: 27-44.
58a. Jeffrey A. Mattes and Diane Martin, *Human Nutrition: Applied Nutrition* (1981) 36A: 131-133.
58b. A.L. Luhby et al., *American Jrl. of Clinical Nutrition* (1971) 24: 684. Cited by James L. Webb, *Jrl. of Reproductive Medicine* (1980) 25, no. 4: 150-156.
58c. Kilmer S. McCully, *Amer. Jrl. of Clinical Nutrition* (1975) 28: 542-549.
58d. G. LeLord et al., *Rev. Neurol.* (1978) 134: 797-801. Cited in ref. 58e.
58e. J. Martineau et al., *Biological Psychiatry* (1981) 16: 627-641.
58f. Kenneth L. Davis et al., *Science* (1985) 227: 1601-1602.
59. K. Folkers, cited in *Nutrition Reviews* (Jan., 1982) 40: 15-16.
59a. K. Folkers et al., *Hoppe-Seyler's Zeitschrift für Physiologische Chemie* (1984) 365, no. 3: 405-414. Cited in *Nutrition Abstracts and Reviews,* Series A (October, 1984) 54, no. 10: 873 (abstract no. 6145).
59b. V. Revuscova et al., *Casopis LeKaru Ceskych* (1982) 121, no. 6: 163-166.
59c. F. deZegher et al., *Lancet* (Aug. 17, 1985): 392-393.
60. John M. Ellis et al., *Res. Commun. in Chem. Path. and Pharm.* (1976) 13, no. 4: 743-756.
61. Karl Folkers et al., *Proc. National Academy of Sciences* (1978) 75, no. 7: 3410-3412.
62. John M. Ellis et al., *Amer. Jrl. of Clinical Nutrition* (1979) 32: 2040-2046.
63. Satoshi Shizukvishi et al., *Biochemical and Biophysical Research* (1980) 95, no. 3: 1126-1130.
64. Alan Gaby and J.V. Wright, *Amer. Family Physician* (1982) 25: 55, 58.
65. S. Pilar, *Canadian Medical Assn. Jrl.* (1983): 536.
66. John A. Kark et al., *Jrl. of Clinical Investigation* (1983) 71: 1224-1229.
66a. Clayton L. Natta and Robert D. Reynolds, *Amer. Jrl. of Clinical Nutrition* (1984) 40: 235-239.
67. G. Delitala et al., *Jrl. of Clinical Endocrinol. Metab.* (1976) 42: 603-606.
67a. A. Isidori et al., *Current Medical Research and Opinion* (1981) 7, no. 7: 475-481.
67b. Durk Pearson and Sandy Shaw, *Life Extension* op. cit. (ref. 42b) pp. 192, 229, 289-290, 477, 483, 509, 771.
68. T.J. Merimee et al., *New England Jrl. of Medicine* (1969) 280, no. 26: 1434-1438.
68a. Kikuo Kasai et al., *Acta Endocrinologica* (1980) 93: 282-286.
68b. N.J. Benevenga and R.D. Steele, *Annual Review of Nutrition* (1984) 4: 157-181.
68c. Roman J. Kutsky, *Handbook of Vitamins and Hormones* (New York: Van Nostrand Reinhold Co., 1973) p. 124.
68d. Thomas K. Koch et al., *New England Jrl. of Medicine* (Sept. 19, 1985) 313, no. 12: 731-733.
68e. Clarence J. Gibbs et al., *New England Jrl. of Medicine* (Sept. 19, 1985) 313, no. 12: 734-738.
68f. *FDA Consumer* (July-August, 1985): 5.
68g. Gina Kolata, *Science* (October 3, 1986) 22-24.
68h. William Regelson, *Science* (Jan. 2, 1987) 235: 14-15.
68i. Mitchell E. Geffner et al., *Lancet* (Feb. 15, 1986): 343-347.
69. G. Delitala et al., *Jrl. of Clinical Endocrinol. Metab.* 1977) 45: 1019-1022.
70. Constanzo Morietti et al., *New England Jrl. of Medicine* (Aug. 12, 1982) 307: 444.
71. T. Tolis et al., *Jrl. of Clinical Endocrinology and Metabolism* (1979) 44: 1197-1199.
72. John H. Richardson and Marsha Chenman, *Jrl. of Sports Medicine* (1981) 21: 119-120.

73. Guy E. Abraham et al., *Annals of Clinical and Laboratory Science* (1981) 11: 333-336.
73a. C.M. Lee and J.E. Leklem, *Annals of Clinical and Laboratory Science* (1984) 14, no. 1: 151-154.
74. R. Prasad et al., *Ann. Nutr. Metab.* (1982) 26: 324-330.
75. Fred Rosen et al., *Vitamins and Hormones* (1964) 22: 609-641, at 610.
75a. M.L. Littman et al., *Proceedings of the Society for Experimental Biology and Medicine* (1963) 113: 667-674.
76. H.G. Petering et al., *Cancer Research* (1964) 24: 367-372.
77. W. Korytnyk and P.G.G. Potti, *Jrl. of Medicinal Chemistry* (1977) 20, no. 4: 567-572.
78. George P. Tryfiates et al., *Jrl. of Nutrition* (1978) 108: 417-420.
79. Dennis M. DiSorbo and Gerald Litwack, *Nutrition and Cancer* (1982) 3, no. 4: 216-222.
79a. Dennis M. DiSorbo and Larry Nathanson, *Nutrition and Cancer* (1983) 5, no. 1: 10-15.
79aa. Dennis M. DiSorbo, Richard Wagner, Jr. and Larry Nathanson, *Nutrition and Cancer* (1985) 7, nos. 1 and 2: 43-52.
79b. J. Dozi-Vassiliades et al., *Mutation Research* (1983) 124: 175-178.
79c. Larry Nathanson in *Medical World News* (1985) 26, no. 3: 174.
80. *Drug Interaction Index,* ed. Ben R. Gant and Thomas D. Gant (Vancouver B.C., Canada: Meditec Publ., 1973) p. D-11.
81. D. Scaglione and A. Vecchione, *Acta Vitaminol. Enzymol.* (1982) 4, no. 3: 207-214.
82. G. Tolis et al., *Jrl. of Clinical Endocrinology and Metabolism* (1977) 44: 1197-1199.
83. Fumio Shimura et al., *Jrl. of Nutritional Science and Vitaminology* (1983) 29: 533-544.
84. Edward J. Calabrese, *Nutrition and Environmental Health,* vol. 1 (New York: Wiley Interscience, 1980).
85. Victor Herbert, *Jrl. of the Amer. Pharmaceutical Assn.* (Dec., 1977) NS17, no. 12: 764-766.
86. Irwin E. Liener, *Toxic Constituents of Plant Foodstuffs,* 2nd ed., (New York: Academy Press, 1980) p. 447.
87. Henry M. Middleton III et al., *Amer. Jrl. of Clinical Nutrition* (1984) 39: 54-61.
87a. M.G. Brush and Marta Perry, *Lancet* (June 15, 1985): 1399.
88. R. Bieganowski and W. Friedrich, *FEBS Letters* (1979) 97: 325-326.
88a. Bernd Elsenhans and Irwin H. Rosenberg, *Biochemistry* (1984) 23: 805-808.
89. David M. Greenberg, *Western Jrl. of Medicine* (April, 1975) 122: 345-348.
89a. J.C. Linnell and D. M. Mathews, *Clinical Science* (1984) 66: 113-121.
89b. I. Chanarin, in *Vitamins in Medicine,* vol. 1, 4th ed., ed. by Brian M. Barker and David Bender, (London: William Heinemann Medical Books, 1980) p. 176.
89c. Dwight Landis Evans et al., *Amer. Jrl. of Psychiatry* (1983) 140: 218-221.
89d. H. Baker et al., *Jrl. of Neuroscience Research* (1984) 11: 419-435.
90. Martin G. Cole and Jaroslav F. Prchal, *Age and Ageing* (1984) 13: 101-105.
90a. E. Busch, *Animal Breed. Abstr.* (1957) 25: 147, cited in ref. 90b.
90b. Alan A. Watson, *Lancet* (Sept. 29, 1962): 644.
90c. Ralph Carmel and Gerald S. Bernstein, *Jrl. of Clinical Investigation* (1984) 73: 868-872.
90d. F. Fernandes-Costa et al., *American Jrl. of Clinical Nutrition* (1985) 41: 784. Cited in the *Jrl. of the American Dietetic Assn.* (1985) 85, no. 8: 1019.
90e. A. Hanck and H. Weiser, *Internationale Zeitschrift für Vitamin und Ernahrungs Forschung* (1985) 27: 189-206.
91. F.R. Ellisard and S. Nasser, *British Jrl. of Nutrition* (1973) 30: 277.
92. Tin-May-Than et al., *British Jrl. of Nutrition* (1978) 40: 269-273.
93. Elizabeth Jacob et al., *Physiological Reviews* (1980) 60: 918-960.
93a. Barry Herzlich and Victor Herbert, *American Jrl. of Gastroenterology* (1984) 79: 489-493.
93b. *Harrison's Principles of Internal Medicine* , ed. Kurt J. Isselbacker et al. (New York: McGraw Hill Book Co., 1980) p. 1519.
94. W. Veeger et al., *New England Jrl. of Medicine* (1962) 267: 1341-1344.
95. J.T. Henderson et al., *Lancet* (Aug. 2, 1972): 241-243.

96. Victor Herbert, *Amer. Jrl. of Clinical Nutrition* (1973) 26: 77-88.
97. J. Michael Poston and Brian A. Hemmings, *Jrl. of Bacteriology* (Dec., 1979) 140, no. 3: 1013-1016.
98. Alfred Doscherholmen, *JAMA* (Nov. 3, 1978) 240, no. 19: 2045.
99. Ronald L. Searcy, *Diagnostic Chemistry* (New York: McGraw Hill Book Co., 1969) p., 576.
100. Louise F. Gray and Louise J. Daniel, *Jrl. of Nutrition* (1959) 67: 623-639.
101. Allen Dong and Stephen C. Scott, *Ann. Nutr. Metab.* (1982) 26: 209-216.
102. R.W. Cullen and S.M. Oace, *Nutrition Reviews* (1979) 37: 116-118.
103. *Nutrition Reviews* (1983) 41: 304-305.
104. Ibid: 306-307.
104a. Louis F. Wertalik et al., *JAMA* (1972) 221, no. 12: 1371-1374.
105. Victor Herbert, *Amer. Jrl. of Clinical Nutrition* (1973) 26: 77-88.
105a. D.V. Frost et al., *Science* (1952) 116: 119-121.
105b. D.V. Frost et al., *Abst. 118th Mtg. Am. Chem. Soc.,* Chicago (Sept., 1950): 70C. Cited in ref. 105a.
105c. N.R. Trenner et al., *Jrl. Amer. Pharm. Assoc.,* Scientific Edition, (1950) 39: 361. Cited in ref. 105a.
106. E.M. Stapert et al., *Jrl. Amer. Pharmaceutical Assn., Scientific Edition* (1954) 43, no. 2: 87-90.
107. A.J. Rosenberg, *Jrl. Biological Chemistry* (1956) 219: 951-956.
107a. Hastings H. Hutchins et al., *Jrl. of the Amer. Pharmaceutical Assn.,* (1956) 45: 806-808.
108. Victor Herbert, *JAMA* (Oct. 14, 1974) 230, no. 2: 241.
109. Victor Herbert, *Amer. Jrl. of Clinical Nutrition* (March, 1976) 29, no. 3: 235-236.
110. Harold L. Newmark et al., *Amer. Jrl. of Clinical Nutrition* (June, 1976) 29, no. 6: 645-649.
111. Victor Herbert, *Amer. Jrl. of Clinical Nutrition* (Feb., 1978) 31, no. 2: 253-258.
112. Martin Marcus, *Amer. Jrl. of Clinical Nutrition* (Aug., 1981) 34: 1622-1623.
112a. H.P.C. Hogenkamp, *Amer. Jrl. of Clinical Nutrition* (1980) 33: 1-3.
112b. Victor Herbert, *Nutrition Today* (Jan./Feb. 1984) 9, no. 1: 34.
112c. Victor Herbert and Elizabeth Jacob., *JAMA* (1975) 232, no. 3: 246.
112d. Shirley Ekvall et al., *Amer. Jrl. of Clinical Nutrition* (1981) 34: 1356-1361.
112e. John D. Hines, *JAMA* (1975) 234, no. 1: 24.
112f. Mary Ann Sestili, *Seminars in Oncology* (1983) 10, no. 3: 299-304.
113. *Nutrition Reviews* (1979) 37, no. 2: 45-46.
113a. Haruki Kondo et al., *Jrl. of Clinical Investigation* (May, 1981) 67: 1270-1283.
113b. Haruki Kondo et al., *Jrl. of Clinical Investigation* (Oct. 1982) 70: 889-898.
113c. J. Fred Kolhouse and Robert H. Allen, *Jrl. of Clinical Investgation* (Dec., 1977) 60: 1381-1392.
113d. J. Fred Kolhouse et al., *New England Jrl. of Medicine* (1978) 299, no. 15: 785-792.
113e. Mitchell Binder et al., *Analytical Biochemistry* (1982) 125: 253-258.
113f. B. Mackler, V. Herbert et al., *Clinical Research* (1984) 32: 490A.
114. Victor Herbert et al., *New England Jrl. of Medicine* (July 22, 1982) 307, no. 4: 255-256.
115. Nina V. Mayasishcheva et al., *Biochimica et Biophysica Acta* (1979) 588: 81-88.
115a. R.H. Allen in *Abstracts of the Joint Meeting of the 18th Congress of the International Society of Hematology, Montreal, Canada, August 16-22, 1980,* p. 53. Cited in ref. 114.
116. Victor Herbert and George Drivas, *JAMA* (Dec. 17, 1982) 248, no. 23: 3096-3097.
116a. V. Herbert et al., *Clinical Research* (1984) 32: 544A.
116b. Victor Herbert et al., *Transactions of the Assn. of American Physicians* (1984) 97: 161-171.
117. C.N. Ugwu and F.J. Gibbins, *Age and Ageing* (1981) 10: 196-197.
118. A. Dupre et al., *Cutis* (Aug., 1979) 24: 210-211.

119. Robert S. Hillman in *Goodman and Gilman's The Pharmacological Basis of Therapeutics*, 6th ed., ed. Alfred G. Gilman, Louis S. Goodman and Alfred Gilman (New York: MacMillan, 1980).

119a. David A. Knapp et al., *American Pharmacy* (1984) 24, no. 1: 4-5.

120. A.D. Ostryanina, cited by Raymond J. Shamberger and Charles E. Willis, *Nutrition in Cancer* , ed. Jan van Eys et al. (New York: Medical and Scientific, 1978) p. 240.

121. L.A. Poirier et al., *Proc. Amer. Assn. Cancer Research, Soc. of Clinical Oncology* (March, 1974) 15:51.

121a. Punya Temcharoen et al.,*Cancer Research* (1978) 38: 2185-2190.

122. Ralph Carmel and Leopoldo Eisenberg,*Cancer* (1977) 40, no. 3: 1348-1353.

122a. J.C. Linnell and D.M. Mathews in *Vitamin B₁₂: Proceedings of the 3rd European Symposium on Vitamin B₁₂ and Intrinsic Factor,* ed. B. Zagalak and W. Friedrick (Berlin: W. de Gruyter, 1979) pp. 1101-1111. Cited in ref. 89a.

122b. Robert F. Schilling, *JAMA* (March 28, 1986) 255, no. 12: 1605-1606.

122c. A.C.M. Kroes et al., *Leukemia Research* (1984) 8, no. 3: 441-448.

122d. Yasuhiko Kano et al., *Cancer Research* (1983) 43: 1493-1496.

122e. Norio Shimizu et al., *Nippon Gan Chiryo Gakkai Shi, Jrl. of the Japanese Society for Cancer Therapy* (1985) 20, no. 1: 40-46.

122f. D. Branca et al., *International Jrl. for Vitamin and Nutrition Research* (1984) 54: 211-216.

123. Roman J. Kutsky, *Handbook of Vitamins, Minerals and Hormones* (New York: Van Nostrand Reinhold, 1981) p. 110.

123a. E. Ralli et al., *Vitamins and Hormones* (1953) 11: 133-155. Cited in ref. 123d.

123b. J. Szorady,*Acta Paediatr. Acad. Sci. Hung.,* vol. IV, 1963. Cited in ref. 123d.

123c. Christopher Nice et al., *Jrl. of Sports Medicine* (1984) 24: 26-29.

123d. R.G. Early and B. Carlson, *Int. Z. Angew. Physiol.* (1969) 17: 43-50. Cited in ref. 123c.

123e. D. Litoff et al., *Medicine and Science in Sports and Exercise* (1985) 17, no. 2: 287.

123f. J.F. Grenier et al., *Acta Vitaminol Enzymol.* (1982) 4: 81-85.

124. Marc Aprahamian et al., *American Jrl. of Clinical Nutrition* (1985) 41: 578-589.

124a. Ashton L. Welsh, *Archives of Dermatology* (1954) 70: 181-198.

124b. General Practitioner Research Group,*Practitioner* (Feb. 1980) 224: 208-211.

125. Joseph J. Barboriak et al., *Jrl. of Nutrition* (1957) 63: 591-599.

125a. J. Vittek and B.L. Slomiany, *Experientia* (1984) 40: 104-106.

126. Thomas S. Gardner, *Jrl. of Gerontology* (1948) 3, no. 1: 1-8.

127. Thomas S. Gardner, *Jrl. of Gerontology* (1948) 3, no. 1: 9-13.

128. Roger J. Williams, *Nutrition Against Disease* (New York: Pitman Publ. Corp., 1971) pp. 141-142.

129. Richard B. Pelton and Roger J. Williams, *Proc. of the Soc. of Experimental Biology and Medicine* (1958) 99: 632-633.

130. Roger J. Williams, *Nutrition In A Nutshell* (New York: Doubleday, 1963).

131. H.P. Morris and S. W. Lippincott, *Jrl. Nat. Cancer Institute* (1941) 2: 47-54.

132. J.A. Crim et al., *Cancer Research* (1967) 27: 1109-1114.

132a. Lyn Howard et al., *Jrl. of Nutrition* (1974) 104: 1024-1032.

133. A. Stewart Truswell,*British Medical Jrl.*(July 27, 1985) 291: 263-266, at 264.

133a. L. Elsborg et al.,*Internat. Jrl. Vit. Nutri. Res.* (1983) 53: 321-329.

133b. Benjamin T. Burton, *Human Nutrition* (New York: McGraw Hill Book Co., 1976) pp. 115-116.

133ba. Bola O.A. Osifo, *Acta Haematologica* (1984) 71: 299-303.

133c. D. Parratt, *Proc. Nutri. Soc.* (1980) 39: 133-140.

133d. M.J. Bober, *British Medical Jrl.*(April 21, 1984) 288: 1234.

134. *Lancet* (June 7, 1975): 1283-1284.

134a. E.H. Reynolds and G. Stramentinoli,*Psychological Medicine* (1983) 13: 705-710.

135. Carl C. Pfeiffer, *Mental and Elemental Nutrients* (New Canaan, Conn.: Keats Publ. Co., 1975) pp. 469-472.
136. K.M. Laurence et al., *British Medical Jrl.* (May 9, 1981) 282: 1509-1511.
136a. Patricia Blessing, *Jrl. of the American Dietetic Assn.* (Sept., 1985) 85, no. 9: 1133. Cited from *News & Features from NIH* (1985) 85, no. 5: 8.
137. G. M. Stirrat, *Lancet* (Mar. 13, 1982): 625-626.
138. R. W. Smithells et al., *Lancet* (May 7, 1983): 1027-1031.
138a. J. Mark Elwood, *Canadian Medical Jrl.* (1983) 129: 1088-1092.
138b. Bolo O.A. Osifo et al., *Jrl. of the Neurological Sciences* (1985) 68: 185-190.
138c. O.R. Hommes and E.A.M.T. Obbens, *Jrl. of the Neurological Sciences* (1972) 16: 271-281. Cited in ref. 138b.
139. Richard R. Streiff, *JAMA* (Oct. 5, 1970) 214, no. 1: 105-108.
140. Lars Ovesen, *Drugs* (1979) 18: 278-298.
140a. D.W. Dawson, *British Jrl. of Obstetrics and Gynaecology.* (1982) 89: 678-680.
141. Richard I. Vogel et al., *Jrl. of Oral Medicine* (1978) 33, no. 1: 20-22.
141a. Angela R.C. Pack, *Jrl. of Clinical Peridontology* (1984) 11: 619-628.
141b. Richard F. Branda and John W. Eaton, *Science* (1978) 201: 625-626.
142. Isobel W. Jennings, *Vitamins in Endocrine Metabolism* (Springfield, Il.: CC. Thomas, 1970).
142a. Charles D. Gerson et al., *Gastroenterology* (1971) 61, no. 2: 224-227.
142b. J.R. Bertino, *Cancer* (May, 1979) 43, no. 5 supp. 2137-2142.
142c. Heyke Diddens et al., *Cancer Treatment Reviews* (1984) 11, supp. A: 37-41.
142d. Yashuhiko Kano et al., *Cancer Research* (1981) 41: 4698-4701.
142e. Enrico Mini et al., *Cancer Research* (1985) 45: 325-330.
142f. Ian W. Taylor et al., *Cancer Research* (1985) 45: 978-982.
142g. Jan H. Schornagel et al., *Biochemical Pharmacology* (1984) 33, no. 20: 3251-3255.
142h. Harry J. Iland et al., *Cancer Research* (1985) 45: 3962-3968.
143. Philip L. Bailin et al., *JAMA* (1975) 232: 359-362.
143a. John H. Klippel and John L. Decker, *New England Jrl. of Medicine* (1985) 312, no. 13: 853-854.
143b. John A. Reidy et al., *Mutation Research* (1983) 122: 217-221.
143c. John A. Reidy and Andrew T.L. Chen, *Human Genetics* (1984) 68: 189-190.
143d. Xin-Zhi Li et al., *Mutation Research* (1986) 173: 131-134.
143e. Grant R. Sutherland, *American Jrl. of Human Genetics* (1979) 31: 125-135.
144. William A. Check, *JAMA* (Aug. 15, 1980) 244, no. 7: 633-634.
145. Charles E. Butterworth and Denise Norris, *Amer. Jrl. of Clinical Nutrition* (1983) 37, no. 2: 332-333.
145a. E.W. Nelson et al., *Amer. Jrl. of Clinical Nutrition* (1978) 31: 82-87, cited by Paul E. MacCosbe and Kathleen Toomey, *Clinical Pharmacy* (1984) 3: 116-117.
145b. T. del Ser Quijano et al., *Epilepsia* (1983) 24: 588-596.
145c. V.A. Lawrence et al., *Jrl. of Laboratory and Clinical Medicine* (1984) 103: 944-948.
146. Alfred Zettner et al., *Annals of Clinical and Laboratory Science* (1981) 11: 516-524.
147. Joseph R. DiPalma and David M. Ritchie, *Ann. Rev. of Pharmacol. Toxicol.* (1977) 17: 133-148.
147a. Richard Hunter et al., *Lancet* (Jan. 10, 1970): 61-63.
147b. Lajla Hellström, *Lancet* (Jan. 9, 1971): 59-61.
147c. P.C. Wilson et al., *Clinical Research* (1983) 31, no. 4: 760A.
147d. D.B. Milne et al., *American Jrl. of Clinical Nutrition* (1984) 39: 535-539.
147e. L. Wada et al., *Federation Proceedings* (March 5, 1986) 45, no. 4: 1081 (abstract no. 5391).
147f. Mukunda D. Mukherjee et al., *American Jrl. of Clinical Nutrition* (1984) 40: 496-507.
147g. Carl C. Pfeiffer, *Mental and Elemental Nutrients* (New Canaan, Comm.: Keats Publishing Co., 1975) p. 168.
147h. A. Wu et al., *British Jrl. of Haematology* (1975) 29: 469-478.

148. C.J.D. Zarafonetis, *Jrl. Investigative Dermatol.* (1950) 15: 399. As cited by Franklin Bicknell and Frederick Prescott, *The Vitamins in Medicine,* op. cit. (ref. 20), p. 137.

148a. W.A. Krehl in *Modern Nutrition in Health and Disease,* 5th ed., ed. Robert S. Goodhart and Maurice E. Shils (Philadelphia: Lea & Febiger, 1973) pp. 946-947.

148b. Else Kierkegaard and Birgit Nielsen, *Ugeskrift for Laeger* (1979) 141, no. 30: 2052-2053.

148c. Derek Meyers, *Med. Jrl. Australia* (June 11, 1977) 1, no. 24: 887.

148d. *Facts and Comparisons* (St. Louis, MO: J.B. Lippincott Co., 1986) p. 360.

148e. P.J. Osgood, et al., *Jrl. Invest. Dermatology* (1982) 79: 354-357, cited by Sophie Worobec, *JAMA* (1984) 251, no. 18: 2348. Also *Chemical Abstracts* (1982) 97: 211652e.

149. Franklin Bicknell and Frederick Prescott,*The Vitamins in Medicine,* op. cit. (ref. 20) p. 137.

150. Benjamin S. Frank and Philip Miele, *Doctor Frank's No-Ageing Diet: Eat and Grow Younger* (New York: Dial Press, 1976).

150a. William W.K. Zung et al., *Psychosomatics* (1974) 15: 127-131.

150b. Edwin J. Olsen, *Jrl. of Gerontology* (1978) 33, no. 4: 514-520.

150c. Israel Zwerling et al., *Jrl. of the American Geriatrics Society* (1975) 23, no. 8: 355-359.

150d. Adrian Ostfeld et al., *Jrl. of the American Geriatrics Society* (1977) 25, no. 1: 1-19.

150e. *Physicians' Desk Reference* , 39th ed. (Oradell, N.J.: Medical Economics Co., 1985) pp. 3003-3004.

150f. Robert S. Goodhart in *Modern Nutrition in Health and Disease,* 5th ed., ed. Robert S. Goodhart and Maurice E. Shils (Philadelphia: Lea & Febiger, 1973) pp. 262-264.

151. Albert E. Winegrad and Douglas A. Greene, *New England Jrl. of Medicine* (1976) 295, no. 25: 1416-1421.

151a. Bruce J. Holub, *Canadian Jrl. of Physiology and Pharmacology* (1984) 62: 1-8.

151b. Douglas A. Greene et al., *Jrl. of Clinical Investigation* (1975) 55: 1326-1336.

151c. K.R.W. Gillon and J.N. Hawthorne, *Life Sciences* (1983) 32: 1943-1947.

151d. David A. Simmons et al., *Transactions of the Assn. of Amer. Physicians* (1982) 95: 292-298.

151e. Cathryn E. Stokes et al.,*Biochimica et Biophysica Acta* (1983) 753: 136-138.

152. Ghafoorunissa, *Indian Jrl. of Experimental Biology* (Sept., 1976) 14: 564-566.

152a. C. Pholpramool et al., *Jrl. of Reproduction and Fertility* (1982) 66: 547-553.

152b. Anthony J. Barak and Dean J. Tuma,*Life Sciences* (1983) 32, no. 7: 771-774.

153. *Recommended Dietary Allowances,* 98th ed. (Washington, D.C., National Academy of Sciences, 1980) p. 181.

154. Arthur C. Guyton, *Textbook of Medical Physiology, 5th ed.,* (Philadelphia: W.B. Saunders Co., 1976) p. 615-616.

154a. I.A. Boyd and C.L. Pathak,*Jrl. of Physiology* (1965) 176: 191-204.

154b. John H. Growdon et al.,*New England Jrl. of Medicine* (1977) 297: 524-527.

154c. Kenneth L. Davis et al., *Life Sciences* (1976) 19: 1507-1515.

154d. Lewis I. Gidez, *Jrl. of Lipid Research* (1984) 25: 1430-1436.

155. Gordon S. Rosenberg and Kenneth L. Davis, *Amer. Jrl. of Clinical Nutrition* (Oct., 1982) 36: 709-720.

156. B.M. Cohen et al., *Amer. Jrl. Psychiatry* (1982) 139: 1162-1164.

156a. Gina Bari Kolata, *Science* (Jan 5., 1979) 203: 36-38.

157. Andre Barbeau in *Choline and Lecithin in Brain Disorders,* vol. 5 of *Nutrition and the Brain,* ed. Andre Barbeau, John H. Growdon and Richard J. Wurtman (New York: Raven Press, 1979) pp. 263-271.

157a. Jan Volavka et al.,*Biological Psychiatry* (1983) 18, no. 10: 1175-1179.

158. Raymond Levy, *Lancet* (Oct. 28, 1978): 944-945.

159. Raymond Levy, *Lancet* (Sept. 18, 1982): 671-672.

160. Paz Chuaqui and Raymond Levy,*British Jrl. of Psychiatry* (1982) 140: 464-469.

160a. George A. Vroulis et al., *Age* (Oct. 1983) 6, no. 4: 136.

160aa. Bruce L. Miller et al., *Life Sciences* (1986) 38: 485-490.

160ab. E.F. Domino et al., in *Alzheimer's Disease: A Report of Progress in Research*, ed. S. Corkin, K.L. Davis, J.H. Growdon, E. Usdin and R. Wurtman (New York: Raven Press, 1982) pp. 393-398.

160b. N. Sitaram et al., *Life Sciences* (1978) 22: 1555-1560.

160c. N. Sitaram et al., *Science* (July 21, 1978) 201: 274-276.

160d. Kenneth L. Davis et al., *Archives of Neurology* (1980) 37: 49-52.

160e. Edith L. Cohen and Richard J. Wurtman, *Science* (1976) 191: 561-562.

160f. Dean R. Haubrich and A. Barbara Pflueger, *Life Sciences* (1979) 24: 1083-1090.

161. Roger J. Williams, *Nutrition Against Disease* op. cit. (ref. 128) p. 181.

161a. Tomiko Ageta et al., *Jrl. of Chromatography* (1985) 343: 186-189.

162. G. Klatskin et al., *Jrl. Experimental Medicine* (1954) 605-614.

163. Adrianne E. Rogers et al., *Drug-Nutrient Interactions* (1981) 1, no. 1: 3-14.

163a. Emanuel Rubin and Charles S. Lieber, *New England Jrl. of Medicine* (1974) 290, no. 3: 128-135.

163b. C.S. Lieber and L.M. DeCarli, *Jrl. of Medical Primatology* (1974) 3: 153-163.

163c. Charles S. Lieber et al., *Proc. National Academy of Sciences* (1975) 72, no. 2: 437-441.

163d. Steven H. Zeisel et al., *Nutrition and the Brain*, ed. A. Barbeau, J.H. Growdon and R.J. Wurtman (New York: Raven Press, 1979) pp. 47-55.

163e. Rodolfo Roberto Brenner, *Drug Metabolism Reviews* (1977) 6, no. 2: 155-211 at 156-157.

164. Lynn Wecker et al., *Drug-Nutrient Interactions* (1982) 1: 125-130.

165. L.J. Bottecelli et al., *Commun. Psychopharmacology* (1977) 1: 519-523.

165a. Madelyn Hirsh Fernstrom in *Nutritional Pharmacology*, ed. Gene A. Spiller (New York: Alan R. Liss, 1981) p. 14.

166. Irvin E. Liener in *Toxic Constituents of Plant Foodstuffs*, ed. Irvin E. Liener (New York: Academic Press, 1969) p. 429.

166a. A.A. Oduduga and A.J. Ogunleye, *Nutrition Reports International* (Aug., 1985) 32, no. 2: 407-418.

166b. Richard J. Wurtman et al., *Lancet* (July 9, 1977): 68-69.

167. Margaret Cobb et al., *Nutrition and Metabolism* (1980) 24: 228-237.

168. Marian T. Childs et al., *Atherosclerosis* (1981) 38: 217-228.

168a. Carlos Krumdieck and C.E. Butterworth, *American Jrl. of Clinical Nutrition* (1974) 27: 866-876.

168b. J.R. Murphy, *Jrl. of Laboratory and Clinical Medicine* (1962) 60: 86. Cited in ref. 168a.

168c. C.W.M. Adams and R.J. Morgan, *Jrl. Pathol. Bacteriol* (1967) 94: 73. Cited in ref. 168a.

168d. C.W. M. Adams, et al., *Jrl. Pathol. Bacteriol* (1967) 94: 77. Cited in ref. 168a.

168e. Madelyn J. Hirsch et al., *Metabolism* (1978) 27, no. 8: 953-960.

168f. John L. Wood and Richard G. Allison, *Federation Proceedings* (1982) 41: 3015-3021.

169. A. Munnich et al., *Lancet* (Aug. 1, 1981): 263.

169a. B. Wolf et al., *Jrl. of Inherited Metabolic Disease* (1985) 8, supp. 1: 53-58.

169b. E.R. Baumgartner et al., *Jrl. of Inherited Metabolic Disease* (1985) 8, supp. 1: 59-64.

169c. K. Bartlett et al., *Jrl. of Inherited Metabolic Disease* (1985) 8, supp. 1: 46-52.

170. Morton J. Cowan et al., *Lancet* (July 21, 1979): 115-118.

171. P.H. Brooks et al., *Veterinary Record* (1977) 101: 46-50.

172. H.E. Sauberlich, *Annals of the N.Y. Academy of Sciences* (1980) 355: 80-97.

173. Brendan M. Charles et al., *Lancet* (July 21, 1979): 118-120.

174. A.R. Johnson et al., *Nature* (May 15, 1980) 285: 159-160.

175. Franklin Bicknell and Frederick Prescott, *The Vitamins in Medicine*, op. cit. (ref. 20) p. 130.

176. I.I. Kaplin, *Amer. Jrl. of Medical Science* (1939) 33: 1681, cited by Franklin Bicknell and Frederick Prescott, ibid, p. 131.

176a. R.P. Bhullar and K. Dakshinamurti, *Jrl. of Cellular Physiology* (1985) 123, no. 3: 425-430. Abstracted in *Nutrition Abstracts and Reviews,* Series A (1985) 55, no. 10: 719 (abstract no. 6291).

176b. Jean-Pierre Bonjour, *Annals of the New York Academy of Sciences* (1985) 447: 97-104.

177. Ruth Okey, *Jrl. of Biological Chemistry* (Sept.-Oct., 1946) 165: 383-4.

177a. *The Merck Index,* 10th ed., ed. Martha Windholz (Rahway, N.J.: Merck & Co., 1983), p. 1006.

177b. U.S. patent no. 2,464,240.

178. Victor Herbert, *Amer. Jrl. of Clinical Nutrition* (1979) 32: 1541-1544.

179. V. Herbert et al., *Blood* (1978) 52, supp. 1: 252.

179a. Mark D. Gelernt and Victor Herbert, *Nutrition and Cancer* (1982) 3, no. 3: 129-133.

180. Neville Colman et al., *Proc. of the Soc. for Experimental Biology and Medicine* (1980) 164, no. 1: 9-12.

180a. Marvin A. Friedman, *Bulletin of Environmental Contamination & Toxicology* (1975) 13, no. 2: 226-232.

181. Victor Herbert, *Amer. Jrl. of Clinical Nutrition* (1979) 32: 1541-1549.

182. L. Barnes, *Physician and Sportsmedicine* (1979) 7: 17-18.

183. Robert N. Girandola et al., *Biochemical Medicine* (1980) 24: 218-222.

183a. D.G. Black and A.A. Sucec, *Medicine and Science in Sports and Exercise* (1981) 13: 93.

183b. M. Harpaz et al., *Medicine and Science in Sports and Exercise* (1985) 17, no. 2: 287.

184. G. Lynis Dohm et al., *Biochemical Medicine* (1982) 28: 77-82.

184a. Michael E. Gray and Larry W. Titlow, *Medicine and Science in Sports and Exercise* (1982) 14, no. 6: 424-427.

185. Charles D. Graber et al., *Jrl. of Infectious Diseases* (Jan., 1981) 143: 101-104.

186. P.W. Stacpoole et al., *New England Jrl. of Medicine* (1979) 300: 372.

187. U.S. patent no. 2, 985,664.

187a. Thomas Cairns et al., *Analytical Chemistry* (1978) 50, no. 2: 317-322.

188. Catherine Fenselau et al., *Science* (Nov. 11, 1977) 198: 625-627.

189. Elaine Robinson, "Cyanogenesis in Plants," *Biological Reviews* (1930) 5: 126-141.

190. Eric E. Conn in *Toxicants Occurring Naturally in Foods,* op. cit. (ref. 9C).

191. Ernst T. Krebs, Jr., *Jrl. of Applied Nutrition* (Fall-Winter, 1970).

192. J.L. Ambrus et al., *Clinical Pharmacology and Therapeutics* (May-June, 1967) 8, no. 3: 362-368.

193. S. Avakian, *Clinical Pharmacology and Therapeutics* (Feb. 24, 1964) 5, no. 6: 712-715.

194. Jonathan Yavelow et al., *Cancer Research* (1983) supp. 49: 2454s-2459s.

194a. Walter Troll and Rakoma Wiesner, *Prostate* (1983) 4: 345-349.

194b. Aaron S. Abramovitz et al., *Jrl. of Biological Chemistry* (1983) 258, no. 24: 15153-15157.

195. Glenn D. Kittler, *Laetrile—Control for Cancer* (New York: Astor-Honor, 1963).

196. Victor Herbert, *Nutrition Cultism: Facts and Fictions* (Philadelphia: George F. Stickley Co., 1980).

197. Victor Herbert, *Amer. Jrl. of Clinical Nutrition* (May, 1979) 32: 1121-1158.

198. Irving J. Lerner, *CA—A Cancer Jrl. for Clinicians* (1981) 31, no. 2: 91-95.

199. O.L. Ekpechi et al., *Nature* (June 11, 1966) 210: 1137-1138.

199a. I.B. Umoh et al., *Annals of Nutrition and Metabolism* (1985) 29: 319-324.

199b. D.M. Greenberg, *Western Jrl. of Medicine* (1975) 122: 345-348.

200. Irvin E. Liener, *Toxic Constituents of Plant Foodstuffs,* op. cit. (ref. 9).

201. Ali K. Osman et al., *Ann. Nutr. Metab.* (1983) 27: 14-18.

202. A. Keith Brewer, *Jrl. of the International Academy of Preventive Medicine* 5, no. 2: 29-53.

202a. M. Von Ardenne, *Advances in Pharmacology and Chemotherapy* (1972) 10: 339-380, at 341.

202b. A. Keith Brewer, *Cytobios* (1979) 24: 99-101.

203. R.D. Montgomery in *Toxic Constituents of Plant Foodstuffs*, ed. Irvin E. Liener, op. cit. (ref. 166) p. 149.

203a. M. Kochi et al., paper accepted for presentation at the 12th International Cancer Congress, Buenos Aires, Oct. 5-11, 1978. Cited by ref. 204.

204. Setsuo Takeuchi et al., *Agric. Biol. Chem.* (1978) 42, no. 7: 1449-1451.

204a. Mutsuyuki Kochi et al., *Cancer Treatment Reports* (1980) 64, no. 1: 21-23.

204b. Erik O. Pettersen et al., *European Jrl. of Cancer and Clinical Oncology* (1983) 19, no. 7: 935-940.

204c. Erik O. Pettersen et al., *European Jrl. of Cancer and Clinical Oncology* (1983) 19, no. 4: 507-514.

204d. Akoko Ishida et al., *Cancer Research* (1983) 43: 4216-4220.

204e. Raymond Taetle and Stephen B. Howell, *Cancer Treatment Reports* (1983) 67, no. 6: 561-566.

205. Mathew M. Ames et al., *Research Communications in Chemical Pathology and Pharmacology,* (Oct., 1978) 22, no. 1: 175-185.

206. John Jee et al., *Jrl. of Pharmaceutical Sciences* (1978) 67, no. 3: 438-444.

206a. J. Paul Davignon, *New England Jrl. of Medicine* (1977) 297, no. 24: 1355-1356.

207. *Federal Register* (Aug. 5, 1977) 42, no. 151: 39768-39806.

208. David M. Greenberg, *Cancer* (Feb. 15, 1980) 45: 799-807.

209. Richard E. Heikila and Felicitas S. Cabbat, *Life Sciences* (1980) 27: 659-662.

210. Wilma K. Mechstroth and Leon M. Dorfman, *Biochemical Pharmacology* (1980) 29: 3307-3309.

211. Kanematsu Sugiura, quoted by Barbara J. Culliton, *Science* (Dec. 7, 1973) 182: 1000-1003.

211a. C. Chester Stock et al., *Jrl. of Surgical Oncology* (1978) 10: 89-123 at 122.

211b. Harold W. Manner, *The Death of Cancer* (Evanston, Il.: Advanced Century Publ. Corp., 1978) pp. 170-176. Also various issues of the *National Health Federation Bulletin.*

212. Ernst Krebs, Jr., *Public Scrutiny* (July-Aug., 1981).

213. Marjorie Sun, *Science* (May 15, 1981) 212: 758-759.

214. Charles G. Moertel et al., *New England Jrl. of Medicine* (Jan. 28, 1982) 306, no. 4: 201-206.

215. *New England Jrl. of Medicine* (July 8, 1982) 307: 118-120.

216. K.M. Birch and F. Schütz, *British Jrl. of Pharmacology* (1946) 1: 186-193. Cited by Donald R. Harkness and Sandra Roth in *Progress in Hematology* (1975) 9: 157-184.

217. E. Hurst, *The Poison Plants of New South Wales* (Sydney, Australia: New South Wales Poison Plants Committee, 1942).

218. James W. Sayre and Sukru Kaymakcalan, *New England Jrl. of Medicine* (May 21, 1964) 270, no. 21: 1113-1115.

219. Victor Herbert, *Amer. Jrl. of Clinical Nutrition* (Jan., 1979) 32: 96-98.

219a. Ronald C. Backer and Victor Herbert, *JAMA* (1979) 241, no. 18: 1891.

220. Edward J. Calabrese, *Medical Hypotheses* (1979) 5: 995-997.

220a. Tapan K. Basu, *Canadian Jrl. Physiol. Pharmacol.* (1983) 61: 1426-1430.

221. A.W. Blyth, *Poisons: Their Effects and Detection* (New York: D. Van Nostrand, 1906).

222. *Medical World News* (Jan. 9, 1978).

223. Kenneth B. Liegner et al., *JAMA* (Dec. 18, 1981) 246: 2841-2842.

224. Eric S. Schmidt et al., *JAMA* (Mar. 6, 1978) 39: 943-947.

225. Kathleen T. Braico et al., *New England Jrl. of Medicine* (Feb. 1, 1979) 300: 238-240.

226. Edward J. Calabrese, *Medical Hypotheses* (1979) 5: 1045-1049.

227. Calvin C. Willhite, *Science* (Mar. 19, 1982) 215: 1513-1515.

954 The Reverse Effect

228. Donald R. Harkness and Sandra Roth, *Progress in Hematology,* vol. IX, ed. Elmer B. Brown (New York: Grune and Stratton, 1975).
228a. Jon Bremer, *Physiological Reviews* (1983) 63, no. 4: 1420-1480.
229. *Nutrition Reviews* (1981) 39, no. 11: 400-402.
230. Peggy Borum, *Annual Review of Nutrition* (1983) 3: 233-259.
230a. Brian Leibovitz, *Carnitine: The Vitamin BT Phenomenon* (New York: Dell Publishing Co., 1984).
230b. Robert E. Keith, *JAMA* (March 7, 1986) 255, no. 9: 1137.
230c. Nongnuj Tanphaichitr, *International Jrl. of Fertility* (1977) 22: 85-91.
231. J.C. Soufir et al., *International Jrl. of Andrology* (1984) 7: 188-197.
232. Peggy R. Borum and Sandra G. Bennett, *Jrl. of the American College of Nutrition* (1986) 5: 177-182.
233. D. Rudman et al., *Jrl. of Clinical Investigation* (1977) 60: 716-723. Cited in ref. 232.
234. R.K. Fuller and C.L. Hoppel, *Hepatology* (1983) 3: 554-558. Cited in ref. 232.

Chapter 6—541 References

1. Ibn Batuta, as cited by M. Collis, *Marco Polo* (New York: James Laughlin, 1960) p. 137.
1a. IUPAC-IUB Commission on Biochemical Nomenclature, *Biochim. Biophys. Acta* (1965) 107: 4. Cited by Gerald M. Jaffe in *Handbook of Vitamins*, ed. Lawrence J. Machlin New York: Marcel Dekker, Inc., 1984) p. 204.
2. R.E. Hughes, *Proc. Royal Soc. Medicine* (1977) 70: 86-89.
3. Irwin Stone, *The Healing Factor—"Vitamin C" Against Disease* (New York: Grossett & Dunlap, 1972).
3a. Irwin Stone, *Medical Hypotheses* (1979) 5: 711-722.
3b. I.B. Chatterjee, *World Review of Nutrition and Dietetics* (1978) 30: 69-87.
3c. S. Shah and N. Nath, *Jrl. of Biochemistry & Biophysics* (1985) 22: 43-48.
4. Irwin Stone, *Jrl. of the International Academy of Metabology* (March, 1974).
5. *Nutrition Reviews* (Oct., 1982) 40: 310-316.
6. Edward J. Calabrese, *Medical Hypotheses* (1982) 8: 173-175.
7. Irwin Stone, *American Laboratory* (April, 1974) 6, no. 4: 38.
7a. Y. Mizushima et al., *Experientia* (1984) 40: 359-361.
8. I.B. Chatterjee, Natarajan Subramanian et al., *Annals of the N.Y. Academy of Sciences* (1975) 258: 24-47.
8a. Nutrition Reviews (1982) 40, no. 10: 289-292.
9. Y. Kagawa et al., *Jrl. Biochem., Tokyo* (1962) 51: 197-203.
10. Y. Kagawa et al., *Biochim. Biophys. Acta* (1961) 51: 413-415.
11. Emil Ginter, *World Rev. Nutr. Dietet* (1979) 33: 104-141.
12. Robert B. Rucker and Michael A. Dubick, *Amer. Jrl. of Clinical Nutrition* (July, 1981) 34, no. 7: 1450-1451.
12a. Miriam Rosin et al., *Cancer Letters* (1980) 8: 299-305.
13. Muge Cummings, *Amer. Jrl. of Clinical Nutrition* (Feb., 1981) 34: 297-298.
14. E.M. Baker et al., *Proc. of the Soc. Experimental Biology and Medicine* (1962) 109: 737.
15. Roger J. Williams and Gary Deason, *Proc. of the National Academy of Sciences* (June, 1967) 57, no. 6: 1638-1641.
16. C. Kalyan Bagchi, *Indian Medical Gazette* (1952) 87, no. 5: 198-200.
17. R. Rajalakshmi et al., *Acta Paediatrica Scandinavica* (1965) 54: 375-382.
18. R. Rajalakshmi et al., *Current Science* (1967) 36, no. 2: 45-46.
19. Linus Pauling, *Vitamin C and the Common Cold* (San Francisco: W.H. Freeman, 1976).
19a. F.R. Klenner, *Jrl. of Applied Nutrition* (1971) 23: 61-88. Cited in ref., 19b.
19b. Robert R. Cathcart, III, *Medical Hypotheses* (1981) 7: 1359-1376.
20. *The Merck Manual,* 13th ed., ed. Robert Berkow, Rahway, N.J.: Merck, Sharp and Dohme Research Labs, 1977) p. 34.
20a. Ibid., 14th ed. (1982) p., 190.
21. Thomas C. Chalmers, *Amer. Jrl. of Medicine* (April, 1975) 58: 532-536.
22. Alan B. Carr et al., *Medical Jrl. of Australia* (Oct. 17, 1981): 411-412.
23. K. Mary Clegg and Jennifer M. MacDonald, *Amer. Jrl. of Clinical Nutrition* (1975) 28: 973-976.
24. A. Murata et al., *Agr. Biol. Chem.* (1971) 35: 294.
24a. A. Murata in *Proceedings of the First Intersect. Congr. Internat. Assoc. Microbiol. Soc.,* ed. T. Hasegawa (Tokyo: Science Council of Japan, 1975) pp. 432-436. Cited by Akura Murata et al., *Jrl. Nutr. Sci. Vitaminol.* (1983) 29: 721-724.
25. Natarajan Subramanian et al., *Biochem. Pharmacol.* (1973) 22: 1671-1673.
26. C. Alan B. Clemetson, *Jrl. of Nutrition* (1980) 110: 662-668.
26a. *Blakiston's Gould Medical Dictionary,* 3rd ed., by Arthur Osol (New York: McGraw Hill Co., 1972) p. 702.
26b. Itarv Yamamoto and Hitoshi Ohmori, *Jrl. Pharm. Dyn.* (1981) 4: 15-19.

956 The Reverse Effect

26c. Lawrence R. De Chatelet et al., *Antimicrobial Agents and Chemotherapy* (1972) 1, no. 1: 12-16.

26d. Elizabeth B. Finley, *Amer. Jrl. of Clinical Nutrition* (1983) 37: 553-556.

27. Darrel van Campen and Earl Cross, *Jrl. of Nutrition* (1968) 95: 617-622.

27a. Elizabeth B. Finley and Florian L. Cerklewski, *Amer. Jrl. of Clinical Nutrition* (1983) 37: 563-556.

28. B.K. Nandi et al., *Biochemical Pharmacology* (1974) 23: 643-647.

29. R. Hume and Elspeth Weyers, *Scottish Medical Jrl.* (1973) 18: 3-7.

30. C.W.M. Wilson, *Annals of the N.Y. Academy of Sciences* (1975) 258: 529-539.

30a. C.W.M. Wilson, *Annals of the N.Y. Academy of Sciences* (1975) 258: 355-376.

30b. Anita J. Thomas et al., *Age and Ageing* (1984) 13: 243-246.

31. Prakash G. Shilorti and K. Seetharam Bhat, *Amer. Jrl. of Clinical Nutrition* (July, 1977) 30: 1077-1081.

32. Charles E. McCall, et al., *Jrl. of Infectious Diseases* (Aug., 1971) 24: 194-198.

33. Bani Basu et al., *Indian Jrl. of Experimental Biology* (May 1977) 15: 352-354.

34. Ralph Golden and Frederick Sargent III, *Archives of Biochemistry & Biophysics* (1952) 39: 138-146.

35. G.N. Schrauzer and W.J. Rhead, *International Jrl. for Vitamin and Nutrition Research* (1973) 43: 201-211.

36. J. Ludvigsson et al., *International Jrl. for Vitamin and Nutrition Research* (1970) 46: 160-165.

37. William F. Geber, et al., *Pharmacology* (1975) 13: 228-233.

38. Benjamin V. Siegel, *Nature* (April 10,., 1975) 254: 531-532.

38a. Bracha Rager-Zisman and Barry R. Bloom, *British Medical Bulletin* (1985) 41, no. 1: 22-27.

39. Benjamin V. Siegel, *Infection and Immunity* (Aug., 1974) 10: 409-410.

40. Helen Dahl and Miklos Degre, *Acta Path. Microbiol. Scand., Section B* (1976) 84: 280-284.

40a. B.V. Siegel and Jane I. Morton, *International Jrl. for Vitamin and Nutrition Research* (1984) 54: 339-342.

41. B.V. Siegel and James I. Morton, *Experientia* (1977) 33: 393-395.

42. Robin C. Fraser et al., *Amer. Jrl. of Clinical Nutrition* (1980) 33: 839-847.

43. Akira Murata et al., *Jrl. of Nutritional Science and Vitaminology* (1975) 21: 261-269.

44. E.M. S. Gatner and R. Anderson, *Clinical and Exper. Immunol.* (1980) 40: 327-335.

45. R. Anderson, *Leprosy Review* (1980) 51: 195-197.

46. Surendra N. Sinha et al., *International Jrl. of Leprosy* (1984) 52, no. 2: 159-162.

47. Fukumi Morishige and Akira Murata, *Jrl. of the International Academy of Preventive Medicine* (1978): 48-56.

48. F.P. McGinn and Judith C. Hamilton, *British Jrl. of Surgery* (1976) 63: 505-507.

49. A. Rebora et al., *Dermatologica* (1980) 160: 106-112.

50. A. Rebora et al., *British Jrl. of Dermatology* (1980) 102: 49-56.

51. W.R. Thomas and P.G. Holt, *Clinical and Exper. Immunol.* (1978) 38: 370-379.

52. R. Anderson and Annette Theron, *South African Medical Journal* (1979) 56: 429-433.

53. W. Prinz et al., *Internat. Jrl. for Vitamin and Nutrition Research* (1977) 47: 248-257.

54. R. Anderson et al., *Amer. Jrl. of Clinical Nutrition* (1980) 33: 71-76.

55. *Lancet* (Feb. 10, 1979): 308.

55a. R.H. Yonemoto in *Modulation and Mediation of Cancer by Vitamins,* ed. F.L. Meyskens and K.N. Prasad (Basel, Switzerland: Karger, (1983) pp. 334-339.

56. W. Byron Smith et al., *Annals of the N.Y. Academy of Sciences* (1979) 258: 329-339.

57. Iancu Gantzea, *Nutrition and Anti-Infectious Defense* (Basel, Switzerland: Karger, 1974) p. 146.

57a. Thomas J. Rogers et al., *Jrl. of Nutrition* (1983) 113: 178-183.

57b. Thomas Rogers and Edward Balish, *Infection and Immunity* (1976) 14, no. 1: 33-38.

57c. Jan Kabelik, *Pharmazie* (1970) 25, no. 4: 266-270 and *Chemical Abstracts* (1970) 73: 83 (item 117195r).

57d. A. Tynecka and Z. Gos, *Chemical Abstracts* (1973) 79: 212 (item 63491n).

57e. Gary S. Moore and Robin D. Atkins, *Mycologia* (1977) 69: 341-348.

57f. Judith A. Appleton and Michael R. Tansey, *Mycologia* (1975) 67: 822-885.

57g. A. Tynecka and Z. Gos, *Acta Microbiol. Polon,* Series B. (1973) 5, no. 22: 51-62.

57h. Moses A. Adetumbi and Benjamin H.S. Lau, *Medical Hypotheses* (1983) 12: 227-237.

57i. T.N. Kaul et al., *Jrl. of Allergy and Clinical Immunology* (1982) 69: 104 (item no. 48).

58. A.A. Hardigree and J.L. Eppler, *Mutation Research* (1978) 58: 231-239.

59. James T. MacGregor and Leonard Jurd, *Mutation Research* (1978) 54: 297-309.

59a. Bruce N. Ames, *Science* (1979) 204: 587-593.

59b. Joseph P. Brown and Paul S. Dietrich, *Mutation Research* (1979) 66: 223-240.

59c. Joseph P. Brown, *Mutation Research* (1980) 75: 243-277.

59d. Hans-Ulrich Aeschbacher et al., *Nutrition and Cancer* (1982) 4, no. 2: 90-98.

59e. G.S. Stoewsand et al., *Federation Proceedings* (March 1, 1984) 43, no. 3: 688 (abstract no. 2356).

59f. C.C.Willhite, *Food Chemistry and Toxicology* (1982) 20, no. 1: 75-79.

60. Lee W. Wattenberg and J. Lionel Leong, *Cancer Research* (1970) 30: 1922-1925.

60a. Joachim Kühnau, *World Review of Nutrition and Dietetics* (1976) 24: 117-191.

60b. K. Morita et al., *Agric. Biol. Chem.* (1978) 42: 1235-1238.

60c. Yochiaki Ito et al., *Mutation Research* (1986) 172: 55-60.

60d. Jae Ho Kim et al., *Cancer Research* (1984) 44: 102-106.

61. C. Sirtori et al., *Pharmacological Research Communications* (1978) 10, no. 9: 809-812.

62. R.E. Hughes and H.K. Wilson in *Progress in Medicinal Chemistry,* vol. 14, ed. G.P. Ellis and G.B. West (Amsterdam: North Holland Publ. Co., 1977) pp. 285-301.

62a. *The Merck Index* 10th ed. (1983): 1226.

62b. *Chicago Medicine* (March 7, 1964).

63. Walter H. Lewis and Memory P.F. Elvin-Lewis, *Medical Botany* (New York: Wiley, 1977).

63a. Faith B. Davis et al., *Cell Calcium* (1983) 4: 71-81.

64. S.D. Varma et al., *Science* (June 20, 1975) 188: 1215-16.

64a. S.D. Varma et al., *Science* (1977) 195: 205-207.

65. J.P. Tayayre and H. Lauressergues, *Arzneimittel Forschung* (1977) 27, no. 6: 1144-1152.

66. J.P. Brown, *Mutation Research* (1980) 75: 243-277.

67. Z. Zloch, *Internat. Jrl. for Vitamin and Nutritoin Research* (1969) 39: 269. Cited by Robert S. Goodhart in *Modern Nutrition in Health and Disease,* 58th ed., ed. by Robert S. Goodhart and Maurice E. Shils (Philadelphia: Lea & Febiger, 1973) p. 259.

67a. Elliott Middleton, Jr. et al., *Jrl. of Immunology* (1981) 127: 546-550.

68. L. Peter Cogan, *Cycles* (July-August, 1973).

68a. R.E. Hope-Simpson, *Nature* (Sept. 14, 1978) 275: 86.

69. *American Jrl. of Psychiatry* (1974) 131: 1251-1266.

70. Kristine Adams, *Amer. Jrl. of Clinical Nutrition* (1981) 34: 1712-1716.

71. David Benton, *Psychopharmacology* (1981) 75: 98-99.

72. G.J. Naylor, *Neuropharmacology* (1980) 19: 1233-1234.

73. Bryant R. Fortner et al., Abstract presented at the 37th Annual Meeting of the Amer. Academy of Allergy, San Francisco, March 7-11, 1981.

74. Stanislaus Ting et al., *Jrl. of Asthma* (1983) 20, no. 1: 39-42.

75. E. Zuskin et al., *Jrl. Allergy Clin. Immunology* (1973) 51: 218-226.

76. L. Puglisi et al., *Advances in Prostaglandin and Thromboxane Research* (1976) 1: 503-506.

76a. C. Brink et al., *Polish Jrl. of Pharmacology and Pharmacy* (1978) 30: 157-166.

77. Richard J. Hargreaves et al., *Toxicology and Applied Pharmacology* (1982) 64: 280-292.

78. R.G. Busnel and A.G. Lehmann, *Behavioural Brain Research* (1980) 1: 351-356.

79. Herbert Sprince et al., *Int. Jrl. Vit. Nutri Res.* (1977) 47, supp. 1G: 185-212.

80. E.M. Baker et al., *Amer. Jrl. of Clinical Nutrition* (1966) 19: 371-378.

81. N. Krasner et al., *Lancet* (1974) 2: 693-695.

81a. Herbert Sprince et al., *Nutrition Reports International* (1978) 17, no. 4: 441-445.

81b. R.G. Busnel and A.G. Lehmann, *Behavioural Brain Research* (1980) 351-356.

82. Virginia Fazio et al., *Amer. Jrl. of Clinical Nutrition* (1981) 34: 2394-2396.

83. M. O'Keane et al., *Jrl. Alcohol* (1972) 7: 6.

84. C.J. Schorah et al., *British Jrl. of Nutrition* (1978) 39: 139-149.

84a. W.S. McCormick, *Archives of Pediatrics* (1952) 69, no. 4: 151-155.

84b. Omer Pelletier, *Annals of the N.Y. Academy of Sciences* (1975) 258: 156-168.

84c. O.S. Hoefel, *Internationale Zeitschrift für Vitamin und Ernahrungsforshung Beiheft* (1983) 24: 121-124.

85. Herbert Sprince et al., *Agents and Actions* (1975) 5, no. 2: 164-173.

85a. Valentine Free and Pat Sanders, *Jrl. of Orthomolecular Psychiatry* (1978) 7, no. 4: 264-270.

85b. Valentine Free and Pat Sanders, *Jrl. of Psychedelic Drugs* (1979) 11, no. 3: 217-222.

85c. Alfred F. Libby and Irwin Stone, *Jrl. of Orthomolecular Psychiatry* (1977) 6, no. 4: 300-308.

85d. Robert E. Willette et al., *Research Communications in Chem. Path and Pharm.* (1983) 42, no. 3. 485-491.

86. Vincent G. Zannoni and Paul H. Sato, *Annals of the N.Y. Academy of Sciences* (1975) 258: 119-131.

86a. V.G. Zannoni et al., *International Jrl. for Vitamin and Nutrition Research* (1977) supp. 16: 99-125.

87. Judith L. Sutton et al., *Biochemical Pharmacology* (1982) 31: 1591-1594.

87a. Judith L. Sutton et al., *British Jrl. of Nutrition* (1983) 49: 27-33.

87b. P.K. Reddi and S.M. Constantinides, *Nature* (1972) 238: 286. Cited in ref. 86c.

87c. K. Rothwell, *Nature* (1974) 252: 69-70.

87ca. Ron Kohen and Mordechai Chevion, paper scheduled to appear in *Free Radical Research Communications* (1985) 1.

87d. Francis J. Peterson et al., *Nutrition Reports International* (1982) 26, no. 6: 1037-1043.

87e. Samuel Schvartsman et al., *Veterinarian and Human Toxicology* (1984) 26, no. 6: 473-475.

87ea. Ron Kohen and Mordechai Chevion, *Biochemical Pharmacology* (1985) 34, no. 10: 1841-1843.

87f. Emil Ginter et al., *Jrl. of Nutrition* (1984) 114: 485-492.

87g. Kamala Krishnaswamy, *Clinical Pharmacokinetics* (1978) 3: 216-240, at 230.

87h. C.S. Catz et al., *Jrl. of Pharmacology and Experimental Therapeutics* (1970) 174: 197-205. Cited in ref. 87g.

87i. G.C. Becking, *Federation Proceedings* (1976) 35: 2480-2485. Cited in ref. 87g.

87j. V.G. Zannoni and P.H. Sato, *Federation Proceedings* (1976) 35: 2464-2469. Cited in ref. 87g.

87k. G.C. Becking, *Canadian Jrl. of Physiology and Pharmacology* (1973) 51: 6-11. Cited in ref. 87g.

87l. A.G. Wade et al., *Biochemical Pharmacology* (1969) 18: 2288-2292. Cited in ref. 87g.

87m. Attallah Kappas et al., *Clinical Pharmacology and Therapeutics* (1976) 20, no. 6: 643-653.

87n. Attallah Kappas et al., *Clinical Pharmacology and Therapeutics* (1978) 23, no. 4: 445-450.

87p. Y.E. Harrison and W.L. West, *Biochem. Pharmacol.* (1971) 20: 2105-2108. Cited in ref. 87n.

87q. E.J. Pantuck et al., *Science* (1975) 187: 744-746. Cited in ref. 87n.

87r. T.C. Campbell and J.R. Hayes, *Pharmacological Reviews* (1974) 26: 171-199. Cited in ref. 87g.

87s. J.C. Son-Lucero et al., *Revue Canadienne de Biologie* (1973) 32 supp.: 69-75. Cited in ref. 87g.

87t. A. Douglas Bender, *Jrl. of the American Geriatrics Society* (1964) 12: 114-134.

87u. D.J. Smithard and M.J.S. Langman, *British Jrl. of Pharmacology* (1978) 5: 181-185.

88. James Greenwood, Jr., *Medical Annals of the Dist. of Columbia* (1964) 33: 274-276.

89. M. Smethurst et al., *Acta Vitaminologica et Enzymologica* (1981) N.S. 3, no. 1: 8-11.

89a. T.K. Basu et al., *Acta Vitaminologica et Enzymologica* (1978) 32: 45-49.

89b. G. Ungar, *Nature* (June 6, 1942) 149: 637-638.

90. John A. Wolfer et al., *Surgery, Gynecology and Obstetrics* (1947) 84: 1-15.

90a. Nancy King and Cleon W. Goodwin, Jr., *Jrl. of the Amer. Dietetic Assn.* (1984) 84, no. 8: 923-925.

91. William W. Coon, *Surgery, Gynecology and Obstetrics* (1962) 114: 522-534.

92. Thomas T. Irvin and Dilip K. Chattopadhyay, *Surgery, Gynecology and Obstetrics* (1978) 147: 49-55.

93. T.V. Taylor, *Lancet* (Sept. 7, 1974): 544.

94. W.M. Ringsdorf, Jr., and E. Cheraskin, *Oral Surgery* (1982) 53: 231-236.

94a. David H. Klasson, *New York State Jrl. of Medicine* (1951) 51: 2388-2392.

95. E.S. Wilkins and M.G. Wilkins, *Experientia* (1979) 35: 244-246.

95a. J.F. Rinehart et al., *Proc. of the Society for Experimental Biology and Medicine* (1936) 35, no. 2: 347-350.

95b. Edith R. Schwartz, *Internationale Zeitschrift für Vitamin und Ernahrungsforschung* (1984) 26: 141-146.

96. C. Alan B. Clemetson, *Jrl. of Nutrition* (1980) 110: 662-668.

97. Victor D. Herbert, *Jrl. of the Amer. Pharmaceutical Assn.* (Dec., 1977) 17, no. 12: 764-766.

98. W.A. Cochrane, *Canadian Medical Assn. Jrl.* (Oct. 23, 1965) 93, no. 17: 893-899.

99. E.P. Samborskaja and T.C. Ferdman, *Bulletin of Experimental Biology and Medicine* (1966) 62, no. 8: 96-98. English Translation published in 1967: 934-935.

100. Archie Kalokerinos, cited by James O. Woolliscroft, *DM—Disease-a-Month* (1983) 29, no. 5: 17-18.

101. Constance Spittle, *Amer. Heart Jrl.* (Sept., 1974) 88: 387-388.

102. Constance Spittle, *Jrl. of Clinical Pathology* (1973) 27: 513.

103. E. Ginter, *International Jrl. for Vitamin and Nutrition Research* (1979) 49: 406-412.

104. George V. Vahouny, *Federation Proceedings* (1982) 41: 2801-2806.

104a. James N. Thomas et al., *British Jrl. of Nutrition* (1984) 51: 339-345.

105. Irma H. Ullrich et al., *Amer. Jrl. of Clinical Nutrition* (1982) 36: 1-9.

105a. R.E. Hughes, *Human Nutrition: Clinical Nutrition* (1986) 40C: 81-86.

105b. R.F. Hughes and E. Jones, *Annals of Human Biology* (1985) 12: 325-332. Cited in ref. 105a.

106. C.J. Bates, *Lancet* (Sept. 17, 1977): 611.

107. Virginia E. Peterson, *Amer. Jrl. of Clinical Nutrition* (1975) 28: 584-587.

108. Gregory E. Johnson and S. Scott Obenshain, *Amer. Jrl. of Clinical Nutrition* (Oct., 1981) 34: 2088-2091.

109. Abdur R. Khan and Frank A. Seedarnee, *Atherosclerosis* (1981) 39: 89-95.

110. V.D. Joshi et al., *Ind. Jrl. Physiol. Pharmacy* (Oct.--Dec., 1981) 25: 348-350.

111. M.L. Burr et al., *Human Nutrition: Clinical Nutrition* (1982) 36C: 135-139 and 399-400.

111a. Eunsook T. Koh, *Oklahoma State Medical Assn. Jrl.* (1984) 77: 197-182.

111b. Mitsuki Yoshioka et al., *International Jrl. for Vitamin and Nutrition Research* (1984) 54: 343-347.

111ba. F. Erden et al., *Acta Vitaminologica et Enzymologica* (1985) 7, no. 1-2: 131-138.

111c. Hilary M. Dobson et al., *Scottish Medical Jrl.* (1984) 29: 176-182.

112. David E. Holloway et al., *Biochemical and Biophysical Research Communications* (Oct. 30, 1981) 102: 1283-1289.

960 The Reverse Effect

113. S.K. Kamath et al., *Federation Proceedings* (1978) 36: 1114.
113a. N. Saha and Py Tan, *Singapore Medical Jrl.* (1983) 24, no. 3: 150-151.
114. G.W. Evans, *Physiology Reviews* (1979) 53: 535.
115. David B. Milne et al., *Amer. Jrl. of Clinical Nutrition* (1981) 34: 2389-2393.
116. S. Kamath et al., *Federation Proceedings* (1978) 37: 589.
117. Johan R. Beetens and Arnold G. Herman, *British Jrl. of Pharmacology* (1983) 80: 249-254.
118. Emil Ginter, *Lancet* (Nov. 27, 1971): 1198-1199.
119. D. Kritchevsky et al., *Experientia* (1984) 40: 350-351.
120. Bandaru S. Reddy et al., in *Mechanisms of Tumor Promotion and Carcinogens* (vol. 2 of *Carcinogenesis—A Comprehensive Survey*) ed. T.L. Slaga, A. Sivak and R.K. Boutwell (New York: Raven Press, 1978).
121. B.I. Cohen et al., *Proceedings of the Amer. Cancer Research/Amer. Society of Clinical Oncology* (1978) 19: 48.
122. Dimitrios A. Linos et al., *Lancet* (Aug. 22, 1981): 379-381.
123. David E. Holloway and Jerry M. Rivers, *Jrl. of Nutrition* (1981) 111: 412-424.
124. D.E. Holloway and J.M. Rivers, *Jrl. of Nutrition* (1984) 114: 1370-1376.
124a. K. Jahan et al., *Bangladesh Medical Research Council Bulletin* (1984) 10, no. 1: 24-28.
124b. S. Banic, *Nature* (1975) 258: 153-154.
124c. G. Petroutsos and Y. Pouliquen, *Ophthalmic Research* (1984) 16: 185-189.
125. Michele Virno et al., *Eye, Ear, Nose and Throat Monthly* (1967) 46: 1502-1508.
126. Michele Virno, *Amer. Jrl. of Ophthalmology* (1966) 62: 824-833.
127. Von C. Hilsdorf, *Klinische Monatsblatter für Augenheilkunde* (1967) 150: 352-358.
128. E. Linner, *Acta Ophthalmologica* (1964) 42: 932-933.
128a. Von M. Gnädinger and J. Willome, *Klinische Monatsblatter für Augenheilkunde* (1968) 153: 352-356.
128b. R. Esilä et al., *Acta Ophthalmologica* (1966) 44: 631-636.
128c. Sumner L. Fishbein and Seymour Goodstein, *Annals of Ophthalmology* (1972) 4: 487-491.
128d. Claus W. Jungeblut, *Jrl. of Experimental Medicine* (1935) 62: 517-521.
128e. Claus W. Jungeblut, *Jrl. of Experimental Medicine* (1937) 65: 127-146.
128f. Claus W. Jungeblut, *Jrl. of Experimental Medicine* (1939) 70: 315-331.
128g. Fred R. Klenner, *Med. & Surg.* (1949) vol. 3, no. 7, cited by W.J. McCormick, *Archives of Pediatrics* (1952) 69, no. 4: 151-155.
128h. Albert B. Sabin, *Jrl. of Experimental Medicine* (1939) 69: 507-515.
128i. John A. Toomey, *American Jrl. of Diseases of Children* (1937) 53: 1202-1208.
128j. Douglas K. Reilly et al., *Advances in Neurology* (1983) 37: 51-60.
129. Roman J. Kutsky, *Handbook of Vitamins and Hormones* (New York: Van Nostrand Reinhold, 1973) p., 195.
130. Von W. Losert et al., *Arzneimittel Forschung* (1980) 30: 21-22.
131. K. Solanki et al., *Intl. Jrl. for Vitamin and Nutrition Research* (1981) 51: 186-187.
132. H. Goldenberg, *Biochem. and Biophysical Research Comm.* (1980) 94: 721-726.
132a. John w. Patterson, *Jrl. of Biological Chemistry* (1950) 183: 81-88.
133. C. Alan B. Clemetson, *Medical Hypothesess* (1976) 2: 193-194.
133a. Peter M.H. Kroneck et al., in *Ascorbic Acid: Chemistry, Metabolism, and Uses*, ed. Paul A. Seib and Bert M. Tolbert (Washington, D.C.: American Chemical Society, 1982) pp. 223, 224.
134. Robert Ryer III et al., *Jrl. of Clinical Nutrition* (1954) 2: 97-132 and 179-194. Name subsequently changed to *Amer. Jrl. of Clinical Nutrition*.
135. K.E. Sarji et al., *Thrombosis Research* (1979) 15: 639-650.
136. E.G. Knox, *Lancet* (1973) 1: 1465.
137. C. Cordova et al., *Atherosclerosis* (1982) 41: 15-19.
138. Morimitsu Nishikimi, *Biochemical and Biophysical Research Communications* (1975) 63, no. 2: 463-468.

139. Pi-Tai Chou and Ahsan U. Khan, *Biochemical and Biophysical Research Communications* (1983) 115, no. 3: 932-937.

139a. Benton H.J. Bielski and Helen W. Richter, *Annals of the N.Y. Academy of Sciences* (1975) 258: 231-237.

139b. R.W. Fessenden and N.C. Verma, *Biophysical Jrl.* (1978) 24: 93-101.

139c. V.N.R. Kartha and S. Krishnamurthy, *International Jrl. for Vitamin and Mineral Research* (1978) 48: 38-43.

139d. Shambhu d. Varma et al., *Proceedings of the National Academy of Sciences* (1979) 76, no. 7: 3504-3506.

139e. J. Blondin et al., *Federation Proceedings* (March 1, 1986) 45, no. 3: 478 (abstract no. 1886).

140. J.A. Vinson et al., *Nutrition Reports International* (April, 1986) 33, no. 4: 665-668.

140a. Daniel T. Organisciak et al., *Investigative Ophthalmology and Visual Science* (1985) 26: 1580-1588.

140b. Zong-Yi Li et al., ibid: 1589-1598.

141. G.T. Terezhalmy et al., *Oral Surgery* (Jan., 1978) 45, no. 1: 56-62.

141a. Johanna Odrich, *New York State Dental Jrl.* (1983) 49: 676, 678.

141b. Tetsuo Nakamoto and Mark McCroskey, *Jrl. of Theoretical Biology* (1984) 108: 163-171.

141c. Tawfik M.A. ElAttar et al., *Prostaglandins, Leukotrienes and Medicine* (1982) 9: 25-34.

141d. J.P. Gutai et al., *American Jrl. of Cardiology* (1981) 48: 899-902. Cited in Wanju S. Dai et al., *American Jrl. of Epidemiology* (1981) 114, no. 6: 804-816.

141e. Ronald Ross et al., *Jrl. of the National Cancer Institute* (1986) 76, no. 1: 45-48.

141f. Roy C. Page and Hubert E. Schroeder, *Periodontitis in Man and Other Animals* (Basel, Switzerland: Karger, 1982) pp. 253-260.

141g. Amid I. Ismail et al., *Jrl. of the American Dental Assn.*, (Dec., 1983) 107: 927-931.

141h. S.N. Woolfe et al., *Jrl. of Clinical Periodontology* (1984) 11: 159-165.

141i. John L. Giunta, *Jrl. of the American Dental Assn.* (1983) 107: 253-256.

141j. John L. Giunta, cited in *Tufts University Diet and Nutrition Letter* (1984) 2, no. 4: 8.

142. James L. Dannenberg, *Jrl. of the Amer. Dental Assn.* (1982) 105: 172-173.

143. Chester Siegel et al., *Jrl. of Periodontology* (1982) 53: 453-455.

143a. K. Schmidt et al., *International Jrl. for Vitamin and Nutrition Research* (1983) 53: 77-86.

144. Libuse Stankova et al., *Annals of the N.Y. Academy of Sciences* (1975) 258: 238-242.

145. R.E. Hughes, *Proceedings of the Royal Society of Medicine* (1977) 70: 86-89.

145a. Ron B. H. Wills et al., *Jrl. of Agricultural and Food Chemistry* (1984) 32: 836-838.

146. L. Hammerstrom, *Acta Physiol. Scand.* (1966) supp. 289: 1-70.

147. Reynold Spector and A.V. Lorenzo, *Amer. Jrl. of Physiology* (1973) 225: 757-763.

148. G.R. Martin and Christyna E. Mecca, *Archives of Biochemistry and Biophysics* (1961) 93: 110-114.

149. Sven Erik Sjöstrand, *Acta Physiologica Scandinavica* (1970) supp. 356: 5-79.

149a. A.B. Rathi et al., *Acta Vitaminol. Enzymol.* (1984) 6, no. 2: 97-102.

150. I. Yamazaki et al., *Jrl. of Biological Chemistry* (1960) 235: 2444-2449.

151. I. Yamazaki et al., *Biochimica et Biophysica Acta* (1961) 60: 62-69.

151a. Carl Lagercrantz, *Acta Chem. Scand.* (1964) 18, no. 2: 562.

152. E.M. Baker et al., *Amer. Jrl. of Clinical Nutrition* (1966) 19, no. 6: 371-378.

153. Rikuro Sasaki et al., *Tohuku Jrl. of Experimental Medicine* (1982) 36: 113-119.

154. Rikuro Sasaki et al., *Jrl. of Gerontology* (1983) 38, no. 1: 26-30.

155. B. Leibovitz and B.V. Seigel, *Jrl. of Gerontology* (1980) 35: 45-56.

155a. S. Som et al., *Acta Vitaminol. Enzymol.* (1983) 5, no. 4: 243-250.

155b. Marina Scarpa et al., *Biochimica et Biophysica Acta* (1984) 801: 215-219.

155c. Y. Inada et al., *Biochemical and Biophysical Research Communications* (1985) 130, no. 1: 182-187.

155d. Hon-Wing Leung et al., *Biochimica et Biophysica Acta* (1981) 664: 266-272.

156. H. Abramson, *Jrl. of Biological Chemistry* (1949) 178: 178-183.

156a. Gottfried Haase and W.L. Dunkley, *Jrl. of Lipid Research* (1969) 10: 561-567.

156b. E.D. Wills, *Biochemical Jrl.* (1969) 113: 315-324.

156c. Subal Bishayee and A.S. Balasubramanian, *Jrl. of Neurochemistry* (1971) 18: 909-920.

157. O.P. Sharma and C.R. Krishna Murti, *Jrl. of Neurochemistry* (1976) 27: 299-301, at 300.

158. A.A. Barber, *Lipids* (1966) 1: 146-151.

159. A. Seregi et al., *Experientia* (1978) 34: 1056-1057.

159a. G.B. Kovachich and O.P. Mishra, *Experimental Brain Research* (1983) 50: 62-68.

159b. Ikuo Abe et al., *Sci. Rep. Res. Inst. Tokoku Univ.* (1979) 26, nos. 3 and 4: 39-45.

160. Athos Ottolenghi, *Archives of Biochemistry and Biophysics* (1959) 79: 355-363.

160a. John M.C. Gutteridge et al., *Biochemical Jrl.* (1979) 184: 469-472.

160b. Elizabeth H. Thiele and Jesse W. Huff, *Archives of Biochemistry and Biophysics* (1960) 88: 203-207.

160c. F. Edmund Hunter, Jr. et al., *Jrl. of Biological Chemistry* (1964) 239, no. 2: 604-613.

160d. Walter C. Brogan, III et al., *Environmental Health Perspectives (1981) 38: 105-110.*

160e. Albert W. Girotti et al., *Photochemistry and Photobiology* (1985) 41, no. 3: 267-276.

160f. Peter J. Hornsby and Joseph F. Crivello, *Molecular and Cellular Endocrinology* (1983) 30: 1-20.

160g. E.D. Wills in *Oxidative Stress,* ed. Helmut Sïes (New York: Academic Press, 1985) pp., 197-218, at 210.

160h. M.J. Barnes and E. Kodiecek, *Vitamins and Hormones* (1972) 30: 1-43. Cited in ref. 160g.

161. Linda H. Chen, *Amer. Jrl. of Clinical Nutrition* (June, 1981) 34: 1036-1041.

162. H.S. Loh et al., *Clinical Pharmacology and Therapeutics* (1974) 16: 390-408.

163. H.S. Loh and C.W.M. Wilson, *Lancet* (Jan. 16, 1971): 110-112.

163a. Masao Igarashi, *International Jrl. of Fertility* (1977) 22: 168-173.

163aa. Brian T. Miller and Theodore J. Cicero, *Life Sciences* (1986) 39: 2447-2454.

163b. Jan Kabrt, *Acta Universitatis Carolinae Medica* (1982) 28, no. 5/6: 345-368.

164. Joseph R. Prohaska and Dean A. Cox, *Jrl. of Nutrition* (1983) 113: 2623-2629.

165. Edwin C. Jungck et al., *Federation Proceedings* (1977) 6: 139.

166. P.K. Paul and P.N. Duttagupta, *Indian Jrl. of Experimental Biology* (Jan., 1978) 16: 18-21.

167. Andres Carballeira et al., *Metabolism* (Dec., 1974) 23, no. 12: 1175-1184.

168. P.F. Jackisch, *Chemical and Engineering News* (1971) 49: 86.

169. G.N. Schrauzer and W.J. Rhead, *International Jrl.: Vitamin and Nutrition Research* (1973) 73: 201-211.

170. N.J. Chinoy and R.P. Buch, *Indian Jrl. of Experimental Biology* (Oct., 1977) 15: 921-922.

170a. A. Srivastava et al., *Andrologia* (1983) 15, no. 5: 431-435.

171. Earl B. Dawson et al., cited by Elizabeth Rasche Gonzalez, *JAMA* (May 27, 1983) 249, no. 20: 2747, 2751.

171a. M.H. Briggs, *Lancet* (Sept. 22, 1973): 677-678.

172. M.H. Briggs, *Lancet* (1973) 2: 1083.

173. A.E. Kitabchi, *Nature* (1967) 215: 1385-1386.

174. A.E. Kitabchi and W.C. Duckworth, *Amer. Jrl. of Clinical Nutrition* (1970) 23: 1012-1014.

174a. J. Richardson, *Medical Hypothesess* (1985) 17: 399-402.

174b. Qi-Wen Xie, *American Jrl. of Chinese Medicine* (1982) 9: 298-304.

175. Abbas E. Kitabchi et al., *Jrl. of Biological Chemistry* (1973) 248: 835-840.

176. Kyutaro Shimizu, *Biochimica et Biophysica Acta* (1970) 210: 333-340.

176a. Ingemar Björkhem et al., *Jrl. of Lipid Research* (1978) 19: 695-704.

177. Vallerie A. Wilbur and Brian L. Walker, *Lipids* (1978) 13: 116-120.

178. Willy A. Behrens and Rene Madere, *Jrl. of Nutrition* (April, 1980) 110, no. 4: 720-724.
179. Ingemar Björkhem et al.,*Jrl. of Lipid Research* (1978) 19: 695-704.
180. Stephen J. Pintauro and James G. Bergan,*Jrl. of Nutrition* (1982) 112: 584-591.
180a. D.A. Bailey et al., *Internat. Jrl. for Vitamin and Nutrition Research* (1970) 40: 435-441.
180b. George O. Gey, *JAMA* (1970) 211, no. 1: 105.
180c. H.W. Kirchoff, *Nutrio et Dieta* (1969) 11: 184-192.
181. R.E. Hughes et al., *British Jrl. of Nutrition* (1980) 43: 385-387.
182. H. Howald , B. Segesser and W.F. Körner, *Annals of the N.Y. Academy of Sciences* (1975) 258: 458-464.
182a. R. Buzina and K. Suboticanec, *Internationale Zeitschrift für Vitamin und Ernahrungsforschung* (1985) 27: 157-166.
183. R.V. Krishnamoorthy, *Proceedings of the Indian Academy of Sciences,* Section B (1969) 70, no. 1: 1-8.
183a. K. Suboticanec-Buzina et al., *International Jrl. for Vitamin and Mineral Research* (1984) 54: 55-60.
183b. Robert E. Keith and Elizabeth Merrill,*Jrl. of Sports Medicine* (1983) 23: 253-256.
183c. Melvin H. Williams,*Nutritional Aspects of Human Physical and Athletic Performance* (Springfield, IL: Charles C. Thomas, 1976).
184. T.K. Basu, *Chem-Biol. Interactions* (1977) 16: 247-250.
185. Edward Calabrese, *Nutrition and Environmental Health,* vol. 1, titled *The Vitamins* (New York: Wiley, 1980) p. 261.
185a. S.S. Epstein and Y. Bishop, *Environmental Research* (1977) 14: 187-193.
185b. Robert A. Roth and Lizabeth A. Dotzlaf,*Fundamental and Applied Toxicology* (1981) 1: 386-388.
186. Sidney S. Mirvish et al.,*Science* (1972) 177: 65-68.
186a. Joseph B. Guttenplan, *Nature* (July 28, 1977) 268: 368-370.
186b. E.P. Norkus and W.A. Kuenzig, *Carcinogenesis* (1985) 6, no. 11: 1593-1598.
186c. H.J. O'Connor et al., *Carcinogenesis* (1985) 6, no. 11: 1675-1676.
187. Thomas H. Jukes, *Food Nutrition News* (Oct.-Nov., 1976).
187a. Thomas H. Jukes, *New England Jrl. of Medicine* (Aug. 25, 1977) 297: 427-430.
188. *Wonderful Water For You!* (an undated advertising brochure of Mountain Valley Water, Hot Springs, Ark.).
188a. W.J. Mergens et al., from *N-Nitroso Compounds: Analysis, Formation and Occurrence,* ed. E.A. Walker, M. Castegnaro, L. Griciuti and M. Borzsonyi (Lyon, France: IARC Scientific Publications, 1980) pp. 259-267.
188b. Anders Kallner et al.,*Amer. Jrl. of Clinical Nutrition* (1979) 32: 530-539.
188c. Jean T. Snook et al., *Amer. Jrl. of Clinical Nutrition* (1983) 37: 532-539.
188d. D. Hornig et al., *International Jrl. for Vitamin and Nutrition Research* (1980) 50: 309-314.
188e. B.J. Rathbone et al., *Proc. of the Nutrition Society* (1986) 45, no. 2: 69A.
188f. D.H. Fine et al., from *N-Nitroso Compounds: Analysis, Formation and Occurrence* op. cit. (ref. 188c) pp. 541-548.
188g. Andre E.M. McLean et al., *Carcinogenesis* (1982) 3, no. 6: 707-709.
188h. Joseph B. Guttenplan,*Cancer Research* (1978) 38: 2018-2022.
189. J.H. Weisburger, *Internationale Zeitschrift für Vitamin und Ernahrungsforschung* (1985) 27: 381-402.
189a. C.L. Leuchtenberger et al., *Jrl. of Cell Biology* (1976) 70: 44A, abstract 132.
189b. K.N. Prasad and B.N. Rama in*Modulation and Mediation of Cancer by Vitamins,* ed. F.L. Meyskens and K.N. Prasad (Basel, Switzerland: Karger, 1983) pp. 244-257.
189c. C.W.M. Wilson, *Annals of the New York Academy of Sciences* (1975) 258: 355-376. Cited in ref. 189b.
190. W.M. Orr,*Biochemistry* (1967) 6: 2995-2999.

190a. K. Yamafuji et al., *Zeitschrift für Krebsforsching and Linische Onkologie* (1971) 76: 1-7.

190b. Kedar N. Prasad et al., *Proc. of the National Academy of Sciences* (1979) 76, no. 2: 829-832.

190c. L. Benade et al.,*Oncology* (1969) 23: 33-43. Cited in ref., 190b.

190d. F.S. Liotti et al., *Jrl. of Cancer Research and Clinical Oncology* (1984) 108: 230-232.

191. N. Bishun et al., *Oncology* (1978) 35: 160-162.

191a. N. Bishun et al., *Cytobios* (1979) 25: 29-36.

192. Stanley Bram et al., *Nature* (1980) 284: 629-631.

193. William F. Benedict et al., *Cancer Research* (1980) 40: 2796-2801.

193a. William F. Benedict et al., *Cancer Research* (1982) 42: 1041-1045.

193b. Sylvia Wassertheil-Smoller et al., *Amer. Jrl. of Epidemiology* (1981) 114, no. 5: 714-724.

193c. N. Pavic et al., *Medical Hypotheses* (1984) 15: 433-436.

193d. Seymour L. Romney et al., *American Jrl. of Obstetrics and Gynecology* (1985) 151, no. 7: 976-980.

194. Jerome L. DeCosse et al., *Surgery* (1975) 78: 608-612.

195. T. Logue and D. Frommer, *Gastroenterological Society of Australia* (Oct., 1980) 10, no. 5: 588.

195a. Frank E. Jones et al., *Jrl. of Surgical Oncology* (1984) 25: 54-60.

196. M. Eymard Poydock et al., *Experimental Cell Research* (1979) 47: 210-217.

196a. G. Kallistratos et al., *Naturwissenshaften* (1984) 71: 160-161.

196b. J.U. Schlegel et al.,*Jrl. of Urology* (1970) 103: 155-159.

196c. Mark S. Soloway et al., *Jrl. of Urology* (1975) 113, no. 4: 483-486.

197. I.A. Sadek and N. Abdelmegid,*Oncology* (1982) 39: 399-400.

197a. Wolcott B. Dunham et al., *Proc. National Academy of Sciences* (1982) 79: 7532-7536.

197b. David G. Morrison et al., *Nutrition and Cancer* (1981) 3, no. 2: 81-85.

198. L. Benade et al., *Oncology* (1969) 23: 33-43.

198a. Richard F. Wagner et al., *International Jrl. of Dermatology* (1984) 23, no. 7: 453-457.

198b. S. Bram et al., *Nature* (1980) 284: 629. Cited in ref., 198a.

198c. G.L. Fisher et al., *Cancer* (1981) 47: 1838. Cited in ref., 198a.

198d. P.G. Parsons and L.E. Morrison,*Cancer Research* (1982) 42: 3783. Cited in ref., 198a.

198e. J.M. Varga and L. Airoldi, *Life Sciences* (1983) 32: 1559. Cited in ref., 198a.

198f. Carleen Moore et al., *Pharmacologist* (1979) 21: 233.

199. Frances E. Knock et al., *Physiol. Chem and Physics* (1981) 13: 325-333.

199a. Wolcott B. Dunham et al., *Proceedings of the National Academy of Sciences* (Dec., 1982) 79: 7532-7536.

199b. Linus Pauling et al., *Proceedings of the National Academy of Sciences* (August, 1985) 82: 5185-5189.

200. Ewan Cameron and Linus Pauling, *Proceedings of the National Academy of Sciences* (Oct., 1976) 73, no. 10: 3685-3689.

200a. William D. DeWys, *Your Patient & Cancer* (May, 1982): 31, 35-36.

201. Robert H. Yonemoto et al., *Proceedings of the Amer. Assn. of Cancer Research* (1976) 17: 288.

202. E.I. Creagan et al., *New England Jrl. of Medicine* (1979) 301: 687-690.

203. Michael Jaffey,*Medical Hypotheses* (1982) 8: 49-84.

203a. Charles G. Moertel et al.,*New England Jrl. of Medicine* (1985) 312, no. 3: 137-141.

203b. Robert E. Wittes, *New England Jrl. of Medicine* (1985) 312, no. 3: 178-179.

203c. Linus Pauling, *How to Live Longer and Feel Better* (New York: W.A. Freeman Co., 1986) pp., 194-195, and 234.

203d. L. Pauling and E. Cameron, Press Release cited in the *International Clinical Nutrition Review* (1985) 5, no. 4: 163-165, at 164.

203e. Linus Pauling and Charles Moertel, *Nutrition Reviews* (Jan., 1986) 44, no. 1: 28-32.

203f. G. Meadows and R. Abdallah, *Federation Proceedings* (March 5, 1986) 45, no. 4: 1077 (abstract no. 5369).

204. Arthur W. Nienhuis, *New England Jrl. of Medicine* (Jan. 15, 1981) 304: no. 3: 170-171.

204a. H. Peter Roeser, *Seminars in Hematology* (1983) 20, no. 2: 91-100.

204b. B. Halliwell and J.M.C. Gutteridge, *Molecular Aspects of Medicine* (1985) 8: 89-193, at 137.

205. W.M. Orr, *Biochemistry* (Oct., 1967) 6: 2995-2999.

205a. Allan J. Davison et al., *Jrl. of Biological Chemistry* (1986) 261, no. 3: 1193-1200.

205b. Eilat Shinar et al., *Jrl. of Biological Chemistry* (1983) 258, no. 24: 14778-14783.

206. M.E. Briggs et al., *Lancet* (1973) 2: 201.

206a. Karl-Heinz Schmidt et al., *Amer. Jrl. of Clinical Nutrition* (1981) 34: 305-311.

206b. Howard Posner, *Annals of Internal Medicine* (Oct., 1984) 101, no. 4: 571-572.

207. R. Swartz, *Annals of Internal Medicine* (Oct., 1984) 101, no. 4: 572.

207a. Charles J. McAllister et al., *JAMA* (Oct. 5, 1984) 252, no. 13: 1684.

207b. P. Malathi and J. Ganguly, *Biochemical Jrl.* (1964) 92: 527-531.

207c. Yuk-Chow Ng et al., *Biochemical Pharmacology* (1985) 34, no. 14: 2525-2530.

207d. Petr Svoboda and Bedrich Mosinger, *Biochemical Pharmacology* (1981) 30: 427-432, at 430.

207e. Diane L. Bray and George M. Briggs, *Jrl. of Nutrition* (1984) 114: 920-928.

208. M.H. Briggs, *Nature* (1972) 238: 277.

209. M.H. Briggs, *British Medical Jrl.* (Dec. 5, 1981) 283: 1547.

209a. N. Subramanian, *Life Sciences* (1977) 20: 1479-1484.

210. John W. Dunne et al., *Life Sciences* (1983) 33: 1511-1517.

211. Thienchai Udomrath et al., *Blood* (Mar., 1977) 49: 471-475.

212. S. Basu et al., *Biochemical and Biophysical Research Communications* (1979) 90, no. 4: 1335-1340.

213. Vernon C. Bode, *Jrl. of Molecular Biology* (1967) 26: 125-129.

214. H.F. Stich et al., *Nature* (April 22, 1976) 260: 722-724.

215. Hirohisa Omura et al., *Jrl. Nutr. Sci. Vitaminol.* (1978) 24: 185-194.

215a. E.P. Norkus et al., *Mutation Research* (1983) 183-191.

216. Eiji Kimoto et al., *Cancer Research* (1983) 43: 824-828.

217. H.F. Stich et al., *Cancer Research* (Oct., 1979) 39: 4145-4151.

218. Miriam P. Rosin et al., *Cancer Letters* (1980) 8: 299-305.

219. H.F. Stich et al., *Food and Cosmetic Toxicology* (1980) 18: 497-501.

220. W. Donald MacRae and H. F. Stich, *Toxicology* (1979) 13: 169-174.

220a. Harlow K. Fischman et al., *Biological Psychiatry* (1984) 19, no. 3: 319-327.

221. S. M. Galloway and R.B. Painter, *Mutation Research* (1979) 60: 321-327.

222. G. Speit et al., *Mutation Research* (1980) 78: 273-278.

222a. G. Krishna et al., *Cancer Research* (June, 1986) 46: 2670-2674.

223. Yoshihide Suwa, *Mutation Research* (1982) 102: 383-391.

223a. J. Fielding Douglas and James Huff, *Jrl. of Toxicology and Environmental Health* (1984) 14: 605-609.

224. J.A. Migliozzi, *British Cancer Jrl.* (1977) 35: 448-453.

224a. Chan H. Park, *Cancer Research* (1985) 45: 3969-3973.

224b. C.H. Park, in *Modulation and Mediation of Cancer by Vitamins,* ed. F.L. Meyskens and K. Prasad (Basel, Switzerland: Karger, 1983) pp. 266-269. Cited in ref. 224a.

224c. C.H. Park et al., *Experimental Hematology* (1980) 8: 853-859. Cited in ref. 224a.

224d. C.H. Park et al., *Cancer Research* (1980) 70: 1062-1065.

224e. Herbert F. Pierson et al., *Cancer Research* (Oct., 1985) 45: 4727-4731.

224f. Toni Huwyler et al., *Immunology Letters* (1985) 10: 173-176.

225. H.A.J. Schut et al., *Molecular Pharmacology* (1978) 14: 682-692.

226. Saeko Sakai et al., *Cancer Research* (1978) 38: 2059-2067.

227. S. Banic, *Cancer Letters* (1981) 11: 239-242.

228. S.S. Mirvish et al., *Cancer Letters* (1976) 2: 101-108.

229. D.J. Korpatnick and H.F. Stich, *Biochemical and Biophysical Research Communications* (1980) 92, no. 1: 292-298.

230. Miriam P. Rosin et al., *Mutation Research* (1980) 72: 533-537.

230a. Shyh-Horng Chiou, *Jrl. of Biochemistry* (1984) 96: 1307-1310.

230b. Nathan A. Berger et al., *Jrl. of Clinical Investigation* (1985) 75: 702-709.

231. Thomas P. Stossel, *Jrl. of Immunology* (1982) 128: 2770-2772.

232. David E. Amacher and Simone C. Paillet, *Cancer Letters* (1981) 14: 151-158.

233. R.J. Shamberger et al., *Proceedings of the National Academy of Sciences* (1973) 70, no. 5: 1461-1463.

234. Kedar N. Prasad, *Life Sciences* (1980) 27: 278-280.

235. Hisayuki Kanamori et al., *Chem. Pharm. Bull.—Tokyo* (1980) 28: 3143-3144.

235a. Samuel M. Cohen et al., *Cancer Research* (1979) 39: 1207-1217.

235b. M.E. Trulson and H.W. Sampson, *Jrl. of Nutrition* (1986) 116: 1109-1115. Cited by C. Wayne Callaway, *JAMA* (Oct. 17, 1986) 256, no. 15: 2097-2099.

236. C.J. Schorah, *Proceedings of the Nutrition Society* (1981) 400: 151.

237. Jennie C. Brand, *Lancet* (Oct. 16, 1982): 873.

237a. D.S. Rathore, *Progressive Horticulture* (1984) 16, no. 1/2: 159-160. Cited in *Nutrition Abstracts and Reviews* (1985) Series A, 55, no. 11: 772.

237aa. O.O. Keshinro, *Nutrition Reports International* (1985) 31, no. 2: 381-387.

237b. S. Boyd Eaton and Melvin Konner, *New England Jrl. of Medicine* (1985) 312, no. 5: 283-298.

238. James D. Cook and Elaine Monsen, *Amer. Jrl. of Clinical Nutrition* (1977) 30: 235-241.

239. Leif Hallberg and Lena Rossander, *Amer. Jrl. of Clinical Nutrition* (1982) 35: 502-539.

239a. Linda H. Chen and Richard R. Thacker, *Federation Proceedings* (March 1, 1984) 43, no. 3: 394.

240. M.A.M. Hussain et al., *Lancet* (May 7, 1977): 977-979.

241. S.H. Rubin et al., *Jrl. of Pharmaceutical Sciences* (1976) 65: 963-968.

242. R.E. Vickery, *International Surgery* (1973) 58: 422-423.

243. E. Stewart Allen, *Current Therapeutic Research* (1969) 11, no. 12: 745-749.

244. Susanne Yung et al., *Jrl. of Pharmaceutical Sciences* (1982) 71, no. 3: 282-285.

245. J.T.L. Nicholson and F.W. Chornock, *Jrl. of Clinical Investigation* (1942) 21: 505-509.

246. J.S. Stewart and C.C. Booth, *Clinical Science* (1949) 27: 15-22.

246a. M.D.D. Bell et al., *Lancet* (Jan. 12, 1985): 71-73.

247. H.S. Loh et al., *Clinical Pharmacology and Therapeutics* (1974) 16: 390-408.

247a. F. Sadoogh-Abasian and D.F. Evered, *British Jrl. of Nutrition* (1979) 42: 15-20.

247b. U. Moses and F. Weber, *International Jrl. for Vitamin and Nutrition Research* (1984) 54: 47-53.

248. Thomas N. Imfeld, *Identification of Low Caries Risk Dietary Components* (Basel, Switzerland: Karger, 1983) pp. 142-164, at 155.

248a. C.M. Schweizer et al., *SSO* (1978) 8: 497. Cited in ref. 248.

248b. W.M. Cort, *Food Technology* (1974) 28: 60-66.

248ba. J.C. Bauernfeind, *Internationale Zeitschrift für Vitaminforschung* (1985) 27: 307-333.

248c. O. Garth Fitzhugh and Arthur A. Nelson, *Proceedings of the Society For Experimental Biology and Medicine* (1946) 61: 195-198.

249. *Kirk-Othmer Encyclopedia of Chemical Technology*, 2nd ed. (New York: Interscience Publishing, Inc., 1963) vol. 2, p. 594.

250. Ibid, 3rd ed. (1978) vol. 3.

251. *Code of Federal Regulations,* Title 21, (Washington, D.C.: Office of the Federal Register, 1982) p. 365, item no. 182.3149.

252. J.E.W. Davies et al., *Experimental Gerontology* (1977) 12, no. 5/6: 215-216.

252a. Harold R. Massie et al., *Gerontology* (1984) 30: 371-375.

253. L.H. Chen and M.L. Chang, *Internat. Jrl. for Vitamin and Nutrition Research* (1978) 29: 87-91.

253a. Lydi Sterrenberg et al., *Toxicology Letters* (1985) 25: 153-159.

254. L.H. Chen and M.L. Chang, *Jrl. of Nutrition* (1978) 108: 1616-1620.

255. Linda H. Chen and Richard R. Thacker,*Nutrition Research* (1984) 4: 657-664.

255a. G. Kelly and B.M. Watts, *Food Research* (1957) 22: 308-315. Cited in ref. 248ba.

255b. B.M. Watts and M. Faulkner, *Food Technology* (1954) 8: 158-161. Cited in ref. 248ba.

256. E.D. Wells, *Biochemical Jrl.* (1969) 113: 315-324.

257. O.P. Sharma and C.R. Krishna Murti, *Jrl. of Neurochemistry* (1976) 27: 299-301, at 301.

258. Harry B. Demopoulos et al.,*Acta Physiologica Scandinavica* (1980) supp. 492: 91-119.

259. Rolando F. Del Maestro,*Acta Physiologica Scandinavica* (1980) supp. 492: 142.

260. B.K. Nandi et al., *Jrl. of Nutrition* (1973) 103: 1688-1695.

260a. H.R. Massie et al., *Experimental Gerontology* (1976) 11: 37-41.

261. Howard B. Stein et al., *Annals of Internal Medicine* (1976) 84: 385-388.

262. William E. Mitch et al., *Clinical Pharmacology and Therepeutics* (1981) 29: 318-321.

263. D.P. Garrick et al., *Lancet* (Oct. 15, 1977): 820-821.

264. Solomon Garb, *Laboratory Tests in Common Use* (New York: Springer Pub. Co., 1976).

265. *CRC Handbook Series in Nutrition and Food,* Section E vol. 1, ed. Miloslav Rechcigl (Cleveland, Ohio: CRC Press, 1978) p. 68.

265a. Gerald A. Maguire and Christopher P. Price, *Clinical Chemistry* (1983) 29, no. 10: 1810-1812.

265b. Frances Talaska Fischbach, *A Manual of Laboratory Diagnostic Tests,* 2nd ed. (Philadelphia: J.B. Lippincott Co., 1984) pp. 832, 833, 842, 855, 856, 859.

266. Grace Y. Lo and Frank Konishi,*Amer. Jrl. of Clinical Nutrition* (1978) 31: 1397-1399.

266a. C.W.M. Wilson, *Annals of the N.Y. Academy of Sciences* (1975) 258: 355-376.

266b. Richard Harkness, *Drug Interactions Handbook* (Englewood Cliffs, N.J.: Prentice Hall, 1984) p. 41.

266c. U. Johansson and B. Akesson, *International Jrl. for Vitamin and Mineral Research* (1985) 55: 197-204.

267. Francis J. Peterson et al., *Nutrition Reports International* (Dec., 1982) 26: 1037-1043.

268. David B. Milne and Stanley T. Omaye, *International Jrl. for Vitamin and Nutrition Research* (1980) 50: 301-308.

269. Eric W. Martin, *Hazards of Medication* (Philadelphia: J.B. Lippincott Co., 1971) p. 231.

269a. Ibid, p. 829.

269b. Richard Harkness, *Drug Interactions Handbook,* op. cit. (ref. 266b) pp. 327.

270. George Rosenthal, *JAMA* (March 8, 1971) 215: 1671.

270a. George V. Rebec et al., *Science* (Jan. 25, 1985) 227: 438-440.

271. Anders Kallner et al., *Amer. Jrl. of Clinical Nutrition* (Mar., 1979) 32: 530-539.

272. Emil Ginter, *Amer. Jrl. of Clinical Nutrition* (Mar., 1980) 33: 538-539.

273. Emil Ginter, *World Review of Nutrition and Dietetics* (1979) 33: 104-141.

274. Jerry A. Tillotson and Richard J. O'Connor,*Amer. Jrl. of Clinical Nutrition* (1981) 34: 2397-2404.

275. J.E.W. Davies et al., *Proc. of the Nutrition Society* (1976) 5: 117A-117B.

276. Rhiannon S. Williams and R.E. Hughes, *British Jrl. of Nutrition* (1972) 28: 167. Cited by ref. 275.

277. T. Giza and J. Weclawowizc, *Int. Z. Vitam. Ernahrungforsch* (1960) 30: 327-332. Cited in ref. 282.

278. E. Cheraskin and W.M. Ringsdorf, Jr., *Int. Z. Vitam. Ernahrungsforch* (1968) 38: 114-117. Cited in ref. 282.

279. E. Cheraskin and W.M. Ringsdorf, Jr., *Int. Z. Vitam. Ernahrungsforsch* (1968) 38: 120-122. Cited in ref. 282.
280. W.M. Ringsdorf, Jr. and E. Cheraskin, *Quint. Inter.* (1978) 12: 81-85. Cited in ref. 282.
281. P.J. Leggott et al., *Jrl. of Dental Research* (1986) 65: 131-134. Cited in ref. 282.
282. *Nutrition Reviews* (Oct., 1986) 44, no. 10: 328-330.

Chapter 7—1413 References

1. Charles H. Hill and Gennard Matrone, *Federation Proceedings* (1970) 29, no. 4: 1474-1481.
1a. Hugh McA. Taggart et al., *Lancet* (Feb. 27, 1982): 475-478.
2. L.J. Deftos, *New England Jrl. of Medicine* (1980) 302: 1351-1353.
3. Seizo Yoshikawa et al., cited by Joan Arehart-Treichel, *Science News* (Aug. 22, 1983) 124: 140-141.
3a. *Geriatrics* (June, 1985) 40, no. 6: 23.
3aa. A. Pecile et al., *Experientia* (1975) 31: 332-333, as cited by Carla Bazzani et al., *Life Sciences* (1984) 34: 461-466.
3b. Robert D. Tiegs, et al., *New England Jrl. of Medicine* (1985) 312: 1097-1100.
3c. John D. Bauer, *Clinical Laboratory Methods* (St. Louis, Mo.: C.V. Mosby Co., 1982) p. 508.
3d. *Longevity Letter* (March, 1985) 3, no. 5: 9.
3e. Graham A. MacGregor, *Hypertension* (1985) 7: 628-637 at 632.
3f. *Cell Calcium* (1985) 6.
3g. W.P.T. James et al., *Lancet* (March 25, 1978): 638-639.
3h. Arthur C. Guyton, *Textbook of Medical Physiology,* 5th ed. (Philadelphia: W.B. Saunders Co., 1976) pp. 891-892.
3i. Joseph A. Johnston, *American Jrl. of Diseases of Children* (1944) 67: 265-274.
3j. Carroll E. Gross et al., *Lancet* (June 16, 1984): 1328-1330.
4. B. Sarkadi et al., *Haematologia* (1981) 14: 121-136.
5. Peter F. Hull et al., *Endocrinology* (1981) 109: 1677-1682.
6. Wai Yiu Cheung, *Federation Proceedings* (1982) 41: 2253-2257.
7. *The Role of Calcium in Biological Systems,* vol. III., ed. Leopold J. Anghileri and Anne Marie Tuffet-Anghileri (Boca Raton, Fla: CRC Press, 1982) pp. 3-44.
8. Laurence S. Bradham et al., *Biochemica et Biophysica Acta* (1970) 201: 250-260.
9. Richard D. Estensen et al., *Infection and Immunity* (1976) 13: 146-151.
10. G.M. Grodsky and L.L. Bennett, cited by S.L. Howell, *Biochemical Society Transactions* (1977) 5: 875-879.
10a. T. Verde et al., *Jrl. of Applied Physiology* (1982) 53, no. 6: 1540-1545.
10b. J.M. Lopes et al., *Jrl. of Applied Physiology* (1983) 54, no. 5: 1303-1305.
10c. C.J. Estler et al., *Psychopharmacology* (1978) 58: 161-166.
10d. Robert C. Schnackenberg, *American Jrl. of Psychiatry* (1973) 130, no. 7: 796-798.
11. R. Rahamimoff et al.,. in *Calcium Transport in Contraction and Secretion,* ed. E. Carafoli et al., (New York: Academic Press, 1982) pp. 253-259.
12. Mats Hammer et al., *Acta Obstet. Gynecol. Scand.* (1981) 60: 345-347.
13. H. Rottka et al., *Internat. Jrl. for Vitamin and Nutrition Research* (1981) 51: 373-379.
14. Jerzy Wrobel, *Acta Biochimica Polonica,* English Edition (1980) 27: 249-255.
15. Jerzy Wrobel, *Acta Physiol. Pol.* (1981) 32: 407-417.
16. J. Wrobel and G. Nagel, *Experientia* (Feb., 1979) 35: 1581-1582.
17. Hun Ki Min et al., *Federation Proceedings* (1966) 25: 917-921.
17a. Horace M. Perry III et al., *Calcified Tissue International* (1986) 38: 115-118.
17b. M. Markowitz et al., *Science* (1981) 213: 672-674. Cited in ref. 17a.
17c. W. Jubiz et al., *Jrl. of Clinical Investigation* (1972) 51: 2040. Cited in ref. 17a.
17d. Alice Kahn, *Medical Self-Care* (Winter, 1984) 27: 40-46.
18. *Biochemistry Correlations,* ed. Thomas M. Devlin (New York: Wiley, 1982) p. 1228.
19. J.R. Bullamore et al., *Lancet* (Sept. 12, 1970): 535-537.
20. *Nutrition Reviews* (1984) 40, no. 1: 27-28.
21. Harry W. Daniell, *Archives of Internal Medicine* (1976) 136: 298-304.
22. Robert P. Heaney et al., *American Jrl. of Clinical Nutrition* (1982) 36: 986-1013.
22a. Frances A. Tylavsky, *Federation Proceedings* (1984) 43, no. 3: 469.

22b. William A. Peck, cited in *Tufts University Diet & Nutrition Letter* (1984) 2, no. 4: 1-2.

22c. Stanton H. Cohn et al., *Calcified Tissue International* (1986) 38: 9-15.

22d. *High Technology* (June, 1986) 6, no. 6: 6.

23. *Food and Nutrition News* (Oct.-Nov., 1975).

24. W. A. Wallace, *Lancet* (June 25, 1983): 1413-1414.

25. Robert P. Heaney, *Western Jrl. of Medicine* (1981) 134: 74-75.

26. Louis V. Avioli, *Federation Proceedings* (1981) 40: 2418-2422.

26a. S. Boyd Eaton and Melvin Konner, *New England Jrl. of Medicine* (1985) 312, no. 5: 282-289.

27. R.P. Heaney, *Jrl. of Clinical Investigation* (1977) 60: 1135-1140.

28. Guy E. Abraham, *Jrl. of Applied Nutrition* (1982) 34: 69-73.

28a. L. Nilas et al., *British Medical Jrl.* (1984) 289: 1103-1106.

28b. R.P. Heaney and R.R. Recker, *American Jrl. of Clinical Nutrition* (1986) 43: 299-305.

29. J.C. Gallagher et al., *Jrl. of Clinical Investigation* (1979) 64: 729-736.

30. Hector F. DeLuca, *Annals of the N.Y. Academy of Sciences* (1980) 355: 1-17.

31. Herta Spencer et al., *Amer. Jrl. of Clinical Nutrition* (1982) 36: 776-787.

31a. Anthony Horsman et al., *New England Jrl. of Medicine* (Dec. 8, 1983) 309: 1405-1407.

32. Elizabeth Rasche Gonzalez, *JAMA* (Aug. 6, 1982) 248, no. 5: 513-514.

33. Robert R. Recker et al., *Annals of Internal Medicine* (Dec., 1977) 87: 649-655.

34. C.J. Lee et al., *Amer. Jrl. of Clinical Nutrition* (1981) 34: 819-823.

34a. John F. Aloia et al., *American Jrl. of Medicine* (1985) 78: 95-100.

34b. "Osteoporosis," *National Institutes of Health Consensus Development Conference Statement* (1984) 5, no. 3. Cited in ref. 34c.

34c. Gina Kolata, *Science* (August 1, 1986) 233: 519-520.

35. K.R. Hightower and V.N. Reddy, *Investigative Ophthalmology and Visual Science* (1982) 22: 263-267.

35a. B.K. Davis, *Proc. of the Society for Experimental Biology and Medicine* (1978) 157: 54-56.

35b. C.Y. Hong et al., *Lancet* (Dec. 22/29, 1984): 1449-1451.

35c. Tu Lin, *Jrl. of Andrology* (1984) 5, no. 3: 201-205.

35d. John H. Richardson et al., *Jrl. of Sports Medicine and Physical Fitness* (1980) 20: 149-151.

36. Ferris Pitts, Jr. and James J. McClure, *New England Jrl. of Medicine* (Dec. 21, 1967) 277: 1329-1336.

37. DeWayne Ashmead, *The Interpretation of Mineral Analysis of Hair* (Clearfield, Utah: Albion Laboratories, undated) p. 59.

38. Herta Spencer et al., *Amer. Jrl. of Clinical Nutrition* (Dec., 1978) 31: 2167-2180.

38a. J.H. Cummings et al., *Amer. Jrl. of Clinical Nutrition* (1979) 32: 2086-2093.

38b. George W. Bo-Linn et al., *Jrl. of Clinical Investigation* (1984) 73: 640-647.

38c. Susan E. Kelly et al., *Gastroenterology* (1984) 87: 596-600.

38d. Jia-Ju Zheng et al., *American Jrl. of Clinical Nutrition* (1985) 41: 243-245.

39. G.W. Hepner et al., *Amer. Jrl. of Digestive Diseases* (1976) 21: 527-532.

40. E.L. Krawitt, *Jrl. of Lab. and Clin. Medicine* (1975) 85: 665-671.

41. E.L. Krawitt, *Calcified Tissue Research* (1975) 18: 119-124. Name subsequently changed to *Calcified Tissue International*.

42. Lindsay H. Allen, *Amer. Jrl. of Clinical Nutrition* (April, 1982) 35: 783-808.

43. Milan Korcok, *JAMA* (1982) 247, no. 8: 1106, 1112.

44. J.F. Aloia, *Annals of Internal Medicine* (1978) 89: 356-358, cited by MIlan Korcok (ref. 43).

44a. Victor S. Schneider and Janet McDonald, *Calcified Tissue Int.* (1984) 36: S151-S154.

44b. G. Donald Whedon, ibid: S146-S150.

44c. J.J. Vitale et al., *Amer. Jrl. of Clinical Nutrition* (1959) 7: 13-22.

44d. Alan J. Fleischman et al., *Jrl. of Nutrition* (1967) 91: 151-158.

44e. A.I. Fleischman et al., *Jrl. of Nutrition* (1966) 88: 255-260.
44f. Marvin L. Bierenbaum et al., *Lipids* (1972) 7, no. 3: 202-206.
44g. Terry L. Bazzarre et al., *Nutrition Reports International* (1983) 28, no. 6: 1225-1232.
45. H. Yacowitz et al., *British Medical Jrl.* (May 22, 1965): 1352-1354.
45a. S. Renaud et al., in *Nutrition in the 80's: Constraints on Our Knowledge,* ed. Nancy Selvey and Philip L. White (New York: Alan R. Liss, Inc., 1981) pp. 361-381.
46. Yoshinori Itokawa, *Jrl. of Applied Physiology* (1974) 37: 835-839.
47. S. Ayachi, *Metabolism* (Dec., 1979) 78: 1234-1238.
48. David A. McCarron et al., *Science* (July 16, 1982) 217: 267-269.
49. Herbert G. Langford and Robert L. Watson, *Amer. Clin. Climatol. Assoc.* (1972) 83: 125-133.
50. David A. McCarron, *New England Jrl. of Medicine* (July 22, 1982) 307: 226-228.
50a. David A. McCarron et al., *Science* (June 29, 1984) 224: 1392-1398.
51. David A. McCarron, *Hypertension* (1980) 2: 162-168.
52. David A. McCarron, *Life Sciences* (1982) 30: 683-689.
53. Scott Ackley et al., *Amer. Jrl. of Clinical Nutrition* (1983) 38: 457-461.
53a. Mario R. Garcia-Palmieri et al., *Hypertension* (1984) 6: 322-328.
53b. David A. McCarron et al., *Clinical Research* (1984) 32, no. 2: 335A.
53c. Jose M. Belizan et al., *JAMA* (1983) 249, no. 9: 1161-1165.
53d. A.R. Whorton et al., *Lipids* (1984) 19, no. 1: 17-24.
54. Stanley M. Garn and Frances A. Larkin, *Science* (1983) 219: 112.
54a. Stephen Seely (1981) *Medical Hypotheses* 7: 907-918.
54b. Robert E. Popham et al., *Medical Hypotheses* (1983) 12: 321-329.
55. Hugo Kesteloot and Joozef Geboers, *Lancet* (April 10, 1982): 813-815.
55a. Harvey W. Gruchow et al., *JAMA* (1985) 253, no. 11: 1567-1570.
56. Mordecai P. Blaustein, *Amer. Jrl. of Physiology* (1977) 232, no. 3: C165-C173.
57. Manfred Blum et al., *JAMA* (1977) 237: 262-263.
57a. John H. Laragh and Mark S. Pecker, cited by Gina Kolata, *Science* (Aug. 17, 1984) 225: 705-706.
57b. John H. Laragh and Mark S. Pecker, *Annals of Internal Medicine* (1983) 95 (Part 2): 735-743.
57c. Andreas P. Niarchos and John H. Laragh, *Modern Concepts of Cardiovascular Disease* (1980) 49, no. 8: 43-48, at 47.
57d. Lawrence M. Resnick, John P. Nicholson and John H. Laragh, *Jrl. of Cardiovascular Pharmacology* (1985) 7, supp. 6: S187-S193.
58. Tony Christensson, *Lancet* (May 8, 1982): 1076.
59. A.K. Sangal and D.G. Beevers, *Lancet* (Aug. 28, 1982): 493.
59a. Paul Erne et al., *New England Jrl. of Medicine* (1984) 310, no. 17: 1084-1088.
59b. Frank F. Vincenzi, *Proc. of the Western Pharmacology Society* (1968) 11: 58-60.
59c. Paul W. Davis and Frank F. Vincenzi, *Life Sciences* (1971) 10, Part II: 401-406. Also discussed by R.H. Wasserman in *Metabolic Pathways,* 3rd ed., vol. 4, entitled *Metabolic Transport,* ed. Lowell E. Hokin (New York: Academic Press, 1972) pp. 355-357.
59d. H.G. McKercher et al., *Calcified Tissue International* (1985) 37: 602-604.
60. *New England Jrl. of Medicine* (Dec. 9, 1982) 307: 1525-1526.
61. William T. Clusin et al., *Lancet* (Feb. 5, 1983): 272-274.
61a. Kenneth L. Baughman, *American Jrl. of Medicine* (Feb. 28, 1986) 80, supp. 2B: 46-50.
62. Jane Kangilaski and Gail McBride, *JAMA* (1982) 247, no. 4: 1911-1917.
63. J.G. Lewis, *Adverse Drug Reaction Bulletin* (Aug., 1981) 89: 324-327.
64. Raymond J. Winquist et al., *Federation Proceedings* (1981) 40: 2852-2854.
65. D. Lynn Morris, *JAMA* (1983) 249: 3212-3213.
65a. David McCall et al., *Current Problems in Cardiology* (August, 1985) 10, no. 8: 3-68 (entire issue).
65b. Matthias Schramm and Robertson Towart, *Life Sciences* (1985) 37: 1843-1860.
65c. Dennis W. Schneck, *Rational Drug Therapy* (May, 1985) 19, no. 5: 1-6.

66. Henry A. Schroeder, *JAMA* (1960) 172: 1902-1908.
66a. Luciano C. Neri and Helen L. Johansen, *Annals of the New York Academy of Sciences* (1978) 304: 203-219.
66b. Denham Harman, *Age* (1984) 7: 111-131 at 115.
67. Marvin L. Bierenbaum et al., *Lancet* (May 3, 1975): 1008-1010.
67a. A. Richey Sharrett and Manning Feinleib,*Lancet* (July 12, 1975): 76.
67b. Marvin L. Bierenbaum, *Lancet* (July 12, 1975): 76.
68. L.C. Neri et al., *Lancet* (April 29, 1972): 931-934.
69. F.W. Stitt et al., *Lancet* (Jan. 20, 1973): 122-126.
70. A.A. Allen, cited by MIldred S. Seelig,*Amer. Jrl. of Clinical Nutrition* (Jan., 1974) 27: 59-79.
71. Mildred Seelig, *ibid.*
71a. J.R. Marier and L.C. Neri, *Magnesium* (1985) 4: 53-59.
71b. J. Durlach et al.,*Magnesium* (1985) 4: 5-15.
72. Earl B. Dawson et al.,*American Jrl. of Clinical Nutrition* (1978) 31: 1188-1197.
72a. George W. Comstock, *American Jrl. of Epidemiology* (1979) 110, no. 4: 375-400.
73. Fayez K. Ghishan et al., *Pediatric Research* (1982) 16: 566-568.
74. O.W. Vaughan and L.J. Filer, Jr., *Jrl. of Nutrition* (1960) 71: 10-14.
75. Adelle Davis, *Let's Get Well* (New York: Harcourt, Brace & World, Inc. 1965) p. 321.
75a. A.R.P. Walker, *American Jrl. of Clinical Nutrition* (June, 1986) 43: 969-971.
75b. S.M. Garn et al., *Ecol. Food Nutr.* (1980) 9: 135-138. Cited in ref. 75a.
75c. S.C. Stecksen-Blicks et al., *Acta Odontologica Scandinavica* (1985) 43: 59-67. Cited in ref. 75a.
75d. A.R.P. Walker et al., *Community Dentistry and Oral Epidemiology* (1981) 9: 37-43. Cited in ref. 75a.
75e. A.S. Richardson et al.,*Community Dentistry and Oral Epidemiology* (1977) 5: 227-230. Cited in ref. 75a.
76. Helen M. Linkswiler, *Federation Proceedings* (1981) 40: 2429-2433.
77. June L. Kelsay et al., *Amer. Jrl. of Clinical Nutrition* (Sept., 1979) 32: 1876-1880.
78. K.W. Heaton and E. W. Pomare, *Lancet* (Jan. 12, 1974): 49-50.
79. W. van Dokkum et al., *British Jrl. of Nutrition* (1982) 47: 451-460.
79a. N.-G. Asp, *British Jrl. of Nutrition* (1981) 46: 385-393.
79b. A.S. Truswell and Ruth M. Kay,*Lancet* (Feb. 14, 1976): 367.
79c. R.W. Kirby et al., *Amer. Jrl. of Clinical Nutrition* (1981) 106: 555, cited by David Kritchevsky,*Nutrition Reports International* (1984) 29, no. 6: 1353-1359.
79d. R.J. Heine et al., *Annals of Nutrition and Metabolism* (1984) 28: 201-206.
79e. A. Wise and D.J. Gilburt, *Food and Cosmetic Toxicology* (1980) 18: 643-648.
79f. S. Viola et al., *Nutrition Reports International* (1970): 367-375. Cited in ref. 79e.
80. John G. Reinhold et al., *Lancet* (Feb. 10, 1973): 283-288.
81. A.R. Walker et al.,*Biochemical Jrl.* (1948) 42: 452-462.
82. K.M. Henry and S.K. Kon,*Biochemical Jrl.* (1945) 39: 117-122.
83. Lindsay H. Allen,*Amer. Jrl. of Clinical Nutrition* (April 1982) 35: 783-808.
83a. David M. Slovik, *Special Topics in Endocrinology and Metabolism* (1983) 5: 83-148.
83b. Joseph T. Judd et al., *Seminars in Oncology* (1983) 10, no. 3: 273-280.
84. *Chemical & Engineering News* (Feb. 11, 1974) 52, no. 6: 14.
85. James L. Robinson and Debra B. Dombrowski, *Nutrition Research* (1983) 3: 407-415.
85a. Roberta P. Durschlag & James L. Robinson, *Journals of Nutrition* (April, 1980) 110, no. 4: 822-828.
85b. A. Denda et al., *Federation Proceedings* (1985) 44, no. 5: 1672.
85c. Robert R. Recker, *New England Jrl. of Medicine* (1985) 313, no. 2: 70-73.
85d. Richard Eastell, *New England Jrl. of Medicine* (Dec. 5, 1985) 313, no. 23: 1481-1482.
85e. Michael J. Nicar and Charles Y.C. Pak,*Jrl. of Clinical Endocrinology and Metabolism* (1985) 61, no. 2: 391-393.
85f. R.C. Puche et al., *Hormone and Metabolic Research* (1985) 17: 244-246.

85g. Eric S. Orwall, *Annals of Internal Medicine* (1982) 97, no. 2: 242-248.

86. O.J. Malm, *Scandinavian Jrl. of Clinical and Lab. Investigation* (1958) 10, supp. 36: 166-172.

87. Food and Drug Admin., cited in *Consumers Reports* (Sept., 1982) 47, no. 9: 478-479.

88. Per Rasmussen and Gro Ramsten Wesenberg, *Acta Odontologica Scandinavica* (1981) 39: 313-319.

89. H.J. Roberts, *New England Jrl. of Medicine* (Feb. 12, 1981) 304: 423.

90. H.J. Roberts, *New England Jrl. of Medicine* (May 28, 1981) 304: 1367.

91. *FDA Drug Bulletin* (April, 1982) 12, no. 1: 5-6.

92. Ivan Stockley, *Drug Interactions* (St. Louis, Mo.: Mosby Co., 1981) pp. 2 and 9.

92a. *The Pill Book,* ed. Lawrence D. Chilnick (Toronto, Canada: Bantam Books, 1982) pp. 205, 298.

93. A.B. Clarkson, Jr. and B.O. Amole, *Science* (June 18, 1982) 216: 1321-1323.

94. Herta Spencer, *Age* (1981) 4: 140.

94a. Richard Harkness, *Drug Interactions Handbook* (Englewood Cliffs, N.J.: Prentice Hall, 1984) p. 332.

95. Robert P. Heaney and Robert R. Recker, *Jrl. of Lab. and Clin. Medicine* (1982) 99: 40-55.

95a. Linda K. Massey and Tracy A. Berg, *Nutrition Research* (1985) 5: 1281-1284.

95b. James K. Yeh et al., *Jrl. of Nutrition* (1986) 116: 273-280.

96. Hector F. DeLuca, *Harvey Lectures* (1980) series 75: 333-379.

96a. Robert P. Heaney and Robert R. Recker, *Annals of Internal Medicine* (1985) 103: 516-521.

96b. Hunter Heath III and C. Wayne Callaway, *Annals of Internal Medicine* (Dec., 1985) 103, no. 6 (part I): 946-947.

96c. G.A. Reinhart and D.C. Mahan, *Jrl. of Animal Science* (1985) 61, suppl. no. 1: 298. Cited in *Nutrition Reviews* (Nov., 1985) 43: no. 11: 345-346.

96d. D.D. Hall et al., *Jrl. of Animal Science* (1985) 61, supp. no. 1: 298. Cited in *Nutrition Reviews* (Nov., 1985) 3, no. 11: 345-346.

97. B. Fleischhans, *Vnitri Lek* 27, no. 1: 98-102.

98. *American Pharmacy* (May, 1979) 19, no. 5: 23-24.

98a. Don R. Swanson, *Longevity Letter* (1985) 3, no. 5: 10.

98b. Marielle Gascon-Barre et al., *Annals of Nutrition and Metabolism* (1985) 29: 289-296.

99. Geoffrey J. Cleghorn and David L. Tudehope, *Australian Pediatric Jrl.* (1981) 17: 298-299.

99a. Lloyd T. Iseri and James H. French, *American Heart Jrl.* (1984) 108, no. 1: 188-193.

100. W.E. Criss and S. Kakiochi, *Federation Proceedings* (1982) 41: 2289-2291.

101. John L. Farber in *Progress in Liver Diseases,* vol. 7, ed. Hans Popper and Fenton Shaffner (New York: Grune and Stratton, 1982) pp. 347-360.

102. John L. Farber, *Life Sciences* (1981) 29: 1289-1295.

102a. H.L. Newmark et al., *Jrl. of the National Cancer Institute* (1984) 72, no. 6: 1323-1325.

102b. Michael J. Wargovich et al., *Carcinogenesis* (1983) 4, no. 9: 1205-1207.

102c. C.F. Tam and R.L. Walford, *Jrl. of Immunology* (1980) 125: 1665-1670. Cited by Ira T. Lott in *Annals of the New York Academy of Sciences* (1982) 396: 15-27.

103. Robert W. Mercer and Philip B. Dunham, *Biochimica et Biophysica Acta* (1981) 648: 63-70.

104. H. Luoma and T. Nuuja, *Caries Research* (1977) 11: 100-108.

105. David A. McCarron, *New England Jrl. of Medicine* (1982) 307: 226-228.

106. Sverker Ljunghall and Hans Hedstrand, *British Medical Jrl.* (Feb. 26, 1977): 553-554.

107. David B. N. Lee and Charles R. Kleeman, *Clinical Digest* (1976) 5, no. 3: 1-6.

107a. A. Srivastava et al., *Andrologia* (1983) 15, no. 5: 431-435.

108. Eric Reiss et al., *Jrl. of Clinical Investigation* (1970) 49: 2146-2149.

109. B.E.C. Nordin and Russell Fraser, *Lancet* (April 30, 1960): 947-951.

110. A. Hogan, *Jrl. of Nutrition* (1950) 41: 203-212.

111. Robert P. Heaney and Robert R. Recker, *Jrl. of Laboratory and Clinical Nutrition* (1982) 99: 46-55.

112. Herta Spencer et al., *Jrl. of Nutrition* (1978) 108: 447-457.

112a. Sally A. Schuette and Helen M. Linkswiler, *Jrl. of Nutrition* (1982) 12: 338-349.

112b. C.R. Anand and H.M. Linkswiler, *Jrl. of Nutrition* (1974) 104: 695-700. Cited by ref. 112a.

112c. H.M. Linkswiler et al., *Transactions of the New York Academy of Sciences* (1974) series 2, 36: 333-340. Cited by ref. 112a.

112d. Y. Kim and H.M. Linkswiler, *Jrl. of Nutrition* (1979) 109: 1399-1404. Cited by ref. 112a.

112e. M. Hegsted and H.M. Linkswiler, *Jrl. of Nutrition* (1981) 111: 241-251. Cited by ref. 112a.

112f. M. Hegsted et al., *Jrl. of Nutrition* (1981) 111: 553-562. Cited by ref. 112a.

112g. H.C. Sherman, *Jrl. of Biological Chemistry* (1920) 44: 21-27.

113. R.S. Goldsmith and S.H. Ingbar, *New England Jrl. of Medicine* (1966) 174: 1-7.

114. R.S. Goldsmith et al., *Jrl. of Clin. Endocrinology* (1976) 43: 523-532.

115. John G. Reinhold, *Jrl. of Nutrition* (1976) 106: 493-503.

116. Suzanne M. Snedeker et al., *Jrl. of Nutrition* (1982) 112: 136-143.

117. D.A. Isenberg et al., *Lancet* (Jan. 2, 1982): 55.

118. Karl L. Insogna, *JAMA* (Dec. 5, 1980) 244, no. 22: 2544-2546.

118a. J.M. Cam et al., *Clinical Science and Molecular Medicine* (1976) 51: 407-414.

118b. Marion D. Francis et al., *Science* (1969) 165: 1264-1266.

118c. C.J. Preston et al., *British Medical Jrl.* (Jan. 11, 1986) 292: 79-80.

119. A. Chiarenza and C. Gallope, *Contact Dermatitis* (1981) 7: 846-847.

120. M.C. Steele and F. A. Ive, *British Jrl. of Dermatology* (1982) 106: 477-479.

120a. Makin D. Maines and Attallah Kappas, *Science* (1977) 198: 1215-1221.

120b. Martin O'Connell et al., *Biochemical Jrl.* (1986) 234: 727-731.

120c. David B. Staab et al., *Jrl. of Nutrition* (1984) 114: 840-844.

120d. *Nutrition Reviews* (1984) 42, no. 4: 167-168.

121. E.J. Underwood, *Trace Elements in Human and Animal Nutrition,* 4th ed. (New York: Academic Press, 1977) p. 16.

122. James M. Stengle and Arthur L. Schade, *British Jrl. of Haematology* (1957) 3: 107-124.

123. Giorgio Casale et al., *Age and Ageing* (1981) 10: 115-118.

124. K. Hoyer, *Acta Med. Scand.* (1944) 119: 562-576 and 577-585.

125. W.F. Wiltink et al., *Clinica Chimica Acta* (1973) 49: 99-104.

126. Bernard E. Statland et al., *Clinical Biochemistry* (1976) 9: 26-29.

127. Rita Long et al., *Clinical Chemistry* (1978) 24: 842.

127a. H.S. Lo and C.W.M. Wilson, *International Jrl. of Vitamin and Nutrition Research* (1971) 41: 253-258. Cited in ref. 127b.

127b. C.W.M. Wilson in *Chronobiology,* ed. Lawrence E. Scheving, Franz Halberg and John E. Pauly (Tokyo, Japan: Igaku Shoin, 1974) pp. 249-255.

128. M. Staubli, *Schweizerische Medicinische Wochensehrift* (1981) 111: 1394-1398.

129. Committee on Iron Deficiency, Council on Foods and Nutrition, *JAMA* (Feb. 5, 1968) 203, no. 6: 407-412.

130. *British Medical Jrl.* (1978) 2: 1317.

130a. Stephen S. Entman et al., *Amer. Jrl. of Obstetrics and Gynecology* (1982) 143: 398-404.

130b. S.M. Ross et al., *South African Medical Jrl.* (1981) 60: 698-701.

130c. *Nutrition Survey—Republic of Paraguay, May-August, 1965,* National Center for Chronic Disease Control, Public Health Service, Bethesda, Md. (Washington, D.C.: U.S. Govt. Printing Office, 1967) pp. 221-227, 241.

130d. Robert E. Hodges et al., *Amer. Jrl. of Clinical Nutrition* (1978) 31: 876-885.

130e. Robert E. Hodges et al., *Annals of the N.Y. Academy of Sciences* (1980) 355: 58-61.

131. J.M. White, *Lancet* (Sept. 8, 1984): 573.
132. O. Giardini et al., *Acta Vitaminologica et Enzymologica* (1985) 7, no. 1-2: 55-60.
132a. James A. Halsted, *American Jrl. of Clinical Nutrition* (1968) 21, no. 12: 1384-1393.
132b. R.S. Lourie et al., *Children* (1963) 10: 143. Cited in ref. 132a.
132c. Kenneth Redman, *Quarterly Jrl. of Crude Drug Research* (1980) 18, no. 4: 153-157.
132d. Benjamin H. Ershoff and Sol Bernick, *Jrl. of Dental Research* (1968) 47, no. 2: 260-271.
133. Erick Dillman et al., *Amer. Jrl. of Physiology* (1980) 239: R377-R381.
134. R.K. Chandra and A.K. Suraya, *Jrl. of Pediatrics* (1975) 86: 899-902.
135. R.K. Chandra et al., *Iron Metabolism*, Ciba Foundation Symposium 51-new series (New York: Elsevier-Excerpta Medica, 1977) pp. 249-268.
136. Akio Shiraishi and Tadashi Arai, *Sabouraudia* (1979) 17: 79-83.
137. J.J. Bullen et al., *Current Topics in Microbiology and Immunology* (1978) 80: 1-35.
138. *Lancet* (Aug. 10, 1974): 325-326.
139. J. Fletcher et al., *Jrl. of Infectious Diseases* (1975) 131, no. 1: 44-50.
139a. J.M. Higgs and R.S. Wells, *British Jrl. of Dermatology* (1972) 86: 88. Cited by James R. Humbert and Linda L. Moore, *Jrl. of Pediatric Gastroenterology and Nutrition* (1983) 2, no. 3: 403-406.
140. J.J. Bullen et al., *British Medical Jrl.* (1972) 1: 69-75.
141. J.J. Bullen, *Reviews of Infectious Diseases* (1981) 3: 1127-1138.
142. Joseph J. Vitale et al., *Advances in Experimental Medicine and Biology* (1977) 91: 229-242.
142a. Selwyn A. Breizman et al., *Advances in Experimental Medicine and Biology* (1981) 35: 155-181.
142b. S.H. Kon, *Medical Hypotheses* (1978) 4: 445-471.
143. Raymond J. Bergeron et al., *Jrl. of Nutrition* (1985) 115: 369-374.
143a. D.B. Clement and L.L. Sawchuk, *Sports Medicine* (1984) 1: 65-74.
143b. A. Hunding et al., *Acta Med. Scand.* (1981) 209: 1637-1640, cited by ref. 143c.
143c. Edward Colt and Budd Heyman, *Jrl. of Sports Medicine* (1984) 24: 13-17.
143d. Edwin W. Hirsch, *Impotence and Frigidity* (New York: Citadel Press 1966)
143e. Darrell R. van Campen and Ross M. Welch, *Jrl. of Nutrition* (1980) 110: 1618-1621. Cited in *Nutrition Reviews* (Jan., 1986) 44, no. 1: 22-24.
144. B.C. Mehta et al., *Indian Jrl. of Medical Sciences* (1980) 34: 107-110.
144a. Michael B. Jacobs, *JAMA* (July 27, 1984) 252, no. 4: 481-482.
145. C. Martinez-Torres and M. Layrisse, *Clinics in Haematology* (June, 1973) 2, no. 2: 339-352.
146. *Nutrition Reviews* (Sept., 1973) 31, no. 9: 275-277.
146a. Bonnie M. Anderson et al., *Amer. Jrl. of Clinical Nutrition* (1981) 34: 1042-1048.
146b. H. Peter Roeser, *Seminars in Hematology* (1983) 20, no. 2: 91-100.
146c. Elizabeth Finley and Florian Cerklewski, cited in *Science News* (Oct. 29, 1983) 124, no. 18: 281.
146d. Judith L. Sutton et al., *Biochemical Pharmacology* (1982) 31, no. 8: 1591-1594.
147. James D. Cook and Elaine R. Monsen, *Amer. Jrl. of Clinical Nutrition* (Feb., 1977) 30: 235-241.
148. Carl V. Moore in *Modern Nutrition in Health and Disease,* 5th ed., ed. Robert S. Goodhart and Maurice E. Shils (Philadelphia: Lea & Febiger, 1973) pp. 301-302.
149. Luis A. Mejia and Guilermo Arroyave, *Amer. Jrl. of Clinical Nutrition* (June 1982) 36: 87-93.
150. Luis A. Mejia et al., *Jrl. of Nutrition* (1979) 109: 129-137.
151. Leif Hallberg and Lena Rossander, *Human Nutrition: Clinical Nutrition* (1982) 36A: 116-123.
152. Maureen O'Keane et al., *Jrl. of Alcohol* (1972) 7: 6-11.
153. Thein-Than et al., *Amer. Jrl. of Clinical Nutrition* (1975) 28: 1348.
154. Karen S. Simpson et al., *Amer. Jrl. of Clinical Nutrition* (1981) 34: 1469-1478.

155. J. Edward Hunter, *Jrl. of Nutrition* (1981) 111: 841-843.

156. W. Frolich in *Nutritional Bioavailability of Iron,* ed. Constance Kies (Washington, D.C.: American Chemical Soc., 1982) pp. 163-171.

157. S.J. Fairweather-Tait, *British Jrl. of Nutrition* (1982) 47: 243-249.

157a. Abdullah M. Thannoun et al., *Federation Proceedings* (1985) 44, no. 5: 1673 (item 7385).

158. D.L. McWhinnie and A.J. Mack, *Human Nutrition: Clinical Nutrition* (1982) 36C: 315-318.

159. R.J. Dobbs and I. McLean Baird, *British Medical Jrl.* (1977) 1641-1642.

160. James D. Cook et al., *Amer. Jrl. of Clinical Nutrition* (1981) 34: 2622-2629.

161. Josephine Miller and Ifendu Nnanna, *Jrl. of Nutrition* (1983) 113: 1169-1175.

162. E. R. Morris and F.E. Green, *Jrl. of Nutrition* (1972) 102: 901-908.

163. Jean Bowering et al., *Jrl. of Nutrition* (1977) 107: 1687-1693.

164. Wim van Dokkum et al., *Annals of Nutrition and Metabolism* (1983) 27: 361-369.

164a. Leif Hallberg et al., *Human Nutrition: Applied Nutrition* (1986) 40A: 97-113.

165. C. Kies and L. McEndree in *Nutritional Bioavailability of Iron,* op. cit (ref. 156) pp. 183-198.

165a. Hadar Merhav et al., *American Jrl. of Clinical Nutrition* (1985) 41: 1210-1213.

166. Timothy A. Morck et al., *Amer. Jrl. of Clinical Nutrition* (1983) 37: 416-420.

167. Leif Halberg, *Annual Reviews of Nutrition* (1981) 1: 123-147.

168. E.D. Willis, *Biochimica et Biophysica Acta* (1965) 98: 238-251.

169. David N.S. Kerr and Stanley Davidson, *Lancet* (Sept. 6, 1958): 489-492.

170. Paul Seligman et al., cited in *Tufts University Diet & Nutrition Letter* (1984) 1, no. 12: 1.

170a. Mary A. O'Neil-Cutting and William H. Crosby, *JAMA* (March 21, 1986) 255, no. 11: 1468-1470.

171. Norton J. Greenberger, *Amer. Jrl. of Clinical Nutrition* (1973) 26: 104-112.

171a. Richard Harkness, *Drug Interactions Handbook,* op. cit. (ref. 94a) p. 19.

171b. Ananda S. Prasad et al., *Amer. Jrl. of Clinical Nutrition* (1975) 28: 377-384.

171c. Erica P. Frassinelli-Gunderson and Sheldon Margen, *American Jrl. of Clinical Nutrition* (1985) 41: 703-712.

172. Manabu Kunimoto et al., *Biochimica et Biophysica Acta* (1981) 646: 169-178.

173. John J. Dougherty et al., *Jrl. of Nutrition* (1981) 111: 1784-1796.

174. Young H. Lee et al., *Jrl. of Nutrition* (1981) 111: 2195-2202.

175. David K. Melhorn and Samuel Gross, *Jrl. of Laboratory and Clinical Medicine* (Nov., 1969) 74, no. 1: 789-802.

176. R.G. Kay, *Jrl. of Human Nutrition* (1981) 35: 25-36.

176a. Osaki Shigemasa et al., *Jrl. of Biological Chemistry* (1966) 241, no. 12: 2746-2751.

177. David R. Blake et al., *Lancet* (Nov. 21, 1981) 1142-1144.

178. B. Sweder van Asbeck et al., *British Medical Jrl.* (1982) 284: 542-544.

178a. Adrian Bomford and Roger Williams, *Quarterly Jrl. of Medicine* (1976) New Series, XLV, 180: 611-623.

178b. D.R. Blake et al., *Annals of the Rheumatic Diseases* (1983) 42: 89-93. Cited in ref. 178c.

178c. B. Halliwell and J.M.C. Gutteridge, *Molecular Aspects of Medicine* (1985) 8: 89-193, at 139.

179. James L. Robotham, *Amer. Jrl. of Diseases of Children* (1980) 134: 875-879.

180. Jerome L. Sullivan, *Lancet* (June 13, 1981): 1293-1294.

180a. Walter J. Decker et al., *Veterinary and Human Toxicology* (1981) 23, supp. 1: 33-34.

180b. L.E. Bottiger and L.A. Carlson, *British Medical Jrl.* (Sept.23, 1972): 731-733.

180c. P.C. Elwood et al., *Lancet* (Mar. 21, 1970): 589-591.

181. Eugene D. Weinberg, *Science* (May 31, 1974) 184: 952-956.

182. Ronald J. Elin and Sheldon M. Wolff, *Jrl. of Immunology* (1974) 112: 737-745.

182a. James N. Fordham, *JAMA* (1985) 254, no. 8: 1006-1008.

183. Jessie R. Ashe et al., *Amer. Jrl. of Clinical Nutrition* (1979) 32: 286-291.
184. Maurice E. Shils in *Modern Nutrition in Health and Disease,* 5th ed., op. cit., p. 287.
185. Mildred S. Seelig, *Amer. Jrl. of Clinical Nutrition* (1964) 14: 342-390.
186. T.W. Anderson et al., in *Magnesium in Health and Disease,* ed. Marc Cantin and Mildred S. Seelig (Menlo Park, Ca.: Sprectrum Publ., 1980) p. 515-521.
187. I. Szelenyi in *World Review of Nutrition and Dietetics,* vol. 17, ed. Geoffrey H. Bourne (New York: S. Karger, 1973) pp. 189-224.
188. Ahmad S. Teebi, *Lancet* (Mar. 26, 1983): 701.
189. Peter W. Flatman and Virgilio L. Lew, *Jrl. of Physiology* (1982) 315: 421-446.
190. R.K. Rude and F.R. Singer, *Annual Review of Medicine* (1981) 32: 245-259.
191. G.K. Eichhorn, cited in *Chemical and Engineering News* (Sept. 10, 1973) 51, no. 37: 12.
192. Edmund B. Flink in *Magnesium in Health and Disease,* op. cit. (ref. 186) pp. 865-882.
193. P. McNair et al., *Diabetes* (1978) 27: 1075-1077.
194. G. Stendig-Lindberg and E. Hultman in *Magnesium in Health and Disease,* op. cit. (ref. 186), pp. 791-800.
194a. C.S. Anast et al., *Science* (Aug. 18, 1972) 177: 606-608.
195. Guy E. Abraham, *Jrl. of Applied Nutrition* (1982) 34: 69-73.
195a. Burton M. Altura and Bella T. Altura, *Magnesium* (1985) 4: 245-271, at 262.
195b. Herbert E. Parker, *Nutrition Reports International* (Oct., 1985) 32, no. 4: 983-990.
196. Robert Whang et al., *Acta Medica Scandinavica,* supp. (1981) 647: 139-144.
196a. Robert Whang et al., *Jrl. of the American College of Nutrition* (1982) 1: 317-322.
197. T. Dyckner and P.O. Wester, *British Medical Jrl.* (June 11, 1983) 286: 1847-1849.
198. J. Mendiola, Jr. et al., in *Magnesium in Health and Disease,* op. cit. (ref. 186), pp. 573-579.
199. Warren Wacker and Bert L. Vallee, *New England Jrl. of Medicine* (1958) 259: 431-438.
200. Hebbel E. Hoff et al., *Amer. Jrl. of Physiology* (1939) 127: 722-730.
200a. Burton M. Altura et al., *Science* (1984) 223: 1315-1317.
200b. *Nutrition Reviews* (1984) 42, no. 6: 235-236.
200c. F.P. Cappuccio et al., *British Medical Jrl.* (1985) 291: 235-238.
201. D. Lehr et al., in *Magnesium in Health and Disease* , op. cit, (ref. 186) pp. 499-506.
202. Joachim Manthey et al., *Circulation* (1981) 64: 722-729.
203. L.T. Iseri and A.R. Bures, *Magnesium in Health and Disease,* op. cit. (ref. 186) pp. 599-563.
204. Michelle Speich et al., *Clinical Chemistry* (1980) 26: 1662-1665.
205. Thomas Dyckner and Per Ola Wester, *Acta Medica Scandinavica,* supp. 647 (1981): 163-169.
206. R.P.C. Bigg and R. Chia, *Medical Jrl. of Australia* (April 4, 1981) 1: 346-348.
206a. Lloyd T. Iseri et al., *Western Jrl. of Medicine* (1983) 138, no. 6: 823-828.
207. Leon Cohen, *JAMA* (May 27, 1983) 249: 2808-2810.
208. Robert K. Rude et al., *Jrl. of Clinical Endocrinology and Metabolism* (1985) 61, no. 5: 933-940.
208a. R.B. Singh et al., *Acta Cardiologica* (1981) 36: 411-429.
209. L. Cohen and R. Kitzes, *JAMA* (1983) 249: 2808-2810.
210. James A. Landauer, *JAMA* (1984) 251: 730.
211. L. Cohen, *JAMA* (1984) 251: 730.
211a. Bella T. Altura and Burton M. Altura, *Neuroscience Letters* (1980) 323-327.
211b. Bella T. Altura and Burton M. Altura, *Magnesium* (1982) 1: 277-291.
211c. Bella T. Altura and Burton M. Altura, *Magnesium* (1984) 3: 195-211.
211d. Burton M. Altura, *Magnesium* (1985) 4: 169-175.
211e. Jerry K. Aikawa, *Magnesium: Its Biological Significance* (Boca Raton, Fla.: CRC Press, 1981) p. 41.
211f. H.Sandvad Rasmussen, *Lancet* (Feb. 1, 1986): 234-236.

212. H.J. Holtmeier and M. Kuhn, *Magnesium in Health and Disease*, op. cit. (ref. 186) pp. 671-677.
213. N.E. Johnson and C. Philipps, *Magnesium in Health and Disease*, op. cit (ref. 186) pp. 827-831.
214. J. Aleksandrowicz and J. Stachura, *Magnesium in Health and Disease*, op. cit. (ref. 186) pp. 225-231.
215. Jerome M. Blondell, *Medical Hypotheses*, (1980) 6: 863-871.
216. F.M. Parsons and G.A. Young, *Magnesium in Health and Disease* , op. cit. (ref. 186) pp. 233-239.
216a.. Betty J. Mills et al., *Jrl. of Nutrition* (1984) 114: 739-745.
216b. J. Eisinger and J. Dagorn, *Magnesium* (1986) 5: 27-32.
217. G. Johansson et al., *Scandinavian Jrl. of Urology and Nephrology*, supp. 53 (1980): 125-130.
218. G. Johansson et al., *Jrl. of Urology* (1980) 124: 770-774.
218a. G. Johansson et al., *Jrl. of the American College of Nutrition* (1982) 1: 179-185.
219. P.C. Hallson et al., *Clinical Science* (1982) 62: 17-19.
220. Hans Göran Tiselius et al., *Urological Research* (1980) 8: 197-200.
221. Walther Wunderlich, *Urological Research* (1981) 9: 157-161.
222. J. Thomas et al., *Magnesium in Health and Disease*, op. cit. (ref. 186) pp. 479-483.
223. E.g. Huf, cited in *CRC Handbook Series in Nutrition and Food, Section E: Nutritional Disorders,* vol. 1, ed. Miloslav Rechcigl (Cleveland, Ohio: CRC Press, 1977) p. 114.
224. D.A. Levison et al.,*Lancet* (March 27, 1982): 704-705.
224a. John P. Elliott, *American Jrl. of Obstetrics and Gynecology* (1983) 147, no. 3: 277-284.
225. Joan L. Caddell, *Lancet* (Aug. 2, 1972): 258-262.
226. Josef Lämmle, *Medical Tribune* (July 3, 1969).
226a. Elyett Gueux et al.,*Jrl. of Nutrition* (1984) 114: 1479-1483
227. M. Santillana et al., *Jrl. Internat. Vitaminol. Nutr.* (1974) 44: 327-346.
227a. R. Eliasson and C. Lindholmer, *Investigative Urology* (1972) 9, no. 4: 286-289.
227b. Thaddeus Mann, *The Biochemistry of Semen and of the Male Reproductive Tract* (London: Methuen & Co., Ltd., 1964) p. 187.
227c. S. Dalterio et al., *Life Sciences* (1985) 37: no. 15: 1425-1433.
228. P. Larvor, *Magnesium in Health and Disease,* op. cit. (ref. 186) pp. 201-224.
228a. F.C.M. Driessens and R.M.H. Verbeeck, *Calcified Tissue International* (1985) 37: 376-380.
228b. C. Robinson et al., *Caries Research* (1981) 15: 70-77.
228c. S. Thiradilok and F. Feagin, *Jrl. of Medical Science* (1978) 15: 144-148. Cited in ref. 228b.
229. Matti Knuuttila et al., *Scandinavian Jrl. of Dental Research* (Aug., 1980) 88: 513-516.
229a. P. Gron et al., *Arch. Oral Biol.,* cited in P. Gron and G.J. Van Campen, *Helvetica Ondontologica Acta* (1967) 11: 71-74.
230. H. Luoma et al., *Magnesium in Health and Disease,* op. cit. (ref. 186) pp. 344-354.
231. Warren E. C. Wacker and Bert L. Vallee, *New England Jrl. of Medicine* (1958) 259: 475-482.
231a. John P. Mordes and Warren E. C. Wacker,*Pharmacological Reviews* (1978) 29, no. 4: 273-300.
232. F.W. Heaton et al.,*Lancet* (Oct. 20, 1962): 802-805.
232a. George H. Hitchings and Elvira A. Falco, *Science* (1946) 104: 568-569.
232b. R. Eliasson and C. Lindholmer,*Investigative Urology* (1972) 9, no. 4: 286-289.
232c. Garry F. Gordon, *Osteopathic Annals* (1983) 11: 38-59.
232d. G. Andermann and M. Dietz, *European Jrl. of Drug Metabolism and Pharmocokinetics* (1982) 7, no. 3: 233-239.
233. R.D. Lindeman, *Magnesium in Health and Disease,* op. cit (ref. 186) pp. 381-399.
233a. J.W. Coburn et al., *Magnesium in Health and Disease,* op. cit., pp. 267-273.

233b. Björn Ahlborg et al., *Acta Phyisiologica Scandinavica* (1968) 74: 238-245.

233c. A. de Hann et al., *Int. Jrl. of Sports Medicine* (1985) 6: 44-49.

234. Richard Harkness, *Drug Interactions Handbook*, op. cit. (ref. 94a) p. 225.

234a. Richard M. Ratzen et al., *Geriatrics* (Sept., 1980) 35: 75-86.

234b. Burton M. Altura and Bella T. Altura, *Federation Proceedings* (1981) 40, no. 12: 2672-2679.

235. Noel W. Solomons, *Amer. Jrl. of Clinical Nutrition* (1982) 35: 1048-1075.

236. Jerry L. Phillips and Parviz Azari, *Cellular Immunology* (1974) 10: 31-37.

236a. *British Medical Jrl.* (April 4, 1981) 282: 1098-1099.

237. *Interpretation Guide* (West Chicago, Il.: Doctors' Data, Inc., April, 1982) p. 10.

237a. John H. Richardson and Pamela D. Drake, *Jrl. of Sports Medicine and Physical Fitness* (1979) 19: 133-134.

237b. Nanaya Tamaki et al., *Jrl. of Nutritional Science and Vitaminology* (1983) 29: 655-662.

238. Dusanka Mikac-Devic, *Advances in Clinical Chemistry* (1970) 13: 271-333.

239. William H. Strain and Walter J. Pories in *Zinc Metabolism*, ed. Ananda S. Prasad (Springfield, IL.: Charles C. Thomas, 1966) pp. 363, 392.

240. M.H. Briggs et al., *Experientia* (1972) 28: 406-407.

241. William H. Strain and Walter J. Pories in *Zinc Metabolism*, op. cit. (ref. 239) pp. 370-371.

241a. K. Michael Hambridge, *Amer. Jrl. of Clinical Nutrition* (1979) 32: 2532-2539.

242. M.H.N. Golden, *Human Nutrition: Clinical Nutrition* (1982) 36C: 185-202.

243. K.C. Verma et al., *Acta Dermatovener* (1980) 60: 337-340.

244. L. Mathers Dunbar and J. Martyn Bailey, *Jrl. of Biological Chemistry* (1975) 250: 1152-1153.

245. S.C. Cunnane, *Progress in Lipid Research* (1981) 20: 601-603.

246. M.S. Manku et al., *Endocrinology* (1979) 104: 774-779.

247. B.L. O'Dell in *Trace Element Metabolism in Man and Animals*, ed. J.M. Gawthorne, J. McC. Howell and C.L. White (Berlin: Springer-Verlag, 1982) p. 321.

248. S.C. Cunnane and D.F. Horrobin, *Proc. Soc. Exp. Biol. Med.* (1980) 164: 583-588.

249. Y.S. Huang et al., *Atherosclerosis* (1982) 41: 193-207.

250. R.F. Borgman et al., *Royal Soc. Health Jrl.* (Feb., 1982) no. 1: 1-2.

251. William H. Strain and Walter J. Pories, *Zinc Metabolism*, op. cit. (ref. 239) pp. 371-372.

252. Philip L. Hooper et al., *JAMA* (1980) 244, no. 17: 1960-1961.

253. L. Klevay, *Archives of Internal Medicine* (1978) 138: 1127-1128.

254. L. Murthy and H. Petering, *Jrl. of Agriculture and Food Chemistry* (1976) 24, no. 4: 808-811.

255. Philip L. Hooper and Philip J. Garry, *Amer. Jrl. of Clinical Nutrition* (1981) 34: 120-121.

256. Peter W.F. Fisher and Maurice W. Collins, *Amer. Jrl. of Clinical Nutrition* (1981) 34: 595-598.

256a. M. Katya-Katya et al., *Nutrition Research* (1984) 4: 633-638.

256b. Stephen F. Crouse et al., *JAMA* (1984) 256, no. 8: 785-787.

257. Ayhan O. Cavdar, *Lancet* (Feb. 6, 1982) 339-340.

258. Lucille S. Hurley and Shyy-Hwa Tao, *Amer. Jrl. of Physiology* (1972) 222: 322-375.

259. Lucille S. Hurley and Shyy-Hwa Tao, *Jrl. of Nutrition* (1975) 105: 220-225.

260. Peter A. Simkin, *Lancet* (Sept. 11, 1976) 2: 539-542.

261. L. Coulston and P. Dandona, *Diabetes* (1980) 29: 665-667.

262. James M. May and Charles S. Contoreggi, *Jrl. of Biological Chemistry* (1982) 257: 4362-4368.

263. C.H. Cho et al., *Pharmacology* (1978) 17: 32-38.

264. Donald J. Frommer, *Medical Jrl. of Australia* (Nov. 22, 1975): 793-796.

264a. Knut Haeger and Erik Lanner, *VASA* (1974) 3: 77-81.

980 The Reverse Effect

264b. S.L. Wallace et al., *Dental Survey* (Sept., 1978): 16, 18, 21, 22.

264c. Carol E. Williamson et al., *Jrl. of Periodontology* (March, 1984) 55, no. 3: 170-174.

264d. Adon A. Gordus et al., *NSF Trace Contaminants Conference* (Conference held in 1973; published in 1974) 1: 463-487. Also *Chemical Abstracts* (1975) 83: 1747z.

264e. D. Oberleas et al., *Psychopharmacology Bulletin* (1971): 35.

265. Karl E. Bergmann et al., *Amer. Jrl. of Clinical Nutrition* (1980) 33: 2145-2150.

265a. Karl E. Bergmann and Renate L. Bergmann, *American Jrl. of Clinical Nutrition* (1985) 42, no. 2: 343-344, followed by a reply from Mari S. Golab et al.: 344-345.

266. Gary S. Assarian and Donald Oberleas, *Clinical Chemistry* (1977) 23, no. 9: 1771-1777.

267. S.B. Deeming and C.W. Weber, *Amer. Jrl. of Clinical Nutrition*, (1977) 30: 2047-2052.

268. L.M. Klevay, *Archives of Internal Medicine* (1978) 138: 1128.

269. Bo Bergman and Rune Söremark, *Jrl. of Nutrition* (1968) 94: 6-12.

269a. Noel W. Solomons in *Zinc and Copper in Medicine,* ed. Zeynel A. Karciouglu and Rauf M. Sarper (Springfield, IL: Charles C. Thomas, 1980) pp. 224-275 at 249.

269b. S. Kumar and K.S.J. Rao, *Nutr. Metab.* (1974) 17: 231, cited in ref. 269a.

269c. Ananda S. Prasad, *Jrl. of the American College of Nutrition* (1985) 4: 591-598.

270. Robert B. Bradford and K. Michael Hambridge, *Lancet* (Feb. 16, 1980): 363.

271. Thomas H. Maugh II, *Science* (Dec. 22, 1978) 202: 1271-1273.

271a. H. Kikkawa et al., *Science* (1955) 121: 43-47.

271b. M.H. Briggs et al., *Experientia* (1972) 28: 406-407.

272. Philip S. Gentile et al., *Pediatric Research* (1981) 15: 123-127.

273. G.D. Renshaw, *Medical Science and the Law* (1976) 16, no. 1: 37-39.

274. Yu S. Ryabukhin in *Hair, Trace Elements and Human Illness,* ed. A.C. Brown and Robert G. Crounse (New York: Praeger Pubs., 1980) p. 12.

275. Jerrold L. Abraham, *Lancet* (Sept. 4, 1982): 554-555.

275a. D. Clink, unpublished Senior Honors Chemistry Thesis, University of Michigan, 1974. Cited by ref. 275b.

275b. Adon A. Gordus et al., *Proc. of the Second International Conference on Nuclear Methods in Environmental Research,* held at the University of Missouri, 1974 (United States Energy Research and Development Admin., 1974) pp. 198-205.

275c. Adon A. Gordus et al., *Proceedings of the First Annual NSF Trace Elements Conference, 1973.* Edited by W. Fulkerson, W.D. Shultz and R.I. Van Hook (Springfield, Va.: NTIS, 1974) pp. 463-487. Cited in *Chemical Abstracts* (1975) 83: 172 (abstract no. 1747z).

276. Ewin A. Eads and Charles E. Lambdin, *Environmental Research* (1973) 6: 247-252.

277. Jose G. Dorea and Sueli Essado Pereira, *Jrl. of Nutrition* (1983) 113: 2375-2381.

277a. Stephen Barrett, *JAMA* (1985) 254, no. 8: 1041-1045.

277b. P.J. Barlow et al., *Lancet* (Dec. 7, 1985): 1297.

277c. William J. Walsh, *JAMA* (May 16, 1986) 255, no. 19: 2603.

277d. George Hickok, ibid.

277e. Robert S. Waters, *JAMA* (May 16, 1986) 255, no. 19: 2604.

277f. Stephen Barrett, ibid.

278. William R. Beisel, *Medical World News* (Feb. 7, 1977): 57-60.

279. B.L. Vallee, *Physiol. Reviews* (1959) 39: 443-490.

280. Milos Chvapil et al., *Proc. of the Soc. for Experimental Biology and Medicine* (1972) 14: 642-646.

280a. Gerard Marx and Pierre Hopmeier, *American Jrl. of Hematology* (1986) 22: 347-353.

280b. Ananda S. Prasad, *Zinc Metabolism* (Springfield, IL: Charles C. Thomas, 1966) p. 390.

281. Pamela J. Fraker et al., *Jrl. of Nutrition* (1977) 107: 1889-1895.

282. Pamela J. Fraker et al., *Proc. of the National Academy of Sciences* (Nov., 1978) 11: 5660-5664.

283. Michael H.N. Golden et al., *Lancet* (June 10, 1978): 1226-1228.

284. Jean Duchateau et al., *Amer. Jrl. of Clinical Nutrition* (1981) 34: 88-93.
285. Gianni Marone et al., *Jrl. of Pharmacology and Exper. Therapeutics* (1981) 217: 292-298.
286. Jean Duchateau et al., *Amer. Jrl. of Medicine* (1981) 70: 1001-1004.
287. B.D. Korant et al., *Nature* (April 12, 1974) 248: 588-590.
287a. George A. Eby et al., *Antimicrobial Agents and Chemotherapy* (1984) 25, no. 1: 20-24.
288. *Nutrition Reviews* (1980) 38: 287-289.
289. Pamela J. Fraker et al., *Jrl. of Nutrition* (1982) 112: 1224-1229.
290. *Nutrition Reviews* (1979) 37: 234-235.
290a. Narendra K. Mathur et al., *International Jrl. of Leprosy* (1984) 52, no. 3: 331-338.
291. David R. Soll et al., *Infection and Immunity* (1981) 32: 1139-1147.
292. Ananda Prasad et al., in *Clinical Applications of Recent Advances in Zinc Metabolism*, ed. Ananda Prasad, Ivor E. Dreosti and Basil S. Hetzel (New York: A.R. Liss, 1982) p. 109.
293. Fred Willmott et al., *Lancet* (May 7, 1983): 1053.
294. John N. Krieger and Michael F. Rein, *Jrl. of Infectious Diseases* (Sept., 1982) 146, no. 3: 341-345.
295. Richard S. Beach et al., *Science* (Oct. 29, 1982) 218: 469-471.
295a. Ranjit Kumar Chandra, *JAMA* (Sept. 21, 1984) 252, no. 11: 1443-1446.
296. Ananda S. Prasad in *Zinc Metabolism,* op. cit., pp. 250-303.
297. K. Michael Hambridge et al., *Pediatric Research* (1972) 6: 868-874.
298. Noel W. Solomons et al., *Pediatric Research* (1976) 10: 923-927.
299. Phylis B. Moser et al., *Nutrition Research* (1982) 2: 585-590.
300. John Patrick, *Lancet* (Jan. 16, 1982): 169-170.
301. Harold H. Sandstead et al., *Amer. Jrl. of Clinical Nutrition* (May, 1967) 20: 422-442.
302. Ananda S. Prasad, *Amer. Jrl. of Clinical Nutrition* (1969) 22: 1215-1221.
303. Lucille S. Hurley, *Amer. Jrl. of Clinical Nutrition* (Oct., 1969) 21, no. 10: 1332-1339.
304. Bert L. Vallee, *Physiological Reviews* (1959) 39: 443-490.
304a. Lucy D. Antoniou et al., *Lancet* (Oct. 29, 1977): 895-898.
304b. William H. Goldiner et al., *Jrl. of the American College of Nutrition* (1983) 2: 157-162.
305. *Clinical, Biochemical and Nutritional Aspects of Trace Elements, ed.* Ananda S. Prasad (New York: A.R. Liss, 1982) p. 21.
306. T.R. Hartoma, *Acta Physiol. Scand.* (1977) 101: 336-341.
307. T. Riita Hartoma et al., *Lancet* (Nov. 26, 1977): 1125-1126.
308. Joel L. Marmar et al., *Fertility and Sterility* (1975) 26, no. 11: 1057-1063.
308a. Ali A. Abbasi et al., *Jrl. of Lab. and Clin. Med.* (1980) 96: 544-550.
309. J.G. Bieri and E.L. Prival, *Jrl. of Nutrition* (1966) 89: 55, cited by Lawrence J. Machlin and Edda Gabriel, *Annals of the New York Academy of Sciences* (1980) 355: 98-108.
309a. Prithiva Chanmugam et al., *Jrl. of Nutrition* (1984) 114: 2066-2072.
309b. Prithiva Chanmugam et al., *Jrl. of Nutrition* (1984) 114: 2073-2079.
310. Sudesh K. Mahajan et al., *Annals of Internal Medicine* (1982) 97: 357-361.
310a. M. Chvapil, *Medical Clinics of North America* (1976) 60: 799. Cited by Ananda S. Prasad, *American Jrl. of Hematology* (1979) 6: 77-87.
311. F.K. Habib, *Preventive Medicine* (1980) 9: 650-656.
312. G. Randolph Schrodt et al., *Cancer* (1964) 17: 1555-1566.
313. Ferenc Györkey et al., *Cancer Research* (1967) 27, part 1: 1348-1354.
313a. F.K. Habib, *Jrl. of Steroid Biochemistry* (1978) 9: 403-407.
313b. F.K. Habib et al., *Prostate* (1984) 5, no. 3: 359.
314. Rodney V. Anderson, *Medical Aspects of Human Sexuality* (1982) 16, no. 9: 25, 29.
315. Robert H. Rhamy, *JAMA* (Aug. 26, 1983) 250, no. 8: 1099-1100.

982 The Reverse Effect

315a. Thaddeus Mann, *The Biochemistry of Semen and of the Male Reproductive Tract,* (London: Methuen & Co., 1964) pp. 183-184.

315b. *Ibid,* p. 185.

316. A.M. Barclay. Paper presented at the annual meeting of the Society for Psychophysiological Research, New Orleans, La., Nov., 1970.

317. A.M. Barclay, *Jrl. of Experimental Research in Personality* (1970) 4: 233-238.

318. A.M. Barclay, *Social Psychology* (1971) 17: 244-249.

319. Sakari Kellokumpu and Hannu Rajaniemi, *Biology of Reproduction* (1981) 24: 298-305.

320. S. Aonuma et al., *Jrl. of Reproduction and Fertility* (1981) 63: 463-466.

320a. Reuben J. Mapletoft, *Biotechnology* (Feb., 1984): 149-160.

321. O. Johnson and R. Eliasson, *Int. Jrl. of Andrology* (1978) 1: 485-488.

322. O. Johnson and R. Eliasson, *Int. Jrl. of Fertility* (1974) 19: 56-62.

323. W.R. Sutton and Victor E. Nelson, *Proc. Soc. for Experimental Biology and Medicine* (1937) 36: 211-213.

324. Vernon E. Wendt et al., in *Zinc Metabolism,* op. cit. (ref. 239) pp. 395-410.

325. G. Frithz and G. Ronquist, *Acta Medica Scandinavica* (1979) 205: 647-649.

326. Peter W. F. Fischer and Maurice W. Collins, *Amer. Jrl. of Clinical Nutrition* (1981) 34: 595-597.

327. Denis M. Medeiros et al., *Nutrition Research* (1983) 3: 51-60.

327a. William R. Harlan et al., *JAMA* (1985) 253, no. 4: 530-534.

328. Joachin Manthey et al., *Circulation* (1981) 64: 722-729.

329. Stephen J. Kopp et al., *Science* (Aug. 27, 1982) 217: 837-839.

330. James F. Riodan and Bert V. Vallee in *Trace Elements in Human Health and Disease,* vol. 1, ed. Ananda S. Prasad (New York: Academic Press, 1976) p. 243.

331. Janet T. McDonald and Sheldon Margen, *Amer. Jrl. of Clinical Nutrition* (1980) 33: 1096-1102.

332. Janet T. McDonald and Sheldon Margen, *Amer. Jrl. of Clinical Nutrition* (1979) 32: 823.

333. *Wall Street Jrl.* (Dec. 31, 1982): 7.

334. J.L. Greger and A.H. Geissler, *Amer. Jrl. of Clinical Nutrition* (1978) 31: 633-637.

335. Sudesh K. Mahajan et al., *Amer. Jrl. of Clinical Nutrition* (1980) 33: 1517-1521.

336. Robert I. Henkin et al., *Amer. Jrl. of Medical Sciences* (1976) 272: 285-299.

336a. Robert I. Henkin, *Biological Trace Element Research* (1984) 6: 263-280.

336b. W.W. Dinsmore et al., *Lancet* (May 4, 1985): 1041-1042.

336c. D. Bryce-Smith and R.I.D. Simpson, *Lancet* (Aug. 11, 1984): 350.

336d. Michele Garrett-Laster et al., *Human Nutrition: Clinical Nutrition* (1984) 38C: 203-214.

337. Kaare Weismann and Hans K. Hagdrup, *Acta Dermatovener, Stockholm* (1981) 61: 444-447.

338. Kaare Weismann, *Acta Dermatovener, Stockholm* (1977) 57: 88-89.

339. Grosvener W. Bissel et al., *JAMA* (1971) 215: 1666-1667.

340. Andre Barbeau, *Medical World News* (Sept. 7, 1973).

340a. H. George Ketola, *Jrl. of Nutrition* (1979) 109: 965-969.

340b. *Nutrition Reviews* (March, 1986) 44, no. 3: 118-120.

341. G.L. Brewer et al., *Jrl. of Laboratory and Clinical Medicine* (1977) 90: 549-554.

342. *Nutrition Reviews* (July, 1983) 41, no. 7: 217-219.

342a. Ananda S. Prasad and Zafrallah T. Cossack, *Archives of Internal Medicine* (1984) 100: 367-371.

342b. M. Cassandra Matustik et al., *Jrl. of the Amer. College of Nutrition* (1982) 1: 331-336.

342c. Pierre Reding et al., *Lancet* (Sept. 1, 1984): 493-495.

343. R.I. Henkin in *Newer Trace Elements in Nutrition,* ed. Walter Mertz and W.E. Comatzer (New York: Marcel Dekker, 1971) pp. 282-312.

344. R.D. Bhattacharya, *Panminerva Medica* (1979) 21: 201-203.

345. Morton K. Schwartz, *Cancer Research* (1975) 35: 3481-3487.
346. O. Guillard et al., *Biomedicine* (1979) 31: 193-194.
347. M.G. Ioskovich, *Biological Abstracts* (1973) 55: 46207.
347a. N.T. Davies, *Jrl. of Plant Foods* (1978) 3: 113-121. Cited by P.J. Aggett and N.T. Davies, *Jrl. of Inherited Metabolic Disease* (1983) 6, supp. 1: 22-30.
348. John J. Miller, *The Miller Message* (July, 1974).
348a. Dorothy Latta and Michael Liebman, *Nutrition Reports International* (1984) 30, no. 1: 141-149.
349. J.L. Greger and S.M. Snedeker, *Jrl. of Nutrition* (1980) 110: 2243-2253.
350. Leslie M. Klevay, *Advances in Nutritional Research* (1977) 1: 227-252.
351. *Nutrition Reviews* (1982) 40, no. 3: 76-77.
352. Herta Spencer et al.,*Jrl. of Nutrition* (1965) 86: 169-177.
353. Donald Oberleas and Barbara F. Harland, *Jrl. of the American Dietetic Assn.* (1981) 79: 433-436.
354. Frank W. Hogarth, *Jrl. of Human Nutrition* (1981) 35: 379-382.
354a. Herta Spencer et al., *Amer. Jrl. of Clinical Nutrition* (1984) 40: 1213-1218.
355. A. Pecoud et al., *Clinical Pharmacology and Therapeutics* (1975) 17: 469-474.
356. Brittmarie Sandstrom et al., *Amer. Jrl. of Clinical Nutrition* (1980) 33: 739-745.
357. Gary W. Evans and Elaine C. Johnson, *Pediatric Research* (1980) 14: 876-880.
358. L.S. Hurley and B. Lönnerdal, *Nutrition Reviews* (1982) 40, no. 3: 65-71.
359. Eric w. Ainscough et al., *Amer. Jrl. of Clinical Nutrition* (1980) 33: 1314-1315.
360. Noel W. Solomons, *Amer. Jrl. of Clinical Nutrition* (1982) 35: 1048-1075.
361. Bonnie M. Anderson et al.,*Amer. Jrl. of Clinical Nutrition* (1981) 34: 1042-1048.
362. S.L. Wolman et al., cited by M.H.N. Golden, *Human Nutrition: Clinical Nutrition* (1982) 36C: 185-202.
362a. Leslie M. Klevay, *Jrl. of the American College of Nutrition* (1984) 3: 149-158.
363. *Clinical, Biochemical and Nutritional Aspects of Trace Elements,* op. cit (ref. 305) p. 497.
364. Ananda S. Prasad et al.,*JAMA* (Nov. 10, 1978) 240, no. 10: 2166-2168.
364a. Melody D. Festa et al.,*American Jrl. of Clinical Nutrition* (1985) 41: 285-292.
365. C.T. Settlemire and G. Matrone, *Jrl. of Nutrition* (1967) 92: 159-164.
365a. Peter W.F. Fischer et al., *Amer. Jrl. of Clinical Nutrition* (1984) 40: 743-746.
365b. Kenneth H. Neldner,*Archives of Dermatology* (1980) 116: 39-40.
366. G.N. Schrauzer, *Bioinorganic Chemistry* (1977) 7: 35-56, at 46-49.
367. E.L. Andronikashvili,*Cancer Research* (1974) 34: 271-274.
367a. Daniel T. Minkel et al., *Cancer Research* (1979) 39: 2451-2456.
368. K.B. Olson et al., *Cancer* (1958) 11: 554-561. Cited by M.K. Schwartz, ref. 345.
368a. L.D. McBean et al., *Amer. Jrl. of Clinical Nutrition* (1972) 25: 672-676. Cited by M. K. Schwartz, ref. 345.
368b. I.L. Mulay et al., *Jrl. National Cancer Institute* (1971) 47: 1-13. Cited by M.K. Schwartz, ref. 345.
368c. A.E. Schwartz et al., *Surgery* (1974) 76: 325-329. Cited by M.K. Schwartz, ref. 345.
369. J. Borovansky et al.,*Neoplasma* (1980) 27: 247-252.
370. Gamal N. Gabrial et al., *Jrl. of the National Cancer Institute* (1982) 68: 785-789.
371. L.Y.Y. Fong and P.M. Newberne,*Jrl. of the National Cancer Institute* (1978) 61: 145-150.
371a. Louise Y.Y. Fong et al., *Jrl. of the National Cancer Institute* (1984) 72, no. 2: 419-425.
371b. K. Wallenius et al., *Int. Jrl. of Oral Surgery* (1979) 8: 56-62.
371c. Moon K. Song et al., *Jrl. of the National Cancer Institute* (1984) 72, no. 3: 647-652.
372. Richard S. Beach et al.,*Nutrition and Cancer* (1982) 3: 172-191.
373. Walter J. Pories, *Annals of the New York Academy of Sciences* (1972) 199: 265-273.
373a. Committee on Diet, Nutrition and Cancer, *Diet, Nutrition and Cancer* (Washington, D.C.: National Academy Press, 1982) p. 10.

373b. J. Cecil Smith, Jr. et al., *Science* (1976) 193: 496-498.

374. Judith Turnland and Sheldon Margen, *Age* (Oct., 1978) 1: 159-160.

374a. D.F. Horrobin and S.C. Cunnane, *Medical Hypotheses* (1980) 6: 277-296, at 281-284.

375. Herta Spencer et al., in *Trace Elements in Human Health and Disease,* op. cit. (ref. 330) pp. 345-359.

375a. Leslie S. Valberg et al., *American Jrl. of Clinical Nutrition* (1984) 40: 536-541.

376. N.F. Adham and M.K. Sung, *Nutrition and Metabolism* (1980) 24: 281-290.

377. Herta Spencer et al., *Jrl. of Nutrition* (1965) 86: 169-177.

378. George J. Brewer and Ulana L. Bereza in *Clinical, Biochemical and Nutritional Aspects of Trace Elements,* op. cit. (ref. 305) p. 213.

378a. George J. Brewer, *American Jrl. of Hematology* (1980) 8: 231-248.

379. Dusanka Mikac-Devic, *Advances in Clinical Chemistry* (1970) 13: 271-333.

379a. Benjamin M. Sahagian et al., *Jrl. of Nutrition* (1967) 93: 291-300.

379b. Fayez K. Ghishan et al., *American Jrl. of Clinical Nutrition* (1986) 43: 258-262.

379c. Richard Harkness, *Drug Interactions Handbook,* op. cit. (ref. 94a) p. 20.

380. Noel W. Solomons and Robert A. Jacob, *Amer. Jrl. of Clinical Nutrition* (1981) 34: 475-482.

380a. Doron Garfinkel, *Medical Hypotheses* (1986) 19: 117-137.

380b. A.S. Prasad, *American Jrl. of Hematology* (1979) 6: 77. Cited in ref. 380a.

380ba. Anne W. Thorburn et al., *British Medical Jrl.* (1986) 292: 1697-1699. Cited by Alexander Grant, *Healthwise* (Oct., 1986) 9, no. 10: 1.

380c. Alta M. Engstrom and Rosemary C. Tobelmann, *Annals of Internal Medicine* (1983) 98, part 2: 870-872.

381. Alber J. Tuyns, *Nutrition and Cancer* (1983) 4, no. 3: 198-205.

382. Ailsa Goulding and Dianne Campbell, *Jrl. of Nutrition* (1983) 113: 1409-1414.

383. H.E. Wardener et al., *Lancet* (Feb. 21, 1981): 411-412.

384. L. Poston et al., *Clinical Research* (Mar. 14, 1981) 282: 847-849.

385. John M. Hamlyn et al., *Nature* (Dec. 16, 1982) 300: 650-652.

386. Fuminori Masugi et al., *Japanese Circulation Jrl.* (Sept., 1985) 49: 980-983.

387. A.M. Heagerty et al., *Lancet* (Mar. 12, 1983): 591.

388. Belding H. Scribner, *JAMA* (July 15, 1983) 250: 388-389.

388a. Arthur C. Guyton, *Medical Physiology,* 6th ed. (Philadelphia: W.B. Saunders Co., 1981) p. 267.

389. David L. Longworth et al., *Clinical Pharmacol. Ther.* (1980) 27: 544-546.

389a. David Robertson et al., *Circulation* (1979) 59, no. 4: 637-643.

389b. David Robertson et al., *New England Jrl. of Medicine* (1978) 298, no. 4: 181-186.

389c. David Robertson et al., *Jrl. of Clinical Nutrition* (1981) 67: 1111-1117.

389d. C.A. Farleigh et al., *Nutrition Research* (1985) 5: 815-826.

389e. Jacqueline J.M. Castenmiller et al., *American Jrl. of Clinical Nutrition (1985) 41:* 52-60.

390. Theodore W. Kurtz and R. Curtis Morris, Jr., *Science* (Dec. 9, 1983) 222: 1139-1141.

390a. T.A. Kotchen et al., *Ann. Int. Med.* (1983) 98, part 2: 817.

390b. Shirley A. Whitescarver et al., *Science* (March 30, 1984) 223: 1430-1432.

390c. R.J. Shneidman and D.A. McCarron, *Clinical Research* (1984) 32, no. 2: 236A.

390d. S.A. Hahn et al., *Clinical Research* (1984) 32, no. 1: 36A

390e. Theodore W. Kurtz and R.C. Morris, Jr., *Life Sciences* (1985) 36: 931-929.

390f. Haralambos Gavras, *Hypertension* (1986) 8: 83-88.

390g. Belding H. Scribner, *JAMA* (July 15, 1983) 250, no. 3: 388-389.

390h. N.G. Levinsky and G.A. Alexander in *The Kidney,* ed. B.M. Bremner and F.L. Rector (Philadelphia: Saunders, 1976) pp. 806-837, cited by J.D. Swales, *Lancet* (May 31, 1980): 1177-1179.

390i. Hans Kaunitz and Ruth Ellen Johnson, *Proceedings of the Soc. for Experimental Biology and Medicine* (1972) 141: 875-878.

391. Gina Kolata, *Science* (1985) 228: 167-168.

391a. Shirley A. Whitescarver et al., *Science* (1985) 228: 352.

391b. John C. Passmore, Shirley A. Whitescarver et al., *Hypertension* (1985) 7, supp. I: I 115-I 120.

391c. Shirley A. Whitescarver et al., *Hypertension* (1986) 8: 56-61.

392. Robert Harris cited by Nicholas Wade,*Science* (June 24, 1977) 196: 1421-1422.

392a. Charles E. Lawrence et al.,*Jrl. National Cancer Institute* (March, 1984) 72, no. 3: 563-568.

392b. Robert J. Morin and Peter Barna, *Longevity Letter* (1986) 4, no. 3: 2-4.

393. J.R. Meier et al., *Mutation Research* (1983) 118: 25-41.

394. Thomas H. Maugh II, *Science* (April 24, 1981) 212: 431.

394a. Council on Environmental Quality, Drinking Water and Cancer: *Review of Recent Findings and Assessment of Risks* (Washington, D.C.: Supt. of Documents, 1980).

395. Thomas H. Maugh II, *Science* (Feb. 13, 1981) 211: 694.

396. G.S. Moore et al., *Jrl. of Environmental Pathology and Toxicology* (1980) 4: 465-470.

397. W. G. Honer et al., *Mutation Research* (1980) 78: 137-144.

398. Jeffrey R. Haag and Richard G. Gieser, *JAMA* (May 13, 1983) 249, no. 18: 2507-2508.

398a. P.T. Penny, *British Medical Jrl.* (1983) 287: 461-462.

398b. James E. Greer, *Southern Medical Jrl.* (March, 1984) 77, no. 3: 297-298, 301.

398c. Alan B. Levy, *Psychosomatics* (Sept., 1986) 27, no. 9: 665-666.

399. W.W. Douglas et al., *Jrl. of Physiology* (1967) 191: 107-121.

400. Stanley J. Birge, Jr.,*Science* (April 14, 1972) 176: 168-170.

400a. Halvor N. Christensen, *Nutrition Reviews* (1984) 42, no. 7: 237-242.

401. Vincent W. Dennis and Peter C. Brazy in *Homeostasis of Phosphate and Other Minerals,* ed. Shaul G. Massry et al., (New York: Plenum Press, 1978) p. 79.

401a. Michael W. Pariza, *JAMA* (Mar. 16, 1984) 251, no. 11: 1455-1458.

402. David F. Bohr, *Hypertension* (1981) 3, supp. II: II 160-II 165.

403. Lewis K. Dahl et al., *Nature* (1963) 198: 1204.

404. James Weiffenbach et al., *Jrl. of Dental Research* (March, 1981) 60, special issue A: abstract 1223.

404a. M. Uhaii and E. Timonen in *Hypertension in Children and Adolescents* (New York: Raven Press, 1981) pp. 287-291, cited by Julie R. Ingelfinger,*JAMA* (July 15, 1983) 250, no. 3: 389-390.

404aa. David A. McCarron, *Hypertension* (1985) 7: 607-627.

404ab. Graham A. MacGregor,*Hypertension* (1985) 7: 628-637.

404b. J.J. Brown et al.,*Lancet* (Aug. 25, 1984): 456.

404c. N. Gledhill, *Sports Medicine* (1984) 1: 177-180.

404d. D.P.M. MacLaren and G.D. Morgan, *Proceedings of the Nutrition Society* (1985) 44, no. 1: 26A.

404e. Harvey G. Klein, *New England Jrl. of Medicine* (1985) 312, no. 13: 854-856.

404f. Allan J. Ryan, *Physician and Sports Medicine* (1985) 13, no. 4: 45.

405. S. Heyden and C.G. Hames,*Nutrition Metabolism* (1980) 24, supp. 1: 50-64.

406. David M. Harlan and George V. Mann, *Amer. Jrl. of Clinical Nutrition* (Feb., 1982) 35: 250-257.

406a. Giuseppe A. Sagnella and Graham A. MacGregor, *Amer. Jrl. of Clinical Nutrition* (1984) 40: 36-41.

407. Ernest Beutler et al., *New England Jrl. of Medicine* (Sept. 29, 1983) 309, no. 13: 756-760.

407a. Mark F. McCarty, *Medical Hypotheses* (1984) 13: 451-463.

408. R.W. Hubbard et al., *Jrl. of Applied Physiology* (1981) 51, no. 1: 8-13.

409. S.B. Olsson, *Acta Medica Scandinavica* (1981) supp. 647: 33-37.

410. Mark F. McCarty, *Medical Hypotheses* (1981) 7: 591-597.

410a. Freeman W. Cope, *Physiological Chemistry and Physics* (1978) 10: 465-467.

410b. Janet Treasure and David Ploth, *Hypertension* (1983) 5: 864-872.

411. Graham A. MacGregor et al.,*Lancet* (Sept. 11, 1982): 567-570.

412. Osamu Iimura et al., *Clinical Science* (1981) 61: 71s-80s.
412a. A. Mark Richards et al., *Lancet* (April 7, 1984): 757-761.
412b. Alan J. Silman, *Lancet* (May 26, 1984): 1189.
412c. Stephen J. Smith et al., *British Medical Jrl.* (1985) 290: 110-113.
412d. Norman M. Kaplan et al., *New England Jrl. of Medicine* (1985) 312, no. 12: 746-749.
412e. Kay-Tee-Khaw et al., *Amer. Jrl. of Clinical Nutrition* (1984) 39: 963-968.
413. Orna Ophir et al., *Amer. Jrl. of Clinical Nutrition* (1983) 37: 755-762.
414. Y.C. Ko, *Nutrition Reports International* (Dec., 1983) 28, no. 6: 1375-1383.
415. Ray M. Acheson and D.R.R. Williams, *Lancet* (May 28, 1983): 1191-1193.
415a. Olov Lindahl et al., *British Jrl. of Nutrition* (1984) 52: 11-20.
416. Ian L. Rouse et al., *Lancet* (Jan. 18, 1981): 5-10.
417. Mark S. Paller and Stuart L. Linas, *Hypertension* (1982) 4, supp. III: III 20-III 26.
417a. L. Tobian et al., *Stroke* (Nov.-Dec, 1985) 16, no. 6: 1058-1059.
417b. Barbara Chipperfield and John R. Chipperfield, *Lancet* (Oct. 6, 1979): 709-712.
418. Burton M. Altura and Bella T. Altura, *Magnesium* (1985) 4: 226-244 and 245-271, at 247.
418a. Richard L. Tannen, *Annals of Internal Medicine* (1983) 98, part 2: 773-780.
418b. James W. Anderson, *Annals of Internal Medicine* (1983) 95, part 2: 842-846.
418c. Walter Kempner, *American Jrl. of Medicine* (1948) 4: 545-577.
418d. David A. McCarron et al., *Nutrition Today* (July/August, 1984): 14-23.
418e. Mitsuki Yoshioka et al., *International Jrl. for Vitamin and Nutrition Research* (1985) 55: 301-307.
419. K.C. Srivastava et al., *Prostaglandins, Leukotrienes and Medicine* (1984) 13: 227-235.
419a. I.S. Cohen, *Experientia* (1983) 39: 1280-1282.
419b. A. Berthelot and J. Esposito, *Jrl. of the Amer. College of Nutrition* (1983) 4: 343-353.
419c. L.C. Chesley et al., *Jrl. Clinical Investigation* (1958) 37: 1362-1372, cited by Berthelot and Esposito (ref. 419b).
419d. G.F. DiBona, *Amer. Jrl. Physiology* (171) 221: 53-57, cited by Berthelot and Esposito (ref. 419b).
419e. M. Cantin, *Lab. Invest.* (1970) 558-559, cited by Berthelot and Esposito (ref. 419b).
420. Denis M. Madeiros et al., *Nutrition Research* (1983) 3: 51-60.
420a. Denis M. Madeiros and Barbara J. Brown, *Biological Trace Element Research* (1983) 5: 165-174.
421. Mark F. McCarty, *Medical Hypotheses* (1981) 7: 271-283.
421a. Toru Yamagami et al., *Research Communications in Chemical Pathology and Pharmacology* (1976) 14, no. 4: 721-727.
421b. Toru Yamagami and Nobuhiko Shibata, *Research Communications in Chemical Pathology and Pharmacology* (1975) 11, no. 2: 273-288.
421c. Karl Folkers et al., *Research Communications in Chemical Pathology and Pharmacology* (Jan., 1981) 31, no. 1: 129-140.
421d. Philip C. Richardson et al., in *Biomedical and Clinical Aspects of Coenzyme Q*, vol. 3, ed. K. Folkers and Y. Yamamura (Amsterdam: Elsevier/North Holland Biomedical Press, 1981) pp. 229-234.
421e. Yoshifumi Iwamoto et al., in *Biomedical and Clinical Aspects of Coenzyme Q*, vol. 3, op. cit. (ref. 421d) pp. 109-119.
421f. Toru Yamagami et al., in *Biomedical and Clinical Aspects of Coenzyme Q*, vol. 2, ed. K. Folkers and Y. Yamamura (Amsterdam: Elsevier Scientific Publ. Co., 1977) pp. 231-242.
421g. Harry B. Demopoulos and Eugene S. Flamm in *Biomedical and Clinical Aspects of Coenzyme Q*, vol. 3 op. cit. (ref. 421d) pp. 373-384.
421h. H.B. Demopoulos et al., *Acta Physiol. Scand.* (1980) suppl. 492: 91-119, cited in ref. 421.
421i. Alan F. Sved, *Proc. National Academy of Sciences* (1979) 76, no. 7: 3511-3514.

421j. Alan F. Sved, *Jrl. of Pharmacology and Experimental Therapeutics* (1982) 221, no. 2: 329-333.
422. Timothy J. Maher and Richard J. Wurtman, *New England Jrl. of Medicine* (Nov. 3, 1983) 309, no. 18: 1125.
422a. Dag S. Thelle et al., *New England Jrl. of Medicine* (June 16, 1983) 308, no. 24: 1454-1457.
422b. *Lancet* (Dec. 7, 1985): 1283-1284.
422c. J.D. Kark et al., *British Medical Jrl.* (Sept. 14, 1985) 291: 699-704.
423. Arthur L. Klatsky et al., *New England Jrl. of Medicine* (1977) 296: 1194-1200.
423a. Arthur L. Klatsky, *Annual Review of Nutrition* (1982) 2: 51-71.
424. Denis M. Medeiros, *Nutrition Reports International* (Oct., 1982) 26: 563-568.
425. S. Freestone and L.E. Ramsay, *Clinical Science* (1982) 63: 403s-405s.
426. H.P.T. Ammon et al., *British Jrl. Clin. Pharmacology* (1983) 15, no. 6: 701-706.
427. P.B. Dews, *Ann. Rev. Nutri.* (1982) 2: 323-341.
428. David Robertson et al., *Amer. Jrl. of Medicine* (July, 1984) 77: 54-60.
429. Charles A. Bertrand et al., *New England Jrl. of Medicine* (1978) 299: 315-316.
430. A.L. Klatsky et al., *JAMA* (1973) 226: 540-543, cited by David Robertson et al., ref. 428.
431. C.H. Hennekens et al., *New England Jrl. of Medicine* (1976) 294: 633-636, cited by David Robertson et al., ref. 428.
432. T.R. Dawber et al., *New England Jrl. of Medicine* (1974) 291: 871-874.
432a. Paul Pentel, *JAMA* (Oct. 12, 1984) 252, no. 14: 1898-1903.
433. Prince McCann et al., *Federation Proceedings* (1983) 42: 989.
434. Ruben D. Bunag et al., *Hypertension* (1983) 5: 218-225.
434a. Beverly A. Clevidence et al., *Biochemical Medicine* (1981) 25: 186-197.
434b. Harry G. Preuss and Richard D. Fournier, *Life Sciences* (1982) 30: 879-886.
434c. S.R. Srinivasan et al., *American Jrl. of Clinical Nutrition* (1980) 33: 561-569.
435. Denis M. Medeiros and Robert F. Borgman, *Nutrition Research* (1982) 2: 455-466.
435a. P.J. Palumbo et al., *American Jrl. of Clinical Nutrition* (1977) 30: 394-401.
435b. Carlos A. Camargo et al., *JAMA* (1985) 253, no. 19: 2854-2857.
436. J.B. Saunders, *Lancet* (Sept. 26, 1981): 653-656.
436a. M.J. Ashley and J.G. Rankin, *Australian and New Zealand Jrl. of Medicine* (1979) 9: 201-206.
436b. Richard P. Donahue et al., *JAMA* (May 2, 1986) 256, no. 17: 2311-2314.
436c. Joyce A. D'Antonio et al., *Cancer* (1986) 57: 1798-1802.
437. Michael H. Criqui et al., *Hypertension* (1981) 3: 557-565.
438. J.F. Potter and D. G. Beevers, *Lancet* (Jan. 21, 1984) 119-122.
439. Victoria Cairns et al., *Hypertension* (1984) 6: 124-131.
439a. I.B. Puddey et al., *Lancet* (Nov. 16, 1985): 1119-1120.
439b. John R. Taylor et al., *Alcoholism: Clinical and Experimental Research* (1984) 8, no. 3: 283-286.
440. N. Conway, *British Heart Jrl.* (1968) 30: 638-644.
440a. M.A. Ireland et al., *Clinical Science* (1984) 66: 643-648.
441. R.C. Reitz et al., *Progress in Lipid Research* (1981) 20: 209-213.
442. M.S. Manku et al., *Prostaglandins in Medicine* (1979) 3: 119-128.
443. Cynthia Baum-Baicker, *Drug and Alcohol Independence* (1985) 15: 207-227.
443a. Vecihi Batuman et al., *JAMA* (July 7, 1983) 309: 17-21.
443b. Denis M. Medeiros and Lynn K. Pellum, *Bulletin of Environmental Contamination and Toxicology* (1984) 32: 525-532.
443c. R.G. Wilcox et al., *Clinical Research* (Sept. 18, 1982) 285: 767-769.
443d. W. Larry Kenney and Edward J. Zambraski, *Sports Medicine* (1984) 1: 459-473.
444. Efrain Reisin, *New England Jrl. of Medicine* (1978) 298: 1-6.
445. J. Edwin Wood and James R. Cash, *Annals of Internal Medicine* (1939) 13: 81-90.
446. Benjamin N. Chiang et al., *Circulation* (1969) 39: 403-421.

446a. P. Berchtold et al., *Biomedicine and Pharmacotherapy* (1983) 37: 251-258.
446b. Dorothy Blair et al., *Amer. Jrl. of Epidemiology* (1984) 119, no. 4: 526-540.
446c. Neill Cohen and Walter Flamenbaum, *American Jrl. of Medicine* (Feb., 1986) 80: 177-181.
446d. Christopher L. Melby, *Nutrition Research* (1985) 5: 1077-1082.
447. G. M. Saunders and Huldah Bancroft, *Amer. Heart Jrl.* (1942) 23: 410-423.
448. M. Colgan, *New Zealand Jrl. of Medicine* (Jan. 28, 1981) 93: 49-51.
448a. Sue A. Thomas, *Public Health Reports* (1984) 99, no. 1: 77-84.
448b. Erika Friedman et al., *Psychosomatic Medicine* (1982) 44, no. 6: 545-553.
448c. Kenneth L. Malinow et al., *Psychosomatic Medicine* (1986) 48, no. 1/2: 95-101.
449. W. Stewart Agras, *Psychosomatic Medicine* (Sept., 1982) 44, no. 2: 389-395.
449a. Michael F. O'Rourke, *Australian New Zealand Jrl. of Medicine* (1983) 13: 84-90.
449b. Yukiko Shimizu et al., *Stroke* (1984) 15, no. 5: 839-846.
449ba. C.M. Fisher, *Lancet* (Dec. 14, 1985): 1349.
449bb. Alan Gilston, *Lancet* (Jan. 25, 1986): 209.
449bc. Lawrence E. Ramsay and Patrick C. Waller, *Lancet* (Oct. 11, 1986) 854-856.
449c. Betsy C. Little et al., *Lancet* (April 21, 1984): 865-867.
449d. Bernard L. Frankel et al., *Psychosomatic Medicine* (1978) 40, no. 4: 276-293.
449e. James P. Henry, *Psychosomatic Medicine* (1978) 40, no. 4: 273-275.
449f. Iris B. Goldstein et al., *Psychosomatic Medicine* (1984) 46, no. 5: 398-414.
449g. Herbert Benson, *New England Jrl. of Medicine* (1977) 296, no. 20: 1152-1156.
449h. Chandra Patel, *Jrl. of the Royal College of General Practitioners* (1976) 26: 211-215.
449i. Dean Ornish et al., *JAMA* (1983) 249, no. 1: 54-59.
449j. Norman M. Kaplan, *Annals of Internal Medicine* (1985) 102: 359-373.
449k. Michael J. Horan et al., *Hypertension* (Sept.-Oct., 1985) 7, no. 5: 818-823.
450. John W. Rowe, *New England Jrl. of Medicine* (Nov. 17, 1983) 309: 1246-1247.
451. S. Rajala et al., *Lancet* (Aug. 27, 1983): 520-521.
451a. *Chronobiologia* (1984) 11, no. 3.
452. Philip R. J. Burch, *Lancet* (Oct. 8, 1983): 852-853.
453. J.R.A. Mitchell, *Lancet* (Nov. 26, 1983): 1248.
453a. Patrick Lavin, *Archives of Internal Medicine* (Jan., 1986) 146: 66-68.
453b. Hypertension-Stroke Cooperative Study Group, *JAMA* (1974) 229, no. 4: 409-418.
453c. J.D. Spence et al., *Clinical Science and Molecular Medicine* (1978) 55: 399s-402s.
453d. *Physicians Desk Reference*, 38th ed. (Oradell, N.J.: Medical Economics Co., 1984) p. 842 and 39th ed. (1985) p. 845.
453e. Steven M. Reppert et al., *Science* (1981) 213: 1256-1257.
453f. E. Cotlove et al., *Amer. Jrl. of Physiology* (1951) 167: 665, cited by Edmund B. Flink in *Potassium: Its Biological Significance*, ed. Robert Whang (Boca Raton, Florida; CRC Press, 1983) p. 98.
454. M.R. Laker, *Lancet* (Dec. 11, 1982): 1338.
455. Chris Lecos, *FDA Consumer* (Feb. 22, 1983): 21-22.
456. M.S. Harris, *Jrl. of Pharmaceutical Sciences* (1981) 70, no. 4: 391-394.
456a. Edmund B. Flink in *Potassium: Its Biologic Significance*, ed. Robert Whang (Boca Raton, Florida: CRC Press, 1983) pp. 37-44.
456b. R.D. Lindeman and J.A. Pederson in *Potassium: Its Biologic Significance*, ed. Robert Whang (Boca Raton, Florida: CRC Press, 1983) pp. 45-75, at 65.
457. D.H. Lawson, *Quarterly Jrl. of Medicine*, New Series (1974) 43, no. 171: 433-440.
458. William H. Bay and Judith A. Hartman, *New England Jrl. of Medicine* (1983) 308: 1166-1167.
459. J. Arnold et al., *Jrl. of Pharmaceutical Sciences* (1980) 69, no. 12, 1416-1418.
460. R.G. Faber et al., *British Jrl. of Medicine* (Aug. 16, 1975): 436-437.
461. F.G. McMahon, *British Jrl. of Medicine* (July 19, 1975): 162.
462. J. Wrobel et al., *Acta Biochimica Polonica* (1973) 20: 249-257.

463. Ronald L. Weinsier and C.E. Butterworth,*Handbook of Clinical Nutrition* (St. Louis: Mosby, 1981) p. 204.

464. M. Linnoila et al.,*Drugs* (1979) 18: 293.

465. Charles V. Wetli and Joseph H. Davis, *JAMA* (Sept. 22, 1978) 240, no. 13: 1339.

466. *Drug Interaction Index,* ed. Ben R. Gant and Thomas D. Gant (Vancouver, B.C., Canada: Meditec Publ., 1973).

466a. Jerome P. Kassirer and John T. Harrington, *New England Jrl. of Medicine* (1985) 312, no. 12: 785-787.

467. Gina Kolata, *Science* (Oct. 22, 1982) 218: 361-362.

468. John T. Harrington et al., *Jrl. of Medicine* (Aug., 1982) 73: 155-159.

469. Olle Hansson, *Lancet* (Dec. 3, 1983): 1309.

469a. *Drug Facts and Comparisons* (St. Louis, Mo.: Facts and Comparisons, Inc., 1985) p. 35.

469b. Ibid., p. 36.

470. Ronald J. Kallen et al., *JAMA* (May 10, 1975) 235: 2125-2126.

471. Edward L. Snyder et al., *New England Jrl. of Medicine* (Feb. 6, 1975) 292: 320.

472. Ali Haddad and Evan Strong,*New England Jrl. of Medicine* (May 15, 1975) 292: 1082.

473. Donald McCaughan, *Lancet* (March 3, 1984): 513-514.

474. H. John Reineck, *Comprehensive Therapy* (Nov., 1981) 7: 12-21.

475. Orville J. Stone, *Medical Times* (Dec., 1971) 99: 143-155.

476. Ernest Newbrun et al.,*Caries Research* (1980) 14: 75-83.

477. Bernhard A. Eskin, *Transactions of the N.Y. Academy of Sciences* (Dec., 1970) 31: 911-947.

478. George Thomas Beatson,*Lancet* (July 18, 1896): 162-165.

479. Bernhard A. Eskin, *Advances in Exper. Medicine and Biology* (1977) 91: 293-304.

479a. G. Norris Bollenback,*Nutrition Today* (Jan./Feb., 1986): 25-27.

480. J. Wolff and I.L. Chaikoff, *Jrl. of Biological Chemistry* (1948) 172: 855-856.

480a. J. Wolff, I.L. Chaikoff et al., *Endocrinology* (1949) 45: 504-513.

481. Frederick L. Trowbridge et al., *Pediatrics* (1975) 56: 82-90.

482. Frederick L. Trowbridge, *Amer. Jrl. of Clinical Nutrition* (1975) 28: 712-716.

483. Jan Wolff, *Amer. Jrl. of Medicine* (1969) 47: 101-124.

484. J. Wolff and I.L. Chaikoff, *Endocrinology* (1948) 42: 468-471.

485. Jane Teas, *Medical Hypotheses* (1981) 7: 601-613.

486. Jane Teas, *Nutrition and Cancer* (1983) 4, no. 3: 217-222.

486a. Jane Teas et al., *Cancer Research* (1984) 44: 2758-2761.

486b. Masato Ohshima and Jerrold M. Ward,*Cancer Research* (Feb., 1986) 46: 877-883.

486c. Bandaru S. Reddy et al., *Nutrition and Cancer* (1985) 7, no 1 and 2: 59-64.

487. G.I. Vidor in *CRC Handbook Series in Food and Nutrition, Section E,* vol. 1, op. cit. (ref. 223).

487a. Committee on Dietary Allowances, Food and Nutrition Board, *Recommended Dietary Allowances,* 9th ed. (Washington, D.C.:*National Academy of Sciences,* 1980) p. 148.

487b. J. Wolff, *American Jrl. of Medicine* (1969) 47: 101. Cited by Marjorie Safran and Lewis E. Braverman, *Obstetrics & Gynecology* (1982) 60, no. 1: 35-40, at 38.

488. Thomas H. Shepard, *Catalog of Teratogenic Agents* (Baltimore, Md.: Johns Hopkins Univ. Press, 1983).

489. J.E. Fulton, Jr. and E. Black, *Dr. Fulton's Step-by-Step Program for Clearing Acne* (New York: Harper and Row, 1983).

490. Marjorie Safran and Lewis E. Braverman, *Obstetrics and Gynecology* (1982) 60, no. 1: 35-40.

491. Lee W. Wattenberg,*Cancer Research* (1975) 35: 3326-3331.

491a. N. Bagchi et al., *Science* (Oct. 18, 1985) 230: 325-327.

491b. C.P. Barsano,*Environmental Health Perspectives* (1981) 38: 71. Cited in ref. 491a.

492. Marshall B. Block and Salvatore J. DeFranceso, *Seminars in Endocrinology and Metabolism* (1979) 36: 510-511.

492a. Robert W. Cullen and Susan M. Oace, *Jrl. of Nutrition Education* (1976) 8: 101-102.

493. Richard F. Gillum, *Amer. Heart Jrl.* (1982) 103: 1084-1085.

494. Daniel S. Bernstein et al., *JAMA* (1966) 198: 499-504.

494a. Olli Simonen and Ossi Laitinen, *Lancet* (Aug. 24, 1985): 432-434.

494b. Jennifer Madans et al., *American Jrl. of Public Health* (1983) 73, no. 3: 296-298.

495. Jenifer Jowsey et al., *American Jrl. of Medicine* (1972) 53: 43-49.

496. O. Grove and B. Halver, *Acta Med. Scand.* (1981) 209: 469-471.

497. Hector F. DeLuca, *Harvey Lectures* (1980) Series 75: 333-379.

497a. Hector F. DeLuca and Heinrich K. Schnoes, *Ann. Rev. Biochem.* (1983) 52: 411-439.

497b. R.A. Corradino et al., *Arch. Biochem. and Biophys.* (1981), 208: 273-277, cited by Hector F. DeLuca and Heinrich K. Schnoes, ibid.

497c. Y. Tanaka et al., *Arch. Biochem and Biophys.* (1980) 199: 473-478, cited by Hector F. DeLuca and Heinrich K. Schoes (ref. 497a).

497d. S. Okamoto et al., *Amer. Jrl. of Physiology,* in press, cited by Hector F. DeLuca and Heinrich K. Schnoes (ref. 497a).

497e. W.A. Rambeck et al., *Annals of Nutrition and Metabolism* (1986) 30: 9-14.

498. John F. Aloia et al., *Jrl. of the Amer. Geriatrics Society* (1982) 30, no. 1: 13-17.

498a. B. Lawrence Riggs et al., *New England Jrl. of Medicine* (1982) 306, no. 8: 446-450.

498b. Joseph M. Lane et al., *Orthopedic Clinics of North America* (1984) 15, no. 4: 729-745.

499. R.G. Van Kesteren et al., *Netherlands Jrl. of Medicine* (1981) 24: 14-16.

499a. John A. Kanis and Pierre J. Meunier, *Quarterly Jrl. of Medicine* (1984) New Series, 53: 145-164.

500. D.S. Berstein et al., *JAMA* (1966) 198: 499-504.

501. H. Luoma et al., *Scand. Jrl. Clin. Lab. Invest.* (1973) 32: 217-224.

502. D.R. Taves, *Nature* (Mar. 23, 1978) 272: 361-362.

502a. Harold S. Fleming and Val S. Greenfield, *Jrl. of Dental Research* (1954) 33, no. 6: 780-788.

503. A.J. Rugg-Gunn et al., *British Medical Jrl.* (1981) 150: 9-12.

503a. J. Afseth et al., *Caries Research* (1984) 18: 134-140.

503b. Hannu Hausen et al., *Community Dentistry and Oral Epidemiology* (1981) 9: 103-107.

504. Henry A. Schroeder, *The Trace Elements and Man* (Old Greenwich, Conn.: Devin-Adair, 1973) p. 15.

505. Thaddeus Mann, *The Biochemistry of Semen and of the Male Reproductive Tract,* op. cit. (ref. 315a) pp. 383-384.

506. I. Rapaport, *Bul. Acad. Nat. Med. Paris* (1959) 143: 367. Cited by Deborah A. Kurtz-Weidinger, ref. 507.

507. Deborah A. Kurtz-Weidinger, *Dental Hygiene* (July, 1982) 56, no. 7: 32-37.

507a. A. Wiseman, *Handbook of Experimental Pharmacology,* XX/2, Chap. 2 (Heidelberg: Springer Verlag, 1970) cited by H.S. Kleiner and D.W. Allmann (ref. 507c).

507b. G. Cimasoni, *Jrl. of Dental Research* (1965) 44: 1134-1144.

507c. H.S. Kleiner and D.W. Allmann, *Archives of Oral Biology* (1982) 27: 107-112.

507d. Arthur C. Guyton, *Textbook of Medical Physiology,* 5th ed., (Philadelphia: W.B. Saunders Co., 1976) pp. 35, 990-991.

507e. Frederick J. Bloomfield and Marjorie M. Young, *Inflammation* (1982) 6, no. 3: 257-267.

508. John Yiamouyiannis, *Fluoride, the Aging Factor* (Delaware, Ohio: Health Action Press, 1983) pp. 60-69, 175-176.

509. Paula Cook-Mozaffari et al., *Jrl. of Epidemiology and Community Health* (1981) 35: 227-244.

509a. C.M. Goodall, *New Zealand Medical Jrl.* (Aug. 27, 1980) 92: 164-167.

510. John S. Neuberger, *Jrl. of the Kansas Medical Society* (1982) 83: 134-139.

511. Irwin H. Herskowitz and Isabel L. Norton, *Genetics* (1963) 48, part 1: 307-310.

512. Alfred Taylor and Nell Carmichael Taylor, *Proc. of the Soc. for Experimental Biology and Medicine* (1965) 119: 252-255.

513. K.C. Kanwar and M. Sengh, *Experientia* (1981) 37: 1328-1329.

514. John J. Miller, testimony before the Special Committee on Fluoridation of the House of Representatives, Michigan State Legislature, Oct. 7, 1963.

514a. D.B. Ferguson, *Nature New Biology* (1971) 231: 159-160.

515. Nicholas C. Leone et al., *Public Health Reports* (1954) 69, no. 10: 925-936.

516. A.E. Martin, *British Dental Jrl.* (Oct. 5, 1965): 312-316.

517. A. Anasuya, *Jrl. of Nutrition* (1982) 112: 1787-1795.

518. Herta Spencer et al., *Annals of the N.Y. Academy of Sciences* (1980) 355: 181-194.

519. Denis English et al., *Blood* (1981) 58, no. 1: 129-134.

520. Jan G. R. Elferink, *Biochemical Pharmacology* (1981) 30: 1981-1985.

521. H.H. Messer et al., *Science* (1972) 177: 893-894.

522. H.H. Messer et al., *Nature New Biology* (Dec. 13, 1972) 240: 218-219.

522a. W.L. Gabler and P.A. Leong, *Jrl. of Dental Research* (1979) 58: 1933-1939.

522b. S.R. Greenberg, *Fluoride* (1982) 15, no. 3: 119-123.

522c. Takeki Tsutsui et al., *Cancer Research* (1984) 44: 938-991.

522d. Takeki Tsutsui et al., *Mutation Research* (1984) 139: 193-198.

522e. Takeki Tsutsui et al., *Mutation Research* (1984) 140: 43-48.

522f. Philip R.N. Sutton, *Medical Hypotheses* (1986) 20: 51.

522g. T. Okamura and T. Matsuhisa, *Jrl. of the Food Hygiene Society of Japan* (6: 382. Cited in ref. 522f.

523. *Chemical Abstracts* (1943) 37: 4818.

524. *Union of South Africa Forestry Science Bulletin* (1973) 236.

525. R. Dalbak et al, *Chemistry* (Sept. 25, 1970).

525a. T.H. Maltzman, *Federation Proceedings* (March 5, 1986) 45, no. 4: 970 (abstract no. 4747).

526. H.J. Wespi, *Schweizerishe Monatsschrift für Zahnheilkunde* (1982) 92: 273-289.

526a. Th. Marthaler, *Schweizerische Monatasschrift für Zahnheilkunde* (1983) 93: 1197-1214.

527. K. Toth and Edit Sugar, *Acta Physiologica Acadamiae Scientiarum Hungaricae, Tomas* (1980) 56, no. 2: 213-218.

527a. Herta Spencer et al., *The Science of the Total Environment* (1981) 17: 1-12.

527b. Ei-Ichiro Ochiai, *Biosystems* (1983) 16: 81-86.

528. William M. Dunlap et al., *Annals of Internal Medicine* (1974) 80: 470-476.

529. Osamu Itoh et al., *Gann* (1981) 72: 673-678.

530. B. Halliwell and J.M. C. Gutteridge, *Lancet* (Sept. 4, 1982): 556.

531. John M.C. Gutteridge, *FEBS Letters* (June, 1983) 157, no. 1: 37-40.

532. Osamu Itoh, *Gann* (1981) 72: 370-376.

533. W. Bohnenkamp and Ulrich Weser, *Biochimica et Biophysica Acta* (1976) 444: 396-406.

534. William J. Bettger et al., *Nutrition Reports International* (1979) 19: 893-900.

535. K.A. Andrewartha and I.W. Caple, *Research in Veterinary Science* (1980) 28: 101-104.

535a. Sofia G. Ljutakova et al., *Archives of Biochemistry and Biophysics* (1984) 235, no. 2: 636-643.

535b. Dawn L. Ellerson and Doris M. Hilker, *Nutrition Reports International* (1985) 32, no. 2: 419-424.

536. Joseph R. Prohaska and O.A. Lukasewycz, *Science* (July 31, 1981) 213: 559-561.

537. L.B. Lee, *Korean Jrl. of Nutrition* (1975) 8.

538. John R.J. Sorenson, *Jrl. of Medicinal Chemistry* (1976) 19, no. 1: 135-148.

538a. John R.J. Sorenson, *Inflammation* (1976) 1, no. 3: 317-331.

538b. John R.J. Sorenson, *Nutrition Research* (1985) supp. 1: 5457-5463.

538c. John R.J. Sorenson and Werner Hangarter, *Inflammation* (1977) 2, no. 3: 217-238.

538d. John R.J. Sorenson, *Progress in Medicinal Chemistry* (1978) 15: 211-260.

539. K.G.D. Allen and L.M. Klevay, *Atherosclerosis* (1978) 29: 81-93.

539a. K.G.D. Allen and L.M. Klevay, *Atherosclerosis* (1978) 31: 259-271.

992 The Reverse Effect

540. Brad W.C. Lau and Leslie M. Klevay, *Jrl. of Nutrition* (1981) 111: 1698-1703.
541. W. Harvey and Kenneth G.D. Allen, *Jrl. of Nutrition* (1981) 111: 1855-1858.
542. Peter W.F. Fischer and Maurice W. Collins, *Amer. Jrl. of Clinical Nutrition* (April, 1981) 34: 595-597.
543. Leslie M. Klevay, *Amer. Jrl. of Clinical Nutrition*, ibid.: 597-598.
543a. Ny Wu et al., *Nutrition Research* (1984) 4: 305-314.
543b. S.C. Croswell and K.Y. Lei, *Jrl. of Nutrition* (1985) 115: 473-482.
543c. Denis M. Medeiros et al., *Federation Proceedings* (March 1, 1984) 43, no. 3: 682 (abstract no. 2325).
543d. Denham Harman, *Jrl. of Gerontology* (1965) 20: 151-153.
543e. Denham Harman, *Circulation* (Oct., 1966) supp. to vols. 33 and 34: III 13-III 14.
544. Robert A. Jacob et al., *Amer. Jrl of Clinical Nutrition* (1978) 31: 477-480.
545. Owen Epstein et al., *Amer. Jrl. of Clinical Nutrition* (1980) 33: 965-967.
546. T. Stephen Davies, Lancet (Oct. 23, 1982): 935.
547. K. Michael Hambridge, *Amer. Jrl. of Clinical Nutrition* (1973) 26: 1212-1215.
547a. Masae Yukawa, *Science of the Total Environment* (1984) 38: 41-54.
548. W.R. Walker and Daphne M. Keets, *Agents and Actions* (1976) 6, no. 4: 454-459.
549. T.B. Fitzpatrick et al., *Science* (1966) 152: 88-89.
550. Jess H. Mottaz and Alvin S. Zelickson, *Advances in Biology of Skin* (1967) 9: 471-489.
551. Henry A. Schroeder, *The Trace Elements and Man*, op. cit. (ref. 504) p. 129.
552. Henry A. Schroeder and Alexis P. Nason, *Jrl. of Investigative Dermatology* (1969) 53, no. 1: 71-78.
552a. Hirosi Yosikawa, *Japanese Jrl. of Medical Science, vol. 2, Biochemistry* (Feb., 1937) 3: 195-196.
553. H. Kikkawa et al., *Science* (1955) 121: 43-47.
554. H. Gross and M.M. Green, *Science* (1955) 122: 330.
555. A. Damon and J. Roen, *Human Biology* (1973) 45: 683-693.
556. G. Lasker and B. Koplan, *Social Biology* (Fall, 1974) 21, no. 3: 290-295.
556a. F.A.J. Thiele, *British Jrl. of Dermatology* (1975) 92: 355-358.
557. Carl C. Pfeiffer, *Mental and Elemental Nutrients* (New Canaan, Conn.: Keats Publ. Co., 1975) p. 336.
558. M.H. Briggs et al., *Experientia* (1972) 28: 406-407.
558a. L.A. Derrick Tovey and G.H. Lathe, *Lancet* (Sept. 14, 1968): 596-600.
558b. Sheila C. Vir et al., *American Jrl. of Clinical Nutrition* (1981) 34: 1479-1483.
559. Thaddeus Mann, *The Biochemistry of Semen and the Male Reproductive Tract*, op. cit. (ref. 315a) p. 283.
560. Sharon Battersby et al., *Fertility and Sterility* (1982) 37: 230-235.
560a. *U.S. Pharmacist* (1985) 10, no. 5: 15. Cited by Alexander Grant, *Healthwise* (Sept., 1985) 8, no. 9: 4.
561. S.S. Riar et al., *Indian Jrl. of Experimental Biology* (1981) 19: 1121-1123.
562. G.L. Fisher et al., *Cancer* (1981) 47: 1838-1844.
563. Ifor D. Capel et al., *Oncology* (1982) 39: 38-41.
563a. Ehad J. Margalioth et al., *Cancer* (1985) 56: 856-859.
564. G.N. Schrauzer et al., *Bioinorganic Chemistry* (1977) 7: 35-56.
564a. G.L. Fisher et al., *Cancer* (1976) 37: 356-363.
565. Ira M. Goldstein et al., *Annals of the N.Y. Academy of Sciences* (1982) 389: 368-379.
566. Edward J. Calabrese et al., *Environmental Research* (1980) 21: 366-372.
567. G.S. Moore and E.J. Calabrese, *Jrl. of Environmental Pathology and Technology* (1980) 4: 271-279.
568. H. Scheinberg and I. Sternlieb, cited by R. Deana et al., *International Jrl. for Vit. Nutr. Res.* (1975) 45: 175-182.
568a. Elizabeth B. Finley and Florian L. Cerlewski, *Amer. Jrl. of Clinical Nutrition* (1983) 37: 553-556.
568b. *Nutrition Reviews* (Sept., 1984) 42, no. 9: 319-321.

569. J.L. Gregor and S.M. Snedeker, *Jrl. of Nutrition* (1980) 110: 2243-2253.
570. Ting-Kai Li and Bert L. Vallee in *Modern Nutrition in Health and Disease, 5th ed.*, ed. Robert S. Goodhart and Maurice E. Shils (Philadelphia: Lea & Febiger, 1973) pp. 388-390.
570a. D. Meissner, *Zeitschrift für die Gesamte Innere Medizin und ihre Grenzgebiete* (1986) 41, no. 4: 114-115. Cited by *Nutrition Abstracts and Reviews, Series A* (Oct., 1986) 56, no. 10: 767-768 (abstract no. 6431).
571. G. I. Drummond et al., *Jrl. of Biological Chemistry* (1971) 246: 4166-4173.
572. John T. McCall, *Amer. Jrl. of Ophthalmology* (1981) 92: 559-567.
572a. David I. Paynter, *Jrl. of Nutrition* (1980) 110: 437-447.
573. L. Hurley in *Clinical, Biochemical and Nutritional Aspects of Trace Elements,* op. cit. (ref. 305) p. 371.
573a. Daret Kasemset and Larry W. Oberley, *Biochemical and Biophysical Research Communications* (1984) 122, no. 2: 682-686.
574. B. Lonnerdal et al., *FEBS Letters* (1979) 108: 51-55.
575. G.L. Everson and R.E. Shrader, *Jrl. of Nutrition* (1968) 94: 89.
575a. K. Hermansen and J. Iversen, *Diabetologia* (1978) 15: 475-479.
575b. Janet E. Merritt and Barry L. Brown, *Cell Calcium* (1984) 5: 159-165.
575c. Ralph R. Cavalieri in *Modern Nutrition in Health and Disease, 5th ed.,* ed. Robert S. Goodhart and Maurice E. Shils (Philadelphia: Lea & Febiger, 1973) p. 389.
576. I.J.T. Davies, *The Clinical Significance of the Essential Biological Metals* (Springfield, Il.: Thomas, 1972) p. 78.
577. Thomas S. Maugh II, *Science* (Dec. 22, 1978) 202: 1271-1273.
577a. Peter E. Sylvester, *British Jrl. of Psychiatry* (1984) 145: 115-120.
577b. P.J. Barlow and P.E. Sylvester, *Nutrition Research* (1985) supp. 1: S379-S381.
577c. Mark F. McCarty, *Medical Hypotheses* (1981) 7: 515-538.
577d. J. Harriett McCoy et al., *Nutrition Reports International* (1979) 19, no. 2: 165-172.
578. I.L. Mulay et al., *Jrl. of the National Cancer Institute* (1971) 47: 1-13, cited by Morton K. Schwartz, *Cancer Research* (1975) 35: 3481-3487.
578a. Larry W. Oberley and Terry D. Oberley, *Jrl. of Theoretical Biology* (1984) 106: 403-422.
579. T. F. Parkinson et al., *Amer. Nuclear Society Transactions* (1979) 32: 172-174.
580. C. Peter Flessel, *Advances in Experimental Medicine and Biology* (1977) 91: 117-128.
581. Frederick S. Archibald and Irvin Fridovich, *Archives of Biochemistry and Biophysics* (1982) 214: 252-263.
582. Vlado Valkovic, *Trace Elements in Human Hair* (New York: Garland, 1977).
583. Louis C. Kervran, *Biological Transformations* (Woodstock, N.Y.: Beckman Pub., 1980).
584. J.L. Hardwick and C.J. Martin, cited by David Beighton, ref. 585.
584a. M.E. Martin et al., *Jrl. of Bacteriology* (1984) 159, no. 2: 745-749.
585. David Beighton, *Microbios* (1980) 28: 149-156.
586. George C. Cotzias, *Medical Clinics of North America* (1976) 60, no. 4: 720-738.
587. Leon Earl Gray, Jr. and John w. Laskey, *Jrl. of Toxicology and Environmental Health* (1980) 6: 861-867.
587a. Richard M. Forbes and John W. Erdman, Jr., *Ann. Rev. Nutri.* (1983) 3: 213-231.
587b. Steven J. Haylock et al., *Jrl. of Inorganic Biochemistry* (1983) 18: 195-211.
587c. Steven J. Haylock et al., *Jrl. of Inorganic Biochemistry* (1983) 19: 105-117.
588. D. Shapcott et al., *Clinical Biochemistry* (1977) 10: 178.
588a. Andrew Szalay, U.S. patent number 4,343,905 (Aug. 10, 1982).
589. Cihad T. Gürson in *Advances in Nutritional Research,* vol. 1, ed. Harold H. Draper (New York: Plenum Press, 1977) p. 48.
590. Robert W. Tuman et al., *Diabetes* (1978) 27: 49-56.
591. Mark F. McCarty, *Medical Hypotheses* (1980) 6: 1177-1189.
591a. Alice E. Hunt et al., *Nutrition Research* (1985) 5: 131-140.

591b. Henry A. Schroeder, *The Trace Elements and Man* (Old Greenwich, Conn.: Devin-Adair Co., 1973) pp. 71-72.

592. H.A. Schroeder et al., *Jrl. of Chronic Diseases* (1970) 23: 123.

593. R.J. Doisy et al., in *Trace Elements in Human Health and Disease,* ed. Ananda S. Prasad, op. cit (ref. 330).

594. Howard A.I. Newman et al., *Clinical Chemistry* (1978) 24: 541-544.

594a. Michel Cote and Denis Shapcott in *Trace Element Metabolism in Man and Animals,* ed. J.M. Gawthorne, J. McC. Howell and C.L. White (Berlin: Springer-Verlag, 1982) pp. 521-525.

595. Abraham S. Abraham et al., *Atherosclerosis* (1982) 41: 371-379.

596. Rebecca Riales and Margaret J. Albrink, *Amer. Jrl. of Clinical Nutrition* (1981) 34: 2670-2678.

596a. J.C. Elwood et al., *Jrl. of the Amer. College of Nutrition* (1982) 1: 263-274.

597. Esther G. Offenbacker and F. Xavïer Pi-Sunyer,*Diabetes* (1980) 29: 919-925.

597a. Gina Kolata, *Science* (Jan. 9, 1987) 235: 163-164.

598. R.F. Borgman et al., *Royal Society of Health Jrl.* (Feb., 1982) 102: 1-2.

599. Richard A. Anderson, *Science of the Total Environment* (1981) 17: 13-29.

600. A.S. Abraham et al., *Gerontology* (1981) 27: 326-328.

601. D. Shapcott et al., *Clinical Biochemistry* (1980) 13: 129-131.

601a. Richard A. Anderson et al., *Biological Trace Element Research* (1984) 6: 327-336.

601b. Richard A. Anderson et al., *Federation Proceedings* (March 5, 1986) 45, no. 4: 471 (abstract no. 4752).

601c. Janet S. Borel et al., *Biological Trace Element Research* (1984) 6: 317-326.

602. Cihad T. Gürson, in *Advances in Nutritional Research,* op. cit. (ref. 589) p. 49.

603. William A. Check, *JAMA* (1982) 247: 3046-3049.

604. A. Leonard and R.R. Lauwerys, *Mutation Research* (1980) 76: 227-239.

605. Gerald E. Baull and David K. Rassin, in *Sulphur in Biology,* Ciba Foundation Symposium 72—New Series (New York: Elsevier, 1979).

606. Daniel P. DeKlerk, *The Prostate* (1983) 4: 73-81.

606a. K. Nakazawa and K. Murata,*Jrl. of International Medical Research* (1978) 6: 217-225.

607. Raymond F. Burk,*Biochemical Pharmacology* (1982) 11, no. 4: 601-602.

608. Kartar Singh et al.,*Indian Jrl. of Ophthalmology* (Dec., 1981) 29: 321-323.

609. L.F. Prescott,*Biochemical Society Transactions* (1982) 10: 84-85.

610. Noriko Tateishi et al.,*Jrl. of Biochemistry* (1981) 90: 1603-1610.

611. Anna M. Novi, *Science* (May 1, 1981) 212: 541-542.

611a. Ian Bremner in *Trace Element Metabolism in Man and Animals,* ed. J.M. Gawthorne, J. McC. Howell and C.L. White (Berlin: Springer-Verlag, 1982) pp. 637-644.

611b. P.D. Whanger et al., in *Trace Element Metabolism in Man and Animals,* ed. J.M. Gawthorne, J. McC. Howell and C.L. White (Berlin: Springer-Verlag, 1982) pp. 660-663.

611c. Kirk B. Nielson et al.,*Jrl. of Biological Chemistry* (1985) 260, no. 9: 5342-5350.

611d. R.J. Cousins, *Jrl. of Inherited Metabolic Disease* (1983) 6, supp. 1: 15-21. (New name is *Jrl. of Inherited Disease).*

611e. Paul J. Thornalley and Milan Vasak, *Biochimica et Biophysica Acta* (1985) 827: 36-44.

611f. *Nutrition Reviews* (Oct., 1985) 43, no. 10: 317-319.

611g. Robert J. Cousins, *Physiological Reviews* (April, 1985) 65, no. 2: 238-309, at 273.

611h. *Nutrition Reviews* (1985) 43, no. 3: 92-94.

612. Fernando Zambrano et al.,*Jrl. of Membrane Biology* (1981) 63: 71-75.

613. Herbert Sprince et al., *Agents and Actions* (1975) 5, no. 2: 164-173.

614. Saxon Graham et al., *Jrl. of the National Cancer Institute* (1978) 61, no. 5: 709-714.

614a. Saxon Graham, *Cancer Research* (1983) 43 supp: 2490s-2413s.

614aa. Kazuyoshi Morita et al., *Agric. Biol. Chem.* (1978) 42, no. 6: 1235-1238.

614ab. Gail E. McKeown-Eyssen and Elizabeth Bright-See,*Nutrition and Cancer* (1984) 6, no. 3: 160-170.

614ac. Chester J. Cavallito and John Hays Bailey, *Jrl. of the American Chemical Society* (1944) 66: 1950-1951.

614ad. Chester J. Cavallito et al., *Jrl. of the American Chemical Society* (1944) 66: 1952-1954.

614b. *The Merck Index,* 10th ed. (Rahway, N.J.: Merck & Co., 1983) item 9843.

614ba. Committee on Dietary Allowances, Food and Nutrition Board, *Recommended Dietary Allowances* (Washington, D.C.: National Academy of Sciences, 1980) p. 184.

614c. K. Seri et al., *Arzneimittel-Forschung* (1979) 29 (II) no. 10: 1517-1520.

614d. John A. Anderson, *Nutrition Reviews* (March, 1984) 42, no. 3: 109-116.

614da. Robert Shapiro, *Mutation Research* (1977) 39: 149-176 at 152.

614db. Stanley I. Wolf and Richard A. Nicklas, *Annals of Allergy* (1985) 54: 420-423.

614e. Howard J. Schwartz, *Jrl. of Allergy and Clinical Immunology* (1983) 71; no. 5: 487-489.

614f. *FDA Drug Bulletin* (1983) 13, no. 2: 11-12.

614g. Dorothy Sogn, *JAMA* (1984) 251, no. 22: 2986-2987.

614h. Alice S. Huang and William M. Fraser, *New England Jrl. of Medicine* (Aug. 23, 1984): 542.

614i. William A. Pryor, *Annals of the New York Academy of Sciences* (1982) 393: 1-22 at 10.

614j. Rhoda Papaioannou and Carl C. Pfeiffer, *Jrl. of Orthomolecular Psychiatry* (1984) 13, no. 2: 105-110.

614k. Bunji Inouye et al., *Toxicology and Applied Pharmacology* (1980) 53: 101-107.

614l. Hikoya Hayatsu and Akiko Miura, *Biochemical and Biophysical Research Communications* (1970) 39, no. 1: 156-160.

615. A.F. Gunnison, *Food and Cosmetics Toxicology* (1981) 9: 667-682.

615a. Yoshihide Suwa et al., *Mutation Research* (1982) 102: 383-391.

616. Dexter B. Northrup and Harland G. Wood, *Jrl. of Biological Chemistry* (1969) 244, no. 21: 5801-5807.

617. Ralph R. Cavalieri in *Modern Nutrition in Health and Disease,* 5th ed., ed. Robert S. Goodhart and Maurice E. Shils op. cit. (ref. 570) pp. 390-391.

617a. John L. Chamberlain III, *Jrl. of Pediatrics* (1961) 59: 81-86.

617b. E. Fischer et al., *Archives Internationales De Pharmacodynamie* (1983) 262: 182-188.

617c. Tadashi Inoue et al., *Mutation Research* (1981) 91: 41-45.

617d. Hajime Mochizuki and Tsuneo Kada, *Mutation Research* (1982) 95: 145-147.

618. Gerald P. O'Hara et al., *Jrl. of Pharmaceutical Sciences* (1971) 60, no. 3: 473-474.

618a. Claes B. Wollheim and Danilo Janjic, *American Jrl. of Physiology* (1984) 246: C57-C68.

618b. Colette N. Thaw et al., *American Jrl. of Physiology* (1984) 247: C150-C155.

618c. Torsten Stenberg and Bo Bergman, *Acta Odontologica Scandinavica* (1983) 41: 149-154.

618d. Joaquin Fontes de Melo et al., *Acta Odontologica Scandinavica* (1985) 43: 69-73.

618e. Jon M. Richards and Norbert I. Swislocki, *Biochemica et Biophysica Acta* (1981) 678: 180-186.

619. *World Health Organization Technical Report No. 532:* 43-48.

619a. X.M. Luo et al., *Federation Proceedings* (1981) 40: 928.

620. J.W. Burrell et al., *Jrl. of the National Cancer Institute* (1966) 36, no. 2: 201-209.

620a. Carl C. Pfeiffer, *Federation Proceedings* (1983) 42, no. 9: 817 (abstract no. 3076).

621. Edward J. Calabrese, *Nutrition and Environmental Health,* vol. 2 (New York: Wiley Interscience, 1980) p. 75.

622. B.E. Braun et al., *Molecular and Cellular Endocrinology* (1982) 26: 177-188.

623. D.A.N. Sirett and J.K. Grant, *Jrl. of Endocrinology* (1982) 92: 95-102.

624. J.W. Thomas and Samuel Moss, *Jrl. of Dairy Science* (1951) 34: 929-934.

625. Linda A. Mauck et al., *Biochemistry* (1982) 21: 1788-1793.

626. Edith M. Carlisle, *Federation Proceedings* (1979) 38: 553.

627. *Scottish Medical Jrl.* (1982) 27: 1-2.

628. Edith M. Carlisle, *Science* (1970) 167: 279-280.

629. Kalus Schwarz, *Federation Proceedings* (1974) 33, no. 6: 1748-1757.

630. Edith M. Carlisle and William F. Alpenfels, *Federation Proceedings* (1980) 39: 1787.

630a. Edith M. Carlisle and William F. Alpenfels, *Federation Proceedings* (March, 1984) 43, no. 3: 680 (abstract 2313).

631. Klaus Schwarz, *Proceedings of the National Academy of Sciences* (1973) 70, no. 5: 1608-1612.

632. Klaus Schwarz, *Lancet* (Feb. 26, 1977): 454-457.

633. T.J. Bassler, *British Medical Jrl.* (April 8, 1978): 919.

634. J. Loeper et al., *Presse Med.* (1966) 74: 865-868.

635. J. Loeper et al., in *Biochemistry of Silicon and Related Problems,* ed. Gerd Bendz and Ingar Lindquist (New York: Plenum Press, 1977): pp. 281-296.

636. J. Loeper et al., *Atherosclerosis* (1979) 33: 397-408.

637. Klaus Schwarz et al., *Lancet* (Mar. 5, 1977): 538-539.

637a. C.H. Becker and A.G.S. Janossy, *Micron* (1979) 10: 267-272.

638. C.H. Becker, *Micron* (1979) 10: 267.

639. Toru Nikaido et al., *Archives of Neurology* (Dec., 1972) 27: 549-554.

640. J.H. Austin in *Biochemistry of Silicon and Related Problems,* op. cit. (ref. 635) pp. 255-268.

641. U.S. patent number 2,943,982.

641a. J. Walter Wilson, *Annals of the New York Academy of Sciences* (1953-1954) 57: 678-683.

641b. D. H. Laughland W.E.J. Phillips, *Canadian Jrl. of Biochemistry and Physiology* (1954) 32, no. 6: 593-599.

642. S. Nadler and S. Goldfischer, *Jrl. of Histochemistry and Cytochemistry* (1970) 18: 368-371.

643. D.A. Levison et al., *Lancet* (Mar. 27, 1982): 704-705.

644. Klaus Schwarz, *Federation Proceedings* (1974) 23, no. 6: 1748-1757.

645. A.W. Varnes and W.H. Strain, *Age* (Oct., 1983) 6, no. 4: 141.

645a. Allen J. Natow, *Cutis* (1986) 37: 328-329

646. Keshan Disease Research Group of the Chinese Academy of Medical Sciences, *Chinese Medical Jrl.* (1979) 92: 471.

646a. A.T. Diplock, *Medical Biology* (1984) 62: 78-80.

646b. P.V. Luoma et al., *Research Communications in Chemical Pathology and Pharmacology* (1984) 46, no. 3: 469-472.

646c. Xiaoshu Chen et al., *Biological Trace Element Research* (1980) 2: 91-107.

646d. Guangqi Yang et al., in *Advances in Nutritional Research,* vol. 6, ed. Harold H. Draper (New York: Plenum Press, 1984) pp. 203-231.

646e. Xu Guang-lu et al., *Nutrition Research* (1985) supp. 1: S187-S192.

647. *Lancet* (Oct. 27, 1979): 889-890.

648. Jukka T. Salonen et al., *Lancet* (July 24, 1982): 175-179.

648a. W.L. Stone et al., *Annals of Nutrition and Metabolism* (1986) 30: 94-103.

649. Raymond F. Burk et al., *Biochemical Pharmacology* (1980) 29: 39-43.

650. J.G. Morris et al., *Science* (Feb. 3, 1984): 491-493.

651. Raymond F. Burk, *Ann. Rev. Nutr.* (1983) 3: 53-70.

652. Nai-Yen Jack Yang and Indrajit Dayalji Desai in *Tocopherol, Oxygen and Biomembranes,* ed. C. de Duve and O. Hayaishi (Amsterdam: Elsevier/North Holland Biomedical Press, 1978) pp. 233-246.

653. L. Juhlin et al., *Acta Dermatovener* (1982) 62: 211-214.

654. R.E. Serfass and H.E. Ganther, *Nature* (June 19, 1975) 255: 640-641.

654a. Kenneth P. McConnell, *Federation Proceedings* (March 5, 1984) 43, no. 4: 793 (abstract no. 2973).

655. Piette-Marie Sinet et al., *Life Sciences* (1979) 24: 29-34.

656. Raymond J. Shamberger et al., *Federation Proceedings* (1978) 37: 261.

657. G.N. Schrauzer, *Bioinorganic Chemistry* (1976) 5: 275-281.

657a. R.J. Shamberger and D.V. Frost, *Canadian Medical Assn. Jrl.* (1969) 100: 682.

657b. Raymond J. Shamberger and Charles E. Willis, *Critical Reviews in Clinical Laboratory Sciences* (1971) 2: 211-221.

657c. G.N. Schrauzer et al., *Bioinorganic Chemistry* (1977) 7: 23-34.

657d. G.N. Schrauzer in *Inorganic and Nutritional Aspects of Cancer,* ed. G.N. Schrauzer (New York: Plenum Press, 1977) pp. 323-344.

657e. Larry C. Clark, *Federation Proceedings* (1985) 44, no. 9: 2584-2589.

657f. Larry C. Clark et al., *Nutrition and Cancer* (1984) 6, no. 1: 13-21.

657g. Julian E. Spallholz et al., *Infection and Immunity* (1973) 8: 841-842.

657h. Julian E. Spallholz et al., *Infection and Immunity* (1973) 8, no. 5: 841-842.

657i. Werner A. Baumgartner, in *Trace Elements in Health and Disease,* ed. N. Kharasch (New York: Raven Press, 1979) pp. 287-305.

658. Gerhard N. Schrauzer and Debra Ishmael, *Annals of Clinical and Laboratory Science* (1974) 4, no. 6: 441-447.

659. G.N. Schrauzer et al., *Bioinorganic Chemistry* (1976) 6: 265-270.

659a. G.N. Schrauzer et al., *Bioinorganic Chemistry* (1978) 8: 387- 396.

659b. R.J. Shamberger, *Proc. of the Amer. Assn. for Cancer Research* (March, 1969) 9: 79 (abstract no. 311).

659c. R.J. Shamberger, *Jrl. of the National Cancer Institute* (1970) 44, no. 4: 931-936.

660. Carmia Borek, *Molecular Interrelations of Nutrition and Cancer,* ed. M.S. Arnott et al., (New York: Raven Press, 1982) pp. 337-350.

661. Daniel Medina et al., *Cancer Research Supp.* (1983) 43: 2460s-2464s.

661a. Henry J. Thompson et al., *Cancer Research* (1984) 44: 2803-2806.

661b. Maryce M. Jacobs, *Cancer Research* (1983) 43: 1646-1649.

661c. Raymond J. Shamberger et al., *Federation Proceedings* (1978) 37: 261.

661ca. Clement Ip, *Jrl. of the National Cancer Institute* (July, 1986) 77, no. 1: 299-303.

661d. Malay Chatterjee and Mihir R. Banerjee, *Cancer Letters* (1982): 187-195.

661e. Daniel Medina and Carol J. Oborn, *Cancer Research* (1984) 44: 4361-4365.

661f. Arthur W. Kilness, *JAMA* (June 27, 1977) 237, no. 26: 2843-2844.

661g. R. Boyne and J. R. Arthur, *Jrl. of Nutrition* (1986) 116: 816-822.

662. Ricardo O. Castillo et al., in *Selenium in Biology and Medicine,* ed. Julian E. Spallholz, John L. Martin and Howard E. Ganther (Westport, Conn.: Avi Publishing, 1981).

662a. L.O. Plantin et al., in *Trace Element Metabolism in Man and Animals,* ed. J.M. Gawthorne, J. McC. Howell and C.L. White (Berlin: Springer-Verlag, 1982) pp. 510-513.

663. Joan M. Braganza, *Lancet* (Nov. 30, 1985): 1238.

663a. H.E. Ganther and M.L. Sunde, *Jrl. of Food Science* (1974) 39: 1-5.

663b. H.E. Ganther et al., *Science* (1972) 175: 1122-1124.

663c. H.E. Ganther et al., (1973) in *Trace Substances in Environmental Health,* ed. Ed. Hemphill (Columbia, Mo.: University of Missouri, 1973), cited by Ganther and Sunde (ref. 663a).

663d. H.E. Ganther, *Environmental Health Perspectives* (1978) 25: 71-76.

663e. Toshima Nobunaga et al., *Toxicology and Applied Pharmacology* (1979) 47: 79-88.

663f. *Nutrition Reviews* (1984) 42, no. 7: 260-262.

664. Richard A. Lawrence et al., *Experimental Eye Research* (1974) 18: 563-569.

664a. W. M. Lewko and W.P. McConnell, *Federation Proceedings* (1982) 41: 623. Cited in ref. 661.

665. I. Ostadalova et al., *Physiologia Bohemoslovaca* (1979) 28: 393-397.

666. I. Ostadalova et al., *Experientia* (Feb. 15, 1978) 34, no. 2: 222-223.

667. Thomas R. Shearer et al., *Investigative Ophthalmology & Visual Science* (1983) 24: 417-423.

668. Kailash C. Bhuyan et al., *Investigative Ophthalmology & Visual Science* (1982) 22, ARVO abstract no. 13: 35.
669. R.W. Grover, *JAMA* (1956) 160: 1397-1398.
670. G. Nanjappa Chetty et al., *International Jrl. of Dermatology* (1981) 20: 119-121.
671. Raymond F. Burk and Daniel G. Brown, cited in *Medical World News* (Dec. 8, 1972) 13, no. 16: 51-53.
672. Eric J. Underwood, *Trace Elements in Human and Animal Nutrition, 4th ed.*, op. cit. (ref. 121) pp. 321-322.
673. Dietrich Behne et al.,*Jrl. of Nutrition* (1982) 12: 1682-1687.
673a. E.C. Segerson et al.,*Jrl. of Animal Science* (1981) 53, no. 5: 1360-1366.
674. K. Alterman, *British Jrl. of Nutrition* (1963) 17: 105.
675. Arthur A. Nelson, *Cancer Research* (April, 1943) 3, no. 4: 230-236.
676. L.A. Cherkes et al., *Experimental Biology & Medicine* (July, 1963) 53, no. 3: 315-317.
677. Henry A. Schroeder and Marian Mitchener, *Jrl. of Nutrition* (Nov., 1971) 101: 1531-1540.
678. Henry A. Schroeder and Marian Mitchener, *Archives of Environmental Health* (June, 1972) 24: 66-71.
679. *Federal Register* (Jan. 8, 1974) 39, no. 5: 1355.
680. Ibid., pp. 1355-1358.
681. K. Nakamuro et al., *Mutation Research* (July, 1976) 40: 177-183.
681a. G. Löfroth and B. Ames, *Environmental Mutagen Society Abstracts,* Annual Meeting, Feb. 13-17, 1977, Colorado Springs, Colorado. Cited in ref. 681b.
681b. C. Peter Flessel in *Advances in Experimental Medicine and Biology* (1977) 91: 117-128, at 125.
682. Makoto Noda et al.,*Mutation Research* (1979) 66: 175-179.
683. Gordon R. Russell et al., *Cancer Letters* (1980) 10: 75-81.
683a. James H. Ray et al., *Mutation Research* (1978) 57: 359-368.
683b. L.W. Lo et al.,*Mutation Research* (1978) 49: 305-312.
683c. Robert F. Whiting et al., *Mutation Research* (1980) 78: 159-169.
683d. *Critical Reviews in Food Science and Nutrition,* ed. Thomas E. Furia (Boca Raton, Florida: CTC Press, 1979) pp. 241, 298.
683e. S. Knuuttila, *Medical Biology* (1984) 62: 110-114.
684. J.R. Spallholz et al., *Proc. Soc. Exper. Biol. and Medicine* (1973) 143: 685-689.
685. J.P. Spallholz et al., *Proc. Soc. Exper. Biol. and Medicine* (1975) 148: 37.
686. Pamela Toy et al., *Research Communications in Chemical Pathology* (July, 1978) 21: 115-131.
687. J.A. Milner et al., in *Selenium in Biology and Medicine*, op. cit. (ref. 662), pp. 146-159.
688. *Selenium in Biology and Medicine*, op. cit. (ref. 662) pp. 531-534.
689. M.L. Scott, cited by D.E. Ulrey, *Selenium in Biology and Medicine*, op. cit. (ref. 662) pp. 176-191, at 182-183.
690. G.F. Combs, Jr. and G.M. Pesti,*Jrl. of Nutrition* (1976) 106: 958-966.
691. L.A. Witting and M.K. Horwitt, *Jrl. of Nutrition* (1964) 84: 351-360.
692. Ivan S. Palmer et al., *Jrl. of Nutrition* (1980) 110: 115-150.
692a. Brad M. Dworkin and William S. Rosenthal,*Lancet* (May 5, 1984): 1015.
692b. H. Korpela et al.,*Nutrition Research* (1985) supp. 1: S424-S425.
693. *Recommended Dietary Allowances*, 9th ed. (Washington, D.C.: National Academy of Sciences, 1980) pp. 162-164.
693a. H. Lithell et al., *Upsala Jrl. of Medical Sciences* (1983) 88: 109-119.
694. Orville A. Levander et al.,*Amer. Jrl. of Clinical Nutrition* (June, 1983) 37: 887-897.
695. Christine D. Thomson et al., *Amer. Jrl. of Clinical Nutrition* (July, 1982) 36: 24-31.
695a. Don R. Swanson, *Longevity Letter* (1986) 4, no. 3: 5-12, at 10.

695b. O.A. Levander et al., *American Jrl. of Clinical Nutrition* (1983) 37: 24-31. Cited in ref. 695a.

695c. C.D. Thomson et al., *American Jrl. of Clinical Nutrition* (1982) 36: 1076-1088. Cited in ref. 695a.

696. Gerhard N. Schrauzer and James E. McGinness, *Trace Substances in Environmental Health* (1979) 13: 64-67.

696a. Kern L. Nuttall, *Medical Hypotheses* (1985) 16: 155-158.

696b. Marja Mutanen and Hannu M. Mykkänen,*Human Nutrition: Clinical Nutrition* (1985) 39C: 221-226.

696c. C.D. Thomson et al., *Proc. of the Nutrition Society* (Jan., 1984) 43: 17A.

696d. Xianmao Luo et al., *American Jrl. of Clinical Nutrition* (1985) 42: 439-448.

697. Klaus Schwarz, *JAMA* (Nov. 28, 1977) 238: 2365.

698. Walter Mertz, *Science* (Sept. 18, 1981) 213: 1332-1338.

699. Kazuhiko Asai, *Organic Germanium, A Medical Godsend* (Tokyo, Japan: Kogakusha, 1977).

700. Masayoshi Kanisawa and Henry A. Schroeder,*Cancer Research* (June, 1967) 27: 1192-1195.

701. Masayoshi Kanisawa and Henry A. Schroeder, *Cancer Research* (April, 1969) 29: 892-895.

701a. H.A. Schroeder et al., *Jrl. of Nutrition* (1968) 96: 37-45.

702. F. Caujolle et al., *Bulletin Des Travaux De La Societe De Pharmacie De Lyon* (1965) 9: 221-235.

703. Nobuko Kumano et al.,*Sci. Rep. Res. Instit. Tohoku Univ.* (1978) 25: 89-95.

704. Bridget T. Hill et al.,*Cancer Research* (June, 1982) 42: 2852-2856.

705. Daniel R. Budman et al.,*Cancer Treatment Reports* (1982) 66: 1667-1668.

705a. Alison M. Badger et al., *Immunopharmacology* (1985) 10: 201-207.

706. Norito Kuga et al., *Acta Path. Jap.* (1976) 26: 63-71.

706a. Iwao Hirono et al., *Jrl. of the National Cancer Institute* (1978) 61, no. 3: 865-869.

707. R.I. Henkin and D.F. Bradley,*Life Sciences* (1970) 9, part II: 701-709.

708. M. Anke et al., *Internat. Arsen-und Nickelsymposium, Jena* (1980) p. 3, cited by M. Kirchgessner et al., *Prog. Clin. Biol. Res.* (1981) 77: 189-197.

709. Forrest H. Nielsen in *Clinical, Biochemical and Nutritional Aspects of Trace Minerals,* op. cit. (ref. 305) pp. 379-404.

709a. Forrest H. Nielsen, *Annual Review of Nutrition* (1984) 4: 21-41.

710. Noel W. Solomons et al.,*Jrl. of Nutrition* (1982) 112: 39-50.

711. G. Rabanyi and A.G.B. Kovach, *Acta Physiologica Academiae Scientiarum Hungaricae* (1980) 55: 345-353.

712. Bertil Magnusson et al., *Scandinavian Jrl. of Dental Research* (1982) 90: 163-167.

712a. David W. Eggleston, *Jrl. of Prosthetic Dentistry* (May, 1984) 51, no. 5: 617-623.

713. J.L. Greger et al., in *Trace Element Metabolism in Man and Animals,* op. cit. (ref. 611a) pp. 101-103.

714. J.M. Barnes and H.B. Stoner, *Pharmaceutical Review* (1970) 11: 211-231.

715. Attallah Kappas and Makin D. Maines, *Science* (1976) 192: 60-62.

716. Morton K. Schwartz,*Cancer Research* (1975) 35: 3481-3487.

716a. George S. Drummond and Attallah Kappas,*Science* (1982) 217: 1250-1252.

716b. *Tin as a Vital Nutrient: Implications in Cancer Prophylaxis and Other Physiological Processes,* ed. Nate F. Cardarelli (Boca Raton, Florida: CRC Press, 1986).

717. A.T. Diplock et al., cited by Leo S. Jensen, *Jrl. of Nutrition* (June, 1979) 105: 769-775.

718. A. Keith Brewer,*Jrl. of the International Academy of Preventive Medicine* 5, no. 2.

719. Arnold S. Relman et al., *Jrl. of Clinical Investigation* (1957) 36: 1249-1256.

720. Ronald R. Fieve and Kay R. Jamieson, *Modern Problems of Pharmacopsychiatry* (1982) 18: 145-163.

720a. Nobutoshi Kobayashi et al., *Gann* (1970) 61: 239-244.

720aa. J.J. Nagyvary et al., *Nutrition Reports International* (1979) 20, no. 5: 677-684.

720b. Andrew J. Adler and Geoffrey M. Berlyne, *American Jrl. of Physiology* (1985) 249: G209-G213.

721. Michael R. Wells and John Savory, *Lancet* (July 2, 1983): 29-34.

722. *Neurotoxicology* (1980) 1, no. 4: 83-88.

723. Daniel P. Perl and Arnold R. Brody, *Science* (April 18, 1980) 208: 297-299.

724. John R. McDermott et al., *Neurology* (June, 1979) 29: 809-814.

724a. J.M. Candy et al., *Lancet* (Feb. 15, 1986): 354-357.

724b. Peter O. Yates and David M. A. Mann, *Lancet* (March 22, 1986): 681.

724c. R.D. West, *Lancet* (1985) 2: 682. Cited in ref. 724d.

724d. Ian J. Deary and A.E. Hendrickson, *Lancet* (May 24, 1986): 1219.

724e. Marsha F. Goldsmith, *JAMA* (April 13, 1984) 251, no. 14: 1805-1812.

724f. Stanley B. Prusiner, *Scientific American* (October, 1984) 251, no. 4: 50-59.

724g. Robert Katzman, *New England Jrl. of Medicine* (April 10, 1986) 314, no. 15: 964-973.

724h. Jurgen Bommer et al., *Lancet* (June 18, 1983): 1390.

725. J.M.C. Gutteridge et al., *Biochimica et Biophysica Acta* (1985) 835: 441-447. Cited in B. Halliwell and J.M.C. Gutteridge, *Molecular Aspects of Medicine* (1985) 8: 89-193, at 137.

725a. Sharon P. Andreoli et al., *New England Jrl. of Medicine* (1984) 310, no. 17: 1079-1084.

725b. Allen C. Alfrey, *New England Jrl. of Medicine* (1984) 310, no. 17: 1113-1115.

725c. A.G. Hocken, *New Zealand Medical Jrl.* (March 28, 1984): 190-192.

725d. Aileen B. Sedman et al., *New England Jrl. of Medicine* (1985) 312, no. 21: 1337-1343.

725e. Herta Spencer and Louis Kramer, *Jrl. of the American College of Nutrition* (1985) 4: 121-128.

726. Steven Levick, *New England Jrl. of Medicine* (July 17, 1980). Cited in ref. 726a.

726a. Doug Henderson, *FDA Consumer* (March, 1982) 16: 11-13.

726b. A. Lione, *Food and Chemical Toxicology* (1983) 21, no. 1: 103-109.

727. Forrest H. Nielsen, *Advances in Nutritional Research,* vol. 3, ed. Harold H. Draper (New York: Plenum Press, 1977) pp. 157-172.

728. Graham Carpenter, *Biochem. and Biophys. Research Communications* (1981) 102: 1115-1121.

729. C.H. Hill in *Trace Elements in Human Health and Disease,* vol. 2, ed. Ananda S. Prasad (New York: Academic Press, 1976) p. 284.

730. T. Romasarma and F.L. Crane, *Current Topics in Cellular Regulation* (1981) 20: 247-302.

731. Torben Clausen et al., *Biochimica et Biophysica Acta* (1981) 646: 261-267.

731a. Shinri Tamura et al., *Jrl. of Biological Chemistry* (1984) 259, no. 10: 6650-6658.

731b. Clayton E. Heyliger et al., *Science* (1985) 227: 1474-1477.

732. Anthony White, *Lancet* (Oct. 17, 1981): 865.

733. A.R. Byrne and L. Kosta, *Science of the Total Environment* (1978) 10: 17-30.

734. Duane R. Myron et al., *Jrl. of Agricultural and Food Chemistry* (1977) 25: 297-300.

735. J.S. Larsen and O. Thomsen, *Basic Research in Cardiology* (1980) 75: 428-432.

736. L.C. Cantley et al., *Jrl. of Biological Chemistry* (1977) 252: 7421-7423.

736a. Robert P. Steffen et al., *Hypertension* (1981) 3: I 173-I 178.

736b. I.S. Cohen, *Experientia* (1983) 39: 1280-1282.

737. D.A.T. Dick et al., *Jrl. of Physiology* (1981) 310: 24P.

738. G.J. Naylor and A. H. W. Smith, *Psych. Med.* (1981) 11: 249-256.

739. H.U. Meisch and H.J. Bielig, *Basic Research in Cardiology* (1980) 75: 413-417.

740. *Lancet* (March 21, 1981): 646-647.

740a. Danuta Witkowska and Jacek Brzezinski, *Polish Jrl. of Pharmacology and Pharmacy* (1979) 31: 393-398.

740b. *Lancet* (Sept. 5, 1981): 511-512.

741. Bohdan R. Nechay et al., *Federation Proceedings* (1986) 45, no. 2: 123-132.

741a. John F. J. Cade, *Medical Jrl. of Australia* (1949) 2: 349-352.

741aa. Solomon H. Snyder, *Science 84* (November, 1984) 5, no. 9: 141-142.

741b. Earl B. Dawson et al., *Diseases of the Nervous System* (1970) 31: 811-820.

742. Earl B. Dawson et al., *Diseases of the Nervous System* (1972) 33: 546-556.

742a. Alex D. Pokorny et al., *Diseases of the Nervous System* (1972) 33: 649-652.

742aa. *The Neurobiology of Lithium,* report on a meeting of the Neurosciences Research Program, *N.R.P. Bulletin,* 1975. Cited by Manfred Eigen and Ruthild Winkler in *Laws of the Game* (New York: Harper and Row, 1983) pp. 304-305.

742b. Michael H. Sheard, *Nature* (1971) 230: 113-114.

742c. M.H. Sheard and G.K. Aghajanian, *Life Sciences* (1970) 9: 285.

742d. *Nutrition Reviews* (1982) 40, no. 10: 293-295.

742e. G.J. Naylor et al., *Lancet* (Nov. 21, 1981): 1175-1176.

742f. G.J. Naylor and A.H.W. Smith, *Psychological Medicine* (1981) 11: 257-263.

742g. Ewen Mac Donald et al., *Lancet* (Oct. 2, 1982): 774.

743. Suzanne Knapp and Arnold J. Mandell, *Science* (May 11, 1973) 180: 645-646.

744. J. Ananth and R. Yassa, *Comprehensive Psychiatry* (1979) 20: 475-482.

745. Jan A. Fawcett, cited in *Chicago Tribune* (May 15, 1983): 1, 8.

745a. E. Ferrari et al., in *Annual Review of Chronopharmacology,* vol. 1, edited by A. Reinberg, M. Smolensky and G. Labrecque (Oxford, England: Pergamon Press, 1984) pp. 407-410.

745b. J. Boyle et al., *British Medical Jrl.* (Jan. 4, 1986) 292: 28.

746. G.R.B. Skinner et al., *Med. Microbiol. Immunol.* (1980) 168: 139-148.

747. G.R.B. Skinner, *Lancet* (July 30, 1983): 288.

747a. B. Shopsin and S. Gershon in *Lithium: Its Role in Psychiatric Research and Treatment,* ed. B. Shopsin and S. Gershon (New York: Plenum Press, 1973) pp. 107-146.

748. Lis Fauerholdt and Per Vendsborg, *Acta Path. Microbiol. Scand.,* Sect. A (1981) 89: 339-341.

748a. Richard Harkness, *Drug Interactions Handbook,* op. cit. (ref. 94a) p. 96.

748b. Jean-Yves Follezou et al., *New England Jrl. of Medicine* (Dec. 19, 1985) 313, no. 25: 1609.

749. Alan Pestronk and Daniel B. Drachman, *Science* (Oct. 17, 1980) 210: 342-343.

750. E. Vinarova et al., *Activitas Nervosa Superior* (1972) supp. 14: 105-107.

751. T.K. Banerji et al., *Life Sciences* (1982) 30: 1045-1050.

751a. Dwane H. Dean and Raymond H. Hiramoto, *Nutrition Reports International* (1984) 30, no. 4: 757-764.

752. M. Kolomaznik et al., *Activitas Nervosa Superior* (1981) supp. 23: 275-276.

753. J. Raboch et al., *Activitas Nervosa Superior* (1981) supp. 23: 274-275.

754. Aaron Gillis, *British Medical Jrl.* (Dec. 16, 1978): 1716.

754a. Joseph Michaeli et al., *JAMA* (April 6, 1984) 251, no. 13: 1680.

755. J. Perez-Cruet and J.T. Dancey, *Experientia* (1977) 33: 646-648.

755a. J.R. King et al., *Psychological Medicine* (1985) 15: 355-361.

756. Norman E. Rosenthal and Frederick K. Goodman, *Annual Reviews of Medicine* (1982) 33: 555-568.

757. R. Bruce Lydiard and Alan J. Gelenberg, *Annual Reviews of Medicine* (1982) 33: 327-344.

757a. Lithium Information Center, Dept. of Psychiatry, University of Wisconsin, Madison, as cited by James W. Jefferson et al., in *Lithium Controversies and Unresolved Issues, Proceedings of the International Lithium Conference, New York, June 5-9, 1976* (Amsterdam, Holland: Excerpta Medica, 1979) pp. 958-963.

757b. James W. Jeffereson, John H. Greist and Deborah L. Ackerman, *Lithium Encyclopedia for Clinical Practice* (Washington, D.C.: American Psychiatric Press, 1983).

757c. Richard Harkness, *Drug Interactions Handbook,* op. cit. (ref. 94a) pp. 319-320.

758. P.L. Oe et al., in *Trace Element Metabolism in Man and Animals,* op. cit. (ref. 611a) pp. 526-529.

759. Rex E. Newnham in *Trace Element Metabolism in Man and Animals,* op. cit. (ref. 611a) pp. 400-402, 611.

760. Ulrich Weser, *Proc. Soc. Exper. Biol. Med.* (1967) 126: 669.

761. Alvin L. Moxon and Kenneth P. DuBois, *Jrl. of Nutrition* (1939) 18: 447-457.

762. Douglas V. Frost, *Advances in Exper. Medicine and Biology* (1977) 91: 259-279.

763. H.F. Smyth, Jr., *Food Cosmet. Toxicol.* (1967) 5: 51-58.

764. Douglas V. Frost, *Chemical and Engineering News* (Oct. 5, 1981): 4.

765. Irene Anundi et al., *FEBS Letters* (Aug., 1982) 145: 285-288.

766. Kenneth P. DuBois et al., *Jrl. of Nutrition* (1940) 19: 477-482. Cited by Edward J. Calabrese in *Nutrition and Environmental Health,* vol. 2, op. cit. (ref. 621) p. 120.

767. O.H. Muth et al., *Amer. Jrl. of Veterinary Research* (Oct., 1971) 32, no. 10: 1621-1623.

768. G.N. Schrauzer et al., *Bioinorganic Chemistry* (1977) 7: 35-56, at 52-53.

768a. K.H. Bauer, *Das Krebsproblem,* 2nd ed. (Berlin: Springer-Verlag, 1963) pp. 784, 811, cited by G.N. Schrauzer et al. (ref. 768).

768b. H. Osswald and K. Goertler, *Verh. Deut. Ges. Path.* (1972) 55: 289, cited by G.N. Schrauzer et al. (ref. 768).

769. G.N. Schrauzer et al., *Bioinorganic Chemistry* (1978) 9: 245-253.

770. Walter Mertz, *Federation Proceedings* (1982) 2807-2812.

771. Gillian R. Paton and A.C. Allison, *Mutation Research* (1972) 16: 332-336.

772. *The Secrets of Spirulina,* ed. Christopher Hills (Boulder Creek, Ca.: Univ. of the Trees Press, 1980) p. 11.

772a. P.N. Saxena et al., *Experientia* (1983) 39: 1077-1083.

773. Forrest H. Nielsen in *Clinical, Biochemical and Nutritional Aspects of Trace Elements,* op. cit. (ref. 305) pp. 379-404.

774. Henry A. Schroeder, *The Trace Elements and Man,* op. cit. (ref. 591b) pp. 166-167.

Chapter 8—106 References

1. Klaus Schwarz in *Clinical Chemistry and Chemical Toxicology of Metals,* ed. Stanley S. Brown (Amsterdam: Elsevier/North-Holland, 1977) p. 3.
1a. Lucius E. Sayre, *A Manual of Organic Materia Medica and Pharmacognosy* (Philadelphia; P. Blakiston's Sons, 1899) p. 30.
2. J.L. Corish, ed. *Health Knowledge,* 2 vols. (New York: Domestic Health Society, 1923) p. 741.
3. Klaus Schwarz, *Federation Proceedings* (1974) 33, no. 6: 1748-1757.
4. M.A. Bray, *British Medical Bulletin* (1983) 39: 249-254.
5. Von Anna M. Reichlmayr-Lais and M. Kirchgessner, *Z. Tierphysiol, Tierernährg u. Futtermittelkde* (1981) 46: 145-150.
6. M. Kirchgessner and Anna M. Reichlmayr-Lais, *Internat. Jrl. Vit. Nutr. Res.* (1981) 51: 421-424.
7. M. Kirchgessner and Anna M. Reichlmayr-Lais, *Trace Element Metabolism in Man and Animals,* ed. J.M. Gawthorne, J. McC. Howell and C.L. White (Berlin: Springer-Verlag, 1982) pp. 390-393.
7a. Anna M. Reichlmayr-Lais and M. Kirchgessner, *Arch. Tierernährung* (1981) 31: 731-737.
7b. H.W. Mielke et al., *American Jrl. of Public Health* (1983) 73: 1366-1369. Cited by ref. 7c.
7c. Howard W. Mielke et al., *Environmental Research* (1984) 34: 64-76.
7d. Carolyn Levitt et al., *JAMA* (Dec. 14, 1984) 252, no. 22: 3127-3128.
7e. C.A. Bache and D. J. Lisk, *Nutrition Reports International* (1984) 30, no. 1: 1-3.
8. John J. Mlller, *The Miller Message* (Aug., 1973) no. 59.
9. D. Kello and K. Kostial, *Environmental Research* (1973) 6: 353.
9a. Dorothy M. Settle and Clair C. Patterson, *Science* (1980) 207: 1167-1176.
10. J. Quarterman and Elaine Morrison, *British Jrl. of Nutrition* (1981) 46: 277-287.
11. Harold G. Petering, *Annals of the N.Y. Academy of Sciences* (1980) 355: 298-308.
11a. C.R.B. Blackburn, *Jrl. of Biological Chemistry* (1949) 178: 855. Cited by John J. Miller, *Jrl. of the International Academy of Preventive Medicine* (Dec., 1976) 3: 8-23, at 18.
12. D. McLean et al., *Science* (Oct. 8, 1976) 194: 199-200.
13. Arthur C. Guyton, *Textbook of Medical Physiology,* 5th ed. (Philadelphia: W.B. Saunders Co., 1976) p. 1076.
14. E.J. Underwood, *Trace Elements in Human and Animal Nutrition,* 4th ed. (New York: Academic Press, 1977) p. 419.
14a. Gary W. Goldstein and Diane Ar, *Life Sciences* (1983) 33: 1001-1006.
14b. Bryan K. Yamamoto and Charles L. Kutscher, *Pharmacology, Biochemistry and Behavior* (1981) 15: 505-512.
14c. Troels Lyngbye et al., *New England Jrl. of Medicine* (Oct. 10, 1985) 313, no. 15: 954-955.
15. David D. Choie et al., *Amer. Jrl. of Pathology* (1972) 66: 265-275.
16. D.G. Beevers et al., *Jrl. of Environmental Pathology and Toxicology* (1980) 4, no. 2-3: 251-260.
16a. S.J. Pocock et al., *British Medical Jrl.* (Oct. 6, 1984) 289: 872-874.
16b. William R. Harlan et al., *JAMA* (1985) 253, no. 4: 530-534.
16c. A.G. Shaper and S.J. Pocock, *British Medical Jrl.* (Oct. 26, 1985) 291: 1147-1149.
17. A.S. Harmuth-Hoene and R. Schlelenz, *Jrl. of Nutrition* (1980) 110: 1774-1784.
17a. F.L. Cerklewski and R.M. Forbes, *Jrl. of Nutrition* (1976) 106: 689-696.
17b. Abraham A. Van Barnveld and Cornelis J.A. Van den Hamer, *Toxicology and Applied Pharmacology* (1985) 79: 1-10.
18. Narayani P. Singh, *Archives of Environmental Health* (May/June 1979): 168-172.

1004 The Reverse Effect

19. A.R. Krall et al., *Magnesium in Health and Disease,* ed. Marc Cantin and Mildred S. Seelig (New York: Spectrum Publications, 1980).
20. Edward J. Calabrese, *Nutrition and Environmental Health,* vol. 2 (New York: Wiley Interscience, 1980).
20a. James C. Barton et al., *Jrl. of Laboratory and Clinical Nutrition* (1978) 92: 536-547.
21. Peter R. Flanagan et al., *Amer. Jrl. of Clinical Nutrition* (1982) 36: 823-829.
22. Gerald R. Bratton, *Medical World News* (May 25, 1981): 3.
22a. Gerald R. Bratton et al., *Toxicology and Applied Pharmacology* (1981) 59: 164-172.
22b. Lyle B. Sasser, Gerald R. Bratton et al., *Jrl. of Nutrition* (1984) 14: 1816-1825.
22c. R.T. Louis Ferdinand et al., *Toxicologist* (1982) 2: 82, cited by ref. 22.
22d. S.J.S. Flora et al., *Zeitschrift für die Gesamte Hygiene* (1984) 7: 409-411.
23. Marcel E. Conrad and James C. Barton, *Gastroenterology* (1978) 74: 731-740.
24. S. Niazi and J. Lim, *Jrl. of Pharmaceutical Sciences* (1982) 71: 1189-1190.
24a. S.J.S. Flora and S.K. Tandon, *Acta Pharmacologica et Toxicologica* (1986) 374-378.
25. A.E. Sobel and M. Burger, *Jrl. of Biochemistry* (1955) 212: 105.
26. C.M. Smith et al., *Jrl. of Nutrition* (1978) 108: 843-847.
27. Katheryn R. Mahaffrey et al., *Amer. Jrl. of Clinical Nutrition* (1982) 35: 1327-1331.
28. F.L. Cerklewski and R.M. Forbes, *Jrl. of Nutrition* (1976) 166: 778-783.
28a. Orville A. Levander et al., *Jrl. of Nutrition* (1977) 107: 378-382.
29. S.J.S. Flora et al., *Acta Pharmacologica et Toxicologica* (1983) 53: 28-32.
29a. Melvin A. Engelman, *Jrl. of the American Dental Assn.* (1963) 66: 122-123.
29b. A.I.B. Fernstrom et al., *British Dental Jrl.* (Sept. 18, 1962) 204-206.
29c. Daniel H. Rosen, *Medical Self-Care* (Fall, 1983): 22-24.
29d. Henry A. Schroeder, *The Trace Elements and Man* (Old Greenwich, Conn.: The Devin-Adair Co., 1973) p. 91.
29e. N.W. Rupp and G.C. Paffenbarger, *Jrl. of the American Dental Assn.* (June, 1971) 82: 1401-1407.
29f. *Consumer Reports* (March, 1986) 51, no. 3: 150-152.
29g. David W. Eggleston, *Jrl. of Prosthetic Dentistry* (May, 1984) 51, no. 5: 617-623.
29h. Magnus Nylander, *Lancet* (Feb. 22, 1986): 442.
29i. Don R. Swanson, *Longevity Letter* (April, 1986) 4, no. 4: 9.
30. Mary M. Gilbert et al., *Jrl. of Toxicology and Environmental Health* (1983) 12: 767-773.
31. J. Alexander et al., *Acta Pharmacol. et Toxicol.* (1974) 45: 387-393.
31a. K. Sumino et al., *Nature* (July 7, 1977) 268: 73-74.
32. Jadwiga Chmielnicka et al., *Bioinorganic Chemistry* (1978) 8: 291-302.
33. Jens C. Hansen and Preben Kristensen, *Toxicology* (1979) 15: 1-17.
34. S. Blackstone et al., *Food and Cosmetic Toxicology* (1979) 12: 511-516.
35. D.R. Murray and R.E. Hughes, *Proc. of the Nutrition Society* (1976) 35: 118A-119A.
35a. Yohko Fujimoto et al., *Research Communications in Chemical Pathology and Pharmacology* (Aug., 1985) 49, no. 2: 267-275.
35b. Eugene F. Ferraro et al., *Calcified Tissue International* (1983) 35: 258-260.
35c. M.E.J. Curzon and P.C. Spector, *Caries Research* (1983) 17: 249-252.
35d. M.E.J. Curzon, P.C. Spector, and H.P. Iker, *Archives of Oral Biology* (1978) 23: 317-321.
36. Ian Bremner, *Trace Element Metabolism in Man and Animals,* ed. J.M. Gawthorne, J.McC. Howell and C.L. White, op. cit., (ref 7), pp. 637-644.
37. K. Schwarz and J. Spallholz, *Federation Proceedings* (1976) 35, no. 3: 255.
38. Ronald H. Jones et al., *Proc. of the Soc. for Exper. Biol. and Med.* (1971) 137: 1231-1236.
39. G.N. Schrauzer et al., *Bioinorganic Chemistry* (1977) 7: 35-56.
40. Henry A. Schroeder, *The Trace Elements and Man,* op. cit., p. 98.
41. D.G. Beevers et al., *Jrl. of Environmental Pathology and Toxicology* (1980) 4, no. 2-3: 251-260.

42. Stephen J. Kopp and Thomas Glonek, *Science* (1982) 217: 837-839.
42a. Aijiroh Tokushige et al., *Hypertension* (1984) 6: 20-26.
42b. H.A. Schroeder, *Jrl. of Chronic Diseases* (1965) 18: 647.
42c. Luciano C. Neri and Helen L. Johansen, *Annals of the N.Y. Academy of Sciences* (1978) 304: 203-219.
42d. E.J. Underwood, *Trace Elements in Human and Animal Nutrition,* op. cit. (ref. 14) p. 252.
42e. Mukta M. Webber, *Nutrition Research* (1986) 6: 35-40.
43. Henry A. Schroeder, *The Trace Elements and Man,* op. cit. (ref. 29d), p. 100.
43a. Roger E. Cramer et al., *Jrl. of the American Chemical Society* (1981) 103, no. 1: 76-81.
44. Benjamin M. Sahagian et al., *Jrl. of Nutrition* (1967) 93: 291-300.
45. Masayoshi Kanisawa and Henry A. Schroeder, *Cancer Research* (1969) 29: 892-895.
46. Maynard B. Chenoweth, *Pharmacological Reviews* (1956) 8: 57-87.
47. Theodore N. Pullman et al., *Annual Review of Medicine* (1963) 14: 175-194.
48. Murray Weiner, *Annals of the N.Y. Academy of Sciences* (1960) 88: 426-510.
49. Arthur E. Martell, *Annals of the N.Y. Academy of Sciences* (1960) 88: 284-292.
50. Harry Forman, *Metal Binding in Medicine,* ed. Marvin J. Seven and L. Audrey Johnson (Philadelphia: Lippincott, 1960) pp. 82-114.
50a. Bruce W. Halstead, *The Scientific Basis of EDTA Chelation Therapy* (Colton, CA: Golden Quill Publishers, Inc., 1979).
51. R.P. Agarwal and D.D. Perrin, *Agents and Actions* (1976) 6: 667-673.
52. Gerald R. Peterson, *JAMA* (1983) 250: 2926.
52a. Louis R. Cantilena, Jr. and Curtis D. Klaassen, *Toxicology and Applied Pharmacology* (1982) 63: 344-350.
53. Mark M. Jones and Mark A. Basinger, *Medical Hypotheses* (1982) 9: 445-453.
53a. J.H. Graziano et al., *Jrl. of Pharmacology and Experimental Therapeutics* (1978) 206, no. 3: 696-700.
53b. H.Vasken Aposhian, *Ann. Rev. Pharmacol. Toxicol.* (1983) 23: 193-215.
53c. *Lancet* (June 9, 1984): 1278-1279.
53d. Teresa Twarog and M. George Cherian, *Toxicology and Applied Pharmacology* (1984) 72: 550-556.
54. Peter M. May and David R. Williams, *FEBS Letters* (1977) 78, no. 1: 134-138.
55. Jack Schubert and S. Krogh Derr, *Nature* (Sept. 28, 1978) 275: 311.
55a. W.H. Beets et al., *Agents and Actions* (1984) 14, no. 2: 283-290.
56. T.J. Baily Gibson, *New Zealand Medical Jrl.* (Jan. 27, 1982): 54-55.

1006 The Reverse Effect

Chapter 9—360 References

1. W.L. Porter in *Autoxidation in Food and Biological Systems,* ed., Michael G. Simic and Marcus Karel (New York: Plenum Press, 1979) p. 327.
1a. M.I. Sololeva, *Khlebopek. Konditer. Prom* (1974) 9: 24, cited by R.J. Sims and J.A. Fioriti in *CRC Handbook of Food Additives,* 2nd ed., vol. 2, ed. Thomas E. Furia (Boca Raton, Florida: CRC Press, 1980) p. 38.
1b. V. Braco et al., *Jrl. of the American Oil Chemists' Soc.* (1981) 58: 688-694.
1c. C.M. Houlihan et al., *Jrl. of the American Oil Chemists' Soc.* (1984) 61, no. 6: 1036-1039.
1d. R.E. Kramer, *Jrl. of the American Oil Chemists' Soc.* (1985) 62, no. 1: 111-113.
2. Winifred M. Cort, *Food Technology* (1974) 28: 60-66.
2a. M.I. Soboleva and I.V. Sirokhman, *Izv. Vyssh. Ucheb. Zaved Pishch. Tekhnol.* (1975) 1: 44, cited by R.J. Sims and J.A. Fioriti in *CRC Handbook of Food Additives,* 2nd ed., vol. 2, ed. Thomas E. Furia, op. cit., p. 38.
2b. S.J. Bishov and A.S. Henick, *Jrl. of Food Science* (1975) 40: 345-348.
2c. A. Bentsath, St. Rusznyak and Albert Szent-Györgyi, *Nature* (1936) 138: 798.
2d. Joachim Kühnau, *World Review of Nutrition and Dietetics* (1976) 24: 117-191.
2e. Emma Jo Lewis and Betty M. Watts, *Food Research* (1958) 23: 274-279.
2f. Fumitaka Hayase and HIromichi Kato, *Jrl. of Nutritional Science and Vitaminology* (1984) 30: 37-46.
2g. R.E. Henze and F.W. Quackenbush, *Jrl. of the American Oil Chemists' Society* (1957) 34, no. 1: 1-4.
2h. K.H. Eberhardt, *Präp Pharm.* (1966) 3, 1: 35. Cited in ref. 160c.
3. Leonard Hayflick, *Drug-Nutrient Interactions* (1985) 4: 13-33.
3a. J. Bjorksten, *Finska Kemists Medd.* (1971) 80, no. 2: 23. Cited in ref. 3.
3b. Sheldon S. Ball et al., *Age* (1985) 8, no. 3: 79.
4. Denham Harman, cited in *Lancet* (Dec. 14, 1968): 1281-1282.
5. Denham Harman, *Jrl. of Gerontology* (Oct., 1968) 23, no. 4: 476.
6. Margaret L. Heidrick et al., *Mechanisms of Ageing and Development* (1980) 13: 367-378.
7. Denham Harman, *Jrl. of the Amer. Geriatrics Soc.* (1976) 23, no. 5: 452.
7a. Dehnam Harman, *Age* (1980) 3: 64-73.
8. Robert R. Kohn, *Jrl. of Gerontology* (1971) 26, no. 3: 378-380.
9. Neal K. Clapp et al., *Jrl. of Gerontology* (1979) 34, no. 4: 497-501.
9a. M. Margaret King and Paul B. McCay, *Cancer Research* (1983) 43 supp: 2485s-2490s.
9b. Paul B. McCay et al., *Cancer Research* (1981) 41: 3745-3748.
9c. Hanspeter Witschi et al., *Jrl. of the National Cancer Institute* (Feb., 1977) 58: 301-305.
10. Denham Harman, *Age* (Oct., 1979) 2: 128-129.
11. Ibid: 109-122.
12. Denham Harman et al., *Jrl. of the American Geriatrics Society* (1977) 25, no. 9: 400-407.
13. A. Comfort et al., *Nature* (Jan. 22, 1971) 229: 254-255.
14. R. Hochschild, *Experimental Gerontology* (1973) 8: 185-191.
14a. R. Hochschild, *Experimental Gerontology* (1973) 8: 177-183.
15. Carl Pfeiffer et al., *Science* (Sept. 27, 1959) 126: 610-611.
16. C.C. Pfeiffer and H.B. Murphree, *Jrl. of Pharmacology and Experimental Therapeutics* (1958) 122: 60A-61A.
16a. Henry B. Murphree et al., *Clinical Pharmacology and Therapeutics* (1960) 1: 303-310.
17. K. Nandy and G.H. Bourne, *Nature* (1966) 210: 313-314.
18. K. Nandy, *Jrl. of Gerontology* (1968) 23: 82-92.
19. A.N. Siakotos et al., *Advances in Experimental Medicine and Biology,* ed. B.W. Volk and S.M. Aronson (New York: Plenum Press, 1972) pp. 53-61.
20. A.N. Siakotos et al., *Biochemical Medicine* (1970) 4: 361-375.

21. *Martindale-The Extra Pharmacopoeia,* 26th ed., ed. Norman W. Blacow (London: The Pharmaceutical Press, 1972) p. 1461.

21a. *Martindale-The Extra Pharmacopoeia,* 28th ed., ed. James E.F. Reynolds (London: The Pharmaceutical Press, 1982) p. 1700.

22. K. Nandy and F.H. Schneider, *Gerontology* (1978) 24, supp. 1: 66-70.

23. Raymond J. Shamberger et al., *Proc. Nat. Acad. Sci.* (1973) 70, no. 5: 1461-1463.

23a. William A. Pryor et al., in *Oxy Radicals and Their Scavenger Systems,* vol 2, ed. Robert A. Greenwald and Gerald Cohen (New York: Elsevier Biomedical, 1983): 185-191, at 185.

24. Richard D. Lippman, *Exp. Gerontology* (1980) 15: 339-351.

25. Karen Brawn and Irwin Fridovich, *Autoxidation in Food and Biological Systems,* ed. Michael G. Simic and Marcus Karel (New York: Plenum Press, 1980) p. 429.

26. Marina Scarpa et al., *Jrl. of Biological Chemistry* (1983) 258: 6695-6697.

26a. J.U. Skaare and T. Henriksen, *Jrl. of the Science of Food and Agriculture* (1975) 26: 1647-1654.

27. Irwin Fridovich, *Advances in Enzymology* (1974) 41: 36-97.

28. Giuseppe Rotilio et al., "Structure and Function Relationships in Biochemical Systems" in *Advances in Exper. Medical Blology,* vol. 148, ed. Francesco Bossa, Emilia Chiancone et al., (New York: Plenum Press, 1982) pp. 155-168.

29. Roger H. Pain, *Nature* (Nov. 17, 1983) 306: 228.

29a. John A. Tainer et al., ibid: 284-287.

29b. William C. Stallings et al., *Jrl. of Biological Chemistry* (Sept. 10, 1984) 259, no. 17: 10695-10699.

29c. Irwin Fridovich, private communication.

29d. Sheri Zidenberg-Cherr et al., *American Jrl. of Clinical Nutrition* (1983) 37: 5-7.

30. S.N. Giri and H.P. Misra, *Medical Biology* (1984) 62: 285-289.

30a. Mathew Walzer, *Jrl. of Immunology* (1927) 14: 143-174.

30b. Andrew L. Warshaw et al., *Laboratory Investigation* (1971) 25, no. 6: 675-684.

30c. C. Andre et al., *European Jrl. of Immunology* (1974) 4: 701-704.

30d. M.W. Smith et al., in *Maternofoetal Transmission of Immunoglobins,* ed. W.A. Hemmings (London: Cambridge University Press, 1976) pp. 381-395.

30e. G. Hemmings et al., *Proc. Royal Soc. of London* (1977) 198B: 439-453.

30f. W.A. Hemmings and E. W. Williams, *Gut* (1978) 19: 715-723.

30g. W.A. Hemmings, *Proc. Royal Soc. of London* (1978) 200B: 175-192.

30h. W.A. Hemmings in *Antigen Absorption by the Gut,* ed. W.A. Hennings (Baltimore: University Park Press, 1978) pp. 37-63.

30i. W.A. Hemmings in *The Biological Basis of Schizophrenia,* ed. Gwynneth Hemmings and W.A. Hemmings (Baltimore: University Park Press, 1978) pp. 239-257.

30j. A.C. Kulangara in *Protein Transmission Through Living Membranes,* ed. W.A. Hemmings (Amsterdam: Elsevier/North Holland Biomedical Press, 1979) pp. 429-430.

30k. J. Siefert et al., ibid, pp. 277-286.

30l. G. Hemmings and W.A. Hemmings, ibid, pp. 269-276.

30m. S.S. Rothmen, *Amer. Jrl. of Physiology* (1980) 238: G391-G402.

30n. W.A. Hemmings, *Medical Hypotheses* (1980) 6: 1209-1213 at 1215-1216.

30o. J.N. Udall et al., *Immunology* (1981) 42: 251-257.

30p. Michael L. G. Gardner, *Quarterly Jrl. of Experimental Physiology* (1982) 67: 629-637.

30q. M. Heyman et al., *Amer. Jrl. of Physiology* (1982) 242: G558-G564.

30r. Patrick J. Gallagher et al. *Atherosclerosis* (1982) 45: 115-127.

30s. Thomas A. Brown et al., *Jrl. of Immunology* (1984) 132, no. 2, 780-782.

30t. Murray Saffran et al., *Science* (Sept. 5, 1986) 233: 1081-1084.

31. Anon., *Nutrition Reviews* (Sept., 1980) 38: 326-327.

31a. Henry J. Forman and Irwin Fridovich, *Jrl. of Biological Chemistry* (1973) 248, no. 8: 2645-2649.

31b. James DiGuiseppi and Irwin Fridovich, *CRC Critical Reviews in Toxicology* (1984) 12, no. 4: 315-342.
31c. Koichi Ishigame and Yoshikazu Nishi, *Clinical Chemistry* (1985) 31, no. 6: 1094-1095.
31d. R. Boyne and J.R. Arthur, *Jrl. of Comparative Pathology* (1981) 91: 271-276. Cited in ref. 31c.
31e. Francoise Hertz and Alex Cloarec,*Life Sciences* (1984) 34: 713-720.
32. Joe M. McCord and Irwin Fridovich, *Jrl. of Biological Chemistry* (1969) 244: 6049.
33. J.M. McCord et al., *Superoxide and Superoxide Dismutases,* ed. A.M. Michelson, J.M. McCord and I. Fridovich (New York: Academic Press, 1977) pp. 129-138.
34. Eugene M. Gregory, *Jrl. of Bacteriology* (1973) 115: 987-991.
35. H. Moustafa Hassan and Irwin Fridovich,*Jrl. of Bacteriology* (1977) 129: 1574-1583.
36. Irwin Fridovich, *Ann. Rev. Pharmacol. Toxicol.* (1983) 23: 239-257.
37. Irwin Fridovich, *Advances in Enzymology* (1974) 41: 36-97.
38. Bo Lönnerdal et al., *FEBS Letters* (1979) 108, no. 1: 51-55.
39. S. Marklund, *Int. Jrl. Biochem.* (1978) 9: 299-306.
40. C.O. Beauchamp and Irwin Fridovich, *Biochimica et Biophysica Acta* (1973) 317: 50-64.
40a. Stefan L. Marklund, *Proc. of the National Academy of Sciences* (Dec., 1982) 79: 7634-7638.
40b. S.L. Marklund, *Medical Biology* (1984) 62: 130-134.
41. G. Rotilio and L. Calabrese, *Superoxide and Superoxide Dismutases,* ed. A.M. Michelson, J.M. McCord and I. Fridovich (New York: Academic Press, 1977) pp. 193-198.
41a. Alessandro Desideri et al.,*Biochimica et Biophysica Acta* (1984) 785: 111-117.
42. D. Tyler, *Biochemistry Jrl.* (1975) 147: 493-504.
43. S. Marklund,*Acta Physiol. Scand.* (1980) supp. 492: 19-23.
43a. R. Fantozzi et al., *International Jrl. of Tissue Reactions* (1985) 7, no. 2: 149-152.
44. I.M. Goldstein et al.,*Jrl. of Biol. Chem.* (1979) 254: 4040-4045.
45. U. Ambanelli et al., *Scad. Jrl. of Rheumatology* (1982) 11: 203-207.
46. Shiro Yamashoji and Goro Kajimoto, *FEBS Letters* (1982) 152: 168-170.
46a. C.E. Weber, *Medical Hypotheses* (1984) 15: 333-348.
46b. Peter L. Chiu et al., *Jrl. of Rheumatology* (1983) 10: 694-700.
46c. John T. McCaffrey et al., *Jrl. of the American Osteopathic Assn* (1983) 83, no. 2: 152-157.
47. Douglas P. Malinowski and Irwin Fridovich, *Biochemistry* (1979) 18: 5909-5923.
48. Karen Brawn and Irwin Fridovich, *Acta Physiol. Scand.* (1980) supp. 492: 9-18.
49. S. Marklund, *Acta Physiol. Scand.* (1980) supp. 492: 19-23.
49a. P.C. Bragt et al., *Inflammation* (1980) 4, no. 3: 289-299.
50. Kuo-Lan Fong et al.,*Jrl. of Biological Chemistry* (1973) 25: 7792-7797.
51. S. Weiss and A. LoBuglio,*Lab. Invest.* (1982) 47: 5-18.
51a. Charles W. Garner, *Lipids* (1984) 19, no. 11: 863-868.
52. L.R. DeChatelet et al., *Antimicrobial Agents and Chemotherapy* (1972) 1: 12-16.
53. U. Benatti et al., *Biochem. and Biophysical Research Communications* (1983) 111: 980-987.
53a. A. Vanella et al., *Gerontology* (1982) 28: 108-113.
53b. Richard G. Cutler in *Free Radicals in Molecular Biology, Ageing and Disease,* ed. Donald Armstrong et al., (New York: Raven Press, 1984) pp. 235-266.
53c. Jerome L. Sullivan, *Gerontology* (1982) 28: 242-244.
53d. Julie M. Tolmasoff, Tetsuya Ono and Richard G. Cutler,*Proc. of the National Academy of Sciences* (1980) 77, no. 5: 2777-2781.
53e. Richard G. Cutler, *Gerontology* (1983) 29: 113-120.
54. Tetsuya Ono and Shigefumi Okada, *Experimental Gerontology* (1984) 19: 349-354.
54a. Michael K. Holland et al., *Biology of Reproduction* (1982) 27: 1109-1118.
54b. Kunihiro Okamura et al., *American Jrl. of Obstetrics and Gynecology* (1984) 149, no. 4: 396-399.

54c. Akira Ono et al., *Nature* (1977) 266: 546-548.

54d. O. Haller et al., *Nature* (1977) 270: 609-611.

55. Bracha Roger-Zisman and Barry R. Bloom, *British Medical Bulletin* (1985) 41, no. 1: 22-27.

55a. B. Halliwell, *Medical Biology* (1984) 62: 71-77.

55b. A.K. Duwe and J.C. Roder, *Medical Biology* (1984) 62: 95-100.

55c. C. Friman et al., *Medical Biology* (1984) 62: 89-90.

55d. A.W. Segal, *Medical Biology* (1984) 62: 81-84.

56. S.J. Weiss et al., *Science* (1983) 222: 625-628.

56a. Samuel T. Test et al., *Jrl. of Clinical Investigation* (Oct., 1984) 74, no. 4: 1341-1349.

57. J.B. Johnston and J.E. Lehmeyer, *Jrl. of Clinical Investigation* (1976) 57: 836-841.

58. William R. Henderson and Michael Kalinger, *Jrl. of Clinical Investigation* (1978) 187-196.

58a. Peter L. Chiu et al., *Jrl. of Rheumatology*, (1983) 10: 694-700.

59. Bernard M. Babior et al., *Jrl. of Clinical Investigation* (1975) 56: 1035-1042.

60. Frederick A. Kuehl, Jr. and Robert W. Egan, *Science* (1980) 210: 978-984.

61. J.V. Bannister et al., *FEBS Letters* (1982) 145: 323-326.

62. Ira M. Goldstein et al., *Jrl. of Clinical Investigation* (1977) 59: 249-254.

63. Gerald Weissman, *Advances in Inflammation Research* (1979) 1: 95-112.

63a. Robert B. Zurier and Donna M. Sayadoff, *Inflammation* (1975) 1, no. 1: 93-101.

63b. P. Bellavite in *Advances in Inflammation Research*, vol. 1, ed. Gerald Weissman, Bengt Samuelsson and Rodolfo Paoletti (New York: Raven Press, 1979) pp. 150-155.

64. Neil M. Bressler et al., *Blood* (1979) 53: 167-178.

65. Henry Rosen and Seymour J. Klebanoff, *Jrl. of Experimental Medicine* (1979) 148, no. 1: 27-39.

66. John T. Cornutte et al., *New England Jrl. of Medicine* (1974) 290, no. 11: 593-597.

67. J. Dwight Stinnett, *Nutrition and the Immune Response* (Boca Raton, Fla.: CRC Press, 1983).

68. E. Siegel and B.A. Sachs, *Jrl. of Endocrinol. Metab.* (1964) 24: 313-318.

69. Stephen J. Weiss et al., *Jrl. of Experimental Medicine* (1978) 147: 316-323.

70. Kuo-Lan Fong et al., *Jrl. of Biological Chemistry* (1973) 248: 7792.

71. Stephen J. Weiss and Albert F. LoBuglio, *Laboratory Investigation* (1982) 47: 5-18.

71a. Peter H. Proctor and Edward S. Reynolds, *Physiological Chemistry and Physics and Medical NMR* (1984) 16: 175-189ff.

72. Stephen J. Weiss and Adam Slivka, *Jrl. of Clinical Investigation* (1982) 69: 255-262.

73. S.J. Klebanoff, *Seminars in Hematology* (1975) 12, no. 2: 117-142.

74. Joe M. McCord, *Science* (1974) 185: 529-531.

75. Robert A. Greenwald and Wai M. Moy, *Arthritis and Rheumatism* (1979) 22, no. 3: 251-259.

76. *Chemical Abstracts* (1979) 91: 208959G.

77. M.I. Salin and J.M. McCord, *Jrl. of Clinical Investigation* (1975) 56: 1319-1323.

78. Stephen J. Weiss, *Jrl. of Biological Chemistry* (1980) 255: 9912-9917.

79. Gidon Czapski and Yael A. Ilan, *Photochemistry and Photobiology* (1978) 28: 651-653.

80. Gerald Cohen, *Photochemistry and Photobiology* (1978) 28: 669-675.

81. Richard B. Johnston, Jr. et al., *Jrl. of Clinical Investigation* (1975) 55: 1357-1372.

81a. B.D. Goldstein et al., *Cancer Letters* (1981) 11: 257-262.

82. Karen Brawn and Irwin Fridovich, *Acta Physiol. Scand.* (1980) supp. 492: 9-18.

82a. Karen Brawn and Irwin Fridovich, *Archives of Biochemistry and Biophysics* (1981) 206, no. 2: 414-419.

83. Ingrid Emerit and Adolf M. Michelson, *Acta Physiol. Scand.* (1980) supp. 492: 59-65.

84. Adolf M. Michelson and K. Puget, *Acta Physiol. Scand.* (1980) supp. 492: 67-80.

85. Rolando F. Del Maestro et al., *Acta Physiol. Scand.* (1980) supp. 492: 43-47.

86. Bernard M. Babior, *New England Jrl. of Medicine* (1978) 298: 659-668.

86a. H.A. Simmonds et al., *Clinical Science* (1985) 68: 561-565.

1010 The Reverse Effect

86b. Harold P. Jones et al., *Biochemical Pharmacology* (1985) 34, no. 20: 3673-3676.

86c. P. Daniel Lew and Thomas P. Stossel, *Jrl. of Clinical Investigation* (Jan, 1981) 67: 1-9.

86d. B. Halliwell and J.M.C. Gutteridge, *Molecular Aspects of Medicine* (1985) 8: 89-193, at 147.

86e. M.G. Battelli et al., *Biochemical Jrl.* (1972) 126: 747-749. Cited in ref. 86d.

86f. E. Della Corte and F. Stirpe, *Biochemical Jrl.* (1972) 126: 739-745. Cited in ref. 86d.

87. Bernard M. Babior, *Jrl. of Laboratory and Clinical Medicine* (1975) 85: 235-244.

87a. Manikkam Suthanthiran et al., *Nature* (1984) 307: 276-278.

87b. Karen P. Burton, *American Jrl. of Physiology* (1985) 248: H 637-H 643.

88. H. Marberger, *Current Therapeutic Research* (1975) 18: 466-475.

89. H.S. Cobble and F.T. Lynd, *Mod. Vet. Practice* (1977) 58: 1009-1012.

90. Jay Brainard et al., *Archives of Ophthalmology* (1982) 100: 1832-1834.

91. K.O. Lewis et al., *Lancet* (July 24, 1982): 188-189.

92. W. Rosenfeld et al., *Dev. Pharmacol. Ther.* (1982) 5: 151-161.

92a. Karen S. Guice et al., *American Jrl. of Surgery* (1986) 151: 163-169.

92b. Karin Przyklenk and Robert A. Kloner, *Circulation Research* (1986) 58, no. 1: 148-156.

93. Larry W. Oberley and Garry R. Buettner, *Cancer Research* (1979) 39: 1141-1149.

94. Thomas W. Kensler et al., *Science* (1983) 21: 75-77.

94a. Bruce N. Ames, *Sciences* (Sept. 23, 1983) 221: 1256-1264, at 1261.

94b. C.M. Hassler and M.R. Bennik, *Federation Proceedings* (March 5, 1986) 45, no. 4: 1087 (abstract 5428).

95. Larry W. Oberley, *Superoxide Dismutase,* vol. II (Boca Raton, Fla: CRC Press, 1982) pp. 127-165.

95a. Larry W. Oberley et al., *Jrl. of the National Cancer Institute* (1983) 71, no. 5: 1089-1094.

96. T.L. Dormandy, *Lancet* (Oct., 19, 1983): 1010-1014.

97. Joe M. McCord and Kenneth Wong, *Oxygen Free Radicals and Tissue Damage,* Ciba Foundation Symposium 65 (Amsterdam, Holland: Excerpta Medica, 1979) p. 345.

98. Klaus M. Goebel et al., *Lancet* (1981): 1015-1017.

98a. Klaus M. Goebel and U. Storck, *American Jrl. of Medicine* (Jan. 1983) 74: 124-128.

99. Ingrid Emerit et al., *Human Genetics* (1980) 55: 341-344.

100. L. Parente, *Prostaglandins* (1982) 23: 725-730.

100a. B. Halliwell and J.M.C. Gutteridge, *Molecular Aspects of Medicine* (1985) 8: 89-193, at 139.

100b. A. Baret, G. Jadot and A.M. Michelson, *Biochemical Pharmacology* (1984) 33: 2755-2760. Cited in ref. 100a.

100c. Sezione di Palma, *Ballettino Della Societa Italiana di Biologia Experimentale* (1982) 58, no. 7: 1079-1085.

101. *Chemical Abstracts* (1979) 90: 52303d.

102. *Chemical Abstracts* (1979) 90: 19873s.

103. A. Vanella et al., *Gerontology* (1982) 28: 108-113.

104. Kozo Utsumi et al., *FEBS Letters* (1977) 79, no. 1: 1-3.

104a. David I. Paynter and Ivan W. Caple, *Jrl. of Nutrition* (1984) 114: 1909-1916.

104b. H. Moustafa Hassan and Irwin Fridovich, *Jrl. of Bacteriology* (1977) 132, no. 2: 505-510.

105. Hans Nohl and Dietmar Hegner, *European Jrl. of Biochemistry* (1978) 82: 563-567.

105a. Kenneth D. Munkres, *Age* (Oct., 1984) 7: 142-143.

106. *Nutrition Reviews* (Sept., 1980) 38: 326-327.

107. J.F. Mattel et al., *Acta Paediatr. Scand.* (1982) 71: 589-591.

108. Anna Jeziorowska et al., *Clinical Genetics* (1982) 22: 160-164.

109. B.W.L. Brooksbank and R. Balazs, *Lancet* (Aug. 16, 1983): 881-882.

109a. Pierre M. Sinet, *Annals of the N.Y. Academy of Sciences* (1982) 396: 83-94.

109b. P.M. Sinet et al., *Acta Paediatrica Scandinavica* (1984) 73: 275-277.

110. M. Habedank and A. Roderwald, *Human Genetics* (1982) 60: 74-77.

110a. G. Anneren and B. Björksten, *Acta Paediatr. Scand.* (1984) 73: 345-348.

110b. Yoram Groner et al., *Annals of the New York Academy of Sciences* (1985) 450: 133-156.

110c. Miriam Schweber, *Annals of the New York Academy of Sciences* (1985) 450: 223-238.

110d. Gina Kolata, *Science* (Dec. 6, 1985) 230: 1152-1153.

110e. Neal R. Cutler et al., *Annals of Internal Medicine* (1985) 103: 566-578.

111. M. Peter Esnouf et al., *Biochemical Jrl.* (1978) 174: 345-348.

112. H. Babich, *Environmental Research* (1982) 29: 1-29.

113. Wallace Snipes et al., *Science* (1975) 188: 64-65.

114. Alec D. Keith et al., *Proc. of the Soc. for Experimental Biology and Medicine* (1982) 170: 237-244.

115. P. Wanda et al., *Antimicrob. Agents Chemother.* (1976) 10: 96-101.

116. V.D. Winston et al., *Amer. Jrl. Veterinary Research* (1980) 41: 391-394.

117. A.L. Branen, *Jrl. of the Amer. Oil Chemists' Soc.* (Feb. 1975) pp. 59-63.

118. *Code of Federal Regulations,* title 21, part 182, subpart D on chemical preservatives, item 182.3173 (Washington, D.C.: Office of the Federal Register National Archives and Records Service, General Services Administration, 1982) p. 365.

119. *Kirk-Othmer Encyclopedia of Chemical Technology,* 2nd ed., vol. 2 (New York: Interscience Encyclopedia, 1963) p. 594.

119a. Al L. Tappel, *Advances in Experimental Medicine and Biology* (1978) 97: 111-131.

119b. B.D. Roebuck et al., *Jrl. of the National Cancer Institute* (1981) 72, no. 6: 1405-1410.

119c. David L. McCormick et al., *Cancer Research* (1984) 2858-2863.

120. W.M. Cort, *Jrl. of the Amer. Oil Chemists' Soc.* (July, 1974) 51: 321-328.

120a. L.W. Wattenberg in *Carcinogenesis, vol. 5, Modifiers of Chemical Carcinogenesis,* ed. T.J. Slaga (New York: Raven Press, 1980) p. 85. Cited by Djurhuus and Lillehaug (ref. 120g).

120b. L.A. Cohen et al., *Jrl. National Cancer Institute* (1984) 72, no. 1: 165-173.

120c. H. Witschi and S. Lock in *Carcinogenesis, vol. 2, Mechanisms of Tumor Promotion and Cocarcinogenesis,* ed. T. J. Slaga, A. Sivak and R.K. Boutwell (New York: Raven Press, 1978) p. 465. Cited by Djurhuus and Lillehaug (ref. 120g).

120d. H.P. Witschi et al., *Toxicology* (1981) 21: 37-45.

120e. H.P. Witschi, ibid: 95-104.

120f. C. Roston, *Food and Chemical Toxicology* (1982) 20: 329-336.

120g. R. Djurhuus and J.R. Lillehaug, *Bulletin of Environmental Contamination and Toxicology* (1982) 29: 115-120.

120h. Alvin M. Malkinson, *Environmental Mutagenesis* (1983) 5: 353-362.

120i. Preben Olsen et al., *Acta Pharmacol. et Toxicol.* (1983) 53: 433-434.

121. Al Tappel et al., *Jrl. of Gerontology* (1973) 28: 415-424.

121a. C.D.H. Evans and J. Hubert Lacey, *British Medical Jrl.* (Feb. 22, 1986) 292: 509-510.

122. W.L. Porter, *Autoxidation in Food and Biological Systems,* ed. Michael G. Simic and Marcus Karel (New York: Plenum Press, 1980) p. 351.

123. Joseph Kanner et al., *Jrl. of Food Science* (1977) 42: 60-64.

123a. H. Kläui and G. Pongracz, in *Vitamin C (Ascorbic Acid),* ed. J.N. Counsell and D.H. Hornig (London: Applied Science Publishers, 1981) pp. 151-168.

124. V.N.R. Kartha and S. Krishnamurthy, *Internat. Jrl. Vitamin and Nutrition Research* (1977) 47: 394-401.

125. Ibid. (1978) 48: 38-43.

126. P. Sanjeev Kumar et al., *Acta Vitaminologica and Enzymologica* (1981) 3 n.s., no. 4: 214-218.

126a. H. Hemilä and M. Wikström, *Scandinavian Jrl. of Immunology* (1985) 21: 227-234.

127. W. Schuller, as cited by L. R. Dugan, *Autoxidation in Food and Biological Systems,* ed. Michael G. Simic and Marcus Karel (New York: Plenum Press, 1980) p. 266.

1012 The Reverse Effect

128. Christopher S. Foote and Robert W. Denny, *Jrl. of the Amer. Chemical Society* (1968) 90: 6033-6035.
129. E.W. Kellogg II and Irwin Fridovich, *Jrl. of Biological Chemistry* (1975) 250: 8812-8817.
130. Norman I. Krinsky and Susan M. Deneke,*Jrl. of the National Cancer Institute* (1982) 69: 205-210.
131. J.E. Packer et al., *Biochem. and Biophys. Research Commun.* (1981) 98: 901-906.
131a. H.W. Renner, *Mutation Research* (1985) 144: 251-256.
131b. Heribert Wefers and Helmut Sies,*Biochemical Pharmacology* (1986) 35, no. 1: 22-24.
131c. Asher Begleiter, *Biochemical Pharmacology* (1985) 34, no. 15: 2629-2636.
131d. W.P. McGuire et al., *Proc. American Assn. of Cancer Research* (1977) 18: 85. Cited in ref. 215 of Chapter 2.
131e. C.E. Myers et al., *Science* (1977) 197: 165. Cited in ref. 215 of Chapter 2.
131f. Y.M. Wang et al., *Cancer Research* (1980) 40: 1022-1027. Cited by Jean Lud Cadet, in *Medical Hypotheses* (1986) 20: 87-94.
131g. J.G.S. Breed et al., *Cancer Research* (1980) 40: 2033-2038. Cited in ref. 131h.
131h. Sheri Zidenberg-Cherr and Carl L. Keen,*Toxicology Letters* (1986) 30: 79-87.
131i. Emilia A. Perez Ripoll et al., *Jrl. of Urology* (1986) 136: 529-531.
131j. Herman Baker et al., *American Jrl. of Clinical Nutrition* (1986) 43: 382-387.
132. Roman J. Kutsky, *Handbook of Vitamins, Minerals and Hormones*, 2nd ed. (New York: Van Nostrand Reinhold, 1981).
133. Karl Ford Nakken, *Strahlentherapie* (1966) 129: 586-595.
134. Bernard D. Goldstein et al.,*Archives of Environmental Health* (1972) 24: 243-247.
135. Karl Ford Nakken and Alexander Hill, *Radiation Research* (1966) 27: 19-31.
136. R.B. Wilson et al., *Experimental and Molecular Pathology* (1973) 18: 357-368.
137. R.J. Shamberger, *Autoxidation in Food and Biological Systems*, ed. Michael G. Simic and Marcus Karel (New York: Plenum Press, 1980) p. 646.
137a. Gian Paolo Littarru et al., in *Biomedical and Clinical Aspects of Coenzyme Q*, vol. 4, ed. K. Folkers and Y. Yamamura (Amsterdam: Alsevier Science Pubs., 1984) pp. 201-208, at 206-207.
137b. Milos Chvapil et al.,*Jrl. of Nutrition* (1974) 104: 434-443.
138. K.A. Andewartha and I.W. Caple, *Research in Veterinary Medicine* (1980) 28: 101-104.
139. R.A. Holman, *Nature* (May 18, 1957): 1033.
140. Kanematsu Sugiura, *Nature* (Nov. 8, 1958): 1311.
140a. T.M. Nicotera et al., *Mutation Research* (1985) 151: 263-268.
141. Richard Heikkila,*Science* (1971) 172: 1257-1258.
142. Raymond J. Shamberger et al.,*Proc. of the National Academy of Sciences* (1973) 70, no. 5: 1461-1463.
143. K.C. Bhuyan et al., *Age* (1981) 4: 141.
143a. John V. Fecondo and Robert C. Augusteyn, *Experimental Eye Research* (1983) 36: 15-23.
144. Simion Oeriu and Elena Vochitu,*Jrl. of Gerontology* (1965) 20: 417-419.
144a. Hansruedi Glatt et al.,*Science* (1983) 220: 961-963.
145. German patent no. 389,912.
146. U.S. patent no. 1,575,529.
147. H.S. Olcott and J. Van der Veen,*Jrl. of Food Science* (1963) 28: 313-315.
148. Luther L. Yaeger and Johann Bjorksten,*Autoxidation in Food and Biological Systems*, ed. Michael G. Simic and Marcus Karel (New York: Plenum Press, 1980) p. 409.
149. L.R. Dugan,*Autoxidation in Food and Biological Systems*, ed. Michael G. Simic and Marcus Karel (New York: Plenum Press, 1980) p. 266.
150. W.L. Porter,*Autoxidation in Food and Biological Systems*, ed. Michael G. Simic and Marcus Karel (New York: Plenum Press, 1980) p. 342.
151. Hans F. Stich et al., *Cancer Letters* (1981) 14: 251-260.
151a. U. Friederich et al., *Mutation Research* (1985) 156: 39-52.

151b. B.A. Kihlman, *Mutation Research* (1974) 26: 53-71.
151c. A. Ronen and M. Marcus, *Mutation Research* (1978) 53: 343-344.
151d. D. Weinstein et al., *Mutation Research* (1972) 16: 391-399. Cited in ref. 151c.
151e. Tatsuhito Yamagami et al., *Surgical Neurology* (1983) 20: 323-331.
151f. J.P. Minton et al., *Cancer* (1983) 51: 1249-1253.
151g. Clifford W. Welsch et al., *International Jrl. of Cancer* (1983) 32: 479-484.
151h. Ayumi Denda et al., *Carcinogenesis* (1983) 4, no. 1: 17-22.
151i. Taisei Nomura, *Cancer Research* (1983) 43: 1342-1346.
151j. K. Rothwell, *Nature* (1974) 252: 69-70.
151k. Abraham Nomura et al., *Jrl. of the National Cancer Institute* (1986) 76: 587-590.
151ka. Lee W. Wattenberg et al., *Cancer Research* (1980) 40: 2820-2823.
151l. Taisei Nomura et al., *Cancer Research* (1983) 43: 5156-5162.
151m. Jacob V. Aranda et al., *Jrl. of Pediatrics* (1983) 103: 975-978.
151n. A.B. Becker et al., *New England Jrl. of Medicine* (1984) 310: 743-746.
151o. Donald C. Rifas, *New England Jrl. of Medicine* (1984) 311: 257.
151p. F. Estelle R. Simons et al., *New England Jrl. of Medicine* (1984) 311: 257.
151q. Kathryn Simmons, *JAMA* (1984) 251, no. 4: 441.
151r. J.L. Ivy et al., *Medicine and Science in Sports and Exercise* (1979) 11, no. 1: 6-11.
151s. D.L. Costill et al., *Medicine and Science in Sports and Exercise* (1978) 10, no. 3: 155-158.
152. K.C.D. Hickman, quoted by Luther L. Yaeger and Johann Bjorksten in *Autoxidation in Food and Biological Systems* ed. Michael G. Simic and Marcus Karel (New York: Plenum Press, 1980) p. 405.
152a. Hisayaki Tanizawa et al., *Chemical and Pharmaceutical Bulletin* (1984) 32, no. 5: 2011-2014.
152b. Charles J. Palenik et al., *Jrl. of Dental Research* (1979) 58, no. 7: 1749.
152c. Paul F. DePaola (Forsythe Dental Center, Boston, Ma.) in a paper presented at the 60th General Session of the International Assn. for Dental Research. From a press release of the Intl. Assn. for Dental Research dated March 18, 1982.
152d. Julia F. Morton, *Quarterly Jrl. of Crude Drug Research* (1972) 12: 1829-1841.
152e. P.K. Reddi and S.M. Constantinides, *Nature* (1972) 238: 286. Cited in ref. 151j.
152f. Hans F. Stich et al., *International Jrl. of Cancer* (1982) 30: 719-724.
152g. Govind J. Kapadia et al., in *Carcinogens and Mutagens in the Environment,* vol. 3, ed. Hans F. Stich (Boca Raton, Florida: CRC Press, 1983) pp. 3-12, at 10.
153. Dan E. Pratt, *Jrl. of Food Science* (1965) 30: 737-741.
154. Irvin E. Liener, *Toxic Constituents of Plant Foodstuffs* ed. Irwin E. Liener (New York: Academic Press, 1969) p. 413.
154a. M. Nagao et al., *Proceedings of the Japanese Cancer Assn., 4th annual meeting,* 1982, p. 67. Cited by ref. 154b.
154b. Ikuko Ueno et al., *Jrl. of Pharmacobiodynamics* (1984) 7: 798-803.
154c. James F. Hatcher and George T. Bryan, *Mutation Research* (1985) 148: 13-23.
154d. Mendel Friedman and G.A. Smith, *Advances in Experimental Medicine and Biology* (1984) 77: 527-544.
154e. James T. MacGregor, *Advances in Experimental Medicine and Biology* (1984) 77: 497-526.
155. Karen Brawn and Irwin Fridovich, *Autoxidation in Food and Biological Systems,* ed. Michael G. Simic and Marcus Karel (New York: Plenum Press, 1980) pp. 434-436.
155a. R. Fink et al., *Lancet* (Aug. 10, 1985): 291-294.
155b. Shinji Kubota, *Alcohol* (1985) 2: 469-472.
155c. C.L. Keen et al., *Nutrition Research* (1985) supp. 1: 564-567.
156. Bruce N. Ames et al., *Proc. of the National Academy of Sciences* (1981) 78: 6858-6862.
157. Robert C. Smith and Lisa Lawing, *Archives of Biochem. and Biophysics* (1983) 223: 166-172.
157a. C. Deby et al., *Biochemical Pharmacology* (1981) 30: 2243-2249.

158. Charles N. Serhan et al., *Prostaglandins* (1984) 27, no. 4: 563-581.
158a. Nobuchika Ogino et al., *Biochemical and Biophysical Research Communications* (1979) 87, no. 1: 194-191.
158b. T. Glazer et al., *Nephron* (1984) 38: 40-43.
158c. J.H. Peters et al., in *Modulation and Mediation of Cancer by Vitamins,* ed. F.L. Meyskens and K.N. Prasad (Basel, Switzerland: Karger, 1983) pp. 104-113.
158d. Mark A. Reynolds et al., *Age* (Oct., 1984) 7: 93-99.
158e. B. Pence and F. Buddingh, *Federation Proceedings* (March 5, 1986) 45, no. 4: 1076 (abstract no. 5363).
159. John W. Armstrong, *The Water of Life* (London: True Health Publ. Co., 1951 and Hackensack, N.J.: Wheman, 1971).
160. C.K. Eapen, *Lancet* (Aug. 6, 1983): 405.
160a. J.T. Solyst et al., *Ann. Nutr. Metab.* (1980) 24: 182-188. Cited by Karan D. Israel et al., *Ann. Nutr. Metab.* (1983) 27: 425-435.
160b. Tong-man Ong et al., *Mutation Research* (1986) 173: 111-115.
160c. F.A. J. Thiele, *British Jrl. of Dermatology* (1975) 92: 355-358.
160d. Yu Chen et al., *Mutation Research* (1986) 164: 71-78.
161. M.A. Boehe and A.L. Branen, *Jrl. of Food Science* (1977) 42, no. 5: 1243-1246.
161a. Denham Harman in *Free Radicals in Molecular Biology, Ageing and Disease,* ed. Donald Armstrong et al., (New York: Raven Press, 1984) pp. 1-12, at 9.
162. Richard D. Lippman, *Age* (Oct., 1983) 6, no. 4: 146.
163. Vergil H. Ferm, *Proc. of the Society for Exper. Biol and Med.* (1964) 116: 675-676.
164. E.W. Kellogg III et al., *Nature* (Oct. 4, 1979) 281: 400-401.
164a. I. Rosenthal, *Experientia* (1983) 39: 718-719.
165. Alan B. Weitberg et al., *New England Jrl. of Medicine* (1983) 308: 26-30.
166. H. Joenje, *Medical Hypotheses* (1983) 12: 55-60.
167. *Bergey's Manual of Determinating Bacteriology,* 8th ed., ed. Robert Earle Buchanan (Baltimore: Williams and Wilkins, 1974).
168. J.K. Clarke, *British Jrl. of Experimental Pathology* (1924) 5: 141-147.
168a. Jose O. Alvarez and Juan M. Navia, *Lancet* (Jan. 11, 1986): 91.
169. Denham Harman, *Age* (1980) 3: 100-102.
170. A.F. McDonagh, *New England Jrl. of Medicine* (1986) 314: 121. Cited in ref. 173.
171. K. Bernhard et al., *Helv. Chim Acta* ((1954) 37: 306. Cited in ref. 173.
172. H. Beer and K. Bernhard, *Chimia* (1959) 13: 291. Cited in ref. 173.
173. Roland Stocker et al. (including Bruce N. Ames), *Science* (Feb. 27, 1987) 235: 1043-1046.

Chapter 10—128 References

1. Sidney Alexander, *Clinical Biochemistry* (1984) 17: 126-131.
2. Edward L. Schneider and John R. Reed,*New England Jrl. of Medicine* (1985) 312, no. 18: 1159-1168, at 1160.
3. Lisa McCann and David S. Holmes, *Jrl. of Personality and Social Psychology* (1984) 46, no. 5: 1142-1147.
4. Roy J. Shephard, *Canadian Medical Assn. Jrl.* (1983) 128: 525-530.
4a. K. Willcutts et al., *Federation Proceedings* (March 7, 1986) 45, no. 4: 972 (abstract no. 4759).
4b. G. Kaminori et al., *Federation Proceedings* (March 7, 1986) 45, no. 4: 972 (abstract no. 4755).
5. Harvey B. Simon, *JAMA* (Nov. 16, 1984) 252, no. 19: 2735-2738.
6. H.P. Rusch and B.E. Kline, *Cancer Research* (1944) 4: 116-118.
7. S.A. Hoffman et al., *Cancer Research* (1962) 22: 597-599.
8. Grant Newton, *Psychological Reports* (1965) 16: 127-132.
9. L.L. Gershbein et al., *Oncology* (1974) 30: 429-435.
9a. F.I. Katch et al., *Research Quarterly for Exercise and Sport* (1984) 55: 242-247. Cited in *Sports Medicine* (1985) 2: 452-453.
9b. B. Gutin et al., *American Jrl. of Medicine* (1985) 79, no. 1: 79-84. Cited in *Nutrition Abstracts and Reviews, Series A* (Feb., 1986) 56, no. 2: 113 (abstract no. 1006).
10. Steven Seely, *Medical Hypotheses* (1980) 6: 873-882.
10a. *Webster's Third New International Dictionary* (Springfield, Mass.: G & C Merriam Co., 1961) p. 1586.
11. R.S. Sohal, cited by William H. Pryor, *Annals of the N.Y. Academy of Sciences* (1982) 398: 1-22.
12. R.S. Sohal et al., *Mechanisms of Ageing and Development* (1984) 26: 75-81.
13. Ben E. Sheffy and Alma J. Williams, *Jrl. of Applied Nutrition* (1983) 35: 116-126.
14. Elizabeth Steinhagen-Thiessen et al., *Age* (Oct., 1983) 6, no. 4: 143-144.
15. Garry D. Wheeler et al., *JAMA* (July 27, 1984) 252, no. 4: 514-516.
15a. William B. Fears et al., *Jrl. of Adolescent Health Care* (1983) 4: 22-24.
16. T.W. Boyden et al., *Fertility and Sterility* (1984) 41: 359-363. Cited in *Sports Medicine* (1984) 1, no. 6: 487.
17. David C. Cumming and Robert W. Rebar, *American Jrl. of Industrial Medicine* (1983) 4: 113-125.
17a. E. Dale and D.H. Gerlach, *Obstetrics and Gynecology* (1979) 54: 47. Cited by Ralph W. Hale, *Clinical Obstetrics and Gynecology* (1983) 26, no. 3: 728-735, at 731.
17b. Richard H. Strauss et al., *JAMA* (Dec. 20, 1985) 254, no. 23: 3337-3338.
17c. J.G. Stewart et al., *Annals of Internal Medicine* (1984) 100: 843-845. Cited in *Sports Medicine* (1985) 2: 305.
17d. Ernst Jokl, *Medicine and Sport* (1977) 10: 129-134.
17e. B. Halliwell and J.M.C. Gutteridge, *Molecular Aspects of Medicine* (1985) 8: 89-193, at 146.
17f. S.R. Grobler et al., *South African Medical Jrl.* (1984) 65: 872-873.
18. Joseph D. Wassersug,*Modern Medicine* (Feb., 1985) 53, no. 2: 21-22, 24.
18a. *Lancet* (June 8, 1985): 1309-1310.
18b. M. Fisher-Williams,*Lancet* (July 20, 1985): 147-148.
19. Gina Maranto, *Discover* (Oct., 1984) 5, no. 10: 19-22.
19a. C.F. Chester and C.P. Conlon, *British Jrl. of Sports Medicine* (1983) 17, no. 4: 143-144.
19b. R. Tyler Frizzell and Gilbert H. Lang,*JAMA* (Feb. 14, 1986) 255, no. 6: 772-774.
19c. T.D. Noakes et al., *Medicine and Science in Sports and Exercise* (1985) 17: 370-375. Cited in ref. 19a.

19d. Raul Artal et al., *Lancet* (Aug. 4, 1984): 258-260.

19e. B.G. Gatmaitan et al., *Jrl. of Experimental Medicine* (1970) 131: 1121-1136. Cited in ref. 5.

19f. Daniel R. Neuspiel, *Mayo Clinical Proceedings* (1986) 61: 226-227.

19g. Heyward L. Nash, *Physician and Sports Medicine* (March 1986) 14, no. 3: 251-253.

20. Allan Bundgaard et al., *Scand. Jrl. Clin. Invest.* (1982) 42: 15-18.

21. Albert L. Sheffer and K. Frank Austen, *Jrl. Allergy and Clinical Immunology* (1984) 73, no. 5, part 2: 699-703.

22. T.H. Lee et al., *Lancet* (March 5, 1983): 520-522.

23. P.H. Howarth and S.L. Holgate, *Lancet* (April 9, 1983): 822.

24. E.R. McFadden, Jr. and R.H. Ingram, Jr., *New England Jrl. of Medicine* (1979) 301, no. 14: 763-769.

25. E.R. McFadden, Jr. and R.H. Ingram, Jr., *New England Jrl. of Medicine* (1984) 311, no. 17: 1127-1128.

26. Allen P. Kaplan, *Jrl. of Allergy and Clinical Immunology* (1984) 73, no. 5, part 2: 704-707.

27. Ellen M. Buchbinder, et al., *JAMA* (Dec. 2, 1983) 250: 2973-2974.

28. James M. Kidd III et al., *Jrl. of Allergy and Clinical Immunology* (1983) 71, no. 4: 407-411.

28a. A. Bundgaard, *Sports Medicine* (1985) 2: 254-266.

29. Thomas R. Friberg and Robert N. Weinreb, *JAMA* (1985) 253, no. 12: 1755-1757.

30. L.A. Kuehn, *Jrl. of Theoretical Biology* (1981) 8: 279-286.

31. S. Corrsin, *Jrl. of Theoretical Biology* (1982) 99: 683-688.

31a. Rudolph H. Dressendorfer et al., *Physician and Sports Medicine* (1985) 13, no. 8, 77-86. Cited by Alexander Grant, *Healthwise* (Sept., 1985) 8, no. 9: 1.

32. Victoria Persky et al., *American Jrl. of Epidemiology* (1981) 114, no. 4: 477-487.

33. Kelvin J.A. Davies et al., *Biochemical and Biophysical Research Communications* (1982) 107: 1198-1205.

34. A.T. Quintanilha, *Biochemical Transactions* (1984) 12: 403-404.

35. L. Packer, *Medical Biology* (1984) 62, 105-109, at 108.

36. Lester Packer and Kathy Fuehr, *Nature* (June 2, 1977) 267: 423.

37. Grace C. Yuan and R. Shihman Chang, *Jrl. of Gerontology* (1969) 4: 82-85.

38. Lester Packer and James R. Smith, *Proc. National Academy of Sciences* (Dec., 1974) 71, no. 12: 4763-4767.

39. Lester Packer and James R. Smith, *Proc. National Academy of Sciences* (April, 1977) 74, no. 4: 1640-1641.

40. Arthur K. Klein et al., *Jrl. of Cell Biology* (1977) 74: 58-67.

41. HiroshiSakagami and Masa-atsu Yamada, *Cell Structure and Function* (1977) 2: 219-227.

42. Robert R. Krohn, *Science* (April 18, 1975) 188: 203.

43. G.M. Martin et al., *Laboratory Investigation* (1970) 23: 86-92.

44. I.L. Cameron, *Jrl. of Gerontology* (1972) 27: 157.

45. James G. Rheinwald and Howard Green, *Nature* (1977) 265: 421-424.

46. R. Holliday, L.I. Huschtscha, G.M. Tarrant and T.B.L. Kirkwood, *Science* (Oct. 28, 1977) 198: 366-372.

47. R. Holliday, L.I. Huschtscha and T.B.L. Kirkwood, *Science* (Sept. 25, 1981) 213: 1505-1508.

48. Leonard Hayflick in *Ageing, Cancer and Cell Membranes*, ed. Carmia Borek, Cecilia M. Fenoglio and Donald West King (New York: George Thieme Verlag and Thieme-Stratton, Inc., 1980) p. 87.

49. C.A. Reznikoff et al., *Cancer Research* (1973) 33: 3231-3238. Cited by ref. 50.

50. A. Macieira-Coelho et al., *Experimental Cell Research* (1976) 100: 228-232.

51. Laura Curatolo et al., *In vitro* (1984) 20, no. 8: 587-601.

52. Jennifer D. Hall et al., *Experimental Cell Research* (1982) 139: 351-359.

53. Dean P. Loven, Duane L. Guernsey and Larry W. Oberley, *International Jrl. of Cancer* (1984) 33: 783-786.

53a. Karl Illmensee and Peter C. Hoppe, *Cell* (1981) 23: 9-18.

53b. Jean L. Marx, *Science* (Jan. 23, 1981) 211: 375-376.

53c. George E. Seidel, Jr., *Jrl. of Experimental Zoology* (1983) 228: 347-354.

53d. Anne McLaren, *Nature* (June 21, 1984) 309: 671-672.

53e. James McGrath and David Solter, *Science* (Dec. 14, 1984) 226: 1317-1319.

54. Gretchen H. Stein and Rosalind M. Yanishevsky, *Experimental Cell Research* (1979) 120: 155-165.

55. Albert Rosenfeld, *The Second Genesis—The Coming Control of Life* (Englewood Cliffs, N.J.: Prentice Hall, 1969).

55a. A. Yabrov, *Medical Hypotheses* (1980) 6: 207-208.

56. *Consumer Reports* (Oct., 1980).

56a. *Science Digest* (June, 1974).

56b. Ranjit Kumar Chandra, *Nutrition Research* (1986) 6: 1-2.

56c. *Nutrition Education in U.S. Medical Schools,* Committee on Nutrition in Medical Education, Food and Nutrition Board, Commission on Life Sciences, National Research Council (Washington, D.C.: National Academy Press, 1985). This book was reviewed in the *American Jrl. of Clinical Nutrition* (April, 1986) 45: 643-644.

56d. Roland L. Weinsier et al., *American Jrl. of Clinical Nutrition* (June, 1986) 43: 959-968.

57. Aileen Brett et al., *Human Nutrition: Applied Nutrition* (1986) 40A: 217-222.

57a. Daphne A. Roe, *Drug-Induced Nutritional Deficiencies* (Westport, Conn.: AVI Publishing Co., 1976).

57b. *Nutrition and Drugs,* ed. Myron Winick (New York: John Wiley and Sons, 1983).

57c. Daphne A. Roe, *Drug-Nutrient Interactions* (1985) 4: 117-135, at 129.

58. Thomas H. Shepard, *Catalog of Teratogenic Agents,* 2nd ed. (Baltimore: Johns Hopkins Univ., 1976).

59. Alan Pestronk and Daniel B. Drachman, *Nature* (1980) 288: 733-734.

60. Oliver Wendell Holmes, *The Professor at the Breakfast Table* (The Riverside Press, 1892) pp. 197-199. Cited by K. Michael Hambridge, *American Jrl. of Clinical Nutrition* (1982) 36: 943-949.

60a. Paul Kurtz, *The Skeptical Inquirer* (1984) 8: 239-246.

60b. Mario Bunge, *The Skeptical Inquirer* (1984) 9: 36-46.

60c. Fred J. Gruenberger, *Science* (1964) 145: 1413-1415.

60d. Petr Skrabanek, *Lancet* (April 26, 1986): 960-961.

61. Gerhard N. Schrauzer, *Medical Hypotheses* (1976) 2: 39-49.

62. Samuel J. Fomon et al., *Proc. Society for Exper. Biology and Medicine* (1983) 173: 190-193.

63. Jorge Chirife and Leon Herszage, *Lancet* (July 17, 1982): 157.

64. B. Bose, *Lancet* (April 24, 1982): 963.

65. F.J. Branicki, *Ann. Royal College Surgeons, England* (1981) 63: 348-352.

66. H. Gordon et al., *Lancet* (Sept. 21, 1985): 663-664.

66a. A. Quataro et al., *Lancet* (Sept. 21, 1985): 664.

66b. Mark K Addison and Juan N. Waterspiel, *Lancet* (Sept. 21, 1985): 665.

66c. Denis Cavanagh and Frank Ostapowicz, *Jrl. of Obstetrics and Gynecology of the British Commonwealth* (1970) 77: 1037-1040.

66d. Jean Louis Trouillet, *Lancet* (July 27, 1985): 180-184.

67. Bonnie Llebman, *Nutrition Action* (Aug., 1981): 11.

67a. C.J. Glueck et al., *American Jrl. of Clinical Nutrition* (1979) 32: 1636-1644.

67b. Fred H. Mattson et al., *Jrl. of Nutrition* (1979) 109: 1688-1693.

67c. Margot J. Mellies et al., *American Jrl. of Clinical Nutrition* (1983) 37: 339-346.

67d. O. Pelletier and M.O. Keith, *Jrl. of the American Dietetic Assn.* (1974) 64: 271-275.

68. Edward J. Cafruny, *Pharmacological Intervention in the Aging Process,* ed. R.C. Adelman, V.J. Cristofalo and J. Roberts (New York: Plenum Press, 1978) p. 225.

69. Helen B. Hiscoe, *New England Jrl. of Medicine* (June 16, 1983) 308, no. 24: 1474-1475.

70. Gary A. Borkan and Arthur H. Norris, *Jrl. of Gerontology* (1980) 35, no. 2: 177-184.

71. Alex Comfort, *Mechanisms of Ageing and Development* (1972) 1: 101-110.

71a. Richard L. Sprott and Edward L. Schneider, *Drug-Nutrient Interactions* (1985) 4: 43-52, at 48.

72. Charles L. Rose and Michel L. Cohen, *Annals of the N.Y. Academy of Sciences* (1977) 301: 671-702.

73. Gary L. Grove, *Archives of Dermatological Research* (1982) 272: 381-385.

74. G.A. Borkan and A. Norris, *Jrl. of Gerontology* (1980) 35: 177-184. Cited in ref. 73.

75. Gary L. Grove et al., *Jrl. of the Society of Cosmetic Chemists* (1981) 32: 15-26.

76. G.L. Grove et al., *British Jrl. of Dermatology* (1982) 107: 393-400.

77. Gary L. Grove and Albert M. Kligman, *Jrl. of Gerontology* (1983) 38, no. 2: 137-142.

78. T.L. Dormandy, *Lancet* (Oct. 29, 1983): 1010-1014, at 1011.

AUTHOR INDEX

This index includes individuals mentioned in the text even if not directly associated with cited references. Reference numbers are used with the author index when precision is fostered, thereby. The letter "n," as is customary, shows that the citation is in a footnote.

Kohen, Ron, 462n (refs. 87ca, 87ea)
Kohn, Robert R., 814
Kohunai, Takashi, 115
Kolata, Gina, 236-237 (ref. 152), 250
(ref. 219), 282, 360n (ref. 68g),
552, 564, 662, 691, 728 (ref.
597a), 840n (ref. 110d)
Kolata, Gina Bari, 399n (ref. 156a)
Kolenick, James J., 257, 260
Kolhouse, J. Fred., 373
Kolomaznik, M., 780
Kon, S.H., 593
Kon, S.K., 572
Kondo, Haruki, 373
Konishi, Frank, 535
Konner, Melvin, 251-252 (refs. 227-
234), 524-525, 537, 549n, 669
Koplan, B., 716
Kopp, Stephen J., 644, 802
Koppang, N., 142n (ref. 63)
Korant, B.D., 635
Korcok, Milan, 556
Kornberg, Arthur, 580
Körner, W.F., 495-498
Korpatnick, D.J., 521
Korpela, H., 760-761
Korpen, C.W., 134 (ref. 149)
Korytnyk, W., 363 (ref. 77)
Koskas, J.P., 161-162 (ref. 228)
Kosta, L., 773
Kostial, K., 791 (ref. 9)
Kotchen, T.A., 661
Kottow, Michael H., 39n
Kovachich, G.B., 485
Kovats, Telegdy, 160-161
Kowalson, Bella, 343
Kraft, Patricia L., 249, 251 (ref.
122c)
Krall, A.R., 795
Kramer, Lois, 772
Kramer, R.E., 810
Krasner, N., 459
Krawitt, E.L., 556
Krazner, E. *See* Berndorfer-Krazner
Krebs, Ernst T., Jr., 409, 412-415,
419-420, 421, 423-424
Krebs, Ernst T., Sr., 412, 414
Krebs, Hans Adolph, 377
Krehl, W.A., 392

Kremer, Joel M., 187n
Krieger, John N., 636 (ref. 294)
Krinsky, Norman I., 852 (ref. 130)
Krishna, G., 520
Krishnamoorthy, R.V., 496-497
Krishna Murthy, P. Bala, 153, 154
Krishnamurthy, S., 101, 228, 482n-
483n
Krishna Murti, C.R., 483, 531
Krishnaswamy, Kamala, 463 (refs.
87g-1, 87r, s)
Kristensen, Preben, 799-800
Kritchevski, David, 33, 224, 241 (ref.
185), 471n, 571n (ref. 79c)
Kriz, Mojmir, 174-176, 180 (ref.
17a), 186
Kroes, M., 376, 388n (ref. 122c)
Krohn, Robert R., 877-879
Kroll, J.S., 354
Kromann, N., 326 (ref. 153)
Kromhout, Daan, 234, 236 (refs.
150, 151)
Krone, C.A., 222n
Kroneck, Peter M.H., 475n (ref.
133a)
Kronfol, Ziad, 28-29
Kruger, Albert, 598
Kruk, Patrica, 142
Krumdieck, Carlos, 404n (refs. 188a-
d)
Krzynowek, Judith, 234n
Kubota, Shinji, 860
Kuehl, Frederick A., Jr., 180n, 181
(ref. 23), 183 (ref. 29), 828 (ref.
60)
Kuehn, L.A., 875
Kuenzig, W.A., 499
Kuga, Norito, 766
Kuhn, M., 612-613
Kuhn, Thomas S., 76-78, 327
Kühnau, Joachim, 811 (ref. 2d), 453n
Kulangara, A.C., 821 (ref. 30j)
Kulwich, Roman, 29 (ref. 87)
Kumano, Nobuko, 765
Kumar, P. Sanjeev, 851
Kumar, Rajiu, 308 (ref. 117)
Kumar, S., 631n (ref. 269b)
Kumashiro, Ryunosuke, 256-257

"Some Men pretend to understand a Book by scouting thro' the Index: as if a Traveller should go about to describe a Palace when he had seen nothing but the Privy."
— Jonathan Swift in *Mechanical Operation of the Spirit* (1704). Cited by Donald E. Knuth in *The Art of Computer Programming*, 2nd ed. (Menlo Park, CA: Addison-Wesley Publ. Co., 1973), p. 617.

The privy, at times, may be the most useful place in the palace.
— Walter A. Heiby

SUBJECT INDEX

If you have difficulty finding an entry, it could be under the major topic but subentered under benefits, dangers, or *reverse effect(s)*. Mineral, vitamin and drug antagonisms are entered under *Mineral-mineral antagonisms, Mineral-vitamin antagonisms, Vitamin-mineral antagonisms,* or *Drug-nutrient interactions*. Cancer entries will be found under the general heading *Cancer* or under *Cancer, specific types*. All *reverse effects*, in addition to appearing under specific topics, are gathered together under *Reverse effects, specific* which follows *Reverse effect, general*.

E

E B Cells, 502
Eczema
  evening primrose oil, 215
  glutathione peroxidase
        deficiency associated
        with, 748
Edema
  aspirin causes, 255
  sodium chloride may cause, 666
  vitamin B_1 may cause, 336-337
EDTA. *See* Ethylene diamine
        tetraacetic acid
Education of physicians, 884-885
Eggs
  avidin, 407
  dangers
    cancer, 229
    vitamin-mineral inhibitors,
        370, 407
Eicosanoids. *See also*
        Leukotrienes;
        Prostaglandins; *and*
        Thromboxanes
  definition, 179-180
Eicosapentenoic acid (EPA). *See
        also* Table 1 (Pages 170-
        171); *and* Fish oils
  dangers
    dementia, senile, 319
    lipid peroxide levels raised,
        318
    platelet count reduced, 315-
        316
    vitamin E status, 236
  fish content varies with algae
        eaten, 320n
  HDL-C/LDL-C benefitted, 240-
        241
  inflammation molified by
        leukotrienes from, 188
  libido, 216n
  low density lipoproteins, 315
  lupus erythematosus benefitted,
        319-320
  meat, 252
  platelet deaggregator, 313, 315
  reverse effect

    bleeding time, aspirin, 326
    rheumatoid arthritis benefitted,
        320
    tests, laboratory, falsified by,
        326
  tumor growth inhibited, 319
Ejaculatory delay
  zinc, 644
Elastin. *See* Collagen
Elderly
  drug metabolism, 83-84
Electricity
  bone formation, 557
  innoculation, 11-12, 12n
  interferon response, 14
  tumor effect, 12
Electromagnetism. *See also*
        Radiation
  reverse effect
    cell glucose, 67, 69
Electron-transport system, 377-
        378
Emphysema
  cadmium from cigarette smoke
        may cause, 804
Encephalopathy
  reverse effect
    bilirubin, 868
Endometrial cancer. *See* Cancer,
        endometrial
Endurance. *See also* Fatigue
  vitamin C, 495
Enteritis. *See* Colitis
Enterocolitis. *See also* Colitis
  vitamin E may cause
        necrotizing, 129
Environmental conditions
  tumors affected by, 15
Eosinophils
  stress affect (animals) on, 21
EPA. *See* Eicosapentenoic acid
Epilepsy
  Dilantin®, 389, 389n, 390
  folic acid, 389
  reverse effect
    vitamin B_6, 354
  water excess dangerous, 61n
  zinc deficiency as cause, 647

How to Give a Gift or Memorial to Your Local Library, and to Libraries of Nearby Colleges and Universities Including your Alma Mater

Here's an idea for persons who wish to add an appropriate "personalized" touch to their giving—as an individual or as a group. A gift of Walter A. Heiby's *The Reverse Effect: How Vitamins and Minerals Promote Health and CAUSE Disease* reflects the taste of the giver or, in the case of memorials, of the individual in whose memory it is given. Moreover, such a gift provides an excellent way for a health-minded organization to help the community. A gift book may also be given in the name of your daughter, son, parent, or other relative in commemoration of a special occasion (e.g., high school or college graduation, birthday, anniversary). A book donation also makes an excellent Christmas or "thank-you" present. (The honored person will point with pride to this book in the library and to the inscription honoring him or her.) A library can use more than one copy of this book should you desire to honor more than one person.

Suggestion: Send your community newspaper a notice of your gift, preferably with a photograph of the person being honored and/or your photo. Perhaps your newspaper would prefer to photograph you making the presentation to the librarian.

Simply write out or send this form to each library:

I would like to establish a gift or memorial. I hearby donate the enclosed sum of $59.50 for the purchase of *The Reverse Effect: How Vitamins and Minerals Promote Health and CAUSE Disease* by Walter A. Heiby (published by: MediScience Publishers, P.O. Box 256A, Deerfield, IL 60015), ISBN 0-938869-01-9.

Please inscribe the inside front cover of this book to show it is a:

☐ gift from the undersigned
☐ memorial in the honor of _____
                              (Name of person honored)
☐ gift in the honor of _____
                              (Name of person honored)

I would like an acknowledgment sent to:

_____
(Relative or friend's name)

_____
(Address)

Signed:_____

Address:_____

City:_____ State:_____ Zip:_____

If you decide against using this form show it to your librarian anyway. Your library might like to adapt it for use in soliciting donations for other books.

1196

"When I get a little money, I buy books; and if any is left, I buy food and clothes."
—Desiderius Erasmus

"A good book, in the language of the booksellers, is a salable one; in that of the curious, a scarce one; in that of men of sense, a useful and instructive one."
—Talbot Wilson Chambers

"The books that help you most are those that make you think the most."
—Theodore Parker

"The best of a book is not the thought which it contains, but the thought which it suggests; just as the charm of music dwells not in the tones but in the echoes of our hearts."
—Oliver Wendell Holmes

"It is one of the more fascinating aspects of the history of science that you could actually make a list of inventions which, if they had been made correctly too early, would have brought science to a standstill. Let me give you a simple example. If Mendeleev had known where to place helium—which was already a known gas by the time that he made the periodic table—the whole table would have been out of kilter. Because he would have had to ask, where are the other gases? Where is argon, krypton, and that whole line of gases?"
—Jacob Bronowski, *A Sense of the Future* (Cambridge, Mass: The MIT Press, 1977) p. 231.

"....the highlights of tomorrow are the unpredictabilities of today."
—Cesar Milstein, *Science* (March 14, 1986) 231: 1261-1268 at 1267.

Every progressive spirit is opposed by a thousand men appointed to guard the past."
—Maurice Maeterlinck, *The Bluebird*.

ORDER FORM

MediScience Publishers
PO Box 256A
Deerfield, IL 60015

Consider the Big Book and the sampler as gifts for scientific and health-minded friends. Why not make your colleagues aware of the *reverse effect* by giving or sending each of them the sampler?

Enclosed is my check or money order (checks on U.S. banks or international money order in U.S. funds if a foreign order) for which please send the following books by Walter A. Heiby. (Sorry, but we cannot accept open account or C.O.D. orders.)

Quantity	Book	Exten.
	Better Health and the Reverse Effect (ISBN 0-938869-03-5). A sampler containing "How to Read Biomedical Literature" and "How to Use the *Reverse Effect* and the *Pleasure Concept*" as well as the associated reference lists from *The Reverse Effect: How Vitamins and Minerals Promote Health and CAUSE Disease*. For use as an introduction to the *reverse effect* and for the guidance of laboratory scientists in designing biomedical experiments. Paperback, each $3.95 ($.26), 4-9 copies, each $3.75 ($.24), 10-99 copies, each $3.50 ($.23), 100 or more, each $3.25 ($.21). *	
	The Reverse Effect: How Vitamins and Minerals Promote Health and CAUSE Disease (ISBN 0-938869-01-9). The First Edition of the big 1216-page volume, cloth bound and Smythe sewn, using acid-free paper to stay white for centuries. Each $59.50 ($3.87); 2-4 copies, each $54.50 ($3.54); 5-9 copies, each $52.50 ($3.41); 10 or more, each $49.50 ($3.22).*	

* All prices postpaid at book rate to USA destinations. Amounts shown in parentheses are sales taxes per book if shipped to an Illinois address. Foreign customers: Please add $2.00 for each sampler ($1.00 each for 10 or more) and $8 for each big book for delivery by surface mail.

Subtotal_____

6 1/2% sales tax (if Ill.)_____

Foreign Postage_____

Total enclosed_____

I understand orders not subject to a quantity discount may be returned for prompt refund. (No return privilege on quantity-discount orders or on foreign orders unless damaged or defective when you receive them.)

Name:_____

Company or Institution:_____

Address:_____

City:_____State:_____Zip:_____

Book Investors: The First Edition of the big book, if ordered in lots of ten or more copies will be autographed by the author, on request, for possible additional value as a long-term investment. Check here if 10 or more copies of the big book are being ordered and autographs are desired ☐ .

"If you require additional copies of this book, we strongly recommend that you purchase them rather than using a photocopier. This is merely in the interests of your own health, since photocopiers have been reported to produce significant amounts of ozone which will peroxidize your lung lipids!" —Barry Halliwell and John M.C. Gutteridge, *Free Radicals in Biology and Medicine* (Oxford, England: Clarendon Press, 1985), p. 223.

COLOPHON

The colophon was an inscription on the last page of a book (or of a manuscript in pre-book times) that gave the name of the printer (or of the scribe) and the date and place of publication. It may also have included the symbol or coat of arms of the printer. The first incunabulum * to include a colophon was the Mainz Psalter of 1457. Its colophon showed the date of publication and the name of its printers, Johann Fust (formerly a partner of Gutenberg) and Peter Schoffer. Later, about 1520, the colophon was moved to the front of the book. Now it has all but disappeared except for the emblem of the publisher that may sometimes appear on the title page or on the book's spine. I think the colophon tradition should be given new life.

Book preparation was done by the dedicated craftsmen and craftswomen at Apollo Books and at Ironwood Press of Winona, Minnesota. Final preparations for camera were skillfully and expeditiously made by Jo Szczesny. Typeface used is Times Roman, composed on an Apple Macintosh Plus personal computer with a General Computer Hyperdrive FX-20, with the output being produced on an Apple Laserwriter Plus laser printer. Software used was Microsoft Word, version 1.2, published by Microsoft, Inc. The book was printed offset in standard black ink on 50 lb. Dynawhite Cougar Opaque Smooth acid-free paper by Walsworth Press, Marceline, Missouri. Endsheet is 90 lb. Mead Endleaf. The volume has been Smythe sewn with C-grade Roxite vellum cloth cover on 98 pt. board. Jacket was printed on 70 lb. Golden Cask gloss enamel.

---

* Any book published before 1501 is termed an incunabulum. The plural is incunabula.